Orthopedic Imaging

A PRACTICAL APPROACH

Orthopedic Imaging

A PRACTICAL APPROACH

FOURTH EDITION

Adam Greenspan, M.D., F.A.C.R.
Professor, Departments of Radiology and Orthopedic Surgery
   University of California, Davis School of Medicine
Chief, Section of Musculoskeletal Imaging
   University of California, Davis Medical Center
   Sacramento, California
Consultant, Shriners Hospital for Children
   Sacramento, California

Foreword by
Michael W. Chapman, M.D.

with illustrations by Laura Pardi Duprey

LIPPINCOTT WILLIAMS & WILKINS
A **Wolters Kluwer** Company

Philadelphia • Baltimore • New York • London
Buenos Aires • Hong Kong • Sydney • Tokyo

Acquisitions Editor: Lisa McAllister
Developmental Editor: Kerry Barrett
Production Editor: Rakesh Rampertab
Manufacturing Manager: Colin Warnock
Cover Designer: Doug Smock
Compositor: Maryland Composition, Inc.
Printer: Quebecor-Kingsport

©2004 by LIPPINCOTT WILLIAMS & WILKINS
530 Walnut Street
Philadelphia, PA 19106-3780 USA
LWW.com
4th—2004 Lippincott Williams & Wilkins
3rd—2000 Lippincott Williams & Wilkins
2nd—1996 Lippincott-Raven Publishers, Philadelphia, PA
1st—1992 Gower Medical Publishers, New York, NY

Printed in the USA

Library of Congress Cataloging-in-Publication Data
Greenspan, Adam.
    Orthopedic imaging: a practical approach/Adam Greenspan; foreword
  by Michael W. Chapman; with illustrations by Laura Pardi Duprey.—4th ed.
      p.; cm.
    Rev. ed. of: Orthopedic radiology. 3rd ed. ©2000.
    Includes bibliographical references and index.
    ISBN 0-7817-5006-7
    1. Radiography in orthopedics. I. Greenspan, Adam. Orthopedic
radiology. II. Title
    [DNLM: 1. Bone and Bones—radiography. 2. Bone Diseases—
  radiography. 3. Bone Neoplasms—radiography. WE 200
  G815a 2004]
  RD734.5.R33G74 2004
  616.7′107572—dc22   2004044191

Care has been taken to confirm the accuracy of the information presented and to describe generally accepted practices. However, the author and publisher are not responsible for errors or omissions or for any consequences from application of the information in this book and make no warranty, expressed or implied, with respect to the currency, completeness, or accuracy of the contents of the publication. Application of this information in a particular situation remains the professional responsibility of the practitioner.

The author and publisher have exerted every effort to ensure that drug selection and dosage set forth in this text are in accordance with current recommendations and practice at the time of publication. However, in view of ongoing research, changes in government regulations, and the constant flow of information relating to drug therapy and drug reactions, the reader is urged to check the package insert for each drug for any change in indications and dosage and for added warnings and precautions. This is particularly important when the recommended agent is a new or infrequently employed drug.

Some drugs and medical devices presented in this publication have Food and Drug Administration (FDA) clearance for limited use in restricted research settings. It is the responsibility of the health care provider to ascertain the FDA status of each drug or device planned for use in their clinical practice.

10 9 8 7 6 5

To my wife Barbara,
my children Michael, Samantha, and Luddy,
and my grandchildren Sydney and Anna, who light up my life

CONTENTS

FOREWORD

In this fourth edition of his text, now retitled *Orthopedic Imaging*, Dr. Greenspan has expanded and improved significantly his very popular and widely used third edition which was entitled *Orthopedic Radiology: A Practical Approach*. Although the third edition contained much material on imaging modalities other than routine radiographs, the change in the title reflects the tremendous advances and innovations that have occurred in imaging over the five years since the last edition was published. Percutaneous, "minimally invasive" treatments and surgical procedures for a host of disorders including those in the musculoskeletal system have been refined and incorporated into daily practice. This evolution is reflected in Dr. Greenspan's discussion of CT-guided radiofrequency thermal ablation of osteoid osteoma as well as other techniques. Sophisticated imaging is not only essential to make many diagnoses but is quickly becoming integrated with many therapies.

This fourth edition continues to be an excellent tool for learning to interpret imaging studies, with an emphasis on conventional radiography, but equally important is essential to the selection of which imaging studies are more appropriate for a given condition and what sequence of imaging studies is most likely to result in a definitive diagnosis at the lowest cost. For example, for a suspected stress fracture of the femoral neck with negative radiographs, should MRI or scintigraphy be ordered? Chapter 1, The Role of the Orthopedic Radiologist, addresses these issues and is essential reading for all practitioners who order imaging studies. Chapter 2, Imaging Techniques in Orthopedics, follows up with detailed information and guidelines to each of the imaging techniques and is required reading for the remainder of the text. Chapter 3, devoted to bone formation and growth, is a cornerstone fur understanding the pathomechanics of many pathological processes affecting osseous structures, whereas Chapters 4 through 33 contain specific information on radiologic imaging of many bone and joint abnormalities, including traumatic, arthritic, neoplastic, infectious, metabolic, endocrinologic, and congenital disorders.

In his preface Dr. Greenspan has thoroughly covered the changes in the fourth edition as compared to the third edition, therefore I will not attempt to enlarge on his description but a few points deserve emphasis. The quality of the images reproduced in the text is outstanding, as Dr. Greenspan has in this edition replaced less clear illustrations with higher quality reproductions. The profuse use of excellent line drawings to augment the images and many tables provides the reader excellent resources for better understanding the material and aides for learning the essentials. While keeping the book in one volume, Dr. Greenspan has added substantially to subjects covered in the third edition and has included many new items such that the text is now comprehensive in its coverage of the musculoskeletal system.

The title will attract radiologists, orthopedic surgeons, physiatrists, and rheumatologists but every practitioner that treats musculoskeletal disorders and orders imaging studies should have access to this text. It is an essential study resource for medical students and for residents in the specialities of radiology and musculoskeletal medicine and surgery. I look forward to seeing the dog-eared and well-worn copies of the third edition in the Department of Orthopedic Surgery at the University of California Davis Medical Center replaced with this excellent updated and expanded fourth edition.

Michael W. Chapman, M.D.
Professor Emeritus of Orthopaedic Surgery
University of California, Davis School of Medicine
Sacramento, California

PREFACE TO THE FIRST EDITION

Orthopedic Radiology: A Practical Approach was written to facilitate the complex process of diagnostic investigation in a broad range of orthopedic disorders. Its underlying concept is threefold: to provide a basic understanding of the currently available imaging modalities used to diagnose many commonly encountered disorders of bones and joints, to help in the choice of the most effective radiologic technique with a view to minimizing the cost of examination as well as the exposure of patients to radiation, and to emphasize the need for providing the orthopedic surgeon with the information required to choose the right therapy. It does not attempt to compete in size and scope with other books on the same subject. Many uncommon entities have been excluded, as have the exact instructions for performing procedures. Likewise, the nature of the volume does not allow inclusion of every detail of a given disorder or full discussion of controversial aspects. These matters are left to the reader's further study of the literature and the many standard and specialized textbooks compiled in the References and Further Readings section at the end of the volume.

As its subtitle states, *Orthopedic Radiology* strives to provide its primary audience, medical students and residents in radiology and orthopedics, with a practical approach to its subject. To this end, crucial information within the text of each chapter has been tabulated in a section entitled "Practical Points to Remember" at the end of the chapter. Numerous original schematic diagrams and tables have been developed, detailing, for example, classifications of fractures, the morphologic features of arthritic and neoplastic disorders, and the positioning of patients for the various standard and special radiographic projections, as well as the most effective radiologic techniques for demonstrating abnormalities. Radiographic reproductions, many of which are accompanied by explanatory, labeled line drawings, have been specially prepared to provide high-quality examples of the classic presentations of a wide spectrum of orthopedic disorders. Moreover, most figure captions are written in a case-study format, which, combined with a system of diagnostic notations (explained in Chapter 1) following each legend is meant to impart an appreciation of the process of radiologic investigations. Although its aim is to teach, *Orthopedic Radiology* should also serve as a convenient reference for physicians interested in bone and joint disorders and those customarily employing radiologic studies in their everyday practice.

Adam Greenspan, M.D., F.A.C.R.

PREFACE

Five years have elapsed since the third edition of this text was released by the publishers. This is a long time when we consider the rapid progress in radiologic imaging and the continued technological advances in this field. These facts prompted a new edition that, in part, reflects the above-mentioned progress, being a very much "overhauled" and improved copy of the previous editions. Because radiologists are now using imaging technologies not connected with an X-ray beam, such as magnetic resonance imaging, ultrasound, and scintigraphy, the older terms "radiography" and "radiology" are often being substituted with a new term, "imaging." Hence, the new title of the book, *Orthopedic Imaging: A Practical Approach*. However, despite the frequent use of these "high-technology" advanced techniques in orthopedic imaging, in this as in the previous editions of this text, the emphasis is placed on conventional radiography which, at least in the eyes of the author, remains a cost-effective modality and plays a fundamental role in the care of patients rendered by orthopedic surgeons and other physicians, and should always be performed first before more sophisticated and advanced imaging techniques are employed. Nevertheless, as in the previous editions, the main objective of this book is to demonstrate the availability of various imaging modalities for evaluation of traumatic, arthritic, neoplastic, infectious, metabolic, and congenital disorders of the musculoskeletal system, and to indicate the effectiveness of specific techniques for specific abnormalities.

There are, however, many changes, additions, and improvements in this edition. The book has received a new design, and color was introduced to better depict the titles and subtitles. As suggested by one of the reviewers of the previous edition, the captions for the illustrations have been improved, with the diagnosis placed at the beginning of the legend in boldface type. Technically suboptimal illustrations have been either deleted or substituted with better-quality images. Outdated text and references have been deleted and replaced with current ones. New tables summarizing the salient features of various disorders have been added. In addition, the text has been revised to include many MRIs, thin-section CTs, and 3-D CT studies.

Several new sections have been added to almost every chapter. For example, in the chapter on imaging techniques the newest information about diagnostic use of positron emission tomography (^{18}FDG PET) was added. In the chapters dealing with trauma, injury to the glenoid and to the glenohumeral ligaments, MRI classification of acromioclavicular joint injury, suprascapular nerve syndrome, injury to the soft tissues of the elbow (including tears of the ligaments), Essex-Lopresti fracture-dislocation, ulnar impingement and ulnar impaction syndromes, and scaphoid dislocations, have been included. New material also consists of injuries to the acetabular labrum, newest advances in MRI of meniscal injuries, navicular bone fractures, sinus tarsi and tarsal tunnel syndromes, Scheuermann disease, and annular tears of the intervertebral disk. In the section dealing with arthritides, recent advances in total joint replacement, updated information on Postel coxarthropathy, newest information on erosive osteoarthritis, and amyloid arthropathy complicating long-term hemodialysis and chronic renal failure have been added. The section on tumors contains new information about the latest advances in imaging of osteoid osteoma and CT-guided radiofrequency thermal ablation of this lesion. Previously omitted facts on intracortical chondroma, Jaffe-Campanacci syndrome, fibrocartilaginous dysplasia of long bones, Mazabraud syndrome, the solid variant of aneurysmal bone cyst (giant cell reparative granuloma), multifocal giant cell tumors, staging of giant cell tumor, epithelioid hemangioma, soft tissue (extraskeletal) osteosarcoma and its differential diagnosis, revised classification of lymphomas, primary leiomyosarcoma of bone, hemangioendothelioma and angiosarcoma of bone, and on lipoma arborescens are now incorporated. In the section on musculoskeletal infections, the role of MRI in diagnosing musculoskeletal infections has been expanded. The section on metabolic disorders incorporates the newest information on imaging techniques for measurement of bone mineral density. In the section on congenital and developmental anomalies, information on Madelung deformity, treatment of congenital hip dysplasia, and material on some of the sclerosing bone dysplasias have been augmented with new material. Again, as in the previous editions, to keep up with the latest developments in musculoskeletal imaging, up-to-date references and suggested readings appear at the end of each chapter.

Despite the increased number of illustrations and the additional text, the single-volume format has been retained. This should facilitate the use of this text by radiologists, orthopedic surgeons, and other physicians interested in application of imaging techniques to musculoskeletal disorders, and should serve as a convenient addition to the multivolume editions of similar books now on the market.

Adam Greenspan, M.D., F.A.C.R.

ACKNOWLEDGMENTS

As the previous editions, this project could not have been completed without the help of many of my friends and colleagues. I am grateful to the many individuals from Lippincott Williams & Wilkins who guided and helped me in the preparation of this text. Especially, many thanks to Lisa McAllister, executive editor, Kerry Barrett, developmental editor, and Rakesh Rampertab, senior production editor, for editorial advice and coordination of the production of this book; to Doug Smock, senior art director, for the beautiful design of the book and its cover; and to Pat Mrozek, project manager, for supervision during the final composition of this text. A special note of acknowledgment goes to Angela Michelier for invaluable secretarial assistance and timely preparation of the manuscript. I also would like to thank Laura Pardi Duprey for preparation of the schematics and drawings, Aaron Peterson for help in creating some of the digital illustrations, Sharon Rule for help in editing some of the sections, and Michael W. Chapman, M.D., for writing the Foreword. Finally, I would like to express my gratitude to all the authors who have given permission to reproduce selected illustrations from their books and publications. They are separately acknowledged on the credit page at the end of the book. Without the conscientious efforts from many of individuals acknowledged here, it would have been impossible to accomplish this task.

INTRODUCTION TO ORTHOPEDIC IMAGING

THE ROLE OF THE ORTHOPEDIC RADIOLOGIST

Spectacular progress has been made and continues to be made in the field of radiologic imaging. The introduction and constant improvements of new imaging modalities—computed tomography (CT) and its spiral (helical) and tridimensional (3-D) variants, digital (computed) radiography (DR, CR) and its variants, digital subtraction radiography (DSR) and digital subtraction angiography (DSA), three-dimensional ultrasound (US), radionuclide angiography and perfusion scintigraphy, positron emission tomography (PET), single-photon emission computerized tomography (SPECT), magnetic resonance imaging (MRI), among others—have expanded the armamentarium of the radiologist, facilitating the sometimes difficult process of diagnosis. These new technologic developments have also brought disadvantages. They have contributed to a dramatic increase in the cost of medical care and have often led clinicians, trying to keep up with new imaging modalities, to order too many frequently unnecessary radiologic examinations.

This situation has served to emphasize the crucial importance of the role of the orthopedic radiologist and the place of conventional radiography. The radiologist must not only comply with prerequisites for various examinations but also, more importantly, screen them to choose only those procedures that will lead to the correct diagnosis and evaluation of a given disorder. To this end, radiologists should bear in mind the following objectives in the performance of their role:

1. To *diagnose an unknown disorder*, preferably by using standard projections along with the special views and techniques obtainable in conventional radiography before using the more sophisticated modalities now available.
2. To perform examinations in the *proper sequence* and to know what should be performed *next* in the radiologic investigation.
3. To demonstrate the determining *radiologic features of a known disorder*, the *distribution* of a lesion in the skeleton, and its *location* in the bone.
4. To monitor the *progress of therapy* and possible *complications*.
5. To be aware of what *specific information* is important to the orthopedic surgeon.
6. To recognize the *limits of noninvasive radiologic investigation* and to know when to *proceed with invasive techniques*.
7. To recognize lesions that require biopsy and those that do not (the "don't touch" lesions).
8. To assume a more active role in therapeutic management, such as performing an embolization procedure, delivering chemotherapeutic material by means of selective catheterization, or performing (usually CT-guided) radiofrequency thermal ablation of osseous lesions (such as osteoid osteoma).

The radiologic diagnosis of many bone and joint disorders cannot be made solely on the basis of particular recognizable radiographic patterns. Clinical data, such as the patient's age, gender, symptoms, history, and laboratory findings, are also important to the radiologist in correctly interpreting an imaging study. Occasionally, clinical information is so typical of a certain disorder that it alone may suffice as the basis for diagnosis. Bone pain in a young person that is characteristically most severe at night and is promptly relieved by salicylates, for example, is so highly suggestive of osteoid osteoma that often the radiologist's only task is finding the lesion. However, in many cases clinical data do not suffice and may even be misleading.

When presented with a patient, the cause of whose symptom is *unknown* (Fig. 1.1) or *suspected* on the basis of clinical data (Fig. 1.2), the radiologist should avoid, as a point of departure in the examination, the more technologically sophisticated imaging modalities in favor of making a diagnosis, whenever possible, on the basis of simple conventional radiographs. This approach is essential not only to maintain cost-effectiveness but also to decrease the amount of radiation to which a patient is exposed. Proceeding first with conventional tech-

nique also has a firm basis in the chemistry and physiology of bone. The calcium apatite crystal, one of the mineral constituents of bone, is an intrinsic contrast agent that gives skeletal radiology a great advantage over other radiologic subspecialties and makes information on bone production and destruction readily available through conventional radiography. Simple observation of changes in the shape or density of normal bone, for example in the vertebrae, can be a deciding factor in arriving at a specific diagnosis (Figs. 1.3 and 1.4).

To aid the radiologist in the analysis of radiographic patterns and signs, some of which may be pathognomonic and others nonspecific, a number of options within the confines of conventional radiography are available. Certain *ways of positioning the patient* when radiographs are obtained allow the radiologist the opportunity to evaluate otherwise hidden anatomic sites and to more suitably demonstrate a particular abnormality. The frog-lateral projection of the hip, for example, is better than the anteroposterior view for imaging the signs of suspected osteonecrosis of the femoral head by more readily demonstrating the crescent sign, the early radiographic feature of this condition (see Figs. 4.58 and 4.59B). The frog-lateral view is also extremely helpful in

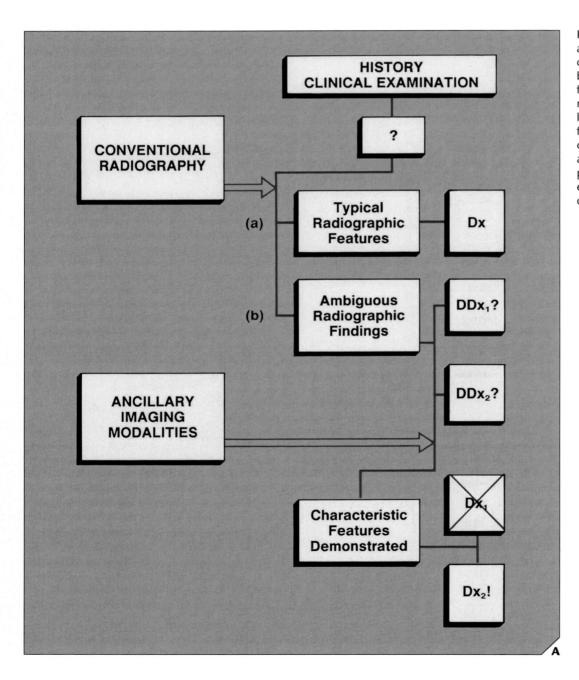

Figure 1.1 Cause of symptoms unknown. (A) and **(B)** The patient's history and the results of the clinical examination, supplied to the radiologist by the referring physician, are not sufficient to form a diagnosis (*?*). On the basis of conventional radiographic studies, (a) the diagnosis is established (*Dx*), or (b) the studies may suggest the differential possibilities (*DDx*). In the latter case, ancillary imaging techniques, such as tomography, arthrography, scintigraphy, computed tomography, or magnetic resonance imaging, among others, are called on to confirm or exclude one of the options.

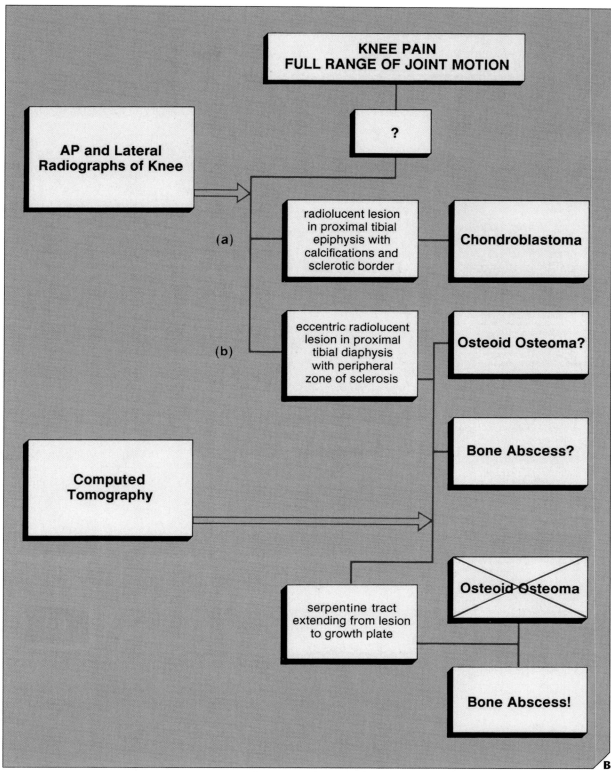

Figure 1.1 *Continued.*

early diagnosis of slipped femoral capital epiphysis (see Fig. 32.30B). Likewise, the application of *special techniques* can help to identify a lesion that is difficult to detect on routine radiographs. Fractures of complex structures such as the elbow, wrist, ankle, and foot are not always demonstrated on the standard projections. Because of the overlap of bones on the lateral view of the elbow, for example, detecting a nondisplaced or minimally displaced fracture of the radial head occasionally requires a special 45-degree angle view (called the radial head–capitellum view) that projects the radial head free of adjacent structures, making an otherwise obscure lesion evident (see Figs. 6.12 and 6.28). Stress radiographic views are similarly useful, particularly in evaluating tears of various ligaments of the knee and ankle joints (see Figs. 9.16, 9.71B, 10.10, 10.11).

An accurate diagnosis depends on the radiologist's acute observations and careful analysis, in light of clinical information, of the radiographic findings regarding the size, shape, configuration, and den-

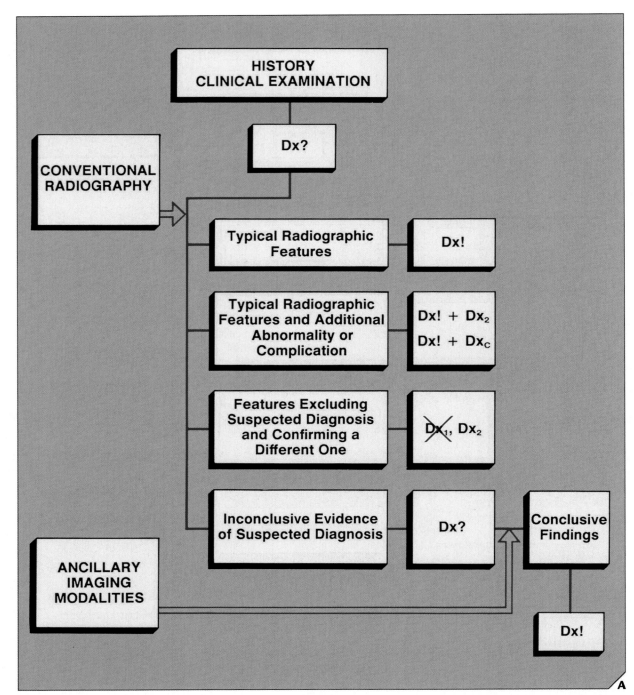

Figure 1.2 Cause of symptoms suspected. (A) and **(B)** From the information supplied by the referring physician, the radiologist may suspect the diagnosis (*Dx?*) and proceed with conventional radiographic studies. The results of the examination may confirm the suspected diagnosis (*Dx!*), reveal an additional abnormality (*Dx!+Dx₂*) or an unsuspected complication *(Dx!+Dxc)*, or exclude the suspected diagnosis and confirm a different one (*Dx₁, Dx₂*). The studies may also show inconclusive evidence of the original suspected diagnosis, in which case ancillary imaging modalities, such as scintigraphy, conventional tomography, computed tomography, or magnetic resonance imaging, among others, are used.

Figure 1.2 *Continued.*

Figure 1.3 Shape and contour of bone. Observation of changes in the shape and contour of a vertebral body on conventional radiographs may disclose critical information leading to a correct diagnosis.

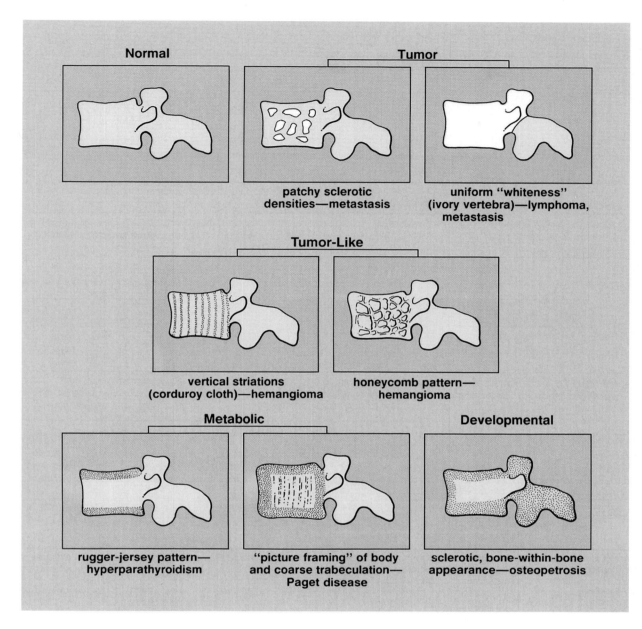

Figure 1.4 Density and texture of bone. Changes in the density and texture of a vertebral body on conventional radiographs may offer useful data for arriving at a diagnosis.

sity of a lesion, its location within the bone, and its distribution in the skeletal system. Until the conventional approach with its range of options fails to provide the radiographic findings necessary for correct diagnosis and precise evaluation of an abnormality, the radiologist need not turn to more costly procedures.

Knowing the *proper sequence* of procedures in radiologic investigation depends, to a great extent, on the pertinent clinical information provided by the referring physician. The choice of modality or modalities for imaging a lesion or investigating a pathologic process is dictated by the clinical presentation as well as by the equipment, availability, physician expertise, cost, and individual patient restrictions. Knowing *where to begin* and *what to do next,* as rudimentary as it may sound, is of paramount importance in reaching a precise diagnosis by the shortest possible route, with the least expense and detriment to the patient. Redundant studies should be avoided. For example, if a patient presents with arthritis and if clinician is interested in demonstrating the distribution of "silent" sites of the disorder, the radiologist should not begin by obtaining radiographs of every joint (a so-called joint survey). It is instead more sensible to perform a scintigraphy and, afterward, to order radiographs of only those areas that show increased uptake of radiopharmaceutical. A simple radionuclide bone scan rather than a broad-ranging bone survey is also a reasonable starting point for investigating other possible sites of involvement when a lesion is detected in a single bone and is suspected of representing

part of a multifocal or systemic disorder, such as polyostotic fibrous dysplasia or metastatic disease. Similarly, if a patient is suspected of having osteoid osteoma around the hip joint and standard radiography has not demonstrated the nidus, a radionuclide bone scan should be performed next to determine the site of the lesion. This should be followed-up by conventional tomography or CT for more precise localization of a nidus in the bone. However, if the routine examination demonstrates the nidus, scintigraphy and conventional tomography can be omitted from the sequence of examination. At this point, only CT scan is required to determine the lesion's exact location in the bone and to obtain specific measurements of the nidus (Fig. 1.5; see also Fig. 17.11). If osteonecrosis (ON) of the femoral head is suspected and the radiographs are normal, MRI should be ordered as the next diagnostic procedure, because it is a more sensitive modality than conventional tomography, CT, or scintigraphy. The text that follows presents many similar situations in which the proper sequence of imaging modalities may dramatically shorten the diagnostic investigation.

Reaching a correct diagnosis does not end the process of radiologic investigation, because the course of treatment often depends on the *identification of distinguishing features of a particular disorder* (Fig. 1.6). For example, the diagnosis of Ewing sarcoma by conventional radiography is only the beginning of a radiologic workup of the patient. The *crucial features* of this tumor must be identified, such as intraosseous and soft-tissue extension (by CT or MRI) and the vascular-

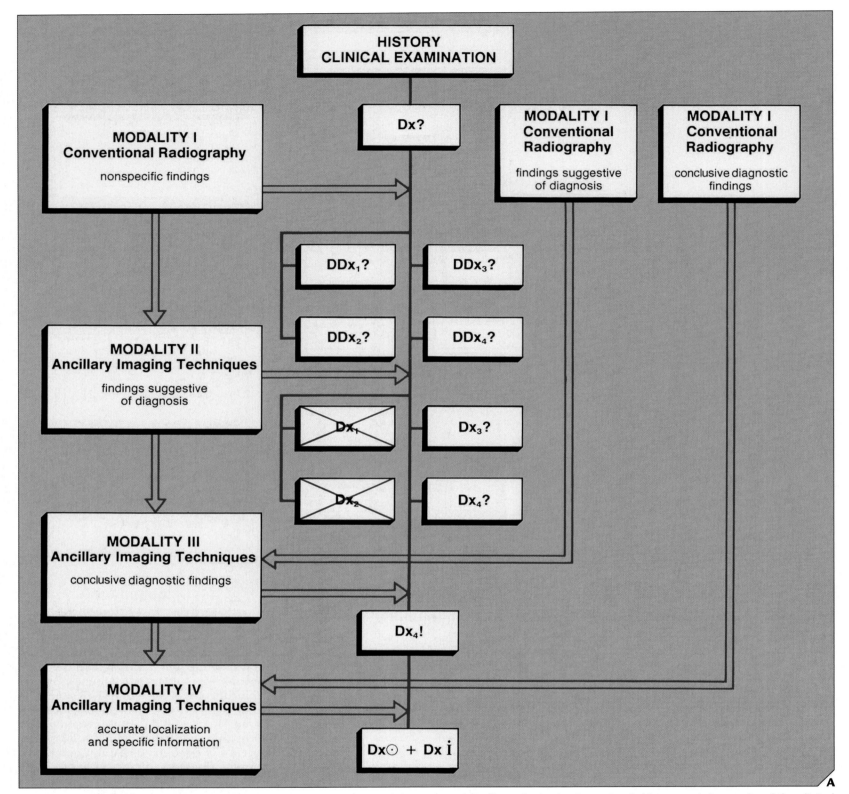

Figure 1.5 Sequence of imaging modalities. (A) and **(B)** A diagnosis is suspected (*Dx?*) on the basis of a patient's history and the results of the clinical examination. The radiologist suggests the proper sequence of imaging modalities, eliminating various disorders in the process and narrowing the differential possibilities to arrive at one correct diagnosis (*Dx!*). An accurate localization (*Dx⊙*) and specific information pertinent to the correct diagnosis (*Dxİ*) are also provided.

Figure 1.5 *Continued.*

B

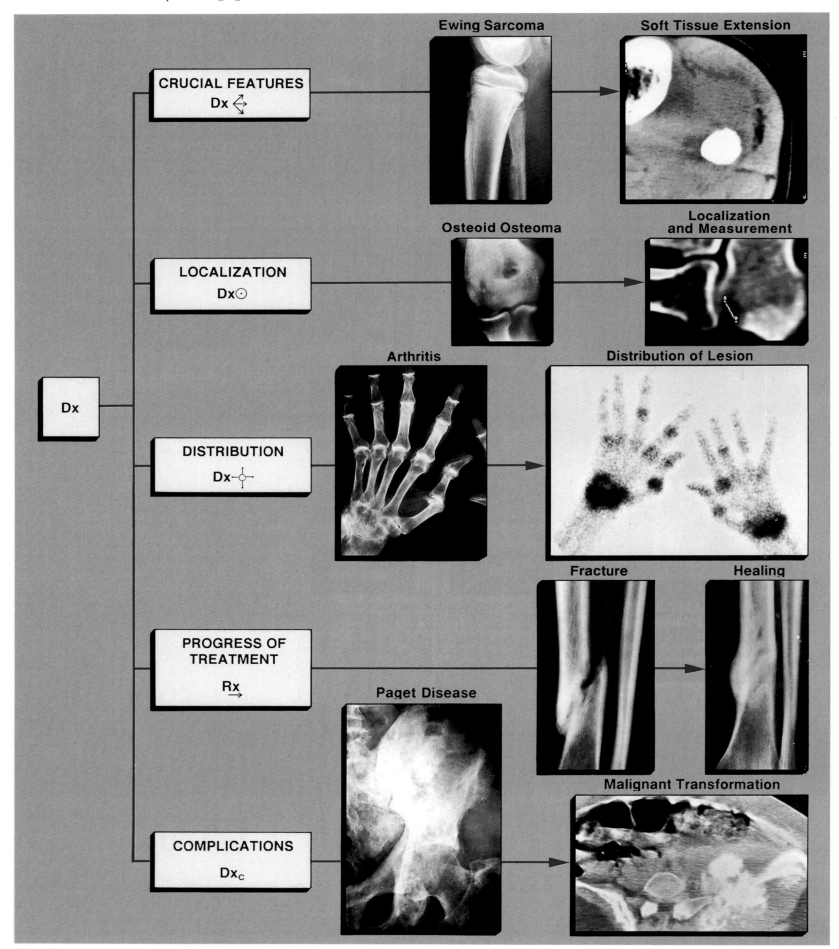

Figure 1.6 Distinguishing features of lesion, progress of treatment, and complications. The diagnosis is known (*Dx*). The clinician is interested in demonstrating: (1) the crucial features of the lesion (*Dx⇆*), i.e., its character, extent, stage, and other pertinent data; (2) the location of the lesion in the bone (*Dx⊙*); (3) the distribution of the lesion in the skeleton (*Dx⊕*); (4) the progress of treatment (*Rx→*); and (5) the emergence of any complications (*Dx_c*).

ity of the lesion (by conventional arteriography or magnetic resonance arteriography [MRA]). Similarly, a diagnosis of osteosarcoma must be followed by determination of the exact extent of the lesion in the bone and the status of bone marrow in the vicinity of the tumor. This can be accomplished by precise measurement of bone marrow density using Hounsfield numbers during CT examination (see Fig. 2.10) or by using MR images with or without contrast enhancement. Diagnosing Paget disease may be an important achievement in the investigation of an unknown disorder, but even more important is the further search for an answer to a crucial question: Is there any sign of malignant transformation? (see Fig. 29.18). *Localization* of a lesion in the skeleton or in a particular bone can frequently be more important than diagnosis itself. The best example of this is, again, the precise localization of the nidus of osteoid osteoma, because incomplete resection of this lesion invariably results in recurrence. Determining the *distribution of a lesion* in the skeleton is helpful in planning the treatment of various arthritides and the management of a patient with metastatic disease. Scintigraphy is an invaluable technique in this respect.

Many of the most important questions put to the radiologist by the orthopedic surgeon concern monitoring the *progress of treatment* and the appearance of possible *complications*. At the stage when the diagnosis is already established, the fate of the lesion, and consequently the patient, must be established. Comparison of earlier radiographic examinations with present findings plays a crucial role at this stage, because it may disclose the dynamics of specific conditions (see Fig. 16.21). Likewise, in monitoring the progress of healing fractures, study of the diagnostic sequence of radiographs complemented by conventional tomography or CT should decide questionable cases. Ancillary imaging techniques such as scintigraphy, CT, and MRI play an essential role in evaluating one of the most serious complications of benign tumors and tumor-like lesions—malignant transformation

that may occur in enchondroma, osteochondroma, fibrous dysplasia, or Paget disease.

Providing the orthopedic surgeon with *specific information* is also an important function of the radiologist at the time when a diagnosis is being established. If, for example, osteochondritis dissecans is diagnosed, the decision on the choice of therapy requires information on the status of the articular cartilage covering the lesion. This information is obtainable by contrast arthrography, alone or combined with CT, or by MRI (see Figs. 6.39–6.41). If the cartilage is intact, conservative treatment should be contemplated; if it is damaged, surgical intervention is the more likely course of treatment. Similarly, in contributing to the plan of treatment of anterior dislocation in the shoulder joint, the radiologist should be aware of the importance to the surgeon of information about the status of the cartilaginous labrum of the glenoid (see Fig. 5.47) and the possible presence of osteochondral bodies in the joint. These features must be confirmed or excluded by arthrography combined with tomography (arthrotomography), CT (computed arthrotomography), or MRI (Fig. 1.7).

Recognizing *the limits of noninvasive radiologic investigation* and knowing when to proceed with *invasive techniques* are as important to arriving at a diagnosis and precise evaluation of a condition as any of the points already mentioned. This situation is best illustrated in the case of tumors and tumor-like bone lesions. Many tumor-like lesions have distinctive radiographic presentations that lead to unquestionable diagnoses on conventional studies. In such cases, invasive procedures such as biopsy are not indicated. This is particularly true of a group of definitely benign conditions commonly called "don't touch" lesions (see Fig. 16.48 and Table 16.10). The name "don't touch" speaks for itself. Conditions such as a bone island (enostosis), posttraumatic juxtacortical myositis ossificans, and a periosteal desmoid are unquestionably benign lesions whose determining features can, with certainty, be demonstrated with the appropriate noninvasive

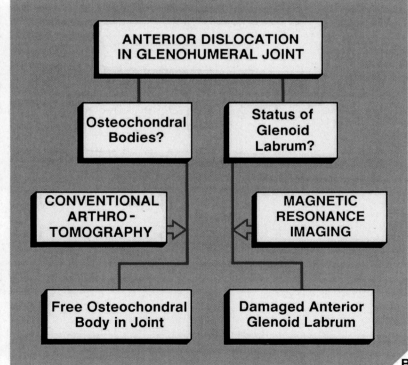

Figure 1.7 Specific information. (A) and **(B)** The diagnosis is known (*Dx*). The radiologist should be aware of the specific information (*i*), for example, regarding the features (*i₁?*) or extent (*i₂?*) of a lesion, which is required by the orthopedic surgeon in planning treatment. The information may also concern the distribution of a lesion and its localization, the progress of treatment, or the emergence of complications. Application of the best radiologic modality for demonstrating the required information is one of the radiologist's primary functions. The modalities may vary depending on the specific information needed.

techniques without the need for histopathologic confirmation. Obtaining a biopsy of such lesions may in fact lead to mistakes in diagnosis and treatment. The histologic appearance of a periosteal desmoid, for example, may exhibit aggressive features resembling a malignant tumor; in inexperienced hands, this can lead to inappropriate treatment. However, there are times when the radiologist faces the situation in which a battery of conventional and sophisticated noninvasive techniques has yielded equivocal information. At this point, there is no shame in saying, "I don't know what it is, but I know a biopsy should be performed" (Fig. 1.8). Fluoroscopy-guided or CT-guided percutaneous biopsy can be performed by the radiologist in the radiology suite, eliminating the use of costly operating-room time and personnel. Occasionally, the radiologist may also assume a more active role in therapeutic management by performing an embolization procedure under image intensification or with CT guidance, or performing radiofrequency thermal ablation of bone lesion. This more interventional role for the radiologist may shorten the length of a patient's hospitalization and be more cost-effective.

In summary, to sufficiently manage the diagnosis and treatment of patients with conditions affecting the musculoskeletal system, the radiologist and the referring physician should be aware of the range of radiologic modalities and their proper uses. This will increase the precision of diagnostic radiologic investigation and reduce the amount of radiation to which a patient is exposed and the cost of hospitalization. The obligation of the radiologist is to:

- Use the conventional radiographic methods, with knowledge of the capabilities and effectiveness of the various techniques, before resorting to more sophisticated modalities.
- Follow a logical sequence of imaging modalities in diagnostic investigation.
- Be as noninvasive as possible at the start, but use invasive techniques if they will shorten the diagnostic pathway.
- Improve communication between the radiologist and the orthopedic surgeon by using the same language and by knowing what the surgeon needs to know about the lesion.
- Provide knowledge to referring physicians about indications, advantages, disadvantages, risks, contraindications, and limitations of the various imaging techniques.

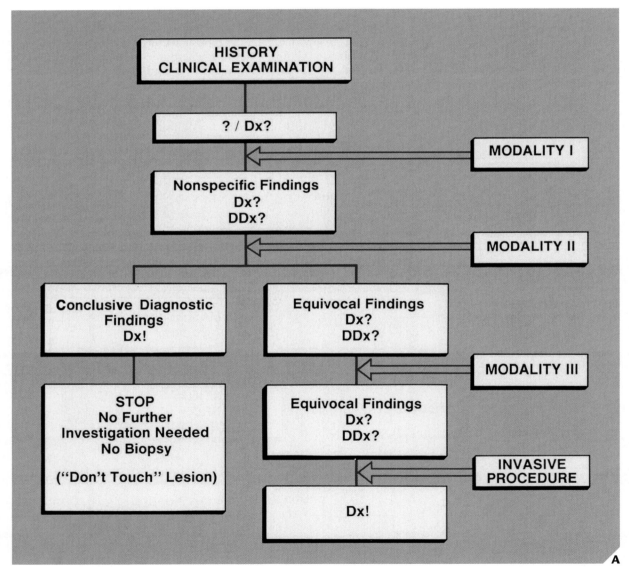

Figure 1.8 Noninvasive versus invasive procedures. (A) and **(B)** The diagnosis is unknown (*?*) or suspected (*Dx?*). Noninvasive radiologic procedures may yield sufficient data to make an unquestionable diagnosis. No further investigation is required, nor is biopsy indicated, particularly if the diagnosis is that of a definitely benign condition commonly called a "don't touch" lesion. However, noninvasive procedures may yield equivocal information at each step in the examination. At this point, proceeding to an invasive procedure such as biopsy is indicated.

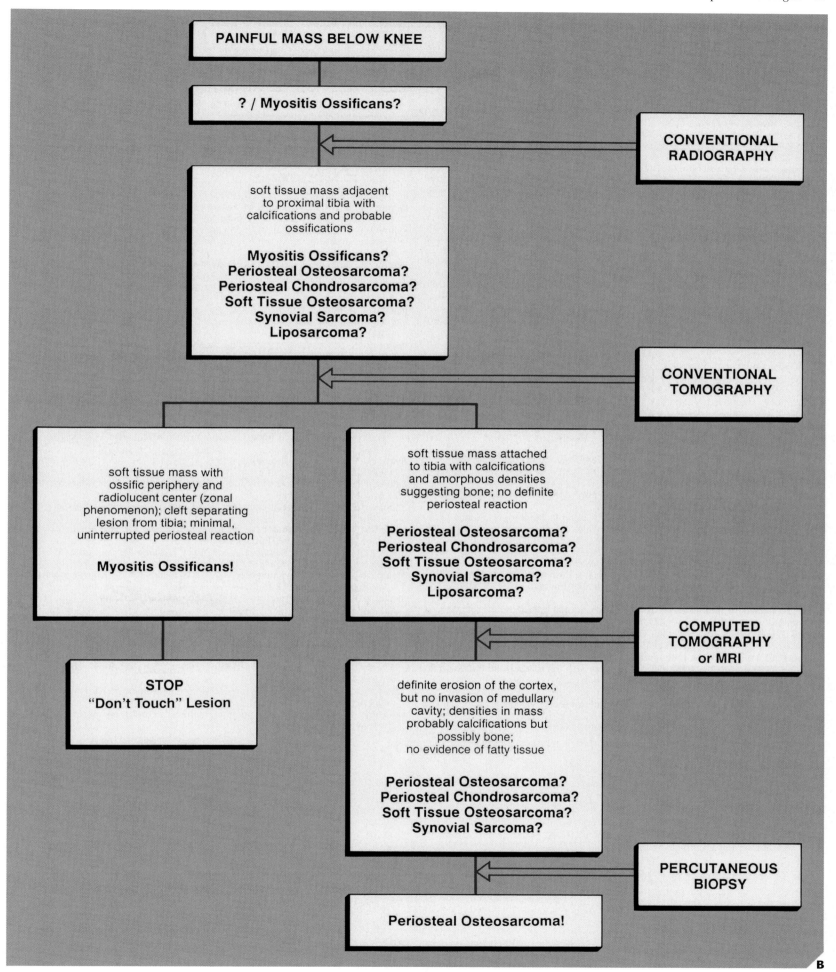

Figure 1.8 *Continued.*

SUGGESTED READINGS

Blackmore CC, Magid DJ. Methologic evaluation of the radiology cost-effectiveness literature. *Radiology* 1997;203:87–91.

Brink JA, Heiken JP, Wang G, McEnery KW, Schlueter FJ, Vannier MW. Helical CT: principles and technical considerations. *Radiographics* 1994;14:887–893.

Brossmann J, Muhle C, Büll CC, et al. Cine MR imaging before and after realignment surgery for patellar maltracking—comparison with axial radiographs. *Skeletal Radiol* 1995;24:191–196.

Cascade PN, Webster EW, Kazerooni EA. Ineffective use of radiology: the hidden cost. *AJR Am J Roentgenol* 1998;170:561–564.

Collier BD, Fogelman I, Brown ML. Bone scintigraphy: Part 2. Orthopedic bone scanning. *J Nucl Med* 1993;34:2241–2246.

Collier BD, Hellman RS, Krasnow AZ. Bone SPECT. *Semin Nucl Med* 1987;17:247–266.

Conway WF, Totty WG, McEnery KW. CT and MR imaging of the hip. *Radiology* 1996;198:297–307.

Delfaut EM, Beltran J, Johnson G, Rousseau J, Marchandise X, Cotten A. Fat suppression in MR imaging: techniques and pitfalls. *Radiographics* 1999;19:373–382

Deutsch AL, Mink JH. Magnetic resonance imaging of musculoskeletal injuries. *Radiol Clin North Am* 1989;27:983–1002.

Fishman EK, Magid D, Ney DR, Chaney EL, et al. Three-dimensional imaging. *Radiology* 1991;181:321–337.

Fishman EK, Wyatt SH, Bluemke DA, Urban BA. Spiral CT of musculoskeletal pathology: preliminary observations. *Skeletal Radiol* 1993;22:253–256.

Foley WD, Wilson CR. Digital orthopedic radiography: vascular and nonvascular. In: Galasko CSB, Isherwood I, eds. *Imaging techniques in orthopedics.* London: Springer-Verlag; 1989:145–158.

Gates GF. SPECT bone scanning of the spine. *Semin Nucl Med* 1998;28:78–94.

Genant HK, Wu CY, van Kuijk C, Nevitt MC. Vertebral fracture assessment using a semiquantitative technique. *J Bone Miner Res* 1993;8:1137–1148.

Gibson DJ. Technology: the key to controlling health care cost in the future. *AJR Am J Roentgenol* 1994;163:1289–1293.

Hamper UM, Trapanotto V, Sheth S, Dejong MR, Caskey CI. Three-dimensional US: preliminary clinical experience. *Radiology* 1994;191:397–401.

Heiken JP, Brink JA, Vannier MW. Spiral (helical) CT. *Radiology* 1993;189:647–656.

Holder LE. Bone scintigraphy in skeletal trauma. *Radiol Clin North Am* 1993;31:739–781.

Holder LE. Clinical radionuclide bone imaging. *Radiology* 1990;176:607–614.

Johnson RP. The role of the bone imaging in orthopedic practice. *Semin Nucl Med* 1997;27:386–389.

Kaplan PA, Matamoros Jr, A, Anderson JC. Sonography of the musculoskeletal system. *AJR Am J Roentgenology* 1990; 155:237–245.

Kumar R, Guinto FC Jr, Madewell JE, Swischuk L, David R. The vertebral body: radiographic configurations in various congenital and acquired disorders. *Radiographics* 1988;8:455–485.

Kuszyk BS, Heath DG, Bliss DF, Fishman EK. Skeletal 3-D CT: advantages of volume rendering over surface rendering. *Skeletal Radiol* 1996;25:207–214.

Levin DC, Spettell CM, Rao VM, Sunshine J, Bansal S, Busheé GR. Impact of MR imaging on nationwide health care costs and comparison with other imaging procedures. *AJR Am J Roentgenol* 1998;170:557–560.

Loehr SP, Pope TL Jr, Martin DF, et al. Three-dimensional MRI of the glenoid labrum. *Skeletal Radiol* 1995;24:117–121.

Magid D, Fishman EK, Sponseller PD, Griffin PP. 2D and 3D computed tomography of the pediatric hip. *Radiographics* 1988;8:901–933.

Manaster BJ. Imaging of the musculoskeletal system. *Acad Radiol* 1995;2:S164–S166.

Margulis AR. Introduction to the algorithmic approach to radiology. In: Eisenberg RL, Amberg JR, eds. *Critical diagnostic pathways in radiology.* Philadelphia: JB Lippincott; 1981.

McDougall IR, Rieser RP. Scintigraphic techniques in musculoskeletal trauma. *Radiol Clin North Am* 1989;27:1003–1011.

McEnery KW, Wilson AJ, Pilgram TK, Murphy WA Jr, Marushack MM. Fractures of the tibial plateau: value of spiral CT coronal plane reconstructions for detecting displacement in vitro. *AJR Am J Roentgenol* 1994;163:1177–1181.

Meschan I, Farrer-Meschan RM. Radiographic positioning, projection, pathology and definition of special terms. In: Meschan I, ed. *Roentgen signs in diagnostic imaging,* vol. 4, 2nd ed. Philadelphia: WB Saunders; 1987.

Mirowitz SA. Fast scanning and fat-suppression MR imaging of musculoskeletal disorders. *AJR Am J Roentgenol* 1993;161:1147–1157.

Moore SG, Bisset GS, Siegel MJ, Donaldson JS. Pediatric musculoskeletal MR imaging. *Radiology* 1991;179:345–360.

Murray IPC, Dixon J. The role of single photon emission computed tomography in bone scintigraphy. *Skeletal Radiol* 1989;18:493–505.

Nelson SW. Some important diagnostic and technical fundamentals in the radiology of trauma, with particular emphasis on skeletal trauma. *Radiol Clin North Am* 1966;4:241–259.

O'Sullivan GS, Goodman SB, Jones HH. Computerized tomographic evaluation of acetabular anatomy. *Clin Orthop* 1992;277:175–181.

Palmer WE, Brown JH, Rosenthal DI. Fat-suppressed MR arthrography of the shoulder: evaluation of the rotator cuff. *Radiology* 1993;188:683–687.

Palmer WE, Caslowitz PL, Chew FS. MR arthrography of the shoulder: normal intraarticular structures and common abnormalities. *AJR Am J Roentgenol* 1995;164: 141–146.

Peterfy CG, Roberts T, Genant HK. Dedicated extremity MR imaging: an emerging technology. *Radiol Clin North Am* 1997;35:1–20.

Petersilge CA. Current concepts of MR arthrography of the hip. *Semin US CT MR* 1997;18:291–301.

Pettersson H, Resnick D. Musculoskeletal imaging. *Radiology* 1998;208:561–562.

Pitt MJ, Speer DP. Radiologic reporting of skeletal trauma. *Radiol Clin North Am* 1990;28:247–256.

Pretorius ES, Scott WW Jr, Fishman EK. Acute trauma to the shoulder: role of spiral computed tomographic imaging. *Emergency Radiol* 1995;2:13–17.

Richardson ML, Frank MS, Stern EJ. Digital image manipulation: what constitutes acceptable alteration of a radiologic image? *AJR Am J Roentgenol* 1995;164: 228–229.

Rogers LF. From the editor's notebook. Imaging literacy: a laudable goal in the education of medical students. *AJR Am J Roentgenol* 2003;180:1201.

Rubin DA, Kneeland JB. MR imaging of the musculoskeletal system: technical considerations for enhancing image quality and diagnostic yield. *AJR Am J Roentgenol* 1994;163:1155–1163.

Ryan PJ, Fogelman I. The bone scan: where are we now? *Semin Nucl Med* 1995;25:76–91.

Seibert JA, Shelton DK, Moore EH. Computed radiography x-ray exposure trends. *Acad Radiol* 1996;3:313–318.

Sheppard S. Basic concepts in magnetic resonance angiography. *Radiol Clin North Am* 1995;33:91–113.

Slone RM, Heare MM, Vander Griend RA, Montgomery WJ. Orthopedic fixation devices. *Radiographics* 1991;11:823–847.

Smith RC, Constable RT, Reinhold C, McCauley T, Lange RC, McCarthy S. Fast spin-echo STIR imaging. *J Comput Assist Tomogr* 1994;18:209–213.

Steinbach LS, Palmer WE, Schweitzer ME. Special focus session—MR arthrography. *Radiographics* 2002;22:1223–1246.

Stoller DW. MR arthrography of the glenohumeral joint. *Radiol Clin North Am* 1997;35:97–116.

Swan JS, Grist TM, Sproat IA, Heiner JP, Wiersma SR, Heisey SM. Musculoskeletal neoplasms: preoperative evaluation with MR angiography. *Radiology* 1995;194:519–524.

Swan JS, Grist TM, Weber DM, Sproat IA, Wojtowycz M. MR angiography of the pelvis with variable velocity encoding and a phased-array coil. *Radiology* 1994;190:363–369.

Thrall JH, Aubrey O. Hampton lecture. Directions in radiology for the next millenium. *AJR Am J Roengenol* 1998;171:1459–1462.

Udupa JK. Three-dimensional imaging techniques: a current perspective. *Acad Radiol* 1995;2:335–340.

IMAGING TECHNIQUES IN ORTHOPEDICS

Choice of Imaging Modality

In this chapter, the principles and limitations of current imaging techniques are described. Understanding the basis of the imaging modalities available to diagnose many commonly encountered disorders of the bones and joints is of utmost importance. It may help determine the most effective radiologic technique, minimizing the cost of examination and the exposure of patients to radiation. To this end, it is important to choose the modality appropriate for specific types of orthopedic abnormalities and, when using conventional techniques (namely, "plain" radiography), to be familiar with the views and the techniques that best demonstrate the abnormality. It is important to reemphasize that conventional radiography remains the most effective means of demonstrating a bone and joint abnormality.

Use of radiologic techniques differs in evaluating the presence, type, and extent of various bone, joint, and soft-tissue abnormalities. Therefore, the radiologist and orthopedic surgeon must know the indications for use of each technique, the limitations of a particular modality, and the appropriate imaging approaches for abnormalities at specific sites. The question, "What modality should I use for this particular problem?" is frequently asked by radiologists and orthope-

dic surgeons alike, and although numerous algorithms are available to evaluate various problems at different anatomic sites, the answer cannot always be clearly stated. The choice of techniques for imaging bone and soft-tissue abnormalities is dictated not only by clinical presentation but also by equipment availability, expertise, and cost. Restrictions may also be imposed by the needs of individual patients. For example, allergy to ionic or nonionic iodinated contrast agents may preclude the use of arthrography; the presence of a pacemaker would preclude the use of magnetic resonance imaging (MRI); physiologic states, such as pregnancy, preclude the use of ionized radiation, favoring, for instance, ultrasound. Time and cost consideration should discourage redundant studies.

No matter what ancillary technique is used, conventional radiograph should be available for comparison. Most of the time, the choice of imaging technique is dictated by the type of suspected abnormality. For instance, if osteonecrosis is suspected after obtaining conventional radiographs, the next examination should be MRI, which detects necrotic changes in bone long before radiographs, tomography, computed tomography (CT), or scintigraphy become positive. In evaluation of internal derangement of the knee, conventional radiographs should be obtained first and, if the abnormality is not obvious, should again be followed-up by MRI, because this modality provides exquisite contrast resolution of the bone marrow, articular cartilage, ligaments, menisci, and soft tissues. MRI and arthrography are currently the most effective procedures for evaluation of rotator cuff abnormalities, particularly when a partial or complete tear is suspected. Although ultrasonography can also detect a rotator cuff tear, its low sensitivity (68%) and low specificity (75% to 84%) make it a less definitive diagnostic procedure. In evaluating a painful wrist, conventional radiographs and trispiral tomography should precede use of more sophisticated techniques, such as arthrotomography or CT–arthrography. MRI may also be performed; however, its sensitivity and specificity in detecting abnormalities of triangular fibrocartilage and various intercarpal ligaments is slightly lower than that of CT–arthrotomography, particularly if a three-compartment injection is used. If carpal tunnel syndrome is suspected, MRI is preferred because it provides a high-contrast difference among muscles, tendons, ligaments, and nerves. Similarly, if osteonecrosis of carpal bones is suspected and the conventional radiographs are normal, MRI would be the method of choice to demonstrate this abnormality. In evaluation of fractures and fracture healing of carpal bones, trispiral tomography and CT are the procedures of choice, preferred over MRI, because of the high degree of spatial resolution. In diagnosing bone tumors, conventional radiography and tomography are still the gold standard for diagnostic purposes. However, to evaluate the intraosseous and soft-tissue extension of tumor, they should be followed by either CT scan or MRI, with the latter modality being more accurate. To evaluate the results of radiotherapy and chemotherapy of malignant tumors, dynamic MRI using gadopentetate dimeglumine (Gd-DTPA) as a contrast enhancement is far superior to scintigraphy, CT, or even plain MRI.

Imaging Techniques

Conventional Radiography

The most frequently used modality for the evaluation of bone and joint disorders, and particularly traumatic conditions, is conventional radiography. The radiologist should obtain at least two views of the bone involved, at 90-degree angles to each other, with each view including two adjacent joints. This decreases the risk of missing an associated fracture, subluxation, and/or dislocation at a site remote from the apparent primary injury. In children, it is frequently necessary to obtain a radiograph of the normal unaffected limb for comparison. Usually the standard radiography comprises the anteroposterior and lateral views; occasionally, oblique and special views are necessary, particularly in evaluating complex structures, such as the elbow, wrist, ankle, and pelvis. A weight-bearing view may be of value for a dynamic evaluation of the joint space under the weight of the body. Special projections, such as those described in the next chapters, may at times be required to demonstrate an abnormality of the bone or joint to further advantage.

Magnification Radiography

Magnification radiography is occasionally used to enhance bony details not well-appreciated on the standard radiographic projections and to maximize the diagnostic information obtainable from a radiographic image. This technique involves a small focal-spot radiographic tube, a special screen–film system, and increased object-to-film distance, resulting in a geometric enlargement that yields magnified images of the bones and joints with greater sharpness and greater bony detail. This technique is particularly effective in demonstrating early changes in some arthritides (see Fig. 12.7) as well as in various metabolic disorders (see Fig. 26.9B). Occasionally, it may be useful in demonstrating subtle fracture lines otherwise not seen on routine projections.

Stress Views

Stress views are important in evaluating ligamentous tears and joint stability. In the hand, abduction–stress film of the thumb may be obtained when gamekeeper's thumb, resulting from disruption of the ulnar collateral ligament of the first metacarpophalangeal joint, is suspected. In the lower extremity, stress views of the knee and ankle joints are occasionally obtained. Evaluation of knee instability caused by ligament injuries may require use of this technique in cases of a suspected tear of the medial collateral ligament, and less frequently in evaluating an insufficiency of the anterior and posterior cruciate ligaments. Evaluation of ankle ligaments also may require stress radiography. Inversion (adduction) and anterior–draw stress films are the most frequently obtained stress views (see Figs. 4.4, 10.10, 10.11).

Scanogram

The scanogram is the most widely used method for limb-length measurement. This technique requires a slit-beam diaphragm with a 1/16-inch opening attached to the radiographic tube and a long film cassette. The radiographic tube moves in the long axis of the radiographic table. During exposure, the tube traverses the whole length of the film, scanning the entire extremity. This technique allows the x-ray beam to intersect the bone ends perpendicularly; therefore, comparative limb lengths can be measured. When a motorized radiographic tube is not available, a modified technique may be used with three separate exposures over the hip joints, knees, and ankles. In this technique, an opaque tape measure is placed longitudinally down the center of the radiographic table. Occasionally, an orthoroentgenogram is obtained. For this technique, the patient is positioned supine with the lower limbs on a 3-foot–long cassette and a long ruler at one side. A single exposure is made, centered at the knees to include the entire length of both limbs and the ruler.

Fluoroscopy and Video Taping

Fluoroscopy is a fundamental diagnostic tool for many radiologic procedures including arthrography, tenography, bursography, arteriography, and percutaneous bone or soft-tissue biopsy. Fluoroscopy combined with videotaping is useful in evaluating the kinematics of joints. Because of the high dose of radiation, however, it is only occasionally used, such as in evaluating the movement of various joints or to detect transient subluxation (i.e., carpal instability). Occasionally, it is used after fractures in follow-up examination of the healing process to evaluate the solidity of the bony union. Fluoroscopy is still used in conjunction with myelography, where it is important to observe the movement of the contrast column in the subarachnoid space; in arthrography, to check proper placement of the needle and to monitor the flow of contrast agent; and intraoperatively, to assess reduction of a fracture or placement of hardware.

Digital Radiography

Digital (computed) radiography is the name given to the process of digital image acquisition using an x-ray detector comprising a photostimulable phosphor imaging plate and an image reader–writer that processes the latent image information for subsequent brightness scaling and laser printing on film (Fig. 2.1). The system works on the principle of photostimulated luminescence. When the screen absorbs x-rays, the x-ray energy is converted to light energy by the process of fluorescence, with the intensity of light being proportional to the energy absorbed by the phosphor. The stimulated light is used to create a digital image (a computed radiograph).

A major advantage of computed radiography over conventional film/screen radiography is that once acquired, the digital image data are readily manipulated to produce alternative renderings. Potential advantages of digitization include contrast and brightness optimization by manipulation of window width and level settings, as well as a

Figure 2.1 Digital radiography. Digital radiograph of the hand without **(A)** and with **(B)** edge enhancement. The bone details and the soft tissues are better appreciated than on the standard radiographs.

variety of image-processing capabilities, quantitation of image information, and facilitation of examination storage and retrieval. In addition, energy subtraction imaging (also called dual-energy subtraction) may be acquired. Two images, acquired either sequentially or simultaneously with different filtration, are used to reconstruct a soft-tissue–only image or a bone-only image.

In digital subtraction radiography, a video processor and a digital disk are added to a fluoroscopy imaging complex to provide online viewing of subtraction images. This technique is most widely used in evaluation of the vascular system, but it may also be used in conjunction with arthrography to evaluate various joints. Use of high-performance video cameras with low noise characteristics allows single video frames of precontrast and postcontrast images to be used for subtraction. Spatial resolution can be maximized using a combination of geometric magnification, electric magnification, and a small anode–target distance. The subtraction technique removes surrounding anatomic structures and thus isolates the opacified vessel or joint, making it more conspicuous.

Nonvascular digital radiography may be used to evaluate various bone abnormalities and, in conjunction with contrast injection, a procedure called digital subtraction arthrography (Fig. 2.2), to evaluate subtle abnormalities of the joints, such as tears of the triangular fibrocartilage or intercarpal ligaments in the wrist, or to evaluate the stability of prosthesis replacement. Digital radiography offers the potential advantages of improved image quality, contrast sensitivity, and exposure latitude, and it provides efficient storage, retrieval, and transmission of radiographic image data. Digital images may be displayed on the film or on a video monitor. A significant advantage of image digitization is the ability to produce data with low noise and a wide dynamic range suitable for window-level analysis in a manner comparable to that used in a CT scanner.

Digital subtraction angiography (DSA), the most frequently used

tear of lunotriquetral ligament

site of a tear of triangular fibrocartilage

leak of contrast to the distal radioulnar joint

Figure 2.2 Digital subtraction arthrography. Digital subtraction arthrogram demonstrates tears of the lunotriquetral ligament and the triangular fibrocartilage complex. **(A)** This image was obtained by subtracting the digitally acquired preinjection image **(B)** from postinjection film. (Courtesy of Dr. B. J. Manaster, Denver, Colorado.)

A   B

Figure 2.3 **Digital subtraction angiography.** Digital radiograph **(A)** and digital subtraction angiogram **(B)** of a 23-year-old man who sustained fractures of the proximal tibia and fibula show disruption of the distal segment of the popliteal artery.

variant of digital radiography, can be used in the evaluation of trauma, bone and soft-tissue tumors, and in general evaluation of the vascular system. In trauma to the extremity, DSA is effectively used to evaluate arterial occlusion, pseudoaneurysms, arteriovenous fistulas, and transection of the arteries (Fig. 2.3). Some advantages of DSA over conventional film techniques are that its images can be studied rapidly and multiple repeated projections can be obtained. Bone subtraction is useful in clearly delineating the vascular structures. In evaluation of bone and soft-tissue tumors, DSA is an effective tool for mapping tumor vascularity.

Tomography

Tomography is a body section radiography that permits more accurate visualization of lesions too small to be noted on conventional radiographs or demonstrates anatomic detail obscured by overlying structures. It uses continuous motion of the radiographic tube and film cassette in opposite directions throughout exposure, with the fulcrum of the motion located in the plane of interest. By blurring structures above and below the area being examined, the object to be studied is sharply outlined on a single plane of focus. The focal plane may vary in thickness according to the distance the x-ray tube travels; the longer the distance (or arc) traveled by the tube, the thinner the section in focus. Newly developed tomographic units can localize the image more precisely and have aided greatly in the ability to detect lesions as small as approximately 1 mm.

The simplest tomographic movement is linear, with the radiographic tube and film cassette moving on a straight line in opposite directions. This linear movement has little application in the study of bones because it creates streaks that often interfere with radiologic interpretation. Resolution of the plane of focus is much clearer when there is more uniform blurring of undesired structures. This requires a multidirectional movement, such as in zonography or in circular tomography, in which the radiographic tube makes one circular motion at a preset angle of inclination. More complex multidirectional hypocycloidal or trispiral movements increase the distance of excur-

sion of the tube and create a varying angle of projection of the x-ray beam during the exposure. These complex movements are more advantageous because they produce even greater blurring and yield the sharpest images. Trispiral tomography is an important radiographic technique in the diagnosis and management of a variety of bone and joint problems. It continues to be one of the tools for examining patients who have sustained trauma to the skeletal system. Its advantages over conventional radiographs include the visualization of subtle fractures (see Figs. 4.5B and 4.6B). It is not only helpful in delineating the fracture line and demonstrating its extent but also helpful in evaluating the healing process (see Fig. 4.43B), posttraumatic complications (see Figs. 4.50B and 4.59C), and bone grafts in the treatment of nonunions. It is also invaluable in evaluating various tumor and tumor-like lesions (for instance, to demonstrate a nidus of osteoid osteoma or to delineate calcific matrix in enchondroma or chondrosarcoma). Small cystic and sclerotic lesions and subtle erosions can also be better demonstrated. As a rule, the tomograms should be interpreted together with a radiograph for comparison.

Computed Tomography

CT is a radiologic modality containing an x-ray source, detectors, and a computer data-processing system. The essential components of a CT system include a circular scanning gantry, which houses the x-ray tube and image sensors, a table for the patient, an x-ray generator, and a computerized data-processing unit. The patient lies on the table and is placed inside the gantry. The x-ray tube is rotated 360 degrees around the patient while the computer collects the data and formulates an axial image, or "slice." Each cross-sectional slice represents a thickness between 0.1 and 1.5 cm of body tissue.

The newest CT scanners use a rotating fan of x-ray beams, a fixed ring of detectors, and predetector collimator. A highly collimated x-ray beam is transmitted through the area being imaged. The tissues absorb the x-ray beam to various degrees depending on the atomic number and density of the specific tissue. The remaining, unabsorbed (unattenuated) beam passes through the tissues and is detected and processed by the computer. The CT computer software converts the x-ray beam attenuations of the tissue into a CT number (Hounsfield units) by comparing it with the attenuation of water. The attenuation of water is designated as 0 (zero) H, the attenuation of air is designated as −1,000 H, and the attenuation of normal cortical bone is +1,000 H. Routinely, axial sections are obtained; however, computer reconstruction (reformation) in multiple planes may be obtained if desired.

The introduction of spiral (helical) scanning was a further improvement of CT. This technique, referred to as volume-acquisition CT, has made possible a data-gathering system using a continuous rotation of the x-ray source and the detectors. It allows the rapid acquisition of volumes of CT data and rendering ability to reformat the images at any predetermined intervals ranging from 0.5 to 10.0 mm. Unlike standard CT, in which up to a maximum of 12 scans could be obtained per minute, helical CT acquires all data in 24 or 32 seconds, generating up to 92 sections. This technology has markedly reduced scan times and has eliminated interscan delay, and hence interscan motion. It also has decreased motion artifacts, improved definition of scanned structures, and markedly facilitated the ability to obtain three-dimensional reconstructions generated from multiple overlapping transaxial images acquired in a single breath hold. Spiral CT allows data to be acquired during the phase of maximum contrast enhancement, thus optimizing detection of a lesion. The data volume may be viewed either as conventional transaxial images or as multiplanar and three-dimensional reformation.

CT is indispensable in the evaluation of many traumatic conditions and various bone and soft-tissue tumors because of its cross-sectional imaging capability. In trauma, CT is extremely useful to define the presence and extent of fracture or dislocation; to evaluate various intraarticular abnormalities, such as damage to the articular cartilage or the presence of noncalcified and calcified osteocartilaginous bodies; and to evaluate adjacent soft tissues. CT is of particular importance in the detection of small bony fragments displaced into the joints after-trauma; in the detection of small displaced fragments of the fractured vertebral body; and in the assessment of concomitant injury to the cord or thecal sac. The advantage of CT over conventional radiography is its ability to provide excellent contrast resolution, accurately measure the tissue attenuation coefficient, and obtain direct transaxial images (see Figs. 11.23C, 11.31, 11.33B and 11.57C). A further advantage is its ability—through data obtained from thin, contiguous sections—to image the bone in the coronal, sagittal, and oblique planes using reformation technique. This multiplanar reconstruction is particularly helpful in evaluating vertebral alignment (Fig. 2.4), demonstrating horizontally oriented fractures of the vertebral body, or evaluating complex fractures of the pelvis, hip (Fig. 2.5), or calcaneus, abnormalities of the sacrum and sacroiliac joints, sternum and sternoclavicular joints, temporomandibular joints, and wrist. Modern CT scanners use collimated fan beams directed only at the tissue layer undergoing investigation. The newest advances in sophisticated software enable three-dimensional reconstruction, which is helpful in analyzing regions with complex anatomy, such as the face, pelvis, vertebral column, foot, ankle, and wrist (Figs. 2.6 to 2.9). New computer systems now permit the creation of plastic models of the area of interest based on three-dimensional images. These models facilitate operative planning and allow rehearsal surgery of complex reconstructive procedures.

CT plays a significant role in the evaluation of bone and soft-tissue tumors because of its superior contrast resolution and its ability to measure the tissue attenuation coefficient accurately. Although CT by itself is rarely helpful in making a specific diagnosis, it can precisely evaluate the extent of the bone lesion and may demonstrate a break through the cortex and the involvement of surrounding soft tissues. Moreover, CT is very helpful in delineating a tumor in bones having complex anatomic structures, such as the scapula, pelvis, and sacrum, which may be difficult to image fully with conventional radiographic techniques or even conventional tomography. CT examination is crucial to determine the extent and spread of a tumor in the bone if limb salvage is contemplated, so that a safe margin of resection can be planned (Fig. 2.10). It can effectively demonstrate the intraosseous extension of a tumor and its extraosseous involvement of soft tissues such as muscles and neurovascular bundles. It is also useful for monitoring the results of treatment, evaluating for recurrence of resected tumor, and demonstrating the effect of nonsurgical treatment such as radiation therapy and chemotherapy.

Occasionally, iodinated contrast agents may be used intravenously to enhance the CT images. Contrast medium directly alters image contrast by increasing the x-ray attenuation, thus displaying increased brightness in the CT images. It can aid in identifying a suspected soft-tissue mass when initial CT results are unremarkable, or it can assess the vascularity of the soft-tissue or bone tumor.

CT has a crucial role in bone mineral analysis. The ability of CT to measure the attenuation coefficients of each pixel provides a basis for accurate quantitative bone mineral analysis in cancellous and cortical bone. Quantitative computed tomography (QCT) is a method for measuring the lumbar spine mineral content in which the average density values of a region of interest are referenced to that of calibration material scanned at the same time as the patient. Measurements are performed on a CT scanner using a mineral standard for simultaneous calibration and a computed radiograph (scout view) for localization. The evaluation of bone mass measurement provides valuable insight into improving the evaluation and treatment of osteoporosis and other metabolic bone disorders.

CT is also a very important modality for successful aspiration or biopsy of bone or soft-tissue lesions, because it provides visible guidance for precise placement of the instrument within the lesion (Fig. 2.11).

Some disadvantages of CT include the so-called average volume effect, which results from lack of homogeneity in the composition of the small volume of tissue. In particular, the measurement of Hounsfield units results in average values for the different components of the tissue. This partial volume effect becomes particularly important when normal and pathologic processes interface within a section under investigation. The other disadvantage of CT is poor tissue characterization. Despite the ability of CT to discriminate among some differences in density, a simple analysis of attenuation values does not permit precise histologic characterization. Moreover, any movement of the patient will produce artifacts that degrade the image quality. Similarly, an area that contains metal (for instance, prosthesis or various rods and screws) will produce significant artifacts. Finally, the radiation dose may occasionally be high, particularly when contiguous and overlapping sections are obtained during examination.

Arthrography

Figure 2.4 CT reconstruction imaging. Sagittal CT reformatted image demonstrates the flexion tear-drop fracture of C-5. It also effectively shows malalignment of the vertebral body and narrowing of the spinal canal. (From Greenspan A, 1992, with permission.)

Arthrography is introduction of a contrast agent ("positive" contrast—iodide solution, "negative" contrast—air, or a combination of both) into the joint space. Despite the evolution of newer diagnostic imag-

Figure 2.5 CT multiplanar imaging. A 62-year-old man sustained a posterior dislocation of the left femoral head. After reduction of dislocation, the anteroposterior radiograph of the left hip showed increased medial joint space and distortion of the medial aspect of the femoral head **(A)**. To evaluate the hip joint further, CT was performed. Coronal **(B)** and sagittal **(C)** reformatted images showed unsuspected fracture of the femoral head, and axial image **(D)** demonstrated a 180-degree rotation of the fractured fragment.

Figure 2.6 CT three-dimensional imaging. Anteroposterior **(A)** and oblique **(B)** three-dimensional CT reformation of the wrist demonstrates a fracture through the waist of the scaphoid bone, complicated by osteonecrosis of the proximal fragment.

Figure 2.9 CT three-dimensional imaging. Three-dimensional CT reformation of the thoracic spine shows sagittal cleft with an anterior defect of T11, a typical appearance of congenital butterfly vertebra.

Figure 2.7 CT three-dimensional imaging. Three-dimensional CT reformation of the elbow shows a fracture of the neck of the radius (*arrow*) and fracture of the olecranon process (*arrowhead*).

ing modalities, such as CT and MRI, arthrography has retained its importance in daily radiologic practice. The growing popularity of arthrography has been partially caused by advances in its techniques and interpretation. The fact that it is not a technically difficult procedure and is much simpler to interpret than ultrasound, CT, or MRI

Figure 2.8 CT three-dimensional imaging. Fracture of the surgical neck of the humerus (*arrow*) and a displaced fracture of the greater tubercle (*short arrow*) are well demonstrated.

makes it very desirable for evaluating various articulations. Although virtually every joint can be injected with contrast, the examination, at the present time, is most frequently performed in the shoulder, wrist, and ankle. It is important to obtain preliminary films prior to any arthrographic procedure, because contrast may obscure some joint abnormalities (i.e., osteochondral body) that can be easily detected on conventional radiographs. Arthrography is particularly effective in demonstrating rotator cuff tear (Fig. 2.12; see Figs. 5.53 and 5.54) and adhesive capsulitis in the shoulder (see Fig. 5.63), and osteochondritis dissecans, osteochondral bodies, and subtle abnormalities of the articular cartilage in the elbow joint (see Fig. 6.38). In the wrist, arthrography retains its value in diagnosing triangular fibrocartilage complex abnormalities (see Fig. 7.23). Recent introduction of the three-compartment injection technique and the combination of arthrographic wrist examination with digital subtraction arthrography (see Fig. 2.2) and postarthrographic CT examination have made this modality very effective when evaluating a painful wrist.

Although arthrography of the knee has been almost completely replaced by MRI, it still may be used to demonstrate injuries to the soft-tissue structures, such as the joint capsule, menisci, and various ligaments (see Fig. 9.61). It also provides important information on the status of the articular cartilage, particularly when subtle chondral or osteochondral fracture is suspected, or when the presence or absence of osteochondral bodies (i.e., in osteochondritis dissecans) must be confirmed (see Figs. 9.46D, 9.50C).

In the examination of any of the joints, arthrography can be combined with tomography (so-called arthrotomography), with CT (CT–arthrography) (Fig. 2.13), or with digitization of image (digital subtraction arthrography) (see Fig. 2.2), thus providing additional information.

There are relatively few absolute contraindications to arthrography. Even hypersensitivity to iodine is a relative contraindication because, in this case, a single contrast study using only air can be performed.

Tenography and Bursography

Occasionally, to evaluate the integrity of a tendon, contrast material is injected into the tendon sheath. This procedure is known as a tenogram (see Figs. 10.13 and 10.71). Since introduction of newer diagnostic modalities, such as CT and MRI, this procedure is seldom

Figure 2.10 **CT measurement of Hounsfield values.** CT evaluation of intraosseous extension of chondrosarcoma is an important part of the radiologic workup of a patient if limb salvage is contemplated. **(A)** Several contiguous axial sections, preferably 1 cm in thickness, of affected and nonaffected limbs are obtained. **(B)** Hounsfield values of the bone marrow are measured to determine the distal extent of tumor in the medullary cavity. A value of +85 indicates the presence of tumor; a value of −48 is normal for fatty marrow. **(C)** The linear measurement is obtained from the proximal articular end of the bone *A* to the point located 5 cm distally to the tumor margin *B*. Point *C* corresponds to the most distal axial section that still shows tumor in the marrow. (From Greenspan A, 1989, with permission.)

Figure 2.11 **CT-guided aspiration biopsy.** Aspiration biopsy of an infected intervertebral disk is performed under CT guidance. **(A)** Measurement is obtained from the skin surface to the area of interest (intervertebral disk). **(B)** The needle is advanced under CT guidance and placed at the site of the partially destroyed disk.

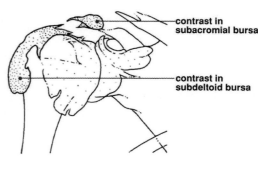

Figure 2.12 Shoulder arthrogram. After injection of contrast into the glenohumeral joint there is filling of subacromial–subdeltoid bursae complex, indicating rotator cuff tear.

contrast in
subacromial bursa

contrast in
subdeltoid bursa

performed. It has relatively limited clinical application, mainly being used to evaluate traumatic or inflammatory conditions of the tendons (such as peroneus longus and brevis, tibialis anterior and posterior, and flexor digitorum longus) of the lower extremity and in the upper extremity to outline the synovial sheaths within the carpal tunnel.

Bursography involves the injection of contrast agent into various bursae. This procedure in general has been abandoned, and only occasionally is the subacromial–subdeltoid bursae complex directly injected with contrast agent to demonstrate partial tears of the rotator cuff.

Angiography

The use of contrast material injected directly into selective branches of the arterial and venous circulation has aided greatly in assessing the involvement of the circulatory system in various conditions and has provided a precise method for defining local pathology. With arteriography, a contrast agent is injected into the arteries and films are made, usually in rapid sequence. With venography, contrast material is injected into the veins. Both procedures are frequently used in evaluation of trauma, particularly if concomitant injury to the vascular system is suspected (see Figs. 2.3 and 4.13).

In evaluation of tumors, arteriography is used mainly to map out bone lesions, demonstrate the vascularity of the lesion, and assess the extent of disease. It is also used to demonstrate the vascular supply of a tumor and to locate vessels suitable for preoperative intraarterial chemotherapy. It is very useful in demonstrating the area suitable for open biopsy, because the most vascular parts of a tumor contain the most aggressive component of the lesion. Occasionally, arteriography can be used to demonstrate abnormal tumor vessels, corroborating findings with radiography and tomography (see Fig. 16.11B). Arteri-

ography is often extremely helpful in planning for limb-salvage procedures, because it demonstrates the regional vascular anatomy and thus permits a plan to be made for the tumor resection. It is also sometimes used to outline the major vessels before resection of a benign lesion (see Fig. 16.12). It can also be combined with an interventional procedure, such as embolization of hypervascular tumors, before further treatment (see Fig. 16.13).

Myelography

During this procedure, water-soluble contrast agents are injected into the subarachnoid space, mixing freely with the cerebrospinal fluid to produce a column of opacified fluid with a higher specific gravity than the nonopacified fluid. Tilting the patient will allow the opacified fluid to run up or down the thecal sac under the influence of gravity (see Figs. 11.16 and 11.48). The puncture usually is performed in the lumbar area at the L2-3 or L3-4 levels. For examination of the cervical segment, a C1-2 puncture is performed (see Fig. 11.16A). Myelographic examination has been almost completely replaced by high-resolution CT and high-quality MRI.

Diskography

Diskography is an injection of contrast material into the nucleus pulposus. Although this is a controversial procedure that has been abandoned by many investigators, under tightly restricted indications and immaculate technique a diskogram can yield valuable information. Diskography is a valuable aid to determine the source of a patient's low back pain. It is not purely an imaging technique, because the symptoms produced during the test (pain during the injection or pain provocation) are considered to have even greater diagnostic value

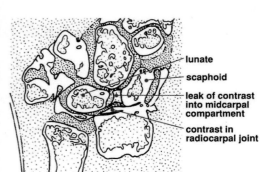

Figure 2.13 CT–arthrography. Coronal CT arthrogram of the wrist demonstrates a subtle leak of contrast from the radiocarpal joint through a tear in the scapholunate ligament, a finding not detected on routine arthrographic examination of the wrist.

lunate

scaphoid

leak of contrast
into midcarpal
compartment

contrast in
radiocarpal joint

than the obtained radiographs. It should always be combined with CT examination (so-called CT–diskogram) (see Figs. 11.49 and 11.50). According to the official position statement on diskography by the Executive Committee of the North American Spine Society in 1988, this procedure "is indicated in the evaluation of patients with unremitting spinal pain, with or without extremity pain, of greater than four months duration, when the pain has been unresponsive to all appropriate methods of conservative therapy." According to the same statement, before a diskogram is performed, the patient should have undergone investigation with other modalities (such as CT, MRI, and myelography) and the surgical correction of the patient's problem should be anticipated.

Ultrasound

Over the past several years, ultrasound has made an enormous impact in the field of radiology and became a useful tool in skeletal imaging. It has several inherent advantages. It is relatively inexpensive, allows comparisons with the opposite normal side, uses no ionizing radiation, and can be performed at bedside or in the operating room. It is a noninvasive modality, relying on the interaction of propagated sound waves with tissue interfaces in the body. Whenever the directed pulsing of sound waves encounters an interface between tissues of different acoustic impedance, reflection or refraction occurs. The sound waves reflected back to the ultrasound transducer are recorded and converted into images.

Various types of ultrasound scanning are available. Most modern ultrasound equipment displays dynamic information in "real time," similar to information that is provided by fluoroscopy. With real-time sonography, the images may be obtained in any scan plane by simply moving the transducer. Thus, imaging may include transverse or longitudinal images and any obliquity can also be produced. Modern probe technology has extended usefulness of ultrasound in orthope-

dic radiology (Fig. 2.14). Higher-frequency transducers of 7.5 and 10 MHz have excellent spatial resolution and are ideal for imaging the appendicular skeleton.

Applications of ultrasound in orthopedics include evaluation of the rotator cuff, injuries to various tendons (for instance, the Achilles tendon), and, occasionally, soft-tissue tumors (such as hemangioma).

The most effective application, however, is in evaluation of the infant hip, for which ultrasound has become the imaging modality of choice. Contributing factors are the cartilaginous composition of the hip, ultrasound's real-time capability for studying motion and stress, absence of ionizing radiation, and relative cost effectiveness. The newest development in this area is the introduction of three-dimensional ultrasound for evaluation of developmental dysplasia of the hip. Three-dimensional sonography provides functional utility in the evaluation of the joint in the added sagittal plane (section image) and craniocaudal projection (revolving spatial image). This technique permits excellent demonstration of the femoral head–acetabulum relationship and femoral head containment (see Figs. 32.16, 32.17). The important advantage of this technique is not only acquisition of images in real time but also subsequent reconstruction and viewing at a workstation, allowing further manipulation of the volume image. This permits extraction of usable measurements and enhancement of the anatomic information obtained from the images.

Ultrasound has recently been applied to certain areas in rheumatic disorders, particularly to detect intraarticular and periarticular fluid collection, and to the differentiation of popliteal fossa masses (e.g., aneurysm versus Baker cyst versus hypertrophied synovium).

More recent ultrasound techniques such as Doppler ultrasound or color-flow imaging, which expresses motion from moving red blood cells in color, have found limited applications in orthopedic radiology. This modality is used mainly to detect arterial narrowing and venous thrombosis. However, there have been a limited number of re-

Figure 2.14 Ultrasound of the shoulder. (A) The bony landmarks (lesser and greater tuberosities, bicipital tendon groove) and **(B)** tendinous structures (supraspinatus) are well outlined.

ports regarding the use of this technology in detecting tumor vascularity within soft-tissue masses.

Scintigraphy (Radionuclide Bone Scan)

Scintigraphy is a modality that detects the distribution in the body of a radioactive agent injected into the vascular system. After an intravenous injection of radiopharmaceutical agent, the patient is placed under a scintillation camera, which detects the distribution of radioactivity in the body by measuring the interaction of gamma rays emitted from the body with sodium iodide crystals in the head of the camera. The photoscans are obtained in multiple projections and may include either the entire body or selected parts.

One major advantage of skeletal scintigraphy over all other imaging techniques is its ability to image the entire skeleton at once (Fig. 2.15). As Johnson remarked, it provides a "metabolic picture" anatomically localizing a lesion by assessing its metabolic activity compared with adjacent normal bone. Bone scan may confirm the presence of the disease, demonstrate the distribution of the lesion, and help evaluate the pathologic process. Indications for skeletal scintigraphy include traumatic conditions, tumors (primary and metastatic), various arthritides, infections, and metabolic bone disease. The detected abnormality may consist of either decreased uptake of bone-seeking radiopharmaceutical (for instance, in the early stage of osteonecrosis) or increased uptake (such as in the case of fracture, neoplasm, a focus of osteomyelitis, etc.). Some structures under normal conditions may show increased activity (such as sacroiliac joints or normal growth plates).

Scintigraphy is a very sensitive imaging modality; however, it is not very specific, and frequently it is impossible to distinguish various processes that can cause increased uptake. Occasionally, however, the bone scan may yield very specific information and even suggest diagnosis, for instance, in multiple myeloma or osteoid osteoma. In the search for myeloma, scintigraphy can distinguish between similar-looking bony metastases because in most myeloma cases, no significant increase in the uptake of the radiopharmaceutical agent occurs; however, in skeletal metastasis, invariably the uptake of the tracer is significantly elevated. In the case of osteoid osteoma, the typical bone scan may demonstrate the so-called double density sign—greater increased uptake in the center, related to the nidus of the lesion, and lesser increased uptake at the periphery, related to the reactive sclerosis surrounding the nidus (Fig. 2.16).

Radionuclide bone scan is an indicator of mineral turnover. Because there is usually an enhanced deposition of bone-seeking radiopharmaceuticals in areas of bone undergoing change and repair, bone scan is useful in localizing tumors and tumor-like lesions in the skeleton. This is particularly helpful in such conditions as fibrous dysplasia, Langerhans cell histiocytosis, or metastatic cancer, in which more than one lesion is encountered, and some may represent a "silent" site of disorder. It also plays an important role in localizing small lesions, such as osteoid osteoma, which may not always be seen on plain-film studies. In most instances radionuclide bone scan cannot distinguish benign lesions from malignant tumors, because increased blood flow with consequently increased isotope deposition and osteoblastic activity will take place in both conditions.

In traumatic conditions, scintigraphy is extremely helpful in the early diagnosis of stress fractures. These fractures may not be seen on conventional radiographs or even on tomographic studies. Scintigraphy is often used to differentiate tibial stress fractures from shin splints. In acute stress fracture hyperperfusion and hyperemia are typically present, and delayed images demonstrate band-like or fusiform uptake in the lesion. Conversely, shin splints are characterized by normal angiographic and blood pool phases with delayed images revealing longitudinally oriented linear areas of increased uptake. Radionuclide bone imaging also has value in diagnosing fractures of the osteopenic bones in elderly patients when routine radiographic examinations appear normal.

In metabolic bone disorders, bone scintigraphy is helpful, for instance, in establishing the extent of skeletal involvement in Paget disease (see Fig. 26.10) and assessing response to treatment. Although it is of no value for patients with generalized osteoporosis, it may occasionally be helpful in differentiating osteoporosis from osteomalacia and multiple vertebral fractures resulting from osteoporosis from those occurring in metastatic carcinoma. Radionuclide bone scan has also been reported to be useful in diagnosis of reflex sympathetic dystrophy syndrome.

Skeletal scintigraphy is frequently used in evaluation of infections. In particular, technetium (Tc) 99m methylene diphosphonate (MDP) and indium (In) 111 are highly sensitive in detecting early and occult osteomyelitis. In chronic osteomyelitis, imaging with gallium

Figure 2.15 Radionuclide bone scan. Scintigraphy obtained in a patient with renal disease and secondary hyperparathyroidism demonstrates several abnormalities: left hydronephrosis secondary to urinary obstruction, resorptive changes of the distal ends of both clavicles, and periarticular soft-tissue calcifications around both shoulders.

A **B**

Figure 2.16 Osteoid osteoma—diagnosis by scintigraphy. A 4-year-old girl had symptoms suggesting a diagnosis of osteoid osteoma; however, a radiograph **(A)** failed to demonstrate the nidus. Scintigraphic examination **(B)** demonstrates a characteristic "double density" sign: more increased uptake in the center is related to the nidus of osteoid osteoma, whereas less increased uptake at the periphery denotes reactive sclerosis.

(Ga) 67 citrate is more accurate in detecting the response or lack of response to treatment than ^{99m}Tc–phosphate bone imaging. For detecting recurrent active infection in patients with chronic osteomyelitis, ^{111}In appears to be the radiopharmaceutical of choice. It must be stressed, however, that because the ^{111}In-labeled leukocytes also accumulate in active bone marrow, the sensitivity for detection of chronic osteomyelitis is reduced. To improve the diagnostic ability of this technique, combined ^{99m}Tc–sulfur colloid bone marrow/^{111}In-labeled leukocyte study has been advocated. The three- or four-phase technique using technetium phosphate tracers can be effectively used to distinguish between soft-tissue infection (cellulitis) and osseous infection (osteomyelitis).

The use of technetium-99m hexamethylpropylene-amine-oxime (HMPAO)–labeled leukocytes for diagnosing infectious processes has recently been advocated. The kinetics and normal distribution of such leukocytes are similar to those of indium 111-labeled white cells. The superior resolution and count density of technetium 99m, however, gives this technique an advantage over the use of indium-labeled leukocytes.

In neoplastic conditions, the detection of skeletal metastasis is probably the most common indication for skeletal scintigraphy. It also is used frequently to determine the extent of a lesion or the presence of so-called skipped lesions or intraosseous metastases. It is not, however, the method of choice to determine the extent of the lesion in

bone. It is important to stress that scintigraphy alone cannot diagnose the type of tumor; however, it may be useful to detect and localize some primary tumors as well as multifocal lesions (such as multicentric osteosarcoma).

Technetium 99m MDP scans are used primarily to determine whether a lesion is monostotic or polyostotic. Such a study is therefore essential in staging a bone tumor. It is important to remember that although the degree of abnormal uptake may be related to the aggressiveness of the lesion, this does not correlate well with histologic grade. Gallium 67 may show uptake in a soft-tissue sarcoma and may help to differentiate a sarcoma from a benign soft-tissue lesion.

Although a bone scan may demonstrate the extent of the primary malignant tumor in bone, it is not as accurate as CT or MRI. It may be useful in the detection of a local recurrence of the tumor and occasionally indicates the response or lack of response to treatment (in the case of radiotherapy or chemotherapy).

In the evaluation of arthritides, a bone scan is extremely helpful in demonstrating the distribution of the lesion in the skeleton and has completely replaced the previously used radiographic joint survey (see Fig. 12.13A). Scintigraphy can determine the distribution of arthritic changes, not only in large and small joints but also in areas usually not detected by standard radiography, such as the sternomanubrial and temporomandibular joints, among others.

With the development of single-photon emission tomography

(SPET) and single-photon emission computed tomography (SPECT), diagnostic precision in evaluating bone and joint abnormalities has increased tremendously. Instrumentation efficacy for SPECT is improving with the introduction of multiple crystal detectors, fan beam and cone beam collimators, detection of a greater fraction of photons, and improved algorithms. In comparison with planar images, SPECT provides increased contrast resolution using a tomographic mode similar to conventional tomography, which eliminates noise from the tissue outside the plane of imaging (Fig. 2.17). It provides not only qualitative information on the uptake of bone-seeking radiopharmaceuticals but also quantitative data.

The principal benefit of SPECT is improvement of lesion detection and anatomical localization, hence producing better diagnostic sensitivity. Bone SPECT has proved particularly useful in the detection of lesions in large and complex anatomic structures, in which it allows removal of overlying and underlying activity from areas of interest. The widest applications have been found in imaging of the spine, pelvis, knees, and ankles. Using SPECT imaging in the spine, for example, lesions can be localized to different parts of the vertebra (i.e., vertebral body, pedicle, articular process, lamina, pars interarticularis, spinous and transverse process). In the knee, SPECT imaging has proved to be highly effective in detection of meniscal tears.

Several bone-seeking tracers are available for scintigraphic imaging. Those most frequently used are as follows:

Diphosphonates

In recent years, there has been remarkable progress in the development of new gamma-emitting diagnostic agents for radionuclide imaging. The radiopharmaceuticals currently in use in bone scanning include the organic diphosphonates, ethylene diphosphonates (HEPD), methylene diphosphonates (MDP), and methane hydroxydiphosphonates (HNDP), all labeled with ^{99m}Tc, a pure gamma-emitter with a 6-hour half-life. MDP is more frequently used, particularly in adults, typically in a dose that provides 15 mCi (555 MBq) of ^{99m}Tc. After intravenous injection of the radiopharmaceutical, approximately 50% of the dose localizes in bone. The remainder circulates freely in the body and eventually is excreted by the kidneys. A gamma camera can then be used in a procedure known as four-phase isotope bone scan. The first phase, the *radionuclide angiogram*, is the first minute after injection when the serial images obtained every 2 seconds demonstrate the radioactive tracer in the major blood vessels. In the second phase, the *blood pool scan*, which lasts from 1 to 3 minutes after injection, isotope is detected in the vascular system and in the extracellular space in the soft tissues before being taken-up by bone. The

Figure 2.17 Effectiveness of SPECT imaging. A 46-year-old woman presented with left hip pain for several months. **(A)** Radiograph demonstrated only minimally advanced degenerative changes of the hip joint. A small radiolucent area in the superior portion of the acetabulum raised some concerns about the diagnosis. **(B)** Conventional radionuclide bone scan in anterior and posterior projections demonstrated a slight increase in the uptake of the tracer localized to the left hip joint. **(C)** SPECT examination was performed. On the tomographic cut at the level of the acetabulae (*inset*), there is an area of increased activity localized to the anterosuperior aspect of the left acetabulum and focal areas of activity related to osteophytes of the femoral head. **(D)** CT examination demonstrating a large degenerative cyst (geod) in the acetabulum in the area corresponding to abnormal uptake of a tracer on SPECT section.

third phase, or *static bone scan,* usually occurs 2 to 3 hours after injection and discloses radiopharmaceutical in the bone. This phase may be divided into two stages. In the first, the isotope diffuses passively through the bone capillaries. In the second stage, the radionuclide is concentrated in bone. The most intense localization occurs in the first and second phases in areas with increased blood flow, and in the third phase, in areas with increased osteogenic activity, increased calcium metabolism, and active bone turnover. The fourth phase is a 24-hour *static image.*

Gallium 67

Gallium 67 citrate is frequently used to diagnose infectious and inflammatory processes in bones and joints. Although the target site of gallium localization is soft tissue, gallium localizes also to some extent in bone because it is incorporated into the calcium hydroxyapatite crystal as a calcium analog, and in bone marrow, because of its behavior as an iron analog. Gallium accumulates in regions of infection because of association with bacterial and cellular debris as well as leukocytes. Because white blood cells migrate to the foci of inflammation and infection, some of the gallium is transported intracellularly to these sites. The sensitivity of ^{67}Ga for abscess detection varies from 58% to 100% and specificity varies from 75% to 99%. The images are usually obtained 6 and 24 hours after the injection of 5 mCi (185 MBq) of this radiopharmaceutical. These images are extremely accurate in following the response to therapy of chronic osteomyelitis and infectious arthritis. In particular, changing activity of ^{67}Ga uptake parallels the patient's clinical course in septic arthritis more closely than the images obtained after injection of technetium-labeled diphosphonate. Over the past few years, there has been a considerable change in the role of gallium imaging in infection. Once the mainstay of radionuclide imaging for infection, gallium scanning has now been supplanted by labeled leukocyte imaging. The gallium 67 citrate scan, however, enhances and complements the diagnostic value of the technetium 99m MDP scan. In conjunction with the latter, gallium scintigraphy has been used to improve the specificity of technetium imaging. For example, sequential technetium–gallium imaging is superior to technetium MDP scintigraphy alone in distinguishing cellulitis from osteomyelitis and in precise localization of infectious foci.

In neoplastic conditions, gallium scan is used to differentiate a sarcoma from a benign soft-tissue lesion.

Indium

The diagnostic advantage of ^{111}In oxine-labeled white blood cells over other bone-seeking radiopharmaceuticals in detecting inflammatory abnormalities in the skeletal system has recently been advocated. Because ^{111}In leukocytes are not usually incorporated into areas of increased bone turnover, indium imaging presumably reflects inflammatory activity only, and early experience has shown it to be specific in detecting abscesses or acute infectious processes, including osteomyelitis and septic arthritis. The sensitivity varies from 75% to 90% and specificity, as recently reported, is approximately 91%. False-negative results are often seen in patients with chronic infections in which there is reduced inflow of circulating leukocytes. False-positive results are seen in patients who have an inflammatory process without infection (such as rheumatoid arthritis mistaken for septic arthritis).

Nanocolloid

Very small particles of ^{99m}Tc-labeled colloid of human serum albumin were tried as a bone marrow imaging agent. Approximately 86% of these particles are 30 nm or smaller, and the remainder are between 30 and 80nm. This nanocolloid has sensitivity for detection of osteomyelitis in the extremities equal to that of indium-labeled leukocytes. The clinical value of this method has not been yet determined.

Immunoglobulins

Recently, radiolabeled human polyclonal IgG has been used as an agent for imaging infection. This labeled immunoglobulin is thought to bind to Fc receptors expressed by cells (macrophages, polymorphonuclear leukocytes, lymphocytes) involved in the inflammatory response. In a study of 128 patients, polyclonal IgG yielded a sensitivity of 91% and specificity of 100%. Polyclonal immunoglobulins have a number of advantages, such as availability in kit form and the fact that they do not require *in vivo* labeling.

Chemotactic Peptides

The same investigators who developed ^{111}In-labeled IgG are also pioneering the use of radiolabeled chemotactic peptides for infection imaging. These are small peptides that are produced by bacteria. They bind to high-affinity receptors on the cell membrane of polymorphonuclear leukocytes and mononuclear phagocytes, stimulating chemotaxis. Rather than using the native peptide, synthetic analogs are created that allow radiolabeling. Small size of ^{111}In-labeled chemotactic peptides allows the component to pass quickly through the vascular walls and enter the site of infection.

Iodine

Iodine 125 is used in a radionuclide technique known as a single-photon absorptiometry (SPA) to determine bone mineral density at peripheral bone sites such as finger and radius. This method measures primarily density of the cortical bone.

Gadolinium

Gadolinium 153 is a radionuclide source in technique dual-photon absorptiometry (DPA), which is also used to calculate bone mineral density. This technique permits measurement of central sites of bone such as the spine and the hip. Gadolinium 153 produces photons at two energy levels, and the images are generated on a whole-body rectilinear scanner. The measurements are obtained for compact and trabecular bone.

Positron Emission Tomography

Positron emission tomography (PET) is a diagnostic imaging technique that allows identification of biochemical and physiologic alterations in the body and assesses the level of metabolic activity and perfusion in various organ systems. The process produces biologic images based on detection of gamma rays that are emitted by a radioactive substance, such as ^{18}F-labeled 2-fluoro-2-deoxyglucose ([18]FDG). One of the main applications of this technique is in oncology, including detection of primary and metastatic tumors and recurrences of the tumors after treatment. Only recently has PET scanning been found to be useful in the diagnosis, treatment, and follow-up of musculoskeletal neoplasms (Fig. 2.18). Although some promising results have been reported in using this technique, detection of bone marrow involvement is still controversial, because physiologic bone marrow uptake and diffuse uptake in reactive changes in bone marrow (such as after chemotherapy) can be observed on FDG PET images. Recently, a significant progress has been made in application of PET scanning in diagnosing infections associated with metallic implants in patients with traumatic conditions.

Magnetic Resonance Imaging

MRI is based on the reemission of an absorbed radio frequency (rf) signal while the patient is in a strong magnetic field. An external magnetic field is usually generated by a magnet with field strengths of 0.2 to 1.5 tesla (T). The system includes a magnet, rf coils (transmitter and receiver), gradient coils, and a computer display unit with digital storage facilities. The physical principals of MRI cannot be discussed here in detail because of space limitations; only a brief overview will be given.

The ability of MRI to image body parts depends on the intrinsic spin of atomic nuclei with an odd number of protons and/or neutrons (for example, hydrogen), thus generating a magnetic moment. Atomic nuclei of tissues placed within the main magnetic field from the usual random alignment of their magnetic poles tend to align

Figure 2.18 Positron emission tomography. (A) A normal whole body PET scan of a 62-year-old woman suspected of having skeletal metastases caused by recently treated breast carcinoma. **(B)** A whole-body PET scan of a 9-year-old girl with Ewing sarcoma of the right ilium shows hypermetabolic tumor in the bone (*lower arrow*) and a metastatic lung nodule (*upper arrow*). **(C)** A whole-body PET scan of a 37-year-old woman with fibrous dysplasia shows multiple skeletal deformities. The lower arrow points to the lesion in proximal femur, and the upper arrow points to a large hypermetabolic focus in the sternum. (**B** and **C** are courtesy of Drs. Frieda Feldman and Ronald van Heertum, New York, NY.)

along the direction of that field. Application of rf pulses causes the nuclei to absorb energy and induces resonance of particular sets of nuclei, which causes their orientation to the magnetic field. The required frequency of the pulse is determined by the strength of the magnetic field and the particular nucleus undergoing investigation. When the rf field is removed, the energy absorbed during the transition from a high- to low-energy state is subsequently released, and this can be recorded as an electrical signal that provides the data from which digital images are derived. Signal intensity refers to the strength of the radio wave that a tissue emits after excitation. The strength of this radio wave determines the degree of brightness of the imaged structures. A bright (white) area in an image is said to demonstrate high signal intensity, whereas a dark (black) area is said to demonstrate a low signal intensity. The intensity of a given tissue is a function of the concentration of hydrogen atoms (protons) resonating within the imaged volume and of the longitudinal and transverse relaxation times, which, in turn, depend on the biophysical state of the tissue's water molecules.

Two relaxation times are described, termed T1 and T2. The T1 relaxation time (longitudinal) is used to describe the return of protons back to equilibrium after application and removal of the rf pulse. T2 relaxation time (transverse) is used to describe the associated loss of coherence or phase between individual protons immediately after the application of the rf pulse. A variety of rf pulse sequences can be used to enhance the differences in T1 and T2, thus providing the necessary image contrast. The most commonly used sequences are spin echo (SE), partial saturation recovery (PSR), inversion recovery (IR), chemical selective suppression (CHESS), and fast scan technique (FS). Spin echo (SE) short repetition times (TR) (800 msec or less) and short echo delay times (TE) (40 msec or less) pulse sequences (or T1) provide good anatomic detail. Long TR (2000 msec or more) and long TE (60 msec or more) pulse sequences (or T2), however, provide good contrast, sufficient for evaluation of pathologic processes. Intermediate TR (1000 msec or more) and short TE (30 msec or less) sequences are known as proton or spin density images. They represent a mixture of T1 and T2 weighting, and although they provide good anatomic details, the tissue contrast is somewhat impaired. IR sequences can be combined with multiplanar imaging to shorten scan time. With a short inversion time (TI), in the range of 100 to 150 msec, the effects of prolonged T1 and T2 relaxation times are cumulative

Table 2.1 **Fat Suppression Techniques**

Methods	Advantages	Disadvantages
Frequency-selective (chemical) fat saturation	Lipid-specific Signal in nonfat tissue unaffected Excellent imaging of small anatomic detail Can be used with any imaging sequence	Occasionally inadequate fat suppression Water signal may be suppressed Inhomogeneities in areas of sharp variations in anatomic structures Increased imaging time
Inversion recovery (STIR)	Excellent contrast resolution Very good for tumor detection Can be used with low-field-strength magnets	Low signal-to-noise ratio Tissue with a short T1 and long T1 may produce the same signal intensity Signal from mucoid tissue, hemorrhage, and proteinaceous fluid may be suppressed
Opposed-phase	Ability to demonstrate small amounts of lipid tissue Simple, fast, and available on every MR imaging system	Fat signal only partially suppressed Suppresses water signal Difficult to detect small tumors imbedded in fat In postgadolinium studies, contrast material may be undetected

and the signal from fat is suppressed. This technique, called short time inversion recovery (STIR), has been useful for evaluating bone tumors. CHESS is a sequence also used for fat signal suppression. In this sequence, the chemical shift artifacts are removed and the high-intensity fat signal is suppressed; thus, the effective dynamic range of signal intensities is increased and contrast depiction of anatomic details is improved.

Fat suppression technique is commonly used in MRI to detect adipose tissue or suppress the signal from adipose tissue. There are three methods to achieve this goal: frequency-selective (chemical) fat saturation, inversion–recovery imaging, and opposed-phase imaging (Table 2.1). Selection of one of these methods depends on the purpose of fat suppression, whether it is used to enhance the contrast or to characterize the tissue and the amount of fat in the tissue under investigation. *Fat saturation* methods are usually chosen for suppression of signal from large amounts of adipose tissue and to provide a good contrast resolution. This technique can be used with any imaging sequence. It is useful to visualize small anatomic details, for example, in postcontrast MR arthrography. *Inversion–recovery* method (such as STIR sequence) allows homogeneous and global fat suppression; however, the generated images have low signal-to-noise ratio, and this technique is not only specific for fat. *Opposed-phase* method is recommended for demonstration of lesions that contain only small amounts of fat. Inability of this technique to detect small tumors embedded in adipose tissue is a main disadvantage.

Recently, fat suppression techniques have been combined with three-dimensional gradient echo imaging, resulting in superior delineation of articular cartilage. The main indication for fat suppression is the assessment of small amounts of bone marrow edema in the subchondral bone, often accompanying osteochondral pathology such as in osteochondral fractures, osteochondritis dissecans, or osteonecrosis.

Fast imaging techniques have become increasingly popular because of a number of advantages compared with much slower SE imaging. In particular, so-called gradient recalled echo (GRE) pulse sequences using variable flip angles (5 to 90 degrees) have gained rapid acceptance in orthopedic imaging, because they represent the most effective means of performing fast MRI. The major advantage is the shortening of imaging time, because the low flip angle rf pulses destroy only a small part of the longitudinal magnetization in each pulse cycle. There are several different types of GRE methods in clin-

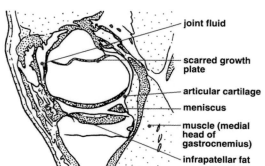

Figure 2.19 MRI of the knee. (A) Sagittal spin echo T1-weighted image (SE; TR 600/TE 20 msec) and **(B)** sagittal MPGR T2*-weighted image (flip angle 30 degrees, TR 35/TE 15 msec) demonstrate various anatomic structures caused by variations in signal intensity of bone, articular cartilage, fibrocartilage, ligaments, muscles, and fat.

quadriceps tendon
cortex
scarred growth plate
posterior cruciate ligament
infrapatellar fat
patellar ligament

joint fluid
scarred growth plate
articular cartilage
meniscus
muscle (medial head of gastrocnemius)
infrapatellar fat

Table 2.2 **MRI Signal Intensities of Various Tissues**

TISSUE	IMAGE	
	T1-WEIGHTED	*T2-WEIGHTED*
Hematoma, hemorrhage (acute, subacute)	Intermediate/High	High
Hematoma, hemorrhage (chronic)	Low	Low
Fat, fatty marrow	High	Intermediate
Muscle, nerves, hyaline cartilage	Intermediate	Intermediate
Cortical bone, tendons ligaments, fibrocartilage, scar tissue	Low	Low
Hyaline cartilage	Intermediate	Intermediate
Red (hematopoietie) marrow	Low	Intermediate
Air	Low	Low
Fluid	Intermediate	High
Proteinaceous fluid	High	High
Tumors (generally)	Intermediate to low	High
Lipoma	High	Intermediate
Hemangioma	Intermediate (slightly higher than muscle)	High

ical use. Each of these methods relies on using a reduced flip angle to enhance signal with short TR. These techniques are known by a variety of acronyms such as FLASH (fast low-angle shot), FISP (fast imaging with steady procession), GRASS (gradient-recalled acquisition in the steady state), and MPGR (multiplanar gradient recalled). Gradient echo sequences are particularly useful in imaging tendons, ligaments, articular cartilage, and loose bodies in the joint. The drawback of this technique is the so-called susceptibility effect, which results in artificial signal loss at the interface between tissues of different magnetic properties. This factor limits the use of gradient echo sequences when imaging patients with metallic hardware.

In most examinations, at least two orthogonal planes should be obtained (axial and either coronal or sagittal), and on many occasions all three planes are necessary. For adequate MRI, surface coils are necessary, because they provide improved spatial resolution. Most surface coils are designed specifically for different areas of the body, such as knee, shoulder, wrist, and temporomandibular joints. Currently, the use of MRI in orthopedic radiology is mainly confined to three areas: trauma, tumors, and infections.

The musculoskeletal system is ideally suited for evaluation by MRI because different tissues display different signal intensities on T1- and T2-weighted images. The images displayed may have a low signal intensity, intermediate signal intensity, or high signal intensity. *Low signal intensity* may be subdivided into signal void (black) and signal

lower than that of normal muscle (dark). *Intermediate signal intensity* may be subdivided into signal equal to that of normal muscle and signal higher than muscle but lower than subcutaneous fat (bright). *High signal intensity* may be subdivided into signal equal to normal subcutaneous fat (bright) and signal higher than subcutaneous fat (extremely bright). High signal intensity of fat planes and differences in signal intensity of various structures allow separation of the different tissue components including muscles, tendons, ligaments, vessels, nerves, hyalin cartilage, fibrocartilage, cortical bone, and trabecular bone (Fig. 2.19). For instance, fat and yellow (fatty) bone marrow display high signal intensity on T1- and intermediate signal on T2-weighted images; hematoma display relatively high signal intensity on T1 and T2 sequences. Cortical bone, air, ligaments, tendons, and fibrocartilage display low signal intensity on T1- and T2-weighted images; muscle, nerves, and hyaline cartilage display intermediate signal intensity on T1- and T2-weighted images. Red (hematopoietic) marrow displays low signal on T1- and low-to-intermediate signal on T2-weighted images. Fluid displays intermediate signal on T1- and high signal on T2-weighting. Most tumors display low-to-intermediate signal intensity on T1-weighted images and high signal intensity on T2-weighted images. Lipomas display high signal intensity on T1- and intermediate signal on T2-weighted images (Table 2.2).

Traumatic conditions of the bones and soft tissues are particularly well suited to diagnosis and evaluation by MRI. Some abnormalities, such as bone contusions or trabecular microfractures, not seen on radiography and CT are well demonstrated by this technique (Fig. 2.20). Occult fractures, which can be missed on conventional x-ray films, become obvious on MR imaging (Fig. 2.21).

Occasionally, MR images may be enhanced by intravenous injection of Gd-DTPA, known as gadolinium, a paramagnetic compound that demonstrates increased signal intensity on T1-weighted images. The mechanism by which gadolinium produces enhancement in MRI is fundamentally different from the mechanism of contrast enhancement in CT. Unlike iodine in CT, gadolinium itself produces no MRI signal. Instead it acts by shortening the T1 and T2 relaxation times of tissues into which it extravasates, resulting in an increase in signal intensity on T1-weighted (short TR/TE) imaging sequences.

Magnetic resonance arthrography has become popular in recent years. The diagnostic accuracy of this technique may exceed that of conventional MRI because the intraarticular structures are better demonstrated if they are separated by means of capsular distention. Such distention can be achieved with intraarticular injection of contrast material such as diluted gadopentetate dimeglumine (gadolinium) or saline. Most commonly a mixture of sterile saline, iodinated contrast agent, 1% lidocaine (or Xylocaine), and gadolinium-DTPA is injected into the joint under fluoroscopic guidance. The generated images are very similar to those obtained of the joint with preexisting joint fluid (joint effusion). In clinical practice magnetic resonance arthrography is predominantly used in the evaluation of shoulder ab-

Figure 2.20 Bone contusion (trabecular injury) (**A**) Coronal T1-weighted MRI of a 44-year-old woman who sustained an injury to her right knee shows area of low signal intensity in the medial femoral condyle. (**B**) On the fast spin-echo inversion recovery (FSE-IR) image, the trabecular injury becomes more conspicuous as a focus of high signal intensity against the low-intensity background of suppressed marrow fat (*arrow*). In another patient, a 35-year-old man, T1-weighted (**C**) and FSE-IR (**D**) coronal MR images show a trabecular injury to the lateral aspect of tibial plateau of the left knee. In a 29-year-old woman, T2-weighted IR with fat saturation coronal MRI (**E**) shows a trabecular injury to the lateral femoral condyle and lateral aspect of the proximal tibia. *(continued)*

Figure 2.20 *Continued.*

normalities, such as internal derangement, glenohumeral joint instability, rotator cuff disorders, or articular cartilage and cartilaginous
labrum abnormalities (Fig. 2.22). Indirect magnetic resonance
arthrography is a procedure in which an intravenous injection of

gadolinium is administered before MRI examination of the joint. This
technique, like magnetic resonance arthrography, may improve detection of rotator cuff tears, labral pathology, and adhesive capsulitis.

Magnetic resonance angiography (MRA) is a technique that

Figure 2.21 Occult fracture of the tibia. A 47-
year-old woman sustained an injury to her left
knee in a car accident. **(A)** Anteroposterior radiograph shows sclerotic area in the proximal tibia,
but no definite fracture is apparent. **(B)** Coronal
and **(C)** axial T1-weighted MR images demonstrate a vertical fracture line extending into the
tibial spines. **(D)** A T2-weighted inversion recovery coronal MRI in addition to the fracture line
shows the tears of the lateral meniscus and lateral
collateral ligament, and joint fluid.

Figure 2.22 Glenoid labrum tear. Magnetic resonance arthrogram of a 26-year-old man who sustained an injury to his right shoulder shows several abnormalities. **(A)** A coronal T1-weighted MR image with fat saturation shows a tear of the inferior cartilaginous labrum of the glenoid. **(B)** An axial T1-weighted MR image with fat saturation shows tears of the anterior and posterior cartilaginous labra associated with stripping of the anterior joint capsule.

helps to visualize blood vessels. Unlike conventional contrast angiography, it does not visualize the blood volume itself but rather depicts a property of blood flow. One of its advantages is that after a three-dimensional MRA data set is collected, one may choose any number of viewing directions. This feature also eliminates vascular overlapping. Numerous pulse sequences have been proposed to produce angiographic contrast. Some rely on the rapid inflow of relaxed blood into the region in which the stationary tissue is saturated. These methods are called time-of-flight (TOF) or flow-related enhancement (FRE). Others, which rely on the velocity-dependent change of phase of moving blood in the presence of a magnetic field gradient, are called the phase-contrast methods. Some methods involve the subtraction of flow-dephased images from flow-compensated images. Applications of MRA in orthopedic radiology include evaluation of the vascular structures in patients with trauma to the extremities and assessment of vascularity of musculoskeletal neoplasms.

Although MRI has many advantages, disadvantages exist as well. These include the typical contraindications of scanning patients with cardiac pacemakers, cerebral aneurysm clips, and claustrophobia. The presence of metallic objects, such as ferromagnetic surgical clips, causes focal loss of signal with or without distortion of image. Metallic objects create "holes" in the image, but ferromagnetic objects cause more distortion. Similar to CT, an average volume effect may be observed in MR images, causing occasional pitfalls in interpretation.

SUGGESTED READINGS

Abdel-Dayem HM. The role of nuclear medicine in primary bone and soft tissue tumors. *Semin Nucl Med* 1997;27:355–363.

Adam G, Drobnitzky M, Nolte-Ernsting CCA, Günther RW. Optimizing joint imaging: MR imaging techniques. *Eur Radiol* 1996;6:882–889.

Aisen AN, Martel W, Braunstein EM, McMillin KI, Phillips WA, Kling TF. MRI and CT evaluation of primary bone and soft tissue tumors. *AJR Am J Roentgenol* 1986;146:749–756.

Allman K, Schafer O, Hauer M, et al. Indirect MR arthrography of the unexercised glenohumeral joint in patients with rotator cuff tears. *Invest Radiol* 1999;34:435–440.

Al Sheikh W, Sfakianakis GN, Mnaymneh W, et al. Subacute and chronic bone infections: diagnosis using In-111, Ga-67, and Tc-99m MDP bone scintigraphy, and radiography. *Radiology* 1985;155:501–506.

Alazraki NP. Radionuclide imaging in the evaluation of infectious and inflammatory disease. *Radiol Clin North Am* 1993;31:783–794.

Alazraki N, Dries D, Datz F, Lawrence P, Greenberg E, Taylor A Jr. Value of a 24-hour image (four-phase bone scan) in assessing osteomyelitis in patients with peripheral vascular disease. *J Nucl Med* 1985;26:711–717.

Alley MT, Shifrin RY, Pelc NJ, Herfkens RJ. Ultrafast contrast-enhanced three-dimensional MR angiography: state of the art. *Radiographics* 1998;18:273–285.

Ammann W, Matheson GO. Radionuclide bone imaging in the detection of stress fractures. *Clin J Sports Med* 1991;1:115–122.

Anderson MW, Greenspan A. State of the art: stress fractures. *Radiology* 1996;199:1–12.

Aoki J, Watanabe H, Shinozaki T, et al. FDG PET of primary benign and malignant bone tumors: standardized uptake value in 52 lesions. *Radiology* 2001;219:774–777.

Aoki J, Watanabe H, Shinozaki T, Takagishi K, Tokunaga M, Koyama Y, Sato N, Endo K. FDG-PET for preoperative differential diagnosis between benign and malignant soft tissue masses. *Skeletal Radiol* 2003;32:133–138.

Arndt WF III, Truax AL, Barnett FM, Simmons GE, Brown DC. MR diagnosis of bone contusions of the knee: comparison of coronal T2-weighted fast spin-echo with fat saturation and fast spin-echo STIR images with conventional STIR images. *AJR Am J Roentgenol* 1996;166:119–124.

Ballinger PW. *Merrill's atlas of radiographic positions and radiologic procedures*, 3rd ed, vol. 1. St Louis: Mosby; 1986.

Beck RN. Radionuclide imaging principles. In: Taveras JM, Ferrucci JT, eds. *Radiology—diagnosis, imaging, intervention*, vol. 1. Philadelphia: JB Lippincott; 1990:1–9.

Becker W, Goldenberg DM, Wolf F. The use of monoclonal antibodies and antibody fragments in the imaging of infectious lesions. *Semin Nucl Med* 1994;24:142–153.

Beltran J, Bencardino J, Mellado J, Rosenberg ZS, Irish RD. MR arthrography of the shoulder: variants and pitfalls. *Radiographics* 1997;17:1403–1412.

Beltran J, Gray LA, Bools JC, Zuelzer W, Weis LD, Unverferth LJ. Rotator cuff lesions of the shoulder: evaluation by direct sagittal CT arthrography. *Radiology* 1986;160:161–165.

Beltran J, Rosenberg ZS, Chandnani VP, Cuomo F, Beltran S, Rokito A. Glenohumeral instability: evaluation with MR arthrography. *Radiographics* 1997;17:657–673.

Bordalo-Rodrigues M, Galant C, Lonneux M, Clause D, Vande Berg BC. Focal nodular hyperplasia of the hematopietic marrow simulating vertebral metastasis on FDG positron emission tomography. *AJR Am J Roentgenol* 2003;180:669–671.

Borders J, Kerr E, Sartoris DJ, et al. Quantitative dual-energy radiographic absorptiometry of the lumbar spine: in vivo comparison with dual-photon absorptiometry. *Radiology* 1989;170:129–131.

Brandt TD, Cardone BW, Grant TH, Post M, Weiss CA. Rotator cuff sonography: a reassessment. *Radiology* 1989;173:323–327.

Brower AC. *Arthritis in black and white*, 2nd ed. Philadelphia: Saunders; 1997.

Brown ML, O'Connor MK, Hung JC, Hayostek RJ. Technical aspects of bone scintigraphy. *Radiol Clin North Am* 1993;31:721–730.

Buckwalter KA, Braunstein EM. Digital skeletal radiography. *AJR Am J Roentgenol* 1992;158:1071–1080.

Buckwalter KA, Rydberg J, Kopecky KK, Crow K, Yang EL. Musculoskeletal imaging with multislice CT. Pictorial Essay. *AJR Am J Roentgenol* 2001;176:979–986.

Burk DL, Mears DC, Kennedy WH, Cooperstein LA, Herbert DL. Three-dimensional computed tomography of acetabular fractures. *Radiology* 1985;155:183–186.

Chhem RK, Cardinal E, Cho KH. Skeletal and superficial soft tissues. In: McGahan JP, Goldberg BB, eds. *Diagnostic ultrasound. A logical approach*. Philadelphia: Lippincott-Raven Publishers; 1998:1115–1134.

Dalinka MK, Boorstein JM, Zlatkin MB. Computed tomography of musculoskeletal trauma. *Radiol Clin North Am* 1989;27:933–944.

Datz FL. Indium-111-labeled leukocytes for the detection of infection: current status. *Semin Nucl Med* 1994;24:92–109.

Datz FL, Morton KA. New radiopharmaceuticals for detecting infection. *Invest Radiol* 1993;28:356–365.

Delfaut EM, Beltran J, Johnson G, Rousseau J, Marchandise X, Cotten A. Fat suppression in MR imaging: techniques and pitfalls. *Radiographics* 1999;19:373–382.

Delpassand ES, Garcia JR, Bhadkamkar V, Podoloff DA. Value of SPECT imaging of the thoracolumbar spine in cancer patients. *Clin Nucl Med* 1995;20:1047–1051.

Derchi LE, Balconi G, DeFlaviis L, Oliva A, Rosso F. Sonographic appearance of hemangiomas of skeletal muscle. *J Ultrasound Med* 1989;8:263–267.

Deutsch AL, Mink JH. Magnetic resonance imaging of musculoskeletal injuries. *Radiol Clin North Am* 1989;27:983–1002.

Dewhirst MW, Sostman HD, Leopold KA, et al. Soft-tissue sarcomas: MR imaging and MR spectroscopy for prognosis and therapy monitoring. *Radiology* 1990;174:847–853.

Disler DG, Recht MP, McCauley TR. MR imaging of articular cartilage. *Skeletal Radiol* 2000;29:367–377.

Erlemann R, Reiser MF, Peters PE, et al. Musculoskeletal neoplasms: static and dynamic Gd-DTPA-enhanced MR imaging. *Radiology* 1989;171:767–773.

Erlemann R, Sciuk J, Bosse A, et al. Response of osteosarcoma and Ewing sarcoma to preoperative chemotherapy: assessment with dynamic and static MR imaging and skeletal scintigraphy. *Radiology* 1990;175:791–796.

Erlemann R, Vassallo P, Bongartz G, et al. Musculoskeletal neoplasms: fast low-angle shot MR imaging with and without Gd-DTPA. *Radiology* 1990;176:489–495.

Errico TJ. The role of diskography in the 1980s. *Radiology* 1989;162:285–286.

Even-Sapir E, Martin RH, Barnes DC, Pringle CR, Iles SE, Mitchell MJ. Role of SPECT in differentiating malignant from benign lesions in the lower thoracic and lumbar vertebrae. *Radiology* 1993;187:193–198.

Farooki S, Seeger LL. Magnetic resonance imaging in the evaluation of ligament injuries. *Skeletal Radiol* 1999;28:61–74.

Feldman F, van Heertum R, Manos C. [18]FDG PET scanning of benign and malignant musculoskeletal lesions. *Skeletal Radiol* 2003;32:201–208.

Ferrucci JT. Imaging algorithms for radiologic diagnosis. In: Traveras JM, Ferrucci JT, eds. *Radiology—diagnosis, imaging, intervention*, vol. 1. Philadelphia: JB Lippincott; 1990:1–79.

Fishman EK. Spiral CT evaluation of the musculoskeletal system. In: Fishman EK, Jeffrey RB Jr, eds. *Spiral CT. Principles, techniques, and clinical applications*. Philadelphia: Lippincott-Raven;1998:273–298.

Fishman EK, Wyatt SH, Bluemke DA, Urban BA. Spiral CT of musculoskeletal pathology: preliminary observations. *Skeletal Radiol* 1993;22:253–256.

Flannigan B, Kursunoglu-Brahme S, Snyder S, et al. MR arthrography of the shoulder: comparison with conventional MR imaging. *AJR Am J Roentgenol* 1990;155:829–832.

Fogelman I, Ryan PJ. Bone scanning in Paget's disease. In: Collier BD Jr, Fogelman I, Rosenthal L, eds. *Skeletal nuclear medicine*. St. Louis: Mosby; 1996:171–181.

Foley WD, Wilson CR. Digital orthopedic radiography: vascular and nonvascular. In: Galasko CSB, Isherwood I, eds. *Imaging techniques in orthopedics*. London: Springer-Verlag; 1989:145–158.

Foo TKF, Sawyer AM, Faulkner WH, Mills DG. Inversion in the steady state: contrast optimization and reduced imaging time with fast three-dimensional inversion-recovery-prepared GRE pulse sequences. *Radiology* 1994;191:85–90.

Fornage BD. Achilles tendon: US examination. *Radiology* 1986;159:759–764.

Fox IM, Zeiger L. Tc-99m-HMPAO leukocyte scintigraphy for the diagnosis of osteomyelitis in diabetic foot infections. *J Foot Ankle Surg* 1993;32:591–594.

Freiberger RH. Introducing arthrography. In: Freiberger RH, Kaye JJ, eds. *Arthrography*. New York: Appleton-Century-Crofts; 1979:1–4.

Freiberger RH, Pavlov H. Knee arthrography. *Radiology* 1988;166:489–492.

Fuchs AW. Cervical vertebrae (part I). *Radiogr Clin Photogr* 1940;16:2–17.

Genant HK, Doi K, Mall JC. Optical versus radiographic magnification for fine-detail skeletal radiography. *Invest Radiol* 1975;10:160–172.

Genant HK, Doi K, Mall JC, Sickles EA. Direct radiographic magnification for skeletal radiology. An assessment of image quality and clinical application. *Radiology* 1977;123:47–55.

Gerscovich EO, Cronan MS, Greenspan A, Jain K, McGahan JP. Developmental dysplasia of the hip (DDH): three-dimensional ultrasound evaluation. Proceedings of the 4th Congress of the International Society for Musculoskeletal Sonography (IS-MUS), Madrid, Spain, 1998:71–74.

Gerscovich EO, Greenspan A, Cronan MS, Karol LA, McGahan JP. Three-dimensional sonographic evaluation of developmental dysplasia of the hip: preliminary findings. *Radiology* 1994;190:407–410.

Goodman PC, Jeffrey RB Jr, Brant-Zawadzki M. Digital subtraction angiography in extremity trauma. *Radiology* 1984;153:61–64.

Greenspan A, Tehranzadeh J. Imaging of infectious arthritis. *Radiol Clin North Am* 2001;39:267–276.

Greenspan A. Tumors of cartilage origin. *Orthop Clin North Am* 1989;20:347–366.

Greenspan A. Imaging modalities in orthopaedics. In: Chapman MW, ed. *Chapman's Orthopaedic Surgery*, 3rd ed. Philadelphia: Lippincott-Williams & Wilkins; 2001:53–74.

Greenspan A, Norman A. The radial head-capitellum view: useful technique in elbow trauma. *AJR Am J Roentgenol* 1982;138:1186–1188.

Greenspan A, Stadalnik RC. A musculoskeletal radiologist's view of nuclear medicine. *Semin Nucl Med* 1997;27:372–385.

Guhlmann A, Brecht Krauss D, Suger G, et al. Fluorine-18-FDG PET and technetium-99m antigranulocyte antibody scintigraphy in chronic osteomyelitis. *J Nucl Med* 1998;39:2145–2152.

Haacke EM, Tkach JA. Fast MR imaging: techniques and clinical applications. *AJR Am J Roentgenol* 1990;155:951–964.

Hamper UM, Trapanotto V, Sheth S, DeJong MR, Caskey CI. Three-dimensional US: preliminary clinical experience. *Radiology* 1994;191:397–401.

Harcke HT, Grisson LE. Performing dynamic sonography of the infant hip. *AJR Am J Roentgenol* 1990;155:837–844.

Harned EM, Mitchell DG, Burk DJ, Vinitski S, Rifkin MD. Bone marrow findings on magnetic resonance images of the knee: accentuation by fat suppression. *Magn Reson Imaging* 1990;8:27–31.

Heiken JP, Brink JA, Vannier MW. Spiral (helical) CT. *Radiology* 1993;189:647–656.

Helgason JW, Chandnani VP, Yu JS. MR arthrography: a review of current technique and applications. *AJR Am J Roentgenol* 1997;168:1473–1480.

Ho C, Sartoris DJ, Resnick D. Conventional tomography in musculoskeletal trauma. *Radiol Clin North Am* 1989;27:929–932.

Hodler J, Fretz CJ, Terrier F, Gerber C. Rotator cuff tears: correlation of sonographic and surgical findings. *Radiology* 1988;169:791–794.

Holder LE. Bone scintigraphy in skeletal trauma. *Radiol Clin North Am* 1993;31:739–781.

Hopper KD, Pierantozzi D, Potok PS, et al. The quality of 3D reconstructions from 1.0 and 1.5 pitch helical and conventional CT. *J Comput Assist Tomogr* 1996;20:841–847.

Hu H, He HD, Foley WD, Fox SH. Four multidetector-row helical CT: image quality and volume coverage speed. *Radiology* 2000;215:55–62.

Hunter JC, Blatz DJ, Escobedo EM. SLAP lesions of the glenoid labrum: CT arthrographic and arthroscopic correlation. *Radiology* 1992;184:513–518.

Jacobson AF. Bone scanning in metastatic disease. In: Collier BD Jr, Fogelman I, Rosenthal L, eds. *Skeletal nuclear medicine*. St. Louis: Mosby; 1996:87–123.

Jadvar H, Conti PS. Diagnostic utility of FDG PET in multiple myeloma. *Skeletal Radiol* 2002;31:690–694.

Johnson RP. The role of bone imaging in orthopedic practice. *Semin Nucl Med* 1997;27:386–389.

Jung H-S, Jee W-H, McCauley TR, Ha K-Y, Choi K-H. Discrimination of metastatic from acute osteoporotic compression spinal fractures with MR imaging. *Radiographics* 2003;23:179–187.

Kapelov SR, Teresi LM, Bradley WG, et al. Bone contusions of the knee: increased lesion detection with fast spin echo imaging with spectroscopic fat saturation. *Radiology* 1993;189:901–904.

Kaplan PA, Anderson MC, Norris MA, Matamoros A Jr. Ultrasonography of post-traumatic soft-tissue lesions. *Radiol Clin North Am* 1989;27:973–982.

Kaplan PA, Matamoros A Jr, Anderson JC. Sonography of the musculoskeletal system. *AJR Am J Roentgenol* 1990;155:237–245.

King AD, Peters AM, Stuttle AWJ, Lavender JP. Imaging of bone infection with labelled white cells: role of contemporaneous bone marrow imaging. *Eur J Nucl Med* 1990;17:148–151.

König H, Sieper J, Wolf KJ. Rheumatoid arthritis: evaluation of hypervascular and fibrous pannus with dynamic MR imaging enhanced with Gd-DTPA. *Radiology* 1990;176:473–477.

Kostakoglu L, Agress Jr H, Goldsmith SJ. Clinical role of FDG PET in evaluation of cancer patients. *Radiographics* 2003;23:315–340.

Krinsky G, Rofsky NM, Weinreb JC. Nonspecificity of short inversion time inversion recovery (STIR) as a technique of fat suppression: pitfalls in image interpretation. *AJR Am J Roentgenol* 1996;166:523–526.

Kuszyk BS, Heath DG, Bliss DF, Fishman EK. Skeletal 3-D CT: advantages of volume rendering over surface rendering. *Skeletal Radiol* 1996;25:207–214.

Lang P, Steiger P, Faulkner K, Glüer C, Genant HK. Osteoporosis. Current techniques and recent developments in quantitative bone densitometry. *Radiol Clin North Am* 1991;29:49–76.

Lang TF, Augat P, Lane NE, Genant HK. Trochanteric hip fracture: strong association with spinal trabecular bone mineral density measured with quantitative CT. *Radiology* 1998;209:525–530.

Levinsohn EM, Palmer AK, Coren AB, Zinberg E. Wrist arthrography: the value of the three compartment injection technique. *Skeletal Radiol* 1987;16:539–544.

Lodge MA, Lucas JD, Marsken PK, et al. A PET Study: 18-FDG uptake in soft tissue masses. *Eur J Nucl Med* 1999;26:22–30.

Love C, Din AS, Tomas MB, Kalapparambath TP, Palestro CJ. Radionuclide bone imaging: an illustrative review. *Radiographics* 2003;23:341–358.

Lund PJ, Nisbet JK, Valencia FG, Ruth JT. Current sonographic applications in orthopedics. *AJR Am J Roentgenol* 1996;166:889–895.

Magid D, Fishman EK. Imaging of musculoskeletal trauma in three dimensions. *Radiol Clin North Am* 1989;27:945–956.

Mao J, Yan H. Fat tissue and fat suppression. *Magn Reson Imaging* 1993;11:385–393.

Massengill AD, Seeger LL, Yao L, et al. Labrocapsular ligamentous complex of the shoulder: normal anatomy, anatomic variation, and pitfalls of MR imaging and MR arthrography. *Radiographics* 1994;14:1211–1223.

McAfee JG. Update on radiopharmaceuticals for medical imaging. *Radiology* 1989;171:593–601.

McCollough CH, Zink FE. Performance evaluation of a multi-slice CT system. *Med Phys* 1999;26:2223–2230.

Meuli RA, Wedeeen VJ, Geller SC, et al. MR gated subtraction angiography: evaluation of lower extremities. *Radiology* 1986;159:411–418.

Mink JH, Deutsch AL. Occult cartilage and bone injuries of the knee: detection, classification, and assessment with MR imaging. *Radiology* 1989;170:823–829.

Mitchell DG, Stolpen AH, Siegelman ES, Bolinger L, Outwater EK. Fatty tissue on opposed-phase MR images: paradoxical suppression of signal intensity by paramagnetic contrast agents. *Radiology* 1996;198:351–357.

Murphey MD, Quale JL, Martin NL, Bramble JM, Cook LT, Dwyer SJ III. Computed radiography in musculoskeletal imaging: state of the art. *AJR Am J Roentgenol* 1992;158:19–27.

Murray IPC, Dixon J. The role of single photon emission computed tomography in bone scintigraphy. *Skeletal Radiol* 1989;18:493–505.

Negendank WG, Crowley MG, Ryan JR, Keller NA, Evelhoch JL. Bone and soft-tissue lesions: diagnosis with combined H-1 MR imaging and P-31 MR spectroscopy. *Radiology* 1989;173:181–188.

Newhouse KE, El-Khoury GY, Buckwalter JA. Occult sacral fractures in osteopenic patients. *J Bone Joint Surg [Am]* 1992;74A:1472–1477.

Ney DR, Fishman EK, Kawashima A, et al. Comparison of helical and serial CT with regard to three-dimensional imaging of musculoskeletal anatomy. *Radiology* 1992;185:865–869.

Palestro CJ, Roumanas P, Swyer AJ, Kim CK, Goldsmith SJ. Diagnosis of musculoskeletal infection using combined In-111 labeled leukocyte and Tc-99m SC marrow imaging. *Clin Nucl Med* 1992;17:269–273.

Palestro CJ, Torres MA. Radionuclide imaging in orthopedic infections. *Semin Nucl Med* 1997;27:334–345.

Palmer WE. MR arthrography: is it worthwhile? *Top Magn Reson Imaging* 1996;8:24–43.

Palmer WE, Brown JH, Rosenthal DI. Rotator cuff: evaluation with fat-suppressed MR arthrography. *Radiology* 1993;188:683–687.

Palmer WE, Brown JH, Rosenthal DI. Labral-ligamentous complex of the shoulder: evaluation with MR arthrography. *Radiology* 1994;190:645–651.

Palmer WE, Caslowitz PL, Chew FS. MR arthrography of the shoulder: normal intraarticular structures and common abnormalities. *AJR Am J Roentgenol* 1995;164:141–146.

Peh WC, Cassar-Pullicino VN. Magnetic resonance arthrography: current status. *Clin Radiol* 1999;54:575–587.

Pennington WT, Mott MP, Thometz JG, Sty JR, Metz D. Photopenic bone scan osteomyelitis: a clinical prospective. *J Pediatr Orthop* 1999;19:695–698

Peterfy CG, Majumdar S, Lang P, van Dijke CF, Sack K, Genant HK. MR imaging of the arthritic knee: improved discrimination of cartilage, synovium, and effusion with pulsed saturation transfer and fat-suppressed T1-weighted sequences. *Radiology* 1994;191:413–419.

Petersein J, Saini S. Fast MR imaging: technical strategies. *AJR Am J Roentgenol* 1995;165:1105–1109.

Petersilge CA, Lewin JS, Duerk JL, Hatem SF. MR arthrography of the shoulder: rethinking traditional imaging procedures to meet the technical requirements of MR imaging guidance. *AJR Am J Roentgenol* 1997;169:1453–1457.

Pettersson H, Resnick D. Musculoskeletal imaging. *Radiology* 1998;208:561–562.

Piraino DW, Davros WJ, Lieber M, et al. Selenium-based digital radiography versus conventional film-screen radiography of the hands and feet: a subjective comparison. *AJR Am J Roentgenol* 1999;172:177–184.

Pretorius DH, Nelson TR, Jaffe JS. 3-dimensional sonographic analysis based on color flow Doppler and gray scale image data: a preliminary report. *J Ultrasound Med* 1992;11:225–232.

Pugh DG, Winkler TN. Scanography of leg-length measurement: an easy satisfactory method. *Radiology* 1966;87:130–133.

Rankin RN, Fenster A, Downey DB, Munk PL, Levin MF, Vellet AD. Three-dimensional sonographic reconstruction: techniques and diagnostic applications. *AJR Am J Roentgenol* 1993;161:695–702.

Ravenel JG, Gordon LL, Pope TL, Reed CE. FDG-PET uptake in occult acute pelvic fracture. *Skeletal Radiol* 2004;33:99–101.

Reed MH. Limb-length discrepancies. In: Reed MH, ed. *Pediatric skeletal radiology.* Baltimore: Williams & Wilkins; 1992:666–668.

Reeder SB, Pelc NJ, Alley MT, Gold GE. Rapid imaging of articular cartilage with steady-state free precession and multipoint fat-water separation. *AJR Am Roentgenol* 2003;180:357–362.

Reinus WR, Hardy DC, Totty WG, Gilula LA. Arthrographic evaluation of the carpal triangular fibrocartilage complex. *J Hand Surg* 1987;12:495–503.

Reuther G, Mutschler W. Detection of local recurrent disease in musculoskeletal tumors: magnetic resonance imaging versus computed tomography. *Skeletal Radiol* 1990;19:85–90.

Rosenberg ZS, Cheung Y. Diagnostic imaging of the ankle and foot. In: Jahss MH, ed. *Disorders of the foot and ankle,* 2nd ed. Philadelphia: WB Saunders; 1991:109–154.

Rubin DA. MR imaging of the knee menisci. *Radiol Clin North Am* 1997;35:21–44.

Rubin RH, Fischman AJ, Callahan RJ, et al. ^{111}In-labeled nonspecific immunoglobulin scanning in the detection of focal infection. *N Engl J Med* 1989;321:935–940.

Rubin RH, Fischman AJ, Needleman NM, et al. Radiolabeled, nonspecific, polyclonal human immunoglobulin in the detection of focal inflammation by scintigraphy: comparison with gallium-67 citrate and technetium-99m labeled albumin. *J Nucl Med* 1989;30:385–389.

Ryan PJ, Fogelman I. The bone scan: where are we now? *Semin Nucl Med* 1995;25:76–91.

Ryan PJ, Taylor M, Grevitt M, Allen P, Shields J, Clarke SE, Fogelman I. Bone single-photon emission computed tomography in recent meniscal tears: an assessment of diagnostic criteria. *Eur J Nucl Med* 1993;20:703–707.

Saloner DA, Anderson CM, Lee RE. Magnetic resonance angiography. In: Higgins CB, Hricak H, Helms CA, eds. *Magnetic resonance imaging of the body,* 2nd ed. New York, Raven Press; 1992:679–718.

Sartoris DJ, Resnick D. Current and innovative methods for noninvasive bone densitometry. *Radiol Clin North Am* 1990;28:257–278.

Sartoris DJ, Sommer FG. Digital film processing: applications to the musculo-skeletal system. *Skeletal Radiol* 1984;11:274–281.

Savelli G, Maffioli L, Maccauro M, De Deckere E, Bombardieri E. Bone scintigraphy and the added value of SPECT (single photon emission tomography) in detecting skeletal lesions. *Q J Nucl Med* 2001;45:27–37.

Schauwecker DS. Osteomyelitis: diagnosis with In-111-labeled leukocytes. *Radiology* 1989;171:141–146.

Schauwecker DS. The scintigraphic diagnosis of osteomyelitis. *AJR Am J Roentgenol* 1992;158:9–18.

Schiesser M, Stumpe KDM, Trentz O, Kossmann T, von Schulthess GK. Detection of metallic implant-associated infections with FDG PET in patients with trauma: correlation with microbiologic results. *Radiology* 2003;226:391–398.

Schirrmeister H, Guhlmann A, Elsner K, et al. Sensitivity in detecting osseous lesions depends on anatomic localization: planar bone scintigraphy versus ^{18}F PET. *J Nucl Med* 1999;40:1623–1629.

Schulte-Altendorneburg G, Gebhard M, Wohlgemuth WA, Fischer W, Zentner J, Wegener R, Balzer T, Bohndorf K. MR arthrography: pharmacology, efficacy and safety in clinical trials. *Skeletal Radiol* 2003;32:1–12.

Sciuk J, Brandau W, Vollet B, et al. Comparison of technetium 99m polyclonal human immunoglobin and technetium 99m monoclonal antibodies for imaging chronic osteomyelitis: first clinical results. *Eur J Nucl Med* 1991;18:401–407.

Seibert JA, Shelton DK, Moore EH. Computed radiography x-ray exposure trends. *Acad Radiol* 1996;4:313–318.

Shapiro R. Current status of lumbar diskography (letter). *Radiology* 1986;159:815.

Shih TT, Huang KM, Li YW. Solitary vertebral collapse: distinction between benign and malignant causes using MR patterns. *J Magn Reson Imaging* 1999;9:635–642.

Shreve PD, Anzai Y, Whal RL. Pitfalls in oncologic diagnosis with FDG PET imaging: physiologic and benign variants. *Radiographics* 1999;19:61–77.

Soble MG, Kaye AD, Guay RC. Rotator cuff tear: clinical experience with sonographic detection. *Radiology* 1989;173:319–321.

Sorsdahl OA, Goodhart GL, Williams HT, Hanna LJ, Rodriguez J. Quantitative bone gallium scintigraphy in osteomyelitis. *Skeletal Radiol* 1993;22:239–242.

Sostman HD, Charles HC, Rockwell S, et al. Soft-tissue sarcomas: detection of metabolic heterogeneity with P-31 MR spectroscopy. *Radiology* 1990;176:837–843.

Steinbach LS, Palmer WE, Schweitzer ME. Special focus session. MR arthrography. *Radiographics* 2002;22:1223–1246.

Streule K, DeShriver M, Fridrich R. ^{99m}Tc-labeled HSA-nanocolloid vs ^{111}In oxine-labeled granulocytes in detecting skeletal septic process. *Nucl Med Commun* 1988;9:59–67.

Stumpe KD, Dazzi H, Schaffner A, von Schulthess GK. Infection imaging using whole-body FDG-PET. *Eur J Nucl Med* 2000;27:822–832.

Sundaram M, McLeod RA. MR imaging of tumor and tumorlike lesions of bones and soft tissues. *AJR Am J Roentgenol* 1990;155:817–824.

Swan JS, Grist TM, Sproat IA, et al. Musculoskeletal neoplasms: preoperative evaluation with MR angiography. *Radiology* 1995;194:519–524.

Totterman S, Weiss SL, Szumowski J, et al. MR fat suppression technique in the evaluation of normal structures of the knee. *J Comput Assist Tomogr* 1989;13:473–479.

Tumeh SS, Aliabadi P, Weissman BN, McNeil BJ. Chronic osteomyelitis: bone and gallium scan patterns associated with active disease. *Radiology* 1986;158:685–688.

Walker CW, Aronson J, Kaplan PA, Molpus WA, Seibert JJ. Radiologic evaluation of limb-lengthening procedures. *AJR Am J Roentgenol* 1991;156:353–358.

Yagei B, Manisals M, Yilmaz E, Ekin A, Ozaksoy D, Kovanlikaya I. Indirect MR arthrography of the shoulder in detection of rotator cuff ruptures. *Eur Radiol* 2001;11:258–262.

Zucherman J, Derby R, Hsu K, et al. Normal magnetic resonance imaging with abnormal discography. *Spine* 1988;13:1355–1359.

BONE FORMATION AND GROWTH

The skeleton is made of cortical and cancellous bone, which are highly specialized forms of connective tissue. Each type of bony tissue has the same basic histologic structure, but the cortical component has a solid, compact architecture interrupted only by narrow canals containing blood vessels (haversian systems), while the cancellous component consists of trabeculae separated by fatty or hematopoietic marrow. Bone is rigid calcified material and grows by the addition of new tissue to existing surfaces. The removal of unwanted bone, called *simultaneous remodeling*, is also a necessary component of skeletal growth. Unlike most tissues, bone grows only by apposition on the surface of an already existing substrate, such as bone or calcified cartilage. Cartilage, however, grows by interstitial cellular proliferation and matrix formation.

Normal bone is formed through a combination of two processes: *endochondral (enchondral) ossification* and *intramembranous (membranous) ossification*. In general, the spongiosa develops by endochondral ossification and the cortex by intramembranous ossification. Once formed, living bone is never metabolically at rest. Beginning in the fetal period, it constantly remodels and reappropriates its minerals along lines of mechanical stress. This process continues throughout life, accelerating during infancy and adolescence. The factors controlling bone formation and resorption are still not well understood, but one fact is clear: bone formation and bone resorption are exquisitely balanced, coupled processes that result in net bone formation equaling net bone resorption.

Most of the skeleton is formed by endochondral ossification (Fig. 3.1), a highly organized process that transforms cartilage to bone and contributes mainly to increasing bone length. Endochondral ossification is responsible for the formation of all tubular and flat bones, vertebrae, the base of the skull, the ethmoid, and the medial and lateral ends of the clavicle. For example, at approximately 7 weeks of embryonic life, cartilage cells (chondroblasts and chondrocytes) produce a hyaline cartilage model of the long tubular bones from the condensed mesenchymal aggregate. The mechanisms leading to calcification of the cartilaginous matrix are not completely understood, but it is generally believed that the promotors of calcification are small membrane-bound vesicles known as matrix vesicles, which are present in the interstitial matrix between the cells. At approximately the ninth week, peripheral capillaries penetrate the model, inducing the formation of osteoblasts. Osseous tissue is then deposited on the spicules of calcified cartilage matrix that remain after osteoclastic resorption, thereby transforming the primary spongiosa into secondary spongiosa.

As this process moves rapidly toward the epiphyseal ends of the cartilage model, a loose network of bony trabeculae containing cores of calcified cartilage is left behind, creating a well-defined line of ad-

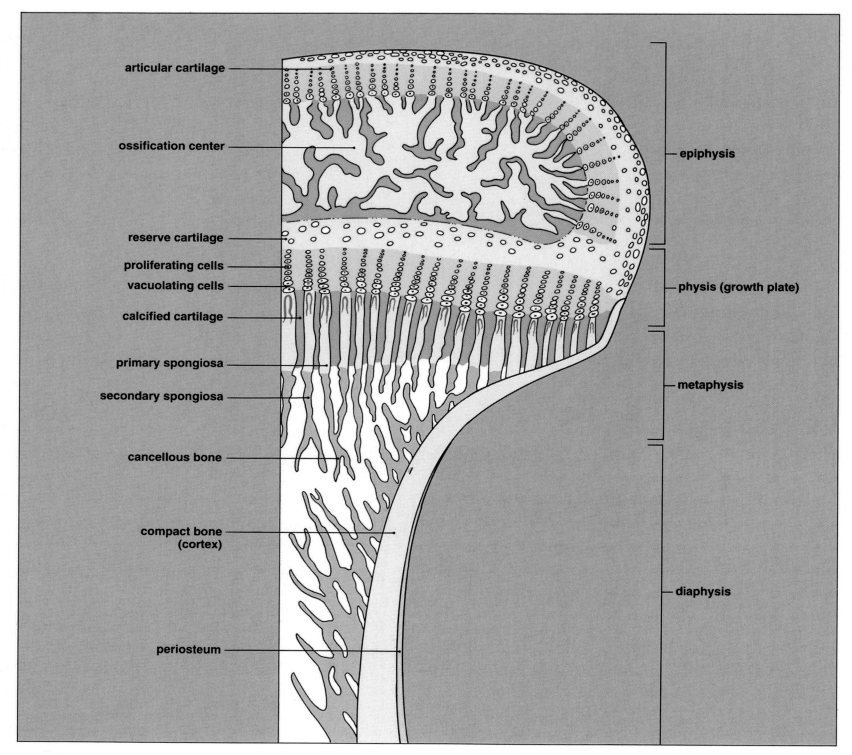

Figure 3.1 Endochondral bone formation. This process occurs at the ossification center, growth plate, and metaphysis. (Modified from Rubin P, 1964, with permission.)

vance. This line represents the growth plate (physis) (Fig. 3.2) and the adjacent metaphysis to which the secondary spongiosa moves as it is formed. The many trabeculae of the secondary spongiosa that are resorbed soon after being formed become the marrow cavity, while other trabeculae enlarge and thicken through the apposition of new bone, although these too eventually undergo resorption and remodeling. Others extend toward the shaft and become incorporated into the developing cortex of the bone, which is formed by intramembra-

nous ossification. At the ends of tubular bones, a similar process is initiated, creating a secondary ossification center in the epiphysis. This nucleus increases in size by the process of maturation and calcification of the cartilage surrounding the secondary center. The peripheral margin of epiphysis termed acrophysis is formed of zones of cell hypertrophy, degeneration, calcification, and ossification, similar to that of the growth plate. Endochondral bone formation is not normally observed after growth plate closure.

epiphyseal bone

epiphyseal vessel (nutrition of growth plate)

end plate

cell proliferation

germinal proliferating cells

palisading

matrix synthesis

hypertrophy

calcification

active calcification

cell degeneration

primary spongiosa

vascular invasion from metaphysis (osteogenesis)

Figure 3.2 Schematic representation of the growth plate. Growth plate during active bone growth. At the top of the diagram, the epiphyseal vessels are supplying nutrition to the germinal proliferating cells. Further down, the cells begin to palisade into vertical columns, and as they approach the metaphysis, the cells undergo hypertrophy and the matrix calcifies. The calcified matrix is then invaded by blood vessels and the primary spongiosa forms. (Modified from Bullough PG, 1992, with permission.)

In intramembranous ossification, bone is formed directly without an intervening cartilaginous stage (Fig. 3.3). Initially, condensed mesenchymal cells differentiate into osteoprogenitor cells, which then differentiate into fibroblasts that produce collagen and fibrous connective tissues, and osteoblasts, which produce osteoid. Beginning at approximately the ninth week of fetal life, the fibrous membrane produced by the fibroblasts forms a periosteal collar and is replaced with osteoid by the action of the osteoblasts. Bones formed by this process include the frontal, parietal, and temporal bones and their squamae; bones of the upper face as well as the tympanic parts of the temporal bone; and the vomer and the medial pterygoid.

Intramembranous ossification also contributes to the appositional formation of periosteal bone around the shafts of the tubular bones, thus forming the cortex of the long and flat bones. This type of bone formation increases bone width. In addition to the periosteal envelope on the outer surface of bone, intramembranous ossification is active in the endosteal envelope covering the inner surface of the cortex and in the haversian envelope at the internal surface of all intracortical canals. These three envelopes are sites of potent cellular activity involving resorption and formation of bone throughout life.

It is interesting to note that the mandible and middle portions of the clavicle are formed by a process that shares features of endochondral and intramembranous ossification. These bones are preformed in cartilage in embryonic life, but they do not undergo endochondral ossification in the conventional manner. Instead, the cartilage model simply serves as a surface for the deposition of bone by connective tissues. Eventually, the cartilage is resorbed and the bones become fully ossified.

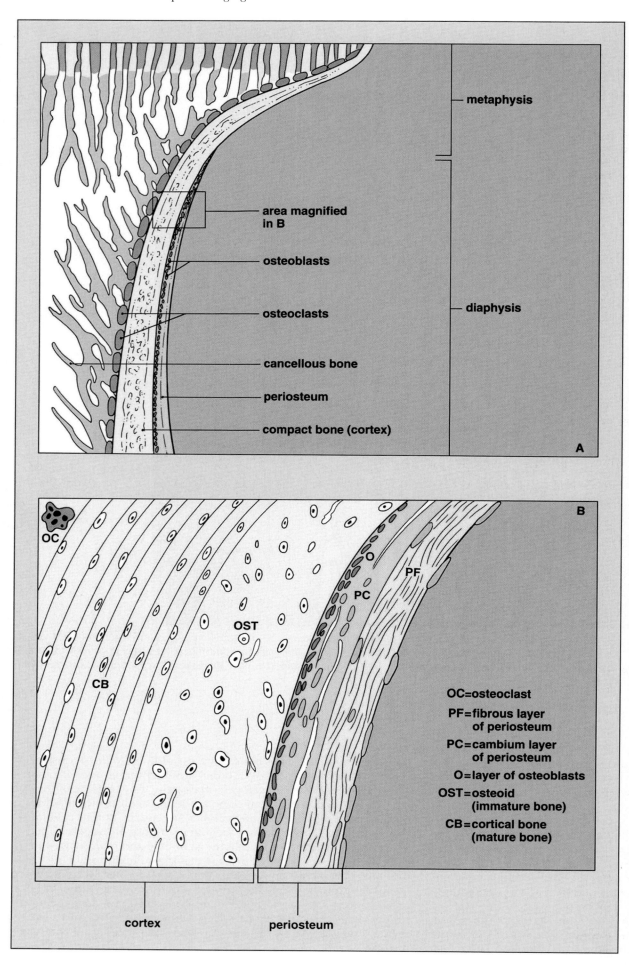

Figure 3.3 Schematic representation of intramembranous ossification. (A) and **(B)** Intramembranous bone formation at the junction of the periosteum and the cortex. Subperiosteal bone formation progress from immature (woven) to more mature bone.

area magnified in B

osteoblasts

osteoclasts

cancellous bone

periosteum

compact bone (cortex)

metaphysis

diaphysis

A

B

OC

O

PF

PC

OST

CB

OC=osteoclast

PF=fibrous layer of periosteum

PC=cambium layer of periosteum

O=layer of osteoblasts

OST=osteoid (immature bone)

CB=cortical bone (mature bone)

cortex

periosteum

SUGGESTED READINGS

Anderson HC. Mechanism of mineral formation in bone. *Lab Invest* 1989;60:320–330.

Aoki J, Yamamoto I, Hino M, et al. Reactive endosteal bone formation. *Skeletal Radiol* 1987;16:545–551.

Bernard GW, Pease DC. An electron microscopic study of initial intramembranous osteogenesis. *Am J Anat* 1969;125:271–290.

Brighton CT. Longitudinal bone growth: the growth plate and its dysfunction. In: Griffin PP, ed. *Instructional course lectures,* vol. 36. Chicago: American Academy of Orthopedic Surgery; 1987:3–25.

Buckwalter JA, Cooper RR. Bone structure and function. In: Griffin PP, ed. *Instructional course lectures,* vol. 36. Chicago: American Academy Orthopedic Surgery; 1987:27–48.

Bullough PG. *Atlas of orthopedic pathology with clinical and radiologic correlations,* 2nd ed. New York: Gower Medical Publishing; 1992:1.2–1.35.

Canalis E, McCarthy T, Centrella M. Growth factors and the regulation of bone remodeling. *J Clin Invest* 1988;81:277–281.

Jaffe HL. *Metabolic, degenerative and inflammatory diseases of bones and joints.* Philadelphia: Lea & Febiger; 1972.

Kirkpatrick JA Jr. Bone and joint growth—normal and in disease. *Clin Rheum Dis* 1981;7:671–688.

Lee WR, Marshall JH, Sissons HA. Calcium accretion and bone formation in dogs. *J Bone Joint Surg [Br]* 1965;47B:157–180.

Oestreich AE. The acrophysis: a unifying concept for enchondral bone growth and its disorders. *Skeletal Radiol* 2003;32:121–127.

Oestreich AE, Crawford AH. *Atlas of Pediatric Orthopedic Radiology,* Stuttgart: Thieme; 1985:17–18.

Posner AS. The mineral of bone. *Clin Orthop* 1985;200:87–99.

Raisz LG, Kream BE. Regulation of bone formation. *N Engl J Med* 1983;309:83–89.

Reddi AH, Anderson WA. Collagenous bone matrix-induced endochondral ossification and hemopoiesis. *J Cell Biol* 1976;69:557–572.

Reed MH. Normal and abnormal development. In: Reed MH, ed. *Pediatric Skeletal Radiology,* Baltimore: Williams & Wilkins; 1992:349–392.

Resnick D, Manolagas SC, Niwayama G. Histogenesis, anatomy, and physiology of bone. In: Resnick D, ed. *Bone and joint imaging.* Philadelphia: WB Saunders; 1989:16–28.

Rubin P. *Dynamic classification of bone dysplasias.* Chicago: Year Book Medical Publishers; 1964:1–23.

Sissons HA. Structure and growth of bones and joints. In: Taveras JM, Ferrucci JT, eds. *Radiology, diagnosis-imaging-intervention,* vol. 5. Philadelphia: JB Lippincott; 1986:1–11.

Sissons HA. The growth of bone. In: *The biochemistry and physiology of bone,* vol. 3, 2nd ed. New York: Academic Press; 1971.

Warshawsky H. Embryology and development of the skeletal system. In: Cruess RL, ed. *The Musculoskeletal system. Embryology, biochemistry, physiology.* New York: Churchill Livingstone; 1982.

TRAUMA

RADIOLOGIC EVALUATION OF TRAUMA

Radiologic Imaging Modalities

The radiologic modalities used in analyzing injury to the musculoskeletal system are as follows:

1. Conventional radiography, including routine views (specific for various body parts), special views, and stress views
2. Digital radiography, including digital subtraction arthrography and angiography (DSA)
3. Fluoroscopy, alone or combined with videotaping
4. Tomography (particularly trispiral tomography)
5. Computed tomography (CT)
6. Arthrography, tenography, and bursography
7. Myelography and diskography
8. Angiography (arteriography and venography)
9. Scintigraphy (radionuclide bone scan)
10. Magnetic resonance imaging (MRI)

Radiography, Fluoroscopy, and Conventional Tomography

In most instances, radiographs obtained in two orthogonal projections, usually the anteroposterior and lateral, at 90 degrees to each other are sufficient (Fig. 4.1). Occasionally, oblique and special views are necessary, particularly in evaluating fractures of complex structures such as the pelvis, elbow, wrist, and ankle (Figs. 4.2 and 4.3). Stress views are important in evaluating ligamentous tears and joint stability (Fig. 4.4).

Certain special modalities are used more often in evaluating different types of injuries in specific anatomic locations. Fluoroscopy and videotaping are useful in evaluating the kinematics of joints. Tomography (zonospiral or trispiral) is useful in confirming the presence of a fracture (Figs. 4.5 and 4.6), delineating the extent of a fracture line and assessing the position of the fragments. It is also valuable in monitoring the progress of healing.

Computed Tomography

CT is essential in the evaluation of complex fractures, particularly in the spinal and pelvic regions (Fig. 4.7). The advantages of CT over conventional radiography are its ability to provide three-dimensional imaging, excellent contrast resolution, and accurate measurement of the tissue attenuation coefficient. The use of sagittal, coronal, and multiplanar reformation provides an added advantage over other imaging modalities.

Figure 4.1 Fracture of the metacarpal bone. (A) Dorsovolar (posteroanterior) view of the hand does not demonstrate a fracture. **(B)** The lateral view reveals a fracture of the third metacarpal bone.

Figure 4.2 Fracture of the radial head. A patient presented with elbow pain after a fall. Anteroposterior **(A)** and lateral **(B)** views are normal; however, the radial head and coronoid processes are not well demonstrated because of bony overlap. A special 45-degree angle view of the elbow **(C)** is used to project the radial head ventrad, free of the overlap of other bones. A short, intraarticular fracture of the radial head is now clearly visible.

Figure 4.3 Fracture of the scapula. (A) Anteroposterior radiograph of the left shoulder shows fracture of the clavicle. Injury to the scapula is not well demonstrated. **(B)** A special "Y" view of the scapula clearly shows the fracture (*arrow*).

Figure 4.4 Tear of the lateral collateral ligament. In most ankle injuries, if a ligamentous tear is suspected, then conventional films should be supplemented by stress views. The standard anteroposterior radiograph of this ankle **(A)** is not remarkable. The same view after application of adduction (inversion) stress **(B)** shows widening of the lateral compartment of the tibiotalar (ankle) joint, indicating a tear of the lateral collateral ligament.

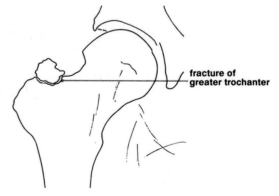

Figure 4.5 Fracture of the greater trochanter. This patient fell out of bed and a fracture of the femoral neck was suspected. The anteroposterior view of the right hip **(A)** is not convincing. Tomographic study **(B)** shows a fracture of the greater trochanter but no fracture of the femoral neck.

Figure 4.6 **Fracture of the hook of the hamate.** A 55-year-old tennis player reported pain in the palm of his left hand in the region of hypothenar. **(A)** Dorsovolar radiograph shows blurred margins of the hook of the hamate (*arrows*), suggestive but not conclusive of a fracture. **(B)** Lateral trispiral tomogram shows obvious fracture at the base of the hamulus (*open arrows*).

Figure 4.7 **Fracture of the sacrum and acetabulum. (A)** Standard anteroposterior view of the pelvis shows obvious fractures of the right obturator ring. **(B)** CT section demonstrates an unsuspected fracture of the sacrum and disruption of the left sacroiliac joint. *(continued)*

Figure 4.7 Fracture of the sacrum and acetabulum *Continued.* **(C)** Axial and **(D)** coronal CT reformatted images in another patient show unsuspected on conventional radiographs fractured fragment displaced into the hip joint. The arrows point to the fracture of the posterior column of the right acetabulum.

Scintigraphy

Radionuclide bone scanning can detect occult fractures or fractures too subtle to be seen on conventional radiographs or tomograms (Fig. 4.8). This technique is also effective in differentiation of tibial stress fractures from shin splints. Scintigraphy occasionally aids in making a differential diagnosis of old-versus-recent fractures and in detecting such complications as early-stage osteonecrosis. However, bone scans seldom provide new information about the status of fracture healing and, in particular, static bone scans fail to separate normally healing fractures from delayed healing fractures or those that result in nonunion. Also, a bone scan cannot indicate the point at which clinical union is established. Scintigraphy is, however, helpful in distinguishing noninfected fractures from infected ones. With osteomyelitis, scanning, using gallium citrate (^{67}Ga) and indium-labeled white blood cells (^{111}In), demonstrates a significant increase in the uptake of the tracer. Because ^{67}Ga is also actively taken-up at the site of a normally healing fracture, but significantly less than that encountered with ^{99m}Tc (technetium) scanning

agents, the combination of ^{67}Ga and ^{99m}Tc methylene diphosphonate (MDP) has been suggested, using the ratio of uptake of ^{67}Ga to ^{99m}Tc to determine whether the fracture is infected. The ratio of ^{67}Ga to ^{99m}Tc MDP should be higher in infected fractures than in noninfected fractures. It is very difficult to differentiate pseudoarthrosis from infection at the fracture site. Standard ^{99m}Tc and ^{67}Ga bone scans are not helpful, because both may be positive for both conditions. In these instances, ^{111}In white blood cell scanning combined with ^{99m}Tc MDP scanning appears to be the best method for determining if a fractured or traumatized bone is infected. For more information regarding recent trials of evaluating infected fractures with new radionuclide agents including immunoglobulins, see Chapter 2.

Arthrography

Arthrography is still used in the evaluation of injuries to articular cartilage, menisci, joint capsules, tendons, and ligaments (Figs. 4.9 and 4.10).

Figure 4.8 Fracture of the femoral neck. (A) Anteroposterior view of the left hip reveals a band of increased density, suggesting a fracture of the femoral neck. **(B)** A bone scan performed after administration of 15 mCi (555 MBq) of ^{99m}TC-labeled methylene diphosphonate shows increased uptake of isotope in the region of the femoral neck, confirming the fracture.

band of increased density

Figure 4.9 Tear of the medial meniscus. In this patient, double-contrast arthrography of the knee shows a horizontal cleavage tear in the posterior horn of the medial meniscus.

Figure 4.10 Tear of the rotator cuff. Single-contrast arthrogram of the right shoulder shows leak of contrast into the subacromial-subdeltoid bursae complex (arrows) diagnostic of full-thickness tear of the supraspinatus tendon.

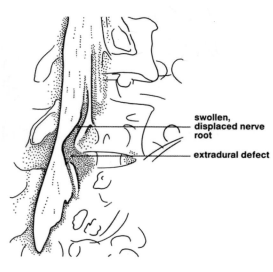

Figure 4.11 Herniation of the lumbar disk. A patient strained his back by lifting a heavy object. Oblique view of the lower lumbosacral spine after injection of metrizamide contrast into the subarachnoid space shows an extradural pressure defect on the thecal sac at the L5-S1 intervertebral space characteristic of disk herniation. Note the markedly swollen, displaced nerve root.

Figure 4.12 Rupture of the annulus fibrosus and disk herniation A spinal needle was placed in the center of the nucleus pulposus and a few milliliters of metrizamide were injected. The leak of contrast into the extradural space indicates a tear of the annulus fibrosus and posterior disk herniation.

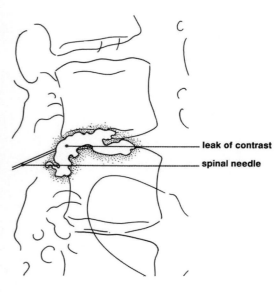

Although virtually every joint can be injected with contrast, the examination is most frequently performed in the knee, shoulder, ankle, and elbow articulations. Tenograms help evaluate injuries to the tendons.

Myelography and Diskography

Myelography, either alone or in conjunction with CT scan, is used to evaluate certain traumatic conditions of the spine (Fig. 4.11). If a disk abnormality is suspected and a myelographic study is not diagnostic, diskography may yield information required for further patient management (Fig. 4.12).

Angiography

Angiography is indicated if concomitant injury to the vascular system is suspected (Fig. 4.13). DSA is preferred because subtraction of the

Figure 4.13 Tear of the femoral artery. A femoral arteriogram was performed to rule out damage to vascular structures by a fractured femur. Transverse fracture of the distal femur resulted in transsection of the superficial femoral artery.

Figure 4.14 Joint effusion. A 64-year-old man sustained injury to the left knee. Axial MRI (multiplanar gradient-recalled, TR 500/TE 15 msec, flip angle 30 degrees) demonstrates a partial tear of the medial retinaculum. Posttraumatic knee effusion shows high signal intensity. Note marked thinning of patellar articular cartilage due to osteoarthritis.

overlying bones results in clear delineation of vascular structures (see Fig. 2.3).

Magnetic Resonance Imaging

MRI plays a leading role in the evaluation of trauma to bone, cartilage, and soft tissue. MRI evaluation of trauma to the knee, particularly abnormalities of the menisci and ligaments, has a high negative predictive value. MRI can be used to screen patients before surgery, so unnecessary arthroscopies are avoided. MRI is probably the only imaging modality that can demonstrate so-called bone contusions. These abnormalities consist of posttraumatic marrow change resulting from a combination of hemorrhage, edema, and microtrabecular injury (see Fig. 2.16). Other subtle abnormalities of various structures and posttraumatic joint effusion can also be well visualized (Fig. 4.14). Similarly, the medial and lateral collateral ligaments, anterior and posterior cruciate ligaments, and tendons around the knee joint can be well demonstrated (see Figs. 9.14, 9.15) and abnormalities of these struc-

tures can be diagnosed with high accuracy. Although occasionally difficult to detect, other types of meniscal injuries, such as bucket-handle tears, tears of the free edge, and peripheral detachments, can be diagnosed. In the shoulder, impingement syndrome and complete and incomplete rotator cuff tears may be effectively diagnosed most of the time (Fig. 4.15). Traumatic lesions of the tendons (such as biceps tendon rupture), traumatic joint effusions, and hematomas are easily diagnosed with MRI. Much more difficult to diagnose is a tear of the cartilaginous labrum. The changes of osteonecrosis at various sites, particularly in its early stage, may be detected by MRI when other modalities, such as conventional radiography, tomography, and even radionuclide bone scan, may be normal. MRI of the ankle and foot has been used in diagnosing tendon ruptures and posttraumatic osteonecrosis of the talus. In the wrist and hand, MRI has been successfully used in early diagnosis of posttraumatic osteonecrosis of the scaphoid. MRI is strongly advocated as the technique of choice in evaluation of abnormalities of the triangular fibrocartilage complex, although arthrography, particularly in conjunction with digital imaging

Figure 4.15 Tear of the rotator cuff. A 60-year-old man presented with right shoulder pain. Oblique coronal T2-weighted MRI (SE; TR 2000/TE 80 msec) demonstrates complete rotator cuff tear. The supraspinatus muscle is retracted medially and no tendon tissue is present in the subacromial space. Joint fluid shows high signal intensity. (From Beltran J, 1990, with permission).

and CT, is also a very effective modality. The greatest use of MRI is for evaluating trauma of the spine, the spinal cord, the thecal sac, and nerve roots, as well as disk herniation (see Fig. 11.89). MRI is also useful in evaluation of spinal ligament injury. Demonstration of the relationship of vertebral fragments to the spinal cord with direct sagittal imaging is extremely helpful, particularly to evaluate injury in the cervical and thoracic area.

Fractures and Dislocations

Fractures and dislocations are among the most common traumatic conditions encountered by radiologists. By definition, a *fracture* is a complete disruption in the continuity of a bone (Fig. 4.16). If only some of the bony trabeculae are completely severed while others are bent or remain intact, the fracture is incomplete (Fig. 4.17). A *dislocation* is a complete disruption of a joint; articular surfaces are no longer in contact (Fig. 4.18). A *subluxation*, however, is a minor disruption of a joint in which some articular contact remains (Fig. 4.19). Proper radiologic evaluation of these conditions contributes greatly to successful treatment by the orthopedic surgeon.

In dealing with trauma, the radiologist has two main tasks:
1. Diagnosing and evaluating the type of fracture or dislocation
2. Monitoring the results of treatment and looking for possible complications.

Diagnosis

The important radiographic principle in diagnosing skeletal trauma is to obtain at least two views of the bone involved, with each view including two joints adjacent to the injured bone (Fig. 4.20). In so doing, the radiologist eliminates the risk of missing an associated fracture, subluxation, and/or dislocation at a site remote from the

Figure 4.17 An incomplete (greenstick) fracture. The ulna is bent and there is a fracture line extending only through the posterior cortex. In the radial fracture some trabeculae remain intact.

apparent primary injury. In children it is frequently necessary to obtain a radiograph of the normal, unaffected limb for comparison.

Radiographic Evaluation of Fractures

The complete radiographic evaluation of fractures should include the following elements: (a) the anatomic *site* and *extent* of a fracture (Fig.

Figure 4.16 A complete fracture. The continuity of the bone is disrupted and there is a narrow gap between the bony fragments.

Figure 4.18 Dislocation. A typical anterior dislocation of the humeral head. The articular surface of the humerus loses contact with the articular surface of the glenoid.

Figure 4.19 Subluxation. There is malalignment of the head of the humerus and the glenoid fossa, but some articular contact remains. Note the associated fracture of the surgical neck of the humerus.

Figure 4.20 Adjacent joints. The radiograph of a suspected fracture of the femoral shaft should include the hip and knee articulations.

SITE AND EXTENT OF FRACTURE

junction of middle and distal thirds of femur

supracondylar

intra-articular

Figure 4.21 Site and extent. Factors in the radiographic evaluation of a fracture: the anatomic site and extent.

4.21); (b) the *type* of fracture, whether it is incomplete, as seen predominantly in children, or complete (Fig. 4.22); (c) the *alignment* of the fragments with regard to displacement, angulation, rotation, foreshortening, or distraction (Fig. 4.23); (d) the *direction* of the fracture line in relation to the longitudinal axis of the bone (Fig. 4.24); (e) the presence of *special features* such as impaction, depression, or compression (Fig. 4.25); (f) the presence of *associated abnormalities* such as fracture with concomitant dislocation or diastasis (Fig. 4.26); and (g) *special types* of fractures that may occur as the result of abnormal stress or secondary to pathologic processes in the bone (Fig. 4.27). The distinction between an *open* (or *compound*) fracture, one in which the fractured bone communicates with the outside environment through an open wound, and a *closed* (or *simple*) fracture, one that does not produce an open wound in the skin, should preferably be made by clinical rather than radiographic examination.

In children the radiographic evaluation of fractures, particularly of the ends of tubular bones, should also take into consideration the involvement of the growth plate (physis). Localization of the fracture line has implications with respect to the mechanism of injury and possible complications. A useful classification of injuries affecting the physis, metaphysis, epiphysis, or all of these structures has been proposed by Salter and Harris (types I to V) and has been expanded by Rang (type VI) and Ogden (types VII to IX) to include four additional types of fractures (Fig. 4.28). Although the injuries described by Rang and Ogden do not directly involve the growth plate, the sequelae of such trauma affect the physis in the same way as the direct injuries described by Salter and Harris. In type VI, which involves only the peripheral region of the growth plate, the injury may not always be associated with a fracture. It may result from a localized contusion, trauma-induced infection, or severe burn. Type VII injury consists of a purely transepiphyseal fracture that, if the epiphysis is not completely ossified, may not even be detectable on the conventional radiograph. Type VIII injury involving the metaphyseal region may be complicated by damage to the blood vessels supplying the growth plate, and in type IX, injury to the periosteum may interfere with the membranous mechanism of bone formation. All such trauma, but particularly types IV and V (see Fig. 4.70), may lead to growth disturbance with consequent limb-length discrepancy.

Indirect Signs as Diagnostic Clues

Although diagnosis of most fractures can be made from conventional radiographs, some subtle, nondisplaced, and hairline fractures may not be apparent at the time of injury. In such instances certain indirect signs of fracture provide useful diagnostic clues.

Soft-Tissue Swelling. Skeletal trauma is always associated with injury to the soft tissues, and in almost all cases of acute fracture there is some radiographic evidence of soft-tissue swelling at the fracture site (Fig. 4.29A). The absence of soft-tissue swelling, however, virtually excludes the possibility of acute fracture (Fig. 4.29B).

Obliteration or Displacement of Fat Stripes. Subtle fractures, particularly in the distal radius, carpal scaphoid, trapezium, and base of the first metacarpal, result in obliteration or displacement of fascial planes. On the lateral view of the wrist, one can detect a radiolucent stripe representing a collection of fat between the pronator quadratus (quadratipronator) and the tendons of the flexor digitorum profundus. Fracture of the distal radius results in a change in the appearance of the *pronator quadratus fat stripe,* which may be anteriorly (volarly) displaced, blurred, or obliterated (MacEwan sign) (Fig. 4.30).

Terry and Ramin have pointed out the usefulness of recognizing the *scaphoid fat stripe,* which is usually visible as a thin radiolucent line paralleling the lateral surface of the scaphoid bone between the radial collateral ligament and the synovial sheath of the abductor pollicis longus and the extensor pollicis brevis. In most fractures of the carpal scaphoid, radial styloid, trapezium, or base of the first metacarpal, the scaphoid fat stripe is obliterated or displaced. This finding is most apparent on the dorsovolar view of the wrist (Fig. 4.31).

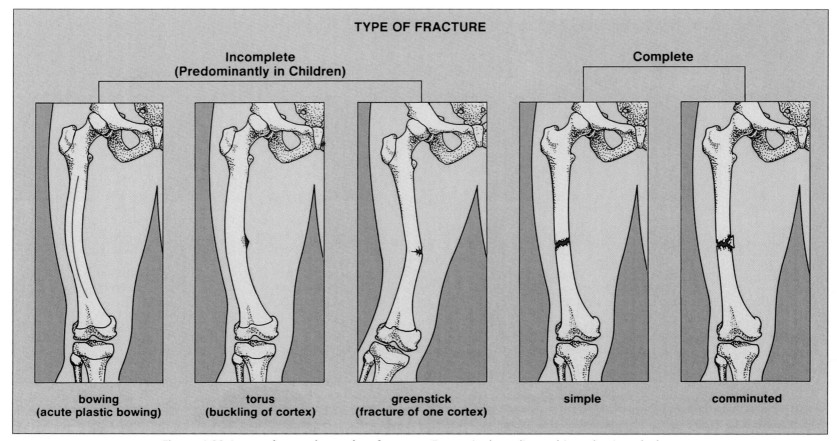

TYPE OF FRACTURE

Incomplete
(Predominantly in Children)

Complete

| bowing (acute plastic bowing) | torus (buckling of cortex) | greenstick (fracture of one cortex) | simple | comminuted |

Figure 4.22 Incomplete and complete fractures. Factors in the radiographic evaluation of a fracture: the type of fracture, incomplete or complete.

ALIGNMENT OF FRAGMENTS

medial
displacement

lateral
displacement

medial angulation
(or lateral
angulation of
distal fragment—
valgus configuration)

lateral angulation
(or medial
angulation of
distal fragment—
varus configuration)

internal rotation

external rotation

overriding with
foreshortening
(bayonet apposition)

distraction

Figure 4.23 Alignment. Factors in the radiographic evaluation of a fracture: the alignment of the fragments.

Figure 4.24 Direction. Factors in the radiographic evaluation of a fracture: the direction of the fracture line.

Figure 4.25 Special features. Factors in the radiographic evaluation of a fracture: special features.

Figure 4.26 Associated abnormalities. Factors in the radiographic evaluation of a fracture: associated abnormalities.

Figure 4.27 Special types. Factors in the radiographic evaluation of a fracture: special types of fractures.

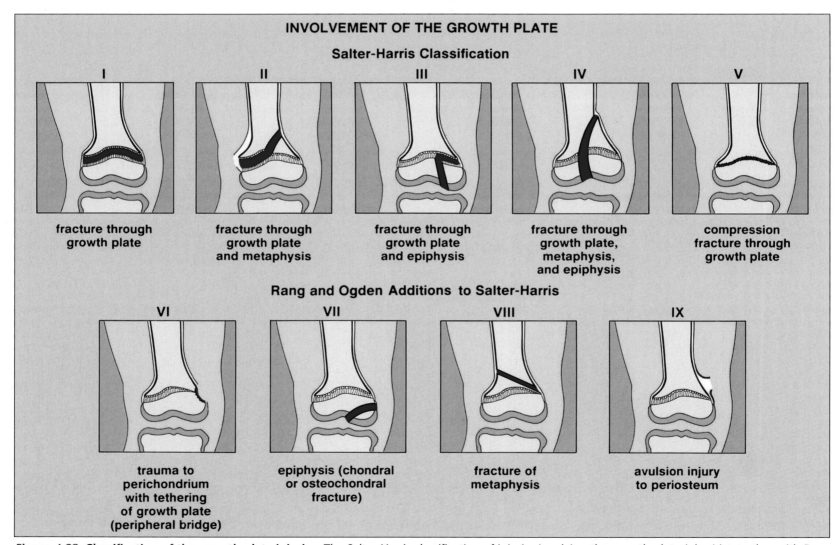

Figure 4.28 Classification of the growth plate injuries. The Salter-Harris classification of injuries involving the growth plate (physis) together with Rang and Ogden additions.

Figure 4.29 Fracture versus ossification center. (A) Dorsoplantar view of the foot reveals prominent soft-tissue swelling localized in the lateral aspect. The radiolucent line at the base of the fifth metatarsal indicates a fracture. **(B)** A similar radiolucent line separates a bony fragment from the base of the fifth metatarsal in another patient who was suspected of sustaining a fracture of this bone. Note the complete lack of soft-tissue swelling. The finding represents a secondary ossification center, not a fracture.

Figure 4.30 Pronator quadratus fat stripe. (A) The fascial plane of the pronator quadratus is demonstrated on the volar aspect of the distal forearm as a radiolucent stripe. **(B)** With fracture of the distal radius, the fat stripe is blurred and volarly displaced secondary to local edema and periosteal hemorrhage.

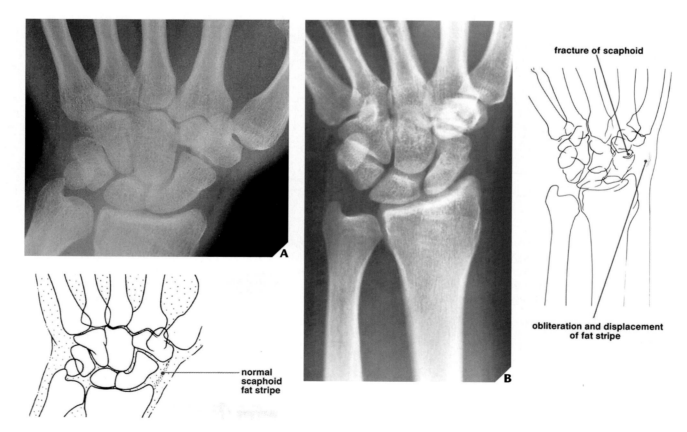

Figure 4.31 Scaphoid fat stripe. (A) Normal scaphoid fat stripe. **(B)** Subtle fracture of the scaphoid resulted in obliteration and radial displacement of the fat stripe.

Periosteal and Endosteal Reaction. The fracture line may not be visible, but the periosteal or endosteal response may be the first radiographic sign of a fracture (Fig. 4.32).

Joint Effusion. This finding, which results in the radiographic appearance of the fat-pad sign, is particularly useful in diagnosing elbow injuries. The posterior (dorsal) fat pad lies deep in the olecranon fossa and is not visible in the lateral projection. The anterior (ventral) fat pad occupies the shallower anterior coronoid and radial fossae and is usually seen as a flat radiolucent strip ventrad to the anterior cortex of the humerus. Distention of the articular capsule by synovial or hemorrhagic fluid causes the posterior fat pad to become visible and also displaces the anterior fat pad, yielding the *fat-pad sign* (Fig. 4.33). When there is a history of elbow trauma and the fat-pad sign is positive, there is usually an associated fracture and every effort should be made to demonstrate it. Even if the fracture line is not demonstrated on multiple films, the patient should be treated for fracture.

Intracapsular Fat–Fluid Level. If a fracture involves the articular end of a bone (particularly a long bone like the tibia, humerus, or femur), blood and bone-marrow fat enter the joint (lipohemarthrosis) and produce a characteristic layering of these two substances on the radiograph: the fat–blood interface, or *FBI sign* (Fig. 4.34) A CT or MRI study can also demonstrate this phenomenon (Figs. 4.35 and 4.36). When the fracture line cannot be demonstrated, diagnosis should be made on the strength of this sign alone.

Double Cortical Line. This finding indicates a subtle but depressed fracture. The actual fracture line may not be apparent, but the double contour of the cortex reflects impaction (Fig. 4.37).

Buckling of the Cortex. Known as the *torus fracture*, this may be the only sign of a tubular bone fracture in children (Fig. 4.38). This finding is sometimes identified more easily on the lateral than on the frontal projection.

Irregular Metaphyseal Corners. This sign, which is secondary to small avulsion fractures of the metaphysis, indicates a subtle injury

Figure 4.32 **Secondary signs of a fracture. (A)** A 49-year-old woman sustained an injury to the lower leg. Anteroposterior radiograph shows periosteal new bone at the medial cortex of the distal third of the tibia just above the malleolus, and more proximally at the lateral aspect. This indirect sign of a fracture represents an early stage of external callus formation. The actual hairline spiral fracture line is barely discernible. **(B)** Example of periosteal callus formation at the medial and lateral cortices of the proximal tibial diaphysis. A transverse band of increased density, visible in the medullary portion of the bone, represents endosteal callus. The fracture line is practically invisible. These features are commonly seen in a stress fracture.

anterior fat pad
posterior fat pad
fracture of radial head

Figure 4.33 Fracture of the radial head. Lateral view of the elbow shows a positive fat-pad sign. The anterior fat pad is markedly elevated and the posterior fat pad is clearly visible in this patient. There is a subtle, nondisplaced fracture of the radial head.

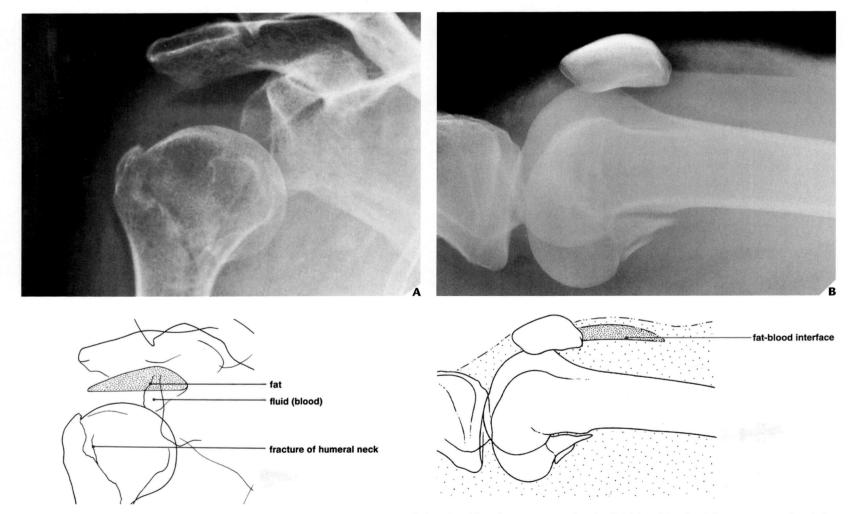

fat
fluid (blood)
fracture of humeral neck

fat-blood interface

A
B

Figure 4.34 Fat-blood interface sign. (A) Erect anteroposterior view of the shoulder demonstrates the fat-fluid level in the joint, an example of the fat–blood interface (FBI) sign. The fracture line extends from the humeral neck cephalad to the greater tuberosity. To demonstrate the FBI sign, the cassette should be positioned perpendicular to the expected fat–fluid level with the central ray directed horizontally. For example, in the shoulder, an upright radiograph (patient standing or sitting) should be obtained. In the knee **(B)**, the patient should be supine and a cross-table lateral view should be performed.

Figure 4.35 Fat–blood interface sign on CT. Axial CT section through the knee joint shows FBI sign in a patient with tibial plateau fracture (not seen on this image).

Figure 4.36 Fat–blood interface sign on MRI. Axial MR image of the knee with the patient in the supine position demonstrates fat–blood interface sign secondary to differential layering of fat mixed with fluid (high signal intensity) and blood (intermediate signal intensity). Note inhomogeneous appearance of blood caused by partial clotting.

Figure 4.37 Fracture of the femur. (A) On the anteroposterior view of the knee, the fracture line is not apparent, but a depressed articular cortex of the lateral femoral condyle projects proximally to the normal subchondral line of the intact segment, producing a double cortical line. **(B)** Lateral radiograph confirms the presence of a subtle fracture of the femoral condyle.

Figure 4.38 Torus fracture. Posteroanterior **(A)** and lateral **(B)** radiographs of the distal forearm demonstrate buckling of the dorsal cortex of the diaphysis of the distal radius. This represents an incomplete torus fracture. Note that the lateral view is more revealing.

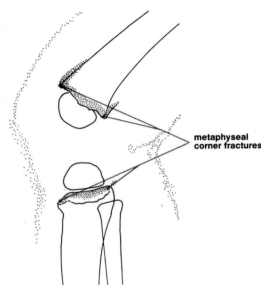

metaphyseal
corner fractures

Figure 4.39 Battered child syndrome. Lateral view of the knee reveals irregular outlines of the metaphyses of the distal femur and the proximal tibia, and subtle corner fractures characteristic of the battered child syndrome.

to the bone caused by a rapid rotary force exerted on the ligaments' insertion. As a result, small fragments of bone are separated from the metaphysis. These *corner fractures* are often present in infants and children who sustain skeletal trauma, and they should be looked for particularly if battered child syndrome, also known as "shaken baby syndrome" or parent–infant trauma syndrome (PITS), is suspected (Fig. 4.39).

Figure 4.40 Anterior dislocation in the hip joint. Anteroposterior view of the left hip shows a typical anterior dislocation of the femoral head. The clue to this diagnosis is the presence of abduction and external rotation of the femur and the position of the femoral head, which is medial and inferior to the acetabulum.

Radiographic Evaluation of Dislocations

Dislocations are more obvious than fractures on conventional radiographs and, consequently, are more easily diagnosed. Some display such a characteristic appearance on frontal projection (anteroposterior view) that this single examination suffices (Fig. 4.40). However, the same principle of obtaining at least two projections oriented at 90 degrees to each other should apply. Supplemental radiographs are occasionally necessary, and in some instances CT is required for exact evaluation of a dislocation.

Monitoring the Results of Treatment

Radiography plays the leading role in monitoring the progress of fracture healing and in detecting any posttraumatic complications. Follow-up radiographs should be taken at regular intervals to evaluate the stage and possible associated complications of fracture healing and other complications that may follow a fracture or dislocation. If radiographs are ambiguous in this respect, CT is the next technique to apply.

Fracture Healing and Complications

Fracture healing depends on many factors: the patient's age, the site and type of fracture, the position of the fragments, the status of the blood supply, the quality of immobilization or fixation, and the presence or absence of associated abnormalities such as infection or osteonecrosis (Table 4.1). Most fractures heal by some combination of endosteal and periosteal callus. Provided that blood supply is adequate, undisplaced fractures and anatomically reduced fractures immobilized with adequate compression heal by *primary union*. In this type of healing, the fracture line becomes obliterated by endosteal (internal) callus. Displaced fractures, i.e., those that are not anatomically aligned or with a gap between fragments, heal by *secondary union*. This type of healing is achieved mainly by excessive periosteal (external) callus, which undergoes full ossification through the stages of granulation tissue, fibrous tissue, fibrocartilage, woven bone, and

Table 4.1 **Factors Influencing Fracture Healing**

PROMOTING	RETARDING
Good immobilization	Motion
Growth hormone	Corticosteroids
Thyroid hormone	Vitamins A and D (high dose)
Calcitonin	Anticoagulants
Insulin Anemia	Anemia
Vitamins A and D	Radiation
Hyaluronidase	Poor blood supply
Anticoagulants	Infection
Electric currents	Osteoporosis
Oxygen	Osteonecrosis
Physical exercise	Comminution
Young age	Old age

compact bone. For the radiologist evaluating follow-up radiographs, the primary indication of bone repair is radiographic evidence of periosteal (external) and endosteal (internal) callus formation (Fig. 4.41). This process, however, may not be radiographically apparent in the early stage of healing. Periosteal response may not be visible on radiographs at sites where there is an anatomic lack of periosteum, for example, in the intracapsular portion of the femoral neck. Likewise, radiographs may not demonstrate endosteal callus formation, because the callus contains only fibrous tissue and cartilage, which are elements that are radiolucent. At this early stage of healing, a fracture may be *clinically united*, that is, show no evidence of motion under stress, yet radiographically the radiolucent band between the fragments may persist (Fig. 4.42A). As the primary temporarily radiolucent callus is gradually converted by the process of endochondral os-

sification to more mature lamellar bone, it is seen on film as a dense bridge (Fig. 4.42B). This constitutes *radiographic union*.

Although conventional radiographs are frequently sufficient to evaluate the progress of fracture healing, routine studies must at times be supplemented by tomography. If a plaster cast, for example, is still in place and obscures the bony details, or if radiographic findings are equivocal (Fig. 4.43), tomographic examination can clarify the status of healing.

Recently, CT with multiplanar reformation proved to be a good method to assess fracture healing. It was, in particular, effective in patients with remaining metallic hardware and those who had multiple surgical procedures including bone grafting. CT with reformation in the coronal and sagittal planes aided surgical planning by providing a more detailed assessment of malalignment and angular deformities, the magnitude of the gap in the bone, and the integrity of the adjacent weight-bearing joints.

In addition to monitoring the progress of callus formation, the radiologist should be aware of radiographic evidence of associated complications of the healing process. These complications are delayed union, nonunion, and malunion. Of the three, *malunion* is the most apparent radiographically and is characterized by union of the bone fragments in a faulty and unacceptable position (Fig. 4.44); surgical intervention is usually the preferred method of treatment in this case.

Delayed union refers to a fracture that does not unite within a reasonable amount of time (16 to 18 weeks), depending on the patient's age and the fracture site. *Nonunion,* however, applies to a fracture that simply fails to unite (Fig. 4.45). Some of the causes of nonunion are listed in Table 4.2. A *pseudoarthrosis* is a variant of nonunion in which there is formation of a false joint cavity with a synovial-like capsule and even synovial fluid at the fracture site; however, some physicians refer to any fracture that fails to heal within 9 months as a pseudoarthrosis

Figure 4.41 Fracture healing. (A). Anteroposterior radiograph of the femur shows a fracture healing predominantly by periosteal callus formation. There is no radiographic evidence of endosteal callus, and the fracture line is still visible. **(B)** Posteroanterior radiograph of the distal forearm demonstrates healing fractures of the radius and ulna. The fracture lines are almost completely obliterated secondary to formation of endosteal callus. Note also the minimal amount of periosteal callus.

Figure 4.42 Clinical versus radiographic union. A 30-year-old woman sustained a fracture of the distal third of the tibia. **(A)** After 3 months of immobilization the plaster cast was removed. The radiograph shows a unilateral periosteal callus from the medial aspect, but the fracture line is still clearly visible. Clinically, however, this fracture was fully united and the patient was allowed to bear weight without a cast. **(B)** One and one-half months later, there is evidence of a dense bridge of periosteal and endosteal callus, indicating radiographic union.

and use the term as a synonym for nonunion. Radiographically, nonunion is characterized by rounded edges; smoothness and sclerosis (eburnation) of the fragment ends, which are separated by a gap; and motion between the fragments (demonstrated under fluoroscopy or on consecutive stress films). To provide adequate evaluation of healing failure, the radiologist needs to distinguish between the three types of nonunion: reactive, nonreactive, and infected (Fig. 4.46).

Reactive (Hypertrophic and Oligotrophic) Nonunion. Radiographically, this type of nonunion is characterized by exuberant bone reaction and resultant flaring and sclerosis of bone ends, the elephant-foot or horse-hoof type (Fig. 4.47). The sclerotic areas do not represent dead bone but the apposition of well-vascularized new bone. Radionuclide bone scan shows a marked increase of isotope uptake at the fracture site. This type of nonunited fracture is usually treated by intramedullary nailing or compression plating.

Nonreactive (Atrophic) Nonunion. With this type of nonunion the radiograph shows an absence of bone reaction at the fragment ends, and the blood supply is generally very scanty (Fig. 4.48). Bone scan shows either minimal or no isotope uptake. In addition to stable internal fixation, such fractures often require extensive decortication and bone grafting.

Infected Nonunion. Radiographic presentation of infected nonunion depends on the infection's activity. Old, *inactive* osteomyelitis shows irregular thickening of the cortex, well-organized periosteal reaction, and reactive sclerosis of cancellous bone (Fig. 4.49), whereas the *active* form shows soft-tissue swelling, destruction of the cortex and cancellous bone associated with periosteal new bone formation, and sequestration (Fig. 4.50). Treatment of infected nonunion depends on the stage of osteomyelitis. Decortication and bone grafting combined with compression plating are used if nonunion is accompanied by inactive osteomyelitis. Treatment of active osteomyelitis involves application of antibiotics and sequestrectomy, usually followed by bone grafting and intramedullary stabilization. Different procedures are individually tailored, depending on the anatomic site and various general and local factors.

Other Complications of Fractures and Dislocations

In addition to the possible complications associated with the process of fracture healing, the radiologist may encounter complications that are not related to that process. Radiographic evidence of the presence of such complications may not show up on immediate follow-up examination, because they may occur weeks, months, or even years after

Figure 4.43 Value of tomography. (A) Conventional radiograph of the lower tibia reveals an oblique fracture of the distal shaft. Although the external callus is well demonstrated, there is a 2-mm gap between the fragments, raising the possibility of nonunion. Supplementary views were also equivocal. **(B)** Tomographic examination demonstrates good bridging of the fragments by periosteal callus from the medial and lateral aspects, confirming radiographic union.

Figure 4.44 Malunion. (A) Anteroposterior radiograph of the leg demonstrates angular malunion. The fracture of the tibia and the segmental fracture of the fibula are solidly united. The distal part of the tibia, however, shows rotation and anterior angulation, and the fractures of the fibula have joined in a bowing deformity. **(B)** The malunion was surgically treated by double osteotomy and internal fixation of the tibia with an intramedullary rod to correct the longitudinal alignment and restore the anatomic axis.

Figure 4.45 Nonunion. A fracture of the proximal fibula failed to unite. Note the gap between the fragments, the complete lack of callus formation, and the rounding of the fragment edges.

Table 4.2 **Causes of Nonunion**

I.	Excess motion (inadequate immobilization)
II.	Gap between fragments
	A. Soft-tissue interposition
	B. Distraction by traction or hardware
	C. Malposition, overriding, or displacement of fragments
	D. Loss of bone substance
III.	Loss of blood supply
	A. Damage to nutrient vessels
	B. Excessive stripping or injury to periosteum and muscle
	C. Free fragments, severe comminution
	D. Avascularity caused by hardware placement
	E. Osteonecrosis
IV.	Infection
	A. Osteomyelitis
	B. Extensive necrosis of fracture margins (gap)
	C. Bone death (sequestrum)
	D. Osteolysis (gap)
	E. Loosening of implants (motion)

Modified from Rosen H, 1993, with permission.

TYPES OF NONUNION

A	B	C	D	E
hypertrophic (elephant foot)	hypertrophic (horse hoof)	oligotrophic	atrophic	infected

Figure 4.46 Complications of fracture. Types of nonunion: reactive (**A–C**); nonreactive (**D**); infected (**E**).

the trauma and sometimes in a location distant from the original site of injury. Consequently, in dealing with patients presenting with a history of fracture or dislocation, radiologists should direct their investigation to areas where these associated complications may occur and should be aware of their radiologic characteristics and appearance.

Disuse Osteoporosis. Mild or moderate osteoporosis, which can be generally defined as a decrease in bone mass, frequently occurs after a fracture or dislocation as a result of disuse of the extremity caused by pain and immobilization in the plaster cast. Other terms often used to describe this condition are demineralization, deossification, bone atrophy, and osteopenia. The latter term is generally accepted as the best description of the nature of this complication.

Radiographically, it is identified by radiolucent areas of decreased bone density secondary to thinning of the cortex and atrophy of the bony trabeculae. It may accompany united as well as nonunited fractures (Fig. 4.51).

Reflex Sympathetic Dystrophy Syndrome. Known also as post-traumatic painful osteoporosis or Sudeck atrophy, reflex sympathetic dystrophy syndrome (RSDS), a severe form of osteoporosis, may occur subsequent to a fracture or even a milder form of injury. It has also been reported as resulting from neurologic or vascular abnormalities unrelated to trauma. Clinically, the patient presents with a painful, tender extremity with hyperesthesia, diffuse soft-tissue swelling, joint stiffness, vasomotor instability, and dystrophic skin changes. Three

Figure 4.47 Reactive nonunion. In hypertrophic nonunion, seen here in the shafts of the tibia and fibula, there is flaring of the bone ends, marked sclerosis, and periosteal response, but no evidence of endosteal callus formation. The gap between the bony fragments persists.

Figure 4.48 Nonreactive nonunion. In atrophic nonunion, seen here at the junction of the middle and distal thirds of the tibia, there is a gap between the fragments, rounding of the edges, and an almost complete lack of bone reaction. Note the malunited fracture of the fibula.

Figure 4.49 Infected nonunion. Nonunion of the fractured distal shaft of the femur with evidence of old, inactive osteomyelitis shows irregular thickening of the cortex, reactive sclerosis of the medullary portion of the bone, and well-organized periosteal reaction.

Figure 4.50 Infected nonunion. (A) Radiograph of a nonunited fracture in the distal shaft of the tibia with associated active osteomyelitis shows thickening of the cortex, sclerosis of the cancellous bone, a gap between the bony fragments, and several sequestra. **(B)** Tomographic examination provides a better demonstration of the multiple sequestra, the cardinal sign of active infection.

Figure 4.51 **Disuse osteoporosis. (A).** Oblique radiograph of the ankle shows a completely united fracture of the distal fibula. Disuse juxta-articular osteoporosis is evident from the thinning of the cortices associated with decreased bone density. **(B)** Anteroposterior view of the knee shows a nonunited fracture of the tibial plateau, with a moderate degree of disuse osteoporosis.

stages have been identified. The initial (or acute) inflammatory stage lasts from 1 to 7 weeks and is characterized by diffuse regional pain, inflammation, edema, and hypothermia or hyperthermia. In the second (or dystrophic) stage, which lasts from 3 to 24 months, the clini-

Figure 4.52 **Sudeck atrophy.** A 35-year-old man sustained fractures of the tibia and fibula, which eventually healed. Subsequently, however, he reported weakness, stiffness, and pain in his foot. Radiographic examination showed changes typical of reflex sympathetic dystrophy syndrome in the foot: rapidly progressive, patchy osteoporosis associated with marked soft-tissue swelling.

cal findings include pain on exercise, increased sensitivity of the skin to pressure and temperature changes, and skin and muscle atrophy. In the final (or atrophic) stage irreversible scleroderma-like skin changes and aponeurotic and tendinous retraction may occur. On the radiograph, RSDS is characterized by soft-tissue swelling and severe, patchy osteoporosis that progresses rapidly (Fig. 4.52). Three-phase technetium bone scan characteristically shows increased blood flow, blood pool, and periarticular increased uptake in the affected areas. These findings are seen in approximately 60% of affected patients.

Volkmann Ischemic Contracture. Developing usually after supracondylar fracture of the humerus, Volkmann contracture is caused by ischemia of the muscles followed by fibrosis. Clinically, it is characterized as the "five Ps" syndrome—pulselessness, pain, pallor, paresthesia, and paralysis. Radiographic examination usually reveals flexion–contracture in the wrist and in the interphalangeal joints of the fingers and hyperextension (or, rarely, flexion) of the metacarpophalangeal joints associated with soft-tissue atrophy (Fig. 4.53).

Posttraumatic Myositis Ossificans. Occasionally after a fracture, dislocation, or even minor trauma to the soft tissues, an enlarging, painful mass develops at the site of injury. The characteristic feature of this lesion includes the clearly recognizable pattern of its evolution, which correlates well with the lapse of time after the trauma. Thus, by the third or fourth week, calcifications and ossifications in the mass begin to develop (Figs. 4.54A and B), and by the sixth to eighth week the periphery of the mass shows definite, well-organized cortical bone (Fig. 4.54C). The important radiographic hallmark of this complication is the presence of the so-called zonal phenomenon. On the radiograph, this phenomenon is characterized by a radiolucent area in the center of the lesion, indicating the formation of immature bone, and by a dense zone of mature ossification at the periphery. In addition, a thin radiolucent cleft separates the ossific mass from the adjacent cortex (Fig. 4.55). These important features help differentiate this condition from juxtacortical osteosarcoma, which may at times appear very similar. It must be stressed, however, that occasionally the focus of myositis ossificans may adhere and fuse with the cortex, mimicking parosteal osteosarcoma on radiographs. In these cases, CT may provide additional information, such as the presence of the zonal phenomenon characteristic of myositis ossificans (Fig. 4.56).

The MRI appearance of myositis ossificans depends on the stage of maturation of the lesion. In the early stage, T1-weighted sequences

Figure 4.53 Volkmann contracture. Having sustained a supracondylar fracture of the humerus that united, a 23-year-old man presented with symptoms typical of Volkmann ischemic contracture. Lateral view of the distal forearm including the wrist and hand shows flexion–contracture in the metacarpopha- langeal and the interphalangeal joints, together with a marked degree of soft-tissue atrophy.

Figure 4.54 Posttraumatic myositis ossificans. (A) A 20-year-old man sustained a transverse fracture at the junction of the middle and distal thirds of the femur. The fracture was treated by open reduction and internal fixation with an intramedullary rod. On the lateral view, obtained 3.5 weeks after injury, an immature focus of myositis ossificans with poorly defined densities in the soft-tissue mass is evident adjacent to the posterior cortex of the femur. **(B)** Maturation of myositis ossificans in a 28-year-old woman who sustained an injury to the thigh 5 weeks before this radiograph was obtained. Note formation of peripheral ossification (*arrows*) and presence of a radiolucent cleft (*open arrows*). **(C)** This radiograph of a 27-year-old man who 1 year previously had sustained a fracture–dislocation in the elbow, which healed, shows a well-organized, mature focus of myositis ossificans. Note the well-developed cortex at the periphery of the osseous mass and the radiolucent gap separating the lesion from the cortex of the humerus.

Figure 4.55 **Posttraumatic myositis ossificans.** A 7-year-old boy presented with a history of trauma 6 weeks before this radiographic examination. The anteroposterior radiograph of the left hip **(A)** demonstrates a lesion that exhibits features of zonal phenomenon characteristic of juxtacortical myositis ossificans. On the frog-lateral projection **(B)** note the cleft separating the ossific mass from the posterolateral cortex.

Figure 4.56 **Posttraumatic myositis ossificans.** A 52-year-old man sustained injury to the lateral aspect of the left thigh 6 months previously. He was concerned about a hard mass he had palpated. **(A)** Radiograph shows an ossific mass adherent to the lateral cortex of the left femur (*arrow*). **(B)** CT scan demonstrates the classic zonal phenomenon of myositis ossificans. Note radiolucent center surrounded by mature cortex.

Figure 4.57 Posttraumatic myositis ossificans. A 41-year-old man presented with a palpable mass over the posterolateral aspect of the proximal right humerus. **(A)** Conventional anteroposterior radiograph of the right shoulder shows calcifications and ossifications overlaying the proximal humerus. **(B)** CT section demonstrates the zoning phenomenon typical of myositis ossificans. The center of the lesion shows a low-attenuation area caused by fatty changes. The cleft separates the mass from the cortex. **(C)** Axial T1-weighted (SE; TR 600/TE 20 msec) MRI shows the center of the lesion to be of high signal intensity, whereas the periphery exhibits low-to-intermediate signal.

usually show a mass that lacks definable borders with homogeneous intermediate signal intensity, slightly higher than that of adjacent muscle. T2-weighted images show the lesion to be of high signal intensity. After intravenous injection of gadopentetate dimeglumine, T1-weighted images show a well-defined peripheral rim of contrast enhancement, but the center of the lesion does not enhance. The more mature lesions show intermediate signal intensity on T1-weighted sequences isointense with adjacent muscle, surrounded by a rim of low signal intensity, which corresponds to peripheral bone maturation. On T2 weighting, the lesion is generally of high signal intensity but may appear inhomogeneous. The rim of low signal is seen at the periphery. Sometimes the focus of myositis ossificans (whether immature or mature) may contain a fatty component, giving the lesion a high intensity signal on T1-weighted images (Fig. 4.57).

Osteonecrosis (Ischemic or Avascular Necrosis). Osteonecrosis, the cellular death of bone tissue, occurs after fracture or dislocation when the bone is deprived of a sufficient supply of arterial blood. However, it is important to recognize that this condition may also develop as a result of factors unrelated to mechanical trauma. Regardless of cause, the pathomechanism of osteonecrosis includes intraluminal vascular obstruction, vascular compression, or disruption of a blood vessel. Among the reported causes of osteonecrosis (other than fracture or dislocation) are the following:

1. *Embolization of arteries.* This may occur in a variety of conditions. It is seen, for example, in certain hemoglobinopathies, such as sickle cell disease, in which arteries are occluded by abnormal red blood cells; in decompression states of dysbaric conditions, such as caisson disease, in which embolization by nitrogen bubbles occurs; or in chronic alcoholism and pancreatitis, when fat particles embolize arteries.
2. *Vasculitis.* Inflammation of the blood vessels may lead to interruption of the supply of arterial blood to the bone, as seen in collagen disorders such as systemic lupus erythematosus.
3. *Abnormal accumulation of cells.* In Gaucher disease, which is characterized by the abnormal accumulation of lipid-containing histiocytes in the bone marrow, or after steroid therapy, which can lead to an increase of fat cells, sinusoidal blood flow may be compromised, resulting in deprivation of blood supply to the bone.
4. *Elevated intraosseous pressure.* This theory, championed by Hungerford and Lennox, suggests that any physiologic or pathologic process that results in increased pressure within the femoral head (which is essentially a sphere of cancellous bone, marrow, and fat surrounded by a cortical shell) may compromise the blood flow and lead to osteonecrosis.
5. *Inhibition of angiogenesis.* Osteonecrosis may result from com-

promise of normal angiogenesis that occurs consistently in bone tissue. This new hypothesis was recently introduced by Smith et al. It is supported by the fact that a number of drugs and mediators, including glucocorticoids, interferons, and other endogenously produced cytokines inhibit angiogenesis. Similar effect was observed in the angiographic studies of the femoral head after administration of steroids.

6. *Mechanical stress.* This causative factor was occasionally attributed to nontraumatic osteonecrosis of the femoral head. The weight-bearing segment of the femoral head is the anterior–superior quadrant, and therefore is under a large mechanical strain. Occlusion of the vessels in this region of the femoral head might be the result of cartilage breakdown secondary to excessive mechanical stress. Support for this hypothesis stems from experiments on rats by Iwasaki and colleagues and Suehiro et al.

7. *Radiation exposure.* Exposure to radiation may result in damage to the vascularity of bone.

8. *Idiopathic.* Often no definite cause can be established, as in the case of spontaneous osteonecrosis that predominantly affects the medial femoral condyle; or in the case of certain osteochondroses such as Legg-Calvé-Perthes disease involving the femoral head, or Freiberg disease affecting the head of the second metatarsal.

Diseases or conditions associated with or leading to osteonecrosis are listed in Table 4.3.

After trauma, osteonecrosis occurs most commonly in the femoral head, the carpal scaphoid, and the humeral head because of the precarious supply of blood to these bones.

Osteonecrosis of the femoral head is a frequent complication after intracapsular fracture of the femoral neck (60% to 75%), dislocation in the hip joint (25%), and slipped capital femoral epiphysis (15% to 40%). In its very early stages, radiographs may appear completely normal; however, radionuclide bone scan may show first decreased and later increased isotope uptake at the site of the lesion, which is a very valuable indication of abnormality. The earliest radiographic sign of this complication is the presence of a radiolucent crescent, which may be seen as early as 4 weeks after the initial injury. This phenomenon, as Norman and Bullough have pointed out, is secondary to the subchondral structural collapse of the necrotic segment and is visible as a narrow radiolucent line parallel to the articular surface of the bone. Radiographically, the sign is most easily demonstrated on the frog-lateral view of the hip (Fig. 4.58), but tomography provides the best modality for imaging the features of the complication itself (Fig. 4.59). Because the necrotic process most of the time does not affect the articular cartilage, the width of the joint space (that is, the radiographic joint space: the width of the articular cartilage of adjoining bones plus the actual joint cavity) is preserved. Preservation of the joint space helps to differentiate this condition from osteoarthritis. In its later stage, osteonecrosis can be readily identified on the anteroposterior view of the hip by a flattening of the articular surface and the dense appearance of the femoral head (Fig. 4.60). The density is secondary to compression of bony trabeculae after microfracture of the nonviable bone, calcification of detritic marrow, and repair of the necrotic area by deposition of new bone, the so-called creeping substitution. Tomographic or CT examination frequently helps to delineate the details of this condition. Ficat and Arlet proposed a classification system of osteonecrosis of the femoral head consisting of four stages, based on radiographic, hemodynamic, and symptomatic criteria (Table 4.4).

A significant breakthrough in identifying osteonecrosis in patients who had normal bone scan results and conventional radiograph results was achieved with MRI. Currently, this modality is considered the most sensitive and specific for the diagnosis and evaluation of osteonecrosis. Its characteristic MRI appearance consists of a circumscribed ovoid area (Fig. 4.61A) or crescent-shaped rim (Fig. 4.61B) of low signal in a subchondral location. This rim corresponds to the interface of repair between ischemic and normal bone consisting mainly

Table 4.3 Diseases or Conditions Associated With or Leading to Osteonecrosis

Trauma
  Fracture of femoral neck
  Dislocation of the femoral head
  Proximal femoral epiphysiolysis
  Slipped capital femoral epiphysis
  Epiphyseal compression
  Fracture of talus
  Fracture of scaphoid
  Kienböck disease
  Vascular injury
  Burns
  Radiation exposure
Hemoglobinopathies
  Sickle cell disease
  Hb S/C hemoglobinopathy
  Hb S/thalassemia
  Polycythemia
Congenital and Developmental Conditions
  Congenital dysplasia of the hip (CDH)
  Ehlers-Danlos syndrome
  Hereditary dysostosis
  Legg-Calvé-Perthes disease
  Fabry disease
Local Infiltrative Lesions
  Gaucher disease
  Neoplastic conditions
  Lymphoproliferative disorders
Metabolic Conditions
  Hypercortisolism
    Corticosteroid medications
    Cushing disease
  Gout and hyperuricemia
  Hyperlipidemia
  Hyperparathyroidism
Dysbaric Disorders
  Caisson disease
Infectious and Inflammatory Conditions
  Osteomyelitis
  Pancreatitis
  Giant cell arteritis
  Systemic lupus erythematosus (SLE)
  Thrombophlebitis
  Acquired immunodeficiency syndrome
  Meningococcemia
Miscellaneous Factors
  Alcohol consumption
  Cigarette smoking
  Chronic renal failure
  Hemodialysis
  Intravascular coagulation
  Organ transplantation
  Pregnancy
  Idiopathic osteonecrosis

of sclerosis and fibrosis. On T2-weighted images, a second inner rim of high signal has been observed (the double line sign) (Fig. 4.61C). It is believed that this appearance represents fibrovascular tissue in the reparative zone. Many authors hypothesize that this finding is pathognomonic for osteonecrosis. Other authors have played-down the importance of this finding, claiming that it may be largely artifactual, representing so-called chemical shift.

Several reports have established the diagnostic sensitivity of MRI in the early stages of osteonecrosis, when radiographic changes are not yet apparent or are nonspecific. MRI has been shown to have 97% sensitivity in differentiating osteonecrotic from normal femoral head and 85% sensitivity in differentiating osteonecrotic femoral head from other disorders of the femoral head, with an overall sensitivity of 91%. MRI appears to be a better predictive test for subsequent

Figure 4.58 Osteonecrosis of the femoral head. The frog-lateral view of the left hip shows the crescent sign (*arrow*) in a 45-year-old woman who sustained hip dislocation 5 weeks earlier.

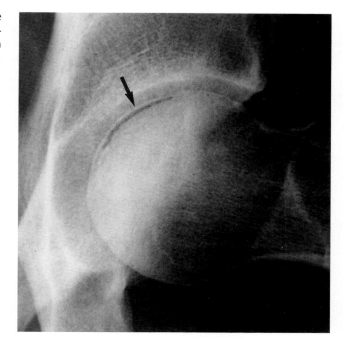

Figure 4.59 Osteonecrosis of the femoral head. (A) A 41-year-old man presented with a history of traumatic dislocation in the left hip joint. On frontal projection, the increased density of the femoral head suggests osteonecrosis, but a definite diagnosis cannot be made. **(B)** The frog-lateral view demonstrates a thin radiolucent line parallel to the articular surface of the femoral head (*arrow*). This represents the crescent sign, a radiographic hallmark of osteonecrosis. **(C)** Tomographic examination confirms the features typical of osteonecrosis: the crescent sign, the dense femoral head, and the preservation of the radiographic joint space indicating intact articular cartilage.

Figure 4.60 Osteonecrosis of the femoral head. A 56-year-old woman sustained an intracapsular fracture of the left femoral neck, which healed after surgical treatment by open reduction and internal fixation. The anteroposterior view shows a Smith-Peterson nail inserted into the femoral neck and head. The fracture line is obliterated. The dense (sclerotic) appearance of the femoral head indicates the development of osteonecrosis.

hemorrhage. If there is enough inflammation, hyperemia, and fibrosis present to replace the fat content of the femoral head (class C or fluid-like), a low-intensity signal with short TR/TE and high-intensity signal with long TR/TE is seen. Finally, in advanced stages, where fibrosis and sclerosis predominate (class D or fibrous-like), low signal intensity is present on both short and long TR/TE images (Table 4.5 and Figs. 4.62 to 4.65). MRI findings correlate well with histologic changes. The central region of high signal intensity corresponds to necrosis of bone and marrow. The low signal of the peripheral band corresponds to the sclerotic margin of reactive tissue at the interface between necrotic and viable bone. As Seiler and coworkers have pointed out, MRI evaluation of osteonecrosis of the femoral head has several advantages: It is noninvasive, does not require ionizing radiation, provides multiplanar images, reflects physiologic changes in the bone marrow, provides excellent resolution of surrounding soft tissues, and makes it possible to evaluate the contralateral femoral head simultaneously.

Osteonecrosis of the carpal scaphoid is a complication commonly seen in 10% to 15% of cases of carpal scaphoid fracture, increasing in incidence to 30% to 40% if there is nonunion. Necrosis generally involves the proximal bone fragment but the distal fragment, although rarely, may also be affected. Evidence of this complication most frequently becomes apparent approximately 4 to 6 months after injury, when radiographic examination shows increased bone density. Although it is most often diagnosed on conventional radiographs, tomographic study (Fig. 4.66), CT (Fig. 4.67), or MRI are indicated when radiographic findings are equivocal.

Only exceptionally scaphoid bone may become osteonecrotic in the absence of fracture. This abnormality is known as Preiser disease.

Osteonecrosis may also develop in the humeral head after a fracture of the humeral neck (Fig. 4.68), but this complication is infrequently seen.

Injury to Major Blood Vessels. A relatively infrequent complication of a fracture or dislocation, injury to the major blood vessels occurs when bone fragments lacerate or completely transect an artery (see Figs. 2.3, 4.13) or a vein, resulting in bleeding, the formation of hematoma, arteriovenous fistula, or a pseudoaneurysm (Fig. 4.69). To demonstrate this abnormality, angiography is the procedure of choice (see Fig. 2.3). This technique is invaluable in visualizing the site of laceration, ascertaining the exact extent of vascular damage, and assessing the status of collateral circulation. It may also be combined with an interventional procedure, such as embolization to control hemorrhage.

Growth Disturbance. A common complication of Salter-Harris type IV and V fractures involving the physis, growth disturbance may result from injury to the growth plate by the formation of an osseous bridge between the epiphysis and metaphysis. As a result of this tethering of the growth plate, localized cessation of bone growth occurs. If the entire physis in a single long bone stops growing, a limb-length

femoral head collapse than radionuclide bone scan. The narrow band-like area of low signal intensity that traverses the femoral head in midcoronal sections present on MRI was a significant indicator of subsequent collapses.

MRI is indispensable in the accurate staging of osteonecrosis, because it reflects the size of the lesion and roughly the stage of the disease. Mitchell and colleagues have described a classification system of osteonecrosis based on alterations in the central region of MR signal intensity in the osteonecrotic focus (Table 4.5). In early stages (class A or fat-like), there is preservation of a normal fat signal, except at the sclerotic reactive margin surrounding the lesion, that manifests as a central region of high signal intensity on short spin-echo (SE) TR/TE images (T1-weighted), and intermediate signal intensity on long TR/TE images (T2-weighted). Later, when there is sufficient inflammation or vascular engorgement, or if subacute hemorrhage is present (class B or blood-like), a high signal intensity is noted on short and long TR/TE images. This signal is similar to that of a subacute

Table 4.4 Osteonecrosis of Femoral Head: Correlation of Clinical Symptoms and Radiologic Findings with Histopathologic Changes Based on Ficat and Arlet classification

Stage	Clinical Symptoms	Radiographic Findings	Scintigraphy	Pathologic Changes	Biopsy
1	None	Normal	Normal	Infarction of weight bearing segments	Necrotic marrow, osteoblasts
2	Mild pain	Increased density of femoral head, normal joint space	Increased uptake	Spontaneous repair	New bone deposition
3	Mild-to-moderate pain	Loss of sphericity and collapse of the femoral head, crescent sign	Increased uptake	Subchondral fracture with collapse, impaction, and fragmentation of the necrotic segment	Dead bone trabeculae and dead marrow cells on both sides of fracture line
4	Moderate pain, assistive devices needed	Joint space narrowing, acetabular changes	Increased uptake	Osteoarthritis	Degenerative changes in articular cartilage

Modified from Chang CC, Greenspan A, Gershwin ME, 1993, with permission.

Figure 4.61 Osteonecrosis of the femoral head demonstrated by MRI.
(A) Coronal T1-weighted (SE; TR 650/TE 25 msec) image shows ovoid area of decreased signal in subchondral location.
(B) Coronal T1-weighted (SE; TR 500/TE 25 msec) image shows a crescent-shaped rim of decreased signal at the weight-bearing segment of the femoral head.
(C) Coronal T1-weighted (SE; TR 650/TE 25 msec) image shows osteonecrotic segment separated from normal bone by low-intensity serpentine border (*arrows*).
(D) Coronal T2-weighted gradient-echo (multiplanar gradient-recalled, TR 500/TE 15 msec, flip angle 15 degrees) image shows the characteristic for osteonecrosis "double-line" sign. Note also high signal of joint fluid.

Table 4.5 Correlation of Magnetic Resonance Imaging Findings with Histologic Changes

Class	MRI Findings	Appearance	Histology
A	Normal fat signal except at the sclerotic margin surrounding the lesion	Fat-like	Premature conversion to fatty marrow within the femoral neck or intertrochanteric region
B	High signal intensity of inner border and low signal intensity of surrounding rim	Blood-like	Bone resorption and replacement by vascular granulation tissue
C	Diffusely decreased signal on T1 and high signal on T2 weighting	Fluid-like	Bone marrow edema
D	Decreased signal on T1- and T2-weighted images	Fibrous	Sclerosis from reinforcement of existing trabeculae at the margin of live bone (i.e., repair tissue interface)

Modified from Chang CC, Greenspan A, Gershwin ME, 1993, with permission.

Figure 4.62 MRI staging of osteonecrosis (class A). (A) Coronal T1-weighted (SE; TR 600/TE 20 msec) image shows preservation of a normal bright signal of fat within the lesion, surrounded by a low-signal-intensity reactive margin in both femoral heads. **(B)** Axial T2-weighted (fast SE; TR 3500/TE 17 msec/Ef) image shows intermediate signal within an osteonecrotic segment, analogous to fat.

Figure 4.63 MRI staging of osteonecrosis (class B). Coronal **(A)** and axial **(B)** T1-weighted (SE; TR 600/TE 20 msec) images show high signal intensity of osteonecrotic segment surrounded by sclerotic margin. **(C)** Coronal T2*-weighted gradient-echo (multiplanar gradient-recalled, TR 500/TE 15 msec, flip angle 15 degrees) image shows high signal in the central portion of the femoral heads.

Figure 4.64 **MRI staging of osteonecrosis (class C). (A)** Axial T1-weighted (SE; TR 600/TE 20 msec) image shows areas of low signal intensity in both femoral heads. **(B)** Coronal T2-weighted (SE; TR 2000/TE 80 msec) image shows a high-signal-intensity area (more pronounced in the left femoral head) surrounded by low-signal margin.

Figure 4.65 **MRI staging of osteonecrosis (class D). (A)** Axial T1-weighted (SE; TR 600/TE 20 msec) and **(B)** coronal T2-weighted (fast SE; TR 3000/TE 136 msec/Ef) images demonstrate sclerotic lesion of late-stage osteonecrosis of the left femoral head that shows low signal intensity on both sequences.

Figure 4.66 **Osteonecrosis of the scaphoid. (A)** Radiograph of the wrist demonstrates a fracture of the carpal scaphoid; however, it is unclear whether the fracture is complicated by osteonecrosis. **(B)** Trispiral tomogram clearly shows nonunion and the presence of osteonecrosis of the distal fragment, together with cystic degeneration. Note also the posttraumatic cyst in the trapezoid bone. The dense spot in the articular end of the ulna represents a bone island. **(C)** In another patient trispiral tomogram shows ununited fracture of the scaphoid and osteonecrosis of the proximal fragment.

Figure 4.67 CT of scaphoid osteonecrosis. A 52-year-old woman sustained a fracture of the scaphoid bone, treated conservatively in a cast. **(A)** Conventional radiograph shows sclerotic changes in the scaphoid, which may be due to healing process or osteonecrosis. **(B)** Coronal reformatted CT shows incompletely healed fracture of the scaphoid complicated by osteonecrosis.

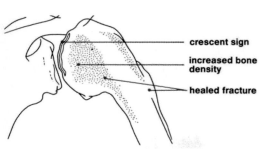

Figure 4.68 Osteonecrosis of the humeral head. Six months after sustaining a fracture of the left humeral neck that united, a 62-year-old man had osteonecrosis of the humeral head, evident on the radiograph from the increased bone density and the collapse of the subchondral segment.

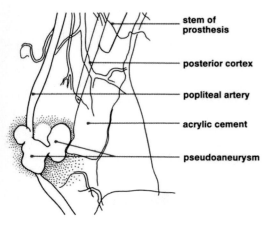

Figure 4.69 Pseudoaneurysm of the popliteal artery. A 30-year-old woman with Gaucher disease and a total hip replacement as a result of osteonecrosis of the femoral head sustained a transverse fracture of the left femoral shaft through the acrylic cement just distal to the stem of the prosthesis. A femoral arteriogram revealed a pseudoaneurysm of the popliteal artery resulting from injury to the vessel by the fractured bone fragment and the acrylic cement. (From Baker ND, 1981, with permission.)

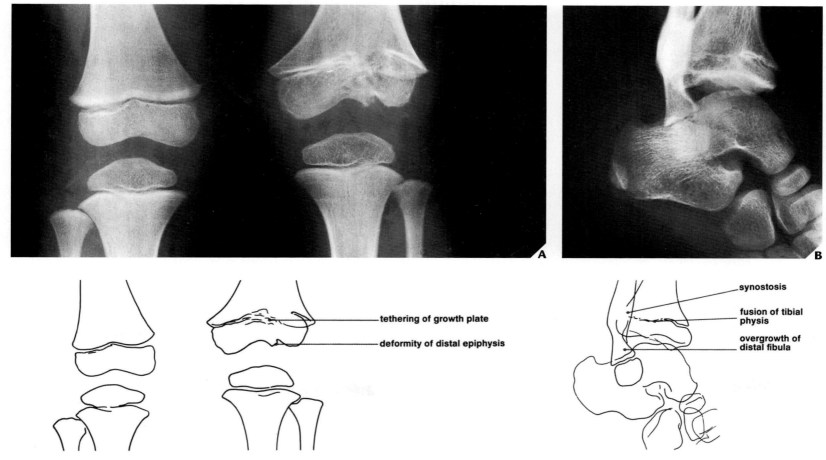

Figure 4.70 Growth disturbance. (A). A 3-year-old boy sustained a fracture of the left distal femur that extended through the growth plate. As a result, the bone at this end prematurely ceased to grow. Anteroposterior radiograph of both knees shows a discrepancy in the length of the femora associated with deformity of the distal epiphysis of the left femur secondary to tethering of the growth plate. **(B)** A 5-year-old girl sustained a Salter-Harris type V fracture of the distal tibia. On the lateral view, a joint deformity is evident as a result of the fusion of the physis of the tibia and overgrowth of the distal fibula. Note also the posttraumatic synostosis of these two bones.

discrepancy will result (Fig. 4.70A). If only one growth plate at the articulations of parallel bones (the radius and ulna or the tibia and fibula) is damaged and ceases to grow, the uninjured bone continues to grow at the normal rate, leading to overgrowth and consequent joint deformity (Fig. 4.70B).

Posttraumatic Arthritis. If a fracture line extends into the joint, the articular surface may become irregular. Such incongruity in the articular surfaces results in abnormal stresses that lead to precocious degenerative changes recognized on the radiograph by narrowing of the joint space, subchondral sclerosis, and formation of marginal osteophytes (Fig. 4.71). A similar complication may also be seen after a dislocation (Fig. 4.72).

Figure 4.71 Posttraumatic osteoarthritis. Dorsovolar **(A)** and lateral **(B)** views of the wrist of a 57-year-old man who had sustained an intraarticular fracture of the distal radius demonstrate residual deformity of this bone and narrowing of the radiocarpal articulation. Trispiral tomogram **(C)** shows, in addition, the multiple subchondral degenerative cysts often seen in posttraumatic arthritis.

Figure 4.72 Posttraumatic osteoarthritis. The anteroposterior radiograph of the right shoulder of a 78-year-old man who presented with a history of several previous dislocations in that joint demonstrates the advanced osteoarthritis resulting from repeated trauma to the articular surfaces of the humeral head and glenoid.

Stress Fractures

Bone is a dynamic tissue that requires stress for normal development. *Stress* is the force or absolute load applied to a bone that may arise from weight-bearing or muscular actions. The force may be of an axial, bending, or torsional nature, and the resulting change in shape of the bone is referred to as *strain. Tensile* forces are produced along the convex side of a bone, while *compressive* forces occur along its concave margin. According to Wolff's law, intermittent forces applied to bone stimulate remodeling of its architecture to withstand the new mechanical environment optimally. Stresses related to daily activities stimulate the remodeling process that, in cortical bone, occurs at the level of the osteon, the basic unit of bone structure. The exact mechanism that activates this process is not known, but some evidence suggests that it may be related to the development of microfractures (Fig. 4.73A). Osteoclastic resorption leading to formation of small resorption areas at the site of microfractures is the initial response to increased stresses; peak bone loss occurs after approximately 3 weeks. These resorption cavities are subsequently filled with lamellar bone, but if bone formation is slow, then the consequent imbalance between bone resorption and bone formation results in weakening of the bone. Periosteal proliferation, endosteal proliferation, or both may produce new bone at the sites of stress in an apparent attempt to buttress the temporarily weakened cortex. Stresses in cancellous bone may result in partial or complete trabecular microfractures (Fig. 4.73B). Microcallus is produced along the complete fractures, and these thickened trabeculae probably account for the sclerosis seen on radiographs when stress injuries occur in cancellous bone. Although microdamage is a physiologic phenomenon, it becomes pathologic when its production greatly exceeds repair. If the inciting activity is not curtailed, repair mechanisms are overwhelmed, which results in accumulation of microdamage and subsequent fatigue fracture of trabecular or cortical bone (see Figs. 4.27 and 4.32B).

Diagnostic imaging has acquired a pivotal role in the assessment of stress injuries to bone because clinical evaluation alone is not definitive. If classic radiographic findings are present, then the diagnosis is straightforward. However, because the underlying pathophysiology is a continuing process rather than a single event, imaging findings are extremely variable and depend on such factors as the type of inciting activity, the bone involved, and the timing of the imaging procedure.

Conventional radiographs play an important role in the workup of a suspected stress fracture and should be the first imaging study obtained. Unfortunately, initial radiographs are often normal, which is not surprising given the degree of microscopic remodeling that occurs in the early stages of stress injury. The sensitivity of early radiographs can be as low as 15%, and follow-up radiographs will demonstrate diagnostic findings in only 50% of cases. The time that elapses between manifestation of initial symptoms and detection of radiographic findings ranges from 1 week to several months, and cessation of physical activity may prevent the development of any radiographic findings.

Initial changes in the cortical bone include subtle ill definition of the cortex ("gray cortex sign") (Fig. 4.74) or faint intracortical radiolucent striations, which are presumably related to the osteoclastic tunneling found early in the remodeling process. These changes may be easily overlooked until periosteal new bone formation and/or endosteal thickening develops in an apparent attempt to buttress the temporarily weakened cortex. As damage increases, a true fracture line may appear (Fig. 4.75). These injuries typically involve the shaft of a long bone and are common in the anterior or posterior cortex of the tibia and in the medial cortex of femur.

Stress injuries in cancellous bone are notoriously difficult to detect. Subtle blurring of trabecular margins and faint sclerotic radiopaque areas may be seen secondary to peritrabecular callus, but a 50% change in bone opacity is required for these changes to be radiographically detectable (Fig. 4.76). With progression of the pathologic process, a readily apparent sclerotic band is seen (Fig. 4.77).

Radionuclide bone scanning has become the gold standard for evaluating stress fractures owing in large part to its ability to demonstrate subtle changes in bone metabolism long before plain radiography can. The most widely used radiopharmaceuticals for imaging of a stress injury are the ^{99m}Tc phosphate analogs; these are taken-up at sites of bone turnover, probably by means of chemiadsorption to the surface of the bone. The degree of uptake depends primarily on the rate of bone turnover and local blood flow, and abnormal uptake may be seen within 6 to 72 hours of injury. The sensitivity of scintigraphy approaches 100%, because only a few false-negative scans have been reported. The classic scintigraphic findings of a stress fracture include a focally intense, fusiform area of cortical uptake, or a transverse band of increased activity (Fig. 4.78). However, the spectrum of findings associated with bone stress is broad, which again reflects the underlying pathophysiologic continuum. Despite its high sensitivity, the specificity of scintigraphy is slightly lower than that of radiography because other conditions such as tumors, infection, bone infarction, and shin splints or periostitis can produce a positive scan. In these instances augmentation of scintigraphy with CT or MRI can be helpful in further diagnostic workup.

CT has a limited role in the diagnosis of stress injuries. It is less sensitive than scintigraphy and radiography in the diagnosis of stress fractures but can be quite useful for better defining an abnormality discovered with another modality (Fig. 4.79). It is well-suited to delineate a fracture line in a location not well-demonstrated on conventional radiography. Longitudinal stress fractures of the tibia occur less frequently than the more typical transverse or oblique varieties, but these may account for up to 10% of tibial stress fractures. These are especially difficult to detect with radiography because of their vertical orientation, and CT has played an important role in diagnosis.

MRI is extremely sensitive in the detection of pathophysiologic changes associated with stress injuries, and it is even more specific than radionuclide scanning. Typical findings in early stress reactions include areas of low signal intensity in the marrow on T1-weighted images that increase in signal intensity with T2 weighting. Fat saturation techniques, such as inversion-recovery (IR) or fast spin-echo (FSE) T2-weighted imaging with frequency-selective fat saturation, are especially useful for identifying these injuries. The increased water content of the associated medullary edema or hemorrhage results in high sig-

PATHOMECHANISM OF STRESS FRACTURE

A. Cortex

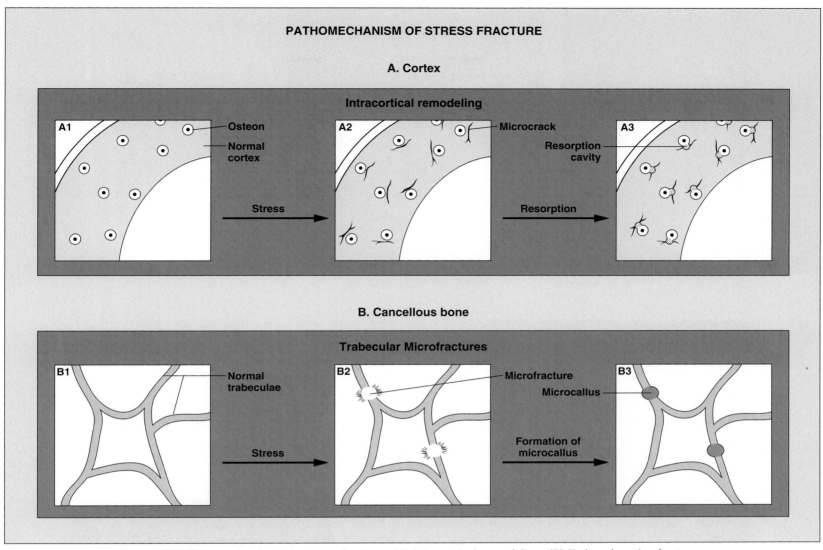

Figure 4.73 Patomechanism of a stress fracture. (A) Intracortical remodeling. **(B)** Trabecular microfractures.

Figure 4.74 Stress fracture. The earliest radiographic changes of stress fracture include "gray cortex" sign consisting of a subtle ill-defined cortical margin *(arrow)*. Compare with a normal definition of the contralateral cortex.

Figure 4.75 Stress fracture. With progression of the pathologic process a cortical fracture becomes visible **(A)**. This finding may be enhanced with a trispiral tomography **(B)**.

Figure 4.76 Stress fracture. The earliest radiographic changes of stress fracture in cancellous bone include subtle blurring of the trabecular margins associated with faint sclerotic areas *(arrow)*.

Figure 4.77 Stress fracture. Typical appearance of a stress fracture in the calcaneus: a vertical band of sclerosis in the posterior aspect of the bone is characteristic of this injury.

Figure 4.78 Scintigraphic presentation of a stress fracture. (A) Fusiform area of increased uptake in medial cortex of the left femur. **(B)** Transverse band of increased uptake in the proximal diaphysis of the left tibia.

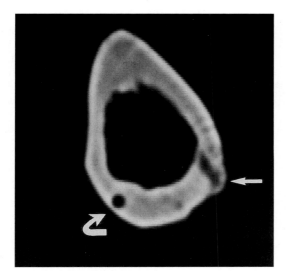

Figure 4.79 CT of the stress fracture. Stress fracture in the tibia *(arrow)* demonstrated by computed tomography. The *curved arrow* points to the nutrient foramen.

nal intensity against the dark background of suppressed fat such that these sequences should maximize sensitivity. On T2-weighted images of more advanced lesions, low intensity bands, contiguous with the cortex, have been seen within the marrow edema; these presumably represent fracture lines (Fig. 4.80). The multiplanar capability of MR provides a further advantage by allowing for optimal demonstration of the fracture line. In some cases, increased signal intensity has also been observed in a juxtacortical and subperiosteal locations. MRI has been advocated as a problem-solving modality, such as in a patient with negative or confusing bone scan. It may secure the diagnosis if the fracture line is identified.

Injury to Soft Tissues

Under normal physiologic circumstances, soft tissues such as muscles, tendons, ligaments, articular menisci, and intervertebral disks are only faintly outlined or not visible at all on conventional radiographs. As a result, only rarely, as in such traumatic conditions as myositis ossificans (see previous discussion) or certain tears of ligaments and tendons, does conventional radiography suffice to demonstrate trauma to the soft tissues (Fig. 4.81). Adequate evaluation of injury to these structures and of the progress of treatment, consequently, re-

Figure 4.81 Soft tissue injury. (A) A common complication of trauma to the muscular structures, myositis ossificans is characterized by the formation of bone in the injured muscle. This condition is apparent on conventional radiography. *(continued)*

quires supplemental studies, which may include stress radiography, arthrography, tenography, bursography, myelography, CT, and MRI.

MRI, in particular, is considered to be the best imaging modality for evaluating traumatic soft-tissue injuries. Differences in signal intensity enable abnormalities of the various structures (muscles, ten-

Figure 4.80 MRI of the stress fracture. (A) Sagittal T1-weighted image shows a diffusely decreased signal in the lateral cuneiform *(arrows)* and a band of signal void in the center of the bone *(curved arrow)*. **(B)** Sagittal fast spin-echo inversion recovery MR image shows increased signal in the cuneiform bone *(arrows)* representing changes due to edema and hemorrhage. The stress fracture remains of low signal intensity *(curved arrow)*.

Figure 4.81 Soft tissue injury *Continued.* **(B)** Calcification of the medial collateral ligament of the knee, known as Pellegrini-Stieda lesion, represents the sequela of traumatic tear of this ligament. **(C)** In certain instances, the tear of a tendon may be diagnosed on radiography. The lateral radiograph of the ankle shows the typical appearance of a torn Achilles tendon.

Figure 4.82 Tear of the Achilles tendon. Sagittal MRI of the ankle (SE; TR 2000/TE 20 msec) shows discontinuity of the Achilles tendon near its insertion to the calcaneus. An inflammatory mass is seen at the rupture site. (From Beltran J, 1990, with permission.)

Figure 4.83 MRI of soft tissue injury. A 14-year-old boy presented with posterior dislocation of the right femoral head. After dislocation was reduced, MRI was performed to assess the injury to the soft tissues. **(A)** Coronal T2*-weighted (multiplanar gradient-recalled TR 500/TE 15 msec, flip angle 15 degrees) sequence shows markedly increased signal surrounding the vastus lateralis and intermedius muscles *(straight arrows)*. Note also the injury involving the medial fascial compartment and gluteal region muscles *(curved arrow)*. **(B)** More posterior coronal section demonstrates increased signal in the gluteus medius and minimus muscles *(straight white arrows)* and the tensor fasciae latae *(curved arrow)*. There is also injury of the obturator internus, obturator externus, and adductor brevis and magnus muscles *(open arrows)*. (From Laorr A, et al., 1995, with permission.)

dons, ligaments, fascias, vessels, and nerves) to be effectively demonstrated. Posttraumatic tenosynovitis, joint effusion, and soft-tissue hematomas are also seen well on MR images. Tears of various ligaments and tendons can be accurately diagnosed; for instance, when evaluating tendon injuries, MRI provides information regarding the location of the tear (whether it is within the tendon, at the tendon insertion, or at the musculotendinous interface), the size of the gap between both tendon ends, the size of the hematoma at the rupture site, and the presence of any inflammatory component (Fig. 4.82).

MRI is invaluable in identifying various injuries to the muscles that may occur during traumatic hip dislocation (Figs. 4.83, 4.84).

Normal skeletal muscle exhibits an intermediate or slightly prolonged T1 relaxation time and a short T2 relaxation time relative to other soft tissues. When muscles are injured, MRI can effectively delineate the variable degrees of strain, contusion, tear, or hematoma, and permits quantification of these injuries. Acute muscle strain gives rise to increased T2 signal intensity, reflecting tissue edema. When an acute muscle tear occurs, muscle shape and architecture appear altered, and signal within the muscle shows an abnormal increase because of intramuscular hemorrhage and edema.

PRACTICAL POINTS TO REMEMBER

[1] When dealing with suspected fractures and dislocations, obtain radiographs in at least two projections at 90 degrees to each other.
[2] To eliminate the risk of missing an associated injury, include the adjacent joints on the film.
[3] When a fracture is suspected, look for associated abnormalities such as:
  • soft-tissue swelling
  • obliteration or displacement of fat stripes
  • periosteal and endosteal reaction
  • joint effusion
  • intracapsular fat-fluid level
  • double cortical line
  • buckling of the cortex
  • irregular metaphyseal corners.
[4] When reporting a fracture, describe:
  • the site and extent
  • the type
  • the direction of the fracture line
  • the alignment of the fragments
  • the presence of impaction, depression, or compression
  • the presence of associated abnormalities
  • whether the fracture is a special type
  • whether the growth plate is involved (in which case the Salter-Harris classification, together with Rang and Ogden additions, provides a useful method of precise evaluation of the injury).

Figure 4.84 MRI of soft tissue injury. In another patient, a 20-year-old man who sustained posterior dislocation in the left hip, a coronal T2*-weighted (multiplanar gradient-recalled; TR 550/TE 15 msec, flip angle 15 degrees) MRI shows disruption and increased signal in the region of the superior and inferior gemelli muscles *(arrows)*. There is also injury to the gluteal muscles *(open arrows)*. (From Laorr A, et al., 1995, with permission.)

[5] When a fracture fails to heal, distinguish between the three types of nonunion:
- reactive (hypertrophic and oligotrophic)
- nonreactive (atrophic)
- infected.

[6] In patients presenting with a history of skeletal trauma, be aware of such possible complications as:
- disuse osteoporosis (mild or moderate)
- reflex sympathetic dystrophy syndrome (RSDS, Sudeck atrophy)
- Volkmann ischemic contracture
- posttraumatic myositis ossificans (the hallmarks of which are the clearly defined pattern of its evolution, the radiographic presence of the zonal phenomenon, and a radiolucent cleft)
- osteonecrosis (the earliest signs may be demonstrated by MRI or later may manifest as an increased uptake of a tracer on scintigraphy; the radiographic hallmark is the radiolucent crescent sign)
- injury to vessels (best demonstrated by digital subtraction angiography)
- growth disturbance
- posttraumatic arthritis.

[7] Regarding juxtacortical myositis ossificans, remember that its MRI appearance depends on the stage of maturation of the lesion:
- in the early stage, T1-weighted images will show a mass of intermediate signal intensity, whereas on T2-weighted images the lesion will be of high signal intensity
- in the mature stage, T1- and T2-weighted images will demonstrate a peripheral rim of low signal intensity corresponding to bone maturation
- the fatty component of the lesion will image as high signal intensity on T1 weighting and as intermediate signal on T2 weighting.

[8] Osteonecrosis can be best staged with MRI. Four classes of osteonecrosis (fat-like; blood-like; fluid-like; and fibrous) correlate well with histopathologic changes in the bone.

[9] Stress fractures should be viewed as the endpoint of a spectrum along which a bone responds to a changing mechanical environment, ranging from excessive remodeling to a frank fracture. In imaging these injuries be aware that:
- initial radiographs are often normal
- the first radiographic abnormality to look for is a subtle poor definition of the cortex ("gray cortex sign")
- radionuclide bone scan is highly sensitive and frequently shows a characteristic fusiform area or transverse band of increased activity
- MRI may show a typical finding of an area of low signal intensity in the bone marrow on T1 weighting that becomes of high signal on T2-weighted images, frequently showing a central low-signal band presumably representing the fracture line.

[10] When dealing with injury to soft tissues, consider using supplemental imaging modalities, including:
- stress radiography
- arthrography
- tenography and bursography
- computed tomography
- magnetic resonance imaging

[11] MRI is an invaluable technique for identifying various injuries to the muscles, tendons, and ligaments. This modality can effectively delineate the variable degrees of strain, contusion, tear, or hematoma, and permits quantification of these injuries.

SUGGESTED READINGS

Adelberg JS, Smith GH. Corticosteroid-induced avascular necrosis of the talus. *J Foot Surg* 1991;30:66–69.

Allard JC, Porter G, Ryerson RW. Occult posttraumatic avascular necrosis of hip revealed by MRI. *Magn Reson Imaging* 1992;10:155–159.

Anderson MW, Greenspan A. State of the art: stress fractures. *Radiology* 1996;199:1–12.

Arger PH, Oberkircher PE, Miller WT. Lipohemarthrosis. *AJR Am J Roentgenol* 1974;121:97–100.

Arndt WF III, Truax AL, Barnett FM, Simmons GE, Brown DC. MR diagnosis of bone contusions of the knee: comparison of coronal T2-weighted fast spin-echo with fat saturation and fast spin-echo STIR images with conventional STIR images. *AJR Am J Roentgenol* 1996;166:119–124.

Assouline-Dayan Y, Chang C, Greenspan A, Shoenfeld Y, Gershwin ME. Pathogenesis and natural history of osteonecrosis. *Semin Arthritis Rheum* 2002;32:94–124.

Athanasian G, Wickiewicz T. Osteonecrosis of the femoral condyle after arthroscopic reconstruction of a cruciate ligament. *J Bone Joint Surg [Am]* 1995;77A:1418–1421.

Baker ND. Pseudoaneurysm—a complication of fracture through cement after total hip replacement. *Orthop Rev* 1981;10:110–111.

Bassett LW, Grover JS, Seeger LL. Magnetic resonance imaging of knee trauma. *Skeletal Radiol* 1990;19:401–405.

Beltran J. *MRI: musculoskeletal system.* Philadelphia: JB Lippincott; 1990.

Beltran J, Burk JM, Herman LJ, Clark RN, Zuelzer WA, Freddy MR, Simon S. Avascular necrosis of the femoral head: early MRI detection and radiological correlation. *Magn Reson Imaging* 1987;5:531–542.

Beltran J, Herman LJ, Burk JM, et al. Femoral head avascular necrosis: MR imaging with clinical-pathologic and radionuclide correlation. *Radiology* 1988;166:215–220.

Blum GM, Crues JV, Sheehan W. MR of occult bony trauma: the missing link. *Appl Radiol* 1993;22:15–21.

Bohrer SP. The fat pad sign following elbow trauma. Its usefulness and reliability in suspecting "invisible" fractures. *Clin Radiol* 1970;21:90–94.

Borden S. Traumatic bowing of the forearm in children. *J Bone Joint Surg [Am]* 1974;56A:611–616.

Caffey J. *Pediatric x-ray diagnosis*, vol. 2, 2nd ed. Chicago: Year Book Medical Publishers; 1973.

Chadwick DJ, Bentley G. The classification and prognosis of epiphyseal injuries. *Injury* 1987;18:157–168.

Chan WP, Liu Y-J, Huang G-S, Jiang C-C, Huang S, Chang Y-C. MRI of joint fluid in femoral head osteonecrosis. *Skeletal Radiol* 2002;31:624–630.

Chang CC, Greenspan A, Gershwin ME. Osteonecrosis: current perspectives on pathogenesis and treatment. *Semin Arthritis Rheum* 1993;23:47–69.

Coleman BG, Kressel HY, Dalinka MK, Schiebler ML, Burk DL, Cohen EK. Radiographically negative avascular necrosis: detection with MR imaging. *Radiology* 1988;168:525–528.

Colwell CW, Robinson C. Osteonecrosis of the femoral head in patients with inflammatory arthritis on asthma receiving corticosteroid therapy. *Orthopedics* 1996;19:941–946.

Cushner FO, Friedman RJ. Osteonecrosis of the femoral head. *Orthop Rev* 1988;17:29–34.

Daffner RH, Pavlov H. Stress fractures: current concepts. *AJR Am J Roentgenol* 1992;159:245–252.

Davidson JK. Dysbaric disorders. Aseptic bone necrosis in tunnel workers and divers. *Clin Rheumatol* 1989;3:1–23.

Davidson JK, Briggs JD. Osteonecrosis and fracture following renal transplantation. *Clin Radiol* 1985;36:27–35.

DeSmet AA. Magnetic resonance findings in skeletal muscle tears. *Skeletal Radiol* 1993;22:479–484.

DeSmet AA, Fisher DR, Heiner JP, Keene JS. Magnetic resonance imaging of muscle tears. *Skeletal Radiol* 1990;19:283–286.

DeSmet AA, Norris MA, Fisher DR. Magnetic resonance imaging of myositis ossificans: analysis of seven cases. *Skeletal Radiol* 1992;21:503–507.

Deutsch AL, Mink JH. Magnetic resonance imaging of musculoskeletal injuries. *Radiol Clin North Am* 1989;27:983–1002.

Deutsch AL, Mink JH, Waxman AD. Occult fractures of the proximal femur: MR imaging. *Radiology* 1989;170:113–116.

Drery P, Sartoris DJ. Osteonecrosis in the foot. *J Foot Surg* 1991;30:477–483.

Eisenberg RL. *Atlas of signs in radiology.* Philadelphia: JB Lippincott; 1984.

Ferlic OC, Morin P. Idiopathic avascular necrosis of the scaphoid—Preiser's disease? *J Hand Surg* 1989;14:13–16.

Ficat RP. Treatment of avascular necrosis of the femoral head. In: Hungerford DS, ed. *The hip: Proceedings of the eleventh open meeting of The Hip Society.* St. Louis: CV Mosby; 1983:279–295.

Ficat RP. Idiopathic bone necrosis of the femoral head: early diagnosis and treatment. *J Bone Joint Surg [Br]* 1985;67B:3–9.

Ficat RP, Arlet J. Ischemia and necrosis of bone. In: Hungerford DS, ed. *Ischemia and necrosis of bone.* Baltimore: Williams & Wilkins; 1980:196.

Ficat RP, Arlet J. Treatment of bone ischemia and necrosis. In: Hungerford DS, ed. *Ischemia and necrosis of bone.* Baltimore: Williams & Wilkins; 1980:171–182.

Frostick SP, Wallace WP. Osteonecrosis of the humeral head. *Clin Rheumatol* 1989;3:651–657.

Genant HK, Kozin F, Bekerman C, McCarty DJ, Sims J. The reflect sympathetic dystrophy syndrome. *Radiology* 1975;117:21–32.

Haajanen J, Saarinen O, Laasonen L, Kuhlback B, Edgren J, Slatis P. Steroid treatment and aseptic necrosis of the femoral head in renal transplant recipients. *Transplant Proc* 1984;16:1316–1319.

Hendrix RW, Rogers LF. Diagnostic imaging of fracture complications. *Radiol Clin North Am* 1989;27:1023–1033.

Herrmann LG, Reineke HG, Caldwell JA. Post-traumatic painful osteoporosis; a clinical and roentgenological entity. *AJR Am J Roentgenol* 1942;47:353–361.

Holt G, Helms CA, Steinbach L, Neumann C, Munk PL, Genant HK. Magnetic resonance imaging of the shoulder: rationale and current applications. *Skeletal Radiol* 1990;19:5–14.

Hungerford DS, Lennox DW. The importance of increased intraoseous pressure in the development of osteonecrosis of the femoral head: implications for treatment. *Orthop Clin North Am* 1985;16:635–654.

Hungerford DS, Zizic TM. Alcoholism associated ischemic necrosis of the femoral head. *Clin Orthop* 1978;130:144–153.

Iannotti JP. Growth plate physiology and pathology. *Orthop Clin North Am* 1990;21:1–17.

Imhof H, Breitenseher M, Trattnig S, et al. Imaging of avascular necrosis of bone. *Eur Radiol* 1997;7:180–186.

Iwasaki K, Hirano T, Sagara K, Nishimura Y. Idiopathic necrosis of the femoral epiphyseal nucleus in rats. *Clin Orthop* 1992;277:31–40.

Jaramillo D, Hoffer FA, Shapiro F, Rand F. MR imaging of fractures of the growth plate. *AJR Am J Roentgenol* 1990;155:1261–1265.

Jelinek JS, Kransdorf MJ. MR imaging of soft-tissue masses. Mass-like lesions that simulate neoplasms. *Magn Reson Imaging Clin North Am* 1995;3:727–741.

Jergesen HE, Khan AS. The natural history of untreated asymptomatic hips in patients who have nontraumatic osteonecrosis. *J Bone J Surg [Am]* 1997;79A:359–363.

Johnston RM, Jones WW. Fractures through human growth plates. *Orthop Trans* 1980;4:295.

Jones DA. Volkmann's ischemia. *Surg Clin North Am* 1970;50:329–342.

Jones G. Radiological appearance of disuse osteoporosis. *Clin Radiol* 1969;20:345–353.

Jones JP, Engleman GP, Najarian JS. Systemic fat embolism after renal transplantation and treatment with corticosteroids. *N Engl J Med* 1965;273:1453–1458.

Kay NRM, Park WM, Bark MB. The relationship between pregnancy and femoral head necrosis. *Br J Radiol* 1972;45:828–831.

Khanna A, Yoon T, Mont M, Hungerford D, Bluemke D. Femoral head osteonecrosis: detection and grading by using a rapid MR imaging protocol. *Radiology* 2000;217:188–192.

Kleinmann P. *Diagnostic imaging of child abuse*. St. Louis: Mosby; 1998.

Koch E, Hofer HO, Sialer G, Marincek B, von Schulthess GK. Failure of MR imaging to detect reflex sympathetic dystrophy of the extremities. *AJR Am J Roentgenol* 1991;156:113–115.

Koo K-H, Ahn I-O, Kim R, et al. Bone marrow edema and associated pain in early stage osteonecrosis of the femoral head: prospective study with serial MR images. *Radiology* 1999;213:715–722.

Kozin F. Reflex sympathetic dystrophy syndrome: a review. *Clin Exp Rheumatol* 1992;10:401–409.

Kransdorf MJ, Meis JM, Jelinek JS. Myositis ossificans: MR appearance with radiologic-pathologic correlation. *AJR Am J Roentgenol* 1991;157:1243–1248.

Kuhlman JE, Fishman EK, Magid D, Scott WW Jr, Brooker AF, Siegelman SS. Fracture nonunion: CT assessment with multiplanar reconstruction. *Radiology* 1988;167:483–488.

Lafforgue P, Dahan P, Chagnaud C, Acquaviva P-C. Early-stage avascular necrosis of the femoral head: MR imaging for prognosis in 31 cases with at least 2 years of follow-up. *Radiology* 1993;187:199–204.

Lang P, Jergesen HE, Moseley ME, Chafetz NI, Genant HK. Avascular necrosis of the femoral head: high-field-strength MR imaging with histologic correlation. *Radiology* 1988;169:517–524.

Langevitz P, Baskila O. Osteonecrosis in patients receiving dialysis: report of two cases and review of the literature. *J Rheumatol* 1990;17:402–406.

Laorr A, Greenspan A, Anderson MW, Moehring HD, McKinley T. Traumatic hip dislocation: early MRI findings. *Skeletal Radiol* 1995;24:239–245.

Laurin NR, Powe JE, Pavlosky WF, Driedger AA. Multimodality imaging of early heterotopic bone formation. *J Can Assoc Radiol* 1990;41:93–95.

Lonergan GJ, Baker AM, Morey MK, Boos SC. From the archives of the AFIP. Child abuse: radiologic-pathologic correlation. *Radiographics* 2003;33:811–845.

Lotke PA, Geker ML. Osteonecrosis of the knee. *J Bone Joint Surg [Am]* 1988;70A:470–473.

MacEwan DW. Changes due to trauma in the fat plane overlying the pronator quadratus muscle. A radiologic sign. *Radiology* 1964;82:879–886.

Mankin HJ. Nontraumatic necrosis of bone (osteonecrosis). *N Engl J Med* 1992;326:1473–1479.

Marcus NO, Enneking WF. The silent hip in idiopathic aseptic necrosis. *J Bone Joint Surg [Am]* 1973;55A:1351–1366.

Markisz JA, Knowles RJR, Altchek DW, Schneider R, Whalen JP, Cahill PT. Segmental patterns of avascular necrosis of the femoral heads: early detection with MR imaging. *Radiology* 1987;162:717–720.

Martin JS, Marsh JL. Current classification of fractures. Rationale and utility. *Radiol Clin North Am* 1997;35:491–506.

Mazet R Jr, Hohl M. Fractures of the carpal navicular. *J Bone Joint Surg [Am]* 1963;45A:82–112.

McDougall IR, Rieser RP. Scintigraphic techniques in musculoskeletal trauma. *Radiol Clin North Am* 1989;27:1003–1011.

Merten DF, Carpenter BLM. Radiologic imaging of inflicted injury in the child abuse syndrome. *Ped Clin North Am* 1990;37:815–837.

Mink JH, Deutsch AL. Occult cartilage and bone injuries of the knee: detection, classification, and assessment with MR imaging. *Radiology* 1989;170:823–829.

Mirzai R, Chang C, Greenspan A, Gershwin ME. Avascular necrosis. *Comp Ther* 1998;24:251–255.

Mirzai A, Chang CC, Greenspan A, Gershwin ME. The pathogenesis of osteonecrosis and the relationship to corticosteroids. *J Asthma* 1999;36:77–95.

Mitchell DG, Joseph PM, Fallon M, et al. Chemical-shift MR imaging of the femoral head: an in vitro study of normal hips and hips with avascular necrosis. *AJR Am J Roentgenol* 1987;148:1159–1164.

Mitchell DG, Kressel HY, Arger PH, Dalinka M, Spritzer CE, Steinberg ME. Avascular necrosis of the femoral head: morphologic assessment by MR imaging, with CT correlation. *Radiology* 1986;161:739–742.

Mitchell DG, Kundel JL, Steinberg MF. Avascular necrosis of the hip: comparison of MR, CT and scintigraphy. *AJR Am J Roentgenol* 1986;147:67–71.

Mitchell DG, Rao VM, Dalinka MK, et al. Femoral head avascular necrosis: correlation of MR imaging, radiographic staging, radionuclide imaging, and clinical findings. *Radiology* 1987;162:709–715.

Moran MC. Osteonecrosis of the hip in sickle cell hemoglobinopathy. *Am J Orthop* 1995;24:18–24.

Müller ME, Allgower M, Schneider R, Willenegger H. *Manual of internal fixation, techniques recommended by the AO Group,* 2nd ed. Berlin: Springer-Verlag; 1979.

Naimark A, Miller K, Segal D, Kossoff J. Nonunion. *Skeletal Radiol* 1981;6:21–25.

Nelson SW. Some important diagnostic and technical fundamentals in the radiology of trauma, with particular emphasis on skeletal trauma. *Radiol Clin North Am* 1966;4:241–259.

Norell H-G. Roentgenologic visualization of the extracapsular fat. Its importance in the diagnosis of traumatic injuries to the elbow. *Acta Radiol* 1954;42:205–210.

Norman A, Bullough P. The radiolucent crescent line—an early diagnostic sign of avascular necrosis of the femoral head. *Bull Hosp J Dis* 1963;24:99–104.

Norman A, Dorfman HD. Juxtacortical circumscribed myositis ossificans: evolution and radiographic features. *Radiology* 1970;96:301–306.

Nuovo MA, Norman A, Chumas J, Ackerman LV. Myositis ossificans with atypical clinical, radiographic, or pathologic findings: a review of 23 cases. *Skeletal Radiol* 1992;21:87–101.

Ogden JA. Skeletal growth mechanism injury patterns. *J Pediatr Orthop* 1982;2:371–377.

Ogden JA. Injury to the growth mechanisms of the immature skeleton. *Skeletal Radiol* 1981;6:237–247.

Ohzono K, Saito M. The fate of nontraumatic avascular necrosis of the femoral head: a radiologic classification to formulate prognosis. *Clin Orthop* 1992;277:73–78.

Ono K, Tohjima T. Risk factors of avascular necrosis of the femoral head in patients with systemic lupus erythematosus under high-dose corticosteroid therapy. *Clin Orthop* 1992;277:89–97.

Pappas JN. The musculoskeletal crescent sign. *Radiology* 2000;217:213–214.

Patton RW, Evans DIK. Silent avascular necrosis of the femoral head in haemophilia. *J Bone Joint Surg [Br]* 1988;70B:737–739.

Petrini F, Amoroso L, Carotti L, Cerioni M, Ravasi E, Lanza R. Myositis ossificans circumscripta: computerized tomography and magnetic resonance findings. *Radiol Med* 1995;90:492–494.

Rang M. *The growth plate and its disorders*. Baltimore: Williams & Wilkins; 1969.

Riley PM, Weiner DS. Hazards of internal fixation in the treatment of slipped capital femoral epiphysis. *J Bone Joint Surg [Br]* 1990;72B:854–858.

Rockwood CA Jr, Green DP. *Fractures in adults*, vol. 1. Philadelphia: JB Lippincott; 1984.

Rockwood CA Jr, Wilkins KE, King RE. *Fractures in children*, vol. 3. Philadelphia: JB Lippincott; 1984.

Rogers LF. *Radiology of skeletal trauma*. New York: Churchill Livingstone; 1992.

Rogers LF. The radiography of epiphyseal injuries. *Radiology* 1970;96:289–299.

Rogers LF, Poznanski AK. State of the art. Imaging of epiphyseal injuries. *Radiology* 1994;191:297–308.

Rosen H. Treatment of nonunions: general principles. In: Chapman MW, ed. *Operative orthopaedics*, 2nd ed. Philadelphia: JB Lippincott; 1993:749–769.

Salter RB. *Textbook of disorders and injuries of the musculoskeletal system*. Baltimore: Williams & Wilkins; 1970.

Salter RB, Harris WR. Injuries involving the epiphyseal plate. *J Bone Joint Surg [Am]* 1963;45A:587–622.

Sclamberg J, Sonin AH, Sclamberg E, D'Sonza N. Acute plastic bowing deformation of the forearm in an adult. *AJR Am J Roentgenol* 1998;170:1259–1260.

Seiler JG III, Christie MJ, Homra L. Correlation of the findings of magnetic resonance imaging with those of bone biopsy in patients who have stage I or II ischemic necrosis of the femoral head. *J Bone Joint Surg [AM]* 1989;71A:28–32.

Shellock FG, Mink J, Deutsch AL. MR imaging of muscle injuries. *Appl Radiol* 1994;23:11–16.

Shimizu K, Moriya H, Akita T, Sakamoto M, Suguro T. Prediction of collapse with magnetic resonance imaging of avascular necrosis of the femoral head. *J Bone Joint Surg [Am]* 1994;76A:215–223.

Shinoda S, Hasegawa Y, Kawasaki S, Tagawa N, Iwata H. Magnetic resonance imaging of osteonecrosis in divers: comparison with plain radiographs. *Skeletal Radiol* 1997;26:354–359.

Shirkhoda A, Armin A-R, Bis KG, Makris J, Irwin RB, Shetty AN. MR imaging of myositis ossificans: variable patterns at different stages. *J Magn Reson Imaging* 1995;5:287–292.

Smith DW. Is avascular necrosis of the femoral head the result of inhibition of angiogenesis? *Med Hypotheses* 1997;49:497–500.

Steinbach LS, Fleckenstein JL, Mink JH. MRI techniques and practical applications. Magnetic resonance imaging of muscle injuries. *Orthopedics* 1994;17:991–999.

Stevens K, Tao C, Lee S-V, et al. Subchondral fractures in osteonecrosis of the femoral head: comparison of radiography, CT, and MR imaging. *AJR Am J Roentgenol* 2003;180:363–368.

Stoller DW, Maloney WJ, Glick JM. The hip. In: Stoller DW, ed. *Magnetic resonance imaging in orthopaedics and rheumatology*. Philadelphia: Lippincott Raven; 1997:93–202.

Suehiro M, Hirano T, Mihara K, Shindo H. Etiologic factors in femoral head osteonecrosis in growing rats. *J Orthop Sci* 2000;5:52–56.

Sugimoto H, Okubu RS, Ohsawa T. Chemical shift and the double-line sign in MRI of early femoral avascular necrosis. *J Comput Assist Tomogr* 1992;16:727–730.

Szabo RM, Greenspan A. Diagnosis and clinical findings of Keinböck's disease. *Hand Clin* 1993;9:399–407.

Takatori Y, Kokubo T, Ninomiya S, Nakamura S, Morimoto S, Kusuba I. Avascular necrosis of the femoral head: natural history and magnetic resonance imaging. *J Bone Joint Surg [Br]* 1993;75B:217–221.

Terry DW Jr, Ramin JE. The navicular fat stripe: a useful roentgen feature for evaluating wrist trauma. *AJR Am J Roentgenol* 1975;124:25–28.

Tervonen O, Snoep G, Stuart MJ, Ehman RL. Traumatic trabecular lesions observed on MR imaging of the knee. *Acta Radiol* 1991;32:389–392.

Thickman D, Axel L, Kressel HY, et al. Magnetic resonance imaging of avascular necrosis of the femoral head. *Skeletal Radiol* 1986;15:133–140.

Thometz JG, Lamdan R. Osteonecrosis of the femoral head after intramedullary nailing of a fracture of the femoral shaft in an adolescent. *J Bone Joint Surg [Am]* 1995;77A:1423–1426.

Trueta J. Nonunion of fractures. *Clin Orthop* 1965;43:23–35.

Trumble TE. Avascular necrosis after scaphoid fracture: a correlation of magnetic resonance imaging and histology. *J Hand Surg [Am]* 1990;15:557–564.

Vande Berg B, Malghem J, Labaisse MA, Noel H, Maldague B. Avascular necrosis of the hip: comparison of contrast-enhanced and nonenhanced MR imaging with histologic correlation. *Radiology* 1992;182:445–450.

Weissman BNW, Sledge CB. *Orthopedic radiology*. Philadelphia: WB Saunders; 1986:1–69.

Wenzel WW. The FBI sign. *Rocky Mount Med J* 1972;69:71–72.

Williams ES, Khreisat S, Ell PJ, King JD. Bone imaging and skeletal radiology in dysbaric osteonecrosis. Clin Radiol 1987;38:589–592.

Williams M, Laredo J-D, Setbon S, et al. Unusual longitudinal stress fractures of the femoral diaphysis: report of five cases. *Skeletal Radiol* 1999;27:81–85.

Zurlo JV. The double-line sign. *Radiology* 1999;212:541–542.

UPPER LIMB I

Shoulder Girdle

Shoulder Girdle

Trauma to the shoulder girdle is common throughout life, but the site of injury varies with age. In children and adolescents, fracture of the clavicle sustained during play or athletic activities is a frequent type of skeletal injury. Dislocations of the shoulder and acromioclavicular separation are often seen in the third and fourth decades of life, whereas fracture of the proximal humerus is commonly encountered in the elderly. Most of these traumatic conditions can be diagnosed on the basis of history and clinical examination, with radiographs obtained mainly to define the exact site, type, and extent of the injury. At times, however, as in posterior dislocation in the glenohumeral joint for example, which is the most commonly missed diagnosis in shoulder trauma, only radiographic examination performed in the proper projections may reveal the abnormality.

Anatomic–Radiologic Considerations

The shoulder girdle consists of bony components—proximal humerus, scapula, and clavicle, forming the glenohumeral and acromioclavicular joints (Fig. 5.1)—and various muscles, ligaments, and tendons reinforcing the joint capsule (Fig. 5.2). The joint capsule inserts along the anatomic neck of the humerus and along the neck of the glenoid. In front, it is reinforced by three glenohumeral ligaments (the superior, middle, and inferior), which converge from the humerus to be attached by the long head of the biceps tendon to the supraglenoid tubercle. The other important ligaments are the acromioclavicular, coracoacromial, and the coracoclavicular (including trapezoid and conoid portions) (Fig. 5.2).

The essential muscles are those that form the rotator cuff (Fig. 5.3). The term rotator cuff is used to describe the group of muscles that envelop the glenohumeral joint, holding the head of the humerus firmly in the glenoid fossa. They consist of the subscapularis anteriorly, the infraspinatus posterosuperiorly, the teres minor posteriorly, and the supraspinatus superiorly (mnemonic SITS). The subscapularis muscle inserts on the lesser tuberosity anteriorly. The insertions of the supraspinatus, infraspinatus, and teres minor muscles are on the greater tuberosity, posteriorly. The supraspinatus tendon covers the superior aspect of the humeral head, inserting on the superior facet of the greater tuberosity. The infraspinatus tendon covers the superior and posterior aspects of the humeral head and inserts on the middle facet, located distal and more posterior to the superior facet. The teres minor is lower in position and inserts on the posteroinferior facet of the greater tuberosity (Fig. 5.3B). In addition, the long head of the biceps with its tendon, which in its intracapsular portion runs through the joint, and the triceps muscle, inserting on the infraglenoid tubercle inferiorly, provide additional support to the glenohumeral joint.

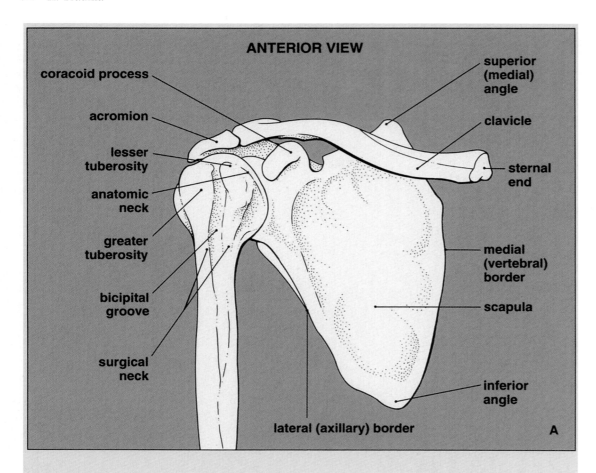

ANTERIOR VIEW

coracoid process

acromion

lesser tuberosity

anatomic neck

greater tuberosity

bicipital groove

surgical neck

superior (medial) angle

clavicle

sternal end

medial (vertebral) border

scapula

inferior angle

lateral (axillary) border

A

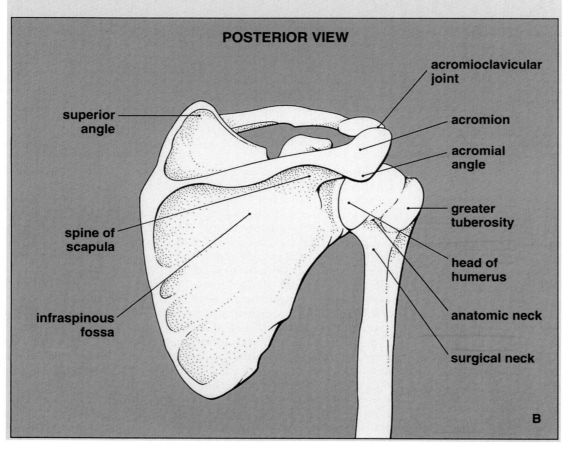

POSTERIOR VIEW

superior angle

spine of scapula

infraspinous fossa

acromioclavicular joint

acromion

acromial angle

greater tuberosity

head of humerus

anatomic neck

surgical neck

B

Figure 5.1 Osseous structures of the shoulder. Anterior **(A)** and posterior **(B)** views of the bony components of the shoulder girdle.

Figure 5.2 Muscles, ligaments, and tendons of the shoulder. Anterior **(A)** and posterior **(B)** views of the muscles, ligaments, and tendons of the shoulder girdle. (Modified from Middleton WD, Lawson TL, 1989, with permission.)

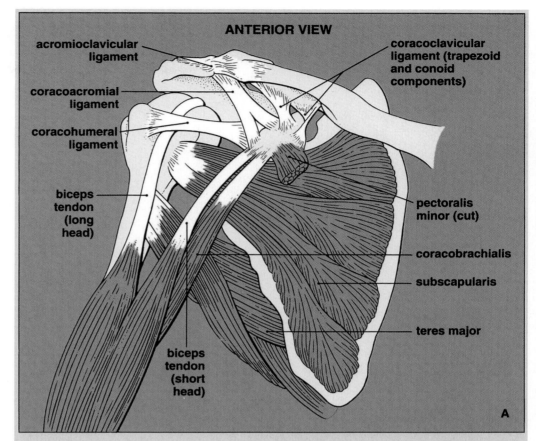

ANTERIOR VIEW

acromioclavicular ligament

coracoclavicular ligament (trapezoid and conoid components)

coracoacromial ligament

coracohumeral ligament

biceps tendon (long head)

pectoralis minor (cut)

coracobrachialis

subscapularis

teres major

biceps tendon (short head)

A

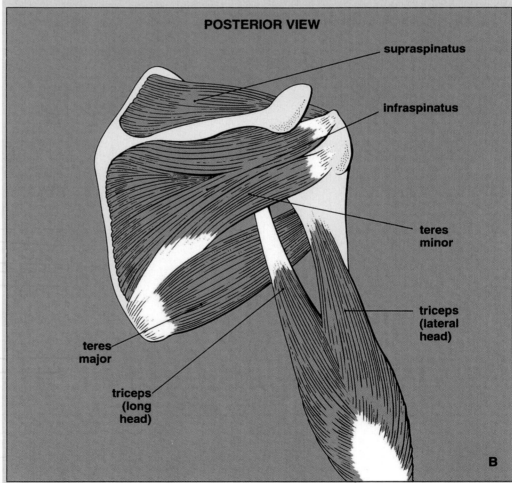

POSTERIOR VIEW

supraspinatus

infraspinatus

teres minor

triceps (lateral head)

teres major

triceps (long head)

B

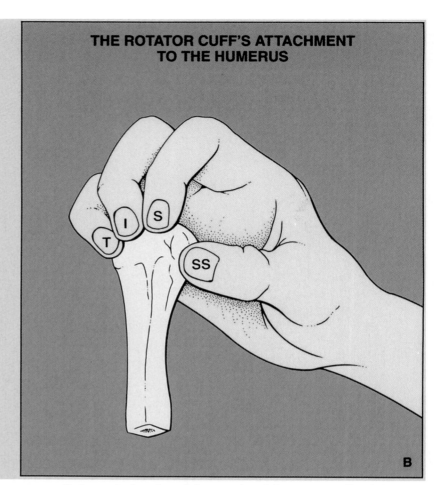

Figure 5.3 Rotator cuff. (A) Schematic of the glenoid fossa (with the humerus removed) shows the location of the muscles of the rotator cuff and the intracapsular portion of the long head of the biceps tendon. **(B)** Four muscles form the "rotator cuff": subscapularis (SS), supraspinatus (S), infraspinatus (I), and teres minor (T). They envelop the joint, blend with the capsule, and grasp their four points of attachment to the humerus, as does the hand in the figure, thus maintaining the integrity of the joint. (Modified from Anderson JE, 1983, with permission.)

Figure 5.4 Anteroposterior view. (A) For the standard anteroposterior projection of the shoulder, the patient may be either supine, as shown here, or erect; the arm of the affected side is fully extended in the neutral position. The central beam is directed toward the humeral head. **(B)** On the film in this projection, the humeral head is seen overlapping the glenoid fossa. The glenohumeral joint is not well demonstrated.

Most trauma to the shoulder area can be sufficiently evaluated on radiographs obtained in the *anteroposterior* projection with the arm in the *neutral* position (Fig. 5.4A) or with the arm *internally* or *externally rotated* to visualize different aspects of the humeral head. The one limitation of these views is that the humeral head is seen overlapping the glenoid, thereby obscuring the glenohumeral joint space (Fig. 5.4). Eliminating the overlap can be accomplished by rotating the patient approximately 40 degrees toward the affected side. This special posterior oblique view, known as the *Grashey projection*, permits the

glenoid to be seen in profile (Fig. 5.5) and is thus particularly effective in demonstrating suspected posterior dislocation. Obliteration of the normally clear space between the humeral head and the glenoid margin on this view confirms the diagnosis (see Figs. 5.48 and 5.50).

Other special views have proved to be useful in evaluating suspected trauma to various aspects of the shoulder. A superoinferior view of the shoulder, known as the *axillary* projection, is helpful in determining the exact relationship of the humeral head and the glenoid fossa (Fig. 5.6), as well as in detecting anterior or posterior disloca-

Figure 5.5 Grashey view. (A). For the anteroposterior view of the shoulder that demonstrates the glenoid in profile (Grashey projection), the patient may be either erect, as shown here, or supine. He or she is rotated approximately 40 degrees toward the side of the suspected injury, and the central beam is directed toward the glenohumeral joint. **(B)** The radiograph in this projection (posterior oblique view) shows the glenoid in true profile. Note that the glenohumeral joint space is now clearly visible.

Figure 5.6 Axillary view. (A) For the axillary view of the shoulder, the patient is seated at the side of the radiographic table, with the arm abducted so that the axilla is positioned over the film cassette. The radiographic tube is angled approximately 5 to 10 degrees toward the elbow, and the central beam is directed through the shoulder joint. **(B)** The film in this projection demonstrates the exact relationship of the humeral head and the glenoid.

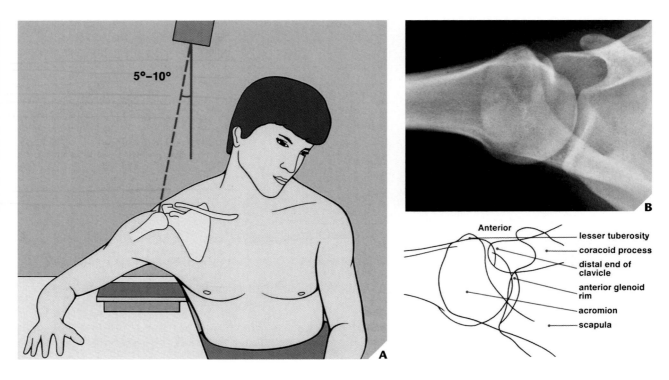

tion. This view, however, may at times be difficult to obtain, particularly if the patient is unable to abduct the arm, in which case a variant of the axillary projection known as the *West Point* view may be similarly effective. In addition to all the benefits of the axillary projection, the West Point view effectively demonstrates the anteroinferior rim of the glenoid (Fig. 5.7). Another useful variant of the axillary projection is the *Lawrence* view. The importance of this projection lies in the fact that it does not require full abduction of the arm, because it can be compensated for by angulation of the radiographic tube (Fig. 5.8). Suspected trauma to the proximal humerus, which can be demon-strated on the anteroposterior or the transscapular projection, may require the *transthoracic lateral* view for sufficient evaluation (Fig. 5.9). Because this projection provides a true lateral view of the proximal humerus, it is particularly valuable in determining the degree of displacement or angulation of the bony fragments (see Fig. 5.27B). When trauma to the bicipital groove is suspected, a *tangent* radiograph of this structure is required (Fig. 5.10). Injury to the acromioclavicular articulation is usually evaluated on the anteroposterior view obtained with a 15-degree cephalad tilt of the radiographic tube (Fig. 5.11). Stress views in this projection, for which weights are strapped to

Figure 5.7 West Point view. (A) For the West Point view of the shoulder, the patient lies prone on the radiographic table, with a pillow placed under the affected shoulder to raise it approximately 8 cm. The film cassette is positioned against the superior aspect of the shoulder. The radiographic tube is angled toward the axilla at 25 degrees to the patient's midline and 25 degrees to the table's surface. **(B)** On the radiograph in this projection, the relationship of the humeral head and the glenoid can be as sufficiently evaluated as on the axillary view, but the anteroinferior glenoid rim, which is seen tangentially, is better visualized.

anteroinferior
glenoid rim

acromion

Figure 5.8 Lawrence view. For the Lawrence variant of the axillary view of the shoulder, the patient lies supine on the radiographic table, with the affected arm abducted up to 90 degrees. The film cassette is positioned against the superior aspect of the shoulder with the medial end against the neck, which places the midportion of the cassette level with the surgical neck of the humerus. The radiographic tube is at the level of the ipsilateral hip and is angled medially toward the axilla. The amount of angulation depends on the degree of abduction of the arm: Less abduction requires increased medial angulation. The central beam is directed horizontally slightly superior to the midportion of the axilla. The Lawrence view demonstrates the same structures as the standard axillary view.

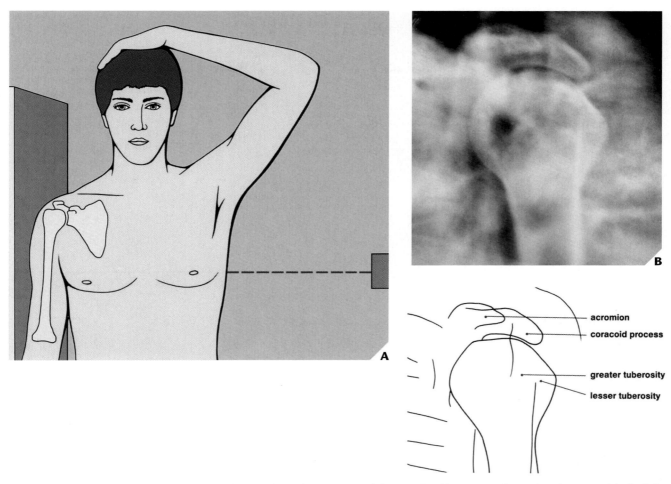

Figure 5.9 Transthoracic lateral view. (A) For the transthoracic lateral projection of the proximal humerus, the patient is erect with the injured arm against the radiographic table. The opposite arm is abducted so that the forearm rests on the head. The central beam is directed below the axilla, slightly above the level of the nipple. **(B)** The film in this projection demonstrates the true lateral view of the proximal humerus.

Figure 5.10 Bicipital groove view. (A) For a tangent film in the superoinferior projection visualizing the bicipital groove (sulcus), the patient is standing and leaning forward, with the forearm resting on the table and the hand in supination. The film cassette rests on the patient's forearm. The central beam is directed vertically toward the bicipital groove, which has been marked on the skin. **(B)** On this view, the bicipital groove is clearly demonstrated.

15°

20°

Figure 5.11 Acromioclavicular view. (A) To evaluate the acromioclavicular articulation, the patient is erect, with the arm of the affected side in the neutral position. The central beam is directed 15 degrees cephalad toward the clavicle. As overexposure of the film will make it difficult to evaluate the acromioclavicular joint properly the radiographic factors should be reduced to approximately 33% to 50% of those used in obtaining the standard anteroposterior view of the shoulder. **(B)** The film in this projection shows the normal appearance of the acromioclavicular joint.

A

B

A

Figure 5.12 Transscapular view. (A) For the transscapular (or Y) projection of the shoulder girdle, the patient is erect, with the injured side against the radiographic table. The patient's trunk is rotated approximately 20 degrees from the table to allow for separation of the two shoulders (*inset*). The arm on the injured side is slightly abducted and the elbow flexed, with the hand resting on the ipsilateral hip. The central beam is directed toward the medial border of the protruding scapula. (This view may also be obtained with the patient lying prone on the radiographic table and the uninjured arm elevated approximately 45 degrees.) **(B)** The film in this projection provides a true lateral view of the scapula, as well as an oblique view of the proximal humerus.

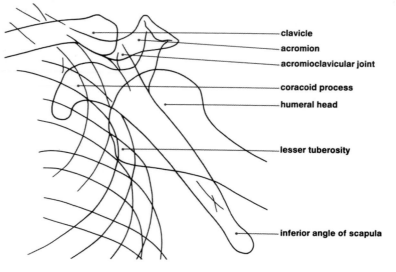

B

- clavicle
- acromion
- acromioclavicular joint
- coracoid process
- humeral head
- lesser tuberosity
- inferior angle of scapula

Figure 5.13 Outlet view. This projection shows the same anatomic structures as demonstrated on the Y view of the shoulder girdle. In addition, coracoacromial arch and space occupied by the rotator cuff are well imaged.

the patient's forearms, are often mandatory, especially in suspected occult acromioclavicular subluxation (see Fig. 5.64). Fracture of the scapula may require a *transscapular* (or *Y*) view for sufficient evaluation (Fig. 5.12). Fracture of the acromion can be adequately evaluated on the shoulder *outlet* view. This projection is obtained similarly to the Y view of the shoulder girdle; however, the central beam is directed toward the superior aspect of the humeral head and is angled approximately 10 to 15 degrees caudad (Fig. 5.13). This view is also effective in demonstration of morphologic types of the acromion (Fig. 5.14; see also Fig. 5.24).

Ancillary imaging techniques are usually used to evaluate injury to the cartilage and soft tissues of the shoulder. The most frequently used modalities are arthrography and magnetic resonance imaging (MRI). Arthrography can be performed using a single- or double-con-

trast technique (Fig. 5.15). In cases of suspected tear of the rotator cuff, for example, a single-contrast arthrogram may reveal abnormal communication between the glenohumeral joint cavity and the subacromial–subdeltoid bursae complex, which is diagnostic of this abnormality (see Fig. 5.53C). Although it is difficult to prescribe for which conditions a single- as opposed to a double-contrast study should be chosen, the latter may be better suited to demonstrate abnormalities of the articular cartilage and capsule, as well as the presence of osteochondral bodies in the joint. A double-contrast study, however, is always indicated when arthrography is to be combined with *CT scan* (computed arthrotomography) for evaluating suspected abnormalities of the fibrocartilaginous glenoid labrum (Fig. 5.16). The effectiveness of this combination lies in the fact that the injected air outlines the anterior and posterior labrum for better demonstration of subtle traumatic changes on CT images. For this study, the patient is placed supine in the CT scanner with the arm of the affected side in the neutral position to allow the air to rise and enhance the outline of the anterior labrum. To evaluate the posterior labrum, the arm is externally rotated (or the patient is positioned prone) to force the air to move posteriorly.

Recent studies have shown the considerable advantage of MRI in the examination of the shoulder. This modality is particularly effective in demonstrating traumatic abnormalities of the soft tissues, such as impingement syndrome, partial and complete rotator cuff tears, biceps tendon rupture, glenoid labrum tears, and demonstration of the traumatic joint effusion. However, the shoulder presents unique difficulties for imaging. Because of space limitations in the magnet, the shoulder cannot be positioned in the center of the magnetic field. This necessitates lateral shift for image centering and scanning a region where the signal-to-noise ratio is relatively low. These problems have been overcome by combining high-resolution scanning with the use of special surface coils. Because the bones and muscles of the shoulder girdle are oriented along multiple nonorthogonal axes, scanning in oblique planes is more effective.

The patient should be positioned in the magnet supine with the arms along the thorax and the affected arm externally rotated. The scanning planes include oblique coronal (along the long axis of the belly of the supraspinatus muscle), oblique sagittal (perpendicular to the course of supraspinatus muscle), and axial (Fig. 5.17). The first two planes are ideal for evaluating all the structures of the rotator cuff; the axial plane is ideal for evaluating the glenoid labrum, bicipital groove, biceps tendon, and subscapularis tendon. Appropriate pulse sequences are critical in displaying normal anatomy and traumatic abnormalities. T1-weighted pulse sequences sufficiently demonstrate the structural anatomy (Figs. 5.17 and Fig. 5.18). Proton density and T2-weighted pulse sequences provide the information necessary to

Figure 5.14 Types of the acromion. On the outlet view of the shoulder, three morphologic types of acromion are well demonstrated. **(A)** Type I (flat). **(B)** Type II (curved). **(C)** Type III (hooked).

Figure 5.15 Arthrography of the shoulder. For arthrographic examination of the shoulder, the patient is positioned supine on the radiographic table, with the unaffected shoulder slightly elevated and the affected arm in external rotation with the palm up. **(A)** With the aid of fluoroscopy, a lead marker is placed near the lower third of the glenohumeral articulation to indicate the site of needle insertion. Under fluoroscopic control 15 mL of positive contrast agent (60% diatrizoate meglumine or another meglumine-type medium) are injected into the joint capsule. The usual study includes supine films of the shoulder in the standard anteroposterior (arm in the neutral position and in internal and external rotation) and the axillary projections. **(B)** A normal arthrogram of the shoulder shows contrast outlining the articular cartilage of the humerus and the glenoid and filling the axillary pouch, the subscapularis recess, and the bicipital tendon sheath.

Figure 5.16 Tear of the glenoid labrum. As the result of an auto accident, a 33-year-old woman sustained an injury to the right shoulder; she presented with pain and limitation of motion in the joint. Standard films of the shoulder were normal. As injury to the cartilaginous labrum was suspected, double-contrast arthrography was performed. Five milliliters of positive contrast agent and 10 mL of room air were injected into the joint capsule. **(A)** This arthrogram shows no evident abnormalities. The subscapularis recess, which is not opacified on this view, was shown later in the study to fill with contrast. **(B)** In conjunction with arthrography, a CT scan of the same shoulder was performed and clearly demonstrates avulsion of the anterior glenoid labrum, a finding not appreciated on the arthrographic study. Note that the avulsed fragment is surrounded by air and shows absorption of the contrast medium. **(C)** The normal appearance of the glenoid labrum is shown for comparison.

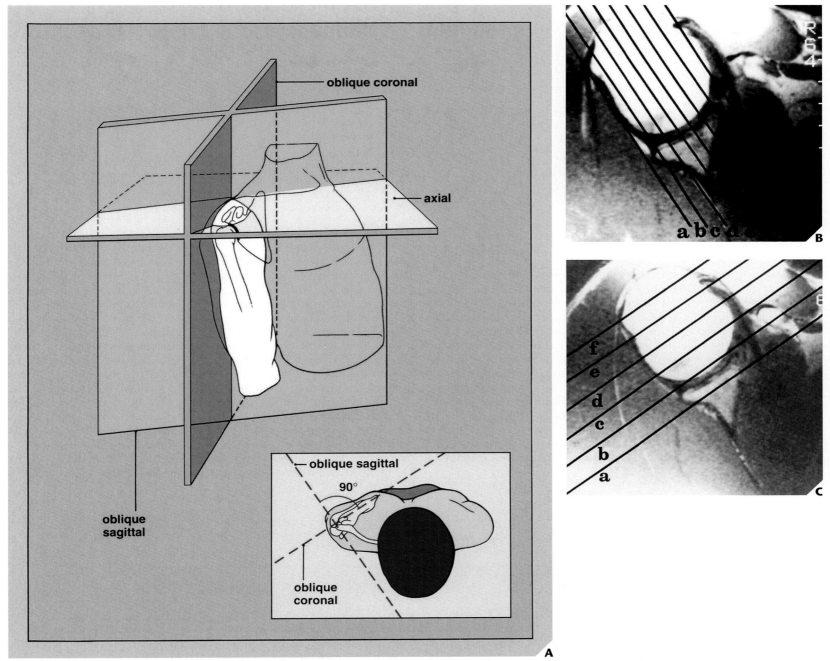

A

Figure 5.17 MRI of the shoulder. (A) Standard planes of MRI sections of the shoulder. **(B)** Oblique coronal sections are obtained parallel to the long axis of the supraspinatus muscle. **(C)** Oblique sagittal sections are obtained perpendicular to the coronal sections. (From Beltran J, 1990, with permission.)

Figure 5.18 MRI of the shoulder. T1-weighted coronal image of the right shoulder demonstrates a normal supraspinatus muscle and tendon attaching to the greater tuberosity of the humerus. (From Holt RG, et al., 1990, with permission.)

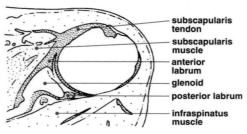

subscapularis
tendon
subscapularis
muscle
anterior
labrum
glenoid
posterior labrum
infraspinatus
muscle

Figure 5.19 MRI of the shoulder. T1-weighted axial image of the left shoulder demonstrates a normal subscapularis muscle and tendon and the infraspinatus muscle. (From Holt RG, et al., 1990, with permission.)

evaluate pathology of rotator cuff, joint space, and bones (see Figs. 5.51, 5.55, and 5.57).

Demonstration of rotator cuff muscles and tendons is greatly facilitated by the use of MRI. The supraspinatus is best demonstrated on oblique coronal and sagittal images, preferably obtained on spin-echo T1-weighted sequences. It is seen as a thick, intermediate-intensity structure, and its tendon inserts on the superolateral aspect of the greater tuberosity of the humerus (Fig. 5.18). The infraspinatus and subscapularis are best demonstrated on axial images as fusiform, intermediate-intensity structures. The infraspinatus tendon inserts distally and more posterior to the supraspinatus on the greater tuberosity, adjacent to the insertion of teres minor. The subscapularis muscle is located anterior to the body of the scapula. It appears on T1-weighted axial images as an intermediate-intensity structure that tapers anteriorly into a low-intensity tendon, where it merges with the anterior aspect of the capsule before inserting on the lesser tuberosity (Fig. 5.19).

The axial images are effective in demonstration of the joint capsule, which is anteriorly reinforced by the anterior glenohumeral ligaments. The capsular complex provides stabilization of the glenohumeral joint. The anterior capsular complex includes the fibrous capsule, the anterior glenohumeral ligaments, the synovial membrane and its recesses, the fibrous glenoid labrum, the subscapularis muscle and tendon, and the scapular periosteum. Three types of anterior capsular insertion have been identified by Zlatkin and colleagues. They are determined by the proximity of insertion to the glenoid margin (Fig. 5.20). In type I, the capsule inserts on the glenoid rim in close proximity to the glenoid labrum. In types II and III, the capsular insertion is further away from the glenoid rim and may reach the scapular neck (Fig. 5.21). The further the anterior capsule inserts from the glenoid margin, the more unstable the glenohumeral joint will be. The posterior portion of the capsule shows no variations and attaches directly to the labrum. The axial images are also effective in demonstration of anterior and posterior cartilaginous

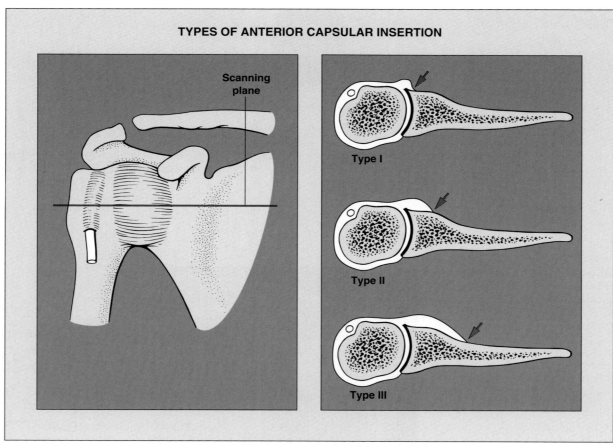

Figure 5.20 Capsule of the shoulder joint. Three types of anterior capsular insertion to the scapula.

Figure 5.21 Capsular insertion to glenoid margin. (A) Axial T1-weighted image after intraarticular injection of gadolinium shows type I of anterior capsular insertion. **(B)** Axial fast spin-echo image with fat saturation and intraarticular gadolinium shows type II of anterior capsular insertion. **(C)** Axial T1-weighted image with fat saturation and intraarticular gadolinium shows type III of anterior capsular insertion.

Figure 5.22 Fibrocartilaginous labrum of the glenoid. (A) Axial T1-weighted and **(B)** axial T2-weighted (multiplanar gradient-recalled) MR images show anterior (*arrows*) and posterior (*curved arrows*) labra as small triangles of low signal intensity.

Figure 5.23 Fibrocartilaginous labrum. Oblique coronal T1-weighted MRI shows a superior (*arrow*) and inferior (*curved arrow*) labra.

Figure 5.24 Variations of the acromial morphology. Schematic representation of morphologic variations of the acromion. **(A)** MRI appearance on oblique sagittal sections. **(B)** Appearance on anatomical specimen.

labrum of the glenoid, which are seen as two small triangles of low signal intensity that are located anteriorly and posteriorly to the glenoid margin (Fig. 5.22). The superior and inferior aspects of the labrum are best demonstrated on the oblique coronal sections (Fig. 5.23). There are numerous imaging variations of the morphology of the cartilaginous labrum. The most common shape is triangular as illustrated in Fig. 5.22. The second most common shape is round. The other morphologic variations include the flat labrum and the cleaved or notched labrum. On rare occasions the anterior and posterior labrum may be absent. Furthermore, there are appearances resembling labral tears, such as undercutting of the labrum by hyaline cartilage, sublabral holes or recesses, and Buford complexes (see Fig. 5.62).

The sagittal images are useful in demonstration of morphologic variations of the acromion. Three types of acromion have been identified by Bigliani and coworkers. Type I shows a flat undersurface, type II a curved undersurface, and type III a hooked undersurface (Figs. 5.24 and 5.25). Type III acromion is considered to be associated with tears of the rotator cuff proximal to the site of insertion of the supraspinatus tendon to the greater tuberosity of the humerus.

In the past decade, direct MR arthrography using injection of contrast solution into the shoulder joint gained worldwide acceptance. This technique is particularly effective for demonstrating labral–ligamentous abnormalities and distinguishing partial-thickness from full-thickness tears of the rotator cuff. A variety of concentrations and mixtures of solutions are used by different radiologists. In our institution, we follow the

recommendation reported by Steinbach and colleagues. We add 0.8 mL of gadopentetate dimeglumine (gadolinium with strength 287 mg/mL) to 100 mL of normal saline solution. Subsequently, we mix 10 mL of this solution with 5 mL of 60% meglumine diatrizoate (iodinated contrast) and 5 mL of 1% lidocaine, which gives a final gadolinium dilution ratio of 1:250. From 12 to 15 mL of this mixture is then injected into the shoulder joint using fluoroscopic guidance in a similar fashion as for conventional shoulder arthrography (see Fig. 5.15). Multiple pre-exercise and postexercise radiographic spot images are obtained in neutral position and in external and internal rotation of the arm. Subsequently, without delay, the patient undergoes MRI examination using similar scanning planes as for a conventional MR study. If glenoid labrum abnormalities are suspected, additional sequences are obtained in so-called ABER (abduction-external rotation) position.

For a summary of the foregoing discussion in tabular form, see Tables 5.1 and 5.2 and Fig. 5.26.

Figure 5.25 Morphologic variations of the acromion. (A) In the sagittal oblique plane, type II acromion shows a mild curved undersurface. **(B)** Type III acromion demonstrates a hooked undersurface (*arrow*).

Table 5.1 Standard and Special Radiographic Projections for Evaluating Injury to the Shoulder Girdle

Projection	Demonstration
Anteroposterior	
Arm in neutral position	Fracture of: Humeral head and neck Clavicle Scapula Anterior dislocation Bankart lesion
Erect	Fat—blood interface (FBI sign)
Arm in internal rotation	Hill-Sacks lesion
Arm in external rotation	Compression fracture of humeral head (trough line impaction) secondary to posterior dislocation
40-degree posterior oblique (Grashey)	Glenohumeral joint space Glenoid in profile Posterior dislocation
15-degree cephalad tilt of radiographic tube	Acromioclavicular joint Acromioclavicular separation Fracture of clavicle
Stress	Occult acromioclavicular subluxation Acromioclavicular separation
Axillary	Relationship of humeral head and glenoid fossa Anterior and posterior dislocations Compression fractures secondary to anterior and posterior dislocations Fractures of: Proximal humerus Scapula
West Point	Same structures and conditions as axillary projection Anteroinferior rim of glenoid
Lateral Transthoracic	Relationship of humeral head and glenoid fossa Fractures of proximal humerus
Tangent (Humeral Head)	Bicipital groove
Transscapular (Y)	Relationship of humeral head and glenoid fossa Fractures of: Proximal humerus Body of scapula Coracoid process Acromion
Oblique (outlet)	Coracoacromial arch Rotator cuff outlet

Table 5.2 **Ancillary Imaging Techniques for Evaluating Injury to the Shoulder Girdle**

Technique	Demonstration	Technique	Demonstration

Tomography	Position of fragments and extension of fracture line in complex fractures
	Healing process:
	  Nonunion
	  Secondary infection
		Ultrasound
		
		Arthrography
		Single- or double-contrast
			Rotator cuff tear
			
			Complete rotator cuff tear
			Partial rotator cuff tear

Computed Tomography	Relationship of humeral head and glenoid fossa Multiple fragments in complex fractures (particularly of scapula) Intraarticular displacement of bony fragments in fractures		Abnormalities of articular cartilage and joint capsule* Synovial abnormalities* Adhesive capsulitis Osteochondral bodies in joint* Abnormalities of bicipital tendon*† Intraarticular portion of bicipital tendon*†

Magnetic Resonance Imaging	Impingement syndrome
	Partial and complete rotator cuff tear‡
	Biceps tendon rupture
	Glenoid labrum tears‡
	Glenohumeral instability
	Traumatic joint effusion
		Double-contrast combined with CT	Inferior surface of rotator cuff*†
			All of the above and in addition:
			  Abnormalities of cartilaginous glenoid labrum
			  Osteochondral bodies in joint
			  Subtle synovial abnormalities

* These conditions are usually best demonstrated using double-contrast arthrography.
† These features are best demonstrated on erect films.
‡ These abnormalties are best demostraed on MR arthrography.

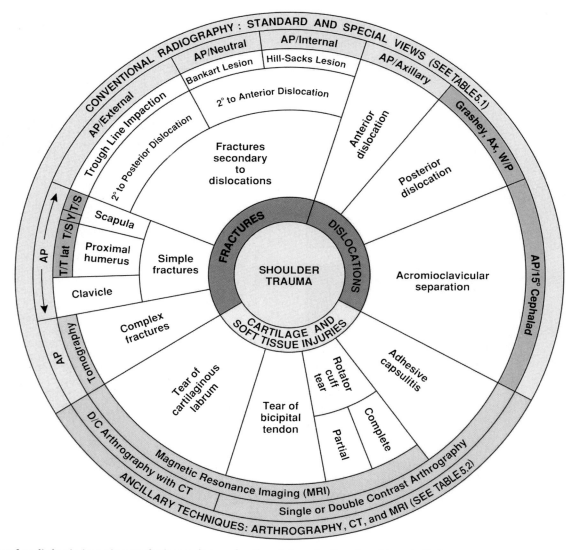

Figure 5.26 Spectrum of radiologic imaging techniques for evaluating injury to the shoulder girdle*
   The radiographic projections or radiologic techniques indicated throughout the diagram are only those most effective in demonstrating the respective traumatic conditions.

Injury to the Shoulder Girdle

Fractures About the Shoulder

Fractures of the Proximal Humerus. Fractures of the upper humerus involving the head, the neck, and the proximal shaft usually result either from a direct blow to the humerus or, as is more often seen in elderly patients, from a fall on the outstretched arm. Nondisplaced fractures are the most common, representing approximately 85% of all such proximal humeral injuries.

The anteroposterior projection is usually sufficient to demonstrate the abnormality, but the transthoracic lateral or the transscapular (or Y) projection may be required to provide a fuller evaluation, particularly of the degree of displacement or angulation of the bony fragments (Fig. 5.27). In cases of comminution, conventional tomography may also need to be used to assess the degree of displacement of the various fragments. The erect anteroposterior radiograph may demonstrate the presence of fat and blood within the joint capsule (the FBI sign of lipohemarthrosis; see Fig. 4.34A), indicating intraarticular extension of the fracture.

Traditional classifications of trauma to the proximal humerus, according to the level of the fracture or the mechanism of injury, have been inadequate to identify the various types of displaced fractures. The four-segment classification described by Neer in 1970 was complex and difficult to follow. He later modified this classification and simplified divisions to various groups. Classification of a displacement pattern depends on two main factors: the number of displaced segments and the key segment displaced. Fractures of the proximal humerus occur between one or all of four major segments: the articular segment (at the level of the anatomic neck), the greater tuberosity, the lesser tuberosity, and the humeral shaft (at the level of the surgical neck). One-part fracture occurs when there is minimal or no displacement between the segments. In two-part fractures, only one segment is displaced. In three-part fractures, two segments are displaced and one tuberosity remaining in continuity with the humeral head. In four-part fractures, three segments are displaced, including both tuberosities. Two-part, three-part, and four-part fractures may or may not be associated with dislocation, either anterior or posterior. The involvement of the articular surface is classified separately into two groups: the anterior fracture–dislocation, termed by Neer as "head splitting," and posterior fracture–dislocation, termed "impression" (Fig. 5.28).

One-part fracture may involve any or all of the anatomic segments of the proximal humerus. There is no or minimal (less than 1 cm) displacement and no or minimal (less than 45 degrees) angulation; the fragments are being held together by the rotator cuff, the joint capsule, and the intact periosteum.

Two-part fracture indicates that only one segment is displaced in relation to the three that remain undisplaced. It may involve the anatomic neck, surgical neck, greater tuberosity, or lesser tuberosity. The two-part fracture involving the anatomic neck of the humerus with displacement of the articular end may be associated with tear of the rotator cuff, and complications such as malunion or osteonecrosis may later develop. In two-part fractures involving the surgical neck of the humerus with displacement or angulation of the shaft, three types may be seen: impacted, unimpacted, and comminuted. These fractures may be associated with either anterior or posterior dislocation. With anterior dislocation, the fracture invariably involves the greater tuberosity; with posterior dislocation, the fracture invariably involves the lesser tuberosity.

Three-part fracture may involve either greater tuberosity or lesser tuberosity and may be associated with anterior or posterior dislocation. Two segments are displaced in relation to two other segments that are not displaced.

Four-part fracture involves the greater and lesser tuberosity in addition to the fracture of the surgical neck, and four major segments are displaced. This may be associated with anterior or posterior dislocation. The four-part fracture is usually associated with impairment of the blood supply to the humeral head, and osteonecrosis of the humeral head is a frequent complication.

Fractures of the Clavicle. A common injury in infancy during delivery, in adolescence caused by a direct blow or fall, and in adulthood as the result of a motor vehicle accident is a fracture of the clavicle, which can be divided into three types according to the anatomic segment involved (Fig. 5.29). The most common site of injury is the middle third of the clavicle, representing 80% of all clavicular fractures. Fractures of the distal (lateral) third (15%) and the proximal (medial) third (5%) are less commonly seen. If displacement is present, the proximal fragment is usually elevated and the distal fragment is displaced medially and caudally. Fractures of the distal third of the clavicle have been classified by Neer into three types (Fig. 5.29B). Type I consists of a fracture without significant displacement and with intact ligaments (Fig. 5.30). Type II fractures are displaced and located between two ligaments: the coracoclavicular ligament, which is detached from the medial segment, and the trapezoid ligament, which remains attached to the distal segment. Type III fracture involves the articular surface, but the ligaments remain intact. The anteroposterior projection of the shoulder usually allows sufficient evaluation of any type of clavicular fracture (Fig. 5.31), but the same

Figure 5.27 Fracture of the proximal humerus. A 60-year-old man fell on a staircase and injured his right arm. **(A)** Anteroposterior radiograph of the shoulder demonstrates a comminuted fracture through the surgical neck of the humerus. The greater tuberosity is fractured, too, but is not significantly displaced. To assess the degree of displacement of the various fragments better the transthoracic lateral view **(B)** was obtained. It demonstrates slight anterior angulation of the humeral head, which in addition is inferiorly subluxed—a finding not well appreciated on the anteroposterior projection.

FOUR-SEGMENT CLASSIFICATION OF FRACTURES OF THE PROXIMAL HUMERUS

Anatomic Segment	One-Part (no or minimal displacement; no or minimal angulation)	Two-Part (one segment displaced)	Three-Part (two segments displaced; one tuberosity remains in continuity with the head)	Four-Part (three segments displaced)
Any or all anatomic aspects				
Articular Segment (Anatomic Neck)				
Shaft Segment (Surgical Neck)		impacted unimpacted comminuted		
Greater Tuberosity Segment				
Lesser Tuberosity Segment				

Fracture—Dislocation	Two-Part (one segment displaced)	Three-Part (two segments displaced; one tuberosity remaining in continuity with the head)	Four-Part (three segments displaced)	Articular Surface
Anterior	fracture of greater tuberosity	fracture of surgical neck and greater tuberosity	fracture of surgical neck and both greater and lesser tuberosity	"head-splitting"
Posterior	fracture of lesser tuberosity	fracture of surgical neck and lesser tuberosity	fractures of surgical neck and both greater and lesser tuberosity	"impression"

Figure 5.28 Neer classification. Fractures of the proximal humerus based on the presence or absence of displacement of the four major fragments that may result from fracture. (Modified from Neer CS II, 1975, with permission.)

TYPES OF CLAVICLE FRACTURES

A. Classification According to Involvement of the Anatomic Segment

I
II
III

I. Proximal third

II. Middle third

III. Distal third

B. Neer Classification of Fractures of the Distal Clavicle

1

2

3

1. Nondisplaced fracture, intact ligaments

2. Displaced interligamentous fracture; conoid ligament torn, trapezoid ligament remains attached to the distal segment

3. Fracture extends to articular surface, ligaments intact

Figure 5.29 Classification of the fractures of the clavicle.

Figure 5.30 Fracture of the acromial end of the clavicle. Type I fracture of the distal third clavicle. There is no displacement of the fractured fragment.

Figure 5.31 Fracture of both clavicles. A 22-year-old man sustained multiple traumas in a motorcycle accident. Anteroposterior view of both shoulders demonstrates a comminuted fracture of the middle third of the right clavicle and a simple fracture of the middle third of the left.

Figure 5.32 Fracture of the sternal end of the clavicle. A 32-year-old woman was injured in a car accident and presented with pain localized to the medial aspect of the right clavicle for the past 3 weeks. **(A)** Anteroposterior radiograph shows questionable lesion of the medial end of the clavicle, however, the abnormality is not well demonstrated. **(B)** A trispiral tomogram clearly shows healing fracture of the medial clavicle.

Figure 5.33 Fracture of the sternal end of the clavicle. A 21-year-old man was assaulted and sustained a direct injury to the left medial clavicle. **(A)** Anteroposterior radiograph is suggestive of a fracture of the medial end of the clavicle, but the fracture line is not well demonstrated. **(B)** A CT section shows a fracture of the left sternal end of the clavicle and associated soft-tissue swelling.

projection obtained with 15-degree cephalad angulation of the radiographic tube may also be useful, particularly in fractures of the middle third of the clavicle. Occasionally, if the diagnosis is in doubt, or if the fracture cannot be well demonstrated on conventional radiography, then trispiral tomography (Fig. 5.32) or CT (Figs. 5.33 and 5.34) might be more effective.

Fractures of the Scapula. Invariably resulting from direct trauma, frequently sustained in motor vehicle accidents or falls from

heights, fractures of the scapula, which constitute approximately 1% of all fractures, 3% of shoulder girdle injuries, and 5% of all shoulder fractures, are classified according to their anatomic locations (Fig. 5.35). Because of their intraarticular extension, fractures of the glenoid rim and glenoid fossa are particularly important. They comprise 10% of all fractures of the scapula; however, fewer than 10% are significantly displaced. Fractures of the *glenoid rim* are subclassified into those involving the anterior portion and those affecting the pos-

Figure 5.34 Fracture of the sternal end of the clavicle. A 34-year-old woman was severely injured in a car accident. **(A)** Anteroposterior radiograph of the right shoulder and upper chest shows multiple rib fractures. The medial portion of the clavicle is not adequately visualized. Axial CT scan **(B)** and coronal reformatted image **(C)** show a comminuted fracture of the sternal end of the right clavicle with anterior displacement and overriding of the fragments.

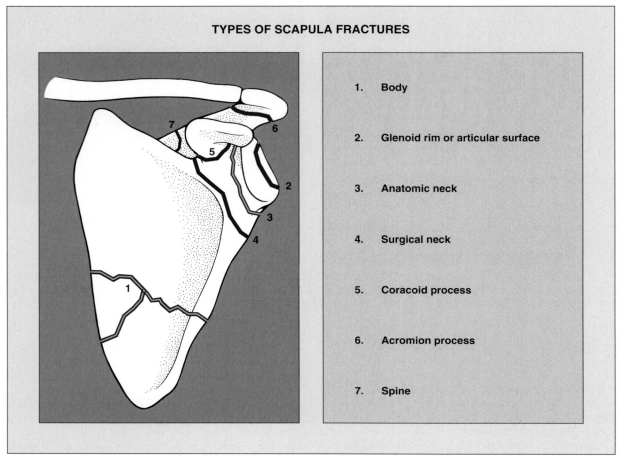

TYPES OF SCAPULA FRACTURES

1. **Body**

2. **Glenoid rim or articular surface**

3. **Anatomic neck**

4. **Surgical neck**

5. **Coracoid process**

6. **Acromion process**

7. **Spine**

Figure 5.35 Fractures of the scapula. Classification of the fractures of the scapula according to anatomic location.

terior segment. Fractures of the *glenoid fossa* are subclassified into injuries involving the inferior segment; transverse disruption of the fossa extending into the vicinity of the suprascapular notch and the coracoid process; central fossa fractures extending across the entire

Figure 5.36 Comminuted fracture of the glenoid. Axial CT section through the shoulder joint shows a comminuted, displaced fracture of the glenoid fossa extending across the entire scapula.

scapula; and combination of the aforementioned fractures, frequently comminuted and displaced (Fig. 5.36).

Scapular fractures may occasionally be evaluated on the anteroposterior view of the shoulder. More commonly, the transscapular (or Y) view may be required, particularly in cases of comminution, because this projection better demonstrates displacement of the fragments (Fig. 5.37). CT scan may also effectively demonstrate the displacement of various segments (Fig. 5.38). Complications, such as injury to the axillary artery or the brachial plexus, are rare.

Dislocations in the Glenohumeral Joint

Anterior Dislocation. Displacement of the humeral head anterior to the glenoid fossa, which usually results from indirect force applied to the arm—a combination of abduction, extension, and external rotation—accounts for approximately 97% of cases of glenohumeral dislocation. It is readily diagnosed on the anteroposterior view of the shoulder (Fig. 5.39), although the Y view is effective as well (Fig. 5.40). CT is equally effective in demonstrating anterior dislocation (Fig. 5.41).

At the time of dislocation, the humeral head strikes the inferior margin of the glenoid, and this may result in compression fracture of one or both of these structures. Fracture most frequently occurs in the posterolateral aspect of the humeral head at the junction with the neck, producing a "hatchet" defect called the *Hill-Sachs lesion;* it is best demonstrated on the anteroposterior projection of the shoulder with the arm internally rotated (Fig. 5.42). Hills-Sachs lesion can also be imaged with CT (Fig. 5.43) or MR. When using the latter modality, either coronal oblique (Fig. 5.44A) or axial (Fig. 5.44B) image reveals this abnormality. Fracture of the anterior aspect of the inferior rim of the glenoid, known as the *Bankart lesion,* is less commonly seen. It may occur secondary to the anterior movement of the humeral head in dislocation and is readily demonstrated on the anteroposterior projection with the arm in the neutral position (Figs. 5.45 and 5.46). When the site of the Bankart lesion is in the cartilaginous labrum, which at

Figure 5.37 **Fracture of the scapula.** A 52-year-old man was injured in a motorcycle accident. **(A)** On the anteroposterior view of the right shoulder, a comminuted fracture of the scapula is evident. Displacement of the fragments, however, cannot be evaluated. **(B)** Transscapular (Y) view demonstrates lateral displacement of the body of the scapula.

Figure 5.38 **Fracture of the scapula.** A 57-year-old woman sustained an injury to the left shoulder in a motorcycle accident. **(A)** Anteroposterior radiograph shows a comminuted fracture of the left scapula. The glenohumeral joint cannot be properly assessed on this study. Two axial CT sections, one at the level of glenohumeral joint **(B)** and the other at the level of body of the scapula **(C)**, and reformatted coronal image **(D)** show to better advantage the configuration of various displaced fragments, as well as an intact glenohumeral joint.

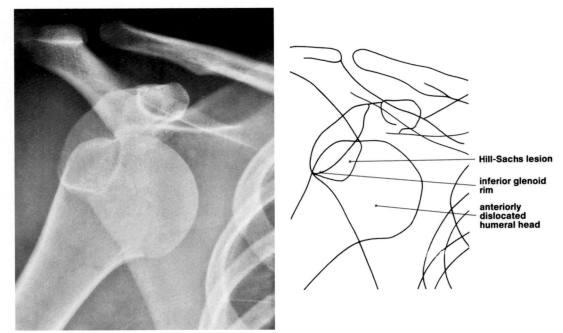

Figure 5.39 Anterior shoulder dislocation. Anteroposterior film of the shoulder shows the typical appearance of anterior dislocation. The humeral head lies beneath the inferior rim of the glenoid.

Figure 5.40 Anterior shoulder dislocation. A dislocation is well demonstrated on this trans-scapular (or Y) projection of the shoulder girdle. An *arrow* is pointing to the empty glenoid fossa. The humeral head *(H)* is medially and anteriorly displaced.

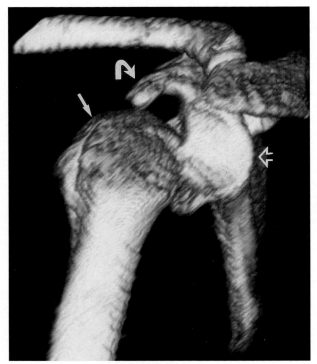

Figure 5.41 Anterior shoulder dislocation. A three-dimensional CT (side view) demonstrates anterior dislocation of the humeral head *(arrow)*. Open arrow points to the empty glenoid fossa, and a curved arrow points to the coracoid process.

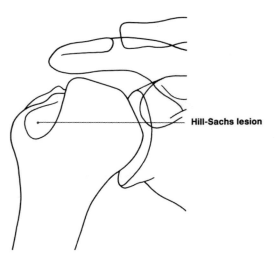

Figure 5.42 Hill-Sachs lesion. Anteroposterior view of the shoulder with the arm internally rotated demonstrates a "hatchet" defect, known as the Hill-Sachs lesion, on the posterolateral aspect of the humeral head.

Figure 5.43 CT of Hill-Sachs lesion. Coronal CT reformatted image shows anterior dislocation in the shoulder joint. The arrow points to the Hill-Sachs lesion.

Figure 5.44 MRI of Hill-Sachs lesion. A 56-year-old woman sustained an anterior shoulder dislocation that has been successfully reduced. A postreduction MRI was performed. Coronal oblique T1-weighted image (A) and gradient-echo MPGR sequence (B) show compression fracture at the posterolateral aspect of the humeral head (arrow). The Hill-Sachs compression is also well demonstrated on the axial gradient-echo MPGR image (C) as a flattening of the posterolateral aspect of the humeral head (open arrow).

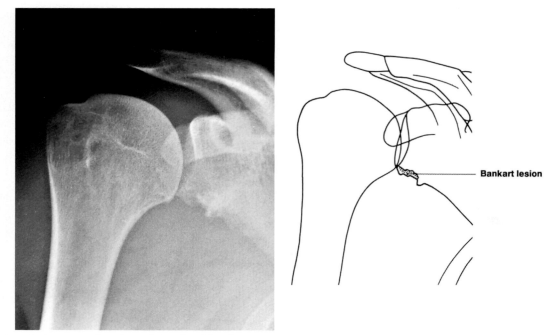

Figure 5.45 Bankart lesion. Anteroposterior view of the shoulder shows compression fracture of the anterior aspect of the inferior portion of the glenoid, known as the Bankart lesion.

Figure 5.46 CT of Hill-Sachs and Bankart lesions. (A) Coronal CT reformatted image and **(B)** three-dimensional CT show Hill-Sachs (*arrow*) and Bankart (*curved arrow*) lesions in a 42-year-old woman with reduced anterior shoulder dislocation.

Figure 5.47 MRI demonstration of Bankart lesion. (A) T1-weighted axial image shows an osseous Bankart lesion *(arrow)* with fracture of the anterior glenoid. **(B)** Proton density axial image shows a detachment of the anteroinferior labrum *(short arrow)*, and a tear of the inferior glenohumeral ligament *(long arrow)*.

times may be detached, it may only be revealed by either computed arthrotomography (see Fig. 5.16) or MRI (Fig. 5.47). The presence of either of these abnormalities is virtually diagnostic of previous anterior dislocation.

Posterior Dislocation. This type of dislocation, which is much less commonly seen—accounting for only 2% to 3% of dislocations in the glenohumeral joint—results from either direct force, such as a blow to the anterior aspect of the shoulder, or indirect force applied to the arm combining adduction, flexion, and internal rotation. Posterior dislocation caused by indirect force most often occurs secondary to accidental electric shock or convulsive seizures. In this type of dislocation, the humeral head lies posterior to the glenoid fossa and usually impacts on the posterior rim of the glenoid.

Making a correct diagnosis is often problematic, because the abnormality can easily be overlooked on the standard anteroposterior film of the shoulder, where the overlapping humeral head and glenoid fossa may be interpreted as normal. It is imperative when dealing with suspected posterior dislocation to demonstrate radiographically the glenoid fossa in profile. This can be performed on the anteroposterior projection by rotating the patient 40 degrees toward the affected side (see Fig. 5.5). Normally, the glenohumeral joint space is clear on this view. Obliteration of the space because of overlap of the humeral head with the glenoid is diagnostic of posterior dislocation (Fig. 5.48). Diagnosis can also be made on the axillary projection, although limited abduction of the arm may make it impossible to obtain this view (Fig. 5.49).

Compression fracture of the anteromedial aspect of the humeral head, known as trough line impaction *(trough sign)*, commonly occurs in posterior dislocation secondary to the impaction of the humeral head on the posterior glenoid rim. This sign refers to a vertical or archlike line within the cortex of the humeral head that projects parallel and lateral to the articular end of this bone. The anteroposterior view of the shoulder with the arm externally rotated readily demonstrates this type of fracture (Fig. 5.50); it is also identifiable on the axillary projection (see Fig. 5.49).

Complications. Anterior or posterior dislocation in the glenohumeral joint may result in complications such as recurrent dislocations, posttraumatic arthritis, and injury to the axillary nerve and axillary artery.

Impingement Syndrome

Impingement syndrome of the shoulder refers to a condition in which the supraspinatus tendon and subacromial bursa are chronically entrapped between the humeral head inferiorly and either the anterior acromion itself, spurs of the anterior acromion or acromioclavicular joint, or the coracoacromial ligament superiorly (coracoacromial arch). Early diagnosis and treatment of impingement syndrome are critical to prevent progression of this condition and improve shoulder function. Frequently, however, clinical signs and symptoms are nonspecific, and the diagnosis is often delayed until a full-thickness defect in the rotator cuff has developed. Only rarely can it be definitely diagnosed based on the clinical findings, characterized by severe pain during abduction and external rotation of the arm. More reliable are radiographic findings associated with this syndrome, including subacromial proliferation of bone, spurring at the inferior aspect of the acromion, and degenerative changes of the humeral tuberosities at the insertion of the rotator cuff.

Neer described three progressive stages of impingement syndrome apparent clinically and at surgery. Stage I consists of edema and hemorrhage and is reversible with conservative therapy. It typically occurs in young individuals engaged in sport activities requiring excessive use of the arm above the head (i.e., swimming). Stage II implies fibrosis and thickening of the subacromial soft tissue, rotator cuff

Figure 5.48 Posterior shoulder dislocation. On the anteroposterior projection of the shoulder obtained by rotating the patient 40 degrees toward the affected side (Grashey view), overlap of the medially displaced humeral head with the glenoid is virtually diagnostic of posterior dislocation.

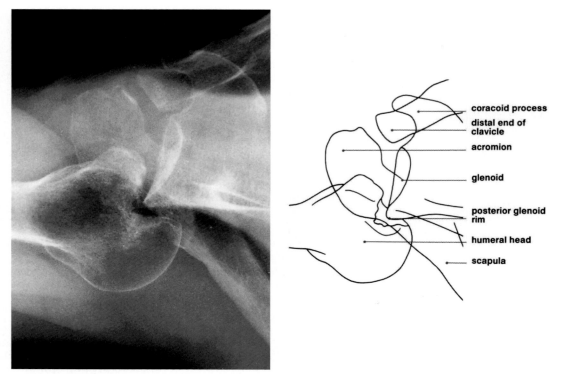

Figure 5.49 Posterior shoulder dislocation. Axillary projection of the shoulder demonstrates posterior dislocation. Note the associated compression fracture of the anteromedial aspect of the humeral head.

tendinitis, and sometimes a partial tear of the rotator cuff. It is manifested clinically by recurrent pain and is often seen in patients 25 to 40 years old. Stage III represents complete rupture of the rotator cuff and is associated with progressive disability. It usually is seen in patients older than 40 years old. Arthrography aids little in the early diagnosis of impingement syndrome, and other ancillary imaging techniques are also unsatisfactory for demonstration of the lesion in the early stages. Because of its high soft-tissue contrast resolution and multiplanar imaging capabilities, MRI is the only technique that can ac-

curately image the early changes of this condition, in particular bursal thickening and effusion (subacromial bursitis), edema, and inflammatory changes of the rotator cuff and its tendons (see Fig. 5.51).

Rotator Cuff Tear

The rotator cuff of the shoulder, a musculotendinous structure about the joint capsule, consists of four intrinsic muscles: the subscapularis, the supraspinatus, the infraspinatus, and the teres minor (see Fig. 5.3). The tendinous portions of the cuff, which converge and fuse to

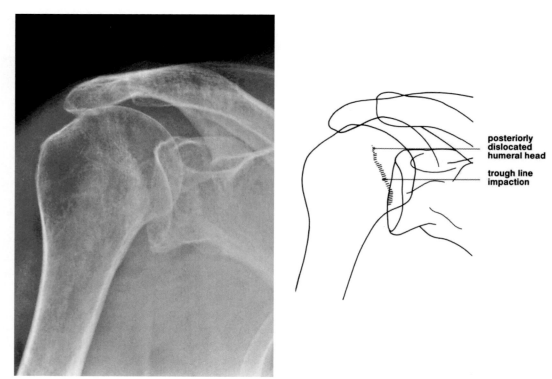

Figure 5.50 Posterior shoulder dislocation. Anteroposterior view of the shoulder demonstrates posterior dislocation in the glenohumeral joint. Note the trough line impaction on the anteromedial aspect of the humeral head.

Figure 5.51 Impingement syndrome. (A) Oblique coronal T1-weighted MR image of early stage of the impingement syndrome. There is slightly increased signal in the critical zone of the supraspinatus tendon. Peribursal fat demarcating the subacromial subdeltoid bursa complex is still intact. (From Holt RG, et al., 1990, with permission.) **(B)** Oblique coronal T1-weighted MR image of stage II impingement syndrome shows a partial tear *(black arrow)* of the supraspinatus tendon. The subacromial–subdeltoid fat line is still preserved *(white arrows)*. **(C)** Oblique coronal T2*-weighted (multiplanar gradient-recalled) image of stage II impingement syndrome demonstrate high-signal-intensity attenuation of the inferior surface of the supraspinatus tendon *(black arrow)*.

form an envelope covering the humeral head, insert into the anatomic neck and tuberosities of the humerus. Tears usually occur in the supraspinatus portion of the cuff, approximately 1 cm from the insertion into the greater tuberosity of the humerus (known as a critical zone).

Injury to the rotator cuff may occur secondary to dislocation in the glenohumeral joint or to sudden abduction of the arm against resistance. It is most commonly seen in patients older than 50 years of age because of normal degenerative changes in the cuff that predispose this structure to rupture after even minor shoulder injuries. Clinically, patients characteristically present with pain in the shoulder and inability to abduct the arm.

Although radiographs of the shoulder are usually insufficient to demonstrate the tear, certain radiographic features characteristic of chronic rotator cuff tear may be present on the anteroposterior view. These include: (a) narrowing of the acromiohumeral space to less than 6 mm; (b) erosion of the inferior aspect of the acromion secondary to cephalad migration of the humeral head; and (c) flattening and atrophy of the greater tuberosity of the humeral head caused by the absence of traction stress by the rotator cuff (Fig. 5.52). Although these findings are usually diagnostic of chronic tear, contrast arthrography may be performed to confirm or exclude the suspected diagnosis. As the intact rotator cuff normally separates the subacromial–subdeltoid bursae complex from the joint cavity, only the glenohumeral joint, the axillary recess, the bursa subscapularis,

and the bicipital tendon sheath should opacify on arthrographic examination (Fig. 5.53A; see also Fig. 5.15B). Opacification of the subacromial–subdeltoid bursae is diagnostic of rotator cuff tear (Fig. 5.53B,C). Occasionally, contrast is seen only in the substance of the rotator cuff, whereas the subacromial–subdeltoid bursae complex remains unopacified, indicating a partial tear of the cuff (Fig. 5.54).

Although arthrography of the shoulder remains the effective technique for evaluating a suspected rotator-cuff tear, MRI is being used more frequently as a noninvasive method to diagnose such a tear. The advantage of MRI over arthrography is not only that it is a noninvasive technique but also that it allows visualization of the osseous and periarticular soft tissue of the shoulder in the coronal, sagittal, axial, and oblique planes. It has proved to be highly sensitive (75% to 92%) and accurate (84% to 94%) for diagnosing full-thickness rotator cuff disruption. Moreover, there is excellent correlation between preoperative assessment of the size of rotator cuff tears by MRI and the measurement at surgery.

Visualization of the rotator cuff is optimal when oblique coronal images are obtained. The MRI findings for rotator cuff tear consist of focal discontinuity of the supraspinatus tendon, tendon and muscle retraction, abnormally increased signal within the tendon, and the presence of fluid in the subacromial–subdeltoid bursa complex (Figs. 5.55, 5.56, and 5.57).

It must be noted, however, that the complex MRI appearance of the rotator cuff can be confounding in the diagnosis of a tear; experi-

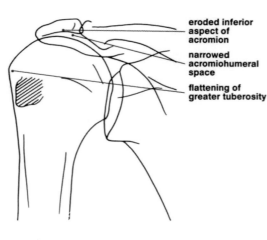

eroded inferior
aspect of
acromion

narrowed
acromiohumeral
space

flattening of
greater tuberosity

Figure 5.52 Chronic rotator cuff tear. The characteristics of chronic rotator cuff tear are identifiable on the anteroposterior view of the shoulder.

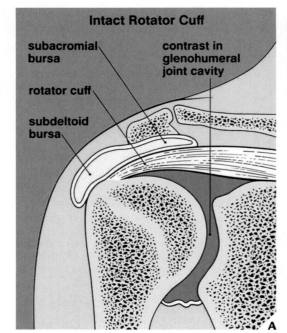

Intact Rotator Cuff

subacromial
bursa

contrast in
glenohumeral
joint cavity

rotator cuff

subdeltoid
bursa

A

Complete Rotator Cuff Tear

contrast in
subacromial–
subdeltoid bursae

B

Figure 5.53 Arthrography of the shoulder joint. The intact rotator cuff **(A)** does not allow communication between the glenohumeral joint cavity and the subacromial–subdeltoid bursae complex. When arthrography is performed for suspected tear of the cuff, opacification of the bursae **(B,C)** indicates abnormal communication between them and the joint cavity, confirming the diagnosis.

C

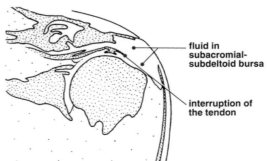

Partial Rotator Cuff Tear

leak of contrast into substance of cuff

subacromial–subdeltoid bursae

tracking of contrast

A

B

Figure 5.54 Partial tear of the rotator cuff. This injury (**A**) allows tracking of contrast into the substance of the cuff (**B**), whereas the subacromial–subdeltoid bursae remain free of contrast.

fluid in subacromial–subdeltoid bursa

interruption of the tendon

Figure 5.55 Full-thickness tear of the supraspinatus tendon. (**A**) Oblique coronal MR image of the left shoulder (multiplanar gradient-recalled T2*-weighted) demonstrates interruption of the supraspinatus tendon and fluid in the subacromial–subdeltoid bursae complex, diagnostic of complete rotator cuff tear. (From Holt RG et al., 1990, with permission.) (**B**) Oblique coronal T2-weighted fat-suppressed MR image of the right shoulder shows a full-thickness tear of the supraspinatus tendon (arrows) and medial retraction of the supraspinatus muscle (*open arrow*).

Figure 5.56 Rotator cuff tear. (A) T2*-weighted (multiplanar gradient-recalled) coronal image shows complete rotator cuff tear with direct communication of fluid between the glenohumeral joint and the subacromial–subdeltoid bursa complex *(arrow)*. **(B)** and **(C)** T2*-weighted (multiplanar gradient-recalled) coronal oblique images show massive rotator cuff tear *(arrows)* with disruption of the supraspinatus *(S)* and infraspinatus *(I)* tendons anteriorly and posteriorly.

ence and total knowledge of normal anatomy are required for correct interpretation. Large tears are well visualized on MR images as areas of discontinuity and irregularity of the rotator cuff tendons, with joint fluid tracking through the cuff defect into the subacromial–subdeltoid bursa complex. With complete rotator cuff tears and retraction of the tendons, the corresponding muscle belly assumes a distorted globular shape that is easily recognized. Chronic tears may result in atrophy of the cuff musculature, manifested on T1-weighted images by a decrease in muscle size and bulk, and by infiltration of the muscle by a band of high-signal-intensity fat. Partial tears may be seen as various

foci of high signal intensity within the homogeneous low signal intensity of the tendon or as irregularity or thinning of the tendon. Obscuration of the subacromial–subdeltoid fat line on T2-weighted images is a sensitive indicator of rotator cuff tears, and increased signal intensity in the same region on T2-weighted sequences corresponds to leakage of joint fluid into the subacromial–subdeltoid bursae complex.

MRI provides the surgeon with critical information regarding size and location of a tear, the specific tendons involved, the degree of musculature atrophy and tendon retraction, and the quality of the

Figure 5.57 Rotator cuff tear. (A) T1-weighted and **(B)** T2*-weighted coronal oblique images show a complete supraspinatus tendon tear with proximal retraction of tendon edge to level of the acromioclavicular joint *(straight arrows)*. Mild fatty atrophy of the supraspinatus muscle *(small curved arrow)* is present.

Figure 5.58 MRI of ALPSA lesion. Axial gradient-echo T2*-weighted MR image shows avulsion of the anterior cartilaginous labrum (*curved arrow*), but the anterior scapular periosteum, although stripped from the bone, remains attached to the labrum (*open arrow*).

torn edges. Such information is invaluable for assessing the feasibility of surgery and the type of necessary repair.

Injury to the Cartilaginous Labrum

Bankart Lesion. Injury to the anterior–inferior cartilaginous labrum, which is usually associated with an avulsion of the inferior glenohumeral ligament from the anterior–inferior glenoid rim, occurs during anterior dislocation in the glenohumeral joint. It may affect only a fibrocartilaginous portion of the glenoid, or it may be associated with a fracture of the anterior aspect of the inferior bony rim of the glenoid (see Fig. 5.45).

POLPSA Lesion. The POLPSA lesion, recently reported as the posterior labrocapsular periosteal sleeve avulsion, consists of avulsion of the attachment of the glenohumeral capsule and the periosteum to which it is attached sustained during posterior shoulder dislocation. Unlike the Bankart lesion, the posterior glenoid labrum is intact, although it is detached from the osseous glenoid.

ALPSA Lesion. The ALPSA lesion is similar to the Bankart lesion. It is an avulsion injury of the anterior labroligamentous periosteal sleeve sustained during anterior dislocation in glenohumeral joint; however, the anterior scapular periosteum does not rupture as it does in the classic Bankart lesion. This results in medial displacement of the labroligamentous structures that also rotate inferiorly on the scapular neck. ALPSA lesion is best seen on axial MRI (Fig. 5.58).

Perthes Lesion. Perthes lesion, originally described by the German surgeon Perthes in 1905, is very similar to ALPSA lesion. The scapular periosteum is intact, however it is stripped medially causing incomplete avulsion of the anterior glenoid labrum. Because avulsed cartilaginous labrum is either not displaced or minimally displaced, conventional MR imaging may not detect this abnormality. The most effective technique to diagnose this lesion is MR arthrography with patient's arm in abduction and external rotation (so-called ABER position) (Fig. 5.59).

Figure 5.59 Perthes lesion. A 32-year-old man had anterior shoulder instability after fall on outstretched hand. **(A)** Axial T1-weighted MR arthrogram with fat saturation shows thickened anterior labrum (*arrows*), but no tear is demonstrated. **(B)** Oblique axial T1-weighted MR arthrogram obtained in ABER (abduction–external rotation) position shows detachment of the anterior labrum from the glenoid (*curved arrow*). (Courtesy of Dr. T.K. Wischer, Basel, Switzerland. Reprinted with permission from Wischer TK, Bredella MA, Genant HK, Stoller DW, Bost FW, Tirman PF. Perthes lesion (a variant of the Bankart lesion): MR imaging and MR arthrographic findings with surgical correlation. *AJR Am J Roentgenol* 2002; 178: 233–237.)

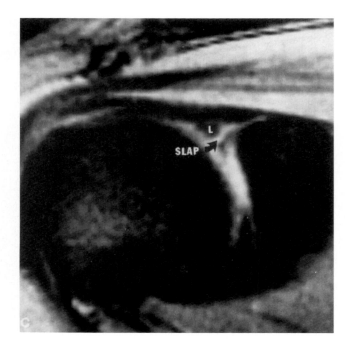

Figure 5.60 MRI of SLAP lesion. A coronal oblique T2*-weighted MRI shows a type II SLAP lesion involving anterior superior glenoid labrum (*L*). Note linear high intensity signal extending across the base of the labrum (*arrow*).

SLAP Lesion. Injury to the superior portion of the cartilaginous glenoid labrum, on either side of the attachment of the long head of the biceps tendon into the labrum at the superior glenoid tubercle, is referred to as SLAP lesion (a superior labral, anterior, and posterior tear) and results from a sudden forced abduction of the arm. It is usually sustained in athletic activities such as tennis, volleyball, or baseball, although occasionally the mechanism of this injury may be a fall on the outstretched arm with the shoulder in abduction and slight forward flexion at the time of impact. SLAP lesions have been classified into four types. Type I is the least common (10%) and consists of a degenerative frayed irregular appearance of the superior portion of the cartilaginous labrum. In this type of injury the labrum remains firmly attached to the glenoid rim. Type II is the most common (40%) and consists of separation of the superior portion of the cartilaginous labrum to the level of the middle glenohumeral ligament, as well as separation of the tendon of the long head of the biceps from the glenoid rim. Type III (30%) consists of a bucket-handle tear of the superior portion of the labrum; however, the attachment site of the tendon of the long head of the biceps is intact. Type IV (15%) consists of the bucket-handle tear of the superior labrum extending into the biceps tendon. MRI findings of SLAP lesion include linear increased signal intensity in the superior portion of the cartilaginous labrum on T2-weighted sequences (Fig. 5.60); on MR arthrography contrast extends into a detached superior portion of the labrum.

GLAD Lesion. Injury to the anteroinferior portion of the cartilaginous glenoid labrum associated with glenolabral articular disruption is referred to as a GLAD lesion. The usual mechanism of this injury is a fall on an outstretched arm in abduction and external rotation resulting in the forced adduction injury to the shoulder where the humeral head strikes against the adjacent articular cartilage of the glenoid. The lesion consists of a superficial tear of the anteroinferior portion of the labrum and is always associated with an inferior flap tear but without evidence of anterior glenohumeral joint instability on physical examination. The deep fibers of the inferior glenohumeral ligament remain attached to the labrum and glenoid rim. A GLAD lesion is effectively diagnosed on MR arthrography. The findings include a nondisplaced tear of the anteroinferior labrum with an adjacent chondral injury, which can range from a cartilaginous flap tear to a depressed lesion of the articular cartilage (Fig. 5.61).

GLOM Lesion. GLOM lesion or GLOM sign (glenolabral ovoid mass) represents an avulsion of a portion of the anterior labrum seen on axial MR image.

Figure 5.61 MRI of GLAD lesion. Axial T2-weighted MR arthrogram of the left shoulder shows a nondisplaced tear of the anteroinferior labrum associated with an osteochondral defect (*arrow*) in a 21-year-old professional ice-hockey player who sustained anterior shoulder dislocation.(Courtesy of Dr. J. Tehranzadeh, Orange, California.)

Figure 5.62 MRI of Buford complex. MR arthrogram shows an absent anterior superior glenoid labrum (*arrow*) and markedly thickened middle glenohumeral ligament (*open arrow*), characteristic features of the Buford complex. This congenital variant can mimic a labral tear. (Courtesy of Dr. L. Steinbach, San Francisco, California.)

Buford Complex. A congenital variant of absence of the anterior superior labrum and marked thickening of the middle glenohumeral ligament that can mimic a labral tear has been termed the Buford complex (Fig. 5.62). MRI appearance of this complex should be differentiated from other normal anatomic variants, such as an isolated detachment of the anterior superior labrum (also known as sublabral foramen or sublabral hole), undercutting of articular cartilage between the labrum and the glenoid cortex, or the presence of a synovial recess (sulcus) interposed between the glenoid rim and the cartilaginous labrum.

Injury to the Glenohumeral Ligaments (GHL)

There are three glenohumeral ligaments located within the anterior portion of the glenohumeral joint that contribute to anterior shoulder stability. The inferior glenohumeral ligament (IGHL) is the thickest structure and extends from the glenoid labrum to the anatomic neck of the humerus. The middle glenohumeral ligament (MGHL) originates at the superior portion of the anterior labrum, and attaches to the base of the lesser tuberosity of the humerus. The superior glenohumeral ligament (SGHL) originates from the superior-anterior labrum and attaches distally to the superior aspect of the lesser tuberosity of the humerus. All of these ligaments may be injured during a traumatic event to the shoulder joint; however, the inferior glenohumeral ligament, the most important stabilizer of the glenohumeral joint, is most commonly traumatized.

HAGL Lesion. Avulsion of the inferior glenohumeral ligament from the anatomic neck of the humerus is referred to as a HAGL lesion. It may be caused by shoulder dislocation, and is often associated with a tear of the subscapularis tendon. This abnormality can be seen on axial, oblique coronal, or sagittal MR images or on MR arthrography.

BHAGL Lesion. Bony humeral avulsion of the glenohumeral ligament (BHAGL) is similar to HAGL, but it is associated with avulsion of a bone fragment from the humerus.

Miscellaneous Abnormalities

Adhesive Capsulitis. Adhesive capsulitis, also referred to as "frozen shoulder," usually results from posttraumatic adhesive inflammation between the joint capsule and the peripheral articular carti-lage of the shoulder. Clinically, it is characterized by pain, stiffness, and limitation of motion in the shoulder joint.

Because radiography, which may only reveal disuse periarticular osteoporosis secondary to this condition, is insufficient to make a diagnosis, single- or double-contrast arthrography is the technique of choice when this abnormality is suspected. The arthrogram usually reveals decreased capacity of the joint capsule, or even complete obliteration of the axillary and subscapular recesses, findings diagnostic of this condition (Fig. 5.63).

Recently, the use of MR imaging has been advocated to diagnose adhesive capsulitis of the shoulder. Emig et al. reported that thickening of the capsule and synovium greater than 4 mm detected on MR studies may be a useful criterion for the diagnosis of this condition.

Acromioclavicular Separation. Injuries to the acromioclavicular joint, which are commonly sustained during athletic activities by individuals between the ages of 15 and 40 years, often result in acromioclavicular separation (dislocation). Various forces may cause injury to the acromioclavicular joint. The most common is a downward blow to the lateral aspect of the shoulder that drives the acromion inferiorly (caudad); others are traction on the arm pulling the shoulder away from the chest wall and a fall on the outstretched hand or on the flexed elbow with the arm flexed forward 90 degrees.

Whatever the mechanism of injury, the degree of damage to the acromioclavicular and coracoclavicular ligaments varies with the severity of the applied force and ranges from *mild sprain* of the acromioclavicular ligament, to *moderate sprain* involving tear of the acromioclavicular ligament, and sprain of the coracoclavicular ligament, with consequent dislocation in the acromioclavicular joint (Table 5.3). It is important to bear in mind, as Rockwood and Green have pointed out, that the major deformity seen in this type of injury is not elevation of the clavicle, but rather downward displacement of the scapula and upper extremity (Fig. 5.64), although some degree of cephalad displacement of the distal end of the clavicle may accompany this type of injury. The clinical symptoms also vary with the severity of the injury; patients may present with symptoms ranging from tenderness, swelling, and slight limitation of motion in the joint to complete inability to abduct the arm.

Suspected acromioclavicular dislocation is readily evaluated on the anteroposterior projection of the shoulder obtained with a 15-de-

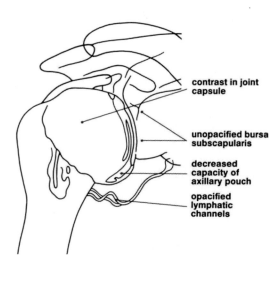

Figure 5.63 Adhesive capsulitis. Double-contrast arthrogram of the shoulder demonstrates the characteristic findings of frozen shoulder. The capacity of the axillary pouch is markedly decreased and the subscapularis recess remains unopacified, whereas the lymphatic channels are filled with contrast secondary to increased intracapsular pressure.

Table 5.3 **Grades of Acromioclavicular Separation**

Grade	Radiographic Characteristics
I (Mild Sprain)	Minimal widening of acromioclavicular joint space, which normally measures 0.3–0.8 cm Coracoclavicular distance within normal range of 1.0–1.3 cm
II (Moderate Sprain)	Widening of acromioclavicular joint space to 1.0–1.5 cm Increase of 25% to 50% in coracoclavicular distance
III (Severe Sprain)	Marked widening of acromioclavicular joint space to 1.5 cm or more and of coracoclavicular distance by 50% or more Dislocation in acromioclavicular joint Apparent cephalad displacement of distal end of clavicle

Figure 5.65 Normal measurements. Schematic diagram shows the normal relation of the coracoid process to the inferior aspect of the clavicle and the normal width of the joint space at the acromioclavicular articulation.

gree cephalad angulation of the radiographic tube (see Fig. 5.11). Often it is necessary to obtain a stress view in this projection by strapping a 5- to 10-pound weight to each forearm. A comparison study of the opposite shoulder is invariably helpful.

Radiographic studies can also be supplemented by quantitating acromioclavicular separation on the basis of the normal relations of the coracoid process, the clavicle, and the acromion (Fig. 5.65). Normally, the distance between the coracoid process and the inferior aspect of the clavicle, known as the coracoclavicular distance, ranges from 1.0 to 1.3 cm; the joint space at the articulation of the clavicle with

the acromion measures 0.3 to 0.8 cm. The degree of widening at these points helps to determine the severity of the injury. An increase, for example, of 0.5 cm in the coracoclavicular distance or a widening of the distance by 50% or more compared with that in the opposite shoulder is characteristic of grade III acromioclavicular separation (Fig. 5.66).

Recently, Antonio and colleagues introduced MRI classification of acromioclavicular joint injury. In *type I injury*, there is a sprain of the acromioclavicular ligament, but the coracoclavicular ligaments are intact. MR imaging shows nonspecific findings. In *type II injury*, there is evidence of rupture of the acromioclavicular ligament, but the coracoclavicular ligament is only sprained. MR imaging shows edema of the coracoclavicular ligament and continuity of its fibers. Acromial end of the clavicle and acromion may show marrow edema. Oblique sagittal MR images are most effective to demonstrate this abnormality. In *type III injury*, there is complete acromioclavicular joint dislocation and the coracoclavicular ligament is ruptured. The deltoid and trapezius muscles may be detached from the distal end of the clavicle. Oblique coronal and sagittal MR images are most effective to diagnose this injury. In *type IV injury*, the acromial end of the clavicle is posteriorly dislocated and the scapula is displaced anteroinferiorly. The most effective MR image to detect this type of injury is in axial orientation. In *type V injury*, the findings are similar to type III, but more severe. The trapezius and deltoid muscle attachments on the clavicle and acromion are completely stripped, and the scapula droops inferiorly. The acromial end of the clavicle is displaced cephalad. Coronal, oblique sagittal, and axial MR images well demonstrate this injury. In the rarest, *type VI injury*, the acromial end of the clavicle is displaced inferiorly towards the acromion and coracoid process.

Posttraumatic Osteolysis of the Distal Clavicle. After injury to the shoulder, such as sprain of the acromioclavicular joint, resorption of the distal (acromial) end of the clavicle may occasionally occur. The osteolytic process, which is associated with mild-to-moderate pain, usually begins within 2 months after the injury. The initial radiographic findings consist of soft-tissue swelling and periarticular osteoporosis. In its late stage, resorption of the distal end of the clavicle results in marked widening of the acromioclavicular joint (Fig. 5.67).

Suprascapular Nerve Syndrome. The suprascapular nerve runs within the spinoglenoid and suprascapular notches of the scapula. It is a mixed motor and sensory nerve that provides motor fibers to the supraspinatus and infraspinatus muscles and carries pain fibers from the glenohumeral and acromioclavicular joints. A rarely diagnosed

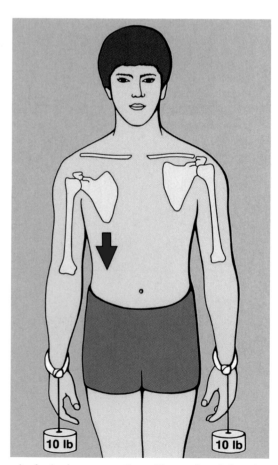

Figure 5.64 Acromioclavicular separation. The major deformity seen in acromioclavicular separation is the downward displacement of the scapula and upper extremity, whereas the position of the clavicle in the affected side remains the same relative to the clavicle in the unaffected side. (Modified from Rockwood CA Jr., Green DP, 1975, with permission.)

Figure 5.66 Acromioclavicular dislocation. (A) Anteroposterior view of shoulder shows apparent cephalad displacement of the distal end of the clavicle and the widening of the acromioclavicular joint and the coracoclavicular distance. The marked deformities seen here, which are characteristic of grade III acromioclavicular separation (severe sprain), are the result of tear of the coracoclavicular and the acromioclavicular ligaments with consequent dislocation in the acromioclavicular joint **(B)**.

clinical entity, a suprascapular nerve syndrome results from entrapment or compromise of this nerve at some point in its path (Fig. 5.68). Most patients report nonspecific pain in the shoulder, neck, anterior chest, or in a combination in these anatomic sites. Later severe weakness and atrophy of the supraspinatus and infraspinatus muscles may occur. A variety of causes of injury or entrapment of the suprascapular nerve have been reported, including fracture of the scapula or humerus, anterior shoulder dislocation, thickening of the transverse scapular ligament, rotator cuff tendonitis, and various malignant and benign tumors. Of the latter, the most commonly encountered mass is a ganglion located in the spinoglenoid notch. The most effective technique to diagnose suprascapular nerve syndrome is MR imaging. This modality can distinguish different etiologic factors responsible for the syndrome and provide anatomic information and demonstrate atrophy of the spinatus muscles. It also can exclude other causes of a shoulder pain, such as rotator cuff tear.

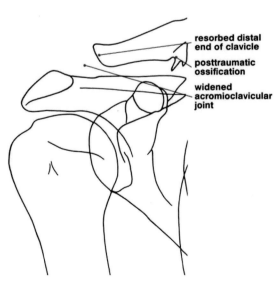

Figure 5.67 Posttraumatic osteolysis. A 50-year-old man who 5 months previously had injured the right shoulder in a fall presented with symptoms of pain while playing tennis. Anteroposterior view of the shoulder shows marked widening of the acromioclavicular joint secondary to resorption of the distal end of the clavicle—radiographic features typical of posttraumatic osteolysis. Note also the posttraumatic ossification at the attachment of the coracoclavicular ligament.

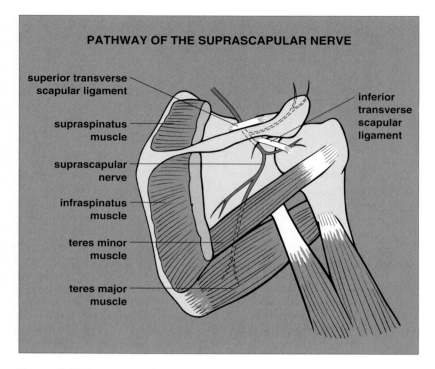

PATHWAY OF THE SUPRASCAPULAR NERVE

superior transverse
scapular ligament

inferior
transverse
scapular
ligament

supraspinatus
muscle

suprascapular
nerve

infraspinatus
muscle

teres minor
muscle

teres major
muscle

Figure 5.68 Suprascapular nerve. Pathway of the suprascapular nerve as seen from the posterior aspect of the right scapula.

PRACTICAL POINTS TO REMEMBER

[1] Fractures of the proximal humerus may be evaluated on the anteroposterior, transscapular, and transthoracic lateral projections. The latter view:
- provides a true lateral image of the proximal humerus
- allows sufficient evaluation of the degree of displacement or angulation of the fragments.

[2] Four-segment Neer classification based on the presence or absence of displacement of the four major fragments is a practical and effective way to evaluate the fractures of the proximal humerus.

[3] Fractures of the scapula, particularly if comminuted and displaced, are best evaluated on the transscapular (or Y) projection. If the diagnosis is in doubt, or the fracture cannot be well demonstrated on conventional radiography, trispiral tomography or CT should be performed.

[4] Neer classification of fractures of the acromial end of the clavicle is based on the site and direction of the fracture line and integrity of the ligaments.

[5] For precise evaluation of the shoulder joint and better demonstration of the glenohumeral articulation, the anteroposterior projection obtained with the patient rotated approximately 40 degrees toward the affected side (Grashey view):
- eliminates the overlap of the humeral head and the glenoid fossa
- allows visualization of the glenohumeral joint space and the glenoid in profile.

[6] The Hill-Sachs lesion, which is best demonstrated on the anteroposterior projection obtained with the arm internally rotated, and the Bankart lesion are virtually diagnostic of previous anterior dislocation.

[7] Compression fracture (trough line sign) of the anteromedial aspect of the humeral head is a common sequela of posterior dislocation. The anteroposterior projection obtained with the arm externally rotated readily demonstrates this finding.

[8] MRI characteristics of impingement syndrome include:
- cystic and sclerotic changes in the greater tuberosity
- perimuscular and peritendinous edema
- thickening of subacromial bursa (or effusion)
- thinning of the supraspinatus tendon
- increased signal intensity in the tendon (on T2 weighting)
- subacromial spur.

[9] Rotator cuff tear may effectively be evaluated by contrast arthrography. Opacification of the subacromial–subdeltoid bursae complex is diagnostic of this injury.

[10] MRI characteristics of rotator cuff tear include:
- discontinuity of the rotator cuff tendons
- high signal intensity within the tendon structure (on T2-weighted images)
- retraction of the musculotendinous junction of spinatus muscles
- atrophy of the supraspinatus muscle and infiltration by fat
- obscuration of the subacromial–subdeltoid fat line (on T1-weighted images)
- fluid in the subacromial–subdeltoid bursae complex.

[11] Oblique sagittal MR images are useful to demonstrate three types of acromion: type 1, flat; type 2, smoothly curved; type 3, hooked.

[12] Axial MR images are useful to demonstrate three types of anterior capsular insertion to the scapula.

[13] ABER position of the arm (abduction and external rotation) is effective to evaluate subtle abnormalities of cartilaginous labrum and labral ligmentous complex during MR arthrography.

[14] Acromioclavicular separation is best demonstrated on the stress anteroposterior projection obtained with a 15-degree cephalad angulation of the radiographic tube and weights strapped to the patient's forearms. The radiographic characteristics of this condition include:
- width of the acromioclavicular joint space
- width of the coracoclavicular distance
- presence or absence of apparent cephalad displacement of the distal end of the clavicle.

[15] Suprascapular nerve syndrome results from entrapment of this nerve caused by a variety of pathological processes including fracture of the scapula or humerus, anterior shoulder dislocation, rotator cuff tendonitis, and benign or maligmant tumors. MRI is the ideal technique to diagnose this syndrome.

SUGGESTED READINGS

Adams JC. *Outline of fractures including joint injuries,* 4th ed. Baltimore: Williams & Wilkins; 1964.

Anderson JE: *Grant's atlas of anatomy,* 8th ed. Baltimore: Williams & Wilkins; 1983.

Antonio GE, Cho JH, Chung CB, Trudell DJ, Resnick D. MR imaging appearance and classification of acromioclavicular joint injury. *AJR Am J Roentgenol* 2003;180:1103–1110.

Arger PH, Oberkircher PE, Miller WT. Lipohemarthrosis. *AJR Am J Roentgenol* 1974;121:97–100.

Bailey RW. Acute and recurrent dislocation of the shoulder. *J Bone Joint Surg [Am]* 1967;49A:767–773.

Bankart A. The pathology and treatment of recurrent dislocation of the shoulder joint. *Br J Surg* 1938;26:23–29.

Beltran J. *MRI musculoskeletal system.* Philadelphia: JB Lippincott; 1990:3.2–3.22; 4.2–4.11.

Beltran J, Bencardino J, Mellado J, Rosenberg ZS, Irish RD. MR arthrography of the shoulder: variants and pitfalls. *Radiographics* 1997;17:1403–1412.

Beltran J, Gray LA, Bools JC, Zuelzer W, Weis LD, Unverferth LJ. Rotator cuff lesions of the shoulder: evaluation by direct sagittal CT arthrography. *Radiology* 1986;160:161–165.

Beltran J, Rosenberg ZS, Chandnani VP, Cuomo F, Beltran S, Rokito A. Glenohumeral instability: evaluation with MR arthrography. *Radiographics* 1997;17:657–673.

Bencardino JT, Beltran J, Rosenberg ZS, et al. Superior labrum anterior-posterior lesions: diagnosis with MR arthrography of the shoulder. *Radiology* 2000;214:267–271.

Bergin D, Schweitzer ME. Indirect magnetic resonance arthrography. *Skeletal Radiol* 2003;10:551–558.

Berquist TH. *Imaging of sports injuries.* Gaithersburg, MD: Aspen Publication, 1992:265–301.

Bigliani LU, Morrison DS, April EW. The morphology of the acromion and its relationship to rotator cuff tears [abstract]. *Orthop Trans* 1986;10:228.

Bigliani LU, Ticker JB, Flatlow EL, Soslowsky LJ, Mow VC. The relationship of acromial architecture to rotator cuff disease. *Clin Sports Med* 1991;10:823–838.

Blum A, Boyer B, Regent D, Simon JM, Claudon M, Mole D. Direct coronal view of the shoulder with arthrographic CT. *Radiology* 1993;188:677–681.

Braunstein EM, O'Connor G. Double-contrast arthrotomography of the shoulder. *J Bone Joint Surg [Am]* 1982;64A:192–195.

Brenner ML, Morrison WB, Carrino JA, et al. Direct MR arthrography of the shoulder: is exercise prior to imaging beneficial or detrimental? *Radiology* 2000;215:491–496.

Bright AS, Torpey B, Magid D, Codd T, McFarland EG. Reliability of radiographic evaluation for acromial morphology. *Skeletal Radiol* 1997;26:718–721.

Brossman J, Stäbler A, Preidler KW, Trudell D, Resnick D. Sternoclavicular joint: MR imaging-anatomic correlation. *Radiology* 1996;198:193–198.

Burk DL Jr, Karasick D, Mitchell DG, Rifkin MD. MR imaging of the shoulder: correlation with plain radiography. *AJR Am J Roentgenol* 1990;154:549–553.

Carrino JA, McCauley TR, Katz LD, Smith RC, Lange RC. Rotator cuff: evaluation with fast spin-echo versus conventional spin-echo MR imaging. *Radiology* 1997;202:533–539.

Carroll KW, Helms CA. Magnetic resonance imaging of the shoulder: a review of potential sources of diagnostic errors. *Skeletal Radiol* 2002;31:373–383.

Carroll KW, Helms CA, Otte MT, Moellken SMC, Fritz R. Enlarged spinoglenoid notch veins causing suprascapular nerve compression. *Skeletal Radiol* 2003;32:72–77.

Cartland JP, Crues JV III, Stauffer A, Nottage W, Ryu RKN. MR imaging in the evaluation of SLAP injuries of the shoulder: findings in 10 patients. *AJR Am J Roentgenol* 1992;159:787–792.

Chandnani VP, Yeager TD, DeBerardino T, et al. Glenoid labral tears: prospective evaluation with MR imaging, MR arthrography, and CT arthrography. *AJR Am J Roentgenol* 1993;161:1229–1235.

Chapman MW. Closed intramedullary nailing of the humerus. *Instr Course Lect AAOS* 1983;32:317–324.

Chung CB, Dwek JR, Feng S, Resnick D. MR arthrography of the glenohumeral joint: a tailored approach. *AJR Am J Roentgenol* 2001;177:217–219.

Cisternino SJ, Rogers LF, Stufflebam BC, Kruglik CG. The trough line: a radiographic sign of posterior shoulder dislocation. *AJR Am J Roentgenol* 1978;130:951–954.

Clark JM, Harryman DT. Tendons, ligaments, and capsule of the rotator cuff. *J Bone Joint Surg [Am]* 1992;74A:713–725.

Cone RO, Resnick D, Danzig L. Shoulder impingement syndrome: radiographic evaluation. *Radiology* 1984;150:29–33.

Cummins CA, Bowen M, Anderson K, Messer T. Suprascapular nerve entrapment at the spinoglenoid notch in a professional baseball pitcher. *Am J Sports Med* 1999;27:810–812.

Cvitanic O, Tirman PFJ, Feller JF, Bost FW, Minter J, Carroll KW. Using abduction and external rotation of the shoulder to increase the sensitivity of MR arthrography in revealing tears of the anterior glenoid labrum. *AJR Am J Roentgenol* 1997;169:837–844.

Davies AM. Review: The current role of computed tomographic arthrography of the shoulder. *Clin Radiol* 1991;44:369–375.

Dépelteau H, Bureau NJ, Cardinal E, Aubin B, Brassard P. Arthrography of the shoulder: a simple fluoroscopically guided approach for targeting the rotator cuff interval. *AJR Am J Roentgenology* 2004;182:329–332.

Deutsch AL, Resnick D, Mink JH, et al. Computed and conventional arthrotomography of the glenohumeral joint: normal anatomy and clinical experience. *Radiology* 1984;153:603–609.

Emig EW, Schweitzer ME, Karasick D, Lubowitz J. Adhesive capsulitis of the shoulder: MR diagnosis. *AJR Am J Roentgenol* 1995;164:1457–1459.

Epstein RE, Schweitzer ME, Frieman BG, Fenlin JM Jr, Mitchell DG. Hooked acromion: prevalence on MR images of painful shoulders. *Radiology* 1993;187:479–481.

Erickson SJ, Cox IH, Hyde JS, Carrera GF, Strandt JA, Estkowski LD. Effect of tendon orientation on MR imaging signal intensity: a manifestation of the "magic angle" phenomenon. *Radiology* 1991;181:389–392.

Erickson SJ, Fitzgerald SW, Quinn SF, Carrera GF, Black KP, Lawson TL. Long bicipital tendon of the shoulder: normal anatomy and pathologic findings on MR imaging. *AJR Am J Roentgenol* 1992;158:1091–1096.

Farin PU, Jaroma H. Acute traumatic tears of the rotator cuff: value of sonography. *Radiology* 1995;197:269–273.

Farley TE, Neumann CH, Steinbach LS, Jahnke AJ, Petersen SS. Full-thickness tears of the rotator cuff of the shoulder: diagnosis with MR imaging. *AJR Am J Roentgenol* 1992;158:347–351.

Farmer KD, Hughes PM. MR arthrography of the shoulder: fluoroscopically guided technique using a posterior approach. *AJR Am J Roentgenol* 2002;178:433–434.

Farooki S, Seeger LL. MR imaging of sports injuries of the shoulder. *Semin Musculoskel Radiol* 1997;1:51–63.

Flannigan B, Kursunoglu-Brahme S, Snyder S, Karzel R, Del Pizzo W, Resnick D. MR arthrography of the shoulder: comparison with conventional MR imaging. *AJR Am J Roentgenol* 1990;155:829–832.

Fritz RC, Helms CA, Steinbach LS, Genant HK. Suprascapular nerve entrapment: evaluation with MR imaging. *Radiology* 1992;182:437–444.

Gagey N, Ravaud E, Lassau JP. Anatomy of the acromial arch: correlation of anatomy and magnetic resonance imaging. *Surg Radiol Anat* 1993;15:63–70.

Garneau RA, Renfrew DL, Moore TE, el-Khoury GY, Nepola JV, Lemke JH. Glenoid labrum: evaluation with MR imaging. *Radiology* 1991;179:519–522.

Gerscovich EO, Greenspan A. Magnetic resonance imaging in the diagnosis of suprascapular nerve syndrome. *Can Assoc Radiol J* 1993;44:307–309.

Goldman AB. Double contrast shoulder arthrography. In: Freiberger RH, Kaye JJ, eds. *Arthrography.* New York: Appleton-Century-Crofts; 1979:165–188.

Gor DM. The trough line sign. *Radiology* 2002;224:485–486.

Goss TP. Fractures of the scapula. In: Moehring HD, Greenspan A, eds. *Fractures— diagnosis and treatment.* New York: McGraw-Hill; 2000:207–216.

Goss TP. The scapula: coracoid, acromial and avulsion fractures. *Am J Orthop* 1996;25:106–115.

Graichen H, Bonel H, Stammberger T, et al. Three-dimensional analysis of the width of the subacromial space in healthy subjects and patients with impingement syndrome. *AJR Am J Roentgenol* 1999;172:1081–1086.

Griffith JF, Antonio GE, Tong CWC, Ming CK. Anterior shoulder dislocation: quantification of glenoid bone loss with CT. *AJR Am J Roentgenol* 2003;180:1423–1430.

Guntern DV, Pfirrmann CWA, Schmid MR, Zanetti M, Binkert CA, Schneeberger AG, Hodler J. Articular cartilage lesions of the glenohumeral joint: diagnostic effectiveness of MR arthrography and prevalence in patients with subacromial impingement syndrome. *Radiology* 2003;226:165–170.

Haygood TM, Langlotz CP, Kneeland JB, Iannotti JP, Williams GR Jr, Dalinka MK. Categorization of acromial shape: interobserver variability with MR imaging and conventional radiography. *AJR Am J Roentgenol* 1994;162:1377–1382.

Haynor DR, Shuman WP. Double contrast CT arthrography of the glenoid labrum and shoulder girdle. *Radiographics* 1984;4:411–421.

Hendrix RW. Imaging of fractures of the shoulder girdle and upper extremities. In: Moehring HD, Greenspan A, eds. *Fractures—Diagnosis and Treatment.* New York: McGraw-Hill; 2000:33–46.

Herzog RJ. Magnetic resonance imaging of the shoulder. *J Bone Joint Surg [Am]* 1997;79A:934–953.

Hill HA, Sachs MD. The grooved defect of the humeral head. A frequently unrecognized complication of dislocations of the shoulder joint. *Radiology* 1940;35:690–700.

Hodler J, Kursunoglu-Brahme S, Snyder SJ, et al. Rotator cuff disease: assessment with MR arthrography versus standard MR imaging in 36 patients with arthroscopic confirmation. *Radiology* 1992;182:431–436.

Holt RG, Helms CA, Steinbach L, Neumann C, Munk PL, Genant HK. Magnetic resonance imaging of the shoulder: rationale and current applications. *Skeletal Radiol* 1990;19:5–14.

Hunter JC, Blatz DJ, Escobedo EM. SLAP lesions of the glenoid labrum: CT arthrographic and arthroscopic correlation. *Radiology* 1992;184:513–518.

Jacobson JA, Lin J, Jamadar DA, Hayes CW. Aids to successful shoulder arthrography performed with a fluoroscopically guided anterior approach. *Radiographics* 2003;23:373–379.

Jee W-H, McCauley TR, Katz LD, Matheny JM, Ruwe PA, Daigneault JP. Superior labral anterior posterior (SLAP) lesions of the glenoid labrum: reliability and accuracy of MR arthrography for diagnosis. *Radiology* 2001;218:127–132.

Jordan LK, Kenter K, Griffiths HL. Relationship between MRI and clinical findings in the acromioclavicular joint. *Skeletal Radiol* 2002;31:516–521.

Kaplan PA, Bryans KC, Davick JP, Otte M, Stinson WW, Dussault RG. MR imaging of the normal shoulder: variants and pitfalls. *Radiology* 1992;184:519–524.

Kaplan PA, Helms CA, Dussault R, Anderson MW, Major NM. *Musculoskeletal MRI.* Philadelphia: WB Saunders; 2001:175–223.

Kaplan PA, Resnick D. Stress-induced osteolysis of the clavicle. *Radiology* 1986;158:139–140.

Keats TE, Pope TL Jr. The acromioclavicular joint: normal variation and the diagnosis of dislocation. *Skeletal Radiol* 1988;17:159–162.

Kilcoyne RF. Imaging choices in the shoulder impingement syndrome. *Appl Radiol* 1993;22:59–62.

Kilcoyne RF, Shuman WP, Matsen FA III, Morris M, Rockwood CA. The Neer classification of displaced proximal humeral fractures: spectrum of findings on plain radiographs and CT scans. *AJR Am J Roentgenol* 1990;154:1029–1033.

Killoran PJ, Marcove RC, Freiberger RH. Shoulder arthrography. *AJR Am J Roentgenol* 1968;103:658–668.

Klein MA, Miro PA, Spreitzer AM, Carrera GF. MR imaging of the normal sternoclavicular joint: spectrum of findings. *AJR Am J Roentgenol* 1995;164:391–393.

Kleinman PK, Kanzaria PK, Goss TP, Pappas AM. Axillary arthrotomography of the glenoid labrum. *AJR Am J Roentgenol* 1984;141:993–999.

Kneeland JB, Middleton WD, Carrera GF, et al. MR imaging of the shoulder: diagnosis of rotator cuff tears. *AJR Am J Roentgenol* 1987;149:333–337.

Kornguth PJ, Salazar AM. The apical oblique view of the shoulder: its usefulness in acute trauma. *AJR Am J Roentgenol* 1988;151:539–541.

Kreitner K-F, Botchen K, Rude J, Bittinger F, Krummenauer F, Thelen M. Superior labrum and labral-bicipital complex: MR imaging with pathologic-anatomic and histologic correlation. *AJR Am J Roentgenol* 1998;170:599–605.

Kursunoglu-Brahme S, Resnick D. Magnetic resonance imaging of the shoulder. *Radiol Clin North Am* 1990;28:941–954.

Kwak SM, Brown RR, Trudell D, Resnick D. Glenohumeral joint: comparison of shoulder positions at MR arthrography. *Radiology* 1998;208:375–380.

Lee JHE, van Raalte V, Malian V. Diagnosis of SLAP lesions with Grashey-view arthrography. *Skeletal Radiol* 2003;32:388–395.

Legan JM, Burkhard TK, Goff WB II, et al. Tears of the glenoid labrum: MR imaging of 88 arthroscopically confirmed cases. *Radiology* 1991;179:241–246.

Liou JTS, Wilson AJ, Totty WG, Brown JJ. The normal shoulder: common variations that simulate pathologic conditions at MR imaging. *Radiology* 1993;186:435–442.

Loehr SP, Pope TL Jr, Martin DF, et al. Three-dimensional MRI of the glenoid labrum. *Skeletal Radiol* 1995;24:117–121.

Ly JQ, Beall DP, Sanders TG. MR imaging of glenohumeral instability. *AJR Am J Roentgenol* 2003;181:203–213.

Mason BJ, Kier R, Bindleglass DF. Occult fractures of the greater tuberosity of the humerus: radiographic and MR imaging findings. *AJR Am J Roentgenol* 1999;172:469–473.

Massengill AD, Seeger LL, Yao L, et al. Labrocapsular ligamentous complex of the shoulder: normal anatomy, anatomic variations, and pitfalls of MR imaging and MR arthrography. *Radiographics* 1994;14:1211–1223.

McCauley TR, Pope CF, Jokl P. Normal and abnormal glenoid labrum: assessment with multiplanar gradient-echo MR imaging. *Radiology* 1992;183:35–37.

McGlynn FJ, El-Khoury GY, Albright JP. Arthrotomography of the glenoid labrum in shoulder instability. *J Bone Joint Surg [Am]* 1982;64A:506–518.

McNiesh LM, Callaghan JJ. CT arthrography of the shoulder: variations of the glenoid labrum. *AJR Am J Roentgenol* 1987;149:963–966.

Meyer SJF, Dalinka MK. Magnetic resonance imaging of the shoulder. *Orthop Clin North Am* 1990;21:497–513.

Middleton WD, Lauson TL. *Anatomy and MRI of the joints.* New York: Raven Press; 1989.

Miner Haygood T, Langlotz CP, Kneeland JB, Iannotti JP, Williams GR Jr, Dalinka MK. Categorization of acromial shape: interobserver variability with MR imaging and conventional radiography. *AJR Am J Roentgenol* 1994;162:1377–1382.

Mink JH, Harris E, Rappaport M. Rotator cuff tears: evaluation using double-contrast shoulder arthrography. *Radiology* 1985;157:621–623.

Mirowitz SA. Normal rotator cuff: MR imaging with conventional and fat-suppression techniques. *Radiology* 1991;180:735–740.

Mitchell MJ, Causey G, Berthoty DP, Sartoris DJ, Resnick D. Peribursal fat plane of the shoulder: anatomic study and clinical experience. *Radiology* 1988;168:699–704.

Mohana-Borges AVR, Chung CB, Resnick D. Superior labral anteroposterior tear: classification and diagnosis on MRI and MR arthrography. *AJR Am J Roentgenol* 2003;181:1449–1462.

Mohana-Borges AVR, Chung CB, Resnick D. MR imaging and MR arthrography of the postoperative shoulder: spectrum of normal and abnormal findings. *Radiographics* 2004;24:69–85.

Monu JUV, Pope TL Jr, Chabon SJ, Vanarthos WJ. MR diagnosis of superior labral anterior posterior (SLAP) injuries of the glenoid labrum: value of routine imaging without intraarticular injection of contrast material. *AJR Am J Roentgenol* 1994;163:1425–1429.

Morrison DS, Bigliani LU. The clinical significance of variation in acromial morphology [abstract]. *Orthop Trans* 1987;11:234.

Müller ME, Allgower M, Schneider R, Willenegger H. *Manual of internal fixation, techniques recommended by the AO Group,* 2nd ed. Berlin: Springer-Verlag; 1979.

Murphey MD. Computed radiography in the musculoskeletal imaging. *Semin Roentgenol* 1997;32:64–76.

Neer CS. Displaced proximal humeral fractures. I. Classification and evaluation. *J Bone Joint Surg [Am]* 1970;52A:1077–1089.

Neer CS, Rockwood CA. Fractures and dislocations of the shoulder. In: Rockwood CA, Green DP, eds. *Fractures.* Philadelphia: JB Lippincott; 1973:585.

Neer CS II. Four-segment classification of displaced proximal humeral fractures. *Instr Course Lect AAOS* 1975;24:160–168.

Neer CS II. Impingement lesions. *Clin Orthop* 1983;173:70–77.

Neer CS II, Rockwood CA Jr. Fractures and dislocations of the shoulder. In: Rockwood CA, Green DP, eds. *Fractures in adults.* Philadelphia: JB Lippincott; 1983:677.

Neumann CH, Holt RG, Steinbach LS, Jahnke AH Jr, Petersen SA. MR imaging of the shoulder: appearance of the supraspinatus tendon in asymptomatic volunteers. *AJR Am J Roentgenol* 1992;158:1281–1287.

Neumann CH, Petersen SA, Jahnke AH. MR imaging of the labral-capsular complex: normal variations. *AJR Am J Roentgenol* 1991;157:1015–1021.

Neviaser TJ. The anterior labroligamentous periosteal sleeve avulsion lesion: a cause of anterior instability of the shoulder. *Arthroscopy* 1993;9:17–21.

Neviaser TJ. The GLAD lesion: another cause of anterior shoulder pain. *Arthroscopy* 1993;9:22–23.

Norwood LA, Barrack R, Jackobson KE. Clinical presentation of complete tears of the rotator cuff. *J Bone Joint Surg [Am]* 1989;71A:499–505.

Palmer WE, Brown JH, Rosenthal DI. Labral-ligamentous complex of the shoulder: evaluation with MR arthrography. *Radiology* 1994;190:645–651.

Palmer WE, Brown JH, Rosenthal DI. Rotator cuff: evaluation with fat-suppressed MR arthrography. *Radiology* 1993;188:683–687.

Palmer WE, Caslowitz PL, Chew FS. MR arthrography of the shoulder: normal intraarticular structures and common abnormalities. *AJR Am J Roentgenol* 1995;164:141–146.

Parsa M, Tuite M, Norris M, Orwin J. MR imaging of rotator cuff tendon tears: comparison of T2*-weighted gradient-echo and conventional dual-echo sequences. *AJR Am J Roentgenol* 1997;168:1519–1524.

Patten RM, Spear RP, Richardson ML. Diagnostic performance of magnetic resonance imaging for the diagnosis of rotator cuff tears using supplemental images in the oblique sagittal plane. *Invest Radiol* 1994;29:87–93.

Pavlov H, Freiberger RH. Fractures and dislocations about the shoulder. *Semin Roentgenol* 1978;13:85–96.

Peh WCG, Farmer THR, Totty WG. Acromial arch shape: assessment with MR imaging. *Radiology* 1995;195:501–505.

Pennes DR. Shoulder joint: arthrographic CT appearance. *Radiology* 1990;175:878–879.

Perthes G. Über Operationen bei habitueller Schulterluxation. *Dtsch Z Chir* 1906;85:199–227.

Pretorius ES, Scott WW Jr, Fishman EK. Acute trauma to the shoulder: role of spiral computed tomographic imaging. *Emerg Radiol* 1995;2:13–17.

Quinn SF, Sheley RC, Demlow TA, Szumowski J. Rotator cuff tendon tears: evaluation with fat-suppressed MR imaging with arthroscopic correlation in 100 patients. *Radiology* 1995;195:497–501.

Rafii M, Firooznia A, Golimbu C, Minkoff J, Bonamo J. CT arthrography of capsular structures of the shoulder. *AJR Am J Roentgenol* 1986;146:361–367.

Rafii M, Firooznia H, Golimbu C, Weinreb J. Magnetic resonance imaging of glenohumeral instability. *MRI Clin North Am* 1993;1:87–104.

Rafii M, Firooznia H, Sherman O, et al. Rotator cuff lesions: signal patterns at MR imaging. *Radiology* 1990;177:817–823.

Rafii M, Minkoff J. Advanced arthrography of the shoulder with CT and MR imaging. *Radiol Clin North Am* 1998;36:609–633.

Recht MP, Resnick D. Magnetic resonance-imaging studies of the shoulder. Diagnosis of lesions of the rotator cuff. *J Bone Joint Surg [Am]* 1993;75A:1244–1253.

Reinus WR, Shady KL, Mirowitz SA, Totty WG. MR diagnosis of rotator cuff tears of the shoulder: value of using T2-weighted fat-saturated images. *AJR Am J Roentgenol* 1995;164:1451–1455.

Resnick D. Shoulder pain. *Orthop Clin North Am* 1983;14:81–97.

Resnick D. Shoulder arthrography. *Radiol Clin North Am* 1981;19:243–253.

Resnick D. Internal derangements of joints. In: Resnick D, ed. *Diagnosis of bone and joint disorders,* vol. 5, 3rd ed. Philadelphia: WB Saunders; 1995:2899–3228.

Resnik CS, Deutsch AL, Resnick D, et al. Arthrotomography of the shoulder. *Radiographics* 1984;4:963–976.

Richards RD, Sartoris DJ, Pathria MN, Resnick D. Hill-Sachs lesion and normal humeral groove: MR imaging features allowing their differentiation. *Radiology* 1994;190:665–668.

Rogers LF. The shoulder and humeral shaft. In: Rogers LF, ed. *Radiology of skeletal trauma,* 2nd ed. New York: Churchill Livingstone; 1992:732–740.

Sanders TG, Tirman PFJ, Linares R, Feller JF, Richardson R. The glenolabral articular disruption lesion: MR arthrography with arthroscopic correlation. *AJR Am J Roentgenol* 1999;172:171–175.

Schulte-Altedorneburg G, Gebhard M, Wohlgemuth WA, Fischer W, Zentner J, Wegener R, Balzer T, Bohndorf K. MR arthrography: pharmacology, efficacy and safety in clinical trials. *Skeletal Radiol* 2003;32:1–12.

Seeger LL, Gold RH, Bassett LW. Shoulder instability: evaluation with MR imaging. *Radiology* 1988;168:695–697.

Seeger LL, Gold RH, Bassett LW, Ellman H. Shoulder impingement syndrome: MR findings in 53 shoulders. *AJR Am J Roentgenol* 1988;150:343–347.

Shuman WP. Gladolinium MR arthrography of the rotator cuff. *Semin Musculoskel Radiol* 1998;2:377–384.

Simons P, Joekes E, Nelissen RGHH, Bloem JL. Posterior labrocapsular periosteal sleeve avulsion complicating locked posterior shoulder dislocation. *Skeletal Radiol* 1998;27:588–590.

Singson RD, Feldman F, Bigliani LU. CT arthrographic patterns in recurrent glenohumeral instability. *AJR Am J Roentgenol* 1987;149:749–753.

Singson RD, Hoang T, Dan S, Friedman M. MR evaluation of rotator cuff pathology using T2-weighted fast spin-echo technique with and without fat suppression. *AJR Am J Roentgenol* 1996;166:1061–1065.

Slivka J, Resnick D. An improved radiographic view of the glenohumeral joint. *J Can Assoc Radiol* 1979;30:83–85.

Smith AM, McCauley TR, Jokl P. SLAP lesions of the glenoid labrum diagnosed with MR imaging. *Skeletal Radiol* 1993;22:507–510.

Snyder SJ, Karzel RP, Del Pizzo W, Ferkel RD, Friedman MJ. SLAP lesions of the shoulder. *Arthroscopy* 1990;6:274–279.

Steinbach LS. Rotator cuff disease. In: Steinbach LS, Tirman PFJ, Peterfy CG, Feller JF, eds. *Shoulder magnetic resonance imaging.* Philadelphia: Lippincott–Raven Publishers; 1998:99–133.

Stevens KJ, Preston BJ, Wallace WA, Kerslake RW. CT imaging and three-dimensional reconstructions of shoulders with anterior glenohumeral instability. *Clin Anat* 1999;12:326–336.

Stiles RG, Otte MT. Imaging of the shoulder. *Radiology* 1993;188:603–613.

Stiles RG, Resnick D, Sartoris DJ, Anare MP. Rotator cuff disruption: diagnosis with digital arthrography. *Radiology* 1988;168:705–707.

Stoller DW, Fritz RC. Magnetic resonance imaging of impingement and rotator cuff tears. *MRI Clin North Am* 1993;1:47–63.

Stoller DW, Genant HK. The joints. In: Moss AA, Gamsu G, Genant HK, eds. *Computed tomography of the body with magnetic resonance imaging,* 2nd ed. Philadelphia: WB Saunders; 1992:435–475.

Tirman PFJ. Glenohumeral instability. In: Steinbach LS, Tirman PFJ, Peterfy CG, Feller JF, eds. *Shoulder magnetic resonance imaging.* Philadelphia: Lippincott–Raven Publishers; 1998:135–167.

Tirman PFJ, Bost FW, Garvin GJ, et al. Posterosuperior glenoid impingement of the shoulder: findings at MR imaging and MR arthrography with arthroscopic correlation. *Radiology* 1994;193:431–436.

Tirman PFJ, Feller JF, Palmer WE, Carroll KW, Steinbach LS, Cox I. The Buford complex—a variation of normal shoulder anatomy: MR arthrographic imaging features. *AJR Am J Roentgenol* 1996;166:869–873.

Tirman PFJ, Palmer WE, Feller JF. MR arthrography of the shoulder. *MRI Clin North Am* 1997;5:811–839.

Torchia ME. Fractures of the humeral head and neck. In: Moehring HD, Greenspan A, eds. *Fractures—diagnosis and treatment.* New York: McGraw-Hill; 2000:217–224.

Tuite MJ, DeSmet AA, Norris MA, Orwin JF. MR diagnosis of labral tears of the shoulder: value of T2*-weighted gradient-recalled echo images made in external rotation. *AJR Am J Roentgenol* 1995;164:941–944.

Tuite MJ, Rubin D. CT and MR arthrography of the glenoid labroligamentous complex. *Semin Musculoskel Radiol* 1998;2:363–375.

Tung GA, Hou DD. MR arthrography of the posterior labrocapsular complex: relationship with glenohumeral joint alignment and clinical posterior instability. *AJR Am J Roentgenol* 2003;180:369–375.

Turner PJ, O'Connor PJ, Saifuddin A, Williams J, Coral A, Butt WP. Prone oblique positioning for computed tomographic arthrography of the shoulder. *Br J Radiol* 1994;67:835–839.

Vanarthos WJ, Ekman EF, Bohrer SP. Radiographic diagnosis of acromioclavicular joint separation without weight bearing: importance of internal rotation of the arm. *AJR Am J Roentgenol* 1994;162:120–122.

Wenzel WW. The FBI sign. *Rocky Mount Med J* 1972;69:71–72.

Willemsen UF, Wiedemann E, Brunner U, et al. Prospective evaluation of MR arthrography performed with high-volume intraarticular saline enhancement in patients with recurrent anterior dislocations of the shoulder. *AJR Am J Roentgenol* 1998;170:79–84.

Williams MM, Snyder SJ, Buford D. The Buford complex—the cordlike middle glenohumeral ligament and absent anterosuperior labrum complex: a normal anatomic capsulolabral variant. *Arthroscopy* 1994;10:241–247.

Wischer TK, Bradella MA, Genant HK, Stoller DW, Bost FW, Tirman PFJ. Perthes lesion (a variant of the Bankart lesion): MR imaging and MR arthrographic findings with surgical correlation. *AJR Am J Roentgenol* 2002;178:233–237.

Workman TL, Burkhard TK, Resnick D, et al. Hill-Sachs lesion: comparison of detection with MR imaging, radiography, and arthroscopy. *Radiology* 1992;185:847–852.

Yang HP, Ji YL, Sung HM, Jong HM, Bo KY, Sung HH, Resnick D. MR arthrography of the labral capsular ligamentous complex in the shoulder: imaging variations and pitfalls. *AJR Am J Roentgenol* 2000;175:667–672.

Yao L, Seeger LL. Imaging of the shoulder. *Curr Opin Orthop* 1991;2:168–172.

Yu JS, Ashman CJ, Jones G. The POLPSA lesion: MR imaging findings with arthroscopic correlation in patients with posterior instability. *Skeletal Radiol* 2002;31:396–399.

Yu JS, Greenway G, Resnick D. Osteochondral defect of the glenoid fossa: cross-sectional imaging features. *Radiology* 1998;206:35–40.

Zaneti M, Weishaupt D, Jost B, Gerber C, Hodler J. MR imaging for traumatic tears of the rotator cuff: high prevalence of greater tuberosity fractures and subscapularis tendon tears. *AJR Am J Roentgenol* 1999;172:463–467.

Zlatkin MB, Bjorkengren AG, Gylys-Morin V, Resnick D, Sartoris DJ. Cross-sectional imaging of the capsular mechanism of the glenohumeral joint. *AJR Am J Roentgenol* 1988;150:151–158.

Zlatkin MB, Dalinka MK, Kressel HY. Magnetic resonance imaging of the shoulder. *Magn Reson Q* 1989;5:3–22.

Zlatkin MB, Iannotti JP, Roberts MC, et al. Rotator cuff tears: diagnostic performance of MR imaging. *Radiology* 1989;172:223–229.

UPPER LIMB II

Elbow

Elbow

Trauma to the elbow is commonly encountered in all age groups but is particularly common in childhood when children, as toddlers, often sustain elbow injuries. Play and athletic activities in childhood and young adolescence are also frequent occasions of trauma. Although history and clinical examination usually provide clues to the correct diagnosis, radiologic examination is indispensable in determining the type of fracture or dislocation, the direction of the fracture line, and the position of the fragments, and also in evaluating concomitant soft-tissue injuries.

Anatomic–Radiologic Considerations

The elbow articulation, a compound synovial joint, comprises the humeroulnar (ulnatrochlear), the humeroradial (radiocapitellar), and the proximal radioulnar joints (Fig. 6.1). It is a hinged articulation with approximately 150° of flexion from a completely extended position. The flexion and extension movements in the elbow occur in the ulnatrochlear and radiocapitellar joints. The biceps, brachioradialis, and brachialis muscles are the primary elbow flexors, while the triceps is the extensor of the elbow joint (Fig. 6.2). Rotational movement occurs as the head of the radius, held tightly by the annular ligament of the ulna, rotates within the ulna's radial notch. The proximal and distal radioulnar joints allow 90° of pronation and supination of the forearm. The stability of the joint is ascertained by the group of ulnar-collateral ligaments medially and radial-collateral ligaments laterally (Fig. 6.3). The ulnar-collateral ligament consists of the anterior bundle, which extends from the anteroinferior aspect of the medial epicondyle to the medial coronoid margin; the posterior bundle, which extends from the posteroinferior aspect of the medial epicondyle to the medial olecranon margin; and the transverse bundle, which extends over the notch between the coronoid process and olecranon. The radial collateral ligament is thinner than the ulnar collateral ligament and inserts in the annular ligament, which in turn encircles the radial head and attaches to the anterior and posterior margins of the radial notch of the ulna. A fibrous capsule deep within the ligament structures surrounds the elbow joint. The anterior joint capsule and synovium insert proximally to the coronoid and radial fossae at the anterior aspect of the humerus. The posterior joint capsule attaches to the humerus just proximal to the olecranon fossa.

When trauma to the elbow is suspected, radiographs are routinely obtained in the anteroposterior and lateral projections, occasionally supplemented by internal and external oblique views.

The *anteroposterior* projection usually suffices to demonstrate injury to the medial and the lateral epicondyles, the olecranon fossa, the capitellum, the trochlea, and the radial head (Fig. 6.4). It also reveals an important anatomic relation of the forearm to the central axis of

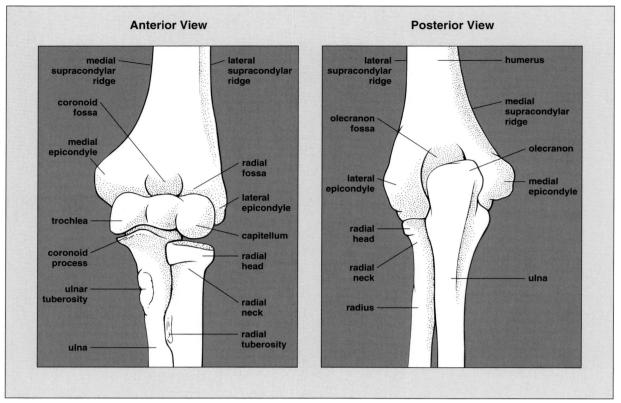

Figure 6.1 Osseous structures of the elbow. Anterior and posterior views of the distal humerus and proximal radius and ulna.

the arm known as the *carrying angle* (Fig. 6.5). Normally, the long axis of the forearm forms a valgus angle of 15° with the long axis of the arm; the forearm is thus angled laterally, that is, away from the central axis of the body.

On the anteroposterior view in children, it is essential to recognize the four secondary ossification centers of the distal humerus:

those of the capitellum, the medial and the lateral epicondyles, and the trochlea. The usual order in which these centers appear and the age at which they become radiographically visible are important factors in the evaluation of injuries to the elbow (Fig. 6.6). Displacement of any of these centers serves as a diagnostic indicator of the type of fracture or dislocation. For example, the medial epicondyle always os-

Figure 6.2 Muscles of the elbow. Anterior and posterior views of the muscles of the elbow joint.

Figure 6.3 Ligaments of the elbow. Medial and lateral views of the ligaments of the elbow joint.

Medial View

Lateral View

Figure 6.4 Anteroposterior view. (A) For the anteroposterior view of the elbow, the forearm is positioned supine (palm up) on the radiographic table, with the elbow joint fully extended and the fingers slightly flexed. The central beam is directed perpendicularly toward the elbow joint. **(B)** The film in this projection demonstrates the medial and the lateral epicondyles, the olecranon fossa, the capitellum, and the radial head. The coronoid process is seen en face, and the olecranon overlaps the trochlea.

Figure 6.5 Carrying angle. The angle formed by the longitudinal axes of the distal humerus and the proximal ulna constitutes the carrying angle of the forearm. Normally, there is a valgus angle of 15°.

Figure 6.6 Ossification centers of the distal humerus. The secondary centers of ossification of the distal humerus usually appear in the following order: the capitellum at 1 to 2 years of age, the medial epicondyle at 4 years of age, the trochlea at 8 years of age, and the lateral epicondyle at 10 years of age.

sifies before the trochlea. If radiographic examination in a child between ages 4 and 8 years reveals a bony structure in the region of the trochlea (that is, before this center of ossification should appear) and shows no evidence of the ossification center of the medial epicondyle, then it must be assumed that the ossification center of the medial epicondyle has been avulsed and displaced into the joint (Fig. 6.7).

The *lateral* view of the elbow allows sufficient evaluation of the olecranon process, the anterior aspect of the radial head, and the humeroradial articulation. It is limited, however, in the information it can provide, particularly with respect to the posterior half of the radial head and the coronoid process, because of the overlap of bony structures (Fig. 6.8).

As with the anteroposterior projection, the lateral view in children reveals significant configurations and relations, which, if distorted, indicate the presence of abnormality. The distal humerus in children has an angular appearance resembling a hockey stick, the angle of which normally measures approximately 140°. Loss of this configuration occurs in supracondylar fracture (Fig. 6.9). Rogers has pointed out, in addition, the importance of the position of the capitellum relative to the distal humerus and the proximal radius. He found that a line drawn along the longitudinal axis of the proximal radius passes through the center of the capitellum and that a line drawn along the anterior cortex of the distal humerus and extended downward through the articulation intersects the middle third of the capitellum (Fig. 6.10). Disruption of this relation serves as an important indication of the possible presence of fracture or dislocation. Finally, regardless of the patient's age, displacement of the normal positions of the fat pads of the elbow also provides a useful diagnostic clue to the presence of fracture. Normally, the posterior fat pad, which lies deep in the olecranon fossa, is not visible on the lateral view. When it becomes visible and the anterior fat pad appears displaced—the positive fat-pad sign (Fig. 6.11; see Fig. 4.33)—demonstration of the fracture line should be undertaken.

The *radial head-capitellum* view is a variant of the lateral projection, which was introduced by the author in 1982. As it overcomes the major limitation of the standard lateral view by projecting the radial head ventrad, free of overlap by the coronoid process, it has proved to be a particularly effective technique. In addition to the radial head, it also clearly demonstrates the capitellum, the coronoid process, the humeroradial and humeroulnar articulations (Fig. 6.12), and subtle fractures of these structures that may be obscure on other projections (see Figs. 6.27, 6.28, and 6.32).

Other modalities may also be necessary for sufficient evaluation of injury to the elbow. Single-contrast or, preferably, double-contrast arthrography, commonly combined with tomography *(arthrotomography)* or CT, has proved effective in visualizing subtle chondral fractures, osteochondritis dissecans, synovial and capsular abnormalities, and osteochondral bodies in the joint. In general, indications for elbow arthrography include detection of the presence, size, and number of intraarticular osteochondral bodies; determination of whether

Figure 6.7 Fracture of the medial epicondyle. Displacement of the ossification center of the medial epicondyle secondary to fracture (**A**) and (**B**) may mimic the normal appearance of the ossification center of the trochlea (**C**).

Figure 6.8 **Lateral view. (A)** For the lateral projection of the elbow, the forearm rests on its ulnar side on the radiographic cassette, with the joint flexed 90°, the thumb pointing upward, and the fingers slightly flexed. The central beam is directed vertically toward the radial head. **(B)** The film in this projection demonstrates the distal shaft of the humerus, the supracondylar ridge, the olecranon process, and the anterior aspect of the radial head. The articular surface and posterior aspect of the radial head are not well demonstrated on this view because of overlap by the coronoid process. The capitellum is also obscured by the overlapping trochlea.

Figure 6.9 **Supracondylar fracture. (A)** Lateral view of the elbow joint in a 3-year-old child shows the normal hockey-stick appearance of the distal humerus. *(continued)*

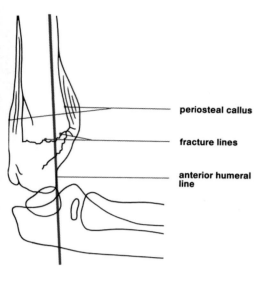

periosteal callus

fracture lines

anterior humeral
line

Figure 6.9 Supracondylar fracture *Continued.* **(B)** Loss of this configuration, as seen in this film in a 3.5-year-old girl who sustained trauma to the elbow 4 weeks before this radiographic examination, serves as an important landmark in recognizing supracondylar fracture of the distal humerus. Note also that the anterior humeral line falls anterior to the capitellum, indicating extension injury (see Fig. 6.10).

calcifications around the elbow joint are intraarticular or extraarticular; evaluation of the articular cartilage; evaluation of juxta-articular cysts if they are communicating with the joint; evaluation of the joint capacity; and evaluation of various synovial and capsular abnormalities. Single-contrast arthrography is preferable when evaluating synovial abnormalities and intraarticular osteochondral bodies, because double contrast may result in air bubbles in the joint. Double-contrast arthrography, however, provides more detailed information; in particular, the articular surface and synovial lining are better delineated and the small details can be better visualized (Fig. 6.13). Frequently, in conjunction with elbow arthrography, conventional tomography may be used in a procedure called arthrotomography (Fig. 6.14) or CT examination (CT arthrography) (Fig. 6.15) can be performed. If

conventional tomographic examination alone is performed, trispiral cuts are preferred, because the thinner sections obtainable by this method provide overall better detail—as, for example, in localizing multiple fragments in comminuted fractures.

Axial CT images of the extended elbow are occasionally effective in demonstrating traumatic abnormalities. They are, however, difficult to obtain in the traumatized patient, and except for visualization of the proximal radioulnar joint and ulnatrochlear articulation, they are not frequently used. Occasionally, these sections can demonstrate osteochondral fractures of the radial head and assess the integrity of the proximal radioulnar joint. However, Franklin and colleagues noted that axial CT images of the flexed elbow (so-called coronal sections) provide an ideal plane for evaluation of the olecranon fossa and

Figure 6.10 Landmarks of the elbow joint. In children, the normal position of the capitellum relative to the distal humerus and the proximal radius is determined by the portions of the capitellum intersected by two lines: Line *(a)* coincident with the longitudinal axis of the proximal radius, passes through the center of the capitellum; and line *(b)* parallel to the anterior cortex of the distal humerus intersects the middle third of the capitellum. Disruption of this relation indicates the possible presence of abnormality (see Figs. 6.9B and 6.25B).

Figure 6.11 Fat-pad sign. Lateral radiograph of the elbow joint shows positive anterior *(arrow)* and posterior *(curved arrow)* fat-pad sign. Open arrow points to the subtle fracture of the radial head.

Figure 6.12 **Radial head–capitellum view. (A).** For the radial head—capitellum projection of the elbow, the patient is seated at the side of the radiographic table, with the forearm resting on its ulnar side, the elbow joint flexed 90°, and the thumb pointing upward. The central beam is directed toward the radial head at a 45° angle to the forearm. **(B)** The film in this projection shows the radial head projected ventrad, free of overlap by the coronoid process, which is also well demonstrated. This projection is also effective in evaluating the capitellum and the humeroradial and humeroulnar articulations.

Figure 6.13 **Arthrography of the elbow joint. (A)** For arthrographic examination of the elbow, the patient's forearm is positioned prone on the radiographic table, with the joint flexed 90° and the fingers lying flat. The joint is entered from the lateral aspect between the radial head and capitellum, and under fluoroscopic control 2 mL of positive contrast agent (60% diatrizoate meglumine) and 8 to 10 mL of room air are injected into the radiocapitellar joint. (The *red dot* marks the point of needle entrance.) Conventional films or tomograms may then be obtained in the standard projections (see Figs. 6.14 and 6.38). **(B, C)** On the elbow arthrogram, one can distinguish anterior, posterior, and annular recesses of the joint capsule. Articular cartilage of the radial head and capitellum is also well demonstrated.

Figure 6.14 **Arthrography of the elbow joint.** Arthrotomography through the ulnar—trochlear articulation (**A**) demonstrates the coronoid recess, and through the radiocapitellar articulation (**B**) demonstrates the annular (periradial), anterior, and posterior recesses of the joint capsule.

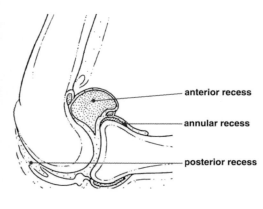

the space between the trochlea and olecranon process posteriorly, as well as the radius and capitellum, and trochlea and coronoid process anteriorly. Axial scans through the flexed elbow also allow additional demonstration of the proximal radius in its long axis.

MRI examination effectively demonstrates traumatic abnormalities of the elbow joint and surrounding soft tissues. Axial, sagittal, and coronal planes are routinely used for elbow imaging. The axial plane is ideal to display the anatomic relationship of the proximal radioulnar joint and the head of the radius. Various tendons, muscles, annular ligament, and neurovascular bundles are also effectively imaged. On coronal images, the trochlea, capitellum, and radial head are well

demonstrated, as well as the various tendons, ligaments, and muscles around the elbow (Fig. 6.16A). On the sagittal plane, the ulnatrochlear and radiocapitellar articulations are well seen, and the biceps, triceps, and brachialis muscle groups are well demonstrated in their long axis. The biceps tendon and anconeus muscles are also well imaged (Fig. 6.16B, C).

MR arthrography is occasionally performed, mainly to evaluate synovial abnormalities and integrity of the joint capsule and ligaments. In addition, subtle intraarticular loose bodies can be detected with this technique and stability of osteochondral fracture or osteochondritis dissecans of the capitellum can be assessed. Similar to one used for shoul-

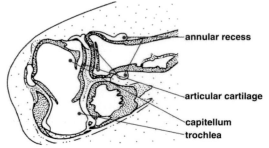

Figure 6.15 **CT arthrography of the elbow.** Postarthrography coronal CT scan of the elbow joint clearly demonstrates the annular recess and the outline of the lateral extension of the joint capsule. The articular cartilage is also well demonstrated.

Figure 6.16 Normal MRI anatomy of the elbow joint. On the coronal section **(A)**, note the anatomic relationship of bony, muscular, and tendinous structures. On the sagittal sections **(B)** and **(C)** the muscular structures (brachialis muscle, anconeus muscle), tendons (triceps tendon, biceps tendon), and bones (distal humerus, olecranon process, and radial head) are well demonstrated. (From Beltran J, 1990, with permission.)

der MR arthrography, concentration of gadolinium mixed with normal saline, iodinated contrast agent, and lidocaine is prepared and a total of up to 10 mL of fluid is injected into the elbow joint. Lateral approach, identical to the technique for conventional elbow arthrography (see Fig. 6.13), is preferred. Coronal, sagittal, and axial images are obtained using fat-suppressed spin echo sequences (Fig. 6.17).

For a summary of the preceding discussion in tabular form, see Tables 6.1 and 6.2 and Figure 6.18.

Figure 6.17 MR arthrography of the elbow. (A) Coronal T1-weighted fat-suppressed image show the anterior band of the ulnar collateral ligament (*arrow*) and the radial collateral ligament (*curved arrow*). The joint is outlined by bright contrast agent. C = capitellum, T = trochlea, RH = radial head. (B) Sagittal T1-weighted fat-suppressed image obtained through the medial part of the elbow joint shows anterior (*arrow*) and posterior (*open arrow*) recesses. T = trochlea, O = olecranon, BM = brachialis muscle, TM = triceps muscle. (C) Sagittal T1-weighted fat-suppressed image obtained through the lateral part of the elbow joint shows attachment of the joint capsule to the proximal radius (*arrow*) and its posterior extent (*open arrows*). C, capitellum; RH, radial head.

Table 6.1 Standard and Special Radiographic Projections for Evaluating Injury to the Elbow

Projection	Demonstration

Anteroposterior	Supra-, trans-, and intercondylar fractures of distal humerus
	Fractures of:
	    Medial and lateral epicondyles
	    Lateral aspect of capitellum
	    Medial aspect of trochlea
	    Lateral aspect of radial head
	Valgus and varus deformities
	Secondary ossification centers of distal humerus

Lateral	Supracondylar fracture of distal humerus
	Fractures of:
	    Anterior aspect of radial head
	    Olecranon process
	Complex dislocations in elbow joint
	Dislocation of radial head
	Fat-pad sign

External Oblique	Fractures of:
	    Lateral epicondyle
	    Radial head

Internal Oblique	Fractures of:
	    Medial epicondyle
	    Coronoid process

Radial Head—Capitellum	Fractures of:
	    Radial head
	    Capitellum
	    Coronoid process
	Abnormalities of humeroradial and humeroulnar articulations

Table 6.2 Ancillary Imaging Techniques for Evaluating Injury to the Elbow

Technique	Demonstration

Tomography	Complex fractures about the elbow joint, particularly to assess position of fragments in comminution
	Healing process:
	    Nonunion
	    Secondary infection

Arthrography Single- or double-cartilage contrast (usually augmented by tomography)	Subtle abnormalities of articular cartilage Capsular ruptures Synovial abnormalities Chondral and osteochondral fractures Osteochondritis dissecans Osteochondral bodies in joint
Computed Tomography Alone or combined with double-contrast arthrography	Same as for arthrography
Magnetic Resonance Imaging	Abnormalities of the ligaments*, tendons, and muscles Capsular ruptures* Joint effusion Synovial cysts* Hematomas Subtle abnormalities of bones (e.g., bone contusion) Osteochondritis dissecans* Epiphyseal fractures (in children)

*These abnormalties are best demonstrated on MR arthrography.

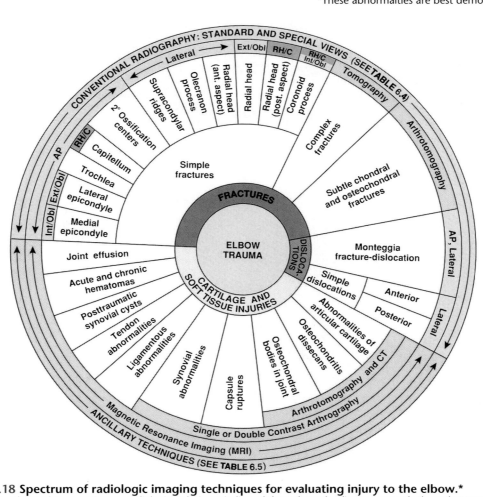

Figure 6.18 Spectrum of radiologic imaging techniques for evaluating injury to the elbow.*
The radiographic projections or radiologic techniques indicated throughout the diagram are only those that are the most effective in demonstrating the respective traumatic conditions.

Injury to the Elbow

Fractures About the Elbow

Fractures of the Distal Humerus. Because the nomenclature of the various structures of the distal humerus used in different anatomy and surgery textbooks is not uniform, confusion has arisen regarding the classification of fractures of the distal humerus. To clarify the picture, a simplified anatomic division of the distal humerus is shown in Fig. 6.19. The significance of the distinction between the articular and extraarticular parts of the distal humerus lies in its importance to diagnosis, treatment, and prognosis. For example, as Rockwood and Green contended, fracture involving only the articular portion of the distal humerus usually results in loss of motion, but not loss of stability, whereas fracture of an entire condyle—that is, both articular and extraarticular portions—usually leads to restriction of motion and instability.

Based on the structure involved, fractures of the distal humerus can be classified as supracondylar, transcondylar, and intercondylar, as well as fractures of the medial and the lateral epicondyles, the capitellum, and the trochlea. The Müller classification is recommended, because it is a practical one based on a distinction between intraarticluar and extraarticular fractures (Fig. 6.20). Usually, such injuries pose no diagnostic problems in adults and are readily evaluated on the anteroposterior and lateral projections of the elbow (Figs. 6.21 and 6.22). Only occasionally may tomographic examination need to be performed to localize comminuted fragments (Fig. 6.23).

In children, however, diagnosis may be problematic because of the presence of the secondary centers of ossification and their variability. Nevertheless, the anteroposterior and lateral projections usually suffice to demonstrate the abnormality, although the fracture line is occasionally more difficult to evaluate on the anteroposterior than on the lateral view. In children between the ages of 3 and 10 years, supracondylar fracture is the most common type of elbow fracture. Extension injury, caused by a fall on the outstretched hand with the elbow hyperextended, is present in 95% of such cases, and characteristically the distal fragment is posteriorly displaced (Fig. 6.24). In the flexion type of injury caused by a fall on the flexed elbow, which occurs in only 5% of cases of supracondylar fracture, the distal fragment is anteriorly and upwardly displaced. Identifying supracondylar fracture on the lateral projection is usually facilitated by recognition of the loss of the normal hockey-stick appearance of the distal humerus and displacement of the capitellum relative to the line of the anterior cortex of the humerus. A positive fat-pad sign is invariably present (Fig. 6.25).

Whatever the age of the patient, it is important in fracture of the distal humerus to demonstrate and evaluate fully the type of injury, the extension of the fracture line, and the degree of displacement, because the method of treatment varies accordingly. When difficulties in interpretation of the type of fracture and the degree of displacement arise, it may be helpful to obtain films of the contralateral normal elbow for comparison.

Complications. The most serious complications of supracondylar fracture are Volkmann ischemic contracture (see Fig. 4.53) and malunion. The latter commonly results in a varus deformity of the elbow, known as cubitus varus.

Fractures of the Radial Head. Fracture of the radial head is a common injury that results, in most cases, from a fall on the outstretched arm and, only rarely, from a direct blow to the lateral aspect of the elbow.

Radial head fractures have been classified by Mason into three types: type I, undisplaced fractures; type II, marginal fractures with displacement (including impaction, depression, and angulation); and type III, comminuted fractures involving the entire head. Later DeLee, Green, and Wilkins suggested adding type IV, fractures of the radial head in association with elbow dislocation (Fig. 6.26). All these fractures can be adequately demonstrated on the anteroposterior and lateral films of the elbow. However, because nondisplaced or minimally displaced fractures may go undetected on these projections, the radial head—capitellum view should be included in the routine radiographic examination to detect occult injuries and to evaluate the degree of displacement (Figs. 6.27 and 6.28). Determination of the exact extension of the fracture line (that is, whether it is extraarticular or intraarticular) and the degree of displacement is crucial to deciding the course of treatment. CT examination plays an important role in this assessment (Fig. 6.29). Nondisplaced or minimally displaced fractures are usually treated conservatively by use of splints or casts, until healing allows active mobilization of the elbow. However, cleavage fracture of the radial articular surface involving one-third or one-half the head with displacement greater than 3 to 4 mm usually indicates the need for open reduction and internal fixation; this is particularly true in younger individuals. Excision of the radial head is the procedure of choice when comminution and displacement of the radial head are present (Fig. 6.30).

Essex-Lopresti Fracture—Dislocation. This complex injury comprises comminuted fracture of the radial head and neck with or without distal extension of fracture line, tear of the interosseous membrane of the forearm, and dislocation in the distal radioulnar joint (Fig. 6.31). This is an unstable injury that, because of bipolar loss of

Figure 6.19 Anatomic structures of the distal humerus. A simplified anatomic division of the structures of the distal humerus.

FRACTURES OF THE DISTAL HUMERUS

Extra-articular—Epicondylar, Supracondylar

avulsion of medial
and/or lateral epicondyle

simple supracondylar fracture

comminuted
supracondylar fracture

Intra-articular—Transcondylar

fracture of trochlea

fracture of capitellum

Intra-articular—Bicondylar, Intercondylar

Y-shaped bicondylar fracture

Y-shaped intercondylar fracture
with supracondylar comminution

complex comminuted fracture

Figure 6.20 Fractures of the distal humerus. Classification of fractures of the distal humerus on the basis of extraarticular and intraarticular extension. (From Müller ME, et al., 1979.)

Figure 6.21 Supracondylar fracture. A 27-year-old man fell from the ladder and onto his outstretched arm. Anteroposterior **(A)** and lateral **(B)** radiographs show a simple supracondylar fracture of the humerus with posterior displacement of the distal fragment.

Figure 6.22 Fracture of the distal humerus. A 25-year-old man sustained a complex intraarticular fracture of the distal humerus in a motorcycle accident. Anteroposterior **(A)** and lateral **(B)** views clearly demonstrate the extension of the fracture lines and the position of the various fragments. The capitellum is separated, laterally displaced, and subluxed; the lateral supracondylar ridge is avulsed and anterolaterally displaced, and the medial epicondyle is externally rotated and medially displaced. *(continued)*

B

Figure 6.22 **Fracture of the distal humerus** *Continued.*

A   **B**

Figure 6.23 **Tomography of the distal humerus fracture.** After a fall from a tree, a 20-year-old woman sustained a comminuted intraarticular fracture of the distal humerus, which was revealed on the standard anteroposterior **(A)** and lateral **(B)** projections of the elbow. However, the inadequate quality of the conventional studies caused by marked soft-tissue swelling, joint effusion, and the clinical condition of the patient (pain and limitation of motion in the joint) made full evaluation of the injury impossible. Anteroposterior **(C)** and lateral **(D)** tomograms were obtained to evaluate the complex deformity. The capitellum is completely separated, medially rotated, and posteriorly displaced; the medial supracondylar ridge is avulsed; and the trochlea and the medial epicondyle are separated from the distal humerus and medially displaced. A bony fragment from the ridge of the coronoid fossa is anteriorly displaced. *(continued)*

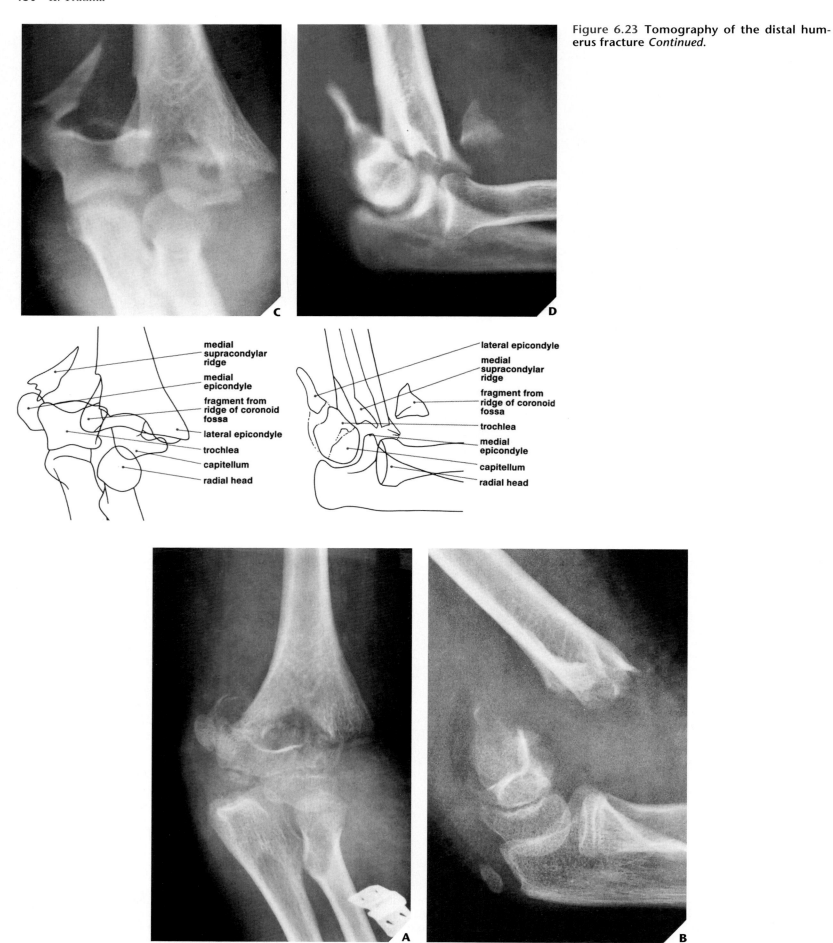

Figure 6.23 **Tomography of the distal humerus fracture** *Continued.*

medial supracondylar ridge
medial epicondyle
fragment from ridge of coronoid fossa
lateral epicondyle
trochlea
capitellum
radial head

lateral epicondyle
medial supracondylar ridge
fragment from ridge of coronoid fossa
trochlea
medial epicondyle
capitellum
radial head

Figure 6.24 Displaced supracondylar fracture. A 9-year-old boy fell off his bicycle and onto his outstretched hand. Anteroposterior **(A)** and lateral **(B)** views of the elbow show supracondylar fracture of the distal humerus with posteromedial displacement of the distal fragment. Note the increase in the valgus angle of the forearm on the anteroposterior view.

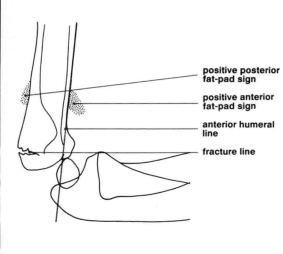

positive posterior
fat-pad sign

positive anterior
fat-pad sign

anterior humeral
line

fracture line

Figure 6.25 Nondisplaced supracondylar fracture. A 3-year-old girl fell on the street. On the anteroposterior view (**A**), the fracture line is practically invisible, whereas on the lateral view (**B**) it is more obvious. There is a positive posterior fat-pad sign, and the anterior fat pad is also clearly displaced. Note that the anterior humeral line intersects the posterior third of the capitellum, indicating slight anterior angulation of the distal fragment.

radial support at both sites (elbow and wrist), requires unique and tailored treatment. In most patients, interfragmentary fixation of radial head fracture is performed, or, in case of severe comminution, silastic radial head prothesis may be indicated to maintain length and stability. Chronic Essex-Lopresti injury with irreducible proximal migration of the radius may require ulnar shortening to restore neutral ulnar variance.

Fracture of the Coronoid Process. Rarely occurring as an isolated injury, fracture of the coronoid process is most often associated with posterior dislocation in the elbow joint. It is, therefore, important in cases of elbow injury to exclude the possibility of fracture of the coronoid process, because undiagnosed it may fail to unite, leading to instability and recurrent subluxation in the joint. The anteroposterior and lateral projections are usually insufficient to evaluate the coronoid process because of overlap of structures on these views. Demonstration of injury is best made on the radial head—capitellum projection (Fig. 6.32) and occasionally on the internal oblique view.

Fracture of the Olecranon. Olecranon fractures usually result from a direct fall on the flexed elbow, and this mechanism frequently produces comminution and marked displacement of the major fragments. An indirect mechanism, like a fall on the outstretched arm, produces an oblique or transverse fracture with minimal displacement. The fracture is usually well demonstrated on a lateral projection of the elbow (Figs. 6.33 and 6.34).

A number of classifications have been developed to evaluate an olecranon fracture. Colton classified olecranon fractures as undisplaced, and displaced, the latter group being subdivided into avulsion fractures, oblique and transverse fractures, comminuted fractures, and fracture—dislocations.

Another practical classification has been developed by Horne and Tanzer, who classified these fractures by their location apparent on the lateral radiographs (Fig. 6.35). Type I fractures are subdivided into two groups: (A) oblique, extraarticular fractures of the olecranon tip and (B) transverse intraarticular fractures originating on the proximal third of the articular surface of olecranon fossa. Type II fractures are transverse or oblique fractures originating on the middle third of the articular surface of olecranon fossa. These fractures also are subdivided into two groups: (A) single fracture line and (B) two fracture lines, one proximal (transverse, or oblique) and the second, more distal, extending posteriorly. Type III fractures involve the distal third of

the olecranon fossa and may be either transverse or oblique. Most fractures are type II.

As far as treatment is concerned, nondisplaced fractures are usually treated conservatively, whereas displaced fractures are most often treated by open reduction and internal fixation.

Osteochondritis Dissecans of the Capitellum

This condition, also referred to as Panner disease, is considered to be related to trauma, namely to repeated exogenous injuries to the elbow. Valgus strain of the elbow in throwing sports such as baseball and football has been implicated as one causative factor. Apparently during the throwing motion, the capitellum is subjected to compression and to shear forces. It most frequently affects the right elbow in right-handed children and adolescents, the majority of whom are males.

In the early stage of the disease, anteroposterior and lateral films may show no significant abnormality (Fig. 6.36 A,B); the only radiographic sign of early-stage Panner disease may become apparent on the radial head—capitellum view with the finding of subtle flattening of the capitellum (Fig. 6.36C). As the condition progresses, the lesion, consisting of a detached segment of subchondral bone with overlying cartilage, gradually separates from its bed in the capitellum. Before separation, the lesion is called "in situ;" after separation, the osteochondral fragment becomes a "loose" body in the joint (Fig. 6.37). Because sometimes more than one fragment is discharged into the joint, osteochondritis dissecans may be mistaken for idiopathic synovial (osteo)chondromatosis, a nontraumatic condition that is a form of synovial metaplasia. In this condition, multiple cartilaginous bodies that are regular in outline and usually uniform in size are seen in the joint (see Fig. 23.2).

One of the radiologic procedures for evaluating osteochondritis dissecans is arthrotomography, which localizes the defect in the cartilaginous surface of the capitellum and distinguishes an in situ lesion from the more advanced stage of the disease (Fig. 6.38). This information is crucial for the orthopedic surgeon, because the in situ lesion may be treated conservatively, whereas surgical intervention may be required if the osteochondral fragment has been partially separated from its bed or discharged into the joint. MRI may also effectively demonstrate the lesion (Fig. 6.39) and provide information about its stability (Fig. 6.40). Type I lesions are intact (in situ), with no fragment displacement; type II lesions are slightly displaced, and the ar-

Figure 6.26 Mason classification of fractures of the radial head.

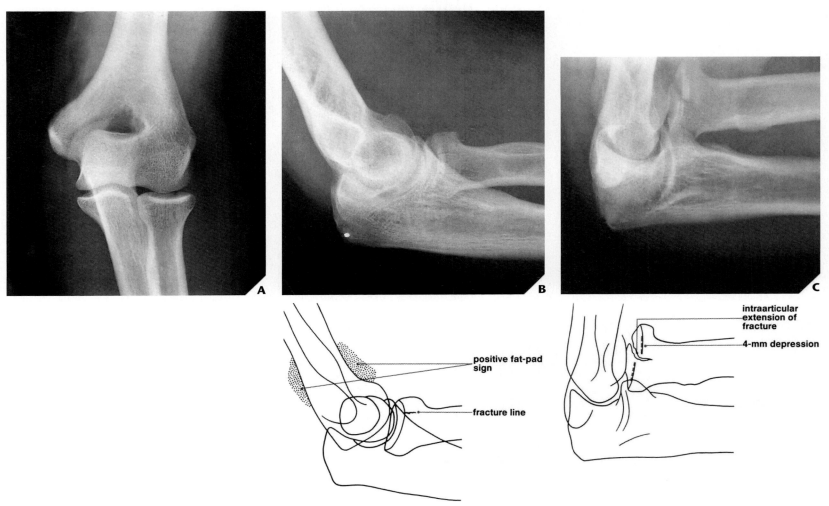

Figure 6.27 Fracture of the radial head. Anteroposterior **(A)** and lateral **(B)** films of the elbow show what appears to be a nondisplaced fracture of the radial head. On the radial head–capitellum view **(C)**, however, intraarticular extension of the fracture line and 4-mm depression of the subchondral fragment are clearly demonstrated. (From Greenspan A, Norman A, 1983, with permission.)

Figure 6.28 Fracture of the radial head. Standard lateral view of the elbow **(A)** demonstrates a fracture of the radial head, but bony overlap prevents exact evaluation of the extent of the fracture line and the degree of displacement. Radial head—capitellum view **(B)** reveals it to be a displaced articular fracture involving the posterior third of the radial head. (From Greenspan A, et al., 1984, with permission.)

Figure 6.29 CT of a fracture of the radial head. (A) Conventional lateral radiograph of the elbow shows a displaced fracture of the radial head (*arrows*). **(B)** Oblique coronal CT shows posterolateral displacement of the fractured fragment, although anatomic orientation is somewhat ambiguous on this image (rh, radial head; f, displaced fractured fragment; c, capitellum; o, olecranon; mt, medial trochlea; lt, lateral trochlea; cp, coronoid process). **(C)** Three-dimensional CT reconstruction image (viewed from the lateral aspect) demonstrates the spatial orientation of the fracture. The arrow points to the posterolaterally displaced fragment, and curved arrow indicates defect in the radial head.

Figure 6.30 Fracture of the radial head. Anteroposterior **(A)** and lateral **(B)** radiographs of the elbow show a markedly comminuted and displaced fracture of the radial head. Excision of the entire radial head would most likely be necessary.

Figure 6.31 Essex-Lopresti fracture—dislocation. The cruciate elements of this injury comprise comminuted fracture of the radial head, ruptured interosseous membrane, and dislocation in the distal radioulnar joint.

ESSEX-LOPRESTI FRACTURE–DISLOCATION

fractured radial shaft

ruptured interosseous membrane

comminuted radial head fracture

widening of the distal radioulnar joint

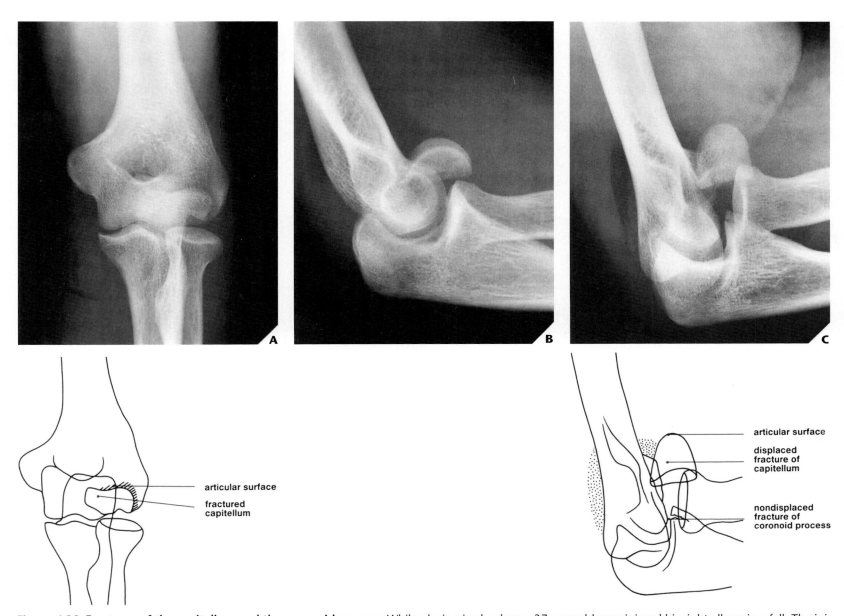

articular surface

fractured capitellum

articular surface

displaced fracture of capitellum

nondisplaced fracture of coronoid process

Figure 6.32 Fractures of the capitellum and the coronoid process. While playing ice hockey, a 37-year-old man injured his right elbow in a fall. The initial anteroposterior **(A)** and lateral **(B)** radiographs show a fracture of the capitellum with anterior rotation and displacement. Note the typical "half-moon" appearance of the displaced capitellum on the lateral view. On the radial head-capitellum film **(C)**, an unsuspected, nondisplaced fracture of the coronoid process is evident. (B and C from Greenspan A, Norman A, 1982, with permission.)

Figure 6.33 Olecranon fracture. A 41-year-old man fell on his flexed elbow and sustained a type II B comminuted olecranon fracture well demonstrated on this lateral radiograph.

Figure 6.34 Olecranon fracture. A 52-year-old woman fell on her outstretched arm and sustained a type III olecranon fracture, effectively demonstrated on the lateral view of the elbow. Note the positive anterior and posterior fat pad sign.

Figure 6.35 Classification of olecranon fractures. (Modified from Horne JG, Tanzer TL, 1981, with permission.)

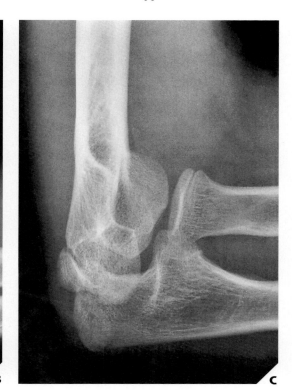

A   B   C

Figure 6.36 Osteochondritis dissecans of the capitellum. A 13-year-old boy who was very active in little league baseball reported pain in his right elbow for several months. Anteroposterior (**A**) and lateral (**B**) films of the elbow demonstrate no abnormalities. On the radial head—capitellum view (**C**), subtle flattening of the capitellum may indicate early-stage osteochondritis dissecans. (From Greenspan A, Norman A, 1982, with permission.)

flattening of capitellum

Figure 6.37 Osteochondritis dissecans of the capitellum. A 15-year-old boy, an active baseball player, reported pain in his right elbow for several months. Anteroposterior view of the elbow (**A**) reveals a radiolucent defect in the capitellum suggesting osteochondritis dissecans; the lateral view (**B**) is normal. Radial head-capitellum projection (**C**) demonstrates not only the full extent of the lesion in the capitellum but also the osteochondral bodies in the joint—a sign of advanced-stage Panner disease. (From Greenspan A, et al., 1984, with permission.) *(continued)*

A

radiolucent defect in capitellum

Figure 6.37 Osteochondritis dissecans of the capitellum *Continued.*

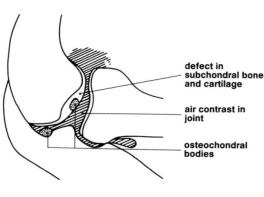

Figure 6.38 Osteochondritis dissecans of the capitellum. Lateral arthrotomogram of the elbow demonstrates defects in the subchondral segment of the capitellum and in the overlying cartilage. Loose osteochondral bodies are present, one located posteriorly in the ulnartrochlear compartment and the other anteriorly in the radiocapitellar compartment. The findings represent advanced-stage osteochondritis dissecans.

Figure 6.39 MRI of osteochondritis dissecans of the capitellum. A 16-year-old baseball player presented with pain in the right elbow for 6 months. The MR sagittal sections (SE sequences; TR 2000/TE 20 msec, TR 2000/TE 80 msec) demonstrate an area of intermediate signal intensity on proton-weighted image **(A)** and high signal intensity on T2-weighted image **(B)**, surrounded by a band of low signal intensity. The articular cartilage is intact. The findings are typical for in situ lesion of osteochondritis dissecans (Panner disease). (From Beltran J, 1990, with permission.)

Figure 6.40 MRI of osteochondritis dissecans of the capitellum. (A) A sagittal T1-weighted MR image shows a linear focus of decreased signal (*open arrow*) at the anterior aspect of the capitellum. **(B)** A sagittal STIR image shows generalized increased signal surrounding a well-defined cystic-appearing focus *(arrows)* in the anterior aspect of the capitellum, consistent with osteochondritis dissecans. **(C)** A sagittal T2*-weighted gradient-echo image reveals a displaced osteochondral body *(open arrow)*.

ticular surface is damaged; type III lesions show detachment of the osteochondral fragment (Fig. 6.41).

Dislocations in the Elbow Joint

Simple Dislocations. The standard method of classifying elbow dislocations is based on the direction of displacement of the radius and the ulna in relation to the distal humerus. Three main types of dislocation can be distinguished as those affecting: (A) both the radius and the ulna, which may be dislocated posteriorly, anteriorly, medially, or laterally (or in a manner combining posterior or anterior with medial or lateral displacement); (B) the ulna only, which may be anteriorly or posteriorly displaced; and (C) the radius only, which may be anteriorly, posteriorly, or laterally dislocated.

Posterior and posterolateral dislocations of the radius and the ulna are by far the most common types. They account for 80% to 90% of all dislocations in the joint (Fig. 6.42). Isolated dislocation of the radial head, however, is a rare occurrence; it is more commonly associated with fracture of the ulna (see "Monteggia Fracture-Dislocation").

Dislocations are easily diagnosed on the standard anteroposterior and lateral films of the elbow.

The presence of dislocation should signal the possibility of an associated fracture of the ulna, which may be overlooked when radiographic examination is focused only on the elbow. For this reason, if dislocation in the elbow joint is suspected, it is mandatory to include the entire forearm on the anteroposterior and lateral films; conversely, in cases of suspected ulnar fracture, radiographs should include the elbow joint. From a practical point of view, it is important, particularly in adults, to obtain two separate films, one centered over the elbow joint and the other over the site of the suspected ulnar fracture. Care should be taken to center the films properly, because dislocation of the radial head can easily be missed on improperly centered films.

Monteggia Fracture—Dislocation. The association of fracture of the ulna with dislocation of the radial head is known by the eponym Monteggia fracture—dislocation. It usually results from forced pronation of the forearm during a fall or a direct blow to the posterior as-

Figure 6.41 MRI of osteochondritis dissecans of the capitellum. A 16-year-old boy with chronic pain in the elbow underwent magnetic resonance (MR) arthrography. **(A)** Coronal and **(B)** sagittal fat-saturation T1-weighted (SE; TR 650/TE 17 msec) MR arthrogram demonstrates osteochondritis dissecans of the capitellum with completely separated, loose osteochondral body (type III lesion).

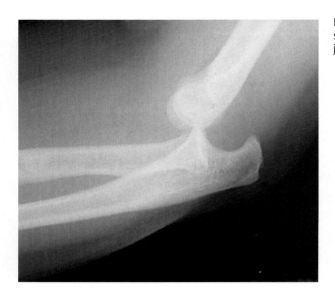

Figure 6.42 Elbow dislocation. Lateral radiograph shows most common type of dislocation in the elbow joint—both radius and ulna are posteriorly displaced.

BADO CLASSIFICATION OF MONTEGGIA FRACTURE-DISLOCATION

Type I

Type II

Type III

Type IV

Figure 6.43 Monteggia fracture—dislocation. The Bado classification of Monteggia fracture—dislocation is based on the four types of abnormalities usually resulting from forced pronation of the forearm. These may occur during a fall or as a result of a direct blow to the posterior aspect of the ulna.

Figure 6.44 Monteggia fracture—dislocation. Lateral radiograph of the elbow joint and proximal third of the forearm shows type I Monteggia fracture—dislocation; anteriorly angulated fracture is at the proximal third of the ulna, associated with anterior dislocation of the radial head.

pect of the ulna. Four types of this abnormality have been described (Fig. 6.43), but the features of the classic description are most commonly (in 60% to 70% of cases) seen: fracture at the junction of the proximal and middle thirds of the ulna, with anterior angulation associated with anterior dislocation of the radial head (type I). It is identifiable on physical examination by marked pain and tenderness about the elbow and displacement of the radial head into the antecubital fossa. The other types, which Bado has described, are as follows:

Type II: Fracture of the proximal ulna with posterior angulation and posterior or posterolateral dislocation of the radial head
Type III: Fracture of the proximal ulna with lateral or anterolateral dislocation of the radial head; type II and type III injuries account for approximately 30% to 40% of Monteggia fractures
Type IV: Fractures of the proximal ends of the radius and the ulna, with anterior dislocation of the radial head (this is the least common type)

The anteroposterior and lateral projections are sufficient to provide a full evaluation of these abnormalities (Figs. 6.44 and 6.45).

Injury to the Soft Tissues

Lateral Epicondylitis (Tennis Elbow). Lateral epicondylitis, first described by Runge in 1878, affects approximately 3% of adults, usually between the ages of 35 and 55. The symptoms include pain of insidious onset, aggravated by activity, at the lateral aspect of the elbow joint. This condition is often diagnosed in tennis players, golfers, and carpenters. The pathomechanism of this abnormality is based on repetitive stress on muscles and tendons adjacent to the lateral aspect of the distal humerus, particularly during excessive pronation and supination of the forearm when the wrist is extended. This results in mucoid degeneration and reactive granulation of the extensor tendons, primarily the extensor carpi radialis brevis tendon, leading to avascularity and calcification of the tendon at its insertion on the lateral epicondyle.

Figure 6.45 Monteggia fracture—dislocation. Anteroposterior **(A)** and lateral **(B)** views of the elbow that include the proximal third of the forearm demonstrate the typical appearance of type III Monteggia fracture—dislocation; fracture is at the proximal third of the ulna, associated with anterolateral dislocation of the radial head.

Figure 6.46 Lateral epicondylitis. A 46-year-old woman presented with chronic pain at the lateral aspect of the elbow. A coronal T2-weighted fat-suppressed MRI shows partial tearing of fibers of the extensor tendons from epicondylar attachment (*arrow*) and soft tissue edema (*open arrows*). The curved arrow points to the joint effusion. (Courtesy of Dr. A. Gentili, San Diego, California)

Conventional radiographs are frequently normal, although soft tissue swelling and calcification can sometimes by observed adjacent to the lateral epicondyle. MRI is useful for assessment of damage to the tendons and evaluation of associated abnormalities of the ligaments (Fig. 6.46). Not uncommonly, MRI may show avulsion of the extensor carpi radialis brevis tendon from the lateral epicondyle and associated bone marrow edema. In some patients, MR imaging demonstrates increased signal within the anconeus muscle.

Tears of the Radial (Lateral) Collateral Ligament Complex (RCLC). The radial collateral ligament complex consists of the radial collateral ligament, the annular ligament, the accessory collateral ligament, and the posterolateral (lateral ulnar) collateral ligament. The first three ligaments provide lateral stability of the elbow joint and prevent varus deformation. The latter ligament provides posterolateral stabilization of the joint. Chronic repetitive microtrauma that results in varus stress may lead to a sprain or to disruption of the RCLC, both of which can be diagnosed with MRI. A sprain appears as a thinning or thickening of the ligament associated with high signal intensity within or adjacent to this structure. A complete tear manifests as discontinuation of the fibers or a defect in the ligament. These abnormalities may also be seen in association with lateral epicondylitis (see previous).

Tears of the Ulnar (Medial) Collateral Ligament Complex (UCLC). The ulnar collateral ligament complex consists of the anterior, posterior, and transverse ligaments. These ligaments provide medial stability to the elbow joint and prevent valgus deformation. The most important of the three bands is the anterior portion, which originates on the inferior aspect of the medial epicondyle and inserts on the medial edge of the coronoid process at the sublime tubercle. UCLC injury commonly occurs in athletes, particularly in baseball pitchers and, less commonly, in javelin throwers, handball players, arm wrestlers, and tennis players. MRI findings include abnormal signal and interruption of the continuity of the fibers or defect in the ligament (in complete rupture) or thickening of the ligament and foci of calcification or ossification (in chronic injury).

MR arthrography can distinguish between partial and complete tears of the ulnar collateral ligament. Recently, DeSmet and colleagues have recommended the use of dynamic sonography with valgus stress to assess injury to the ulnar collateral ligament in baseball pitchers. This technique uniquely demonstrates the medial joint laxity and instability when measurements of the degree of joint widening during valgus stress of the elbow are obtained.

PRACTICAL POINTS TO REMEMBER

[1] On the anteroposterior projection of the elbow:
 • observe the normal 15° valgus carrying angle formed between the arm and the forearm
 • (in the child) recognize the four secondary ossification centers of the distal humerus and the age at which they appear: capitellum at 1 to 2 years, medial epicondyle at 4 years, trochlea at 8 years, and lateral epicondyle at 10 years.

[2] On the lateral view of the elbow:
 • note the normal angular (hockey-stick) appearance of the distal humerus; the angle measures approximately 140°; loss of this angle occurs in supracondylar fracture
 • evaluate the position of the capitellum relative to the longitudinal axis of the proximal radius and the anterior humeral line
 • pay attention to the presence or absence of the fat-pad sign; if this sign is positive in a patient with an elbow injury, then fracture should always be considered

[3] The radial head—capitellum projection is very useful in evaluating elbow trauma and should always be obtained as part of a routine study.

[4] Arthrotomography is an important technique in selected cases of elbow injury. The procedure helps to visualize:
 • subtle chondral and osteochondral fractures
 • osteochondritis dissecans
 • synovial and capsular abnormalities
 • osteochondral bodies in the joint.

[5] MR arthrography of the elbow joint is useful to evaluate synovial abnormalities, integrity of the joint capsule and ligaments, and to detect intraarticular loose bodies.

[6] Supracondylar fracture of the distal humerus (usually of the extension type) is very common in children. The lateral film showing loss of the hockey-stick appearance of the distal humerus is diagnostic. If the lateral projection is equivocal, then obtain a film of the contralateral (normal) elbow for comparison.

[7] Fracture of the radial head is common in adults. It is important to demonstrate:
 • the type of fracture
 • the extension of the fracture line
 • the degree of articular displacement.
 This information determines whether a conservative or a surgical course of treatment is indicated.

[8] Fracture of the coronoid process is usually occult and is most often associated with posterior dislocation in the elbow joint. If unrecognized, it may fail to unite, leading to recurrent subluxation or dislocation in the joint. The radial head—capitellum view is best suited to demonstrate it.

[9] Fractures of the olecranon are best demonstrated on the lateral view. They are classified into three types, according to the origin of the fracture line at the articular surface of the olecranon fossa.

[10] The orthopedic management of osteochondritis dissecans requires demonstrating the status of the articular cartilage of the capitellum and determining the stability of the osteochondral fragment. Arthrotomography, MRI, or MR arthrography are the procedures of choice.

[11] In every case of ulnar fracture, look for associated dislocation of the radial head; conversely, in every case of dislocation, look for fracture of the ulna (Monteggia fracture—dislocation). Proper radiographic technique for imaging these often-missed injuries

requires, in adults, obtaining two separate films that include the elbow joint and the forearm: one centered over the joint and the other over the mid-forearm. In children, a single film that includes the elbow joint and the entire forearm suffices.

[12] Essex-Lopresti fracture—dislocation is a complex, unstable injury that comprises comminuted fracture of the radial head and neck, tear of the interosseous membrane of the forearm, and dislocation in the distal radioulnar joint.

[13] Lateral epicondylitis (or tennis elbow) is most effectively evaluated with MR imaging. This technique may show avulsion of the extensor carpi radialis brevis tendon from the lateral epicondyle and associated bone marrow edema.

SUGGESTED READINGS

Anderson SE, Otsuka N, Steinbach LS. MR imaging of pediatric elbow trauma. *Semin Musculoskeletal Radiol* 1998;2:185–198.

Awaya H, Schweitzer ME, Feng SA, et al. Elbow synovial fold syndrome: MR imaging findings. *AJR Am J Roentgenol* 2001;177:1377–1381.

Bado JL. The Monteggia lesion. Springfield, IL: CC Thomas; 1962.

Beltran J, Rosenberg ZS. MR imaging of pediatric elbow fractures. *MRI Clin North Am* 1997;5:567–578.

Berquist T. Elbow and forearm. In: Berquist T, ed. *MRI of the musculoskeletal system*, 3rd ed. Philadelphia: Lippincott–Raven Publishers; 1996:609–672.

Bianco AJ. Osteochondritis dissecans. In: Morrey BF, ed. *The elbow and its disorders.* Philadelphia: WB Saunders; 1985:254–259.

Bledsoe RC, Izenstark JL. Displacement of fat pads in disease and injury of the elbow: a new radiographic sign. *Radiology* 1959;73:717–724.

Bohrer SP. The fat pad sign following elbow trauma: its usefulness and reliability in suspecting "invisible" fractures. *Clin Radiol* 1970;21:90–94.

Boyd H, McLeod A. Tennis elbow. *J Bone Joint Surg [Am]* 1973;55-A:1183–1187.

Brodeur AE, Silberstein MJ, Graviss ER. *Radiology of the pediatric elbow.* Boston: Hall Medical; 1981.

Bunnell DH, Fisher DA, Bassett LW, Gold RH, Ellman H. Elbow joint: normal anatomy on MR images. *Radiology* 1987;165:527–531.

Carrino JA, Morrison WB, Zou KH, Steffen RT, Snearly WN, Murray PM. Noncontrast MR imaging and MR arthrography of the ulnar collateral ligament of the elbow: prospective evaluation of two-dimensional pulse sequences for detection of complete tears. *Skeletal Radiol* 2001;30:625–632.

Chapman MW. Closed intramedullary nailing of the humerus. *Instr Course Lect AAOS* 1983;32:317–324.

Coel M, Yamada CY, Ko J. MR imaging of patients with lateral epicondylitis of the elbow (tennis elbow): importance of increased signal of the anconeus muscle. *AJR Am J Roentgenol* 1993;161:1019–1021.

Colton CL. Fractures of the olecranon in adults: classification and management. *Injury* 1973;5:121–129.

Cone RO, Szabo R, Resnick D, Gelberman R, Taleisnik J, Gilula LA. Computed tomography of the normal radioulnar joints. *Invest Radiol* 1983;18:541–545.

Cotten A, Boutin RD, Resnick D. Normal anatomy of the elbow on conventional MR imaging and MR arthrography. *Semin Musculoskeletal Radiol* 1998;2:133–140.

Cotten A, Jacobson J, Brossmann J, et al. Collateral ligaments of the elbow: conventional MR imaging and MR arthrography with coronal oblique plane and elbow flexion. *Radiology* 1997;204:806–812.

Daniels DL, Mallisee TA, Erickson SJ, Boynton MD, Carrera GF. Radiologic-anatomic correlations. The elbow joint: osseous and ligamentous structures. *Radiographics* 1998;18:229–236.

DeLee JC, Green DP, Wilkins KE. Fractures and dislocations of the elbow. In: Rockwood CA Jr, Green DP, eds. *Fractures in adults*, vol. I, 2nd ed. Philadelphia: JB Lippincott; 1984:559–652.

De Smet AA, Winter TC, Best TM, Bernhardt DT. Dynamic sonography with valgus stress to assess elbow ulnar collateral ligament injury in baseball pitchers. *Skeletal Radiol* 2002;31:671–676.

Eto RT, Anderson PW, Harley JD. Elbow arthrography with the application of tomography. *Radiology* 1975;115:283–288.

Fowles JV, Sliman N, Kassab MT. The Monteggia lesion in children. Fracture of the ulna and dislocation of the radial head. *J Bone Joint Surg [Am]* 1983;65A:1276–1282.

Franklin PD, Dunlop RW, Whitelaw G, Jacques E Jr, Blickman JG, Shapiro JH. Computed tomography of the normal and traumatized elbow. *J Comput Assist Tomogr* 1988;12:817–823.

Fritz RC. The elbow. In: Deutsch AL, Mink JH, eds. *MRI of the musculoskeletal system. A teaching file*, 2nd ed. Philadelphia: Lippincott–Raven Publishers; 1997:77–148.

Fritz RC. Magnetic resonance imaging of the elbow. *Semin Roentgenol* 1995;30:241–264.

Fritz RC, Steinbach LS, Tirman PF, Martinez S. MR imaging of the elbow: an update. *Radiol Clin North Am* 1997;35:117–144.

Gaary E, Potter HG, Altchek DW. Medial elbow pain in the throwing athlete: MR imaging evaluation. *AJR Am J Roentgenol* 1997;168:795–800.

Greenspan A, Norman A. The radial head-capitellum view: useful technique in elbow trauma. *AJR Am J Roentgenol* 1982;138:1186–1188.

Greenspan A, Norman A. The radial head-capitellum view: another example of its usefulness [letter]. *AJR Am J Roentgenol* 1982;139:193.

Greenspan A, Norman A. Letter to the editor [Reply]. *AJR Am J Roentgenol* 1983;140:1273.

Greenspan A, Norman A, Rosen H. Radial head-capitellum view in elbow trauma: clinical application and radiographic-anatomic correlation. *AJR Am J Roentgenol* 1984;143:355–359.

Holtz P, Erickson SJ, Holmquist K. MR imaging of the elbow: technical considerations. *Semin Musculoskeletal Radiol* 1998;2:121–131.

Horne JG, Tanzer TL. Olecranon fractures: a review of 100 cases. *J Trauma* 1981;21:469–472.

Janarv PM, Hesser U, Hirsch G. Osteochondral lesions in the radiocapitellar joint in the skeletally immature: radiographic, MRI, and arthroscopic findings in 13 consecutive cases. *J Pediatr Orthop* 1997;17:311–314.

Kohn AM. Soft tissue alterations in elbow trauma. *AJR Am J Roentgenol* 1959;82:867–874.

Mirowitz SA, London SL. Ulnar collateral ligament injury in baseball pitchers: MR imaging evaluation. *Radiology* 1992;185:573–576.

Mitsunaga MM, Adishian DA, Bianco AJ Jr. Osteochondritis dissecans of the capitellum. *J Trauma* 1982;22:53–55.

Morrey BF. Anatomy of the elbow joint. In: Morrey BF, ed. *The elbow and its disorders,* 2nd ed. Philadelphia: WB Saunders; 1993:16–52.

Morrey BF, An KN. Articular and ligamentous contributions to the stability of the elbow joint. *Am J Sports Med* 1983;11:315–319.

Müller ME, Allgower M, Schneider R, Willenegger H. *Manual of internal fixation, techniques recommended by the AO Group,* 2nd ed. Berlin: Springer-Verlag; 1979.

Murphy BJ. MR imaging of the elbow. *Radiology* 1992;184:525–529.

Murphy WA, Siegel MJ. Elbow fat pads with new signs and extended differential diagnosis. *Radiology* 1977;124:659–665.

Nelson SW. Some important diagnostic and technical fundamentals in the radiology of trauma, with particular emphasis on skeletal trauma. *Radiol Clin North Am* 1966;4:241–259.

Norell HG. Roentgenologic visualization of the extracapsular fat. Its importance in the diagnosis of traumatic injuries to the elbow. *Acta Radiol* 1954;42:205–210.

Peiss J, Adam G, Cassser R, Vohahn R, Gunther RW. Gadopentetate-dimeglumine-enhanced MR imaging of osteonecrosis and osteochondritis dissecans of the elbow: initial experience. *Skeletal Radiol* 1995;24:17–20.

Reckling FW, Peltier LF. Riccardo Galeazzi and Galeazzi's fracture. *Surgery* 1965;58:453–459.

Rogers LF. Fractures and dislocations of the elbow. *Semin Roentgenol* 1978;13:97–107.

Rogers LF, Malave S Jr, White H, Tachdjian MO. Plastic bowing, torus and greenstick supracondylar fractures of the humerus: radiographic clues to obscure fractures of the elbow in children. *Radiology* 1978;128:145–150.

Rosenberg ZS, Beltran J, Cheung Y, Broker M. MR imaging of the elbow: normal variant and potential diagnostic pitfalls of the trochlear groove and cubital tunnel. *AJR Am J Roentgenol* 1995;164:415–418.

Rosenberg ZS, Bencardino J, Beltran J. MRI of normal variants and interpretation pitfalls of the elbow. *Semin Musculoskeletal Radiol* 1998;2:141–153.

Sauser DD, Thordarson SH, Fahr LM. Imaging of the elbow. *Radiol Clin North Am* 1990;28:923–940.

Schwartz ML, Al-Zahrani S, Morwessel RM, Andrews JR. Ulnar collateral ligament injury in the throwing athlete: evaluation with saline-enhanced MR arthrography. *Radiology* 1995;197:297–299.

Singson RD, Feldman F, Rosenberg ZS. Elbow joint: assessment with double-contrast CT arthrography. *Radiology* 1986;160:167–173.

Smith FM. Children's elbow injuries: fractures and dislocations. *Clin Orthop* 1967;50:7–30.

Sonin AH, Tutton SM, Fitzgerald SW, Peduto AJ. MR imaging of the adult elbow. *Radiographics* 1996;16:1323–1336.

Steinbach LS, Palmer WE, Schweitzer ME. Special focus session. MR arthrography. *Radiographics* 2002;22:1223–1246.

Steinbach LS, Schwartz ML. Elbow arthrography. *Radiol Clin North Am* 1998;36:635–649.

Stoller DW. The elbow. In: Stoller DW, ed. *Magnetic resonance imaging in orthopedics & sports medicine.* Philadelphia: JB Lippincott; 1993:633–682.

Stoller DW, Genant HK. The joints. In: Moss AA, Gamsu G, Genant HK, eds. *Computed tomography of the body with magnetic resonance imaging,* 2nd ed. Philadelphia: WB Saunders; 1992:435–475.

Takahara M, Ogino T, Takagi M, Tsuchida H, Orui H, Nambu T. Natural progression of osteochondritis dissecans of the humeral capitellum: initial observations. *Radiology* 2000;216:207–212.

Tehranzadeh J, Kerr R, Amster J. Magnetic resonance imaging of tendon and ligament abnormalities. Part 1. Spine and upper extremities. *Skeletal Radiol* 1992;21:1–9.

Weston WJ. Elbow arthrography. In: Dalinka MK, ed. *Arthrography.* New York: Springer-Verlag; 1980.

CHAPTER 7

UPPER LIMB III

Distal Forearm, Wrist, and Hand

Distal Forearm

Injury to the distal forearm, caused predominantly (90% of cases) by a fall on the outstretched hand, is common throughout life but is most common in the elderly. The type of injury usually sustained is fracture of the distal radius or ulna, the incidence of which substantially exceeds that of dislocation in the distal radioulnar and radiocarpal articulations. Although history and physical examination usually provide important information regarding the type of injury, radiographs are indispensable in determining the exact site and extent; in several types of fractures, only adequate radiographic examination can lead to a correct diagnosis.

Anatomic–Radiologic Considerations

Radiographs obtained in the posteroanterior and lateral projections are usually sufficient to evaluate most injuries to the distal forearm (Figs. 7.1 and 7.2). On each of these views, it is important to appreciate the normal anatomic relations of the radius and the ulna for a complete evaluation of trauma.

The posteroanterior view of the distal forearm reveals anatomic variations in the length of the radius and the ulna, known as *ulnar variance* or *Hulten variance*. As a rule, the radial styloid process exceeds the length of the articular end of the ulna by 9 to 12 mm. At the site of articulation with the lunate, however, the articular surfaces of the radius

and the ulna are on the same level, yielding *neutral ulnar variance* (Fig. 7.3). Occasionally, the ulna projects more proximally—*negative ulnar variance* (or ulna minus variant); or more distally—*positive ulnar variance* (or ulna plus variant) (Fig. 7.4). Wrist position is an important determinant of ulnar variance. The generally accepted standard position is a posteroanterior view obtained with the wrist flat on the radiographic table, neutral forearm rotation, and with the elbow flexed 90° and the shoulder abducted 90°. The posteroanterior radiograph also reveals an important anatomic feature of the radius known as the *radial angle* (also called the *ulnar slant* of the articular surface of the radius), which normally ranges from 15° to 25° (Fig. 7.5).

The lateral view of the distal forearm demonstrates another significant feature, the *volar tilt* of the articular surface of the radius (known variously as the *dorsal angle, palmar facing,* or *palmar inclination*). The tilt normally ranges from 10° to 25° (Fig. 7.6).

Both these measurements have practical importance to the orthopedic surgeon in assessing displacement and the position of fragments after fracture of the distal radius. They can also help the surgeon to decide between closed and open reduction, as well as assist in follow-up examinations.

Ancillary imaging techniques are occasionally required for evaluating trauma to the distal forearm and wrist. Arthrographic examination (Fig. 7.7) may need to be performed in cases of suspected injury to the triangular fibrocartilage complex (TFCC), which consists of the triangular fibrocartilage (articular disk), the meniscus homolog, the

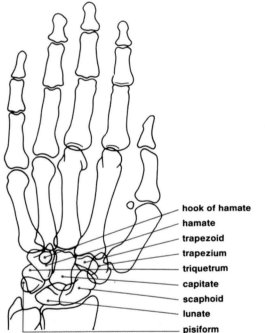

hook of hamate
hamate
trapezoid
trapezium
triquetrum
capitate
scaphoid
lunate
pisiform

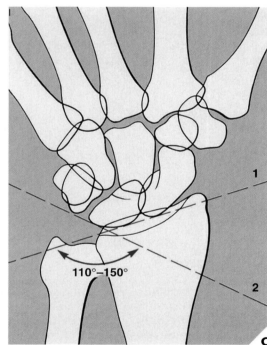

110°–150°

Figure 7.1 Dorsovolar (posteroanterior) view of the distal forearm, wrist, and hand. For the purpose of classification, a distinction is made between traumatic conditions involving the distal forearm, the wrist, and the hand. From a radiologic perspective, however, the positioning of the limb for posteroanterior and lateral films of the wrist area (that is, the distal forearm and the carpus) and the hand is essentially the same. **(A)** For the posteroanterior (dorsovolar) view of the wrist and the hand, patients are seated with the arm fully extended on the radiographic table. The portion of the limb from the distal third of the forearm to the fingertips rests prone on the film cassette. Whether the wrist area or the hand is the focus of evaluation, the hand usually lies flat (palm down), with the fingers slightly spread. The point toward which the central beam is directed, however, varies. For the wrist, the beam is directed toward the center of the carpus; for the hand, the beam is directed toward the head of the third metacarpal bone. For better demonstration of the wrist area, the patient's fingers may be flexed to cause the carpus to lie flat on the film cassette (*inset*). **(B)** On the film in this projection, the distal radius and the ulna, as well as the carpal and metacarpal bones and phalanges, are well demonstrated. The thumb, however, is seen in an oblique projection; the bases of the second to fifth metacarpals partially overlap. In the wrist, there is also overlap of the pisiform and the triquetrum, as well as the trapezium and trapezoid bones. **(C)** On this projection, a carpal angle can be determined. It is formed by two tangents, the first drawn against the proximal borders of the scaphoid and lunate (1), the second drawn against the proximal borders of the triquetrum and lunate (2). The angle measures normally between 110° and 150°, showing considerable deviation with age, sex, and race.

hamate
trapezium
capitate
triquetrum
scaphoid
lunate

Figure 7.2 Lateral view of the wrist and hand. (A) For the lateral projection of the wrist area and the hand, the patient's arm is fully extended and resting on its ulnar side. The fingers may be fully extended or, preferably, slightly flexed (*inset*), with the thumb slightly in front of the fingers. For evaluation of the wrist area, the central beam is directed toward the center of the carpus, while for the hand it is directed toward the head of the second metacarpal. **(B)** On the film in this projection, the distal radius and the ulna overlap, but the relation of the longitudinal axes of the capitate, the lunate, and the radius can sufficiently be evaluated (see Fig. 7.66). Although the metacarpals and the phalanges also overlap, dorsal or volar displacement of a fracture of these bones can easily be detected (see Fig. 4.1). The thumb is imaged in true dorsovolar projection. **(C)** A more effective way of imaging the fingers in the lateral projection is to have the patient spread the fingers in a fan-like manner, with the ulnar side of the fifth phalanx resting on the film cassette. The central beam is directed toward the heads of the metacarpals. **(D)** On the film in this projection, the overlap of the phalanges commonly seen on the standard lateral view is eliminated. The interphalangeal joints can readily be evaluated.

Figure 7.3 **Neutral ulnar variance.** **(A)** As a rule, the radial styloid process rises 9 to 12 mm above the articular surface of the distal ulna. This distance is also known as the radial length. **(B)** At the site of articulation with the lunate, the articular surfaces of the radius and the ulna are on the same level.

Figure 7.4 **Negative and positive ulnar variance.** **(A)** Negative ulnar variance. The articular surface of the ulna projects 5 mm proximal to the site of radiolunate articulation. **(B)** Positive ulnar variance. The articular surface of the ulna projects 8 mm distal to the site of radiolunate articulation.

Figure 7.5 **Ulnar slant.** The ulnar slant of the articular surface of the radius is determined, with the wrist in the neutral position, by the angle formed by two lines: one perpendicular to the long axis of the radius at the level of the radioulnar articular surface (a) and a tangent connecting the radial styloid process and the ulnar aspect of the radius (b).

Figure 7.6 **Palmar inclination.** The palmar inclination of the radial articular surface is determined by measuring the angle formed by a line perpendicular to the long axis of the radius at the level of the styloid process (a) and a tangent connecting the dorsal and volar aspects of the radial articular surface (b).

Figure 7.7 Arthrography of the wrist. (A) For arthrographic examination of the radiocarpal joint, the wrist is positioned prone on a radiolucent sponge to open the joint for needle insertion. Under fluoroscopic control, the joint is entered using a 22-gauge needle at a point lateral to the scapholunate ligament. (The red dot marks the site of puncture.) Two or 3 mL of contrast (60% diatrizoate meglumine) is injected, and posteroanterior (dorsovolar), lateral, and oblique films are obtained. Posteroanterior **(B)** and lateral **(C)** views show contrast filling the radiocarpal compartment, the prestyloid and volar radial recesses, and the pisotriquetral space. Intact triangular fibrocartilage does not allow contrast to enter the distal radioulnar joint, and intact intercarpal ligaments prevent leak of contrast into the intercarpal articulations.

Figure 7.8 Triangular fibrocartilage complex. The triangular fibrocartilage complex (TFCC) includes the triangular fibrocartilage, radioulnar ligament, ulnocarpal ligament, extensor carpal ulnaris tendon sheath, and meniscus homolog. It is located between the distal ulna and the proximal carpal row, stabilizes the distal radioulnar joint, and functions as a cushion of compressing axial forces. The triangular fibrocartilage attaches medially to the fovea of the ulna and laterally to the lunate fossa of the radius.

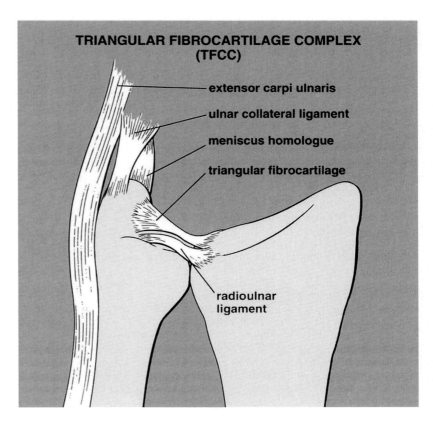

Table 7.1 **Standard Radiographic Projections for Evaluating Injury to the Distal Forearm**

Projection	Demonstration
Posteroanterior	Ulnar variance
	Carpal angle
	Radial angle
	Distal radioulnar joint
	Colles fracture
	Hutchinson fracture
	Galeazzi fracture—dislocation
Lateral	Palmar facing of radius
	Pronator quadratus fat-stripe
	Colles fracture
	Smith fracture
	Barton fracture
	Galeazzi fracture—dislocation

dorsal and volar radioulnar ligaments, and the ulnar collateral ligament (Fig. 7.8). Because the radiocarpal cavity into which contrast is injected normally does not communicate with the distal radioulnar joint, opacification of this compartment indicates a tear of the triangular fibrocartilage (see Fig. 7.23). In a small percentage of cases, a false-positive result may be caused by a normal anatomic variant allowing communication between the radiocarpal compartment and the distal radioulnar joint.

For a summary in tabular form of the standard radiographic projections and ancillary imaging techniques used to evaluate trauma to the distal forearm, see Tables 7.1 and 7.2.

Injury to the Distal Forearm

Fractures of the Distal Radius

Colles Fracture. The most frequently encountered injury to the distal forearm, *Colles fracture,* usually results from a fall on the outstretched hand with the forearm pronated in dorsiflexion. It is most commonly seen in adults older than age 50 years and more often in women than in men. In the classic description of this injury, known in the European literature as the *Pouteau fracture,* the fracture line is extraarticular, usually occurring approximately 2 to 3 cm from the articular surface of the distal radius. In many cases, the distal fragment is

Table 7.2 **Ancillary Imaging Techniques for Evaluating Injury to the Distal Forearm**

Technique	Demonstration
Arthrography	Radiocarpal articulation
	Tear of triangular fibrocartilage complex
Arteriography	Concomitant injury to the arteries of the forearm
Radionuclide Imaging (scintigraphy, bone scan)	Subtle fractures of radius and ulna
Computed Tomography	Fracture healing and complications of healing
	Soft-tissue injury (muscles, tendons)
Magnetic Resonance Imaging	Soft-tissue injury
	Subtle fractures and bone contusion of radius and ulna
	Tear of triangular fibrocartilage complex
	Abnormalities of various tendons, ligaments, and muscles
	Injury to the interosseous membrane

radially and dorsally displaced and shows dorsal angulation, although other variants in the alignment of fragments may also be seen (Fig. 7.9). Commonly, there is an associated fracture of the ulnar styloid process. It should be noted that some authors (e.g., Frykman) include intraarticular extension of the fracture line, as well as an associated fracture of the distal end of the ulna, under this eponym (Fig. 7.10, Table 7.3).

Radiographs in the posteroanterior and lateral projections are sufficient to demonstrate Colles fracture. The complete evaluation on both views should take note of the status of the radial angle and the palmar inclination, as well as the degree of foreshortening of the radius secondary to impaction or bayonet-type displacement (Figs. 7.11, 7.12, and 7.13). CT scanning may provide additional information concerning the exact position of displaced fragments (Fig. 7.14).

Complications. At the time of fracture, concomitant injury to the median and ulnar nerves may occur. Lack of stability of the fragments during healing may result in loss of reduction, but delayed union and nonunion are very rarely seen. As a sequela, posttraumatic arthritis may develop in the radiocarpal articulation.

Barton and Hutchinson Fractures. Both these fractures are intraarticular fractures of the distal radius. The classic *Barton fracture* affects the dorsal margin of the distal radius and extends into the radiocarpal articulation (Fig. 7.15); occasionally, there may also be an associated dislocation in the joint. When the fracture involves the volar margin of the distal radius with intraarticular extension, it is known as a *reverse* (or *volar*) *Barton fracture* (Fig. 7.16). Because in both variants the fracture line is oriented in the coronal plane, it is best demonstrated on the lateral or oblique projections.

The *Hutchinson fracture* (also known as chauffeur's fracture—a name derived from the era of hand-cranked automobiles when direct trauma to the radial side of the wrist was often sustained from recoil of the crank) involves the radial (lateral) margin of the distal radius, extending through the radial styloid process into the radiocarpal articulation. Because of the sagittal orientation of the fracture line, the posteroanterior view is better suited to diagnose this type of injury (Fig. 7.17).

Smith Fracture. Usually resulting from a fall on the back of the hand or a direct blow to the dorsum of the hand in palmar flexion, a Smith fracture consists of a fracture of the distal radius, which sometimes extends into the radiocarpal joint, with volar displacement and angulation of the distal fragment (Fig. 7.18). Because the deformity in this fracture is the opposite of that seen in a Colles injury, it is often referred to as a reverse Colles fracture; it is, however, much less common than Colles. There are three types of Smith fracture, defined on the basis of the obliquity of the fracture line (Fig. 7.19), which is best assessed on the lateral projection. Types II and III are usually unstable and may require surgical intervention.

Galeazzi Fracture–Dislocation. This abnormality, which may result indirectly from a fall on the outstretched hand combined with marked pronation of the forearm or directly from a blow to the dorsolateral aspect of the wrist, consists of a fracture of the distal third of the radius, sometimes extending into the radiocarpal articulation and an associated dislocation in the distal radioulnar joint. Characteristically, the proximal end of the distal fragment is dorsally displaced, commonly with dorsal angulation at the fracture site; the ulna is dorsally and ulnarly (medially) dislocated. Two types of Galeazzi injury have been identified. In type I, the fracture of the radius is extraarticular in the distal third of the bone (Fig. 7.20). In type II, the radius fracture is usually comminuted and extends into the radiocarpal joint (Fig. 7.21).

Posteroanterior and lateral films are routinely obtained when this injury is suspected, but the lateral view clearly reveals its nature and extent (Figs. 7.20B and 7.21B).

Piedmont Fracture. An isolated fracture of the radius at the junction of the middle and distal thirds without associated disruption of the distal radioulnar joint is known as the Piedmont fracture. This injury is also called "fracture of necessity," because open reduction

**COLLES FRACTURE: VARIANTS
IN ALIGNMENT OF FRAGMENTS**

volar   dorsal

impaction without
displacement

simple dorsal
displacement

dorsal displacement
and dorsal angulation

radial (lateral) displacement

radial (lateral) displacement
and radial angulation

Figure 7.9 Colles fracture. Five variants of displacement and angulation of the distal fragment in Colles fracture. Some of these patterns may occur in combinations, yielding complex deformity.

and internal fixation are necessary to achieve an acceptable functional result. If this fracture is treated conservatively with closed reduction and cast application, then the interosseous space may be compromised because of muscle action, resulting in loss of pronation and supination after the bone union is completed.

Essex-Lopresti Fracture–Dislocation. This fracture, which affects the radial head and is associated with tear of the interosseous membrane of the forearm and dislocation in the distal radioulnar joint, was discussed in Chapter 6.

Ulnar Impingement Syndrome. Ulnar impingement syndrome is caused by a short distal ulna that impinges on the distal radius proximal to the sigmoid notch. A short ulna may represent a congenital anomaly, such as negative ulnar variance, or may be the result of premature fusion of the distal ulnar growth plate secondary to previous trauma. In most cases, however, it is caused by surgical procedures that involve resection of the distal ulna secondary to trauma, rheumatoid arthritis, or correction of a Madelung deformity. The clinical symptoms of the ulnar impingement syndrome consist of ulnar-sided wrist pain and limitation of motion in the radiocarpal joint. In addi-

tion, patients experience discomfort during pronation and supination of the forearm. On radiography, the characteristic changes of this abnormality include a short ulna and scalloping of the medial aspect of the distal radius in cases of negative ulnar variance or premature fusion of the distal ulnar growth plate, or radial scalloping and radioul-

Table 7.3 Frykman Classification of Distal Radius Fractures

Radius Fracture	Distal Ulna Fracture	
Location	*Absent*	*Present*
Extraarticular	I	II
Intraarticular (radiocarpal joint)	III	IV
Intraarticular (radioulnar joint)	V	VI
Intraarticular (radiocarpal and radioulnar joints)	VII	VIII

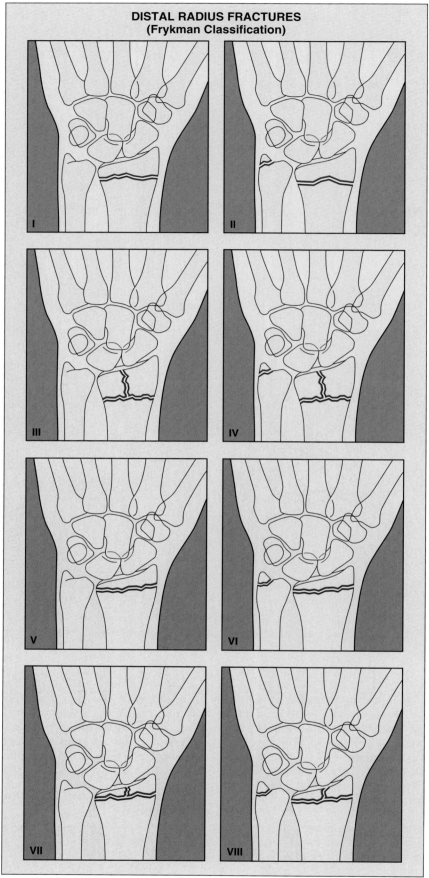

Figure 7.10 Distal radius fractures. Frykman classification of distal radius fractures according to the location of fracture line (intraarticular versus extraarticular) and association of distal ulna fracture.

Figure 7.11 Colles fracture. Posteroanterior **(A)** and lateral **(B)** views of the distal forearm demonstrate the features of Colles fracture. On the posteroan-terior projection, a decrease in the radial angle and an associated fracture of the distal ulna are evident. The lateral view reveals the dorsal angulation of the distal radius, as well as a reversal of the palmar inclination. On both views, the radius is foreshortened secondary to bayonet-type displacement. The frac-ture line does not extend to the joint (Frykman type II).

Figure 7.12 Intraarticular fracture of the dis-tal radius. Posteroanterior radiograph of the dis-tal forearm **(A)** and trispiral tomogram **(B)** show Frykman type IV fracture. The fracture extends into the radiocarpal joint, the distal radioulnar joint is spared, and there is an associated fracture of the ulnar styloid.

Figure 7.13 Intraarticular fracture of the distal radius. Posteroanterior **(A)** and oblique **(B)** radiographs of the distal forearm show Frykman type VI fracture. The fracture line extends into the distal radioulnar joint and in addition there is a fracture of the ulnar styloid.

Figure 7.14 CT of intraarticular fracture of the distal radius. **(A)** Posteroanterior radiograph shows intraarticular fracture of the distal radius. The fracture appears to be nondisplaced. **(B)** Coronal CT and **(C)** three-dimensional CT reformatted images demonstrate displacement (arrow) and depression (curved arrow) of the fractured fragments.

Figure 7.15 Barton fracture. Schematic **(A)** and oblique radiograph **(B)** show the typical appearance of Barton fracture. The fracture line in the coronal plane extends from the dorsal margin of the distal radius into the radiocarpal articulation.

Figure 7.16 Reverse Barton fracture. Schematic (A), oblique radiograph (B), and lateral trispiral tomogram (C) show the reverse (or volar) Barton fracture; the fracture line is also oriented in the coronal plane, but extends from the volar margin of the radial styloid process into the radiocarpal joint.

Figure 7.17 Hutchinson fracture. Schematic (A) and dorsovolar radiographs (B) showing classic appearance of Hutchinson fracture. The fracture line in the sagittal plane extends through the radial margin of the radial styloid process into the radiocarpal articulation.

Figure 7.18 Smith fracture. Posteroanterior (A) and lateral (B) films of the distal forearm show the typical appearance of Smith fracture. Volar displacement of the distal fragment is clearly evident on the lateral view.

Figure 7.19 Smith fracture. The three types of Smith fracture are distinguished by the obliquity of the fracture line. Volar displacement of the distal fragment is characteristic of all three types. **(A)** In Smith type I, the fracture line is transverse, extending from the dorsal to the volar cortices of the radius. **(B)** The oblique fracture line in type II extends from the dorsal lip of the distal radius to the volar cortex. **(C)** Type III, which is almost identical to the reverse Barton fracture (see Fig. 7.16), is an intraarticular fracture with extension to the volar cortex of the distal radius.

Figure 7.20 Galeazzi fracture–dislocation. Posteroanterior **(A)** and lateral **(B)** radiographs of the distal forearm show type I Galeazzi fracture–dislocation. The simple fracture of the radius affects the distal third of the bone, and the proximal end of the distal fragment is dorsally displaced and angulated. In addition, there is dislocation in the distal radioulnar joint.

Figure 7.21 Galeazzi fracture–dislocation. Posteroanterior **(A)** and lateral **(B)** projections of the distal forearm demonstrate the two components of Galeazzi fracture–dislocation type II. The posteroanterior view clearly reveals the fracture of the distal radius, which in this case is a comminuted fracture extending into the radiocarpal joint. The distal fragment has a slight lateral angulation. Note also the associated comminuted fracture of the ulnar styloid process and the dislocation in the radioulnar joint. These features are also seen on the lateral projection, but this view provides in addition a better demonstration of the dorsal dislocation of the distal ulna.

nar convergence in cases of distal ulnar resection. Before these findings become obvious on conventional radiologic studies, MRI may be helpful in early recognition of this condition.

Ulnar Impaction Syndrome. Also known as the ulnolunate abutment syndrome, the ulnar impaction syndrome is a well-recognized entity clinically characterized by ulnar-sided wrist pain and limitation of motion in the radiocarpal joint. It is frequently associated with the positive ulnar variance. The pathologic mechanism of this syndrome is linked to altered and increased forces transmitted across the ulnar side of the wrist, leading to compression of the distal ulna on the medial surface of the lunate bone. This causes development of degenerative changes in the cartilage covering both bones. In addition, frequent association of the tear of the triangular fibrocartilage has been reported. In cases of excessive ulnar length, dorsal subluxation of the ulna is present compromising supination of the forearm. MRI is the most effective technique for diagnosis of this syndrome and demon-

stration of pathologic changes in the affected bones and surrounding soft tissues. MR imaging reveals bone marrow edema of the distal ulna and lunate, subchondral sclerosis and cyst formation, and destruction of the cartilage. Associated abnormalities, such as tears of the triangular fibrocartilage and lunotriquetral ligament, are also well imaged (Fig. 7.22). Treatment of this condition includes TFCC debridement and ulnar shortening.

Injury to the Soft Tissue at the Distal Radioulnar Articulation

One of the most common sequelae of injury to the distal radioulnar articulation is tear of the TFCC. Tear may occur as the result of fractures such as those described in the preceding sections or independently after injury to the distal forearm and wrist.

Radiographs in the standard projections are invariably normal regarding the status of the triangular cartilage, particularly if there is no

Figure 7.22 Ulnar impaction syndrome. (A) Coronal T1-weighted MR image shows a positive ulnar variance and sclerosis of the proximal ulnar aspect of the lunate (*arrow*). **(B)** Coronal T1-weighted MRI obtained slightly more volarly and **(C)** corresponding T2*-weighted image demonstrate subchondral cysts (straight arrows) and involvement of triquetrum (*curved arrows*). Note also disruption of the triangular fibrocartilage.

Figure 7.23 Wrist arthrogram. A single-contrast arthrogram of the wrist shows leak of contrast into the space occupied by the triangular cartilage, with characteristic filling of the distal radioulnar compartment, confirming a tear of the triangular fibrocartilage complex (compare with Fig. 7.7B).

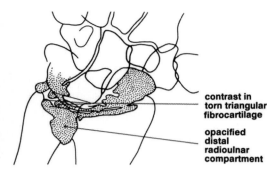

contrast in
torn triangular
fibrocartilage

opacified
distal
radioulnar
compartment

evidence of fracture or dislocation on which to base suspicion of soft-tissue injury. When it is suspected, however, a single-contrast arthrogram of the wrist can confirm or exclude the diagnosis. Normally, contrast fills the radiocarpal compartment, the prestyloid and volar radial recesses, and the pisotriquetral space (see Fig. 7.7). The presence of contrast in the distal radioulnar compartment or at the site of the triangular cartilage indicates a tear (Fig. 7.23).

Until recently, arthrography has been the procedure of choice for evaluation of TFCC. Currently, it is generally believed that in the diagnosis of TFCC abnormalities, MRI approaches arthrography in accuracy. The advantage of MRI is its noninvasiveness and ability to image the entire fibrocartilage substance, whereas arthrography is limited to evaluation of the surface of this structure only. On coronal T1-weighted MR images, the normal TFCC appears as a biconcave band of homogeneous low signal intensity extending across the space between the distal ulna, medial aspect of distal radius, and triquetrum and lunate bones (see Figs. 7.8 and 7.26). Tears of the TFCC manifest as discontinuities and fragmentation of this structure. The torn fibrocartilage becomes irregular in contour and is interrupted by high signal intensity areas on T2-weighted images (Fig. 7.24). However, one of the recent studies published by Haims and colleagues, questions the sensitivity of MR imaging in diagnosing peripheral tears of the trian-

gular fibrocartilage. In this respect, the authors reported the sensitivity of MRI of only 17%, with a specificity of 79%, and accuracy of 64%.

Wrist and Hand

Considered as a functional unit, the wrist and hand are the most common sites of injury in the skeletal system. Fractures of the metacarpals and phalanges, however, by far predominate in incidence over fractures and dislocations in the carpal bones and joints, which constitute approximately 6% of all such injuries. In most instances, history and physical examination provide valuable information on which to base a suspected diagnosis, but radiographic findings derived from films obtained in at least two projections at 90° to each other (see Fig. 4.1) are essential to determine a specific diagnosis of injury to these sites.

Anatomic–Radiologic Considerations

Trauma to the wrist and hand usually can be sufficiently evaluated on conventional radiographs in the dorsovolar (posteroanterior) and lateral projections (see Figs. 7.1 and 7.2). However, determination of the exact extent of damage to the different carpal bones forming the complex structure of the wrist may require supplemental studies specific for the various anatomic sites. These special views include the following:

1. Dorsovolar obtained in ulnar deviation of the wrist for evaluation of the scaphoid bone, which appears foreshortened on the standard dorsovolar projection as a result of its normal volar tilt (Fig. 7.25)
2. Supinated oblique for visualizing the pisiform bone and the pisotriquetral joint (Fig. 7.26)
3. Pronated oblique for imaging the triquetral bone, the radiovolar aspect of the scaphoid, and the radial styloid process (Fig. 7.27)
4. Carpal–tunnel for demonstrating the hook of the hamate, the pisiform, and the volar aspect of the trapezium (Fig. 7.28).

A full assessment of traumatic conditions and their sequelae may also require ancillary imaging techniques. Among the most commonly performed are conventional tomography, most often in the form of thin-section trispiral cuts, for detecting occult fractures; fluoroscopy combined with videotaping for evaluation of wrist kinematics and joint instability; arthrography and magnetic resonance imaging (MRI) for determining soft-tissue injuries such as capsular and tendinous ruptures; and radionuclide bone scan for detecting subtle fractures and early complications of fracture healing. Computed tomography (CT) has evolved as a versatile tool and adjunctive procedure for imaging various traumatic abnormalities of the wrist. In many institutions, this technique virtually replaced conventional tomography, because it is easier to perform, is faster, and has a lower radiation dose. After standard axial sections are obtained, reformation images in additional imaging planes can be acquired and three-dimensional (3-D) reconstruction can be performed (see Fig. 2.6A, B). CT can be combined with arthrography (see Fig. 2.13) or can be enhanced by intra-

Figure 7.24 Tear of the triangular fibrocartilage complex. Coronal T2*-weighted GRASS image of the left wrist shows a full-thickness tear of the TFCC. The triangular fibrocartilage is torn and displaced from the ulnar styloid (*arrow*). Moderate amount of fluid is seen in the distal radioulnar joint (*curved arrow*).

Figure 7.25 Ulnar deviation. (A) For the dorsovolar view of the wrist in ulnar deviation, the forearm rests flat on the radiographic table with the anterior surface down and the elbow flexed 90°. The hand, lying flat on the film cassette, is ulnarly deviated. The central beam is directed toward the carpus. **(B)** The film in this projection demonstrates the scaphoid free of the distortion because of its normal volar tilt when the wrist is in the neutral position.

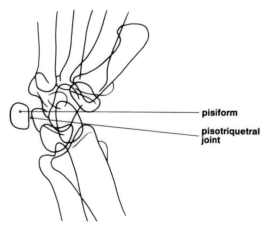

Figure 7.26 Supinated oblique view. (A) For the supinated oblique view of the wrist, the hand resting on its ulnar side on the film cassette is tilted approximately 30° to 35° toward its dorsal surface. The outstretched fingers are held together, with the thumb slightly abducted. The central beam is directed toward the center of the wrist. **(B)** The film in this projection demonstrates the pisiform bone and the pisotriquetral joint.

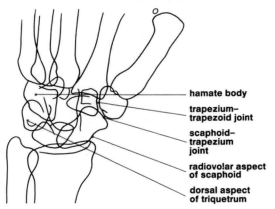

Figure 7.27 Pronated oblique view. (A) For the pronated oblique view of the wrist, the hand resting on its ulnar side on the film cassette is tilted approximately 40° to 45° toward its palmar surface. The slightly flexed fingers are held together, with the thumb in front of them. The central beam is directed toward the center of the carpus. **(B)** The film in this projection demonstrates the dorsal aspect of the triquetrum, the body of the hamate, the radiovolar aspect of the scaphoid, and the scaphoid—trapezium and trapezium—trapezoid articulations.

venous contrast material. It is effective in demonstrating subluxation in the distal radioulnar joint and in evaluating so-called humpback deformity of the scaphoid, osteonecrosis of the lunate (Kienböck disease), and fractures of the hook of the hamate, among other abnormalities. Axial sections are obtained after positioning the patient prone with the arm extended above the head. One- or 2-mm contiguous sections are acquired, preferably using a spiral (helical) technique. Direct coronal sections can also be obtained with the wrist in maximal volar flexion or dorsal extension.

Arthrography still remains an effective procedure for evaluating the TFCC abnormalities and tears of various intercarpal ligaments. In general, single-contrast arthrography using positive contrast agents is performed. However, if postarthrographic CT examination is to be performed, double-contrast arthrography using air is preferable. The introduction of the three-compartment injection technique and combining the arthrographic wrist examination with digital technique and postarthrographic CT examination make this modality a procedure of choice in evaluating a painful wrist. A complete arthrographic

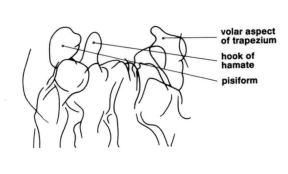

Figure 7.28 Carpal–tunnel view. (A) For the carpal—tunnel view of the wrist, the hand is maximally dorsiflexed by means of the patient's opposite hand or a strap, with the palmar surface of the wrist resting on the film cassette. The central beam is directed toward the cup of the palm at approximately a 15° angle. **(B)** The film in this projection demonstrates an axial view of the hook of the hamate, as well as the pisiform bone and the volar margin of the trapezium.

CARPAL JOINT COMPARTMENTS

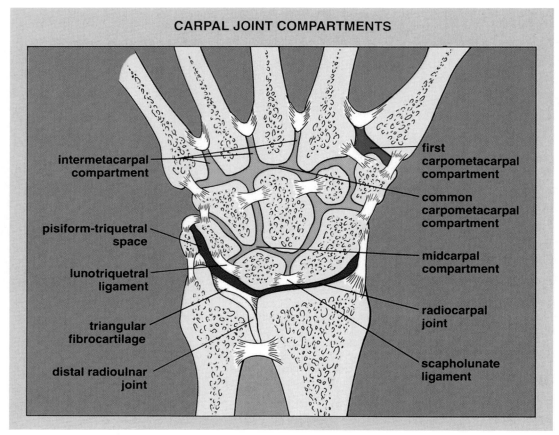

intermetacarpal
compartment

first
carpometacarpal
compartment

common
carpometacarpal
compartment

pisiform-triquetral
space

midcarpal
compartment

lunotriquetral
ligament

radiocarpal
joint

triangular
fibrocartilage

distal radioulnar
joint

scapholunate
ligament

Figure 7.29 Compartments of the carpus. Carpal joint compartments are separated from one another by various interosseous ligaments.

evaluation of the wrist requires opacification of the midcarpal compartment, radiocarpal compartment, and distal radioulnar joint. These three compartments are normally separated from one another by various interosseous ligaments and in the case of distal radioulnar joint, by the TFCC (Fig. 7.29). Flow of contrast from one compartment to another indicates a defect in one of these ligaments. Unidirectional contrast flow through the ligament defects, associated with a small flap acting as a valve, has been reported and may be overlooked if the contrast is injected on only one side of the defect. For this reason, the separate injection of all three compartments is preferable. It has to be stressed, however, that defects in the ligaments may occasionally be found in normal, asymptomatic subjects; therefore, their significance remains uncertain.

More recently, digital subtraction arthrography has been advocated by Resnick and Manaster as an effective way to demonstrate subtle leaks of contrast. The advantages of digital subtraction arthrography include not only shortening of examination time but also decrease in concentration of contrast agent and more precise localization of defects in intercarpal ligaments, particularly when the defects are multiple (see Fig. 2.2).

MRI has become a very promising imaging modality for evaluation of the wrist and hand (Fig. 7.30). To achieve optimum quality examination, the use of a dedicated local (surface) radiofrequency coil and limited field of view is recommended. This technique may image not only abnormalities of the soft tissues, including various muscles, tendons, interosseous ligaments, and triangular fibrocartilage but also bony abnormalities such as occult fractures and early osteonecrosis, particularly of the lunate and scaphoid. It is also very useful in imaging the carpal tunnel (Fig. 7.31) and detecting the subtle abnormalities of carpal tunnel syndrome (Fig. 7.32).

The coronal plane is the best to demonstrate the interosseous ligaments of the proximal carpal row (scapholunate and lunatotriquetral ligaments) and the TFCC. These structures exhibit a low-intensity

lunotriquetral
interosseous
ligament

scapholunate
interosseous
ligament

triangular
fibrocartilage

Figure 7.30 MRI of the wrist. Coronal T2-weighted MR image (gradient-echo pulse sequence) of the wrist demonstrates distal radius and ulna and carpal bones. The proximal interosseous ligaments and the triangular fibrocartilage are clearly delineated. (From Beltran J, 1990, with permission.)

Figure 7.31 MRI of the wrist. Proton density-weighted spin-echo axial MR image (TR 2000/TE 20 msec) through the carpal tunnel demonstrates the various structures. Note the median nerve, displaying intermediate signal intensity and flexor retinaculum imaged with low signal intensity. (From Beltran J, 1990, with permission.)

signal on T1- and T2-weighted sequences (see Fig. 7.30). In this plane, various intrinsic and extrinsic dorsal and volar ligaments of the wrist (Fig. 7.33) are also seen. In the sagittal plane, all flexor and extensor tendons with their respective insertions are clearly depicted, as well as some of the ligaments including the radioscaphocapite, radiolunatotriquetral, and dorsal radiolunate (Fig. 7.34). In the axial plane, various ligaments and tendons are shown in cross-sections; their anatomic relationship to the bone structures, arteries, and nerves can be evaluated effectively (Fig. 7.35). This plane is also ideal for imaging of the Guyon canal. This anatomic structure is located on the volar aspect of the wrist, medially to the carpal tunnel, between the pisiform bone and the hook of the hamate (Fig. 7.36). It is bounded by the flexor retinaculum from the dorsal aspect, hypothenar musculature from the medial aspect, and by fascia from the volar aspect. It contains the ulnar vein, ulnar artery, and ulnar nerve.

Ancillary techniques such as stress films and arthrography may also need to be used for evaluation of disruption or displacement of the ligaments of the hand, particularly in gamekeeper's thumb. For a summary in tabular form of the standard and special radiographic projections, as well as the ancillary techniques used to evaluate trauma to the wrist and hand, see Tables 7.4 and 7.5 and Fig. 7.37.

Injury to the Wrist

Fractures of the Carpal Bones

Fracture of the Scaphoid Bone. Fractures of the scaphoid (or carpal navicular) are the second most common injuries of the upper limb, exceeded in frequency only by fractures of the distal radius, and they comprise 2% of all fractures. Of all fractures and dislocations in the carpus, this fracture is the most common, accounting for 50% to 60% of such injuries. They frequently occur in young adults (ages 15 to 30) after falls on the outstretched palm of the hand. Scaphoid fractures can be classified according to direction of the fracture line (Fig. 7.38), the degree of stability of the fragments, and the location of the fracture line. From a diagnostic perspective, the latter is a more prac-

Figure 7.32 Carpal tunnel syndrome. A 21-year-old woman with clinically diagnosed carpal tunnel syndrome underwent MRI examination of her right wrist. Proton density-weighted **(A)** and T2-weighted **(B)** axial images demonstrate an increased signal of the median nerve and thickened synovium surrounding the flexor tendons in the carpal tunnel. Note the volar bowing of the flexor retinaculum and the absent fat plane between the deep flexor tendons and the more dorsal radiolunatotriquetral ligament. (From Beltran J, 1990, with permission.)

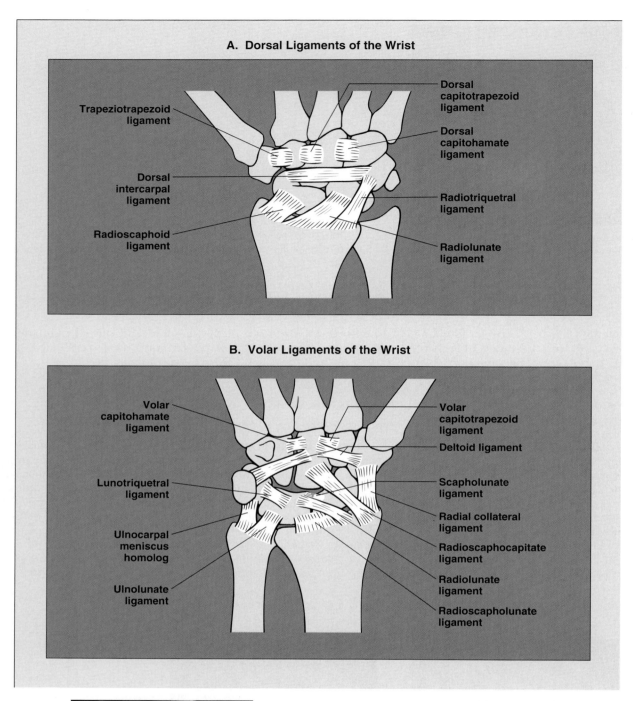

A. Dorsal Ligaments of the Wrist

Trapeziotrapezoid ligament

Dorsal capitotrapezoid ligament

Dorsal capitohamate ligament

Dorsal intercarpal ligament

Radioscaphoid ligament

Radiotriquetral ligament

Radiolunate ligament

B. Volar Ligaments of the Wrist

Volar capitohamate ligament

Volar capitotrapezoid ligament

Deltoid ligament

Lunotriquetral ligament

Scapholunate ligament

Ulnocarpal meniscus homolog

Radial collateral ligament

Radioscaphocapitate ligament

Ulnolunate ligament

Radiolunate ligament

Radioscapholunate ligament

Figure 7.33 **Ligaments of the wrist.** Schematic representation of dorsal **(A)** and volar **(B)** ligaments of the wrist.

Radioscaphocapitate ligament

Dorsal intercarpal ligament

Figure 7.34 MRI of the wrist. Sagittal MRI through the wrist from the mid aspect **(A)**, **(B)** to the ulnar aspect **(C)**, **(D)**. The volar and dorsal radiolunate components of the radioscapholunate ligaments are well demonstrated. The radiolunatotriquetral ligament is seen volar to the capitate—lunate articulation. The radioscaphocapitate ligament is seen inserting at the volar and proximal one third of the capitate bone. (From Beltran J, 1990, with permission.) *(continued)*

Figure 7.34 **MRI of the wrist.** *Continued.*

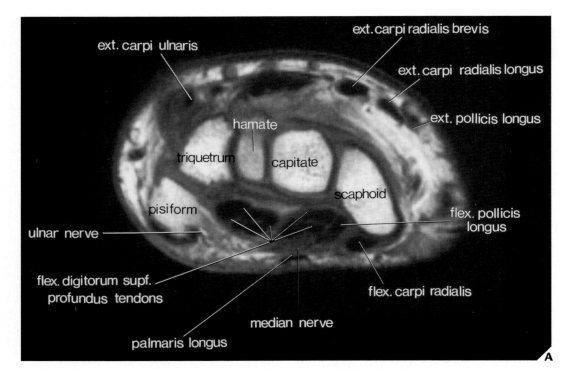

Figure 7.35 **MRI of the wrist.** Axial T1-weighted MR images through the proximal **(A)** and distal **(B)** carpus effectively demonstrate various anatomic structures of the wrist.

In image A:
ext. carpi ulnaris
ext. carpi radialis brevis
ext. carpi radialis longus
hamate
ext. pollicis longus
triquetrum
capitate
scaphoid
pisiform
flex. pollicis longus
ulnar nerve
flex. digitorum supf. profundus tendons
flex. carpi radialis
median nerve
palmaris longus

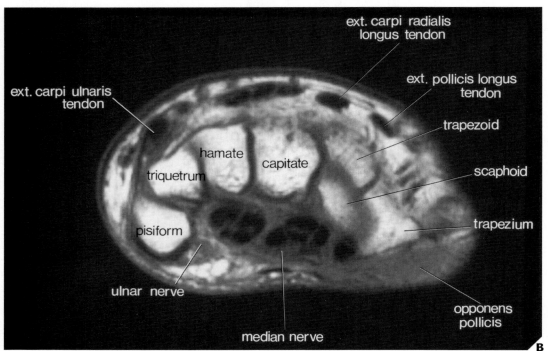

In image B:
ext. carpi radialis longus tendon
ext. carpi ulnaris tendon
ext. pollicis longus tendon
trapezoid
hamate
capitate
triquetrum
scaphoid
pisiform
trapezium
ulnar nerve
median nerve
opponens pollicis

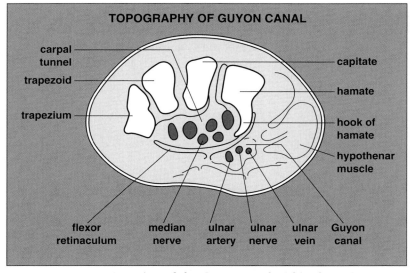

Figure 7.36 Location of the Guyon canal within the wrist.

TOPOGRAPHY OF GUYON CANAL
carpal tunnel
trapezoid
trapezium
capitate
hamate
hook of hamate
hypothenar muscle
flexor retinaculum
median nerve
ulnar artery
ulnar nerve
ulnar vein
Guyon canal

Table 7.4 **Standard and Special Radiographic Projections for Evaluating Injury to the Wrist and Hand**

Projection	Demonstration	Projection	Demonstration

Dorsovolar	Carpal bones
	Three carpal arcs
	Eye of the hamate
	Scaphoid fat stripe
	Radiocarpal articulation
	Metacarpals
	Phalanges
	Carpometacarpal, metacarpophalangeal, and interphalangeal joints
	Scapholunate dissociation:
	Terry-Thomas sign
	Scaphoid signet-ring sign
	Fractures of:
	   Scaphoid
	   Capitate
	   Lunate
	   Metacarpals
	   Phalanges
	Bennett and Rolando fractures in ulnar deviation
		Oblique (hand)
		
		Supinated Oblique (wrist)
		
		Pronated Oblique (wrist)
		
		Body of Hamate Fractures
		
		Carpal—Tunnel
		
		Abduction—Stress (thumb)
			Fractures of:
			   Metacarpals
			   Phalanges
			Boxer's fracture
			Pisotriquetral joint
			Pisiform fractures
			Dorsal aspect of triquetrum and triquetral fractures
			Radiovolar aspect of scaphoid
			Articulations between:
			   Scaphoid and trapezium
			   Trapezium and trapezoid
			Volar aspect of trapezium
			Fractures of:
			   Hook of the hamate
			   Pisiform
			Gamekeeper's thumb

In ulnar deviation	Scaphoid fractures		

Lateral	Longitudinal axial alignment of third metacarpal, capitate, lunate, and radius
	Fractures of:
	   Triquetrum
	   Metacarpals
	   Phalanges
	Carpal dislocations:
	   Lunate
	   Perilunate
	   Midcarpal
	Dislocations of metacarpals and phalanges		

Table 7.5 **Ancillary Imaging Techniques for Evaluating Injury to the Wrist and Hand**

Technique	Demonstration	Technique	Demonstration
Fluoroscopy/Videotaping	Kinematics of wrist and hand Carpal instability Transient carpal subluxations	*Tomography* (usually trispiral) Projections:	

Radionuclide Imaging (scintigraphy, bone scan)	Subtle chondral and osteochondral fractures
	Fracture healing and complications (e.g., infection, osteonecrosis)
		Dorsovolar
		  Lateral
		  Oblique
			Fractures of carpal bones, particularly scaphoid and lunate
			Rolando fracture
			Keinböck disease

Arthrography (single-contrast)	Tear of:
	   Intercarpal ligaments
	   Ulnar collateral ligament (gamekeeper's thumb)
			Fracture healing and complications (e.g., nonunion and osteonecrosis)

Magnetic Resonance Imaging	Guyon canal
	Carpal tunnel syndrome
	Injury to the soft tissues
	Subtle fractures
	Osteonecrosis
		Lateral
		  Carpal—tunnel
		  Flexion—extension
		
		Computed Tomography
			Fractures of hook of the hamate
			Stability of scaphoid fracture
			Subtle fractures, particularly of hook of the hamate
			Humpback deformity of scaphoid
			Fracture healing and complications

Figure 7.37 Spectrum of radiologic imaging techniques for evaluating injury to the distal forearm, wrist, and hand.*
The radiographic projections or radiologic techniques indicated throughout the diagram are only those that are the most effective in demonstrating the respective traumatic conditions.

Figure 7.38 Scaphoid fractures. Russe classified fractures of the scaphoid bone according to the direction of the fracture line.

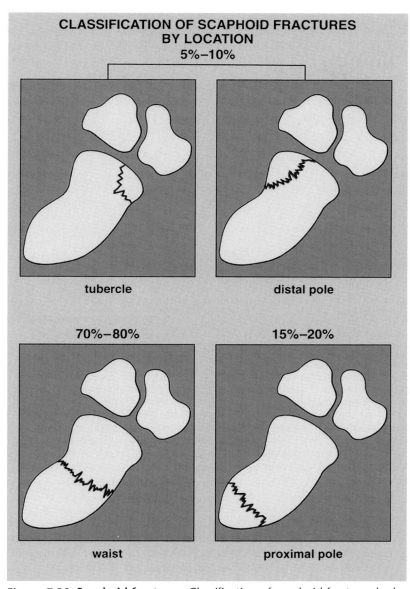

CLASSIFICATION OF SCAPHOID FRACTURES BY LOCATION

5%–10%

tubercle

distal pole

70%–80%

15%–20%

waist

proximal pole

Figure 7.39 Scaphoid fractures. Classification of scaphoid fractures by location of the fracture line.

tical way of classifying fractures of the scaphoid (5% to 10% of which occur in the tuberosity and distal pole, 15% to 20% in the proximal pole, and 70% to 80% in the waist), because it has prognostic value (Fig. 7.39). Fractures of the tuberosity (extraarticular) and distal pole usually result from a direct trauma and rarely cause any significant clinical problems. Fractures of the waist, if there is no displacement or carpal instability, display a good healing pattern in more than 90% of cases. Fractures involving the proximal pole have a high incidence of nonunion and osteonecrosis.

When fracture of the scaphoid is suspected, standard radiographs are routinely obtained in the dorsovolar, dorsovolar in ulnar deviation, oblique, and lateral projections, and these conventional studies usually suffice to demonstrate the abnormality. When they fail to do so, however, thin-section trispiral tomography has proved very effective (Fig. 7.40). This technique is equally helpful in monitoring the progress of healing of scaphoid fractures and in detecting posttraumatic complications, especially when routine follow-up films are unconvincing (Fig. 7.41). Likewise, CT is effective in this respect (Figs. 7.42 and 7.43; see also Fig. 4.67A,B). In particular, so-called humpback deformity of the scaphoid after a fracture (in which the proximal fragment dorsiflexes and the distal fragment undergoes palmar flexion, resulting in dorsal apical angulation of the scaphoid) can be well evaluated by this modal-

ity (Fig. 7.44). In the past decade, MR imaging became the technique of choice to diagnose subtle fractures of the carpal bones and to detect various complications, including osteonecrosis. In particular, MRI is very effective in demonstrating a fracture line that is not apparent on conventional radiographs (Fig. 7.45).

Complications. Delayed diagnosis and consequently delayed treatment of scaphoid fracture may lead to complications such as nonunion, osteonecrosis, and posttraumatic arthritis, the first two of which are the most commonly seen. Although occasionally both fragments of the scaphoid may become necrotic, osteonecrosis usually affects the proximal fragment (see Fig. 7.47) and only rarely the distal pole because of the good supply of blood to this part of the bone. Osteonecrosis most frequently becomes apparent 3 to 6 months after the

Figure 7.40 Scaphoid fractures. A 28-year-old man sustained an injury to his left wrist; pain persisted for 3 weeks. Dorsovolar **(A)** and lateral **(B)** films show periarticular osteoporosis, but no fracture line is evident. On a thin-section trispiral tomogram in the lateral projection **(C)**, a fracture of the scaphoid becomes apparent.

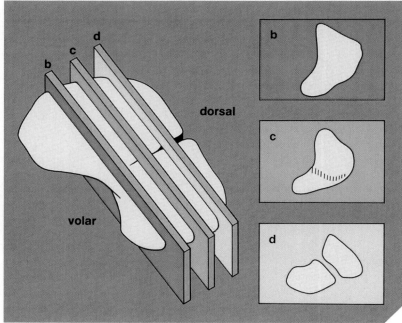

Figure 7.41 Healed scaphoid fracture. On follow-up examination of a 27-year-old man who had undergone a bone grafting procedure for nonunion of a scaphoid fracture, a radiograph in the dorsovolar projection **(A)** suggests persistence of nonunion and graft failure. For fuller evaluation, trispiral tomography using 1-mm thin sections was performed. The sections from the volar aspect of the bone **(B)**, **(C)**, demonstrate good union and success of the graft. Although a gap is evident on the dorsal section **(D)**, it has no clinical significance, only giving the impression of nonunion. The reason for this is illustrated in the schematic diagram **(E)**, in which the planes through the scaphoid (*b, c, d*) correspond to the sections on the tomograms **(B)**, **(C)**, **(D)**.

Figure 7.42 CT of healed scaphoid fracture. A 56-year-old man was treated conservatively for a scaphoid fracture with closed reduction and cast application. **(A)** Dorsovolar radiograph of the wrist shows a radiolucent line *(arrow)* suggestive of a nonunion. **(B)** Oblique coronal CT image demonstrates, however, complete union *(curved arrow)*.

Figure 7.43 CT of ununited scaphoid fracture. Coronal **(A)** and sagittal **(B)** CT images show nonunion of a scaphoid fracture. Note sclerotic edges and gap between the fractured fragments.

Figure 7.44 Humpback deformity. A sagittal reformatted CT image shows a humpback deformity of a fractured scaphoid. Note palmar flexion of the distal fragment (*arrow*) and dorsal apex angulation (*curved arrow*).

injury when the affected fragment shows evidence of increased density. Because conventional radiography may at times fail to demonstrate this feature, CT or trispiral tomographic examination is recommended as a valuable aid (Fig. 7.46). Patients with delayed union or nonunion are more prone to osteonecrosis, but healing may sometimes occur despite it (Fig. 7.47). Tehranzadeh and colleagues introduced lateral flexion–extension complex motion tomography to evaluate the healing process after scaphoid fractures and, in particular, the stability of the fractured fragments. The examination includes acquisition of neutral lateral tomographic views followed by lateral tomograms, first with full flexion and then with full extension of the wrist. This technique diagnosed all of the healed or stable fractures and was significant in the detection of motion between the fracture fragments of unstable scaphoid fractures in 93% of all cases. In recent years, however, CT scanning almost completely replaced conventional tomography, becoming a very useful technique in demonstrating scaphoid fractures and complications, particularly osteonecrosis and nonunion (see Fig. 7.43). Nonunion is usually treated surgically by bone grafting. If this approach fails, then the scaphoid may be excised and replaced by prosthesis (Fig. 7.48).

Fracture of the Triquetral Bone. Although fracture of the triquetrum is not uncommon, it can easily be missed if proper radiographic examination is not performed. In most cases, triquetral fracture is best demonstrated on the lateral and pronated oblique projections of the wrist. However, as overlapping bones on these views may at times obscure the fracture line, tomographic examination in the lateral projection may be required to confirm the diagnosis. Radionuclide bone scan can also be a valuable aid in localizing the site of trauma when fracture is suspected and routine films are normal (Fig. 7.49).

Fracture of the Hamate Bone. An infrequent type of wrist injury—accounting for approximately 2% of all carpal fractures—fracture of the hamate most often results from a direct blow to the volar aspect of the wrist. This is particularly true in fractures of the hook of the hamate (or hamulus), which together with fractures of the hamate body constitute the two groups of hamate injuries. Most hamulus fractures occur in sports activities requiring the use of a racket, club, bat, or similar implement that may cause direct injury to the palmar aspect of the wrist.

Figure 7.45 MRI of scaphoid fracture. A 27-year-old man fell on ice and presented with snuffbox tenderness. Dorsovolar (**A**) in ulnar deviation and oblique (**B**) radiographs (as well as conventional dorsovolar and lateral views, not shown here) were normal. Coronal T1-weighted (**C**) and coronal fat-suppressed T2-weighted (**D**) MR images show fracture of the proximal pole of the scaphoid (*arrows*).

oddly shaped
distal pole

fracture of
scaphoid

posttraumatic
arthritis

Figure 7.46 Scaphoid fracture complicated by osteonecrosis. On follow-up examination of a 40-year-old man who had sustained a fracture of the scaphoid, which was treated by immobilization for 3 months, the dorsovolar film **(A)** shows persistence of the fracture line, an oddly shaped distal scaphoid pole, and evidence of posttraumatic arthritis of the radioscaphoid compartment of the radiocarpal joint. To determine the potential cause of nonunion and the extent of arthritis, trispiral tomography **(B)** was performed, revealing unsuspected osteonecrosis of the distal fragment. (From Sherman SB, et al., 1983, with permission.)

Figure 7.47 Healed scaphoid fracture and osteonecrosis. Trispiral tomogram **(A)** in the dorsovolar projection shows a dense proximal segment of the scaphoid indicative of osteonecrosis. Note that the fracture is fully united. In another patient, a coronal CT **(B)** shows healed fracture of the scaphoid with osteonecrosis of the proximal fragment.

Figure 7.48 Scaphoid prosthesis. A 35-year-old man sustained a fracture of the scaphoid. Nonunion was complicated by osteonecrosis. The bone was excised and silastic prosthesis inserted. Note the smoothness of the margins of the prosthesis, as well as its ivory-like homogeneous density and lack of trabecular pattern.

Figure 7.49 Fracture of triquetrum. A 45-year-old man, having fallen on his outstretched hand, presented with localized tenderness on the dorsal aspect of the wrist. Dorsovolar **(A)** and lateral **(B)** radiographs of the wrist are normal. Radionuclide bone scan **(C)**, which was performed to localize the possible site of trauma reveals increased uptake of the tracer on the ulnar side of the carpus, suggesting fracture. Tomographic examination in the lateral projection **(D)** unequivocally demonstrates triquetral fracture. The tomographic appearance of the normal triquetrum **(E)** is shown for comparison.

Fractures of the hamate body, which may extend either ulnarly or radially to the hamulus, usually are readily demonstrated on the standard views of the wrist. The lateral and pronated oblique radiographs are preferable, particularly in detecting fractures that may be oriented in the coronal plane (Fig. 7.50).

Fractures of the hamulus, however, are not apparent on routine studies and consequently may go undiagnosed. As an aid to recognizing hamulus fracture on the standard dorsovolar view of the wrist, Norman and colleagues have identified the *eye sign*. The sign derives its name from the dense, oval, cortical ring shadow that is normally seen over the hamate on the dorsovolar projection. This "eye" of the hamate is actually the hook of the hamate seen on end. Although in most cases the absence or indistinct outline of the cortical shadow or the presence of sclerosis suggests the diagnosis of hamulus fracture, a film of the op-

posite wrist should be obtained for comparison (Fig. 7.51A, B). Confirmation of the diagnosis and evaluation of the type, site, and extent of the fracture may be made on the carpal–tunnel projection (Fig. 7.51C). This view may also be effective when the suspected fracture is distal to the base of the hook and, as a result, the eye of the hamate may still be visible (Fig. 7.52). The carpal–tunnel view, however, is not always definitively diagnostic, because the degree of dorsiflexion of the wrist required for this projection (see Fig. 7.28) is often limited because of pain, particularly in patients with acute or subacute fractures. Limited dorsiflexion may cause the anterior margins of the capitate and the pisiform to overlap and obscure the fracture line (Fig. 7.52B). In such cases, trispiral tomographic studies in the lateral and carpal–tunnel projections (Fig. 7.52C, D) are usually diagnostic. CT axial sections of the wrist with sagittal reformation are equally effective.

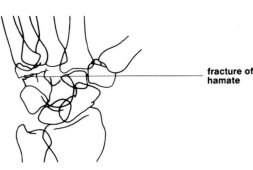

Figure 7.50 Fracture of the hamate. On the pronated oblique view of the wrist, a fracture of the hamate body is clearly evident.

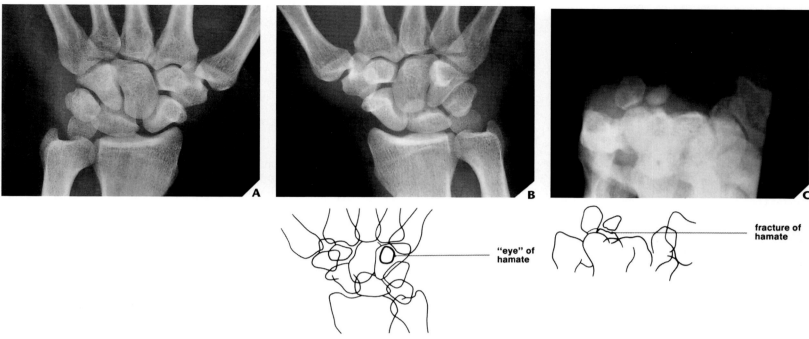

Figure 7.51 **Fracture of the hook of the hamate.** Having injured his right wrist while playing golf, a 36-year-old man presented with symptoms of pain in his palm on pressure, weakness of grasp, and occasional paresthesia of the little finger. The tenderness was limited to the area over the hook of the hamate. On the dorsovolar view of the wrist **(A)**, the oval cortical shadow normally seen projecting over the hamate is not visible, suggesting fracture. On a comparison study of the left wrist **(B)**, the eye of the hamate is clearly seen. Fracture of the hamate, suggested by the disappearance of the cortical shadow of the hamate in the right wrist, is confirmed on the carpal–tunnel projection **(C)**.

Figure 7.52 **Fracture of the hook of the hamate.** After falling on the palm of his right hand, a 66-year-old man reported pain in the palm, numbness, and weakness in the fingers innervated by the ulnar nerve. No obvious abnormalities are seen on the dorsovolar view of the wrist **(A)**; the eye of the hamate is clearly discernible. On the conventional carpal–tunnel view **(B)**, obtained without the maximum degree of dorsiflexion caused by pain, the pisiform partially overlaps the hamulus. A short radiolucent line is evident, however, at the base of the hamulus, but the diagnosis of fracture cannot be made conclusively. Trispiral tomograms in the lateral **(C)** and carpal–tunnel **(D)** projections unquestionably demonstrate a fracture of the hook of the hamate distal to the base. The normal appearance of the hamulus on, respectively, the same projections **(E)**, **(F)** is shown for comparison. **(A, B, D):** (From Greenspan A, et al., 1985, with permission.)

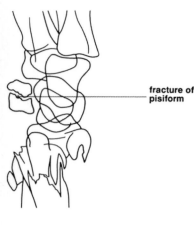

fracture of pisiform

Figure 7.53 Fracture of the pisiform. A 66-year-old woman sustained a crush injury to the left wrist in a motor vehicle accident. Routine films in the dorsovolar, lateral, and oblique projections revealed comminuted fractures of the distal radius and the ulna. To exclude the possibility of associated carpal fractures, especially in view of the severity of the injury seen on the routine studies, a film in the supinated oblique projection was obtained. The view clearly demonstrates, in addition, a fracture of the pisiform.

Fracture of the Pisiform Bone. Fracture of the pisiform is rare. It usually results from direct injury to the wrist as, for example, from a fall on the outstretched hand or use of the hand as a hammer to strike an object. It may be an isolated injury or may coexist with fractures of other bones (Fig. 7.53). Radiographs in the supinated oblique and carpal–tunnel projections are best suited to demonstrate the abnormality.

Fracture of the Capitate Bone. An uncommon type of carpal injury, accounting for only 1% to 3% of carpal fractures, fracture of the capitate usually occurs in association with other injuries to the carpus, particularly fracture of the scaphoid and perilunate dislocation. It usually results from a fall on the outstretched hand, with hyperdorsiflexion of the hand causing impingement of the bone against the distal radius; it may also result from a direct blow to the wrist. The waist (or neck) of the capitate is the most common site of fracture. The dorsovolar view of the wrist usually demonstrates the abnormality (Fig. 7.54A), although the lateral view may be helpful in determining rotation or displacement of the fragment. Trispiral tomography is useful in outlining the details of the fracture and determining the stage of healing (Fig. 7.54B).

Fracture of the Lunate Bone. Usually the result of a fall on the dorsiflexed wrist or a strenuous push on the heel of the hand, fracture of the lunate is a rare type of carpal injury, accounting for less than 3% of all carpal fractures. It is often seen in association with perilunate dislocation but more commonly occurs as a pathologic fracture of necrotic bone secondary to Kienböck disease (see later). The standard views of the wrist, particularly the dorsovolar and lateral projections, are usually sufficient to demonstrate the abnormality, although CT scanning may also be required for a full evaluation.

Kienböck Disease

Single or repeated trauma to the lunate or dislocation of the bone may impair its blood supply and cause it to become necrotic. However, the development of Kienböck disease, as this form of osteonecrosis affecting the lunate is known, may not be solely attributable to extrinsic trauma. Whether the natural history begins with a single simple transverse fracture or numerous compression fractures from repeated compressive strains is still the subject of speculation. An interesting but controversial hypothesis links this condition with negative ulnar variance in individuals whose ulna projects more proximally. They may be predisposed to Kienböck disease because of compression of the lunate against the irregular articular surface created by the discrepancy in radial and ulnar lengths.

Once lunate necrosis begins, an established progressive sequence of events is set in motion. This progression is marked by lunate flattening and elongation, proximal migration of the capitate, scapholunate dissociation, and, finally, osteoarthritis of the radiocarpal joint. This series of changes also forms the basis for the classification of Kienböck disease (Fig. 7.55). Clinically, stage I is indistinguishable from a wrist sprain. Wrist radiographs may be completely normal, and only trispiral tomography or CT may detect a subtle linear fracture. Skeletal scintigraphy may show increased uptake of a radiopharmaceutical tracer by the lunate. MRI may demonstrate the abnormality, displaying decreased signal intensity of lunate on T1-weighted images (Fig. 7.56). As the condition progresses (stage II), the conventional radiographs and trispiral tomographic studies in the dorsovolar and lateral projections show increased density of the lunate accompanied by some degree of flattening on the radial side of this bone (Fig. 7.57). The radionuclide bone scan is invariably positive in this stage. In stage III, the radiographs demonstrate marked decrease in height of the lunate and proximal migration of the capitate (Fig. 7.58). Necrotic and cystic degeneration may lead to further fragmentation and collapse (Fig. 7.59). Scapholunate dissociation is a prominent feature of this stage. Stage IV is marked by almost complete disintegration of the lunate and development of radiocarpal osteoarthritis with typical changes of joint space narrowing, osteophyte formation, subchondral sclerosis, and degenerative cysts (Fig. 7.60).

Merely diagnosing Kienböck disease is not sufficient from the orthopedic point of view; rather, it is essential for the radiologist to demonstrate the integrity of the bone. The reason for this is that at an

Figure 7.54 Fracture of the capitate. A 23-year-old man fell on his outstretched hand. **(A)** Dorsovolar view of the wrist demonstrates a fracture through the neck of the capitate. **(B)** After conservative treatment (3 months of immobilization in a plaster cast), trispiral tomography was performed. On this film, there is clear evidence of lack of union. Note the small necrotic bone fragment, which was not too well demonstrated on the standard projection.

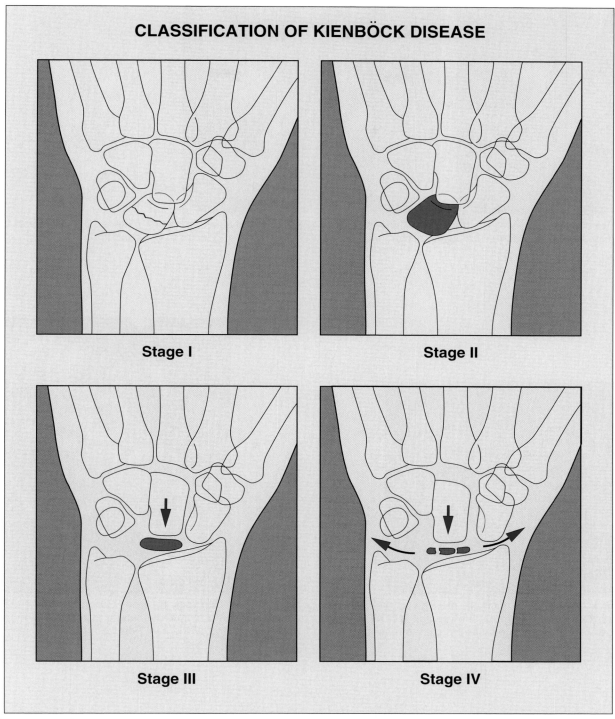

CLASSIFICATION OF KIENBÖCK DISEASE

Stage I

Stage II

Stage III

Stage IV

Figure 7.55 **The four stages of Kienböck disease.** (Modified from Gelberman RH, Szabo RM, 1993, with permission.)

Figure 7.56 Kienböck disease. A 35-year-old man with wrist pain underwent radiologic investigation for Kienböck disease. **(A)** Conventional dorsovolar radiograph of the left wrist is normal. **(B)** Coronal T1-weighted MRI shows low signal intensity of the lunate consistent with osteonecrosis. (Courtesy of Dr. L. Steinbach, San Francisco, CA.)

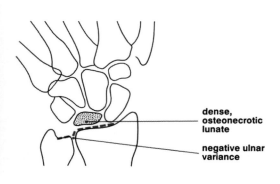

dense,
osteonecrotic
lunate

negative ulnar
variance

Figure 7.57 Kienböck disease. Dorsovolar radiograph **(A)** and tomogram **(B)** of the wrist show the dense, flattened appearance of the lunate characteristic of Kienböck disease. Note the presence of negative ulnar variance, a possible predisposing factor in this condition.

Figure 7.58 Kienböck disease. A 21-year-old man presented with long-standing wrist pain. A dorsovolar radiograph shows stage III of Kienböck disease. Note collapse of osteonecrotic lunate and proximal migration of the capitate.

Figure 7.59 Kienböck disease. Coronal CT of the wrist reveals cystic changes of the osteonecrotic lunate associated with a pathologic fracture. (Courtesy of Dr. L. Friedman, Hamilton, Canada.)

Figure 7.60 Kienböck disease. Stage IV of Kienböck disease is marked by fragmentation and collapse of the lunate, proximal migration of the capitate, rotary subluxation of the scaphoid, and osteoarthritis of the radiocarpal joint.

Figure 7.61 Kienböck disease. (A) Lateral tomogram of the wrist in a patient with Kienböck disease shows the dense appearance of the lunate characteristic of osteonecrosis; there is also clear evidence of cystic degeneration. Because no fracture line is present, the surgeon has the option of performing a revascularization procedure. After triquetrolunate arthrodesis, the dorsovolar view of the wrist in radial deviation **(B)** and a trispiral tomogram **(C)** demonstrate the vascular bone flap bridging the triquetrum and the lunate.

early stage of the disease, in the absence of fracture or fragmentation, a revascularization procedure aimed at restoring circulation to the lunate may prevent further progression of the necrotic process and eventual collapse of the bone (Fig. 7.61). In the event of fracture (Fig. 7.62) or fragmentation (Fig. 7.63) of the lunate, which are best diagnosed on trispiral tomograms in the dorsovolar and lateral projections or on CT, alternatives to revascularization—such as silastic arthroplasty or, in the absence of a collapse deformity, ulnar lengthening or radial shortening—would then have to be considered. In some cases, the latter procedures restoring neutral ulnar variance may allow spontaneous healing of lunate fracture.

Dislocations of the Carpal Bones

The most frequent types of dislocation in the wrist are scapholunate dislocation, perilunate dislocation, midcarpal dislocation, and lunate

dislocation. To understand better the pattern of dislocation of the carpal bones, Johnson stressed the occurrence of the so-called vulnerable zone, the common site of wrist injuries (Fig. 7.64). Two major types of injury are recognized: the lesser arc and greater arc patterns. Lesser-arc injury involves, in sequential stages, rotary subluxation of the scaphoid, perilunate dislocation, midcarpal dislocation, and lunate dislocation, whereas greater-arc injury involves fracture of any of the bones adjacent to lunate associated with dislocations. The wrist ligaments stabilize the carpus to the distal radius and ulna. The radiocapitate and capitotriquetral ligaments are the prime stabilizers of the distal carpal row. The proximal carpal row is stabilized by the volar radiotriquetral, the dorsal radiocarpal, the ulnolunate, the ulnotriquetral, and the ulnar collateral ligaments. The scaphoid is stabilized distally by the radiocapitate and radial collateral ligaments and proximally by the radioscaphoid and scapholunate ligaments (see Fig. 7.33). Mayfield, and later Yeager, Dalinka, and Gilula, stressed the pattern of four sequential stages of lesser-arc injury (Fig. 7.65). Stage I represents a scapholunate dissociation and rotary subluxation of the scaphoid. Stage II represents a dislocation of the capitate known also as perilunate dislocation. Stage III represents midcarpal dislocation, the result of disruption of articulation between the lunate and triquetrum. Stage IV represents a complete lunate dislocation. This pattern follows the progression from the least severe injury, *scapholunate dissociation* (rotary subluxation of the scaphoid), in which there is a tear of the radioscaphoid, palmar radiocapitate, and scapholunate ligaments, to a more severe *perilunate dislocation*, in which there is, in addition, tear of the radiocapitate ligaments, to a still more severe injury, *midcarpal dislocation* (dislocation of the capitate dorsally to the lunate and subluxation, but not complete dislocation, of the lunate),

Figure 7.62 Kienböck disease. (A) On a trispiral tomogram in the dorsovolar projection with the wrist ulnarly deviated, there is no evidence of lunate fracture. **(B)** The lateral view, however, shows clear indication of a fracture line.

Figure 7.63 Kienböck disease. Dorsovolar **(A)** and lateral **(B)** trispiral tomograms of the wrist demonstrate fragmentation of the lunate seen in advanced Kienböck disease.

Figure 7.64 Vulnerable zone of the wrist. The "vulnerable zone" of the carpus is represented by shaded areas. Most fractures, fracture dislocations, and dislocations of the carpal bones occur within it. The lesser arc outlines the "dislocation zone," whereas the greater arc outlines the "fracture—dislocation zone." (Modified from Yeager B, Dalinka M, 1985, with permission.)

with tear of the volar and dorsal radiotriquetral and ulnotriquetral ligaments, to the severest injury, *lunate dislocation,* in which there is a tear of the radiolunate fascicle of the dorsal radiocarpal ligament and of the volar ligaments, leaving the lunate entirely without ligamentous attachments.

An appreciation of two important normal relations of the carpal bones—one seen on the lateral and the other on the dorsovolar view of the wrist—should aid in recognizing the presence of abnormality. The lateral view obtained with the wrist in the neutral position reveals the alignment of the radius, the lunate, the capitate, and the third metacarpal along their longitudinal axes (Fig. 7.66). On the dorsovolar view of the wrist in the neutral position, Gilula has identified three smooth arcs outlining the proximal and distal carpal rows. Arc I joins the proximal articular surfaces of the scaphoid, the lunate, and the triquetrum; arc II outlines the distal concavities of the same bones;

Figure 7.66 Longitudinal axial alignment. On the lateral view of the wrist, the central axes of the radius, the lunate, the capitate, and the third metacarpal normally form a straight line.

arc III is formed by the proximal convexities of the capitate and the hamate (Fig. 7.67). The diagnostic significance of distortion in both these relations is discussed in the sections that follow.

Scapholunate Dissociation. Injury to the scapholunate ligament may result in intercarpal ligament instability that leads to rotary subluxation of the scaphoid, a type of scapholunate dissociation. On the dorsovolar view of the wrist, which alone is sufficient to diagnose this condition, two signs can be seen that indicate its presence.

The first, known in the literature as the *Terry-Thomas sign,* is characterized by a widening of the space between the scaphoid and the lunate, which normally measures no more than 2 mm (Fig. 7.68). Occasionally, this finding is not evident on the dorsovolar view of the wrist in the neutral position but becomes apparent when the wrist is ulnarly deviated (Fig. 7.69).

The other of these signs, the *signet-ring sign,* receives its name from a cortical ring shadow that is normally *not* seen on the scaphoid on the dorsovolar projection with the wrist in the neutral position (see Fig. 7.67). In rotary subluxation of the scaphoid, however, volar tilt and rotation of the scaphoid cause it to appear foreshortened and the bone's tuberosity to be seen on end, producing the characteristic ring shadow (Fig. 7.70A). To rely on this sign as a diagnostic indicator, dorsovolar films must be obtained with the wrist in the neutral position or in ulnar deviation, because in radial deviation of the wrist the scaphoid normally tilts volarly, creating a similar radiographic picture (Fig. 7.70B).

When radiographic findings are normal in cases of suspected injury to the intercarpal ligament complex, fluoroscopy combined with

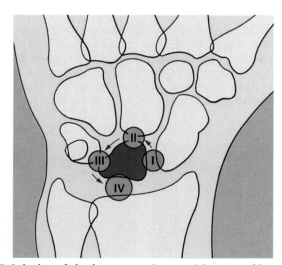

Figure 7.65 Injuries of the lesser arc. Sequential stages of lesser-arc injury. Stage I represents a scapholunate failure that results in a scapholunate dissociation or rotary subluxation of the scaphoid. Stage II represents a capitolunate failure that results in a dislocation of the capitate (perilunate dislocation). Stage III represents a triquetrolunate failure because the articulation between the lunate and triquetrum is disrupted, leading to a midcarpal dislocation. Stage IV represents a complete lunate disruption, caused by dorsal radiocarpal ligament failure. (Modified from Yeager B, Dalinka M, 1985, with permission.)

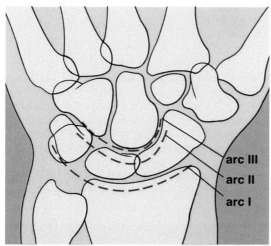

Figure 7.67 Arcs of the carpus. Three smooth arcs outlining the proximal and distal carpal rows are identifiable on the dorsovolar view of the normal wrist.

Figure 7.69 Scapholunate dissociation. (A) On the dorsovolar projection of the wrist in the neutral position, a gap between the scaphoid and the lunate is not well demonstrated. **(B)** On ulnar deviation, however, the gap becomes apparent, indicating scapholunate dissociation.

Figure 7.68 Terry-Thomas sign. Dorsovolar view of the wrist shows an abnormally wide space between the scaphoid and the lunate–the Terry-Thomas sign–indicating scapholunate dissociation caused by tear of the intercarpal ligaments.

Figure 7.70 Signet-ring sign. (A) On the dorsovolar view of the wrist in the neutral position, rotary subluxation of the scaphoid can be recognized by the cortical ring shadow that appears projecting over the scaphoid (compare with Fig. 7.67). This phenomenon is caused by the bone's volar tilt and rotation, which cause it to appear foreshortened and its tuberosity to be seen on end. **(B)** A similar picture can be seen on the dorsovolar view of the wrist in radial deviation, but this apparent ring shadow is caused by the normal volar tilt of the scaphoid exaggerated by radial deviation.

Figure 7.71 Transient subluxation. Having sustained an injury to the wrist 3 months previously, a patient presented with pain and an audible click on ulnar deviation of the wrist. Routine films in the dorsovolar, dorsovolar in ulnar deviation, and oblique projections were normal. Fluoroscopy combined with videotaping confirmed suspected lunate—capitate instability. On ulnar deviation (the *arrow* indicates direction of motion), transient scapholunate dissociation and lunate—capitate subluxation became apparent. Schematic diagrams based on the video sequence show the relationship of the carpal bones before **(A)** and after **(B)** the click. In **(B)**, note the small gap between the lunate and the capitate caused by transient dorsal subluxation of the capitate.

videotaping can sometimes contribute to an evaluation of wrist kinematics and to the diagnosis of carpal instability or transient subluxation (Fig. 7.71). Arthrographic examination of the wrist (Fig. 7.7) is effective when routine radiographic or videofluoroscopic findings are not conclusive. A wrist arthrogram can reveal abnormal communication between the radiocarpal and midcarpal compartments that indicates a tear in the scapholunate or lunotriquetral interosseous ligament complex (Fig. 7.72).

MRI may also demonstrate abnormalities of scapholunate and lunotriquetral ligaments. The scapholunate ligament connects the volar, proximal, and dorsal borders of the scaphoid bone to the lunate bone. On MRI, it appears as a low-signal-intensity structure. The lunotriquetral ligament connects the volar, proximal, and dorsal borders of the lunate bone to the triquetral bone, also exhibiting low signal intensity. Both ligaments blend almost imperceptibly with the articular cartilages of the joint. The tears of these ligaments are diagnosed on MRI when the single or scattered areas of high signal intensity are identified within the structures, or when there is discontinuity of a low-signal-intensity ligament traversed by hyperintense fluid (Fig. 7.73). However, according to Schweitzer and colleagues, when

MRI results were compared with those of arthrography and arthroscopy, they showed sensitivity of only 50%, specificity of 86%, and accuracy of 77% for tears of scapholunate ligament, and 52%, 46%, and 49%, respectively, for lunotriquetral ligament tears. Nonvisualization of the scapholunate ligament was a helpful sign of a tear; however, not seeing the lunotriquetral ligament did not necessarily mean it was torn.

Lunate and Perilunate Dislocations. Dorsovolar and lateral radiographs of the wrist in the neutral position are usually sufficient to

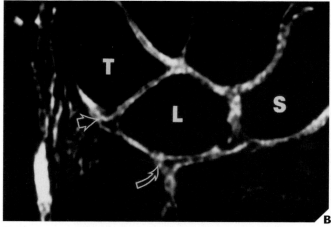

Figure 7.72 Tear of the scapholunate ligament. A 21-year-old man injured his right wrist during a wrestling competition. Standard views, including ulnar deviation of the wrist, were unremarkable. Likewise, videofluoroscopic examination did not reveal significant abnormalities. A wrist arthrogram, however, shows leak of contrast into the midcarpal articulations, indicating a tear in the scapholunate interosseous ligament complex. Note also that the triangular fibrocartilage complex is intact, because no contrast entered the distal radioulnar joint.

Figure 7.73 Tear of the scapholunate and lunotriquetral ligaments. (A) Coronal fat-suppressed T1-weighted image after gadolinium injection to the radiocarpal joint shows a tear of the scapholunate ligament *(arrow)*. L, lunate; C, capitate; S, scaphoid. **(B)** Coronal gradient echo image shows a tear of the lunotriquetral ligament *(arrow)*. There is also a tear of the triangular fibrocartilage *(curved arrow)*. T, triquetrum; L, lunate; S, scaphoid.

Figure 7.74 Lunate dislocation. (A) On the lateral view of the wrist, lunate dislocation is evident from the break in the longitudinal alignment of the third metacarpal and the capitate over the distal radial surface at the site of the lunate, which is volarly rotated and displaced. **(B)** Dorsovolar projection shows a disrupted arc II at the site of the lunate, indicating malalignment. Note also the triangular appearance of the lunate, a finding virtually pathognomonic of dislocation of this bone.

diagnose suspected lunate and perilunate dislocations. As the lateral view clearly demonstrates, the normal alignment of the longitudinal axes of the lunate, the capitate, and the third metacarpal over the distal radial surface, a break at any point in this line is pathognomonic of subluxation or dislocation. Lunate dislocation can thus be recognized when its axis is angled away from the distal radial surface, while the capitate remains in its normal alignment (Fig. 7.74A). Similarly, lunate dislocation can also be identified on the dorsovolar projection by disruption of arc II described by the distal concave surfaces of the scaphoid, the lunate, and the triquetrum, as well as the concomitant triangular appearance of the lunate (Fig. 7.74B).

Perilunate dislocation can be recognized on the lateral view of the wrist by the dorsal or volar angulation of the longitudinal axis of the capitate away from its normal central alignment with the lunate and the distal radial surface. The lunate in this case remains in articulation with the radius, although there may be some degree of tilt of the lunate because of subluxation associated with perilunate dislocation (Fig. 7.75A). On the dorsovolar view, the overlapping of the proximal and distal carpal rows and a break in arcs II and III at the site of the capitate indicate the presence of perilunate dislocation (Fig. 7.75B).

Transscaphoid Perilunate Dislocation. When dislocation of the carpal bones is associated with a fracture, the prefix *trans* indicates which bone is fractured. The most common fracture associated with carpal dislocation is transscaphoid perilunate dislocation. As in the preceding types of carpal dislocations, radiographs in the standard dorsovolar, dorsovolar in ulnar deviation, and lateral projections usually suffice to lead to a firm diagnosis. The normal relations of the carpal bones seen on these views should help to identify the type of abnormality. Although rarely effective in evaluating carpal dislocations,

tomographic examination may be indicated when radiographs of the wrist are equivocal as to which carpal bones are dislocated (Fig. 7.76). Other types of associated fractures are less commonly seen (Fig. 7.77).

Scaphoid Dislocation. Dislocation of scaphoid bone is rare. Two types have been reported: isolated dislocation and dislocation in conjunction with axial carpal disruption. In the former injury, the distal carpal row is normal (Fig. 7.78), whereas in the latter type there is disruption of the distal carpal row and proximal migration of the radial half of the carpus (Fig. 7.79). A common factor of this injury is dorsiflexion and ulnar deviation of the wrist when a sudden force causes a distraction effect on the radial aspect of the wrist, with subsequent ejection of the scaphoid. Isolated dislocations of the scaphoid are generally treated with closed reduction. Dislocations associated with axial carpal disruption mandate open reduction and internal fixation to stabilize the carpus.

Carpal Instability

Various carpal instabilities have been described. The most common include dorsal intercalated segment instability (DISI) and volar intercalated segment instability (VISI).

To explain the carpal instability, Lichtman and colleagues developed the carpal ring theory. The proximal carpal row, which represents intercalated segment, moves as a unit firmly stabilized by interosseous ligaments. Controlled mobility occurs at the scapho-trapezium (radial link) and triquetrohamate (ulnar link) joints (Fig. 7.80). With a break in the ring, either within bony structures or ligaments, the proximal carpal row no longer moves as a unit. The lunate will then tilt either dorsally or volarly in response to this uncontrolled

Figure 7.75 Perilunate dislocation. (A) Lateral radiograph of the wrist demonstrates perilunate dislocation characterized by displacement of the capitate dorsal to the lunate, which, although slightly volarly rotated, remains in articulation with the distal radius. Note the break in the longitudinal alignment of the third metacarpal and the capitate with the lunate and the distal radial surface. On the dorsovolar projection **(B)**, perilunate dislocation is evident from the overlapping proximal and distal carpal rows and the resulting disruption of arcs II and III.

Figure 7.76 Transscaphoid perilunate dislocation. (A) Dorsovolar radiograph of the wrist in ulnar deviation clearly shows scaphoid fracture, but the disruptions in the distal carpal arcs are unclear as to the type of dislocation. The lateral view was also inconclusive. **(B)** Lateral tomogram demonstrates that the capitate is displaced dorsal to the lunate, which remains in articulation with the distal radius–the classic appearance of perilunate dislocation.

Figure 7.77 Transradial, transscaphoid, transtriquetral lunate dislocation. Dorsovolar view of the wrist clearly reveals fractures of the radial styloid process, the scaphoid, and the triquetrum. The wide space separating the proximal and distal carpal rows and the triangular shape of the lunate indicate the possibility of lunate dislocation. Note the disruption in arcs I and II. The lateral view confirmed volar displacement of the lunate and the normal position of the capitate. This abnormality can be described as transradial, transscaphoid, and transtriquetral lunate dislocation.

Figure 7.78 Isolated scaphoid dislocation. Dorsovolar **(A)** and oblique **(B)** radiographs show volar dislocation of the scaphoid. The distal carpal row is not affected and the capitate bone is in anatomic position.

Figure 7.79 Scaphoid dislocation with axial carpal disruption. Dorsovolar radiograph of the wrist shows radial volar dislocation of the scaphoid bone (*curved arrow*) associated with proximal migration of the capitate (*arrow*). Note the interruption of the third arc of the carpus (compare with Fig. 7.67). An open arrow points to the associated fracture of the fourth metacarpal bone.

mobility, manifested by either DISI or VISI (Fig. 7.81). DISI is the most common deformity. It is recognized on the true lateral view of the wrist by dorsal tilt of the lunate, frequently associated with volar (palmar) tilt of the scaphoid (the capitolunate angle measures more than 30°, and the scapholunate angle more than 60°) (Fig. 7.81C). It may be caused by either bony or ligamentous disruption in the ring on the radial side of the wrist. Most commonly, scaphoid fracture with or without nonunion and scapholunate ligamentous dissociation may be the cause of this deformity. VISI is recognized when volar tilt of the lunate is noted on the true lateral view frequently accompanied by dorsal tilt of capitate (the capitolunate angle measures more than 30° and the scapholunate angle less than 30°) (Fig. 7.81D). It is caused by a

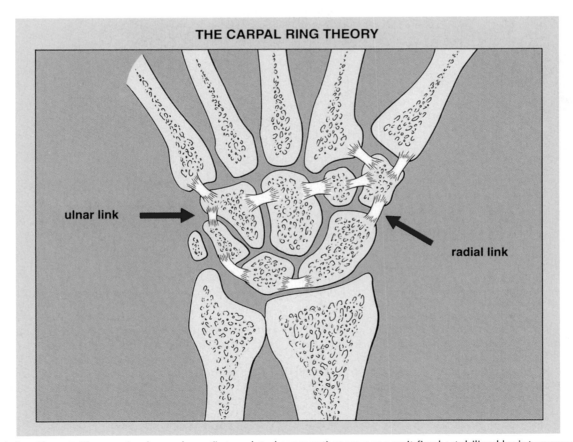

Figure 7.80 The carpal ring theory. The proximal carpal row (intercalated segment) moves as a unit firmly stabilized by interosseous ligaments. *Controlled* mobility occurs at the scaphotrapezium (radial link) and triquetrohamate (ulnar link) joints. A break in the ring, either bony or ligamentous, can produce *uncontrolled* mobility, manifested by either dorsal intercalated segment instability (DISI) or volar intercalated segment instability (VISI). (Modified from Lichtman DM, et al., 1981, with permission.)

SCAPHOLUNATE ANGLE

30°–60°

3MC

3MC = third metacarpal bone
C = capitate
S = scaphoid
L = lunate
R = radius

C

S

L

R

A

in normal wrist the scapholunate
angle is between 30°–60°

CAPITOLUNATE ANGLE

3MC

C

S

L

R

0°–30°

B

in normal wrist the capitolunate
angle is between 0°–30°

DISI AND VISI DEFORMITIES

DISI

Dorsal Intercalated Segment Instability
(Dorsiflexion Carpal Instability)

C   L

C-L ∠ > 30°

S-L ∠ > 60°

S

C

1. dorsal tilt of lunate
2. volar tilt of scaphoid

VISI

Volar Intercalated Segment Instability
(Volarflexion Carpal Instability)

L

C-L ∠ > 30°   C

S-L ∠ < 30°

S

D

1. volar tilt of lunate
2. dorsal tilt of capitate

Figure 7.81 **Dorsal intercalated segment instability (DISI) and volar intercalated segment instability (VISI).** (A) Normal scapholunate angle. The scapholunate angle is formed by the intersection of longitudinal axes of scaphoid and lunate and normally measures from 30° to 60°. (B) Normal capitolunate angle. The capitolunate angle is formed by the intersection of the capitate axis (drawn from the midpoint of its head to the center of its distal articular surface) and the lunate axis (drawn through the center of its proximal and distal poles) and normally measures from 0° to 30°. (C) In DISI, the scapholunate angle measures more than 60° and the capitolunate angle more than 30°. (D) In VISI, the scapholunate angle measures less than 30°, and the capitolunate angle much more than 30°. (Modified from Gilula LA, Weeks PM, 1978, with permission.)

break in the ring on the ulnar side of the wrist. Most frequently, it is ligamentous dissociation and triquetrohamate joint disruption that leads to this deformity. According to McNiesh, when breaks in the ring occur on the radial and ulnar sides as, for instance, in concurrent scapholunate and lunotriquetral ligamentous dissociation, the VISI pattern predominates.

Injury to the Hand

Fractures of the Metacarpal Bones

Bennett and Rolando Fractures. Bennett and Rolando fractures are *intraarticular* fractures that occur at the base of the first metacarpal bone. From the perspective of orthopedic management, it is important to distinguish these from the *extraarticular* types, which are transverse or oblique fractures of the first metacarpal just distal to the carpometacarpal joint (Fig. 7.82). Failure to diagnose and treat properly intraarticular metacarpal fractures may result in protracted pain, stiffness, and posttraumatic arthritis caused by incongruity of articular surfaces.

The *Bennett fracture* is a fracture of the proximal end of the first metacarpal that extends into the first carpometacarpal joint. Usually, a small fragment on the volar aspect of the base of the first metacarpal remains in articulation with the trapezium bone, while the rest of the first metacarpal is dorsally and radially dislocated as the result of pull of the abductor pollicis longus (Fig. 7.83). For this reason, the injury

Figure 7.82 Extraarticular fracture. An extraarticular fracture at the base of the first metacarpal should not be confused with Bennett and Rolando fractures, which are intraarticular.

Figure 7.83 Bennett fracture. A 27-year-old man who was involved in a fist-fight presented with pain localized in the right thenar. Dorsovolar radiograph of the hand **(A)** shows the typical appearance of Bennett fracture. A small fragment at the base of the first metacarpal remains in articulation with the trapezium, while the rest of the bone is dorsally and radially dislocated. The accompanying schematic diagram **(B)** shows the pathomechanics of this injury.

should properly be called a fracture–dislocation. Diagnosis and evaluation of the Bennett fracture are readily made on conventional radiographs of the hand in the dorsovolar, oblique, and lateral projections.

The *Rolando fracture* is a comminuted Bennett fracture; the fracture line may have a Y, V, or T configuration. Because there may be multiple fragments, the routine radiographic projections used to diagnose the Bennett fracture usually need to be supplemented by trispiral tomographic examination to localize comminuted fragments and to exclude the possibility of entrapment of a small bony fragment in the first carpometacarpal joint (Fig. 7.84).

Boxer's Fracture. Boxer's fracture is a fracture of the metacarpal neck with volar angulation of the distal fragment. It may occur in any of the metacarpal bones but is most commonly seen in the fifth metacarpal. The fracture and deformity are sufficiently demonstrated on conventional radiographs of the hand in the dorsovolar and oblique projections (Fig. 7.85). Because comminution frequently accompanies this type of fracture, it is important to determine its extent. Comminution may predispose the fracture after reduction to settle into an angular deformation. The oblique projection usually suffices to determine the extent of comminution (Fig. 7.85B).

Injury to the Soft Tissue of the Hand

Gamekeeper's Thumb Gamekeeper's thumb results from disruption of the ulnar collateral ligament of the first metacarpophalangeal joint, often accompanied by fracture of the base of the proximal phalanx. The abnormality is termed "gamekeeper's thumb" because it was originally seen affecting Scottish game wardens who in-

Figure 7.84 Rolando fracture. (A) Oblique view of the right hand shows a comminuted intraarticular fracture of the proximal end of the first metacarpal–Rolando fracture. To localize the fragments, trispiral tomographic examination **(B)** was performed, revealing a small bone chip entrapped in the trapeziometacarpal joint. *(continued)*

Figure 7.84 Rolando fracture. *Continued.*

bone
fragment in
joint

Figure 7.85 Boxer's fracture. (A) Dorsovolar radiograph of the right hand demonstrates a fracture of the fifth metacarpal with volar angulation of the distal fragment—a simple boxer's fracture. When comminution is present, it is essential for its prognostic value to demonstrate the extent of fracture lines, because such fractures are frequently unstable. The oblique projection **(B)** usually suffices to determine the extent of comminution.

sesamoid
bone

fracture
fragments

Figure 7.86 Gamekeeper's thumb. Having fallen on his hand on the ski slopes, a 38-year-old man presented with pain at the base of his right thumb. Physical examination revealed instability in the first metacarpophalangeal joint. Oblique **(A)** and dorsovolar **(B)** films of the right thumb show a fracture of the base of the proximal phalanx and local soft-tissue swelling—findings associated with gamekeeper's thumb. In another patient, dorsovolar and lateral films of the first phalanx did not show evidence of fracture, but because instability of the first metacarpophalangeal joint was indicated on physical examination, an abduction–stress film of the thumb was obtained **(C)**. The film **(D)** demonstrates subluxation of the joint by the increase to more than 30° in the angle between the first metacarpal and the proximal phalanx of the thumb, confirming gamekeeper's thumb. *(continued)*

Figure 7.86 Gamekeeper's thumb *Continued.*

jured the ulnar collateral ligament because of the method they used to kill rabbits. Currently, because it is more frequently seen in skiing accidents, the term "skier's thumb" is applied. This type of injury can also occur in breakdancers ("breakdancer's thumb"). When ruptured, the torn end of the ulnar collateral ligament can become displaced superficially to the adductor pollicis aponeurosis. This is known as the *Stener lesion.* Standard dorsovolar and oblique films of

the thumb usually suffice to demonstrate the associated fracture (Fig. 7.86A,B), but full evaluation requires an abduction–stress film of the thumb when this condition is suspected. An increase to more than 30° in the angle between the first metacarpal and the proximal phalanx is a characteristic finding in gamekeeper's thumb, indicating subluxation (Fig. 7.86C,D). Arthrographic examination of the thumb may also be performed to assess disruption, displacement, or entrapment of the ulnar collateral ligament (Fig. 7.87).

Recently, MRI has been applied to investigate this injury (Fig. 7.88), particularly to detect a displaced tear of the ulnar collateral ligament (Fig. 7.89). Likewise, ultrasound has proved to be a simple, reliable, and cost-effective tool for recognition of the Stener lesion.

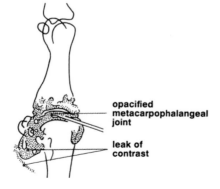

Figure 7.87 Gamekeeper's thumb. An arthrogram of the first metacarpophalangeal joint demonstrates the characteristic findings in gamekeeper's thumb. The leak of contrast along the ulnar side of the head of the first metacarpal indicates a tear of the ulnar collateral ligament. (Courtesy of Dr. D. Resnick, San Diego, CA.)

Figure 7.88 MRI of the gamekeeper's thumb. Coronal T1-weighted **(A)** and coronal STIR **(B)** images show a tear of the ulnar collateral ligament (u) of the first metacarpophalangeal joint (*curved arrows*). The torn ligament is not displaced, maintaining its longitudinal orientation (*small arrows*). **(C)** Coronal fat-suppressed T2-weighted image shows normal appearance of intact ulnar collateral ligament (*arrow*).

Figure 7.88 MRI of the gamekeeper's thumb *Continued.*

Figure 7.89 **MRI of the Stener lesion. (A)** Coronal T1-weighted MR image shows disruption of the ulnar collateral ligament *(arrow)*. The normal low-intensity signal of this structure is not present. **(B)** Coronal T2-weighted MR image shows displacement of the proximal fragment of this ligament away from the joint and its perpendicular rather than longitudinal orientation *(arrow)*, characteristic of the Stener lesion.

PRACTICAL POINTS TO REMEMBER

Distal Forearm

[1] For a full evaluation of trauma on the posteroanterior view of the distal forearm, it is important to recognize:
- ulnar variance: neutral, negative, and positive
- the radial angle, which normally ranges from 15° to 25°
- the radial length.

[2] For a full evaluation of trauma on the lateral view of the distal forearm, it is important to recognize the volar tilt of the articular surface of the radius, which normally ranges from 10° to 25°.

[3] A complete evaluation of the Colles fracture should take into consideration:
- the degree of foreshortening of the radius
- the direction of displacement of the distal fragment
- intraarticular extension of the fracture line
- associated fracture of the ulna.

[4] Learn to distinguish the Colles fracture from the:
- Barton fracture, dorsal and volar types, which are best demonstrated on the lateral projection
- Hutchinson (or chauffeur's) fracture, which is best seen on the posteroanterior view
- Smith fracture, which is best evaluated on the lateral projection.

[5] Frykman classification of distal radius fractures according to the location of fracture line (intraarticular versus extraarticular) and association of distal ulna fracture has a practical prognostic value and serves as a guide to orthopedic management.

[6] With the finding of dislocation in the distal radioulnar articulation, look for an associated radial fracture—Galeazzi fracture–dislocation.

[7] Learn to distinguish ulnar impingement syndrome from ulnar impaction (ulnolunate abutment) syndrome. The first is caused by short distal ulna that impinges on the distal radius. The latter, frequently associated with positive ulnar variance, leads to compression of the distal ulna on the medial surface of the lunate bone.

[8] A common sequela of trauma to the distal radioulnar joint, tear of the triangular fibrocartilage complex can be confirmed or excluded by single-contrast arthrogram of the wrist or MRI examination.

Wrist

[1] If clinical history and physical examination are consistent with scaphoid fracture and routine radiographs appear normal, then trispiral tomography is the next logical step.

[2] CT examination is effective in demonstrating and evaluating so-called humpback deformity of the scaphoid.

[3] Delayed diagnosis and treatment of scaphoid fracture may result in nonunion, osteonecrosis, and posttraumatic arthritis.

[4] Triquetral fracture is best diagnosed on the lateral and pronated oblique views of the wrist. If plain films appear normal, then tomography in the lateral projection can confirm or exclude the diagnosis.

[5] Fractures of the hamate body are best demonstrated on the lateral and pronated oblique projections.

[6] In suspected fracture of the hook of the hamate, look for the oval cortical ring shadow projecting over the hamate on the dorsovolar view of the wrist. If this "eye" of the hamate is absent, indistinctly outlined, or sclerotic, then hamulus fracture is highly probable. Trispiral tomography in the lateral and carpal–tunnel projections is a useful technique in evaluating the hamulus.

[7] Fracture of the pisiform is best demonstrated on the supinated oblique and carpal–tunnel projections.

[8] In Kienböck disease, the choice of surgical procedures depends on a demonstration of the integrity of the lunate. Tomography, preferably trispiral, in two planes is usually indicated. MRI may demonstrate osteonecrosis in the early stages.

[9] Lunate and perilunate dislocations are readily identified on the lateral view by disruption of the normal central alignment of the longitudinal axes of the capitate and lunate over the distal radial surface:
- in lunate dislocation disruption of the alignment occurs at the lunate
- in perilunate dislocation it occurs at the capitate
- in midcarpal dislocation it occurs at the site of both bones

[10] In any type of carpal dislocation, look for an associated fracture.

[11] If intercarpal instability is suspected and routine radiographs are normal, then fluoroscopy combined with videotaping should be the next examination. If ligament tear is suspected, then arthrography or MRI should be performed.

[12] There are two main types of carpal instability: dorsal intercalated segment instability (DISI) and volar intercalated segment instability (VISI).

Hand

[1] Learn to distinguish the Bennett and Rolando fractures—intraarticular fractures occurring at the base of the first metacarpal bone—from extraarticular fractures.

[2] The Bennett fracture involves a dislocation of most of the first metacarpal and is, therefore, a fracture–dislocation.

[3] When evaluating the Rolando fracture—really a comminuted Bennett fracture—exclude the possibility of entrapment of a fragment in the first carpometacarpal joint. Tomography is an essential technique in evaluating comminution.

[4] In the boxer's fracture, comminution of the volar cortex is often present. It is essential to demonstrate its presence radiographically.

[5] In suspected gamekeeper's thumb, obtain an abduction-stress film of the thumb.

[6] Disruption, displacement, or entrapment of the ulnar collateral ligament in gamekeeper's thumb can be evaluated on an arthrogram of the first metacarpophalangeal joint.

[7] MRI is an effective technique to distinguish between a nondisplaced and a displaced tear (Stener lesion) of the ulnar collateral ligament of the first metacarpophalangeal joint.

SUGGESTED READINGS

Abbit PL, Riddervold HO. The carpal tunnel view: helpful adjuvant for unrecognized fractures of the carpus. *Skeletal Radiol* 1987;16:45–47.

Abrahamsson SO, Sollerman C, Lundborg G, Larson J, Egund N. Diagnosis of displaced ulnar collateral ligament of the metacarpophalangeal joint of the thumb. *J Hand Surg [Am]* 1990;15A:457–460.

Adkinson JW, Chapman MW. Treatment of acute lunate and perilunate dislocations. *Clin Orthop* 1982;164:199–207.

Ahn JM, Sartoris DJ, Kang HS, et al. Gamekeeper thumb: comparison of MR arthrography with conventional arthrography and MR imaging in cadavers. *Radiology* 1998;206:737–744.

Alexander AH, Lichtman DM. Kienböck's disease. In: Lichtman DM, ed. *The wrist and its disorders.* Philadelphia: WB Saunders; 1988:329–343.

Andersen JL, Gron P, Langhoff O. The scaphoid fat stripe in the diagnosis of carpal trauma. *Acta Radiol* 1988;39:97–99.

Arkless R. Cineradiography in normal and abnormal wrist. *AJR Am J Roentgenol* 1966;96:837–844.

Aufranc OE, Jones WN, Turner RH. Anterior marginal articular fracture of distal radius. *JAMA* 1966;196:788–791.

Azouz EM. Longitudinal CT of the forearm in children. *J Can Assoc Radiol* 1984;35:388–389.

Bado JL. The Monteggia lesion. *Clin Orthop* 1967;50:71–86.

Barton NJ. Twenty questions about scaphoid fractures. *J Hand Surg [Br]* 1992;17B:289–310.

Beckenbaugh RD, Shives TC, Dobyns JH, Linscheid RL. Kienböck's disease: the natural history of Kienböck's disease and consideration of lunate fractures. *Clin Orthop* 1980;149:98–106.

Beltran J. *MRI: musculoskeletal system.* Philadelphia: JB Lippincott; 1990.

Bennett EH. On fracture of the metacarpal bone of the thumb. *BMJ* 1886;11:12–13.

Berná JD, Chavarria G, Albaladejo F, Meseguer L, Pellicer A, Sánchez-Cañizares MA, Pérez-Flores D. Panoramic versus conventional radiography of scaphoid fractures. *AJR Am J Roentgenol* 2004;182:155–159.

Berger RA. The gross and histologic anatomy of the scapholunate interosseous ligament. *J Hand Surg [Am]* 1996;21A:170–178.

Berger RA, Blair WR, el-Khoury GY. Arthrotomography of the wrist: the triangular fibrocartilage complex. *Clin Orthop* 1983;172:257–264.

Berquist TH. Hand and wrist. In: Berquist TH, ed. *MRI of the musculoskeletal system,* 3rd ed. Philadelphia: Lippincott–Raven Publishers; 1996:673–734.

Berquist TH. Knee. In: Berquist TH, ed. *MRI of the musculoskeletal system,* 3rd ed. Philadelphia: Lippincott–Raven Publishers; 1996:285–409.

Bhalla S, Higgs PE, Gilula LA. Utility of the radial-deviated, thumb-abducted lateral radiographic view for the diagnosis of hamate hook fractures: case report. *Radiology* 1998;209:203–207.

Binkovitz LA, Cahill DR, Ehman RL, Bergquist TH. Magnetic resonance imaging of the wrist: normal cross sectional imaging and selected abnormal cases. *Radiographics* 1988;8:1171–1202.

Biondetti PR, Vannier MW, Gilula LA, Knapp R. Wrist: coronal and transaxial CT scanning. *Radiology* 1987;163:149–151.

Bishop AT, Beckenbaugh RD. Fracture of the hamate hook. *J Hand Surg [Am]* 1988;13A:135–139.

Blair WF, Berger RA, el-Khoury GY. Arthrotomography of the wrist: an experimental and preliminary clinical study. *J Hand Surg [Am]* 1985;10A:350–359.

Bogumill GP. Anatomy of the wrist. In: Lichtman DM, ed. *The wrist and its disorders.* Philadelphia: WB Saunders; 1988:14–26.

Bonzar M, Firrell JC, Hainer M, Mah ET, McCabe SJ. Kienböck disease and negative ulnar variance. *J Bone Joint Surg [Am]* 1998;80A:1154–1157.

Boulas HJ, Milek MA. Hook of the hamate fractures: diagnosis, treatment and complications. *Orthop Rev* 1990;19:518–529.

Bowers WH, Hurst LC. Gamekeeper's thumb: evaluation by arthrography and stress roentgenography. *J Bone Joint Surg [Am]* 1977;59A:519–524.

Breitenseher MJ, Metz VM, Gilula LA, et al. Radiographically occult scaphoid fractures: value of MR imaging in detection. *Radiology* 1997;203:245–250.

Brøndum V, Larsen CF, Skov O. Fracture of the carpal scaphoid: frequency and distribution in a well-defined population. *Eur J Radiol* 1992;15:118–122.

Brismar J. Skeletal scintigraphy of the wrist in suggested scaphoid fracture. *Acta Radiol* 1988;29:101–107.

Brown RR, Fliszar E, Cotten A, Trudell D, Resnick D. Extrinsic and intrinsic ligaments of the wrist: normal and pathologic anatomy at MR arthrography with three-compartment enhancement. *Radiographics* 1998;18: 667–674.

Bryan RS, Dobyns JH. Fractures of the carpal bones other than lunate and navicular. *Clin Orthop* 1980;149:107–111.

Bush CH, Gillespy T III, Dell PC. High-resolution CT of the wrist: initial experience with scaphoid disorders and surgical fusions. *AJR Am J Roentgenol* 1987;149:757–760.

Campbell CS. Gamekeeper's thumb. *J Bone Joint Surg [Br]* 1955;37B:148–149.

Carrino JA, Smith DK, Schweitzer ME. MR arthrography of the elbow and wrist. *Semin Musculoskel Radiol* 1998;2:397–414.

Cerezal L, del Piñal F, Abascal F, Garcia-Valtuille R, Pereda T, Canga A. Imaging findings in ulnar-sided wrist impaction syndromes. *Radiographics* 2002;22:105–121.

Clavero JA, Alomar X, Monill JM, Esplugas M, Golano P, Mendoza M, Salvador A. MR imaging of ligament and tendon injuries of the fingers. *Radiographics* 2002;22:237–256.

Cohen MS. Fractures of the carpal bones. *Hand Clin* 1997;13:587–599.

Cone RO, Szabo R, Resnick D, Gelberman R, Taleisnick J, Gilula L. Computed tomography of the normal radioulnar joint. *Invest Radiol* 1983;18:541–545.

Cone RO, Szabo R, Resnick D, Gelberman R, Taleisnik J, Gilula L. Computed tomography of the normal soft tissues of the wrist. *Invest Radiol* 1983;18:546–551.

Cooney WP, Dobyns JH, Linscheid RL. Complications of Colles' fractures. *J Bone Joint Surg [Am]* 1980:62A;613–619.

Cooney WP III, Linscheid RL, Dobyns JH. Fractures and dislocations of the wrist. In: Rockwood CA, Green DP, Buchholz RW, eds. *Fractures in adults,* vol. 1, 3rd ed. Philadelphia: JB Lippincott; 1991:563–678.

Corfitsen M, Christensen SE, Cetti R. The anatomic fat pad and the radiological "scaphoid fat stripe." *J Hand Surg [Br]* 1989;14B:326–328.

Cristiani G, Cerofolini E, Squarzina PB, et al. Evaluation of ischemic necrosis of carpal bones by magnetic resonance imaging. *J Hand Surg [Br]* 1990;15B:249–255.

Crittenden JJ, Jones DM, Santarelli AG. Bilateral rotational dislocation of the carpal navicular. Case report. *Radiology* 1970;94:629–630.

Culp RW, Lemel M, Taras JS. Complications of common carpal injuries. *Hand Clin* 1994;10:139–155.

Curtis DJ, Downey EF Jr. A simple first metacarpophalangeal stress test. *Radiology* 1983;148:855–856.

Dalinka MK. MR imaging of the wrist. *AJR Am J Roentgenol* 1995;164:1–9.

Dalinka MK, Osterman AL, Kricun ME. Trauma to the carpus. *Contemp Diagn Radiol* 1982;5:1–6.

De Palma AF, Gartland JJ, Dowling JJ. Colles' fracture. *Pa Med* 1966;69:72–75.

Deshmukh SC, Shanahan D, Coulthard D. Distal radioulnar joint incongruity after shortening of the ulna. *J Hand Surg [Br]* 2000;25:434–438.

De Smet L. Ulnar variance: fact and fiction review article. *Acta Orthop Belg* 1994;60:1–9.

Desser ST, McCarthy S, Trumble T. Scaphoid fractures and Kienböck's disease of the lunate: MR imaging with histopathologic correlation. *Magn Reson Imaging* 1990;8:357–361.

Downey EF Jr, Curtis DJ. Patient-induced stress test of the first metacarpophalangeal joint: a radiographic assessment of collateral ligament injuries. *Radiology* 1986;158:679–683.

Duong RB, Nishiyama H, Mantil JC, et al. Kienböck's disease: scintigraphic demonstration in correlation with clinical, radiographic, and pathologic findings. *Clin Nucl Med* 1982;7:418–420.

Egawa M, Asai T. Fracture of the hook of the hamate: report of six cases and suitability of computerized tomography. *J Hand Surg [Am]* 1983;8A: 393–398.

Ellis K. Smith's and Barton's fractures. *J Bone Joint Surg [Br]* 1965;47B:724–727.

Engel J, Ganel A, Ditzian R, Militeanu J. Arthrography as a method of diagnosing tear of the ulnar collateral ligament of the metacarpophalangeal joint of the thumb ("gamekeeper's thumb"). *J Trauma* 1979;19:106–109.

Epner RA, Bowers WH, Guilford WB. Ulnar variance—the effect of wrist positioning and roentgen filming technique. *J Hand Surg [Am]* 1982; 7A: 298–305.

Escobedo EM, Bergman AG, Hunter JC. MR imaging of ulnar impaction. *Skeletal Radiol* 1995;24:85–90.

Fernandez DL, Eggli S. Non-union of the scaphoid: revascularization of the proximal pole with implantation of a vascular bundle and bone-grafting. *J Bone Joint Surg [Am]* 1995;77A:883–893.

Filan SL, Herbert TJ. Avascular necrosis of the proximal scaphoid after fracture union. *J Hand Surg [Br]* 1995;20B:551–556.

Fisher MR, Rogers LF, Hendrix RW. A systematic approach to the diagnosis of carpometacarpal dislocations. *Radiographics* 1982;2:612–627.

Fowler C, Sullivan B, Williams LA, McCarthy G, Savage R, Palmer A. A comparison of bone scintigraphy and MRI in the early diagnosis of the occult scaphoid waist fracture. *Skeletal Radiol* 1998;27:683–687.

Friedman L, Yong-hing K, Johnston GH. Forty degree angled coronal CT scanning of scaphoid fractures through plaster and fiberglass casts. *J Comput Assist Tomogr* 1989;3:1101–1104.

Friedman L, Yong HK, Johnston GH. The use of coronal computed tomography in the evaluation of Kienböck's disease. *Clin Radiol* 1991;44:56–59.

Friedman SL, Palmer AK. The ulnar impaction syndrome. *Hand Clin* 1991;7:295–310.

Gaebler C, Kukla C, Breitenseher M, Trattnig S, Mittlboeck M, Vecsei V. Magnetic resonance imaging of occult scaphoid fractures. *J Trauma* 1996; 41:73–76.

Geissler WB, Freeland AE, Savoie FH, et al. Intracarpal soft-tissue lesions associated with an intra-articular fracture of the distal end of the radius. *J Bone Joint Surg [Am]* 1996;78A:357–364.

Gelberman RH, Salamon PB, Jurist JM, Posch JL. Ulnar variance in Kienböck's disease. *J Bone Joint Surg [Am]* 1975;57A:674–676.

Gelberman RH, Szabo RM. Kienböck's disease. *Orthop Clin North Am* 1984;15:355–367.

Gerwin M. The history of Kienböck's disease. *Hand Clin* 1993;9:385–390.

Gilbert TJ, Cohen M. Imaging of acute injuries to the wrist and hand. *Radiol Clin North Am* 1997;35:701–725.

Gilula LA. Roentgenographic evaluation of the hand and wrist. In: Weeks PM, ed. *Acute bone and joint injuries of the hand and wrist.* St. Louis: Mosby; 1981;3.

Gold RH. Arthrography of the wrist. In: Arndt R-D, Horns JW, Gold RH, eds. *Clinical arthrography.* Baltimore: Williams & Wilkins; 1981.

Goldfarb CA, Yin Y, Gilula LA, Fisher AJ, Boyer MI. Wrist fractres: what the clinican wants to know. *Radiology* 2001;219:11–28.

Goldman AB. The wrist. In: Freiberger RH, Kaye JJ, eds. *Arthrography.* New York: Appleton-Century-Crofts; 1979:227–290.

Golimbu CN, Firoozina H, Melone CP Jr, Rafii M, Weinreb J, Leber C. Tears of the triangular fibrocartilage of the wrist: MR imaging. *Radiology* 1989;173:731–733.

Golimbu CN, Firoozina H, Rafii M. Avascular necrosis of carpal bones. *Magn Reson Imaging Clin North Am* 1995;3:281–303.

Green DP, O'Brien ET. Classification and management of carpal dislocations. *Clin Orthop* 1980;149:55–72.

Green SM, Greenspan A. An expanded imaging approach for diagnosing tears of the triangular fibrocartilage complex. *Bull Hosp Joint Dis Orthop Inst* 1988;48:187–190.

Greenspan A, Posner MA, Tucker M. The value of carpal tunnel trispiral tomography in the diagnosis of fracture of the hook of the hamate. *Bull Hosp Joint Dis Orthop Inst* 1985;45:74–79.

Gundry CR, Kursunoglu-Brahme S, Schwaighofer B, Kang HS, Sartoris DJ, Resnick D. Is MR better than arthrography for evaluating the ligaments of the wrist? In vitro study. *AJR Am J Roentgenol* 1990;154:337–341.

Haims AH, Schweitzer ME, Morrison WB, Deely D, Lange R, Osterman AL, Bednar JM, Taras JS, Culp RW. Limitations of MR imaging in the diagnosis of peripheral tears of the triangular fibrocartilage of the wrist. *AJR Am J Roentgenol* 2002;178:419–422.

Haims AH, Schweitzer ME, Morrison WB, et al. Internal derangement of the wrist: indirect MR arthrography versus unenhanced MR imaging. *Radiology* 2003;227:701–707.

Haramati N, Hiller N, Dowdle J, et al. MRI of the Stener lesion. *Skeletal Radiol* 1995;24:515–518.

Harper MT, Chandnani VP, Spaeth J, Santangelo JR, Providence BC, Bagg MA. Gamekeeper thumb: diagnosis of ulnar collateral ligament injury using magnetic resonance imaging, magnetic resonance arthrography and stress radiography. *J Magn Reson Imaging* 1966;6:322–328.

Helms CA, Major NM. Rapid triple-compartment wrist arthrography with diluted contrast medium. *Can Assoc Radiol J* 1993;44:227–229.

Hergan K, Mittler C, Oser W. Pitfalls in sonography of the gamekeeper's thumb. *Eur Radiol* 1997;7:65–69.

Hergan K, Mittler C, Oser W. Ulnar collateral ligament: differentiation of displaced and nondisplaced tears with US and MR imaging. *Radiology* 1995;194:65–71.

Hinke DH, Erickson SJ, Chamoy L, Timins ME. Ulnar collateral ligament of the thumb: MR findings in cadavers, volunteers, and patients with ligamentous injury (gamekeeper's thumb). *AJR Am J Roentgenol* 1994;163:1431–1434.

Hobby JL, Dixon AK, Bearcroft PWP, Tom BDM, Lomas DJ, Rushton N, Matthewson MH. MR imaging of the wrist: effect on clinical diagnosis and patient care. *Radiology* 2001;220:589–593.

Howard FM. Fractures of the basal joint of the thumb. *Clin Orthop* 1987;220:46–57.

Hunter JC, Escobedo EM, Wilson AJ, Hanel DP, Zink-Brody GC, Mann FA. MR imaging of clinically suspected scaphoid fractures. *AJR Am J Roentgenol* 1997;168:1287–1293.

Hunter TB, Peltier LF, Lund PJ. Radiologic history exhibit. Musculoskeletal eponyms: Who are those guys? *Radiographics* 2000;20:819–836.

Imaeda T, Nakamura R, Miura T, et al. Magnetic resonance imaging in Kienböck's disease. *J Hand Surg [Br]* 1992;14B:12–19.

Imaeda T, Nakamura R, Miura T, Makino N. Magnetic resonance imaging in scaphoid fractures. *J Hand Surg [Br]* 1992;17B:20–27.

Imaeda T, Nakamura R, Shionoya K, Makino N. Ulnar impaction syndrome: MR imaging findings. *Radiology* 1996;201:495–500.

Johnson PG, Szabo RM. Angle measurements of the distal radius: a cadaver study. *Skeletal Radiol* 1993;22:243–246.

Johnston GHF, Freidman L, Kriegler JC. Computerized tomographic evaluation of acute distal radial fractures. *J Hand Surg [Am]* 1992;17A:738–744.

Jonsson K, Jonsson A, Sloth M, Kopylov P, Wingstrand H. CT of the wrist in suspected scaphoid fracture. *Acta Radiol* 1992;33:500–501.

Kang HS, Kindynis P, Brahme SK, et al. Triangular fibrocartilage and intercarpal ligaments of the wrist: MR imaging. *Radiology* 1991;181:401–404.

Kienböck R. Über traumatische Malazie des Mondbeins, und ihre Folgezustande: Entartungsformen und Kompressionsfrakturen. *Fortschr Roentgenstr* 1910;16:77–103.

Kuszyk BS, Fishman EK. Direct coronal CT of the wrist: helical acquisition with simplified patient positioning. *AJR Am J Roentgenol* 1996;166:419–420.

Langer AJ, Gron P, Langhoff O. The scaphoid fat stripe in the diagnosis of carpal trauma. *Acta Radiol* 1988;29:97–99.

Lees VC, Scheker LR. The radiological demonstration of dynamic ulnar impingement. *J Hand Surg [Br]* 1997;22B:448–450.

Levinsohn EM, Palmer AK. Arthrography of the traumatized wrist. Correlation with radiography and the carpal instability series. *Radiology* 1983;146:647–651.

Levinsohn EM, Palmer AK, Coren AB, Zinberg E. Wrist arthrography: the value of three compartment injection technique. *Skeletal Radiol* 1987;16:539–544.

Levinsohn EM, Rosen ID, Palmer AK. Wrist arthrography: value of the three-compartment injection method. *Radiology* 1991;179:231–239.

Lichtman DM, Alexander AH, Mack GR, Gunther SF. Kienböck's disease: update on silicone replacement arthroplasty. *J Hand Surg [Am]* 1982;7A:343–347.

Lichtman DM, Schneider JR, Swafford AF, et al. Ulnar midcarpal instability—clinical and laboratory analysis. *J Hand Surg [Am]* 1991;6A:515–523.

Linkous MD, Gilula LA. Wrist arthrography today. *Radiol Clin North Am* 1998;36:651–672.

Linn MR, Mann FA, Gilula LA. Imaging the symptomatic wrist. *Orthop Clin North Am* 1990;21:515–543.

Louis DS, Buckwalter KA. Magnetic resonance imaging of the collateral ligaments of the thumb. *J Hand Surg [Am]* 1989;14A:739–741.

Louis DS, Huebner J, Hankin F. Rupture and displacement of the ulnar collateral ligament of the metacarpophalangeal joint of the thumb. *J Bone Joint Surg [Am]* 1986;68A:1320–1326.

Malik AM, Schweitzer ME, Culp RW, Osterman LA, Manton G. MR imaging of the type II lunate bone: frequency, extent, and associated findings. *AJR Am J Roentgenol* 1999;173:335–338.

Manaster BJ. Digital wrist arthrography: precision in determining the site of radio-carpal-midcarpal communication. *AJR Am J Roentgenol* 1986;147:563–566.

Manaster BJ. The clinical efficacy of triple-injection wrist arthrography. *Radiology* 1991;178:267–270.

Manaster BJ, Mann RJ, Rubinstein S. Wrist pain: correlation of clinical and plain film findings with arthrographic results. *J Hand Surg [Am]* 1989;14A:466–473.

Mann FA, Wilson AJ, Gilula LA. Radiographic evaluation of the wrist: what does the hand surgeon want to know? *Radiology* 1992;184:15–24.

Mayfield JK. Mechanism of carpal injuries. *Clin Orthop* 1980;149:45–54.

Mayfield JK, Johnson RP, Kilcoyne RF. Carpal dislocations: patho-mechanics and progressive perilunar instability. *J Hand Surg* 1980;5:226–241.

Mayfield JK, Johnson RP, Kilcoyne RF. The ligaments of the human wrist and their functional significance. *Anat Rec* 1976;186:417–428.

McDonald G, Petrie D. Ununited fracture of the scaphoid. *Clin Orthop* 1975;108:110–114.

McMurtry RY, Jupiter JB. Fractures of the distal radius. In: Browner B, Jupiter J, Levine A, Trafton P, eds. *Skeletal trauma*. Philadelphia: WB Saunders; 1991:1063–1094.

McNiesh LM. Unique musculoskeletal trauma. *Radiol Clin North Am* 1987;25:1107–1132.

Merhar GL, Clark RA, Schneider HJ, Stern PJ. High-resolution computed tomography of the wrist in patients with carpal tunnel syndrome. *Skeletal Radiol* 1986;15:549–552.

Mesgarzadeh M, Schneck CD, Bonakdarpour A. Carpal tunnel: MR imaging. Part I. Normal anatomy. *Radiology* 1989;171:743–748.

Mesgarzadeh M, Schneck CD, Bonakdarpour A, Mitra A, Conaway D. Carpal tunnel: MR imaging. Part II. Carpal tunnel syndrome. *Radiology* 1989;171:749–754.

Metz VM. Arthrography of the wrist and hand. In: Gilula LA, Yuming Y, eds. *Imaging of the wrist and hand*. Philadelphia: WB Saunders; 1996.

Metz VM, Mann FA, Gilula LA. Three-compartment wrist arthrography: correlation of pain site with location of uni- and bidirectional communications. *AJR Am J Roentgenol* 1993;160:819–822.

Metz VM, Mann FA, Gilula LA. Lack of correlation between site of wrist pain and location of noncommunicating defects shown by three-compartment wrist arthrography. *AJR Am J Roentgenol* 1993;160:1239–1243.

Milankov M, Somer T, Jovanovic A, Brankov M. Isolated dislocation of the capal scaphoid: two case reports. *J Trauma* 1994;36:752–754.

Morgan WJ, Breen TF, Coumas JM, et al. Role of magnetic resonance imaging in assessing factors affecting healing in scaphoid nonunions. *Clin Orthop* 1997;336:240–246.

Munk PL, Lee MJ, Logan PM, et al. Scaphoid bone waist fractures, acute and chronic: imaging with different techniques. *AJR Am J Roentgenol* 1997;168:779–786.

Munk PL, Vellet AD, Levin MR, Steinbach LS, Helms CA. Current status of magnetic resonance imaging of the wrist. *Can Assoc Radiol J* 1992;43:8–18.

Muren C, Nygren E, Svartengren G. Computed tomography of the scaphoid in the longitudinal axis of the bone. *Acta Radiol* 1990;31:110–111.

Murphy D, Eisenhauer M. The utility of a bone scan in the diagnosis of clinical scaphoid fracture. *J Emerg Med* 1994;12:709–712.

Murray WT, Meuller PR, Rosenthal DI, Jauernek RR. Fracture of the hook of the hamate. *AJR Am J Roentgenol* 1979;133:899–903.

Nakamura R, Imaeda T, Horii E, Miura T, Hayakawa RT. Analysis of scaphoid fracture displacement by three-dimensional computed tomography. *J Hand Surg [Am]* 1991;16A:485–492.

Nakamura T, Yabe Y, Horiuchi Y. Fat suppression magnetic resonance imaging of the triangular fibrocartilage complex: comparison with spin echo, gradient echo pulse sequences and histology. *J Hand Surg [Br]* 1999;24B:22–26.

Newland CC. Gamekeeper's thumb. *Orthop Clin North Am* 1992;23:41–48.

Norman A, Nelson JM, Green SM. Fractures of the hook of the hamate: radiographic signs. *Radiology* 1985;154:49–53.

O'Callaghan BI, Kohut G, Hoogewoud H-M. Gamekeeper thumb: identification of the Stener lesion with US. *Radiology* 1994;192:477–480.

Oneson SR, Scales LM, Timins ME, Erickson SJ, Chamoy L. MR imaging interpretation of the Palmer classification of triangular fibrocartilage complex lesions. *Radiographics* 1996;16:97–106.

Oneson SR, Timins ME, Scales LM, Erickson SJ, Chamoy L. MR imaging diagnosis of triangular fibrocartilage pathology with arthroscopic correlation. *AJR Am J Roentgenol* 1997;168:1513–1518.

Palmer AK. Triangular fibrocartilage complex lesions: a classification. *J Hand Surg [Am]* 1989;14A:495–604.

Palmer AK, Glisson RR, Werner FW. Ulnar variance determination. *J Hand Surg [Am]* 1982;7A:376–379.

Palmer AK, Levinsohn M, Kuzma GR. Arthrography of the wrist. *J Hand Surg [Am]* 1983;8A:15–23.

Palmer AK, Werner FW. The triangular fibrocartilage complex of the wrist: anatomy and function. *J Hand Surg [Am]* 1981;6A:153–162.

Pederzini L, Luchetti R, Soragni O, et al. Evaluation of the triangular fibrocartilage complex tears by arthroscopy, arthrography and magnetic resonance imaging. *Arthroscopy* 1992;8:191–197.

Peltier LF. Eponymic fractures: John Rhea Barton and Barton's fractures. *Surgery* 1953;34:960–970.

Pennes DR, Jonsson K, Buckwalter KA. Direct coronal CT of the scaphoid bone. *Radiology* 1989;171:870–871.

Perlik PC, Guilford WB. Magnetic resonance imaging to assess vascularity of scaphoid nonunions. *J Hand Surg [Am]* 1991;16A:479–484.

Pittman CC, Quinn SF, Belsole R, Greene T, Rayhack J. Digital subtraction wrist arthrography: use of double contrast technique as a supplement to single contrast arthrography. *Skeletal Radiol* 1989;17:119–122.

Posner MA, Greenspan A. Trispiral tomography for the evaluation of wrist problems. *J Hand Surg [Am]* 1988;13A:175–181.

Posner MA, Retaillaud J. Metacarpophalangeal joint injuries of the thumb. *Hand Clin* 1992;8:713–732.

Protas JM, Jackson WT. Evaluating carpal instabilities with fluoroscopy. *AJR Am J Roentgenol* 1980;135:137–140.

Pruitt DL, Gilula LA, Manske PR, Vannier MW. CT scanning with image reconstruction in the evaluation of distal radius fractures. *J Hand Surg [Am]* 1994;19A:720–727.

Quinn SF, Pittman CC, Belsole R, Greene TL, Rayhack JM. Digital subtraction wrist arthrography: evaluation of the multiple-compartment technique. *AJR Am J Roentgenol* 1988;151:1173–1174.

Rayan GM. Scaphoid fractures and nonunions. *Am J Orthop* 1995;24:227–236.

Reinus WR, Hardy DC, Totty WG, Gilula LA. Arthrographic evaluation of the carpal triangular fibrocartilage complex. *J Hand Surg [Am]* 1987;12A:495–503.

Rennie WJ, Finlay DBL. Posttraumatic cystlike defects of the scaphoid: late sign of occult microfracture and useful indicator of delayed union. *AJR Am J Roentgenol* 2003;180:655–658.

Resnick D. Arthrography and tenography of the hand and wrist. In: Dalinka MK, ed. *Arthrography*. New York: Springer-Verlag; 1980.

Resnick D, Danzig LA. Arthrographic evaluation of injuries of the first metacarpophalangeal joint: gamekeeper's thumb. *AJR Am J Roentgenol* 1976;126:1046–1052.

Richards R, Bennett J, Roth J. Scaphoid dislocation with radial axial carpal disruption. *AJR Am J Roentgenol* 1993;160:1075–1076.

Romaniuk CS, Butt WP, Coral A. Bilateral three-compartment wrist arthrography in patients with unilateral wrist pain: findings and implications for management. *Skeletal Radiol* 1995;24:95–99.

Rominger MB, Bernreuter WK, Kenney PJ, Lee DH. MR imaging of anatomy and tears of wrist ligaments. *Radiographics* 1993;15:1233–1246.

Ruby LK, Cooney WP III, An KN, Linscheid RL, Chao EY. Relative motion of selected carpal bones: a kinematic analysis of the normal wrist. *J Hand Surg [Am]* 1988;13A:1–10.

Sanders WE. Evaluation of the humpback scaphoid by computed tomography in the longitudinal axial plane of the scaphoid. *J Hand Surg* 1988;13A:182–187.

Schweitzer ME, Brahme SK, Hodler J, et al. Chronic wrist pain: spin-echo and short tau inversion recovery MR imaging and conventional and MR arthrography. *Radiology* 1992;182:205–211.

Sherman SB, Greenspan A, Norman A. Osteonecrosis of the distal pole of the carpal scaphoid following fracture—a rare complication. *Skeletal Radiol* 1983;9:189–191.

Sides D, Laorr A, Greenspan A. Carpal scaphoid: radiographic pattern of dislocation. *Radiology* 1995;195:215–216.

Smith DK. Scapholunate interosseous ligament of the wrist: MR appearances in asymptomatic volunteers and arthrographically normal wrists. *Radiology* 1994;192:217–221.

Smith DK. Anatomic features of the carpal scaphoid: validation of biometric measurements and symmetry with three-dimensional MR imaging. *Radiology* 1993;187:187–191.

Smith DK. Dorsal carpal ligaments of the wrist: normal appearance on multiplanar reconstructions of three-dimensional Fourier transform MR imaging. *AJR Am J Roentgenol* 1993;161:119–125.

Smith DK, Gilula LA, Amadio PC. Dorsal lunate tilt (DISI configuration): sign of scaphoid fracture displacement. *Radiology* 1990;176:497–499.

Smith DK, Snearly WN. Lunotriquetral interosseous ligament of the wrist: MR appearances in asymptomatic volunteers and arthrographically normal wrists. *Radiology* 1994;191:199–202.

Spaeth HJ, Abrams RA, Bock GW, et al. Gamekeeper thumb: differentiation of nondisplaced and displaced tears of the ulnar collateral ligament with MR imaging. *Radiology* 1993;188:553–556.

Spence LD, Savenor A, Nwachuku I, Tilsley J, Eustace S. MRI of fractures of the distal radius: comparison with conventional radiographs. *Skeletal Radiol* 1998;27:244–249.

Staniforth P. Scaphoid fractures and wrist pain: time for new thinking. *Injury* 1991;22:435–436.

Stark HH, Jobe FW, Boyes JH, Ashworth CR. Fracture of the hook of the hamate in athletes. *J Bone Joint Surg [Am]* 1977;59A:575–582.

Steinborn M, Schürmann M, Staebler A, Wizgall I, Pellengahr C, Heuck A, Reiser M. MR imaging of ulnocarpal impaction after fracture of the distal radius. *AJR Am J Roentgenol* 2003;181:195–198.

Stener B. Displacement of the ruptured ulnar collateral ligament of the metacarpophalangeal joint of the thumb. *J Bone Joint Surg [Br]* 1962;44B:869–879.

Stewart NR, Gilula LA. CT of the wrist: a tailored approach. *Radiology* 1992;183:13–20.

Szabo RM, Greenspan A. Diagnosis and clinical findings of Kienböck's disease. *Hand Clin* 1993;9:399–408.

Taleisnik J. Current concepts review: carpal instability. *J Bone Joint Surg [Am]* 1988;70A:1262–1268.

Tehranzadeh J, Davenport J, Pais MJ. Scaphoid fracture: evaluation with flexion-extension tomography. *Radiology* 1990;176:167–170.

Theumann NH, Pfirrmann CWA, Antonio GE, Chung CB, Gilula LA, Trudell DJ, Resnick D. Extrinsic carpal ligaments: normal MR arthrographic appearance in cadavers. *Radiology* 2003; 226:171–179.

Thorpe AP, Murray AD, Smith FW, Ferguson J. Clinically suspected scaphoid fracture: a comparison of magnetic resonance imaging and bone scinitgraphy. *Br J Radiol* 1996;69:109–113.

Tiel-van Buul MMC, Roolker W, Verbeeten BWB, Broekhuizen AH. Magnetic resonance imaging versus bone scintigraphy in suspected scaphoid fracture. *Eur J Nucl Med* 1996;23:971–975.

Timins ME. Osseous anatomic variants of the wrist: findings on MR imaging. *AJR Am J Roentgenol* 1999;173:339–344.

Timins ME, Jahnke JP, Krah SF, Erickson SJ, Carrera GF. MR imaging of the major carpal stabilizing ligaments: normal anatomy and clinical examples. *Radiographics* 1995;15:575–587.

Timins ME, O'Connell SE, Erickson SJ, Oneson SR. MR imaging of the wrist: normal findings that may simulate disease. *Radiographics* 1996;16:987–995.

Tirman R, Weber ER, Snyder LL, Koonce TW. Midcarpal wrist arthrography for the detection of tears of the scapholunate and lunotriquetral ligaments. *AJR Am J Roentgenol* 1985;144:107–108.

Totterman SM, Miller RJ. MR imaging of the triangular fibrocartilage complex. *MRI Clin North Am* 1995;3:213–227.

Totterman SM, Miller RJ. Triangular fibrocartilage complex: normal appearance on coronal three-dimensional gradient-recalled-echo MR images. *Radiology* 1995;195:521–527.

Totterman SM, Miller RJ. Scapholunate ligament: normal MR appearance on three-dimensional gradient-recalled-echo images. *Radiology* 1996;200:237–241.

Totterman SM, Miller RJ, McCance SE, Meyers SP. Lesions of the triangular fibrocartilage complex: MR findings with a three-dimensional gradient-recalled-echo MR sequence. *Radiology* 1996;199:227–232.

Totterman SM, Miller R, Wasserman B, Blebea JS, Rubens DJ. Intrinsic and extrinsic carpal ligaments: evaluation by three-dimensional Fourier transform MR imaging. *AJR Am J Roentgenol* 1993;160:117–123.

Trumble TE. Avascular necrosis after scaphoid fracture: a correlation of magnetic resonance imaging and histology. *J Hand Surg [Am]* 1990;15A:557–564.

Trumble TE, Irving J. Histologic and magnetic resonance imaging correlations in Kienböck's disease. *J Hand Surg [Am]* 1990;15A:879–884.

Trumble TE, Schmitt SR, Vedder NB. Factors affecting functional outcome of displaced intra-articular distal radius fractures. *J Hand Surg [Am]* 1994;19A:325–340.

Vanden ES, De Smet L, Fabry G. Diagnostic value of arthrography and arthroscopy of the radiocarpal joint. *Arthroscopy* 1994;10:50–53.

Waizenegger M, Barton NJ, Davis TR, Wartie ML. Clinical signs in scaphoid fractures. *J Hand Surg [Br]* 1994;19B:743–747.

White SJ, Louis DS, Braunstein EM, Hankin FM, Greene TL. Capitate-lunate instability: Recognition by manipulation under fluoroscopy. *AJR Am J Roentgenol* 1984; 143:361–364.

Wilson AJ, Gilula LA, Mann FA. Unidirectional joint communications in wrist arthrography: an evaluation of 250 cases. *AJR Am J Roentgenol* 1991;157:105–109.

Wilson AJ, Mann FA, Gilula LA. Imaging the right hand and wrist. *J Hand Surg [Br]* 1990;15B:153–167.

Yeager BA, Dalinka MK. Radiology of trauma to the wrist: dislocations, fracture dislocations, and instability patterns. *Skeletal Radiol* 1985;13:120–130.

Yin Y, Wilson AJ, Gilula LA. Three-compartment wrist arthrography: direct comparison of digital subtraction with nonsubtraction images. *Radiology* 1995;197:287–290.

Yu JS. Magnetic resonance imaging of the wrist. *Orthopedics* 1994;17:1041–1048.

Zanetti M, Hodler J, Gilula LA. Assessment of dorsal or ventral intercalated segmental instability configurations of the wrist: reliability of sagittal MR images. *Radiology* 1998;206:339–345.

Zanetti M, Linkous MD, Gilula LA, Hodler J. Characteristics of triangular fibrocartilage defects in symptomatic and contralateral asymptomatic wrists. *Radiology* 2000;216:840–845.

Zeiss J, Jakab E, Khimji T, Imbriglia J. The ulnar tunnel at the wrist (Guyon's canal): normal MR anatomy and variants. *AJR Am J Roentgenol* 1992;158:1081–1085.

Zinberg EM, Palmer AK, Coren AB, Levinsohn EM. The triple injection wrist arthrogram. *J Hand Surg [Am]* 1988;13A:803–809.

Zlatkin MB, Greenan G. Magnetic resonance imaging of the wrist. *Magn Reson Q* 1992;8:65–96.

LOWER LIMB I

Pelvic Girdle and Proximal Femur

Pelvic Girdle

Fractures involving the structures of the pelvic girdle, which are usually sustained in motor vehicle accidents or falls from heights, represent only a small percentage of all skeletal injuries. Their importance, however, lies in the significant morbidity and mortality associated with them, which is usually caused by accompanying injury to the major blood vessels, nerves, and lower urinary tract. Because the clinical signs of pelvic trauma may not always be obvious, radiographic examination is essential to establish a correct diagnosis. Fractures of the acetabulum constitute approximately 20% of all pelvic fractures, and they may or may not be associated with dislocation in the hip joint. Fractures of the proximal (upper) femur, occasionally referred to as hip fractures, occur frequently in the elderly, often as a result of minimal injury. They are seen more frequently in women than in men (2:1), with intracapsular fractures of the proximal femur having an even higher female-to-male ratio (5:1).

Anatomic–Radiologic Considerations

The main radiologic modalities used in evaluation of traumatic conditions of the pelvic girdle, acetabulum, and proximal femur include conventional radiography and computed tomography (CT). Other an-

cillary techniques are also essential for a complete evaluation of concomitant soft-tissue and pelvic–organ injuries: angiography for the pelvic blood vessels and cystourethrography for the lower urinary tract. Radionuclide bone scan and magnetic resonance imaging (MRI) may also be necessary to disclose subtle fractures of the femoral neck and early stages of posttraumatic osteonecrosis of the femoral head.

The standard and special radiographic projections used to evaluate injury to the pelvic girdle and proximal femur include the anteroposterior view of the pelvis, the anterior and posterior oblique views of the pelvis, the anteroposterior view of the hip, and the frog-lateral view of the hip. At times, the groin-lateral or other special projections may also be required.

Most traumatic conditions involving the sacral wings, the iliac bones, the ischium, the pubis, and the femoral head and neck can be evaluated sufficiently on the *anteroposterior* projection of the pelvis and hip (Fig. 8.1). This view also demonstrates an important anatomic relation of the longitudinal axes of the femoral neck and shaft. Normally, the angle formed by these axes ranges from 125° to 135°. This measurement is valuable in determining displacement in femoral neck fractures. A varus configuration is characterized by a decrease in this angle, and a valgus configuration by an increase in this angle (Fig. 8.2). The anteroposterior view, however, is frequently not sufficient to

Figure 8.1 Anteroposterior view. (A) For the anteroposterior view of the pelvis and hip, the patient is supine with the feet in slight (15°) internal rotation (*inset*), which compensates for the normal anteversion of the femoral neck (see Fig. 8.7B), elongating its image. For a view of the entire pelvis, the central beam is directed vertically toward the midportion of the pelvis; for selective examination of either hip joint, it is directed toward the affected femoral head. **(B)** The radiograph in this projection demonstrates the iliac bones, the sacrum, the pubis, and the ischium, as well as the femoral heads and necks and both the greater and the lesser trochanters. The acetabula are partially obscured by the overlying femoral heads, and the sacroiliac joints are seen en face.

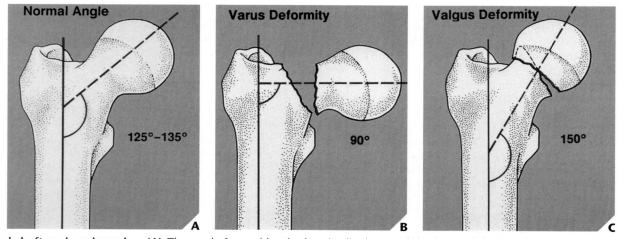

Figure 8.2 Femoral shaft and neck angles. (A) The angle formed by the longitudinal axes of the femoral shaft and neck normally ranges from 125° to 135°. In the evaluation of displacement in femoral neck fractures, a decrease in this angle **(B)** is known as a varus deformity, while an increase **(C)** characterizes a valgus deformity.

Figure 8.3 Ferguson view. (A) For the angled anteroposterior (Ferguson) view of the pelvis, the patient is in the same position as for the standard anteroposterior projection. The radiographic tube, however, is angled approximately 30° to 35° cephalad, and the central beam is directed toward the midportion of the pelvis. **(B)** The radiograph in this projection provides a tangential view of the sacroiliac joints and the sacral bone. The pubic and ischial rami are also well demonstrated.

provide adequate evaluation of the entire sacral bone, the sacroiliac joints, and the acetabulum. Demonstration of the sacroiliac joints requires either a posteroanterior projection, which is obtained to greater advantage with 25° to 30° caudal angulation of the radiographic tube, or an anteroposterior view with 30° to 35° cephalad angulation. The latter projection, known as the *Ferguson* view, is also helpful in more effectively evaluating injury to the sacral bone and the pubic and ischial rami (Fig. 8.3). Oblique projections, known as *Judet* views, are necessary to evaluate the acetabulum. The *anterior (internal) oblique* projection helps delineate the iliopubic (anterior) column and the posterior lip (rim) of the acetabulum (Fig. 8.4). The *posterior (external) oblique* projection delineates the ilioischial (posterior) column and the anterior acetabular rim (Fig. 8.5). Of value in demonstrating the structures of the proximal femur and hip, the *frog-lateral* projection allows adequate evaluation of fractures of the femoral head and the greater and the lesser trochanters (Fig. 8.6). Demonstration of the anterior and posterior aspects of the femoral head as well as the anterior rim of the acetabulum may require a *groin-lateral* projection of the hip, which is particularly useful in evaluating anterior or posterior displacement of fragments in proximal femoral fractures and the degree of rotation of the femoral head. This projection, by providing an almost true lateral image of the proximal femur, also demonstrates an important anatomic feature, the angle of anteversion of the femoral neck, which normally ranges from 25° to 30° (Fig. 8.7).

Ancillary imaging techniques play a crucial role in the evaluation of traumatic conditions of the pelvis and acetabulum, providing essential and often otherwise unobtainable information that helps the orthopedic surgeon determine the method of treatment and assess the prognosis of pelvic and acetabular fractures. Because the surgical management of such fractures is based on the stability of the fragments and the presence or absence of intraarticular extension of the fracture line and intraarticular fragments, CT examination is necessary to provide information that is not available from the standard and special projections of conventional radiography (Fig. 8.8; see also Figs. 8.22B,C, 8.23B–D). In addition to ascertaining the size, number, and position of the major fragments and data about the condition of the weight-bearing parts of the joint and the configuration of the fracture fragments, CT can delineate soft tissue and concomitant injury to soft-tissue structures. However, in cases of severe injury when immediate surgical intervention is required, obtaining CT scans may be time consuming and impractical. In such cases, conventional radiographs can be obtained more quickly, allowing more rapid recognition of the type of injury. CT is particularly effective in the postsurgical assessment of the alignment of fragments and fracture healing.

Figure 8.4 Anterior oblique view. (A) For the anterior oblique (Judet) view of the pelvis, the patient is supine and anteriorly rotated, with the affected hip elevated 45° (*inset*). The central beam is directed vertically toward the affected hip. **(B)** On the radiograph in this projection, the iliopubic (anterior) column (see Fig. 8.19) and the posterior lip of the acetabulum are well delineated.

MRI offers superior capabilities for evaluating traumatic conditions of the hip. In particular, it has been shown to provide a rapid, precise, and cost-effective diagnosis of radiographically occult hip fractures and may help reveal traumatic lesions such as bone contusions (trabecular microfractures) as the cause of hip pain when the history of trauma is unknown. MRI is also effective in diagnosis of posttraumatic osteonecrosis of the femoral head and can identify and quantify the muscle injury and joint effusion/hemarthrosis that invariably accompany traumatic anterior and posterior dislocation in the hip joint.

The urinary system is frequently at risk in pelvic fractures. Bladder injuries have been reported in 6% and urethral injuries in 10% of patients with pelvic fractures. The evaluation of such conditions requires contrast examination of the urinary system by means of intravenous urography (IVP) and cystourethrography. Pelvic arteriography and venography may also be required to evaluate injury to the vascular system. In addition to its diagnostic value, arteriography can be combined with an interventional procedure, such as embolization, to control hemorrhage.

For a summary of the preceding discussion in tabular form, see Tables 8.1 and 8.2 and Fig. 8.9.

Injury to the Pelvis and Acetabulum

The pelvis is a nearly rigid ring essentially comprising three elements: the sacrum and two paired lateral components, each composed of the ilium, the ischium, and the pubis. Because of this configuration and the interrelationship of its components, identification of an apparently solitary fracture should not end the process of radiographic examination. The pelvis should be scrutinized carefully for other fractures of the ring or diastasis in the sacroiliac joints or the pubic symphysis (see Fig. 4.7).

Classification of Pelvic Fractures

Various classification systems have been proposed not only to identify the distinctive appearances of pelvic injuries as an aid to radiographic recognition and diagnosis but also to categorize such injuries as an aid to orthopedic management and prognosis. The latter point is partic-

anterior
acetabular lip

posterior
acetabular lip

posterior column

Figure 8.5 Posterior oblique view. (A) For the posterior oblique (Judet) view of the pelvis, the patient is supine and anteriorly rotated, with the unaffected hip elevated 45° (*inset*). The central beam is directed vertically through the affected hip. **(B)** On the film in this projection, the ilioischial (posterior) column, the posterior acetabular lip, and the anterior acetabular rim are well demonstrated (see Fig. 8.19).

Figure 8.6 Frog-lateral view. (A) For the frog-lateral view of the proximal femur and hip, the patient is supine with the knees flexed, the soles of the feet together, and the thighs maximally abducted. For simultaneous imaging of both hips, the central beam is directed vertically or with 10° to 15° cephalad angulation to a point slightly above the pubic symphysis (*inset*); for selective examination of one hip, it is directed toward the affected hip joint. **(B)** The film in this projection demonstrates the lateral aspect of the femoral head and both trochanters.

Anterior

femoral head

angle of
anteversion

greater
trochanter

lesser trochanter

ischial tuberosity

Figure 8.7 Groin-lateral view. (A) For the groin-lateral view of the hip, the patient is supine with the affected extremity extended and the opposite leg elevated and abducted. The cassette is placed against the affected hip on the lateral aspect, and the central beam is directed horizontally toward the groin with approximately 20° cephalad angulation. **(B)** The film in this projection provides almost a true lateral image of the femoral head, thereby allowing evaluation of its anterior and posterior aspects. It also demonstrates the anteversion of the femoral neck, which normally ranges from 25° to 30°.

true, synovial joint

syndesmotic joint

pubic symphysis
anterior part of acetabulum
femoral head
acetabulum
posterior part of acetabulum

Figure 8.8 CT of the sacroiliac and hip joints. (A) CT section at the level of S-2 demonstrates the true (synovial) sacroiliac joints. **(B)** In this section through the hip joints, the relation of the femoral heads to the acetabula can be evaluated sufficiently. The pubic bone and the pubic symphysis are also well delineated.

Table 8.1 Standard and Special Radiographic Projections for Evaluating Injury to the Pelvis, Acetabulum, and Proximal Femur

Projection	Demonstration	Projection	Demonstration
Anteroposterior	Angle of femoral neck	*Oblique* (Judet views)	
	Radiographic landmarks (lines) relating to acetabulum:	Anterior (internal)	Iliopubic line
	Iliopubic (iliopectineal)		Fractures of:
	Ilioischial		Anterior (iliopubic) column
	Teardrop		Posterior acetabular rim
	Acetabular roof	Posterior (external)	Quadrilateral plate
	Anterior acetabular rim		Fractures of:
	Posterior acetabular rim		Posterior (ilioischial) column
	Varus and valgus deformities		Anterior acetabular rim
	Avulsion fractures	*Frog-Lateral*	Fractures of:
	Malgaigne fracture		Femoral head and neck
	Fractures of:		Greater and lesser trochanters
	Ilium (Duverney)		
	Ischium	*Groin-Lateral*	Angle of anteversion of femoral head
	Pubis		
	Sacrum (in some cases)		Anterior and posterior cortices of femoral neck
	Femoral head and neck		
	Dislocations in hip joint		Ischial tuberosity
With 30°–35° cephalad angulation (Ferguson) (or posteroanterior with or without 25°–30° caudal angulation)	Fractures of:		Rotation and displacement of femoral head in subcapital fractures
	Sacrum		
	Pubis ramus		
	Ischial		
	Injury to sacroiliac joints		

ularly important in pelvic fractures because of the inherent instability of the structures composing the pelvic girdle, their integrity depending entirely on ligamentous support and the stabilizing influence of the sacroiliac joints. Thus, pelvic fractures can be grouped according to whether they significantly detract from the stability of the pelvic ring, with the orthopedic management and prognosis of those fractures identified as stable (Fig. 8.10) differing considerably from that of unstable fractures (Fig. 8.11).

Systems that classify pelvic injuries for the purpose of radiographic diagnosis and orthopedic management using categories other than stable and unstable have also been suggested. Pennal, Tile, and colleagues have elaborated a system based on the direction of the force that produces pelvic injuries. They identified four patterns of force as underlying mechanisms of injury that produce distinctive radiographic appearances:

1. *Anteroposterior compression,* in which the force vector in the anteroposterior or posteroanterior direction produces vertically oriented fractures of the pubic rami and disruption of the pubic symphysis and sacroiliac joints, which often results in bilateral pelvic "dislocation" (sprung pelvis, "open book" injury).

2. *Lateral compression,* in which the lateral force vector often results in horizontally or coronally oriented fractures of the pubic rami, compression fractures of the sacrum, fractures of the iliac wings, and central dislocation in the hip joint as well as varying degrees of pelvic instability caused by displacement or rotation of one or both hemipelves, depending on whether the compressive force is applied more anteriorly or more posteriorly.

3. *Vertical shear,* in which the inferosuperiorly oriented disruptive force, delivered to one or both sides of the pelvis lateral to the midline often as a result of a fall from a height, frequently produces vertically oriented fractures of the pubic rami, sacrum, and iliac wings. Because of significant ligamentous disruption, this type of force is associated with injuries producing severe pelvic instability.

4. *Complex patterns,* in which at least two different force vectors have been delivered to the pelvis, the patterns produced by anteroposterior and lateral compression being the most commonly encountered.

Table 8.2 Ancillary Imaging Techniques for Evaluating Injury to the Pelvis, Acetabulum, and Proximal Femur

Technique	Demonstration	Technique	Demonstration
Tomography (multidirectional)	Position of fragments and extension of fracture line in complex fractures, particularly of pelvis and acetabulum	*Radionuclide Imaging* (scintigraphy, bone scan)	Occult fractures Stress fractures Posttraumatic osteonecrosis
Computed Tomography	Same features as above		
	Weight-bearing parts of joints	*Intravenous Urography* (IVP)	Concomitant injury to ureters, urinary bladder, and urethra
	Sacroiliac joints		
	Intraarticular fragments	*Cystourethrography*	
	Soft-tissue injuries	*Angiography* (arteriography, venography)	Injury to vascular system
MRI	Soft-tissue injuries		
	Posttraumatic osteonecrosis		
	Occult fractures		
	Bone contusions (trabecular microfractures)		

Figure 8.9 Spectrum of radiologic imaging techniques for evaluating injury to the pelvic girdle.*
The radiographic projections or radiologic techniques indicated throughout the diagram are only those that are the most effective in demonstrating the respective traumatic conditions.

This system, which corresponds to the more traditional categorization of pelvic fractures into stable and unstable, has practical value in allowing sufficient evaluation of pelvic injuries to be made on the anteroposterior projection in patients requiring immediate surgical intervention when CT scans would be impractical to obtain. It also provides correlations between the type of force delivered to the pelvis and the concomitant ligamentous and pelvic—organ injury that can be expected. In anteroposterior compression-type injuries, for example, the anterior sacroiliac ligaments, the sacrotuberous—sacroiliac ligament complex, and the symphysis ligaments are damaged. This type of injury may also be associated with urethral and urinary bladder rupture and damage to the pelvic blood vessels. In lateral compression injuries, rupture of the posterior sacroiliac ligament and/or the sacrospinous—sacrotuberous ligament complex may result. Injury to the urinary tract may or may not be present. In vertical shear injuries, the ipsilateral posterior and anterior sacroiliac, the sacrospinous—sacrotuberous, and the anterior symphysis ligaments are usually ruptured. Vertical shear injuries are frequently accompanied by damage to the sciatic nerve and pelvic blood vessels, often resulting in massive

hemorrhage. The discussion that follows, however, focuses on the more traditional pedagogic categories of pelvic trauma.

Fractures of the Pelvis

Avulsion Fractures. Usually involving the anterosuperior or anteroinferior iliac spine or the ischial tuberosity, avulsion fractures, which are classified as stable fractures (Fig. 8.12, see also Fig. 8.10), most commonly occur in athletes as a result of forcible muscular contraction: the *sartorius muscle* and *tensor fasciae latae* in avulsion of the anterosuperior iliac spine; the *rectus femoris muscle* in avulsion of the anteroinferior iliac spine; the *hip rotators* in avulsion of greater trochanter; the *iliopsoas* in avulsion of the lesser trochanter; the *adductors* and *gracilis* in avulsion of pubic bone; and the *hamstrings* in avulsion of the ischial tuberosity. Most fractures of these structures are apparent on a single anteroposterior radiograph of the pelvis (Fig. 8.13). However, confusion in diagnosis may arise when healing occurs by exuberant callus formation, at which time or after full ossification such fractures may be mistaken for neoplasms. Another entity that may mimic avulsion injury to the pelvis is the so-called pelvic digit, a

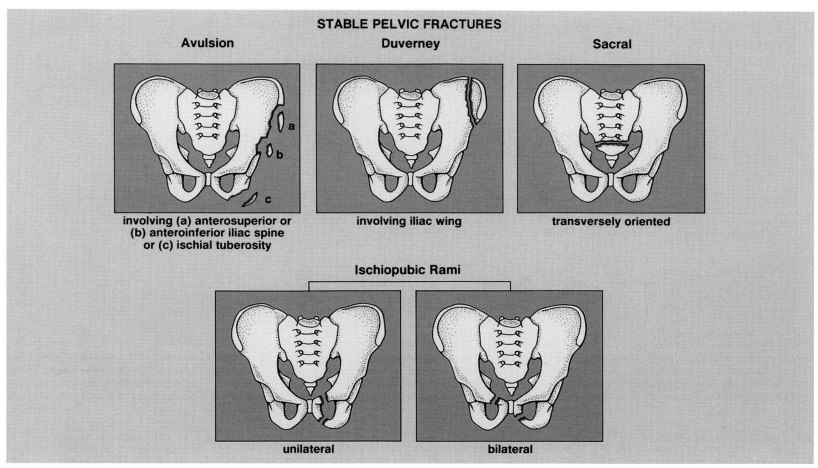

Figure 8.10 Stable pelvic fractures. (Modified from Dunn AW, Morris HD, 1968, with permission.)

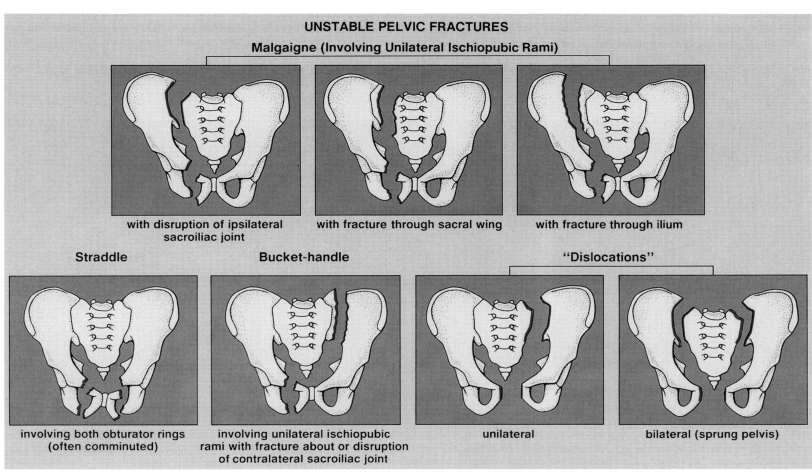

Figure 8.11 Unstable pelvic fractures. (Modified from Dunn AW, Morris HD, 1968, with permission.)

Figure 8.12 Sites of avulsion fractures.

SITES OF AVULSION FRACTURES

iliac crest
(attachment of
abdominal muscles)

anterior superior
iliac spine
(attachment of sartorius
and tensor fasciae latae)

anterior inferior
iliac spine
(attachment of rectus
femoris)

greater trochanter
(attachment of gluteal,
obturator internus,
gemellus, and
piriform muscles)

lesser trochanter
(attachment of
iliopsoas)

body of pubis
and inferior pubic ramus
(attachment of adductors and
gracilis muscles)

ischial tuberosity
(attachment of hamstrings)

congenital anomaly characterized by a bony formation in the soft tissue about the pelvic bones (Fig. 8.14).

Malgaigne Fracture. This unstable injury, involving one hemipelvis, most commonly consists of unilateral fractures of the superior and inferior pubic rami and disruption of the ipsilateral sacroiliac joint (see Fig. 8.11). In the variants of this type of injury, the unilateral fractures of the pubic rami may be accompanied by a fracture through the sacral wing near the sacroiliac joint or through the ilium (see Fig. 8.11). Separation of the pubic symphysis may coexist with such injuries, and cephalad or posterior displacement of the en-

tire hemipelvis may occur. The Malgaigne fracture, which is recognized clinically by shortening of the lower extremity, is readily demonstrated on the anteroposterior radiograph of the pelvis (Fig. 8.15).

Miscellaneous Pelvic Fractures. Injuries other than the Malgaigne fracture are also easily evaluated on radiographs of the pelvis in the standard and special projections or on CT examination. The *Duverney fracture* is a stable fracture of the wing of the ilium without interruption of the pelvic ring (see Fig. 8.10). The *straddle fracture* (see Fig. 8.11) consists of comminuted fractures of both obturator rings

Figure 8.13 Avulsion fractures. A 16-year-old boy was injured during an athletic activity. **(A)** Anteroposterior radiograph of the pelvis shows a crescent-shaped fragment adjacent to the lateral aspect of the iliac wing, which represents the avulsed apophysis of the anterosuperior iliac spine. **(B)** Anteroposterior radiograph of the hip in a 26-year-old runner clearly demonstrates avulsion of the ischial tuberosity. **(C)** As a sequela of avulsion of the ischial tuberosity and injury to the soft tissue in the region, a 28-year-old athlete had ossification of the obturator externus muscle.

Figure 8.14 Pelvic digit. A rare congenital anomaly, the pelvic digit may occasionally be mistaken for avulsion fracture. **(A)** Anteroposterior view of the left hip shows a finger-like, jointed structure attached to the caudal portion of the left ischium. **(B)** Anteroposterior view of the hip in a 55-year-old man with no history of trauma demonstrates a well-formed digit at the site of the anteroinferior iliac spine. (From Greenspan A, Norman A, 1982, with permission.)

Figure 8.15 Malgaigne fracture. A 35-year-old man who was involved in an automobile accident sustained vertical fractures of the left obturator ring and fracture of the ipsilateral iliac bone—a typical Malgaigne injury.

Figure 8.16 Sprung pelvis (bilateral dislocation). A 25-year-old man was involved in a motorcycle accident. Anteroposterior view of the pelvis reveals the typical appearance of pelvic "dislocation." The pubic symphysis is disrupted and markedly widened, and there is widening of both sacroiliac joints.

Figure 8.17 Radiographic landmarks of the hip. (A), (B). On the anteroposterior view of the hip, six lines relating to the acetabulum and its surrounding structures can be distinguished: *a*, iliopubic or iliopectineal (arcuate) line: *b*, ilioischial line, formed by the posterior portion of the quadrilateral plate (surface) of the iliac bone; *c*, teardrop, formed by the medial acetabular wall, the acetabular notch, and the anterior portion of the quadrilateral plate; *d*, roof of the acetabulum; *e*, anterior rim of the acetabulum; and *f*, posterior rim of the acetabulum. Distortion of any of these normal radiographic landmarks indicates the possible presence of abnormality.

(that is, all four ischiopubic rami). In one third of patients with this unstable fracture, bladder rupture or urethral injuries occur. The *bucket-handle* or *contralateral double vertical fracture* involves the superior and inferior ischiopubic rami on one side combined with fracture about or disruption of the sacroiliac joint on the opposite side (see Fig. 8.11). *Fractures of the sacrum,* which may be either transversely or vertically oriented (see Fig. 8.10), may occur alone or, more often, in association with other pelvic injuries, such as the so-called *pelvic dislocations.* The latter are characterized by disruption in one or both sacroiliac joints (unilateral or bilateral "dislocation") associated with separation of the pubic symphysis (Fig. 8.16; see also Fig. 8.11). The anteroposterior projection obtained with 30° cephalad angulation, as well as computed tomography, is helpful in disclosing sacral fractures, which are frequently overlooked.

Figure 8.18 Acetabular fracture. A 32-year-old drug-addicted subject was hit by a car. **(A)** Anteroposterior view of the pelvis shows a comminuted fracture of the right acetabulum, fracture of the right ilium, and diastasis in the pubic symphysis. There is also a fracture of the sacrum with diastasis in the left sacroiliac joint. **(B)** On the anterior oblique projection, the acetabular fracture is seen to involve mainly the anterior pelvic column.

Figure 8.19 Columns of the pelvis. Lateral (**A**) and medial (**B**) views of the pelvis show the division of the bone into anterior and posterior columns, which provides the basis for the traditional classification of acetabular fractures. (Modified from Judet R, et al., 1964, with permission.)

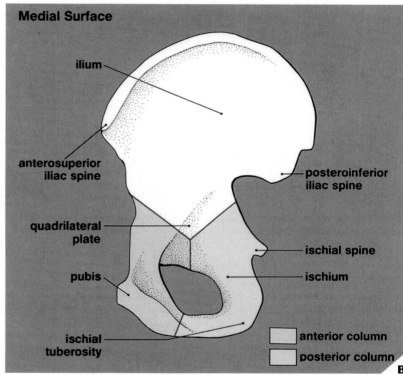

Fractures of the Acetabulum

Evaluation of the acetabulum on conventional radiographs may be difficult because of obscuring overlying structures (Fig. 8.17A). If acetabular fracture is suspected, then radiographs in at least four projections should be obtained: the anteroposterior view of the pelvis, the anteroposterior view of the hip, and the anterior and posterior oblique (Judet) views. Radiography may also need to be supplemented by conventional tomography or CT, as discussed previously.

As an aid to recognizing the presence of abnormality on the anteroposterior projection of the pelvis and hip, Judet, Judet, and Le-

tournel have identified six lines relating to the acetabulum and its immediately surrounding structures (Fig. 8.17). Fracture of the acetabulum usually distorts these radiographic landmarks, allowing a diagnosis to be made on the anteroposterior projection, but an accurate and complete evaluation of the fracture requires that oblique views be obtained (Fig. 8.18). As mentioned, the anterior (internal) oblique projection demonstrates the iliopubic column and the posterior lip of the acetabulum (see Fig. 8.4), and the posterior (external) oblique view images the ilioischial column and the anterior rim of the acetabulum (see Fig. 8.5). These projections, together with the division of the pelvic bone into anterior and posterior columns (Fig. 8.19), provide the basis for the traditional classification of acetabular fractures. This classification has

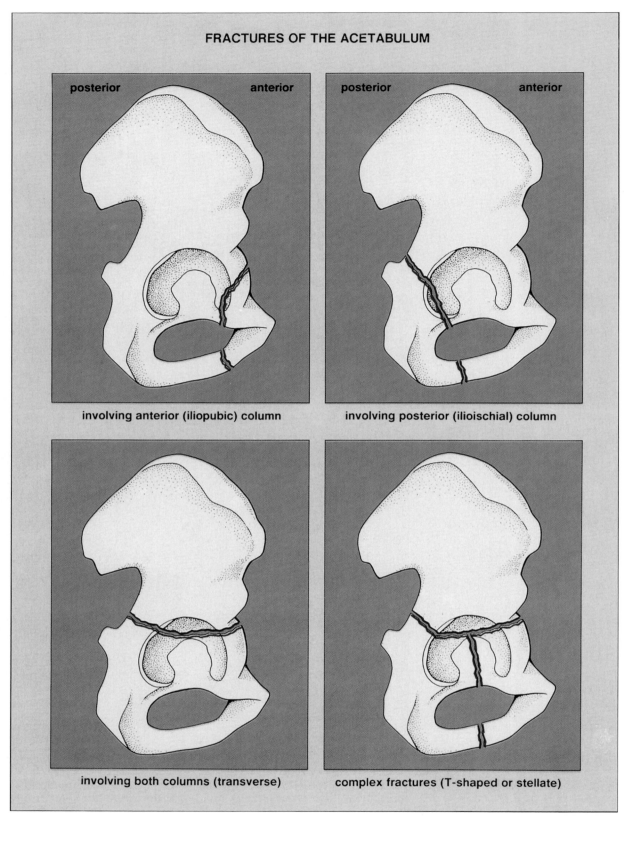

FRACTURES OF THE ACETABULUM

posterior   anterior   posterior   anterior

involving anterior (iliopubic) column   involving posterior (ilioischial) column

involving both columns (transverse)   complex fractures (T-shaped or stellate)

Figure 8.20 Classification of acetabular fractures. In the traditional classification of acetabular fractures, the fracture may involve the anterior column, the posterior column, or both columns. In complex acetabular fractures, both columns are involved and the fracture line may be T-shaped or stellate. (Modified from Letournel E, 1980, with permission.)

been modified by Letournel to include the following types of fractures (Fig. 8.20):

1. Fracture of the iliopubic (anterior) column (rare type of fracture)
2. Fracture of the ilioischial (posterior) column (common type of fracture)
3. Transverse fracture through the acetabulum involving both pelvic columns (common type of fracture)
4. Complex fractures, including T-shaped and stellate fractures,

in which the acetabulum is broken into three or more fragment (the most common type of fracture).

CT plays a leading role in the evaluation of acetabular and pelvic fractures because of its capability of demonstrating the exact position of displaced fragments, which may be trapped within the hip joint, as well as allowing adequate assessment of concomitant soft-tissue injury (Figs. 8.21–8.23). It also requires less manipulation of the patient than the standard radiographic views—a fact especially important in patients with multiple injuries.

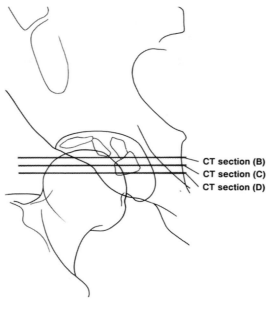

CT section (B)
CT section (C)
CT section (D)

Figure 8.21 CT of the acetabular fracture. As a result of an automobile accident, a 30-year-old woman sustained an injury that was diagnosed on the standard projections as a fracture of the acetabular roof. **(A)** On the posterior oblique projection, the fracture is shown to be comminuted. CT examination was performed, and sections **(B)**, **(C)**, **(D)** show the topographic distribution of the various intraarticular fragments and evidence of infero-lateral subluxation of the femoral head—important information not appreciated on the standard projections.

intraarticular fragments

normal contralateral hip joint

inferolaterally subluxed head

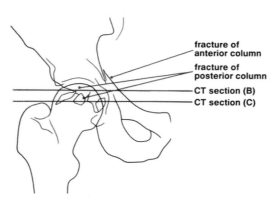

Figure 8.22 **CT of the acetabular fracture.** A 22-year-old man sustained an injury caused by the dashboard during an automobile accident. **(A)** Standard anteroposterior film of the hip shows fractures of the anterior and posterior columns. **(B)**, **(C)** On CT examination, demonstration of the exact extent of the fracture lines and the spatial relationships between the fragments provides crucial information for the orthopedic surgeon in planning open reduction and internal fixation.

fracture of anterior column
fracture of posterior column
CT section (B)
CT section (C)

Figure 8.23 **CT of the acetabular fracture.** After a fall on the street, a 63-year-old man experienced discomfort while walking. **(A)** Standard anteroposterior view of the right hip shows a radiolucent line in the acetabular roof but no other findings indicative of abnormality. Other views of the pelvis were not obtained because the patient refused. With his consent the next day, multiple CT sections **(B)**, **(C)**, **(D)** were obtained, confirming fracture of the acetabular roof. They reveal in addition completely unsuspected fractures of the anterior column and iliac bone, with marked thickening of the obturator internus muscle secondary to hemorrhage and edema.

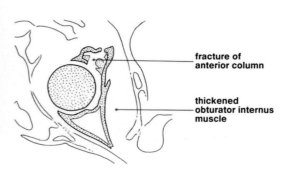

fracture of anterior column

thickened obturator internus muscle

Figure 8.24 MRI of normal acetabular labrum. Coronal fat-suppressed T1-weighted MR arthrographic image shows a normal appearance of the acetabular labrum (*arrow*). Note the triangular shape, smooth contour, and low signal intensity of this structure. [Reprinted with permission from Steinbach LS, Palmer WE, Schweitzer ME. Special focus session. MR arthrography. *Radiographics* 2002; 22: 1223–1246].

Injuries of the Acetabular Labrum

The fibrocartilaginous labrum is directly attached to the osseous rim of the acetabulum. It blends with the transverse ligament at the margins of the acetabular notch. Because the labrum is thicker posterosuperiorly and thinner anteroinferiorly, on cross-section it appears as a triangular structure, similar to the labrum of the scapular glenoid. The acetabular labrum can be injured in conjunction with acetabular fracture, hip dislocation, or even minor trauma to the hip joint. In the latter situation, the clinical symptoms include anterior inguinal pain, limitation of motion in the hip joint, painful clicking, transient locking, and "giving way" of the hip. Onset of pain may be linked to sports activities or to twisting or slipping injury. Conventional radiographs, unless obvious fracture or dislocation is present, are invariably normal. The most effective technique for diagnosis of a pathologic labral condition is MR arthrography. Czerny and colleagues have recently reported a sensitivity of 90% and accuracy of 91% of MR arthrography for detection of labral tears and detachments. The normal labrum appears on axial and coronal images as a triangular structure with low signal intensity on all imaging sequences (Fig. 8.24). A tear of the labrum is diagnosed either when deformity of its contour is present or when a linear diffuse high signal is present. In the most severe cases, the labrum is detached from the acetabulum (Fig. 8.25). Treatment of this condition includes arthroscopic resection of the injured labrum or repair of a tear.

Proximal Femur

Injury to the Proximal Femur

Fractures of the Proximal Femur

When fracture of the proximal femur is suspected, the standard radiographic examination should include at least two projections: the

Figure 8.25 MRI of torn acetabular labrum. **(A)** Axial fat-suppressed T1-weighted MR arthrographic image shows a torn labrum displaced from the acetabular rim (*straight arrow*). **(B)** Sagittal T1-weighted MR arthrographic image shows separation of the torn labral fragment from the underlying articular cartilage (*curved arrow*). **(C)** In another patient, coronal fat-suppressed T1-weighted MR arthrographic image shows a tear of the inferior labrum (*arrow*). [**(A)** and **(B)** reprinted with permission from Steinbach LS, Palmer WE, Schweitzer ME. Special focus session. MR arthrography. *Radiographics* 2002; 22: 1223–1246].

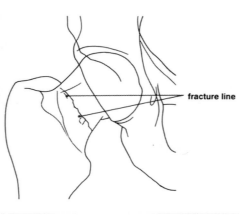

Figure 8.26 Midcervical fracture. In a fall in her bathroom, an 83-year-old woman sustained a typical nondisplaced mid-cervical fracture of the femoral neck, as demonstrated on this anteroposterior view.

Figure 8.27 Basicervical fracture. A 37-year-old man fell from a ladder. **(A)** On the anteroposterior view of the right hip, a displaced basicervical fracture of the femoral neck is evident. The type of displacement, however, cannot be determined with certainty on this film. To obtain this crucial information, tomography was performed. **(B)** On the anterior cut (obtained 14 cm above the level of the radiographic table), the femoral head is sharply outlined. **(C)** On the posterior cut (obtained 7 cm above the table), in contrast to the indistinct contour of the femoral head, the sharp outline of the femoral shaft indicates its posterior displacement.

anteroposterior and the frog-lateral views of the hip (see Figs. 8.1 and 8.6); the groin-lateral radiograph of the hip is also frequently required (see Fig. 8.7). For many nondisplaced and displaced fractures, however, a single anteroposterior view of the hip may suffice (Fig. 8.26). In cases of subtle or impacted fractures, tomographic examination may be necessary and is particularly helpful in determining the type and degree of displacement (Fig. 8.27). Radionuclide bone scan may also need to be called on in questionable cases (see Fig. 4.8B).

Traditionally, fractures of the proximal femur (so-called hip fractures) are divided into two groups: (a) *intracapsular fractures* involving the femoral head or neck, which may be capital, subcapital, transcervical, or basicervical and (b) *extracapsular fractures* involving the trochanters, which may be intertrochanteric or subtrochanteric (Fig. 8.28). The significance of this distinction lies in the greater incidence of posttraumatic complications after intracapsular fracture of the upper femur. The most common complication, osteonecrosis (ischemic or avascular necrosis), occurs in 15% to 35% of patients sustaining intracapsular fractures, but the percentage varies according to the reported series.

The reason for the high incidence of the development of osteonecrosis after fracture of the femoral neck lies in the nature of the blood supply to the proximal femur. The capsule of the hip joint arises from the acetabulum and attaches to the anterior aspect of the femur along the intertrochanteric line at the base of the femoral neck. Posteriorly, the capsule envelops the femoral head and proximal two thirds of the neck. Most of the blood supply to the femoral head is derived from the circumflex femoral arteries, which form a ring at the base of the neck, sending off branches that ascend subcapsularly along the femoral neck to the femoral head. Only a very small portion of the femoral head is supplied by arteries in the ligamentum teres (ligamentum capitis femoris) (Fig. 8.29). Because of this vascular configuration, intracapsular fractures tend to tear the vessels, interrupting the blood supply and leading eventually to osteonecrosis. The trochanteric region, however, is extracapsular and receives an excellent supply of blood from branches of the circumflex femoral arteries and from muscles that attach around both trochanters. Thus, as a rule, intertrochanteric fractures do not lead to osteonecrosis of the femoral head.

Nonunion is also a common complication following fracture of the femoral neck, occurring in 10% to 44% of patients with such fractures. According to Pauwels, the obliquity of the fracture line determines the prognosis. The more oblique the fracture line is, the more likely nonunion will occur (Fig. 8.30).

Intracapsular Fractures. Of the many classifications of femoral neck fractures that have been proposed, the Pauwels and Garden classifications are useful from a practical point of view because they take

FRACTURES OF THE PROXIMAL FEMUR

Intracapsular

capital (uncommon)   subcapital (common)   trans- or midcervical (rare)   basicervical (uncommon)

Extracapsular

intertrochanteric   subtrochanteric

Figure 8.28 Fractures of the proximal femur. Fractures of the proximal femur are traditionally classified as intracapsular and extracapsular.

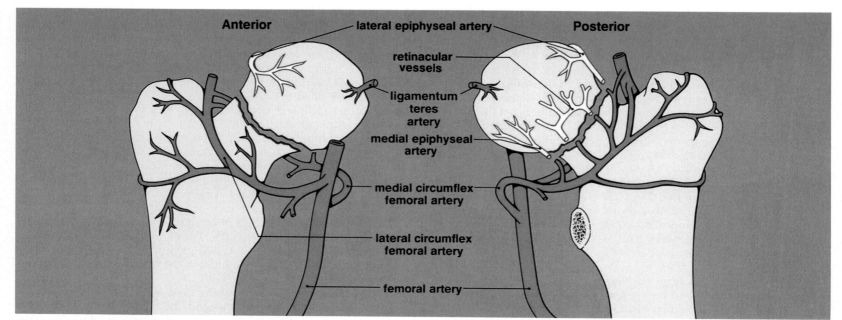

Figure 8.29 Blood supply to the proximal femur. The proximal femur is supplied with blood mainly by the circumflex femoral arteries, branches of which ascend subcapsularly along the femoral neck to the femoral head. Intracapsular fracture of the proximal femur may so severely interrupt the blood supply that osteonecrosis results.

into consideration the stability of the fracture—an important factor in orthopedic management and prognosis.

Pauwels classifies femoral neck fractures according to the degree of angulation of the fracture line from the horizontal plane on the postreduction anteroposterior radiograph, stressing that the closer the fracture line approximates the horizontal, the more stable the fracture and the better the prognosis (Fig. 8.30). Garden, however, proposed a staging system of femoral neck fractures based on displacement of the femoral head before reduction. Displacement in the Garden system is graded according to the position of the principal (medial) compressive trabeculae (Fig. 8.31). His classification of such fractures is divided into four stages (Fig. 8.32):

Stage I   Incomplete subcapital fracture. In this so-called impacted or abducted fracture, the femoral shaft is externally rotated and the femoral head is in valgus. The medial trabeculae of the femoral head and neck form an angle greater than 1808 (Fig. 8.33). This is a stable fracture with a good prognosis.

Stage II   Complete subcapital fracture without displacement. In this complete fracture through the neck, the femoral shaft remains in normal alignment with the femoral head, which is not displaced but rather tilted in a varus deformity so that its medial trabeculae do not align with those of the pelvis. The medial trabeculae of the head form an angle of approxi-

mately 1608 with those of the femoral neck. This is also a stable fracture with a good prognosis.

Stage III Complete subcapital fracture with partial displacement. In this category, the femoral shaft is externally rotated. The femoral head is medially rotated, abducted, and tilted in a varus deformity. The medial trabeculae of the head are out of alignment with those of the pelvis. This fracture is usually unstable, but it may be converted to a stable fracture by proper reduction. The prognosis is not as good as that for stage I and stage II fractures.

Stage IV   Complete subcapital fracture with full displacement. In this type the femoral shaft, in addition to being externally rotated, it is upwardly displaced and lies anterior to the femoral head. Although the head is completely detached from the shaft, it remains in its normal position in the acetabulum. The medial trabeculae are in alignment with those of the pelvis (Fig. 8.34). This is an unstable fracture with a poor prognosis.

This staging of femoral neck fractures has important prognostic value. In following-up 80 patients over 1 year, Garden found complete union in all those graded stages I and II, 93% in those graded stage III, and only 57% in those graded stage IV. Osteonecrosis occurred in only 8% of nondisplaced stage I or stage II fractures but in 30% of displaced stage III or IV fractures.

Figure 8.30 The Pauwels classification of intracapsular fractures. The classification is based on the obliquity of the fracture line: the more the fracture line approaches the vertical, the less stable the fracture, and consequently the greater the chances for nonunion. (Modified from Pauwels F, 1976, with permission.)

Figure 8.31 Trabeculae of the hip. The Garden staging system of femoral neck fractures is based on the three groups of trabeculae that are demonstrable within the femoral head and neck. The principal tensile trabeculae form an arc, extending from the lateral margin of the greater trochanter, through the superior cortex of the neck and across the femoral head, ending at its inferior aspect below the fovea. The principal (medial) compressive trabeculae are vertically oriented, extending from the medial cortex of the neck into the femoral head in a triangular configuration. They are normally aligned with the trabeculae seen in the acetabulum. The secondary (lateral) compressive trabeculae extend from the calcar and lesser trochanter to the greater trochanter in a fan-like pattern. The central area bounded by this trabecular system is known as Ward triangle.

Figure 8.32 The Garden classification of subcapital fractures. The Garden staging of subcapital femoral fractures is based on displacement of the femoral head before reduction. Displacement is graded according to the position of the medial compressive trabeculae. (Modified from Garden RS, 1974, with permission.)

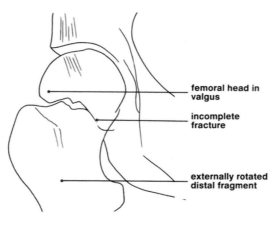

Figure 8.33 Subcapital fracture. After a fall to the floor, a 72-year-old woman sustained a fracture of the right femoral neck. Anteroposterior projection demonstrates a subcapital fracture, which appears to be impacted. The femoral head is in valgus, the distal fragment is externally rotated, and the medial trabeculae of the femoral head and neck form an angle greater than 180°. These features characterize a Garden stage I fracture.

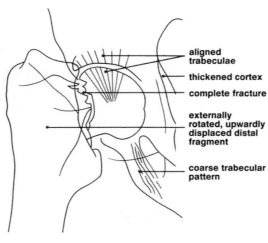

Figure 8.34 Subcapital fracture. After a fall on a subway platform, a 77-year-old woman sustained a fracture of the right femoral neck. Anteroposterior view of the hip shows a complete subcapital fracture with full displacement. The head, which is detached from the neck, is in its normal position in the acetabulum. Note the alignment of the trabeculae in the head and acetabulum. The femoral shaft is upwardly displaced and externally rotated. These features identify this injury as a Garden stage IV fracture. As an incidental finding, note the thickening of the cortex and the coarse trabecular pattern characteristic of Paget disease.

Figure 8.35 Intertrochanteric fracture. (A) Anteroposterior view of the right hip demonstrates a comminuted, three-part intertrochanteric fracture, which can be classified as a Boyd-Griffin type II fracture. **(B)** Anteroposterior projection of the right hip shows a comminuted, multi-part intertrochanteric fracture associated with a subtrochanteric component. This fracture can be classified as a Boyd-Griffin type III fracture. (For the Boyd-Griffin classification of intertrochanteric fractures, see Fig. 8.37.)

Extracapsular Fractures. Frequently resulting from direct injury in a fall, extracapsular fractures occur in an even older age group than do intracapsular fractures. Most of these fractures are intertrochanteric, the major fracture line extending from the greater to the lesser trochanter, and they are usually comminuted. Radiographic diagnosis can usually be made on a single anteroposterior projection of the hip (Fig. 8.35). Rarely, the fracture line may be obscure, requiring oblique projections or even tomography for its demonstration.

As mentioned, extracapsular fractures of the proximal femur, for which several classifications have been developed, can generally be divided into two major subgroups: intertrochanteric and subtrochanteric. Intertrochanteric fractures can be further subdivided according to the number of fragments or the extension of the fracture line. A simple classification of such fractures has been proposed that considers the number of fragments (Fig. 8.36). The two-part fracture in this system is stable, whereas the four-part and multi-part fractures are unstable. Boyd and Griffin have proposed a classification of intertrochanteric fractures according to the presence or absence of comminution and involvement of the subtrochanteric region (Fig. 8.37). Comminution of the posterior and medial cortices has important prognostic value. If comminuted, the fracture is unstable and may require a displacement osteotomy, a procedure particularly important in the treatment of four-part fractures when both trochanters are in-

volved. If there is no comminution, then the fracture is stable and treatment involves fixation with a compression screw.

Subtrochanteric fractures have been classified by Fielding according to the level of the fracture line and by Zickel according to their level, obliquity, and comminution (Fig. 8.38). An important fact about subtrochanteric fractures is their relatively benign course caused by the good supply of blood and adequate collateral circulation to this region of the femur. The occurrence of osteonecrosis of the femoral head and the incidence of nonunion as a result of intertrochanteric and subtrochanteric fractures are very low. The only serious complication to watch for is postoperative infection.

Dislocations in the Hip Joint

Traumatic dislocation of the femoral head is an uncommon injury resulting from a high-energy force and often accompanied by other significant injuries. The injury is caused by a substantial axial force, such as a knee impacting against the dashboard in a motor vehicle accident.

Generally, dislocations in the hip joint can be classified as anterior, posterior, or central (medial). The position of the hip at the moment of impact determines the direction of dislocation: hip flexion, adduction, and internal rotation result in posterior dislocation, and

SIMPLE CLASSIFICATION OF INTERTROCHANTERIC FRACTURES

Two-Part

Three-Part

linear intertrochanteric

with comminution of lesser trochanter

with comminution of greater trochanter

Four-Part

Multipart

with comminution of both trochanters

with comminution of both trochanters and intertrochanteric region

Figure 8.36 Classification of intertrochanteric fractures. The simple classification of intertrochanteric fractures is based on the number of bony fragments.

Figure 8.37 The Boyd-Griffin classification of intertrochanteric fractures. This classification is based on the presence or absence of comminution and the involvement of the subtrochanteric region. (Modified from Boyd HB, Griffin LL, 1949, with permission.)

Figure 8.38 Classification of subtrochanteric fractures. The Fielding classification of subtrochanteric fractures (*top left*) is based on the level of the subtrochanteric region in which the fracture occurs. Type I fractures, the most common type, occur at the level of the lesser trochanter; type II, within the region 2.5 cm below the lesser trochanter; and type III, the least common type, occurs within the region 2.5 cm to 5 cm below the lesser trochanter. The Zickel classification of subtrochanteric fractures takes into consideration the level and obliquity of the fracture line as well as the presence or absence of comminution. (Modified from Fielding JW, 1973; Zickel RE, 1976, with permission.)

Figure 8.39 Anterior hip dislocation. A 19-year-old man sustained an anterior hip dislocation. Note on this anteroposterior radiograph a typical position of the femoral head, which lies inferior and medial to the acetabulum.

hip abduction and external rotation yield anterior dislocation. Posterior dislocation of the femoral head is far more common than anterior dislocation, which constitutes only 5% to 18% of all hip dislocations. It is also more frequently associated with fractures, particularly involving the posterior acetabular rim; anterior dislocation, in contrast, tends to be simple, without associated fracture. A predisposition to traumatic posterior hip dislocation has been suggested for individ-

Figure 8.40 Posterior hip dislocation. A 30-year-old woman sustained a typical posterior hip dislocation in an automobile accident. Note on this anteroposterior projection that the extremity is adducted and the femoral head overlaps the posterior lip of the acetabulum.

Figure 8.41 Central hip dislocation. While riding a bicycle, a 43-year-old man was hit by a truck. Anteroposterior view of the right hip shows a typical central dislocation in the hip associated with a comminuted fracture of the medial acetabular wall. Note the protrusion of the femoral head into the pelvic cavity.

uals with retroversion or decreased anteversion of the femoral neck. Similarly, increased femoral neck anteversion may predispose to traumatic anterior hip dislocation. Dislocations are readily identified on radiographs of the hip in the anteroposterior projection. In *anterior dislocation,* which accounts for only 13% of all hip dislocations, the femoral head is displaced into the obturator, pubic, or iliac region. On the anteroposterior film, the femur is abducted and externally rotated and the femoral head lies medial and inferior to the acetabulum (Fig. 8.39). In *posterior dislocation,* which is the most common type of dislocation, the anteroposterior view reveals the femur to be internally rotated and adducted, while the femoral head lies lateral and superior to the acetabulum (Fig. 8.40). *Central dislocation* (or *central protrusio*) is always associated with an acetabular fracture, with the femoral head protruding into the pelvic cavity (Figs. 8.41 and 8.42).

Dislocation of the femoral head is often accompanied by significant injuries involving the bone and cartilage, the joint space, and the muscles and ligaments surrounding the joint. CT has proved indispensable for identifying fractures associated with hip dislocations, and it remains the best means of detecting cortical disruption. MRI has assumed a highly significant role among imaging modalities, especially because of its superior capabilities in comparison with CT in evaluating cancellous bone, cartilage, muscle, ligaments, and intraarticular fluid. MRI can effectively identify and quantify the muscle injury and joint effusion/hemarthrosis that invariably accompany traumatic anterior and posterior dislocation of the hip (see Figs. 4.83 and 4.84). It is also useful for demonstrating bone contusions, which occur commonly in both types of dislocation, as well as the less common sequelae of acute hip dislocation, including cortical infraction, osteochondral fracture, and tear of the acetabular labrum. It may also be helpful in identifying soft-tissue interposition in the joint space. The real importance of performing MRI after hip dislocation is to identify possible complications such as osteonecrosis of the femoral head.

Traumatic hip dislocations are treated with immediate closed reduction, preferably within 6 hours of injury. Such attention is required

Figure 8.42 Central hip dislocation. A 22-year-old woman was injured in a car accident. **(A)** Anteroposterior radiograph of the right hip shows a complex acetabular fracture associated with a central displacement of the femoral head. **(B)** A coronal CT reformatted image shows medial displacement of the medial acetabular wall and central hip dislocation.

to lower the risk of osteonecrosis, one of the two main complications related to hip dislocation; the other is posttraumatic osteoarthritis.

A recent study found that osteonecrosis developed in only 4.8% of patients whose hip dislocation was reduced within 6 hours, compared with 58.8% of patients whose reduction occurred more than 6 hours after injury. The early detection of osteonecrosis is critical because the initial period offers the greatest chance of preserving joint function with surgical procedures such as drilling, rotational osteotomy, or core decompression with or without vascularized grafting. Posttraumatic osteoarthritis, with an incidence ranging from 17% to 48.8% in different series, has been attributed to the severity of the initial injury, intraarticular loose bodies, and continued heavy work after injury. Simple dislocations have a better prognosis than those with an associated fracture.

PRACTICAL POINTS TO REMEMBER

Pelvis and Acetabulum

[1] Fractures of the pelvis are important because of the high incidence of concomitant injury to:
- major blood vessels
- nerves
- lower urinary tract

[2] Pelvic fractures can be classified for the purposes of radiographic diagnosis and orthopedic management:
- into stable and unstable injuries on the basis of the stability of the fragments
- according to the direction of the force delivered to the pelvis as injuries resulting from anteroposterior compression, lateral compression, vertical shear, or complex pattern

[3] Fractures of the acetabulum are best demonstrated on the anterior and posterior oblique projections (Judet views).

[4] In acetabular fractures it is important to distinguish between:
- fractures of the anterior pelvic column
- fractures of the posterior pelvic column

[5] CT plays an important role in the evaluation of fractures of both the pelvis and acetabulum because of its capability of demonstrating:
- the exact position and configuration of comminuted fragments
- the presence or absence of intraarticular fragments
- injury to the soft tissues

[6] MRI offers superior capabilities for evaluating traumatic conditions of the hip, in particular:
- to diagnose occult fractures and bone contusions (trabecular microfractures)
- to identify and quantify effectively the muscle injury and joint effusion that accompany traumatic hip dislocations

[7] MR arthrography is effective to evaluate injuries to the acetabular labrum, such as tears and detachments.

[8] Intravenous urography (IVP) and cystourethrography are essential in the evaluation of concomitant injury to the lower urinary system.

Proximal Femur

[1] The importance of distinguishing between intracapsular and extracapsular fractures of the proximal femur (hip fractures) lies in the possible complications. Intracapsular fractures of the femoral neck are associated with a higher incidence of non-union and osteonecrosis of the femoral head.

[2] The Garden staging of intracapsular fractures of the femoral neck has practical value in determining stability and prognosis.

[3] The Boyd-Griffin classification of intertrochanteric fractures according to the presence or absence of comminution and involvement of the subtrochanteric region has important prognostic value and serves as a guide to operative management.

[4] Subtrochanteric fractures are classified by:
- Fielding, according to the level of the fracture line
- Zickel, according to the level, obliquity, and comminution of the fracture

[5] MRI is the ideal modality to detect and evaluate early changes of posttraumatic osteonecrosis of the femoral head.

Dislocations in the Hip Joint

[1] Dislocations in the hip joint are classified as anterior, posterior, and central (medial).

[2] Posterior dislocations are more common and are frequently associated with fractures involving the posterior acetabular rim.

[3] Anterior dislocations are rare. On the anteroposterior radiograph, the femur is abducted and externally rotated, and the femoral head lies medial and inferior to the acetabulum.

SUGGESTED READINGS

Aliabadi P, Baker ND, Jaramillo D. Hip arthrography, aspiration, block, and bursography. *Radiol Clin North Am* 1998;36:673–690.

Allard JC, Porter G, Ryerson RW. Occult posttraumatic avascular necrosis of hip revealed by MRI. *Magn Reson Imaging* 1992;10:155–159.

Blundell CM, Parker MJ, Pryor GA, Hopkinson-Woolley J, Bhonsle SS. Assessment of the AO classification of intracapsular fractures of the proximal femur. *J Bone Joint Surg [Br]* 1998;80B:679–683.

Boyd HB, Griffin LL. Classification and treatment of trochanteric fractures. *Arch Surg* 1949;58:853–866.

Brandser E, Marsh JL. Acetabular fractures: easier classification with a systematic approach. *AJR Am J Roentgenol* 1998;171:1217–1228.

Brandser EA, El-Khoury GY, Marsh JL. Acetabular fractures: a systematic approach to classification. *Emerg Radiol* 1995;2:18–28.

Bray TJ. Acetabular fractures: classification and diagnosis. In: Chapman MW, ed. *Operative orthopedics*, vol. 1, 2nd ed. Philadelphia: JB Lippincott; 1993:539–553.

Bray TJ, Templeman DC. Fractures of the femoral neck. In: Chapman MW, ed. *Operative orthopaedics*, vol. 1, 2nd ed. Philadelphia: JB Lippincott; 1993:583–594.

Bucholz RW. The pathological anatomy of Malgaigne fracture-dislocations of the pelvis. *J Bone Joint Surg [Am]* 1981;63A:400–404.

Burgess AR, Tile M. Fractures of the pelvis. In: Rockwood CA Jr, Green DP, Bucholz RW, eds. *Fractures in adults*, vol. 2, 3rd ed. Philadelphia: JB Lippincott; 1991:1399–1479.

Burk DL, Mears DC, Kennedy WH, Cooperstein LA, Herbert DL. Three-dimensional computed tomography of acetabular fractures. *Radiology* 1985;155:183–186.

DeLee JC. Fractures and dislocations of the hip. In: Rockwood CA Jr, Green DP, Bucholz RW, eds. *Fractures in adults*, vol. 2, 3rd ed. Philadelphia: JB Lippincott; 1991:1481–1651.

Coleman BG, Kressel HY, Dalinka MK, Scheibler ML, Burk DL, Cohen EK. Radiographically negative avascular necrosis: detection with MR imaging. *Radiology* 1988;168:525–528.

Combs JA. Hip and pelvis avulsion fractures in adolescents. *Physician Sports Med* 1994;22:41–49.

Conway WF, Totty WG, McEnery KW. CT and MRI imaging of the hip. State of the art. *Radiology* 1996;198:297–307.

Cvitanic O, Henzie G, Skezas N, Lyons J. Minter J. MRI diagnosis of tears of the hip abductor tendons (gluteus medius and gluteus minimus). *AJR Am J Roentgenol* 2004;182: 137–143.

Czerny C, Hofmann S, Neuhold A, et al. Lesions of the acetabular labrum: accuracy of MR imaging and MR arthrography in detection and staging. *Radiology* 1996;200:225–230.

Czerny C, Hofmann S, Urban M, et al. MR arthrography of the adult acetabular-labral complex: correlation with surgery and anatomy. *AJR Am J Roentgenol* 1999;173:345–349.

DeSmet AA. Magnetic resonance findings in skeletal muscle tears. *Skeletal Radiol* 1993;22:479–484.

DeSmet AA, Fisher DR, Heiner JP, Keene JS. Magnetic resonance imaging of muscle tears. *Skeletal Radiol* 1990;19:283–286.

Deutsch AL, Mink JH, Waxman AD. Occult fractures of the proximal femur: MR imaging. *Radiology* 1989;170:113–116.

Dunn AW, Morris HD. Fractures and dislocations of the pelvis. *J Bone Joint Surg [Am]* 1968;50A:1639–1648.

El-Khoury GY, Daniel WW, Kathol MH. Acute and chronic avulsive injuries. *Radiol Clin North Am* 1997;35:747–766.

Ensign MR. Magnetic resonance imaging of hip disorders. *Semin Ultrasound CT MR* 1990;11:288–306.

Erb RE, Steele JR, Nance EP Jr, Edwards JR. Traumatic anterior dislocation of the hip: spectrum of plain film and CT findings. *AJR Am J Roentgenol* 1995;165:1215–1219.

Fielding JW. Subtrochanteric fractures. *Clin Orthop* 1973;92:86–99.

Fitzgerald RH. Acetabular labrum tears: diagnosis and management. *Clin Orthop* 1995;311:60–68.

Fernbach SK, Wilkinson RH. Avulsion injuries of the pelvis and proximal femur. *AJR Am J Roentgenol* 1981;137:581–584.

Garcia-Morales F, Seo GS, Chengazi V, Monu JUV. Collar osteophytes: a cause of false-positive findings in bone scans for hip fractures. *AJR Am J Roentgenol* 2003;181:191–194.

Garden RS. The structure and function of the proximal end of the femur. *J Bone Joint Surg [Br]* 1961;43B:576–589.

Garden RS. Low-angle fixation in fractures of the femoral neck. *J Bone Joint Surg [Br]* 1961;43B:647–663.

Garden RS. Reduction and fixation of subcapital fractures of the femur. *Orthop Clin North Am* 1974;5:683–712.

Ghelman B, Freiberger RH. The adult hip. In: Freiberger RH, Kaye JJ, eds. *Arthrography*. New York: Appleton-Century-Crofts; 1979:189–216.

Goldman AB. Hip arthrography in infants and children. In: Freiberger RH, Kaye JJ, eds. *Arthrography*. New York: Appleton-Century-Crofts; 1979:217–235.

Greenspan A, Norman A. The pelvic digit. *Bull Hosp Joint Dis Orthop Inst* 1984;44:72–75.

Greenspan A, Norman A. The "pelvic digit"—an unusual developmental anomaly. *Skeletal Radiol* 1982;9:118–122.

Guy RL, Butler-Manuel PA, Holder P, Brueton RN. The role of 3-D CT in the assessment of acetabular fractures. *Br J Radiol* 1992;65:384–389.

Haims A, Katz LD, Busconi B. MR arthrography of the hip. *Radiol Clin North Am* 1998;36:691–702.

Hayes CW, Balkissoon AA. Magnetic resonance imaging of the musculoskeletal system. II. The hip. *Clin Orthop* 1996;322:297–309.

Hougaard K, Thomsen PB. Traumatic posterior dislocation of the hip—prognostic factors influencing the incidence of avascular necrosis of the femoral head. *Arch Orthop Trauma Surg* 1986;106:32–35.

Hunter JC, Brandser EA, Tran KA. Pelvic and acetabular trauma. *Radiol Clin North Am* 1997;35:559–590.

Judet R, Judet J, Letournel E. Fractures of the acetabulum: classification and surgical approaches for open reduction—preliminary report. *J Bone Joint Surg [Am]* 1964; 46A:1615–1646.

Kricun ME. Fractures of the pelvis. *Orthop Clin North Am* 1990;21:573–590.

Kyle RF, Campbell SJ. Intertrochanteric fractures. In: Chapman MW, ed. *Operative orthopaedics*, vol. 1, 2nd ed. Philadelphia: JB Lippincott; 1993:595–604.

Laorr A, Greenspan A, Anderson MW, Moehring HD, McKinley T. Traumatic hip dislocation: early MRI findings. *Skeletal Radiol* 1995;24:239–245.

Letournel E. Acetabulum fractures: classification and management. *Clin Orthop* 1980;151:81–106.

Magid D, Fishman EK, Ney DR, Kuhlman JE, Frantz KM, Sponseller PD. Acetabular and pelvic fractures in the pediatric patient: value of two- and three-dimensional imaging. *J Pediatr Orthop* 1992;12:621–625.

Magid D, Fishman EK, Sponseller PD, Griffin PP. 2D and 3D computed tomography of the pediatric hip. *Radiographics* 1988;8:901–933.

Malgaigne JF. The classic-double vertical fractures of the pelvis. *Clin Orthop* 1980;151:8–11.

Martinez CR, DiPasquale TG, Helfet DL, Graham AW, Sanders RW, Ray LD. Evaluation of acetabular fractures with two- and three-dimensional CT. *Radiographics* 1992;12:227–242.

Mears DC. Fracture-dislocation of the pelvic ring. In: Chapman MW, ed. *Operative orthopaedics*, vol. 1, 2nd ed. Philadelphia: Lippincott; 1993:505–538.

Mitchell DG, Rao VM, Dalinka MK, et al. Femoral head avascular necrosis: correlation of MR imaging, radiographic staging, radionuclide imaging, and clinical findings. *Radiology* 1987;162:709–715.

Moehring HD. Hip dislocations and femoral head fractures. In: Chapman MW, ed. *Operative orthopaedics*, vol. 1, 2nd ed. Philadelphia: Lippincott; 1993:571–582.

Nerubay J. Traumatic anterior dislocation of hip joint with vascular damage. *Clin Orthop* 1976;116:129–132.

Oka M, Monu JUV. Prevalence and patterns of occult hip fractures and mimics revealed by MRI. *AJR Am J Roentgenol* 2004;182:283–288.

Olson SA, Matta JM. Surgical treatment of fractures of the acetabulum. In: Browner BD, Jupiter JB, Levine AM, Trafton PG, eds. *Skeletal trauma*, 2nd ed. Philadelphia: WB Saunders; 1990:1181–1222.

Palmer WE. MR arthrography of the hip. *Semin Musculoskel Radiol* 1998;2:349–361.

Pauwels F. *Biomechanics of the normal and diseased hip*. New York: Springer-Verlag; 1976.

Pennal GF, Tile M, Waddell JP, Garside H. Pelvic disruption: assessment and classification. *Clin Orthop* 1980;151:12–21.

Petersilge CA. Chronic adult hip pain: MR arthrography of the hip. *Radiographics* 2000;20:S43–S52.

Petersilge CA. Current concepts of MR arthrography of the hip. *Semin Ultrasound CT MRI* 1997;18:291–301.

Potok PS, Hopper KD, Umlauf MJ. Fractures of the acetabulum: imaging, classification, and understanding. *Radiographics* 1995;15:7–23.

Potter HG, Montgomery KD, Heise CW, Helfet DL. MR imaging of acetabular fractures: value in detecting femoral head injury, intraarticular fragments, and sciatic nerve injury. *AJR Am J Roentgenol* 1993;163:881–886.

Resnik CS, Stackhouse DJ, Shanmuganathan K, Young JWR. Diagnosis of pelvic fractures in patients with acute pelvic trauma. *AJR Am J Roentgenol* 1992;158:109–112.

Richardson P, Young JWR, Porter D. CT detection of cortical fracture of the femoral head associated with posterior hip dislocation. *AJR Am J Roentgenol* 1990;155:93–94.

Rogers LF, Hendrix RW. *Radiology of skeletal trauma*, 2nd ed. New York: Churchill Livingstone, 1992:991–1103.

Saks BJ. Normal acetabular anatomy for acetabular fracture assessment: CT and plain film correlation. *Radiology* 1986;159:139–145.

Schultz E, Miller TT, Boruchov SD, Schmell EB, Toledano B. Incomplete intertrochanteric fractures: *Radiology* 1999;211:237–240.

Scott WW, Magid D, Fishman EK, Riley LH Jr, Brooker AF Jr, Johnson CA. 3-D evaluation of acetabular trauma. *Contemp Orthop* 1987;15:17–24.

Sherlock DA. Traumatic anterior dislocation of the hip. *J Trauma* 1988;28:411–413.

Steinbach LS, Palmer WE, Schweitzer ME. Special focus session. MR arthrography. *Radiographics* 2002;22:1223–1246.

Stevens MA, El-Khoury GY, Kathol MH, Brandser EA, Chow S. Imaging features of avulsion injuries. *Radiographics* 1999;19:655–672.

Sullivan JD, Kahn DS. Formation of a bone and joint following blunt injury to the pelvis. *Clin Orthop* 1979;140:80–84.

Tehranzadeh J, Vanarthos W, Pais MJ. Osteochondral impaction of the femoral head associated with hip dislocation: CT study in 35 patients. *AJR Am J Roentgenol* 1990;155:1049–1052.

Tile M. *Fractures of the pelvis and acetabulum*. Baltimore: Williams & Wilkins; 1984.

White MS. Three-dimensional computed tomography in the assessment of fractures of the acetabulum. *Injury* 1991;22:13–19.

Wiss DA. Subtrochanteric femur fractures. In: Chapman MW, ed. *Operative orthopaedics*, vol. 1, 2nd ed. Philadelphia: JB Lippincott; 1993:605–620.

Yang R-S, Tsuang Y-H, Hang Y-S, Liu T-K. Traumatic dislocation of the hip. *Clin Orthop* 1991;265:218–227.

Young JWR, Burgess AR, Brumback RJ, Poka A. Lateral compression fractures of the pelvis: the importance of plain radiographs in the diagnosis and surgical management. *Skeletal Radiol* 1986;15:103–109.

Young JWR, Resnik CS. Fracture of the pelvis: current concepts of classification. *AJR Am J Roentgenol* 1990;155:1169–1175.

Zickel RE. An intramedullary fixation device for the proximal part of the femur. Nine year's experience. *J Bone Joint Surg [Am]* 1976;58A:866–872.

LOWER LIMB II

Knee

Knee

The vulnerability of the knee, the largest joint in the body, to direct trauma makes knee injuries very common throughout life. Most acute injury to the knee is sustained during adolescence and adulthood, with motor vehicle accidents and athletic activities being the major causing factors. Fractures are much more common than dislocations, but injuries to the cartilaginous and soft-tissue structures, such as tears of the menisci and ligaments, are the most common types of injuries, particularly in older adolescents and younger adults. The symptoms accompanying knee trauma vary according to the specific site of injury and thus constitute important indications of the type of injury. However, clinical history and physical examination are rarely sufficient for making a precise diagnosis. Radiologic examination plays a determining role in diagnosing the various traumatic conditions involving the knee joint.

Anatomic–Radiologic Considerations

Conventional radiographs are the first-line approach to the traumatized knee, and often they are sufficient for evaluating many traumatic conditions of the joint. However, the great incidence of cartilaginous and soft-tissue injuries, occurring either as isolated conditions or in association with fractures, requires the use of ancillary imaging techniques for adequate evaluation of the joint capsule, articular cartilage, menisci, and ligaments.

The standard radiographic examination usually consists of obtaining films of the knee in four projections: the anteroposterior, the lateral, and the tunnel projections, as well as an axial view of the patella. The *anteroposterior* radiograph of the knee allows sufficient evaluation of many of the most important aspects of the distal femur and proximal tibia: the medial and lateral femoral and tibial condyles; the medial and lateral tibial plateaus and tibial spines; and the medial and lateral joint compartments and the head of the fibula (Fig. 9.1). However, the patella is not well demonstrated on this view because it appears superimposed on the distal femur. Proper evaluation of this structure requires a *lateral* projection (Fig. 9.2) on which the relationship of the patella and femur can also be assessed. Proximal (superior) displacement of the patella is called patella alta; distal (inferior) displacement is called patella baja. The length of the patella is measured from its upper pole (base) to the apex. The length of the patellar ligament is measured from its proximal attachment, just above the apex, to the notch on the proximal margin of the tibial tubercle. These two measurements are approximately equal and the normal variation does not exceed 20% (Fig. 9.3). In addition to imaging the patella in profile, the lateral radiograph of the knee allows evaluation of the femoropatellar compartment, the suprapatellar bursa (pouch), and the quadriceps tendon. The femoral condyles overlap on this projection, and the tibial plateaus are demonstrated in profile. Occasionally, a cross-table lateral view of the knee—obtained with the patient

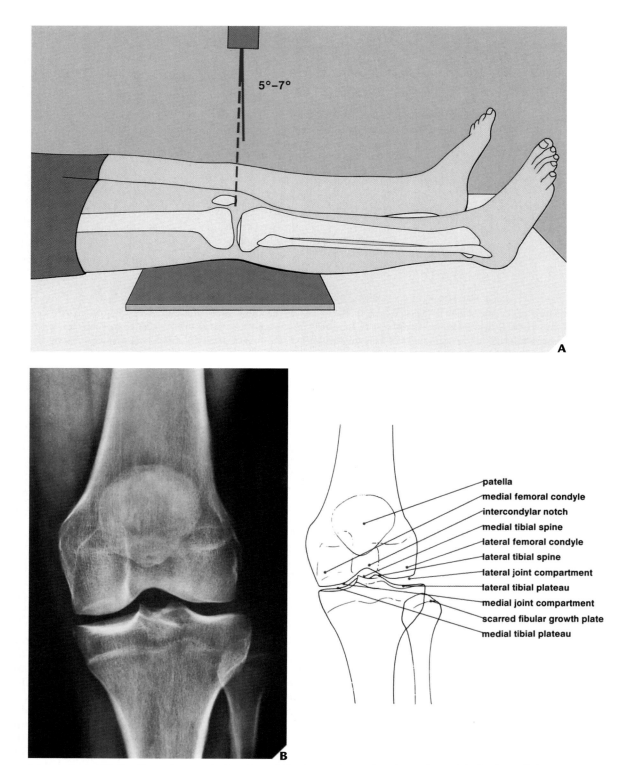

Figure 9.1 Anteroposterior view. (A) For the anteroposterior view of the knee, the patient is supine, with the knee fully extended and the leg in the neutral position. The central beam is directed vertically to the knee with 5° to 7° cephalad angulation. **(B)** The radiograph in this projection sufficiently demonstrates the medial and lateral femoral and tibial condyles, the tibial plateaus and spines, and both the medial and lateral joint compartments. The patella is seen en face as an oval structure between the femoral condyles.

supine, the affected leg extended, and the central beam directed horizontally—may be required to demonstrate the intracapsular fat-fluid level (FBI sign of lipohemarthrosis; see Fig. 4.34B). An angled posteroanterior projection of the knee, known as the *tunnel* (or *notch*) view, is also obtained as part of the standard radiographic examination (Fig. 9.4). This view is useful in visualizing the posterior aspect of the femoral condyles, the intercondylar notch, and the intercondylar eminence of the tibia.

To demonstrate an *axial* view of the patella, various techniques are available. The one most commonly used provides what has been called the *sunrise* view (Fig. 9.5). However, the degree of flexion required to obtain this view results in depressing the patella more deeply within the intercondylar fossa; consequently, the articular surfaces of the femoropatellar joint are not well demonstrated, and subtle subluxations of the patella may not be detected. To overcome this limitation, Merchant and colleagues have described a technique for obtain-

Figure 9.2 Lateral view. (A) For the lateral view of the knee, the patient is lying flat on the same side as the affected knee, which is flexed approximately 25° to 30°. The central beam is directed vertically toward the medial aspect of the knee joint with approximately 5° to 7° cephalad angulation. **(B)** The film in this projection demonstrates the patella in profile, as well as the femoropatellar joint compartment and a faint outline of the quadriceps tendon. The femoral condyles are seen overlapping, and the tibial plateaus are imaged in profile. Note the slight posterior tilt of the tibial plateaus, which normally measures approximately 10°.

ing an axial view of the patella that demonstrates the femoropatellar joint to better advantage (Fig. 9.6). It is particularly effective in detecting subluxations of the patella, because it allows specific measurements to be made of the normal relations of the patella to the femoral condyles. Subtle abnormalities in these relations may not be seen on the standard axial view because of the degree of knee flexion required for that view, which prevents the patella from subluxing.

The measurements of the femoropatellar relations obtainable from Merchant axial projection concern the sulcus angle and the congruence angle (Fig. 9.7). Normally, the *sulcus angle*, which is described by the highest points of the femoral condyles and the deepest point of the intercondylar sulcus, measures approximately 138°. By dissecting this angle with two lines—a reference line drawn from the apex of the patella to the deepest point of the sulcus and a second line from the

FEMOROPATELLAR RELATIONSHIP

PL = patellar ligament
L = patella length

PL ≅ L
±20%

L

PL

Figure 9.3 Femoropatellar relationship. The length of the patella and the patellar ligament are approximately equal; normal variability does not exceed 20%.

40°

40°

A

- intercondylar notch
- notch of popliteal tendon
- medial tibial spine
- lateral tibial spine
- intercondylar eminence

B

Figure 9.4 Tunnel view. (A) For the tunnel (or notch) projection of the knee, the patient is prone with the knee flexed approximately 40°, with the foot supported by a cylindrical sponge. The central beam is directed caudally toward the knee joint at a 40° angle from the vertical. **(B)** The film in this projection demonstrates the posterior aspect of the femoral condyles, the intercondylar notch, and the intercondylar eminence of the tibia.

lowest point of the patellar articular ridge to the deepest point of the sulcus—Merchant and colleagues were able to determine the degree of congruence, or the *congruence angle,* of the femoropatellar joint. When the deepest point of the patellar articular ridge fell medial to the reference line, the angle formed was assigned a negative value; when it fell lateral to the reference line, the angle was designated with a positive value. In 100 normal subjects included in their study, the average congruence angle was −6°. An angle of +16° or greater was found to be associated with various patellofemoral disorders, particularly lateral patellar subluxation (see Fig. 9.40). On occasion, patellofemoral disorders that are more difficult to diagnose may require, as Ficat and Hungerford recommended, additional tangential views obtained with 30°, 60°, and 90° of knee flexion.

Among the ancillary techniques available for the evaluation of injuries to the knee, tomography, arthrography, and magnetic resonance imaging (MRI) provide crucial information. Tomography is especially useful in the evaluation of complex fractures of the distal femur, the tibial plateaus, and the patella. In fractures of the tibial plateaus, it is effective in determining the amount of depression of the

articular surface and in identifying small comminuted fragments that may be displaced into the joint, as well as comminution about the tibial spines, which may indicate avulsion of the cruciate ligaments. Tomography, by its ability to demonstrate the integrity of the anterior cortex, is also helpful in planning a surgical approach to the treatment of tibial plateau fractures.

Arthrography used to be the procedure of choice in evaluating injuries to the soft-tissue structures of the knee, such as the joint capsule, menisci, and ligaments (Fig. 9.8). It is still valuable in examination of the articular cartilage, particularly when subtle chondral or osteochondral fracture is suspected, or when confirmation of the presence or absence of osteochondral bodies in the knee joint is required in suspected osteochondritis dissecans. However, in the evaluation of the menisci, cruciate ligaments, and collateral ligaments, arthrographic examination has been almost completely replaced by MRI.

The medial and lateral menisci (or semilunar cartilages) of the knee are crescent-shaped fibrocartilaginous structures attached, respectively, to the medial and lateral aspects of the superior articular

Figure 9.5 Sunrise view. (A) For an axial (sunrise) view of the patella, the patient is prone, with the knee flexed 115°. The central beam is directed toward the patella with approximately 15° cephalad angulation. **(B)** The radiograph in this projection demonstrates a tangential (axial) view of the patella. Note the deep position of this structure in the intercondylar fossa. The femoropatellar joint compartment is well demonstrated.

Figure 9.6 Merchant view. (A) For the Merchant axial view of the patella, the patient is supine on the table, with the knee flexed approximately 45° at the table's edge. A device keeping the knee at this angle also holds the film cassette. The central beam is directed caudally through the patella at a 60° angle from the vertical. **(B)** On the film in this projection, the articular facets of the patella and femur are well demonstrated.

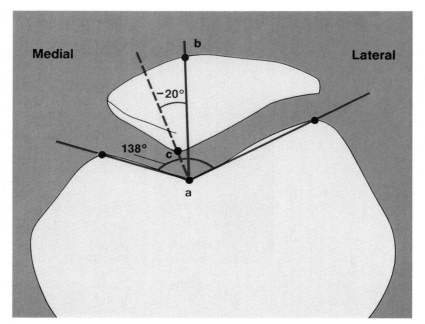

Figure 9.7 Sulcus and congruence angles. Two specific measurements can be obtained from the Merchant axial view: the sulcus angle and the congruence angle. The sulcus angle, formed by lines extending from the deepest point of the intercondylar sulcus *(a)* medially and laterally to the tops of the femoral condyles, normally measures approximately 138°. To determine the congruence angle, the sulcus angle is bisected to establish a reference line *(ba)*, which is drawn to connect the apex of the patella *(b)* with the deepest point of the sulcus *(a)*. In normal subjects, this line is close to vertical. A second line *(ca)* is then drawn from the lowest point on the articular ridge of the patella *(c)* to the deepest point of the sulcus *(a)*. The angle formed by this line and the reference line is the congruence angle. If the lowest point on the patellar articular ridge is lateral to the reference line, then the congruence angle has a positive value; if it is medial to the reference line, as in the present example, then the angle has a negative value. In Merchant's study, the average congruence angle in normal subjects was −6° (SD, ± 11°). (Modified from Merchant AC, et al., 1974, with permission.)

surface of the tibia (Fig. 9.9). Normally, the medial meniscus is visualized on arthrography as a triangular structure intimately attached to the joint capsule and tibial (medial) collateral ligament; its smooth borders are coated by positive-contrast medium and surrounded by injected air. The normal arthrogram shows no air or contrast within the substance of the meniscus or at its periphery (Fig. 9.10A–C). Although the lateral meniscus is structurally very similar to the medial meniscus, it has a very important distinguishing feature. The popliteal muscle's tendon and its sheath pass through a portion of the posterior horn of the lateral meniscus, separating it from the joint capsule. This anatomic site, known as the *popliteal hiatus,* gives an arthrographic impression of separation of the periphery of the lateral meniscus from the capsule; it should not be mistaken for a tear (Fig. 9.10D, E). An important fact to remember is that not all areas of the menisci are well demonstrated by knee arthrography. Only the parts seen tangentially can be assessed accurately. For example, the posterior part of the posterior horn of the lateral meniscus constitutes a blind spot, because it extends deeply into the knee joint (see Fig. 9.9).

The cruciate ligaments of the knee are also structures commonly subject to injury (Fig. 9.11). In the evaluation of these ligaments, arthrography was the procedure of choice before the MRI era and is even now occasionally performed. The radiograph is obtained to best

advantage in the lateral projection with 60° to 80° of knee flexion and with the examiner applying pressure to the posterior aspect of the proximal tibia. When tensed, the anterior cruciate ligament normally projects as a straight line extending from the intercondylar notch to a point approximately 8 mm posterior to the anterior margin of the tibia. The posterior cruciate ligament is seen as a straight or slightly bulging line extending to the posterior margin of the tibial plateau (Fig. 9.12).

In the past decade, MRI of the knee has gained wide acceptance in the diagnosis of traumatic abnormalities, and currently is the method of choice in evaluating various knee structures, particularly the menisci, cruciate ligaments, and collateral ligaments. Routinely, T1-weighted and T2-weighted images are obtained in the sagittal, coronal, and axial planes. The sagittal plane is generally the most effective for evaluation of the cruciate ligaments, menisci, patellar ligament, and quadriceps tendon. Coronal sections are needed for evaluation of the medial and lateral collateral ligaments, as well as the menisci. The axial plane is best to evaluate the patellofemoral joint compartment. The axial plane is also helpful in evaluating the popliteal cysts and their relationship to the surrounding structures of the popliteal fossa.

MR arthrography is effective in evaluating residual or recurrent

Figure 9.8 Arthrography of the knee. For arthrographic examination of the knee, the patient is supine on the radiographic table, with both legs fully extended and in the neutral position. The patella is pulled laterally and rotated anteriorly, and the joint is entered from the lateral aspect at the midpoint of the patella. Before injection of contrast, the joint should be aspirated to avoid dilution of the contrast medium by joint fluid. For a double-contrast study, 40 to 50 mL of room air are injected into the joint, followed by 5 to 7 mL of positive-contrast agent (usually 60% diatrizoate meglumine mixed with 0.3 mL of epinephrine 1: 1000, which delays absorption of the contrast). Radiographs are then obtained in the prone position using the spot-film technique (see Fig. 9.10).

Figure 9.9 Tibial plateau. In the topography of the tibial plateau, the medial meniscus is a C-shaped fibrocartilaginous structure with anterior horn attached anteriorly to the intercondylar eminence of the tibia and with posterior horn inserted into the intercondylar area in front of the attachment of the posterior cruciate ligament. The anterior horn of the lateral meniscus, which is an O-shaped structure, is attached in front of the lateral intercondylar tubercle, and the posterior horn inserts medially into the lateral intercondylar tubercle, in front of the attachment of the posterior horn of the medial meniscus.

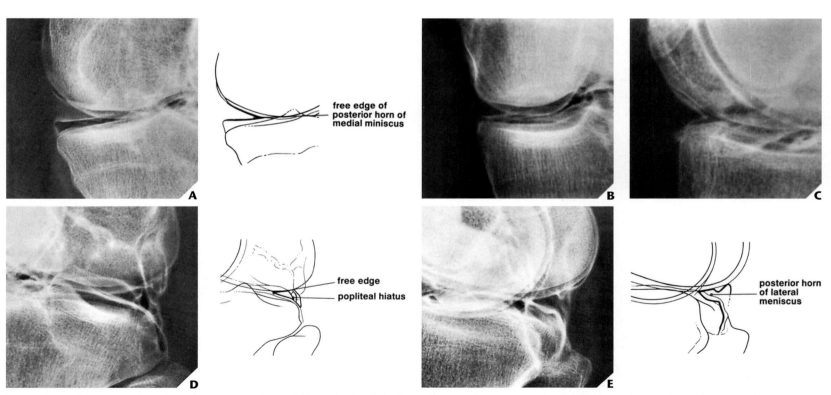

Figure 9.10 Arthrography of the knee. Multiple spot films obtained during arthrographic examination of the knee demonstrate the normal appearance of the medial **(A)**, **(B)**, **(C)** and lateral **(D)**, **(E)** semilunar cartilages. The contrast-outlined margins of the medial meniscus show its triangular shape. The posterior horn **(A)** is longer than the body **(B)** and the anterior horn **(C)**, and the free edge of the meniscus is sharply pointed. Features of the normal lateral meniscus include the gap of the popliteal hiatus, which separates the meniscus from the joint capsule **(D)**. The posterior horn reattaches to the capsule more posteriorly **(E)**. No contrast should be seen within the substance of any aspect of the menisci.

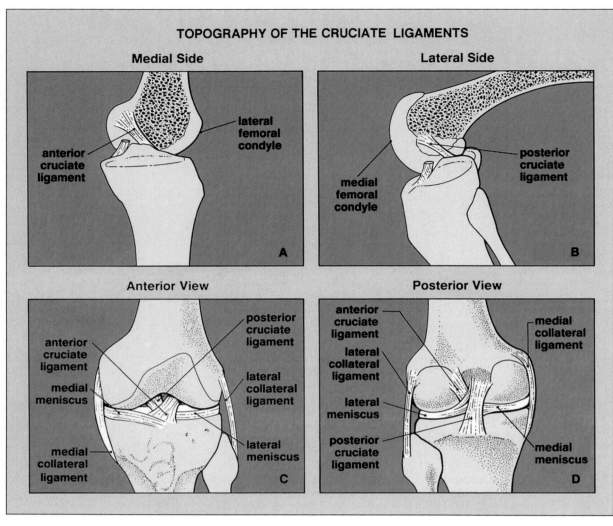

Figure 9.11 The cruciate ligaments. In the topography of the cruciate ligaments of the knee, the anterior cruciate ligament arises on the medial surface of the lateral femoral condyle at the intercondylar notch (**A**) and attaches on the anterior portion of the intercondylar eminence of the tibia (**C**) (see also Fig. 9.9). The posterior cruciate ligament originates on the lateral surface of the medial femoral condyle within the intercondylar notch (**B**) and inserts on the posterior surface of the intercondylar eminence (**D**) (see also Fig. 9.9). Neither cruciate ligament is attached to the tibial tubercles.

meniscal tears after meniscal surgery. It is also a valuable technique to demonstrate loose intraarticular chondral or osteochondral bodies, synovial plicae, and to evaluate the stability of various osteochondral lesions, including osteochondritis dissecans and osteochondral fracture. MR arthrography of the knee is performed by injecting up to 40 mL of diluted gadolinium solution into the joint using the same tech-nique as described for conventional knee arthrography (see Fig. 9.8). Coronal, sagittal, and axial images are obtained, most commonly with fat-suppressed T1-weighted and T2-weighted sequences.

The menisci are seen on MRI as wedge-shaped or bow-tie–shaped structures of uniformly low signal intensity in practically all pulse sequences (Fig. 9.13). The anterior and posterior cruciate ligaments,

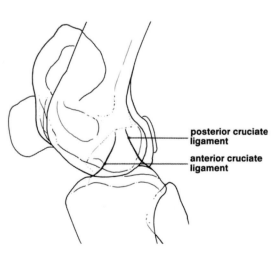

Figure 9.12 Arthrography of the cruciate ligaments. Double-contrast arthrogram of the knee demonstrates the normal appearance of the cruciate ligaments. Note the angle formed by their projectional intersection and their taut appearance. Each ligament can be traced from its origin in the femur to its insertion in the tibia. The boundaries of the cruciate ligaments are sharply outlined because the contrast medium coats their synovial reflexions. The cruciate ligaments are extrasynovial structures; only the anterior surface of the anterior cruciate ligament and the posterior surface of the posterior cruciate ligament are covered by synovium.

like the menisci, are seen as low-signal-intensity structures on all spin echo sequences. The anterior cruciate ligament is straight and fan-shaped (slightly wider at its femoral attachment) and demonstrates low-to-intermediate signal intensity (Fig. 9.14A). The posterior cruciate ligament is arcuate in shape when the knee is in extension or mild flexion and becomes increasingly taut as the knee is flexed. Normally,

it has very low signal intensity (Fig. 9.14B). Anteriorly to the posterior cruciate ligament, one can observe a small bulge produced by the anterior meniscofemoral ligament, also known as the ligament of Humphrey (Fig. 9.14B, C). Posteriorly, a small bulge is created by the posterior meniscofemoral ligament, known as the ligament of Wrisberg (Fig. 9.14D).

Figure 9.13 Appearance of normal menisci on MRI. (A) Anterior and posterior horns of the medial meniscus as seen on sagittal T2*-weighted MPGR sequence (flip angle 30°). **(B)** Anterior and posterior horns of the lateral meniscus as seen on sagittal T2*-weighted MPGR sequence (flip angle 30°). **(C)** Body of the medial meniscus as seen on sagittal spin-echo T1-weighted sequence. **(D)** Anterior and posterior horns of the lateral meniscus as seen on sagittal spin-echo T1-weighted sequence. **(E)** Schematic representation of topography of the medial and lateral menisci and surrounding structures as seen in the midplane of the coronal MRI. (Modified from Firooznia H, 1992, with permission.)

Figure 9.14 Cruciate ligaments. Spin-echo sagittal MR images (TR 2000/TE 20 msec) of the normal cruciate ligaments. **(A)** Anterior margin of the anterior cruciate ligament is straight and well defined; the posterior margin is ill defined because of the oblique orientation of the ligament. **(B)** The posterior cruciate ligament is seen in its entirety, in one plane, from the femoral to the tibial attachments. Observe the small bulge anteriorly produced by the anterior meniscofemoral ligament. **(C)** In this sagittal section, the anterior meniscofemoral ligament of Humphrey is very prominent, simulating a loose body or meniscal fragment. **(D)** Here, meniscofemoral ligaments, both anterior (Humphrey) and posterior (Wrisberg), are prominent. (From Beltran J, 1990, with permission.)

Figure 9.15 Collateral ligaments. (A) Spin-echo coronal MR image (TR 2000/TE 20 msec) of the normal medial collateral ligament. The medial collateral ligament is well defined in this section through the intercondylar notch. The insertion of the posterior cruciate ligament in the inner aspect of the medial femoral condyle is well demonstrated. The menisci are seen as small triangles of low signal intensity. **(B)** Spin-echo coronal MR image (TR 2000/TE 20 msec) of the lateral (fibular) collateral ligament. On this posterior section, note the meniscofemoral ligament, which extends from the posterior horn of the lateral meniscus to the inner surface of the medial femoral condyle. The lateral and medial menisci and posterior cruciate ligament are well demonstrated. (From Beltran J, 1990, with permission.)

The medial collateral ligament consists of two components: superficial and deep. The superficial component, which is the principal medial stabilizer of the knee, arises from the medial femoral epicondyle just below the adductor tubercle and inserts into the medial aspect of the tibia, approximately 5 cm below the joint line. The deep layer of the medial collateral ligament, which is considered part of the fibrous capsule, attaches loosely to the peripheral margin of the body of the medial meniscus. The lateral collateral ligament attaches to the lateral epicondyle of the femur superiorly just above the popliteus groove, in which region it merges with the outer surface of the capsule. From here it extends inferiorly and posteriorly to attach to the anterior portion of the apex of the fibular head. Both collateral ligaments are best demonstrated on the images obtained in the coronal plane. Like the menisci and cruciate ligaments, they also display low signal intensity (Fig. 9.15).

Evaluation of knee instability caused by ligament injuries may require obtaining stress views. These techniques are most commonly performed in cases of suspected injury to the medial collateral ligament (Fig. 9.16; see also Fig. 9.71). They are less frequently performed during the evaluation of insufficiency of the anterior and posterior cruciate ligaments (Fig. 9.17). These examinations should preferably be performed under local anesthesia.

Figure 9.16 Valgus stress. For a stress film of the knee evaluating the medial collateral ligament, the patient is supine, with the knee flexed approximately 15° to 20°. The leg is placed in the device, and the pressure plate is applied against the lateral aspect of the knee. (The *arrows* show the direction of the applied stresses.) Films are then obtained in the anteroposterior projection (see Fig. 9.71B).

Figure 9.17 Anterior-drawer stress. For a stress film of the knee evaluating the anterior cruciate ligament, the patient is placed in the device on his or her side, with the knee flexed 90°. The pressure plate is applied against the anterior aspect of the knee. (The *arrows* show the direction of the applied stresses.) Films are then obtained in the lateral projection.

Arteriography and venography may need to be used in the evaluation of concomitant injury to the vascular system. Computed tomography (CT) is effective in evaluation of tibial plateau fractures, and it is occasionally used to evaluate injury to the cartilage and soft tissues, particularly the menisci and cruciate ligaments. CT used in conjunction with arthrography (computed arthrotomography) is useful in the evaluation of osteochondritis dissecans (see Fig. 9.51C,D) and in detecting nonopaque osteochondral bodies in the knee joint.

For a summary of the preceding discussion in tabular form, see Tables 9.1 and 9.2 and Fig. 9.18.

Injury to the Knee

Fractures About the Knee

Fractures of the Distal Femur. Most often sustained in motor vehicle accidents or falls from heights, fractures of the distal femur are classified according to the site and extension of the fracture line as supracondylar, condylar, and intercondylar. Supracondylar fractures can be further classified as nondisplaced, impacted, displaced, and comminuted (Fig. 9.19). These injuries are usually well demonstrated on the standard anteroposterior and lateral projections of the knee

Table 9.1   Standard and Special Radiographic Projections for Evaluating Injury to the Knee

Projection	Demonstration	Projection	Demonstration

Anteroposterior	Medial and lateral joint compartments
	Varus and valgus deformities
	Fractures of:
	    Medial and lateral femoral condyles
	    Medial and lateral tibial plateaus
	    Tibial spines
	    Proximal fibula
	Osteochondral fracture
	Osteochondritis dissecans (late-stage)
	Spontaneous osteonecrosis
	Pellegrini-Stieda lesion
		Lateral (continued)	Sinding-Larsen-Johansson disease*
			Osgood-Schlatter disease*
			Osteochondral fracture
			Osteochondritis dissecans (late stage)
			Spontaneous osteonecrosis
			Joint effusion
			Tears of:
			    Quadriceps tendon
			    Patellar ligament

Overpenetrated	Bipartiite or multipartite patella Fractures of patella	Stress Cross-table	Tears of cruciate ligaments FBI sign of lipohemarthrosis
Stress	Tear of collateral ligaments	*Tunnel* (posteroanterior)	Posterior aspect of femoral condyles

Lateral	Femoropatellar joint compartment
	Patella in profile
	Suprapatellar bursa
	Fractures of:
	    Distal femur
	    Proximal tibia
	    Patella
		
		Axial (sunrise and
		    Merchant)
			Intercondylar notch
			Intercondylar eminence of tibia
			Articular facets of patella†
			Sulcus angle†
			Congruence angle†
			Fractures of patella
			Subluxation and dislocation of
			    patella†

* These conditions are best demonstrated using a low-kilovoltage/soft-tissue technique.
† These features are better demonstrated on Merchant axial view.

Table 9.2 **Ancillary Imaging Techniques for Evaluating Injury to the Knee**

Technique	Demonstration	Technique	Demonstration

Tomography	Position of fragments and extension of fracture line in complex fractures of:
	  Distal femur
	  Proximal tibia
	  Patella
	Quantification of depression in tibial plateau fractures
	Healing process:
	  Nonunion
	  Secondary infection
		Arthrography (continued)
		
		Computed Tomography and Computed Arthrotomography
			Subtle abnormalities of articular cartilage
			Spontaneous osteonecrosis
			Injuries to:
			  Articular cartilage
			  Cruciate ligaments
			  Menisci
			Osteochondral bodies in joint
			Osteochondritis dissecans

Arthrography
  (usually double-contrast; occasionally single-contrast using air only)
	Meniscal tears
	Injuries to:
	  Cruciate ligaments
	  Medial collateral ligament
	  Quadriceps tendon
	  Patellar ligament
	  Joint capsule
	Chondral and osteochondral fractures
	Osteochondritis dissecans (early and late stages)
	Osteochondral bodies in joint
		Radionuclide Imaging
		  (scintigraphy, bone scan)
		
		Angiography (arteriography, venography)
		Magnetic Resonance Imaging
		
		Magnetic Resonance Arthrography
			Subtle fractures not demonstrated on standard studies
			Early and late stages of:
			  Osteochondritis dissecans
			  Spontaneous osteonecrosis
			Concomitant injury to arteries and veins
			Same as arthrography, computed tomography, and radionuclide imaging
			Residual or recurrent meniscal tears
			Complications after meniscal surgery
			Loose intraarticular bodies
			Synovial plicae
			Stability of osteochondral lesions
			Tears of collateral ligaments

Figure 9.18 Spectrum of radiologic imaging techniques for evaluating injury to the knee.*

*The radiographic projections or radiologic techniques indicated throughout the diagram are only those that are the most effective in demonstrating the respective traumatic conditions.

FRACTURES OF THE DISTAL FEMUR

Supracondylar

nondisplaced   impacted   displaced   comminuted

Condylar   **Intercondylar**

Figure 9.19 Classification of distal femur fractures. Fractures of the distal femur can be classified according to the site and extension of the injury as supracondylar, condylar, and intercondylar fractures.

(Fig. 9.20); however, in rare instances an oblique view of the knee may be needed to evaluate an obliquely oriented fracture line. Tomography may also be required in cases of comminution for a full evaluation of the fracture lines and localization of the fragments (Fig. 9.21), although more recently helical CT with multiplanar and three-dimensional reformation has surpassed conventional tomographic technique.

Fractures of the Proximal Tibia. The medial and lateral tibial plateaus are the most common sites of fractures of the proximal tibia. Because they usually result when the knee is struck by a moving vehi-

joint fluid   fabella

calcified popliteal artery

Figure 9.20 Supracondylar fracture. A 58-year-old man was injured in a motorcycle accident. Anteroposterior **(A)** and lateral **(B)** radiographs of the knee demonstrate a comminuted supracondylar fracture of the distal femur. The extension of the fracture lines and the position of the fragments can be assessed adequately on these standard studies.

Figure 9.21 Supracondylar fracture. A 22-year-old racing car driver was injured in an accident on the track. **(A)** Anteroposterior view of the right knee shows a comminuted fracture of the distal femur. Tomography was performed, and sections in the anteroposterior **(B)** and lateral **(C)** projections demonstrate intraarticular extension of the fracture lines, with split of the condyles and posterior displacement of the distal fragments. The multiple comminuted fragments can be localized.

cle, they are also called "fender" or "bumper" fractures; some, however, may be the result of twisting falls. The Hohl classification gives an overview of six different types of tibial plateau fractures and is useful in correlating the various types of injuries with the applied forces causing them (Fig. 9.22). In the Hohl classification, pure abduction injury results in a nondisplaced split fracture of the lateral tibial plateau (type I) (Fig. 9.23). When axial compression is combined with abduction force, local central depression (type II) and local split depression (type III) fractures occur (Fig. 9.24). Total depression fractures (type IV), which are more commonly seen in the medial tibial plateau because of its anatomic configuration (absence of the fibula), are characterized by lack of comminution of the articular surface. Type V fractures in the Hohl classification, which are infrequently encountered, are local split fractures without central depression involv-

Figure 9.22 The Hohl classification of fractures of the tibial plateau. (Modified from Hohl M, 1967, with permission.)

Figure 9.23 Fracture of the tibial plateau. A 30-year-old man was hit by a car while he was crossing the street. Anteroposterior radiograph (**A**) and tomogram (**B**) show a wedge fracture of the lateral tibial plateau.

Figure 9.24 Fracture of the tibial plateau. Anteroposterior view of the knee shows the appearance of a tibial plateau fracture, which is a combination of wedge and central depression fractures involving the lateral tibial condyle.

Figure 9.25 Fracture of the tibial plateau. Anteroposterior film (**A**) and lateral tomogram (**B**) demonstrate the characteristic appearance of the Y-type bicondylar tibial fracture.

ing the anterior or posterior aspects of the tibial plateau. Comminuted fractures involving both tibial plateaus and having a Y or T configuration (type VI) usually result from vertical compression, such as a fall on the extended leg (Fig. 9.25). Types III and VI are frequently associated with fracture of the proximal fibula.

Fractures of the tibial plateau may not be obvious on the routine radiographic examination of the knee, particularly if there is no depression (Fig. 9.26A, B). In such cases, however, the cross-table lateral projection often reveals the FBI sign, which indicates the presence of an intraarticular fracture (Fig. 9.26C). Demonstration of an obscure fracture line may require oblique projections, but tomographic examination may reveal the fracture line and demonstrate its extension (Fig. 9.26D). If the fracture is depressed, then conventional tomography can also help quantify the degree of depression (Fig. 9.27).

The role of CT in evaluation of tibial plateau fractures has been well established. CT provides optimal visualization of the plateau depression, defects, and split fragments. It also proved more accurate than conventional tomography in assessing depressed and split fractures when they involved the anterior and posterior border of the plateau, and in demonstrating the extent of fracture comminution. According to Rafii and coworkers, the degree of fracture depressions and separation as measured by the computerized technique is often more accurate than measurements obtained from conventional tomograms. Particularly useful are reformatted images in various planes and three-dimensional (3-D) reformation (Figs. 9.28, 9.29, and 9.30). Recently, Kode and coworkers suggested that MRI was equivalent or superior to two-dimensional (2-D) CT reformation for depiction of tibial plateau fracture configuration (Figs. 9.31 and 9.32). The multiplanar capabilities of MRI may facilitate 3-D perception and, in addition, this technique permits assessment of the asso-

ciated injuries to the ligaments and menisci that are not visible on CT scans (Fig. 9.33).

An important feature of tibial plateau fractures is their association with injury to ligaments and the menisci. The structures most at risk are the medial collateral and the anterior cruciate ligaments (see Fig 9.11) and the lateral meniscus (see Fig. 9.9), because lateral tibial plateau fractures usually result from valgus stress (Fig. 9.34).

Moreover, damage to the anterior cruciate ligament may be associated with avulsion of the lateral tibial spine or the anterior intercondylar eminence. Stress views and MRI usually reveal these associated abnormalities. If clinical examination and radiologic studies, including stress views, show ligamentous structures to be intact, then nondisplaced fractures of the tibial plateau can be treated conservatively. In depression-type fractures, however, Larson recommends open reduction in patients whose fractures show 8 mm of articular depression. Generally, surgery is indicated for fractures of the tibial plateau showing articular depression of 10 mm or more.

Complications. The most frequent complications of fractures of the distal femur and the proximal tibia are malunion and posttraumatic arthritis.

Segond Fracture. The Segond fracture is a small-fragment avulsion fracture from the lateral aspect of the proximal tibia just below the level of the tibial plateau, best demonstrated on anteroposterior view of the knee (Fig. 9.35). The mechanism of this injury is internal rotation of the leg associated with varus stress on a flexed knee that creates tension on the lateral capsule and lateral capsular ligament. This, in turn, causes an avulsion fracture at the insertion of this ligament on the lateral tibial plateau. This injury may be associated with capsular tear, a tear of the anterior cruciate ligament, and lateral meniscus tear, resulting in chronic anterolateral knee instability.

Figure 9.26 Fracture of the tibial plateau. While crossing the street, a 38-year-old woman was struck by a car. Anteroposterior (**A**) and lateral (**B**) radiographs show substantial joint effusion, but the fracture line is not clearly seen. (**C**) Cross-table lateral view demonstrates the FBI sign, indicating intraarticular extension of the fracture. (**D**) Tomographic section clearly demonstrates a wedge fracture of the lateral tibial condyle.

blood
fat–blood interface
fat
fracture

Figure 9.27 **Fracture of the tibial plateau.** A 72-year-old woman was injured in an automobile accident. Anteroposterior (**A**) and lateral (**B**) views of the left knee show a depression fracture of the lateral tibial plateau; however, the amount of depression cannot be determined. To do so, anteroposterior (**C**) and lateral (**D**) tomographic sections were obtained. They show 12 mm of articular depression, which mandates surgical treatment to restore the joint surface congruity.

wedge of depression

Figure 9.28 **CT of fracture of the tibial plateau.** A 23-year-old man was injured in a motorcycle accident. The conventional radiographs of the right knee showed fracture of the tibial plateau. (**A**) Axial CT section through the proximal tibia shows a comminuted fracture of the medial tibial plateau. (**B**) Sagittal reformatted image shows that the anterior part of the plateau is mainly affected. (**C**) Coronal reformatted image demonstrates comminution and depression. (**D**) Anterior view of the 3-D reformatted image in addition to depression of the medial anterior tibial plateau shows associated fracture of the proximal fibula. (**E**) Bird's eye view of the 3-D reformatted image shows the spatial orientation of the fracture lines. *(continued)*

Figure 9.28 CT of fracture of the tibial plateau. *Continued.*

Figure 9.29 CT of fracture of the tibial plateau. A 22-year-old man fell down from a tall ladder and injured his right knee. The conventional radiographs demonstrated fracture of the tibial plateau. **(A)** Coronal reformatted CT scan shows extension of the lateral tibial plateau fracture into the tibial shaft. **(B)** Posterior view of the 3-D reformation shows the fracture line, but the interfragmental split is not well demonstrated. **(C)** Anterior view of the 3-D reformation shows the split better. **(D)** Bird's eye view of the 3-D CT scan effectively demonstrates the details of the split and comminution of the tibial plateau.

Figure 9.30 CT of fracture of the tibial plateau. Coronal **(A)** and sagittal **(B)** CT reformatted images show a Hohl type III (displaced, local spit depression) fracture of the lateral tibial plateau. **(C)** 3-D reconstructed image (posterior view) more realistically depicts the features of this injury.

Figure 9.31 MRI of fracture of the tibial plateau. **(A)** T2-weighted (spin-echo, TR 2000/TE 80 msec) coronal image shows a broad-based band of low signal intensity traversing the lateral tibial plateau (*long arrows*). Extensive soft-tissue edema is seen superficial to the iliotibial band (*small arrows*). **(B)** Proton density-weighted (spin-echo, TR 2000/TE 20 msec) sagittal image shows central localized depression of the tibial plateau (*arrow*). The degree of comminution and depression is well depicted.

Figure 9.32 MRI of fracture of the tibial plateau. (A) Coronal gradient echo (MGPR) image shows a tibial plateau fracture (*arrowheads*). **(B)** Sagittal gradient echo (MGPR) image demonstrates the anterior extension of the fracture and evulsion of the tibial spines (*arrowheads*).

Recently, Hall and Hochman described a reverse Segond-type fracture affecting medial tibial plateau, associated with tears of the posterior cruciate ligament, medial collateral ligament, and medial meniscus. The mechanism of this injury and the constellation of radiographic findings are the reverse of that seen with the classic Segond injury complex. The avulsion fracture of the medial tibial plateau is caused by a valgus stress and external rotation of a flexed knee.

Fractures and Dislocations of the Patella. Fractures of the patella, which may result from a direct blow to the anterior aspect of the knee or from indirect tension forces generated by the quadriceps tendon, constitute approximately 1% of all skeletal injuries. Generally, patellar fractures may be longitudinal (vertical), transverse, or comminuted (Fig. 9.36). In the most commonly encountered patellar injury, seen in 60% of cases, the fracture line is transverse or slightly oblique, involving the midportion of the patella. In evaluation of such injury, it is important to recognize what has been called the bipartite or multipartite patella. This anomaly represents a developmental variant of the accessory ossification center or centers of the superolateral margin of the patella and

Figure 9.33 MRI of fracture of the tibial plateau. Sagittal T2-weighted image shows a fracture of the medial tibial plateau (*small black arrows*) associated with a tear of the posterior horn of the medial meniscus (*white arrows*). Joint effusion (*large black arrow*) demonstrates high signal intensity.

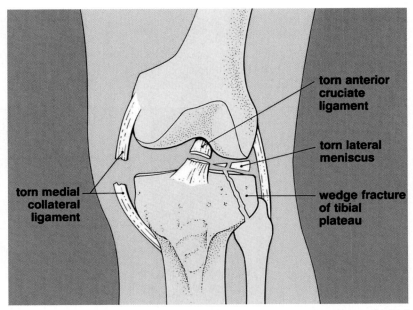

Figure 9.34 Tibial plateau fracture-associated injuries. Lateral tibial plateau fractures, which result from valgus stress, are often associated with tears of the lateral meniscus and the medial collateral and anterior cruciate ligaments.

Figure 9.35 Segond fracture. A 27-year-old woman sustained an injury to her left knee in a skiing accident. Anteroposterior radiograph shows a small fragment of bone evulsed from the lateral aspect of the tibia (*arrow*), characteristic of Segond fracture.

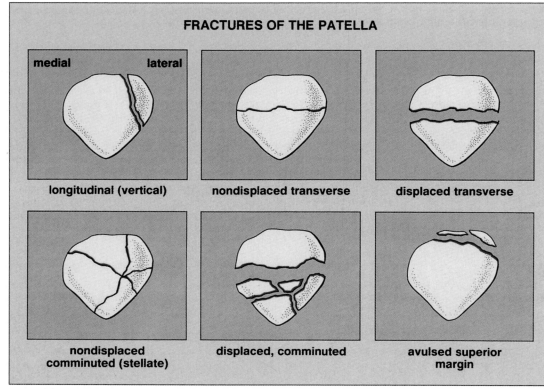

FRACTURES OF THE PATELLA

medial | lateral

longitudinal (vertical)

nondisplaced transverse

displaced transverse

nondisplaced comminuted (stellate)

displaced, comminuted

avulsed superior margin

Figure 9.36 Classification of patellar fractures. (Adapted from Hohl M, Larson RL, 1975, with permission.)

Figure 9.37 Multipartite patella. Anteroposterior (**A**) and axial (**B**) radiographs demonstrate the typical appearance of a bipartite patella. Note the position of the accessory ossification center at the superolateral margin of the patella. (**C**) A tripartite patella was an incidental finding on this overpenetrated anteroposterior film, which was obtained to exclude the possibility of gouty arthritis.

Figure 9.38 Fracture of the patella. After a fall on the stairs, a 63-year-old man presented with severe pain in the anterior aspect of the right knee. Anteroposterior **(A)** and lateral **(B)** radiographs show the typical appearance of fracture of the patella. Note the significant suprapatellar joint effusion.

should not be mistaken for a fracture (Fig. 9.37). Tomography or CT may help distinguish this developmental anomaly from patellar fracture. As an aid to avoid misdiagnosing a bipartite or multipartite patella as a fracture, it is important to keep in mind that the accessory ossification centers are invariably in the upper lateral quadrant of the patella and, if the apparent fragments are put together, they do not form a normal patella. Fracture fragments, however, form a normal patella if they are replaced. Injury to the patella is usually sufficiently demonstrated on the overpenetrated anteroposterior and lateral views of the knee (Fig. 9.38).

Dislocations of the patella, which are usually lateral, result from acute injury and are easily diagnosed on the standard projections of the knee. It is much more difficult to diagnose so-called transient dislocation, referred to the traumatic condition when dislocated patella reduces on its own. Transient dislocation may be associated with hypoplastic trochlear notch of the femur. Although clinical symptoms are helpful, the most accurate diagnostic modality in this respect is MRI. It shows a characteristic pattern of "bone contusion" or trabecular injury on the medial aspect of the patella and anterior lateral femoral condyle (Fig. 9.39). The medial retinaculum is invariably injured, but medial patellar cartilage may or may not show abnormalities. Subluxations of the patella are much more common than true dislocations and usually result from chronic injury. The best radiographic examination for demonstrating patellar subluxation, particularly in subtle cases, is the Merchant axial view (Fig. 9.40).

Figure 9.39 Transient dislocation of the patella. Axial **(A)** and **(B)** coronal T2-weighted fat-suppressed MR images of a 38-year-old woman show characteristic abnormalities of this injury: "bone contusion" on the medial aspect of the patella and lateral femoral condyle (*arrows*) associated with hypoplastic trochlear notch (*open arrow*) and joint effusion (*curved arrows*). Arrowheads are indicating a tear of the medial retinaculum.

Figure 9.40 Subluxation of the patella. A 23-year-old woman experienced occasional knee pain and buckling, particularly while jogging. **(A)** Standard axial view of the patella shows no apparent abnormalities. **(B)** Merchant axial view, however, demonstrates lateral subluxation of the patella. Note the positive congruence angle (see Fig. 9.7).

Sinding-Larsen-Johansson and Osgood-Schlatter Diseases

Sinding-Larsen-Johansson and Osgood-Schlatter diseases are conditions that are seen predominantly in adolescents and are now considered to be related to trauma. They occur at either end of the patellar ligament: Sinding-Larsen-Johansson disease at its proximal end, where it attaches to the lower pole (apex) of the patella; and Osgood-Schlatter disease at its distal end, where it attaches to the tibial tubercle (tuberosity).

Sinding-Larsen-Johansson disease is characterized clinically by local pain and tenderness on palpation and radiographically by separation and fragmentation of the lower pole of the patella, associated with soft-tissue swelling and, occasionally, calcifications at the site of the patellar ligament. This condition is believed to be caused by persistent traction at the cartilaginous junction of the patella and patellar ligament. The lateral radiograph, preferably obtained with a lowkilovoltage/soft-tissue technique, is the single most important examination (Fig. 9.41); in combination with a positive clinical examination, it usually establishes the diagnosis.

Osgood-Schlatter disease, which occurs three-time more frequently in adolescent boys than in adolescent girls, is characterized by fragmentation of the tibial tubercle and soft-tissue swelling anterior to it. In 25% to 33% of all reported cases, the condition is bilateral. As in Sinding-Larsen-Johansson disease, the lateral film, obtained using a soft-tissue technique, is most effective in demonstrating this condition (Fig. 9.42). However, an accurate diagnosis is based on radiographic and clinical findings. Soft-tissue swelling is a fundamental diagnostic feature. On MRI, as Hayes and Conway pointed out, T1-weighted images shows replacement of the normal high-signal infrapatellar fat with an area of decreased signal adjacent to the patellar ligament insertion. The ligament itself may show focal areas of increased signal, depending on the degree of associated tendinitis (Figs. 9.43 and 9.44).

Occasionally, Sinding-Larsen-Johansson and Osgood-Schlatter diseases may coexist. It is important to remember that the presence of multiple ossification centers in the tibial tuberosity and lower pole of the patella may at times mimic these conditions. However, the absence of soft-tissue swelling in such cases allows the distinction to be made.

Injuries to the Cartilage of the Knee

Osteochondral (or chondral) fracture, osteochondritis dissecans, and spontaneous osteonecrosis are three conditions with similar radiologic appearances. They are invariably confused with each other, and in many instances the terms are used interchangeably. They represent, however, three separate orthopedic entities, each with a specific cause and each requiring a specific treatment. Usually, history, physical examination, and radiographic presentation can help distinguish these conditions from one another.

Osteochondral (or Chondral) Fracture. Shearing, rotary, or tangentially aligned impaction forces directed to the knee joint may result in acute injury to the articular end of the femur. The resulting fracture may involve cartilage only—chondral fracture—or cartilage and the underlying subchondral segment of bone—osteochondral

fragmented lower pole of patella

calcification and ossification in patellar ligament

soft tissue swelling

Figure 9.41 Sinding-Larsen-Johansson disease. A 13-year-old boy experienced pain and swelling at the site of the patellar ligament. He had no history of acute trauma. **(A)** Lateral radiograph of the right knee shows fragmentation of the lower pole of the patella and significant soft-tissue swelling associated with calcifications and ossifications of the patellar ligament—findings characteristic of Sinding-Larsen-Johansson disease. **(B)** The normal left knee is shown for comparison.

Figure 9.42 Osgood-Schlatter disease. A 12-year-old boy had severe tenderness over the left tibial tuberosity. The lateral film, obtained with a low-kilovoltage/soft-tissue technique, reveals fragmentation of the tibial tuberosity in association with soft-tissue swelling—characteristic findings in Osgood-Schlatter disease.

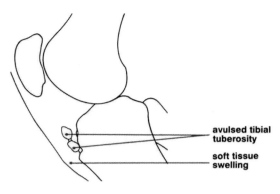

avulsed tibial tuberosity

soft tissue swelling

Figure 9.43 MRI of Osgood-Schlatter disease. T1-weighted **(A)** (spin-echo, TR 700/TE 20 msec) and T2*-weighted **(B)** sagittal images demonstrate focus of decreased signal within normal sharp V-shaped area formed by the patellar ligament and anterior tibia *(arrow).*

Figure 9.44 MRI of Osgood-Schlatter disease. A sagittal T2-weighted image of the knee of a 14-year-old boy demonstrates inflammatory changes along the distal patellar ligament *(arrowheads).*

Figure 9.45 Chondral and osteochondral fracture. A chondral fracture **(A)** affects only the cartilage, whereas an osteochondral fracture **(B)** involves the cartilage and the subchondral segment of bone.

Figure 9.46 Osteochondral fracture. A 22-year-old man dislocated his left patella in a skiing accident. The dislocation was spontaneously reduced, and he did not seek medical attention. Eight months later, he was seen by an orthopedic surgeon for chronic joint effusion and locking of the knee. The standard radiographic examination in the anteroposterior **(A)**, lateral **(B)**, and tunnel **(C)** projections reveal joint fluid, a defect in the lateral femoral condyle, and a large osteochondral body, representing an osteochondral fracture, in the area of the intercondylar notch. Double-contrast arthrography **(D)** confirmed the intraarticular osteochondral body and also showed a defect in the articular cartilage covering the posterolateral aspect of the lateral femoral condyle **(E)**. Note the similarity between this condition and osteochondritis dissecans (see Fig. 9.49). *(continued)*

joint fluid

defect in lateral condyle

osteochondral fragment

Figure 9.46 Osteochondral fracture. *Continued.*

fracture (Fig. 9.45). These fractures, which may occur in either of the femoral or tibial condyles, the tibial plateau, and the patella, may range in severity from minimal indentation of the articular surface to displacement of an osteochondral fragment into the joint. Because a chondral fracture involves only articular cartilage, it can be demonstrated either by arthrography or by MRI. An osteochondral fracture, however, may be seen on conventional radiography, particularly if the fragment has been dislodged. The presence of such a fragment in the joint may be indistinguishable from the radiographic appearance of osteochondritis dissecans (see below). However, a clinical history of acute injury sustained in sports-related activities, such as football, soccer, or skiing, and associated with symptoms such as severe pain, local tenderness, and often joint effusion, is invariably helpful in making a distinction between these similar conditions (Fig. 9.46).

Osteochondritis Dissecans. Osteochondritis dissecans is a relatively common condition, seen predominantly in adolescents and young adults and more often in males than in females, and has recently come to be considered a form of osteochondral fracture caused not by acute but by chronic injury. As in acute osteochondral fractures, shearing or rotary forces applied to the articular surface of the femur result in detachment of a fragment of articular cartilage, often together with a segment of subchondral bone.

Aichroth has pointed out that the separated segment is avascular and this feature distinguishes osteochondritis dissecans from acute osteochondral fracture. In a clinical survey of osteochondritis dissecans in 200 patients, he also determined the distribution of the lesion. The most common location was the lateral aspect of the medial femoral condyle, a non-weight-bearing segment; other sites were less commonly affected (Fig. 9.47). The degree of damage to the articular cartilage, as in acute osteochondral fractures, varies from an in situ osteochondral body, to an osteocartilaginous flap, to complete detachment of an osteochondral segment (Fig. 9.48).

In the early stages of the disease, conventional radiographs in the standard projections usually show no abnormality. The only positive finding may be joint effusion. In more advanced stages of the disease, a radiolucent line is seen separating the osteochondral body from the femoral condyle (Fig. 9.49). For the orthopedic management of this condition, it is important to evaluate the status of the articular cartilage. Double-contrast arthrography can differentiate an in situ lesion from a more advanced lesion, where the osteochondral body is partially or completely detached from its bed (Fig. 9.50). Separation of the fragment mandates surgical intervention. Sometimes, other special techniques may need to be used, such as using only air as a contrast medium, combining arthrography with tomography or CT to demonstrate the presence and distribution of the osteochondral bodies (Fig. 9.51), or performing MRI examination of the knee (Fig. 9.52). For the latter, T1-weighted and T2-weighted images in coronal and sagittal planes are most effective. The lesion usually displays intermediate signal intensity on all sequences and is separated by a narrow zone of low signal intensity from the viable bone. The disruption of articular cartilage is best seen on T2 or T2* (gradient echo) images (Fig. 9.53). When osteochondral body is separated from the host bone by a rim of a high signal intensity on T2-weighted images (a phenomenon that denotes a fluid or granulation tissue), it usually signifies loosening or complete detachment of the necrotic fragment (Fig. 9.54).

Occasionally, a small, disk-shaped secondary ossification center is present on the posterior portion of the femoral condyle; this normal variant should not be mistaken for osteochondritis dissecans. Similarly, during normal ossification of the distal femoral epiphysis, developmental changes may appear as irregularities in the outline of the condyle. The appearance of these irregularities, which are usually posteriorly located and hence best seen on the tunnel projection, may mimic osteochondritis dissecans (Fig. 9.49). This normal variant is usually seen between the ages of 2 and 12.

Figure 9.47 Site of the lesion. Osteochondritis dissecans most frequently affects the medial femoral condyle, the non-weight-bearing portion (the lateral aspect of the condyle and the intercondylar notch), which is the most common site of the lesion. The lateral femoral condyle is much less commonly involved. (Modified from Aichroth P, 1971, with permission.)

Figure 9.48 Stages of osteochondritis dissecans. The spectrum of chronic injury to the articular end of the distal femur (osteochondritis dissecans) ranges from an in situ lesion to a defect in the subchondral bone associated with a dislodged osteochondral body.

Figure 9.49 Osteochondritis dissecans. An 11-year-old boy presented with pain in his right knee for 3 months. Posteroanterior (tunnel) radiograph of the knee shows the typical lesion of osteochondritis dissecans in the medial femoral condyle. A radiolucent line separates the oval in situ body from the femoral condyle. Incidentally, the lateral femoral condyle shows an irregular outline of the weight-bearing segment. This finding represents a developmental variant in ossification and is of no further consequence.

Figure 9.50 Arthrography of osteochondritis dissecans. A 23-year-old man presented with chronic pain in the knee for 4 months. He had no history of acute trauma in recent years. Tunnel **(A)** and lateral **(B)** views show a defect in the subchondral bone at the inferocentral aspect of the lateral femoral condyle and an osteochondral fragment that has been discharged into the joint. Arthrography was performed to evaluate the articular cartilage. The arthrogram **(C)** shows contrast filling the subchondral defect, indicating damage to the articular cartilage.

Figure 9.51 CT-arthrography of osteochondritis dissecans. A 13-year-old boy had pain in his right knee for 8 months. **(A)** Anteroposterior film shows the lesion of osteochondritis dissecans in its classic location, the lateral aspect of the medial femoral condyle. The lesion appears to be still in situ. **(B)** On contrast arthrography, the lesion is shown to be covered by intact articular cartilage from the inferior aspect of the femoral condyle, but computed arthrotomographic sections **(C)**, **(D)** demonstrate that the lesion, located in the anterolateral aspect of the femoral condyle (a portion not protected by articular cartilage), is partial discharged into the joint at the site of the attachment of the posterior cruciate ligament. *(continued)*

site of attachment
of posterior cruciate
ligament

defect in condyle

protruding
osteochondral body

medial tibial spine

Figure 9.51 CT-arthrography of osteochondritis dissecans. *Continued.*

zone of demarcation

in situ
osteochondral body

zone of demarcation

in situ
osteochondral body

intact articular
cartilage

growth plate

Figure 9.52 **MRI of osteochondritis dissecans.** An 11-year-old boy experienced knee pain for 3 months. **(A)** MR image in the coronal plane (spin-echo, TR 1800/TE 20 msec) shows bony fragment well separated from the medial femoral condyle by the low signal intensity line. **(B)** Image in the sagittal plane (spin echo TR 800/TE 20 msec) demonstrates intact articular cartilage overlying the separated fragment, indicating an in situ lesion.

Figure 9.53 MRI of osteochondritis dissecans. (A) Anteroposterior radiograph of the right knee shows a lesion of osteochondritis dissecans in the medial femoral condyle (*arrow*). Coronal **(B)** and sagittal **(C)** T2-weighted fat-suppressed MR images demonstrate the osteochondral body being still in situ (*arrows*), although the articular cartilage is already damaged (*curved arrows*).

Figure 9.54 MRI of osteochondritis dissecans. A loose osteochondral body in the medial femoral condyle is seen on T1-weighted coronal **(A)** and sagittal **(B)** images (*white arrows*). **(C)** On the sagittal T2*-weighted sequence high-signal-intensity fluid (*small arrows*) separates the loose fragment from the viable bone.

Figure 9.55 Spontaneous osteonecrosis. Four weeks before this radiographic examination, a 58-year-old man felt a sharp pain in the right knee when he stepped off a curb. The pain subsided after 1 week but recurred soon afterward. **(A)** Anteroposterior radiograph of the knee shows flattening of the medial aspect of the medial femoral condyle. **(B)** Radionuclide bone scan was performed, and it shows a marked increase in uptake of the tracer in the area of the medial femoral condyle. The features seen in both studies characterize an early stage of spontaneous osteonecrosis.

Figure 9.56 Spontaneous osteonecrosis. A 74-year-old man stepped off a curb and felt a sharp pain in the left knee. Radiographs obtained on the next day were normal. The pain in the knee subsided after 10 days, but 2 months later joint effusion developed, which was aspirated. He was given a series of three intraarticular injections of steroids (hydrocortisone), after which most of the symptoms subsided. Four months after the initial injury the symptoms recurred, and at this time the standard radiographic examination was repeated. Anteroposterior projection shows a large radiolucent defect surrounded by a zone of sclerosis in the weight-bearing segment of the medial femoral condyle. The lesion represents spontaneous osteonecrosis.

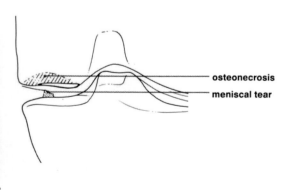

Figure 9.57 Spontaneous osteonecrosis. A 63-year-old woman missed a step while descending the staircase and felt a sharp pain in the left knee. The radiographic examination performed 3 days later showed only moderate osteoporosis, which was not related to trauma. Three months later she was reexamined for persistent pain and accumulation of fluid in the joint. **(A)** Anteroposterior radiograph of the knee shows spontaneous osteonecrosis in the weight-bearing portion of the medial femoral condyle. Double-contrast arthrography was performed to evaluate any possible injury to the menisci. The arthrogram **(B)** demonstrates a vertical tear of the medial meniscus at the site of the osteonecrotic lesion.

Figure 9.58 Normal appearance of suprapatellar bursa. The suprapatellar bursa normally appears on the lateral view of the knee as a radiodense strip just posterior to the quadriceps tendon.

Spontaneous Osteonecrosis. Characterized by acute onset of pain, spontaneous osteonecrosis of the knee is a distinct clinicopathologic entity with a predilection for the weight-bearing segment of the medial femoral condyle. It occurs in older adults, frequently in their sixth and seventh decades of life, and should not be mistaken for adult onset of osteochondritis dissecans. Although the cause is obscure, certain factors such as trauma, intraarticular injection of steroids, and possibly tear of the meniscus, as Norman and Baker have pointed out, may play a role in the pathogenesis of this condition.

The earliest radiologic sign of this condition is an increased uptake of isotope on radionuclide bone scan; radiographically, the earliest indication is a minimal degree of flattening of the femoral condyle (Fig. 9.55). Later, usually 1 to 3 months after the sudden onset of symptoms, radiographs may show a subchondral focus of radiolucency. As the condition progresses, the lesion may be seen radiographically as a subchondral osteolytic (necrotic) focus surrounded by a sclerotic margin representing a zone of repair (Fig. 9.56). Fre-

quently, these lesions are accompanied by meniscal tears and, for this reason, either contrast arthrography or MRI should always be performed if spontaneous osteonecrosis is suspected (Fig. 9.57). Some authors postulate that the concentration of stress of the torn meniscus on the articular cartilage may result in local ischemia, thus predisposing to the development of osteonecrosis.

Injury to the Soft Tissues about the Knee

Knee Joint Effusion. Normally, the suprapatellar bursa is apparent on a radiograph of the knee in the lateral projection as a thin, radiodense strip just posterior to the quadriceps tendon (Fig. 9.58). In knee joint effusion, which often occurs secondary to injury elsewhere in the knee, the suprapatellar bursa fills with fluid. Distention of the bursa is evident radiographically as an oval density that obliterates the fat space anterior to the femoral cortex (Fig. 9.59). If there is an associated intraarticular fracture of either the distal femur or the proximal

posterior suprapatellar fat pad
quadriceps tendon
distended suprapatellar bursa
anterior suprapatellar fat pad
infrapatellar joint compartment
infrapatellar fat pad
patellar ligament

A **B**

Figure 9.59 Knee joint effusion. In knee joint effusion, the suprapatellar bursa distends with fluid, thus obliterating the fat space posterior to the quadriceps tendon. (Modified from Hall FM, 1978, with permission.)

tibia, then a cross-table lateral view may demonstrate the FBI sign (see Fig. 9.26C).

Meniscal Injury. Similar to the other fibrocartilaginous structures, the menisci of the knee (see Fig. 9.9) are not visible on conventional radiographs. Contrast arthrography may demonstrate these structures, although MRI has become a standard procedure for evaluating the menisci.

Tear of the medial meniscus is a common injury resulting from physical and sports-related activities. Various types of tears may be encountered (Fig. 9.60). The most common type is a vertical tear, which may be simple or bucket-handle; horizontal tears usually occur in an older age group. The patient usually reports pain and locking of the knee. On clinical examination, there is tenderness along the medial joint line. On arthrography, meniscal tear is recognized as a projection of positive contrast medium or air into the substance of the meniscus or at its periphery (Fig. 9.61). On MRI, the menisci are seen as structures of uniformly low signal intensity. A meniscal tear is identified by the presence of an increased intrameniscal signal that extends to the surface of this structure (Fig. 9.62). A globular or linear focus of increased signal intensity in the meniscus that does not extend to the surface does not represent a tear. The significance of this finding is still unclear. Stoller, Genant, and Beltran believe that these findings represent an area of hyaline or myxoid degeneration within the substance of the meniscus. These abnormalities, known as type I (round focus) and type II (linear area) meniscal lesions (Fig. 9.63A,B), are not seen on arthroscopic examination of the knee. The true tears are designated as type III and type IV lesions (Fig. 9.63C; see also Fig. 9.62). Occasionally, meniscal tears may be associated with meniscal or parameniscal cysts (Fig. 9.64).

The sensitivity and specificity of MR imaging for diagnosis of meniscal tears is high, ranging from 90% to 95% in most studies. As recently reported by Helms, use of the fat suppression technique increases the dynamic range of signal in the menisci, rendering meniscal tears more conspicuous. A number of signs related to specific types of meniscal tears have been identified. Among the most accurate secondary signs of the bucket-handle tear of the medial meniscus are absence of two consecutive "bow-tie" appearances of this meniscus on sagittal images and the so-called double posterior cruciate ligament

sign. The normal body of the medial meniscus, which is usually approximately 9 to 12 mm in width, should appear at least on two sections on the peripheral sagittal images as a bow tie. The presence of only a single bow-tie configuration indicates a displaced bucket-handle tear into the middle part of the knee joint. On more central sagittal sections, the displaced part of the meniscus assumes a posterior cruciate ligament-like configuration, projecting more anteriorly to the posterior cruciate ligament (Fig. 9.65).

Although meniscal tears are best diagnosed on coronal and sagittal MR images, Lee and colleagues recently pointed out the effectiveness of axial fat-saturated fast-spin-echo imaging in demonstrating some tears. In particular, vertical tears and displaced meniscal fragments have been clearly demonstrated with this technique (Fig. 9.66).

Tears of the lateral meniscus are less common (see Fig. 9.66). This has been attributed to the greater degree of mobility of the lateral meniscus because of its rather loose peripheral attachment to the synovium and lack of attachment to the fibular (lateral) collateral ligament. Lateral meniscal tears, however, commonly accompany a developmental anomaly, the so-called discoid meniscus, which according to Kaplan is probably related to an abnormal attachment of its posterior horn to the tibial plateau and repetitive abnormal movements, with subsequent enlargement and thickening of meniscal tissue. The discoid meniscus is recognized clinically by a loud clicking sound on flexion and extension of the knee joint and radiographically on the anteroposterior radiograph by an abnormally wide lateral joint compartment (Fig. 9.67A). Its arthrographic appearance is characterized by the absence of the normally triangular shape of the structure; the meniscus is thicker and wider and projects more deeply into the joint (Fig. 9.67B). On MRI, the discoid meniscus is similar in appearance to the arthrographic image with a lack of normal triangular shape and deep extension into the interior of the joint. On sagittal images, the normal bow-tie configuration of the body of the lateral meniscus is seen on more than two sections when the discoid variant is present (Figs. 9.68 and 9.69). Because of its abnormal shape and thickness, the lateral discoid meniscus is prone to tears (Fig. 9.70).

Meniscal tears may also be associated with fractures of the tibial plateau resulting from direct trauma. In this case, both menisci are equally subject to injury.

Figure 9.60 Spectrum of meniscal injuries. Meniscal injuries can be broadly classified as longitudinal, horizontal, and radial, depending on the plane in which they occur. The left panel represents diagrammatically the radiologic image of the meniscus; the right panel, various tears.

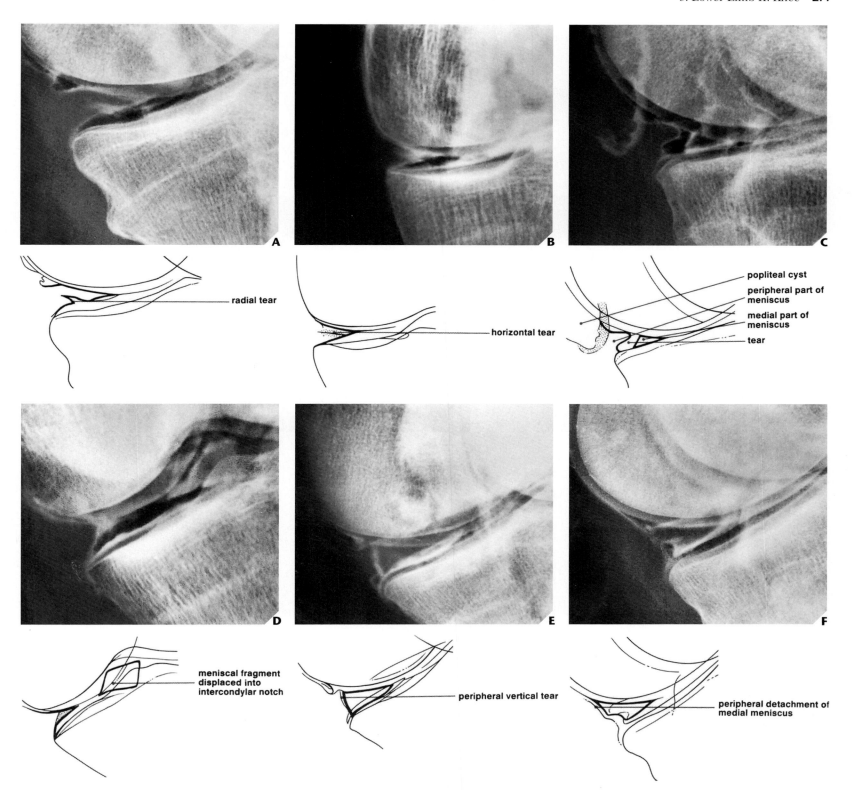

Figure 9.61 Arthrography of the meniscal tears. Arthrographically, meniscal tears are recognized by a projection of contrast medium or air into the substance of the structure or at its periphery. The following spot films demonstrate some of the various types of tears that may affect the medial meniscus: radial (oblique) **(A)** tear of the posterior horn; horizontal **(B)** tear of the body; bucket-handle **(C)** tear of the posterior horn; bucket-handle **(D)** tear of the body with displacement of the fragment into the intercondylar notch; peripheral **(E)** tear of the posterior horn; and peripheral **(F)** detachment of the posterior horn.

Figure 9.62 **Tears of the medial meniscus. (A)** Sagittal spin-echo T1-weighted MR image (SE; TR 700/TE 20 msec) shows a tear of the medial meniscus. Note the high-intensity signal of the tear, which extends into the inferior surface of the meniscus. **(B)** Sagittal T2-weighted MR image (SE; TR 2300/TE 80 msec) shows a tear of the posterior horn of the medial meniscus (*arrow*) extending into the tibial articular surface. **(C)** Sagittal fat-suppressed image obtained after intraarticular administration of a dilute solution of gadopentetate dimeglumine shows a tear of the posterior horn of the medial meniscus.

Figure 9.63 **Meniscal lesions. (A).** Sagittal spin-echo MR image (SE; TR 2000/TE 20 msec) shows a type I lesion of the posterior horn of the medial meniscus. The intrameniscal round lesion does not extend to the articular surface. **(B)** In a type II lesion of the posterior horn of the medial meniscus, the configuration is linear, and as with a type I, the lesion does not extend into the articular surface. **(C)** Schematic representation of various types of meniscal lesions.

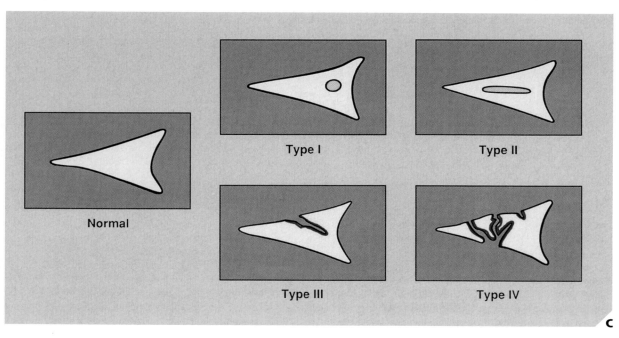

Figure 9.64 Parameniscal cyst. A coronal T2-weighted fat-suppressed MRI shows a tear of the medial meniscus (*arrows*) and a large parameniscal cyst (*curved arrow*).

Figure 9.65 Bucket-handle tear of the medial meniscus. (A) Schematic explanation of absence of the second bow-tie sign of displaced tear (Modified from Helms CA, 2002 with permission). **(B)** Sagittal T2-weighted fat-suppressed MRI shows a "double" posterior cruciate ligament sign. An *arrow* points to the normal posterior cruciate ligament and a *curved arrow* points to the displaced fragment of the medial meniscus that assumed configuration of the posterior cruciate ligament. **(C)** Coronal T2-weighted fat-saturated MR image confirms the presence of a bucket-handle tear of the medial meniscus (*arrows*). A curved arrow points to the medially displaced part of the meniscus. Note also a tear of the medial collateral ligament (*arrowheads*).

Figure 9.66 Tear of the lateral meniscus. (A) An axial fast-spin-echo MRI shows a tear of the posterior horn of the lateral meniscus (*arrow*) in a 38-year-old woman. **(B)** A sagittal MR image confirms the presence of a tear (*arrow*).

Figure 9.67 Arthrography of discoid meniscus. A 20-year-old competition ice skater sustained an injury to her left knee. On physical examination, there was a loud click during movement of the knee joint. **(A)** Anteroposterior view of the knee shows an abnormally wide lateral joint compartment. **(B)** Double-contrast arthrogram demonstrates a discoid meniscus. Note the absence of the normal triangular shape of this structure and its extension deep into the interior of the joint. No tear is apparent.

Figure 9.68 MRI of discoid meniscus. Coronal T1-weighted MR image shows a discoid lateral meniscus in a 17-year-old boy. Note lack of normal triangular shape of this meniscus (*arrows*) and extension into the interior of the joint (*curved arrow*).

Figure 9.69 MRI of discoid meniscus. Coronal **(A)** and sagittal **(B)** T2-weighted fat-suppressed MR images show a discoid lateral meniscus (*arrows*) in an 18-year-old woman.

Figure 9.70 Tear of the discoid meniscus. A 10-year-old boy twisted his right knee during play and experienced severe pain. On physical examination, there was a loud click on flexion–extension of the knee joint. Double-contrast arthrogram demonstrates a tear of the body of a lateral discoid meniscus.

Figure 9.71 **Tear of the medial collateral ligament.** A 24-year-old athlete twisted his knee while throwing the discus during field competition. Physical examination revealed tenderness in the medial aspect of the knee joint and medial instability. **(A)** Anteroposterior radiograph of the knee shows the width of the medial and lateral joint compartments to be normal. **(B)** The same projection obtained after application of valgus stress shows widening of the medial joint compartment, a finding consistent with the clinical diagnosis of tear of the medial collateral ligament. Note also the avulsion of the lateral tibial tubercle, which is occasionally associated with tear of the anterior cruciate ligament.

Ligament and Tendon Injuries. *Tears of the Medial Collateral Ligaments.* The most common injury to the ligaments of the knee is tear of the tibial (medial) collateral ligament. It is diagnosed clinically by instability of the medial joint compartment and radiographically on a stress film of the knee by widening of the medial tibiofemoral joint compartment (Fig. 9.71). It is important to remember that partial or total tear of the medial collateral ligament is almost always associated with tear of the joint capsule, because these two structures are intimately attached to each other.

On arthrographic examination, tear of the medial collateral ligament is characterized by leak of contrast from the joint along its medial aspect (Fig. 9.72). However, in chronic ligament injuries, the leak of contrast may not be demonstrated because the joint capsule has resealed, even though the ligament is disrupted. As the ligament heals, the fibrous tissue may calcify and later ossify, giving a characteristic appearance on the anteroposterior radiograph of the knee known as the Pellegrini-Stieda lesion. The presence of this abnormality is virtually diagnostic of previous tear of the medial collateral ligament (Fig. 9.73; see also Fig. 4.81).

Abnormalities of the medial and lateral collateral ligaments can

be demonstrated effectively with MRI, with coronal T2-weighted sequences being most revealing. These ligamentous injuries are commonly subclassified into three grades. Grade 1 is diagnosed if only a few fibers are disrupted. Grade 2 is diagnosed with disruption of up to 50% of the ligamentous fibers. Grade 3 is a complete tear of the ligament. Sprain of the medial collateral ligament is depicted on MRI as thickening of this structure associated with slightly increased internal signal caused by intraligamentous edema and hemorrhage. Fluid may be present on both sides of the ligament. Partial tear is diagnosed when abnormal increased signal intensity is identified within the ligament substance, extending into the superficial or deep surface. A complete tear exhibits discontinuity of the normally low-signal-intensity ligament structure. It is usually associated with marked thickening and serpentine contours of the affected ligament (Figs. 9.74 and 9.75). The injury to the lateral collateral ligament is best demonstrated on the posterior coronal images. Edema and hemorrhage are seen as ligamentous thickening associated with increased signal intensity on T2-weighted or T2*-weighted images. A complete tear exhibits a wavy contour of the ligament and loss of its continuity (Fig. 9.76).

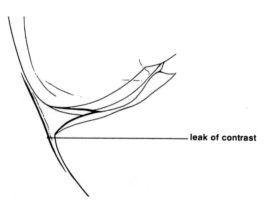

— leak of contrast

Figure 9.72 **Tear of the medial collateral ligament.** A 32-year-old man injured his knee in an automobile accident. Conventional radiographs were unremarkable. Double-contrast arthrogram demonstrates that the medial semilunar cartilage is normal. There is, however, a leak of contrast into the soft tissue along the medial aspect of the joint. This feature is diagnostic of tear of the medial collateral ligament.

Figure 9.73 Pellegrini-Stieda lesion. A 50-year-old man presented with a history of injury, including tear of the medial collateral ligament 3 years previously. Tunnel view of the knee shows the typical appearance of the Pellegrini-Stieda lesion—calcification and ossification at the site of the femoral attachment of the medial collateral ligament (see also Fig. 4.75B).

Tears of the Cruciate Ligaments. Isolated injuries to the cruciate ligaments, which are usually the result of internal rotation of the leg combined with hyperextension, are uncommon. They are more often associated with another ligament injury (usually to the medial collateral ligament) and meniscal tears (usually of the medial meniscus). This association of injuries has been called the "unhappy O'-Donoghue triad." Valgus stress on the knee joint opens the medial joint compartment and may result in tear of the posterior joint capsule as well as the posterior or anterior cruciate ligament. This stress is also responsible for tear of the medial meniscus and medial collateral ligament (Fig. 9.77).

The accuracy of radiographic examinations with respect to injury to the cruciate ligaments has not been completely determined. The standard anteroposterior and lateral radiographs may show a bone fragment, representing the avulsed intercondylar eminence of the tibia, at the site of cruciate insertion (Fig. 9.78). Sometimes, the tear can be diagnosed on double-contrast arthrography, which may demonstrate the posterior cruciate ligament, but not the anterior cruciate ligament—a finding that is regarded as abnormal. This injury is often missed on

Figure 9.75 Grade 3 medial collateral ligament injury. (A) A coronal proton density-weighted (SE; TR 2000/TE 20 msec) image shows amorphous structure of intermediate signal intensity replacing the proximal attachment of the medial collateral ligament (*arrow*). The distal part of the ligament is intact (*curved arrow*). **(B)** A coronal T2-weighted (SE; TR 2000/TE 80 msec) image shows mildly increased signal intensity within the region of the proximal segment of the medial collateral ligament, representing a combination of edema and hemorrhage (*arrow*). The underlying ligament cannot be defined.

imaging examinations that include even the use of arthrotomography and CT. The procedure of choice in these circumstances is MRI.

For MR examination of the anterior cruciate ligament, as Stoller and colleagues advocate, the knee should be placed in 10° to 15° of external rotation to orient the ligament with the sagittal imaging plane. Either 3- or 5-mm thin contiguous sections are routinely obtained in axial, sagittal, and coronal planes. A torn anterior cruciate ligament is demonstrated on MR images by the absence or abnormal course of this structure, abnormal signal intensity within the ligamentous substance, or the presence of an edematous focus (Figs. 9.79 and 9.80). The buckling of the posterior cruciate ligament is an indirect sign of anterior cruciate ligament tear. The best plane to demonstrate these findings is the sagittal plane, and the best pulse sequence is spin-echo T2 weighting or gradient-echo (MPGR) T2* weighting.

Tears of the posterior cruciate ligament are identified on sagittal T1-weighted images by disruption of the integrity of the ligament or by abnormal shape. On T2-weighted images, the tear is demonstrated by the presence of high signal intensity within the ligament, which represents fluid within the tear (Fig. 9.81). As Bassett and coworkers

Figure 9.74 Grade 1 medial collateral ligament injury. A coronal T2-weighted (SE; TR 2000/TE 80 msec) image shows a band of increased signal intensity (*arrows*) representing fluid medially to the intact tibial collateral ligament.

Figure 9.76 Tear of the lateral collateral ligament. Tear of the lateral collateral ligament (*arrows*) can be seen on **(A)** T1-weighted and **(B)** T2*-weighted coronal images.

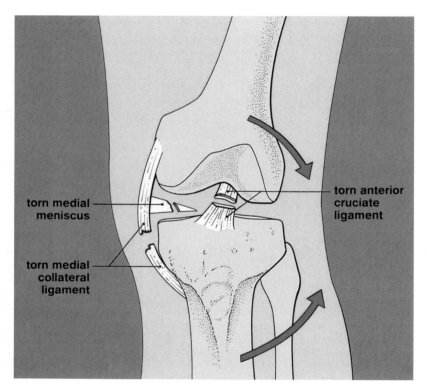

torn medial meniscus

torn medial collateral ligament

torn anterior cruciate ligament

Figure 9.77 Triad of meniscoligamentous injury. The "unhappy O'-Donoghue triad" results from valgus stress on the knee joint that causes the medial joint compartment to open. The triad comprises tears of the medial meniscus and the anterior cruciate and the medial collateral ligaments. (Modified from O'Donoghue DH, 1984, with permission.)

Figure 9.78 Tear of the anterior cruciate ligament. Anteroposterior **(A)** and lateral **(B)** films of the knee in a 38-year-old soccer player show avulsion of the tibial eminence, suggesting tear of the anterior cruciate ligament. The diagnosis was confirmed by arthroscopy.

Figure 9.79 Tear of the anterior cruciate ligament. Sagittal spin-echo T2-weighted MR image (SE; TR 2000/TE 80 msec) shows a tear of the anterior cruciate ligament. Only the proximal part of the ligament at the femoral attachment is well seen. The distal half shows lack of normal low signal intensity caused by swelling and edema (compare with Fig. 9.14A). Arthroscopic examination demonstrated an acute tear of the anterior cruciate ligament at its insertion to the tibia.

Figure 9.80 Tear of the anterior cruciate ligament. (A) Sagittal T1-weighted image shows loss of normal contour of the proximal part of the anterior cruciate ligament (*arrow*). **(B)** Sagittal T2*-weighted image shows hyperintense signal representing hemorrhage within an anterior cruciate ligament at its lateral condylar attachment (*arrow*), characteristic of a ligamentous tear.

Figure 9.81 Tear of the posterior cruciate ligament. (A) Sagittal T1-weighted image shows complete tear of the posterior cruciate ligament. *Open arrow,* area of hemorrhage; *solid arrows,* ligament discontinuity. **(B)** Sagittal T2*-weighted image shows a posterior cruciate ligament tear with edema and hemorrhage (*curved arrow*). The interface between cartilage (*small arrows*) and fluid (*large arrow*) is well demonstrated.

Figure 9.82 Tear of the quadriceps tendon. A 30-year-old man was injured during a football game. Lateral film of the knee shows lack of definition of the quadriceps tendon and the presence of a soft-tissue mass in the suprapatellar region—findings characteristic of quadriceps tendon rupture.

Figure 9.83 Tear of the quadriceps tendon. A lateral radiograph of the knee shows low position of the patella (patella baja) secondary to chronic tear of the quadriceps tendon.

Figure 9.84 Patellar ligamentous-tendinous attachments. Normally, the balance of forces on the patellar ligamentous-tendinous attachments maintains the patella in position (**A**). Tear of the quadriceps tendon causes downward displacement of the patella (**B**). In tear of the patellar ligament, the reverse mechanism occurs (**C**) (see also Fig. 9.3).

Figure 9.85 Tear of the patellar ligament. A 38-year-old woman athlete was injured during a running competition. Anteroposterior **(A)** and lateral **(B)** radiographs of the knee demonstrate an abnormally high position of the patella (patella alta), a finding suggesting tear of the patellar ligament. The diagnosis was confirmed on surgical exploration.

have pointed out, evulsion of the ligament from its tibial attachment is identified on MR images by bone fracture of the posterior tibial plateau and redundancy of the ligament.

Tears of the Quadriceps Tendon and Patellar Ligament. Although ruptures of the quadriceps tendon usually occur in the elderly, they may at times be seen in athletes. A lateral radiograph of the knee may show lack of definition of the quadriceps tendon and widen-ing of its anteroposterior diameter secondary to hemorrhage and edema (Fig. 9.82). Occasionally, the lateral film may also show the patella in a lower-than-normal position secondary to an imbalance in forces on the patellar ligamentous attachments (Fig. 9.83); in tear of the patellar ligament, the reverse of this mechanism occurs (Figs. 9.84 and 9.85). MRI is the procedure of choice for demonstrating and evaluating this injury (Fig. 9.86)

Figure 9.86 Tears of the quadriceps tendon and patellar ligament. **(A)** Sagittal spin-echo proton density MR image (SE; TR 2000/TE 20 msec) shows partial rupture of the quadriceps tendon, represented by edema and hemorrhage (intermediate signal intensity) between the tendon fibers (low signal intensity) *(arrow)*. **(B)** Sagittal spin-echo proton density MR image (SE; TR 2000/TE 20 msec) demonstrates evulsion of the patellar ligament at the insertion into the tibial tuberosity *(arrow)*. (From Beltran J, 1990, with permission.)

PRACTICAL POINTS TO REMEMBER

[1] The posterior aspect of the femoral condyles and the inter-condylar notch are best shown on the tunnel projection of the knee.

[2] Merchant axial projection of the patella, rather than the standard sunrise view, is better suited to evaluate:
- the articular facets of the patellofemoral joint
- subtle patellar subluxations.

[3] In arthrographic examination of the menisci, be aware of:
- the popliteal hiatus at the posterior horn of the lateral meniscus, which is a normal feature that may be confused with a tear
- a blind spot involving the posterior portion of the posterior horn of the lateral meniscus, where a tear can be overlooked.

[4] CT is very effective in assessing depressed and split fractures of tibial plateau and in demonstrating the extent of fracture comminution.

[5] MRI is the modality of choice to evaluate soft-tissue injury around the knee, in particular to the menisci and the cruciate and collateral ligaments. It is also the best modality to image posttraumatic joint effusion, acute and chronic hematomas, and other traumatic abnormalities of the muscular, ligamentous, and tendinous structures.

[6] Tibial plateau fractures are often accompanied by meniscal tear and ligament injury, best demonstrated by MRI.

[7] Segond fracture is a small-fragment avulsion fracture from the lateral aspect of the proximal tibia that frequently is associated with a capsular tear, tear of the anterior cruciate ligament, and tear of the lateral meniscus.

[8] The bipartite or multipartite patella may mimic patellar fracture. To avoid misdiagnosing these developmental anomalies as a fracture, remember that:
- the bipartite or multipartite patella is seen at the superolateral margin of the patella
- the apparent comminuted fragments do not form a whole, as they would in patellar fracture.

[9] Sinding-Larsen-Johansson and Osgood-Schlatter diseases are conditions related to trauma. In both entities, soft-tissue swelling on clinical examination and imaging studies is a fundamental diagnostic feature.

[10] Learn to distinguish three conditions that have very similar radiologic presentations:
- osteochondral fracture, which is an acute injury to the articular cartilage and subchondral bone
- osteochondritis dissecans, which is the result of chronic injury
- spontaneous osteonecrosis, which is characterized by acute onset of pain and has been linked to trauma, corticosteroid injections, and meniscal tear.

    Contrast arthrography, arthrotomography, computed arthrotomography, and MRI are essential techniques in the evaluation of the status of the articular cartilage in each of these conditions.

[11] Tears of the menisci and ligaments of the knee are best demonstrated by MRI. Tears of the medial meniscus are much more common than tears of the lateral semilunar cartilage. The discoid lateral meniscus predisposes this structure to injury.

[12] Bucket-handle tear of the medial meniscus has characteristic MRI appearance:
- on sagittal sections through the body of the medial meniscus, there is only one image of the bow-tie sign
- on more lateral sagittal sections obtained closer to the interior of the knee joint, a double PCL sign may be seen.

[13] Discoid meniscus has characteristic MRI appearance:
- on coronal sections, there is lack of normal triangular shape and deep extension of the meniscus into the interior of the joint
- on sagittal sections through the body of the lateral meniscus, there are more than two images of bow-tie configuration of this structure.

[14] The "unhappy O'Donoghue triad," resulting from valgus stress forces applied to the knee joint, consists of tears of the:
- medial meniscus
- medial collateral ligament
- anterior cruciate ligament.

[15] High position of the patella (patella alta) may indicate a tear of the patellar ligament; low position of the patella (patella baja) may indicate a tear of the quadriceps tendon.

SUGGESTED READINGS

Ahlback S, Bauer GCH, Bohne WH. Spontaneous osteonecrosis of the knee. *Arthritis Rheum* 1968;11:705–733.

Aichroth P. Osteochondritis dissecans of the knee: a clinical survey. *J Bone Joint Surg [Br]* 1971;53B:440–447.

Aichroth P. Osteochondral fractures and their relationship to osteochondritis dissecans of the knee. *J Bone Joint Surg [Br]* 1971;53B:448–454.

Alparslan L, Winalski CS, Boutin RD, Minas T. Postoperative magnetic resonance imaging of articular cartilage repair. *Semin Musculoskelet Radiol* 2001;5:345–363

Anderson SE, Bosshard C, Steinbach LS, Ballmer FT. MR imaging of calcification of the lateral collateral ligament of the knee: a rare abnormality and a cause of lateral knee pain. *AJR Am J Roentgenol* 2003;181:199–202.

Anderson MW, Raghavan N, Seidenwurm DJ, Greenspan A, Drake C. Evaluation of meniscal tears: fast spin-echo versus conventional spin-echo magnetic resonance imaging. *Acad Radiol* 1995;2:209–214.

Apley AG. Fractures of the tibial plateau. *Orthop Clin North Am* 1979;10:61–74.

Applegate GR, Flannigan BD, Tolin BS, Fox JM, Del Pizzo W. MR diagnosis of recurrent tears in the knee: value of intraarticular contrast material. *AJR Am J Roentgenol* 1993;161:821–825.

Araki Y, Yamamoto H, Nakamura H, Tsukaguchi I. MR diagnosis of discoid lateral menisci of the knee. *Eur J Radiol* 1994;18:92–95.

Arger PH, Oberkircher PE, Miller WT. Lipohemarthrosis. *AJR Am J Roentgenol* 1974;121:97–100.

Arnoczky S. Anatomy of the anterior cruciate ligament. *Clin Orthop* 1983;172:19–25.

Auge WK, Kaeding CC. Bilateral discoid medial menisci with extensive intrasubstance cleavage tears: MRI and arthroscopic correlation. *Arthroscopy* 1994;10:313–318.

Bassett LW, Grover JS, Seeger LL. Magnetic resonance imaging of knee trauma. *Skeletal Radiol* 1990;19:401–405.

Beltran J. *MRI: musculoskeletal system.* Philadelphia: JB Lippincott; 1990.

Berlin RC, Levinsohn EM, Chrisman H. The wrinkled patellar tendon: an indication of abnormality in the extensor mechanism of the knee. *Skeletal Radiol* 1991;20:181–185.

Berquist TH. *Imaging of orthopedic trauma,* 2nd ed. New York: Raven Press; 1991.

Berquist TH. *Magnetic resonance imaging of the musculoskeletal system.* New York: Raven Press; 1990.

Bessette GC, Hunter RE. The anterior cruciate ligament. *Orthopedics* 1990;13:551–562.

Bianchi S, Zwass A, Abdelwahab IF, Banderali A. Diagnosis of tears of the quadriceps tendon of the knee: value of sonography. *AJR Am J Roentgenol* 1994;162:1137–1140.

Blackburne JS, Peel TE. A new method of measuring patellar height. *J Bone Joint Surg [Br]* 1977;59B:241–242.

Blankenbaker DG, De Smet AA, Smith JD. Usefulness of two indirect MR imaging signs to diagnose lateral meniscal tears. *AJR Am J Roentgenol* 2002;178:579–582.

Bock GW, Bosch E, Mishra DK, Daniel DM, Resnick D. The healed Segond fracture: a characteristic residual bone excrescence. *Skeletal Radiol* 1994;23:555–556.

Bodne D, Quinn SF, Murray WT, et al. Magnetic resonance images of chronic patellas tendonitis. *Skeletal Radiol* 1988;17:24–28.

Boeree NR, Watkinson AF, Ackroyd CE, Johnson C. Magnetic resonance imaging of meniscal and cruciate injuries of the knee. *J Bone Joint Surg [Br]* 1991;73B:452–457.

Bonamo JJ, Saperstein AL. Contemporary magnetic resonance imaging of the knee: the orthopedic surgeon's perspective. *Magn Reson Imaging Clin North Am* 1994;2:481–495.

Bouffard JA, Dhanju J. Ultrasonography of the knee. *Semin Musculoskeletal Radiol* 1998;2:245–270.

Boutin RD, Januario JA, Newberg AH, Gundry CR, Newman JS. MR imaging features of osteochondritis dissecans of the femoral sulcus. *AJR Am J Roentgenol* 2003;108:641–645.

Brandser EA, Riley MA, Berbaum KS, El-Khoury GY, Bennet DL. MR imaging of anterior cruciate ligament injury: independent value of primary and secondary signs. *AJR Am J Roentgenol* 1996;167:121–126.

Brantigan OC, Voshell AF. Ligaments of the knee joint: the relationship of the ligament of Humphry to the ligament of Wrisberg. *J Bone Joint Surg [Br]* 1946B;28:66–67.

Brown DW, Allman FL Jr, Eaton SB. Knee arthrography: a comparison of radiographic and surgical findings in 295 cases. *Am J Sports Med* 1978;6:165–172.

Buckwalter KA, Pennes DR. Anterior cruciate ligament: oblique sagittal MR imaging. *Radiology* 1990;175:276–277.

Burger RS, Larson RL. Acute ligamentous injury. In: Larson RL, Grana WA, eds. *The knee: form, function, pathology, and treatment.* Philadelphia: WB Saunders; 1993:513–598.

Burk DL Jr, Mitchell DG, Rifkin MD, Vinitski S. Recent advances in magnetic resonance imaging of the knee. *Radiol Clin North Am* 1990;28:379–393.

Campbell SE, Sanders TG, Morrison WB. MR imaging of meniscal cysts: incidence, location, and clinical significance. *AJR Am J Roentgenol* 2001;177:409–413.

Campos JC, Chung CB, Lektrakul N, Pedowitz R, Trudell D, Yu J, Resnick D. Pathogenesis of the Segond fracture: anatomic and MR imaging evidence of an iliotibial tract or anterior band avulsion. *Radiology* 2001;219:381–386.

Capps GW, Hayes CW. Easily missed injuries around the knee. *Radiographics* 1994;14:1191–1210.

Carson WG, James SL, Larson RL, Singer KM, Winternitz WW. Patellofemoral disorders: physical and radiographic evaluation. II. Radiographic examination. *Clin Orthop* 1984;185:178–186.

Chan WP, Peterfy C, Fritz RC, Genant HK. MR Diagnosis of complete tears of the anterior cruciate ligament of the knee: importance of anterior subluxation of the tibia. *AJR Am J Roentgenol* 1994;162:355–360.

Cheung LP, Li KCP, Hollett MD, Bergman AG, Herfkens RJ. Meniscal tears of the knee: accuracy of detection with fast spin-echo MR imaging and arthroscopic correlation in 293 patients. *Radiology* 1997;203:508–512.

Cobby MJ, Schweitzer ME, Resnick D. The deep lateral femoral notch: an indirect sign of a torn anterior cruciate ligament. *Radiology* 1992;184:855–858.

Connolly B, Babyn PS, Wright JG, Thorner PS. Discoid meniscus in children: magnetic resonance imaging characteristics. *Can Assoc Radiol J* 1996;47:347–354.

Coumas JM, Palmer WE. Knee arthrography. Evolution and current status. *Radiol Clin North Am* 1998;36:703–728.

Cross MJ, Waldrop J. The patella index as a guide to the understanding and diagnosis of patello-femoral instability. *Clin Orthop* 1975;110:174–176.

Crotty JM, Monu JU, Pope TJ. Magnetic resonance imaging of the musculoskeletal system. IV. The knee. *Clin Orthop* 1996;330:288–303.

Crues JV III, Mink J, Levy TL, Lotysch M, Stoller DW. Meniscal tears of the knee: accuracy of MR imaging. *Radiology* 1987;164:445–448.

Crues JV III, Ryu R. Knee. In: Stark DD, Bradley WG Jr (eds). *Magnetic Resonance Imaging*. St. Louis: Mosby Year Book; 1992:2355–2423.

Crues JV, Ryu R, Morgan FW. Meniscal pathology: the expanding role of magnetic resonance imaging. *Clin Orthop* 1990;252:80–87.

Crues JV III, Stoller DW. The menisci. In: Mink J, Reicher MA, Crues JV III, Deutsch L (eds). *MR Imaging of the Knee*, 2nd ed. New York, Raven; 1993:91–140.

D'Ambrosia, RD, MacDonald GL. Pitfalls in the diagnosis of Osgood-Schlatter disease. *Clin Orthop* 1975;110:206–209.

Daffner RH, Riemer BL, Lupetin AR, Dash N. Magnetic resonance imaging in acute tendon rupture. *Skeletal Radiol* 1986;15:619–621.

Dalinka MK. Knee arthrography. In: Dalinka MK (ed). *Arthrography*. New York, Springer-Verlag; 1980:1–88.

DeFlaviis L, Nessi R, Scaglione P, Balconi G, Albisetti W, Derchi LE. Ultrasonic diagnosis of Osgood-Schlatter and Sinding-Larson-Johansson disease of the knee. *Skeletal Radiol* 1989;18:193–197.

Delamarter RB, Hohl M, Hopp E. Ligament injuries associated with tibial plateau fractures. *Clin Orthop* 1990;250:226–233.

De Smet A, Graf BK. Meniscal tears missed on MR imaging: relationship to meniscal tear patterns and anterior cruciate ligament tears. *Am J Roentgenol* 1994;162:905–911.

De Smet AA, Fisher DR, Graf BK, Lange RH. Osteochondritis dissecans of the knee: value of MR imaging in determining lesion stabilization and presence of articular cartilage defects. *Am J Roentgenol* 1990;155:549–553.

DeSmet AA, Ilahi OA, Graf BK. Reassessment of the MR criteria for stability of osteochondritis dissecans in the knee and ankle. *Skeletal Radiol* 1996;25:159–163.

De Smet AA, Tuite MJ, Norris MA, Swan JS. MR diagnosis of meniscal tears: analysis of causes of errors. *AJR Am J Roentgenol* 1994;163:1419–1423.

Deutsch AD, Shellock FG, Mink JH. Imaging of the patellofemoral joint: emphasis on advanced techniques. In: Fox J, Del Pizzo W, eds. *The patellofemoral joint*. New York: McGraw-Hill; 1993.

Dietz GW, Wilcox DM, Montgomery JB. Segond tibial condylar fracture: lateral capsular ligament avulsion. *Radiology* 1986;159:467–469.

Dumas J, Edde DJ. Meniscal abnormalities: prospective correlation of double-contrast arthrography and arthroscopy. *Radiology* 1986;160:453–456.

Elstrom J, Pankovich AM, Sassoon H, Rodriguez J. The use of tomography in assessment of fractures of the tibial plateau. *J Bone Joint Surg [Am]* 1976;58A:551–555.

Eqund N. The axial view of the patellofemoral joint. *Acta Radiol Diagn* 1986;27:101–104.

Erickson SJ, Cox IH, Correra GF, Strandt JA, Estokowski LD. Effect of tendon orientation on MR imaging signal intensity: a manifestation of the "magic angle" phenomenon. *Radiology* 1991;181:389–392.

Escobedo EM, Mills WJ, Hunter JC. The "reverse Segond" fracture: association with a tear of the posterior cruciate ligament and medial meniscus. *AJR Am J Roentgenol* 2002;178:979–983.

Eustace S, Hentzen P, Adams J, Harper K, Jara H. Comparison of conventional and turbo spin-echo T1-weighted MR imaging in acute knee trauma. *AJR Am J Roentgenol* 1999;172:1393–1395.

Fairclough JA, Johnson SR. Ski injuries, the significance of flake fractures. *Injury* 1988;19:79–80.

Farley TE, Howell SM, Love KF, Wolfe RD, Neumann CH. Meniscal tears: MR and arthrographic findings after arthroscopic repair. *Radiology* 1991;180:517–522.

Fayad LM, Parellada JA, Parker L, Schweitzer ME. MR imaging of anterior cruciate ligament tears: is there a gender gap? *Skeletal Radiol* 2003;32:639–646.

Ficat RP, Hungerford DS. *Disorders of the patellofemoral joint*. Baltimore: Williams & Wilkins; 1977.

Firooznia H. Knee. In: Firooznia H, Golimbu CN, Rafii M, Rauschning W, Weinreb JC,

eds. *MRI and CT of the musculoskeletal system*. St. Louis: Mosby-Year Book; 1992:661–797.

Firooznia H, Golimbu C, Rafii M. MR imaging of the menisci: fundamentals of anatomy and pathology. *Magn Reson Imaging Clin North Am* 1994;2:325–347.

Fischer SP, Fox JM, Pizzo WD, Friedman MJ, Snyder SJ, Ferkel RD. Accuracy of diagnoses from magnetic resonance imaging of the knee: a multi-center analysis of one thousand and fourteen patients. *J Bone Joint Surg [Am]* 1991;73A:2–10.

Fitzgerald SW, Remer EM, Friedman H, Rogers LF, Hendrix RW, Schafer MF. MR evaluation of the anterior cruciate ligament: value of supplementing sagittal images with coronal and axial images. *AJR Am J Roentgenol* 1993;160:1233–1237.

Franklin JL, Rosenberg TD, Paulos LE, France EP. Radiographic assessment of instability of the knee due to rupture of the anterior cruciate ligament. *J Bone Joint Surg [Am]* 1991;73A:365–372.

Freiberger RH. Meniscal abnormalities. In: Freiberger RH, Kaye JJ, eds. *Arthrography*. New York: Appleton-Century-Crofts; 1979:55–91.

Freiberger RH. Technique of knee arthrography. In: Freiberger RH, Kaye JJ, eds. *Arthrography*. New York: Appleton-Century-Crofts; 1979:5–30.

Freiberger RH, Pavlov H. Knee arthrography. *Radiology* 1988;166:489–492.

Friedman RL, Jackson DW. Magnetic resonance imaging of the anterior cruciate ligament: current concepts. *Orthopedics* 1996;19:525–532.

Fulkerson JP, Hungerford DS. *Disorders of the patellofemoral joint,* 2nd ed. Baltimore: Williams & Wilkins; 1990.

Gentili A, Seeger LL, Yao L, Do HM. Anterior cruciate ligament tear: indirect signs at MR imaging. *Radiology* 1994;193:835–840.

Gilley JS, Gelman MI, Edson DM, Metcalf RW. Chondral fractures of the knee: Arthrographic, arthroscopic, and clinical manifestations. *Radiology* 1981;138:51–54.

Girgis FG, Marshall JL, Al Monajem ARS. The cruciate ligaments of the knee joint: anatomical, functional and experimental analysis. *Clin Orthop* 1975;106:216–231.

Goldman AB, Pavlov H, Rubinstein D. The Segond fracture of the proximal tibia: a small avulsion fracture that reflects ligamentous damage. *AJR Am J Roentgenol* 1988;151:1163–1167.

Graf BK, Cook DA, De Smet AA, Keene JS. "Bone bruises" on magnetic resonance imaging evaluation of anterior cruciate ligament injuries. *Am J Sports Med* 1993;21:220–223.

Grelsamer RP, Meadows S. The modified Insall-Salvati ratio for assessment of patellar height. *Clin Orthop* 1992;282:170–176.

Grelsamer RP, Proctor CS, Bazos AN. Evaluation of patellar shape in the sagittal plane: a clinical analysis. *Am J Sports Med* 1994;22:61–66.

Grover JS, Bassett LW, Gross ML, Seeger LL, Finerman GAM. Posterior cruciate ligament: MR imaging. *Radiology* 1990;174:527–530.

Ha TPT, Li KCP, Beaulieu CF, et al. Anterior cruciate ligament injury: fast spin-echo MR imaging with arthroscopic correlation in 217 examinations. *AJR Am J Roentgenol* 1998;170:1215–1219.

Haims AH, Katz LD, Ruwe PA. MR arthrography of the knee. *Semin Musculoskel Radiol* 1998;2:385–395.

Haims AH, Medvecky MJ, Pavlovich R, Jr, Katz LD. MR imaging of the anatomy of and injuries to the lateral and posterolateral aspects of the knee. *AJR Am J Roentgenol* 2003;180:647–653.

Hall FJ. Arthrography of the discoid lateral meniscus. *AJR Am J Roentgenol* 1977;128:993–1002.

Hall FM. Radiographic diagnosis and accuracy in knee joint effusions. *Radiology* 1975;115:49–54.

Hall FM, Hochman MG. Medial Segond-type fracture: cortical avulsion of the medial tibial plateau associated with tears of the posterior cruciate ligament and medial meniscus. *Skeletal Radiol* 1997;26:553–555.

Hall M. Tibial condylar fractures. *J Bone Joint Surg [Am]* 1967;49A:1455–1567.

Hamada M, Shino K, Kawano K, Araki Y, Matsui Y, Doi T. Usefulness of magnetic resonance imaging for detecting intrasubstance tear and/or degeneration of lateral discoid meniscus. *Arthroscopy* 1994;10:645–653.

Haramati N, Staron RB, Cushin S, Nickoloff EL, Feldman F. Value of the coronal plane in MRI of internal derangement of the knee. *Skeletal Radiol* 1994;23:211–215.

Haramati N, Staron RB, Rubin S, Shreck EH, Feldman F, Kiernan H. The flipped meniscus sign. *Skeletal Radiol* 1993;22:273–277.

Harley JD. An anatomic arthrographic study of the relationships of the lateral meniscus and the popliteus tendon. *AJR Am J Roentgenol* 1977;128:181–187.

Harris RD, Hecht HL. Suprapatellar effusions: a new diagnostic sign. *Radiology* 1970;97:1–4.

Hayes CW, Conway WF. Magnetic resonance imaging of miscellaneous knee joint disorders. In: Bloem JL, Sartoris DJ, eds. *MRI and CT of the musculoskeletal system. A textatlas*. Baltimore: Williams & Wilkins; 1992:442–471.

Heller L, Langman J. The meniscofemoral ligaments of the human knee. *J Bone Joint Surg [Br]* 1964;46B:307–313.

Helms CA. The meniscus: recent advances in MR imaging of the knee. *AJR Am J Roentgenol* 2002;179:1115–1122.

Helms CA, Laorr A, Cannon WD Jr. The absent bow tie sign in bucket-handle tears of the menisci in the knee. *AJR Am J Roentgenol* 1998;170:57–61.

Hess T, Rupp S, Hopf T, Gleitz M, Liebler J. Lateral tibial avulsion fractures and disruptions to the anterior cruciate ligament. A clinical study of their incidence and correlation. *Clin Orthop* 1994;303:193–197.

Hodler J, Haghighi P, Trudell D, Resnick D. The cruciate ligaments of the knee: correlation between MR appearance and gross and histologic findings in cadaveric specimens. *AJR Am J Roentgenol* 1992;159:357–360.

Hohl M. Tibial condylar fractures. *J Bone Joint Surg [Am]* 1967;49A:1455–1467.

Hughston JC, Hergenroeder PT, Courtenay BG. Osteochondritis dissecans of the femoral condyles. *J Bone Joint Surg [Am]* 1984;66A:1340–1348.

Inoue M, Shino K, Hirose H, Horibi S, Ono K. Subluxation of the patella: computed tomography of patellofemoral congruence. *J Bone Joint Surg [Am]* 1988;70A:1331–1337.

Insall J, Salvatti E. Patella position in the normal knee joint. *Radiology* 1971;101:101–104.

Jee W-H, McCauley TR, Kim J-M, Jun DJ, Lee-Y-J, Choi B-G, Choi K-H. Meniscal tear configurations: categorization with MR imaging. *AJR Am J Roentgenol* 2003;180:93–97.

Jensen DB, Johansen TP, Berg-Nielsen A, Henriksen O. Magnetic resonance imaging in evaluation of the sequelae of tibial plateau fractures. *Skeletal Radiol* 1990;19:127–129.

Justice WW, Quinn SF. Error patterns in the MR imaging evaluation of menisci of the knee. *Radiology* 1995;196:617–621.

Kang HS, Resnick D. *MRI of the extremities: an anatomic atlas.* Philadelphia: WB Saunders; 1991.

Kaplan EB. Discoid lateral meniscus of the knee joint. *J Bone Joint Surg [Am]* 1957;39A:77–87.

Kaplan PA, Nelson NL, Garvin KL, Brown DE. MR of the knee: the significance of high signal in the meniscus that does not clearly extend to the surface. *AJR Am J Roentgenol* 1991;156:333–336.

Kaplan PA, Walker CW, Kilcoyne RF, Brown DE, Tusek D, Dussault RG. Occult fracture patterns of the knee associated with anterior cruciate ligament tears: assessment with MR imaging. *Radiology* 1992;183:835–838.

Kaye JJ. Anatomy and arthrography of the normal menisci. In: Freiberger RH, Kaye JJ, eds. *Arthrography.* New York: Appleton-Century-Crofts; 1979:31–53.

Kirsch MD, Fitzgerald SW, Friedman H, Rogers LF. Transient patellar dislocation: diagnosis with MR imaging. *AJR Am J Roentgenol* 1993;161:109–113.

Kode L, Lieberman JM, Motta AO, Wilber JH, Vasen A, Yagan R. Evaluation of tibial plateau fractures: efficacy of MR imaging compared with CT. *AJR Am J Roentgenol* 1994;163:141–147.

Krause BL, Williams JP, Catterall A. Natural history of Osgood-Schlatter disease. *J Pediatr Orthop* 1990;10:65–68.

Kriegsman J. Negative MRI findings in knee injury: clinical implications. *Contemp Orthop* 1991;22:549–555.

Lancourt JE, Cristini JA. Patella alta and patella infera: their etiological role in patellar dislocation, chondromalacia, and apophysitis of the tibial tubercle. *J Bone Joint Surg [Am]* 1975;57A:1112–1115.

Laurin CA, Dussault R, Levesque HP. The tangential x-ray investigation of the patellofemoral joint: x-ray technique, diagnostic criteria and their interpretation. *Clin Orthop* 1979;144:16–26.

Laurin CA, Levesque HP, Dussault R, Labille H, Peides JP. The abnormal lateral patellofemoral angle. *J Bone Joint Surg [Am]* 1978;60A:55–60.

Lecas LK, Helms CA, Kosarek FJ, Garrett WE. Inferiorly displaced flap tears of the medial meniscus: MR appearance and clinical significance. *AJR Am J Roentgenol* 2003;32:619–627.

Lee J. Papakonstantinou O, Brookenthal KR, Trudell D, Resnick DL. Arcuate sign of posterolateral knee injuries: anatomic, radiographic, and MR imaging data related to patterns of injury. *Skeletal Radiol* 2003;32:619–627.

Lee J, Weissman B, Nikpoor N, Aliabodi P, Sosman JL. Lipohemarthrosis of the knee: a review of recent experiences. *Radiology* 1989;173:189–191.

Lee JHE, Singh TT, Bolton G. Axial fat-saturated FSE imaging of the knee: appearance of meniscal tears. *Skeletal Radiol* 2002;31:384–395.

Lerman J, Gray D, Schweitzer M, Bartolozzi A. MR evaluation of the anterior cruciate ligament: value of axial images. *J Comput Assist Tomogr* 1995;19:604–607.

Linden B. The incidence of osteochondritis dissecans in the condyles of the femur. *Acta Orthop Scand* 1976;47:6640–667.

Liu SH, Osti L, Henry M, Bocchi L. The diagnosis of acute complete tears of the anterior cruciate ligament: comparison of MRI, arthrometry and clinical examinations. *J Bone Joint Surg [Br]* 1995;77B:586–588.

Lotke PA, Ecker ML. Current concept review. Osteonecrosis of the knee. *J Bone Joint Surg [Am]* 1988;70A:470–473.

Lotke PA, Ecker ML. Osteonecrosis of the medial tibial plateau. *Contemp Orthop* 1985;10:47.

Lugo-Olivieri CH, Scott WW Jr, Zerhouni EA. Fluid-fluid levels in injured knees: do they always represent lipohemarthrosis? *Radiology* 1996;198:499–502.

Main WK, Scott WN. Knee anatomy. In: Scott WN, ed. *Ligament and extensor mechanism injuries of the knee: diagnosis and treatment.* St. Louis: Mosby–Year Book; 1991;13:32.

McCauley TR, Moses M, Kier R, Lynch JK, Barton JW, Joki P. MR diagnosis of tears of anterior cruciate ligament of the knee: importance of ancillary findings. *AJR Am J Roentgenol* 1994;162:115–119.

Medlar RC, Lynce ED. Sinding-Larsen-Johansson disease. Its etiology and natural history. *J Bone Joint Surg [Am]* 1978;60A:1113–1116.

Merchant AC, Mercer RL, Jacobsen RH, Cool CR. Roentgenographic analysis of patellofemoral congruence. *J Bone Joint Surg [Am]* 1974;56A:1391–1396.

Mesgarzadeh M, Moyer R, Leder DS, et al. MR imaging of the knee: expanded classification and pitfalls to interpretation of meniscal tears. *Radiographics* 1993;13:489–500.

Middleton WD, Lawson TL. *Anatomy and MRI of the joints: a multiplanar atlas.* New York: Raven Press; 1989.

Milgram JW. Radiological and pathological manifestations of osteochondritis dissecans of the distal femur: a study of 50 cases. *Radiology* 1978;126:305–311.

Miller TT, Gladden P, Staron RB, Henry JH, Feldman F. Posterolateral stabilizers of the knee: anatomy and injuries assessed with MR imaging. *AJR Am J Roentgenol* 1997;169:1641–1647.

Miller TT, Staron RB, Feldman F. Patellar height on sagittal MR imaging of the knee. *AJR Am J Roentgenol* 1996;167:339–341.

Mink JH, Deutsch AL. Occult cartilage and bone injuries of the knee: detection, classification, and assessment with MR imaging. *Radiology* 1989;170:823–829.

Mink JH, Deutsch AL. The knee. In: Mink JH, Deutsch AL, eds. *MRI of the musculoskeletal system: a teaching file.* New York: Raven Press; 1990:251–387.

Mink JH, Levy T, Crues JV III. Tears of the anterior cruciate ligament and menisci of the knee: MR imaging evaluation. *Radiology* 1988;167:769–774.

Mink JH, Reicher MA, Crues JV III, Deutsch AL. *MR imaging of the knee,* 2nd ed. New York: Raven Press; 1993.

Moore TM, Harvey JP Jr. Roentgenographic measurement of tibial-plateau depression due to fracture. *J Bone Joint Surg [Am]* 1974;56:155–160.

Muheim G, Bohne WH. Prognosis in spontaneous osteonecrosis of the knee. Investigation by radionuclide scintimetry and radiography. *J Bone Joint Surg [Br]* 1970;52B:605–612.

Murphy BJ, Smith RL, Uribe J, Janecki CJ, Hechtman KS, Mangasarian RA. Bone signal abnormalities in the posterolateral tibia and lateral femoral condyle in complete tears of the anterior cruciate ligament: a specific sign? *Radiology* 1992;182:221–224.

Nachlas IW, Olpp JL. Para-articular calcification (Pellegrini-Stieda) in affections of the knee. *Surg Gynecol Obstet* 1945;81:206–212.

Nance EP Jr, Kaye JJ. Injuries of the quadriceps mechanism. *Radiology* 1982;142:301–307.

Nathan PA, Cole SC. Discoid meniscus: a clinical and pathologic study. *Clin Orthop* 1969;64:107–113.

Newberg AH, Seligson D. Patellofemoral joint: 30 degrees, 60 degrees, and 90 degrees views. *Radiology* 1980;137:57–61.

Nicholas JA, Freiberger RH, Killoran PJ. Double-contrast arthrography of the knee: its value in the management of two hundred and twenty-five knee derangements. *J Bone Joint Surg [Am]* 1970;52A:203–220.

Niitsu M, Anno I, Fukubayashi T, Shimojo H, Kuno SY, Akisada M. Tears of cruciate ligaments and menisci: evaluation with cine MR imaging. *Radiology* 1991;178:859–864.

Norman A, Baker ND. Spontaneous osteonecrosis of the knee and medial meniscal tears. *Radiology* 1978;129:653–660.

O'Donoghue DH. Surgical treatment of injuries to ligaments of the knee. *JAMA* 1959;169:1423–1431.

O'Donoghue DH. Chondral and osteochondral fractures. *J Trauma* 1966;6:469–481.

Ogden JA, Southwick WO. Osgood-Schlatter's disease and tibial tuberosity development. *Clin Orthop* 1976;116:180–189.

Osgood RB. Lesions of the tibial tubercle occurring during adolescence. *Boston Med Surg J* 1903;148:114–117.

Pavlov H. The cruciate ligaments. In: Freiberger RH, Kaye JJ, eds. *Arthrography.* New York: Appleton-Century-Crofts; 1979:93–107.

Pavlov H, Freiberger RH. An easy method to demonstrate the cruciate ligaments by double-contrast arthrography. *Radiology* 1978;126:817–818.

Pope TL Jr. MR imaging of knee ligaments. In: Weissman BN, ed. *Syllabus: a categorical course in musculoskeletal radiology.* Oak Brook, IL: Radiological Society of North America; 1993:197–210.

Quinn SF, Brown TF. Meniscal tears diagnosed with MR imaging versus arthroscopy: how reliable a standard is arthroscopy? *Radiology* 1991;181:843–847.

Quinn SF, Brown TR, Szumowski J. Menisci of the knee: radial MR imaging correlated with arthroscopy in 259 patients. *Radiology* 1992;185:577–580.

Rafii M, Firooznia H, Golimbu C, Bonamo J. Computed tomography of tibial plateau fractures. *AJR Am J Roentgenol* 1984;142:1181–1186.

Rand JA, Berquist TH. The knee. In: Berquist TH, ed. *Imaging of orthopedic trauma.* 2nd ed. New York: Raven Press; 1991:333–432.

Raunest J, Oberle K, Loehnert J, Hoetzinger H. The clinical value of magnetic resonance imaging in the evaluation of meniscal disorders. *J Bone Joint Surg [Am]* 1991;73A:11–16.

Reicher MA, Hartzman S, Duckwiler GR, Bassett LW, Anderson LJ, Gold RH. Meniscal injuries: detection using MR imaging. *Radiology* 1986;159:753–757.

Remer EM, Fitzgerald SW, Friedman H, Rogers LF, Hendrix RW, Schafer MF. Anterior cruciate ligament injury: MR imaging diagnosis and patterns of injury. *Radiographics* 1992;12:901–915.

Resnick D. Internal derangements of joints. In: Resnick D, ed. *Diagnosis of bone and joint disorders,* 3rd ed. Philadelphia: WB Saunders; 1995:2899–3228.

Robertson PL, Schweitzer ME, Bartolozzi AR, Ugoni A. Anterior cruciate ligament tears: evaluation of multiple signs with MR imaging. *Radiology* 1994;193:829–834.

Rogers LF. *Radiology of skeletal trauma,* 2nd ed. New York: Churchill Livingstone; 1992:1199–1317.

Rosenberg ZS, Kawelblum M, Cheung YY, Beltran J, Lehman WB, Grant AD. Osgood-Schlatter lesion: fracture or tendinitis? Scintigraphic, CT, and MR imaging features. *Radiology* 1992;185:853–858.

Roychowdhury S, Fitzgerald SW, Sonin AH, Peduto AJ, Miller FH, Hoff FL. Using MR imaging to diagnose partial tears of the anterior cruciate ligament: value of axial images. *AJR Am J Roentgenol* 1997;168:1487–1491.

Rubin DA, Harner CD, Costello JM. Treatable chondral injuries in the knee: frequency of associated focal subchondral edema. *AJR Am J Roentgenol* 2000;174:1099–1106.

Rubin DA, Kettering JD, Towers JD, Britton CA. MR imaging of knees having isolated and combined ligament injuries. *AJR Am J Roentgenol* 1998;170:1207–1213.

Rubin DA, Kneeland JB, Listerud J, Underberg-Davis SJ, Dalinka MK. MR diagnosis of meniscal tears of the knee: value of fast spin-echo vs conventional spin-echo pulse sequences. *AJR Am J Roentgenol* 1994;162:1131–1135.

Rubin DA, Paletta GA. Current concepts and controversies in meniscal imaging. *Magn Reson Imaging Clin North Am* 2000;8:243–271.

Ruwe PA, McCarthy S. Cost-effectiveness of magnetic resonance imaging. In: Mink JH, Reicher MA, Crues JW, Deutsch AL, ed. *MR imaging of the knee,* 2nd ed. New York: Raven Press; 1993:463–466.

Ruwe PA, Wright J, Randall RL, Lynch JK, Jokl P, McCarthy S. Can MR imaging effectively replace diagnostic arthroscopy? *Radiology* 1992;183:335–339.

Ryu KN, Kim IS, Kim EJ, et al. MR imaging of tears of discoid lateral menisci. *AJR Am J Roentgenol* 1998;171:963–967.

Sartoris DJ, Kursunoglu S, Pineda C, Kerr R, Pate D, Resnick D. Detection of intra-articular osteochondral bodies in the knee using computed arthrotomography. *Radiology* 1985;155:447–450.

Schlatter C. Verletzungen des schnabelförmigen Fortsatzes der oberen Tibiaepiphyse. *Beitr Klin Chir* 1903;38:874–887.

Schlenzka D, Schwesinger G. The height of the patella: an anatomical study. *Eur J Radiol* 1990;11:19–21.

Schneider R, Freiberger RH. Extrameniscal abnormalities. In: Freiberger RH, Kaye JJ, eds. *Arthrography.* New York: Appleton-Century-Crofts; 1979:109–135.

Schweitzer ME, Tran D, Deely DM, Hume EL. Medial collateral ligament injuries: evaluation of multiple signs, prevalence and location of associated bone bruises, and assessment with MR imaging. *Radiology* 1995;194:825–829.

Schweitzer ME, Mitchell DG, Ehrlich SM. The patellar tendon: thickening, internal signal buckling, and other MR variants. *Skeletal Radiol* 1993;22:411–416.

Scotti DM, Sadhu VK, Heimberg F, O'Hara AE. Osgood-Schlatter's disease: an emphasis on soft tissue changes in roentgen diagnosis. *Skeletal Radiol* 1979;4:21–25.

Scuderi C. Rupture of the quadriceps tendon, study of twenty tendon ruptures. *Am J Surg* 1958;95:626–635.

Shankman S, Beltran J, Melamed E, Rosenberg ZS. Anterior horn of the lateral meniscus: another potential pitfall in MR imaging of the knee. *Radiology* 1997;204:181–184.

Shellock FG, Mink JH, Deutsch AL. Patellar tracking abnormalities: clinical experience with kinematic MR imaging in 130 patients. *Radiology* 1989;172:799–804.

Shellock FG, Mink JH, Deutsch AL, Foo TKF. Kinematic MR imaging of the patellofemoral joint: comparison of passive positioning and active movement techniques. *Radiology* 1992;184:574–577.

Shellock FG, Mink JH, Deutsch AL, Foo TKF, Sullenberger P. Patellofemoral joint: identification of abnormalities with active-movement "unloaded" versus "loaded" kinematic MR imaging techniques. *Radiology* 1993;188:575–578.

Shellock FG, Mink JH, Fox JM. Patello-femoral joint: kinematic MR imaging to assess tracking abnormalities. *Radiology* 1988;168:551–553.

Sinding-Larsen MF. A hitherto unknown affection of the patella in children. *Acta Radiol* 1921;1:171–173.

Singson RD, Feldman F, Staron R, Kiernan H. MR imaging of displaced bucket-handle tear of the medial meniscus. *AJR Am J Roentgenol* 1991;156:121–124.

Smillie IS. The congenital discoid meniscus. *J Bone Joint Surg [Br]* 1948;30B:671–682.

Smith D, Totty W. The knee after partial meniscectomy: MR imaging features. *Radiology* 1990;176:141–144.

Sonin AH, Fitzgerald SW, Bresler ME, Kirsch MD, Hoff FL, Friedman H. MR imaging appearance of the extensor mechanism of the knee: functional anatomy and injury patterns. *Radiographics* 1995;15:367–382.

Sonin AH, Fitzgerald SW, Friedman H, Hoff FL, Hendrix RW, Rogers LF. Posterior cruciate ligament injury: MR imaging diagnosis and patterns of injury. *Radiology* 1994;190:455–458.

Sonin AH, Fitzgerald SW, Hoff FL, Friedman H, Bresler ME. MR imaging of the posterior cruciate ligament: normal, abnormal, and associated injury patterns. *Radiographics* 1995;15:551–561.

Stark JE, Siegel MJ, Weinberger E, Shaw DW. Discoid menisci in children: MR features. *J Comput Assist Tomogr* 1995;19:608–611.

Stoller DW. *Magnetic resonance imaging in orthopedics and sports medicine.* Philadelphia: JB Lippincott; 1993.

Stoller DW, Martin C, Crues JV III, Kaplan L, Mink JH. Meniscal tears: pathologic correlation with MR imaging. *Radiology* 1987;163:731–735.

Tung GA, Davis LM, Wiggins ME, Fadale PD. Tears of the anterior cruciate ligament: primary and secondary signs at MR imaging. *Radiology* 1993;188:661–667.

Twaddle BC, Hunter JC, Chapman JR, Simonian PT, Escobedo EM. MRI in acute knee dislocation: a prospective study of clinical, MRI and surgical findings. *J Bone Joint Surg [Br]* 1996;78B:573–579.

Umans H, Wimpfheimer O, Haramati N, Applbaum YH, Adler M, Bosco J. Diagnosis of partial tears of the anterior cruciate ligament of the knee: value of MR imaging. *AJR Am J Roentgenol* 1995;165:893–897.

Vahey TN, Broome DR, Kayes KJ, Shelbourne KD. Acute and chronic tears of the anterior cruciate ligament: differential features at MR imaging. *Radiology* 1991;181:251–253.

Vahey TN, Hunt JE, Shelbourne KD. Anterior translocation of the tibia at MR imaging: a secondary sign of anterior cruciate ligament tear. *Radiology* 1993;187:817–819.

Weber WN, Neumann CH, Barakos JA, Peterson SA, Steinbach LS, Genant HK. Lateral tibial rim (Segond) fractures: MR imaging characteristics. *Radiology* 1991;180:731–734.

Weiss KL, Morehouse HT, Levy IM. Sagittal MR images of the knee: a low-signal band parallel to the posterior cruciate ligament caused by a displaced bucket-handle tear. *AJR Am J Roentgenol* 1991;156:117–119.

Wershba B, Dalinka MK, Coren GS. Double-contrast knee arthrography in the evaluation of osteochondritis dissecans. *Clin Orthop* 1975;107:81–86.

White LM, Schweitzer ME, Weishaupt D, Kramer J, Davis A, Marks PH. Diagnosis of recurrent meniscal tears: prospective evaluation of conventional MR imaging, indirect MR arthrography, and direct MR arthrography. *Radiology* 2002;222:421–429.

Williams JL, Cliff MM, Bonakdarpour A. Spontaneous osteonecrosis of the knee. *Radiology* 1973;107:15–19.

Wright DH, De Smet AA, Norris M. Bucket-handle tears of the medial and lateral menisci of the knee: value of MR imaging in detecting displaced fragments. *AJR Am J Roentgenol* 1995;165:621–625.

Yu JS, Salonen DC, Hodler J, Haghighi P, Trudell D, Resnick D. Posterolateral aspect of the knee: improved MR imaging with a coronal oblique technique. *Radiology* 1996;198:199–204.

Zanetti M, Pfirrmann CWA, Schmid MR, Romero J, Seifert B, Hodler J. Patients with suspected meniscal tears: prevalence of abnormalities seen on MRI of 100 symptomatic and 100 contralateral asymptomatic knees. *AJR Am J Roentgenol* 2003;181:635–641.

Zeiss J, Saddemi SR, Ebraheim NA. MR imaging of the quadriceps tendon: normal layered configuration and its importance in cases of tendon rupture. *AJR Am J Roentgenol* 1992;159:1031–1034.

LOWER LIMB III

Ankle and Foot

Ankle and Foot

The ankle is the most frequently injured of all the major weight-bearing joints in the body. Most victims are young adults injured while participating in athletic activities such as running, skiing, and soccer. Ankle structures susceptible to injury include bones, ligaments, tendons, and syndesmoses; ligaments can be damaged in the absence of fractures. When this occurs, damage to ligaments may go unrecognized on conventional radiographs, with the result that the patient is not properly treated.

The type of fracture usually indicates the mechanism of injury determined, as Kleiger has pointed out, by the position of the foot, the direction and intensity of the applied force, and the resistance of the structures making up the joint. The mechanism of injury may in turn serve as an indicator of which ligament structures are damaged.

Although occasionally meticulous history taking and clinical examination can help determine the mechanism of trauma and predict damage to the various structures, radiologic examination is the key to reliable evaluation of the site and extent of injury. There are two basic types of ankle trauma: inversion injuries and eversion injuries. These, however, may be complicated by internal or external rotation, hyperflexion or hyperextension, and vertical compression forces.

Foot injuries are also common and usually result from direct trauma, such as a blow or a fall from a height; only rarely do such injuries result from indirect forces such as abnormal stress or strain of muscles or tendons. Foot fractures, accounting for 10% of all fractures, are more common than dislocations, which usually are associated with fractures, and occur at the midtarsal, tarsometatarsal, and metatarsophalangeal articulations.

Anatomic–Radiologic Considerations

The ankle joint proper consists of the tibiotalar and distal tibiofibular articulations, the latter a syndesmotic joint rather than a true synarthrodial one. In matters of injury, however, one must consider that the ankle joint acts as a unit with other joints of the foot, particularly the talocalcaneal (subtalar) articulation, where application of stress can have great impact on ankle injuries.

The ankle joint is formed by three bones—the distal tibia and fibula and the talus—and three principal sets of ligaments—the medial collateral (deltoid) ligament; the lateral collateral ligament, consisting of the anterior talofibular, posterior talofibular, and calcaneofibular ligaments; and the syndesmotic complex, a fibrous joint between the distal tibia and fibula (Fig. 10.1). The distal tibiofibular syndesmotic complex, one of the most important anatomic structures in maintaining ankle integrity and stability, consists of three elements: the distal anterior tibiofibular ligament, the distal posterior tibiofibular ligament, and the interosseous membrane.

PRINCIPAL GROUPS OF ANKLE LIGAMENTS

Medial Collateral (Deltoid) Ligament

medial view

tibionavicular band

tibiotalar band

tibiocalcaneal band

Lateral Collateral Ligament

lateral view

posterior talofibular

anterior talofibular

calcaneofibular

Distal Tibiofibular Syndesmotic Complex

lateral view

interosseous membrane

distal posterior tibiofibular

distal anterior tibiofibular

posterior view

interosseous membrane

distal posterior tibiofibular

Figure 10.1 Ligaments of the ankle. Three principal sets of ligaments form the ankle joint: the medial collateral (deltoid) ligament, the lateral collateral ligament, and the distal tibiofibular syndesmotic complex, which is important for maintaining ankle integrity and stability.

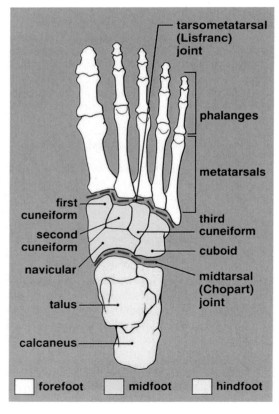

tarsometatarsal (Lisfranc) joint

phalanges

metatarsals

first cuneiform

second cuneiform

navicular

talus

calcaneus

third cuneiform

cuboid

midtarsal (Chopart) joint

☐ forefoot ☐ midfoot ☐ hindfoot

Figure 10.2 Anatomic divisions of the foot. The foot can be viewed as comprising three anatomic parts: the hindfoot, midfoot, and forefoot, separated respectively by the midtarsal (Chopart) and tarsometatarsal (Lisfranc) joints.

From the viewpoint of anatomy and kinetics, the foot is divided into three distinct sections: hindfoot, midfoot, and forefoot. The hindfoot, separated from the midfoot by the midtarsal (or Chopart) joint, includes the talus and calcaneus; the midfoot, separated from the forefoot by the tarsometatarsal (Lisfranc) joint, includes the navicular, cuboid, and three cuneiform bones; and the forefoot includes the metatarsals and phalanges (Fig. 10.2). The muscles attached to the tibia and fibula end in tendons proximal to or at the level of the ankle joint. These tendons insert into the foot (Fig. 10.3).

A word about terminology is in order, because the terminology describing motion of the ankle and foot in the literature is not uniform and confusion has been created about the various mechanisms of ankle and foot injuries. Frequently, but incorrectly, the terms adduction, inversion, varus, and supination have been used interchangeably, as have their counterparts abduction, eversion, valgus, and pronation. However, supination and pronation are more appropriately applied to compound motion. *Supination* consists of adduc- tion and inversion of the forefoot (motion in the tarsometatarsal and midtarsal joints) and inversion of the heel, which assumes a varus configuration (motion in subtalar joint), as well as slight plantar flexion of the ankle (tibiotalar) joint. In *pronation*, compound motion consists of abduction and eversion of the forefoot (motion in the tarsometatarsal and midtarsal joints) and eversion of the heel, which assumes a valgus configuration (motion in the subtalar joint), together with slight dorsiflexion (or dorsal extension) of the ankle (Fig. 10.4).

Adduction properly applies to medial deviation of the forefoot, and *abduction* to lateral deviation of the forefoot, both motions occurring in the tarsometatarsal (Lisfranc) joint; *adduction of the heel* refers to inversion of the calcaneus; and *abduction of the heel* refers to eversion of the calcaneus, both motions occurring in the subtalar joint. *Plantar flexion* refers to caudad (downward) foot motion, *dorsiflexion* to cephalad (upward) foot motion—motions occurring in the ankle (tibiotalar) joint. Varus and valgus should not be used to describe motion but should be reserved for description of ankle or foot position in case of

Figure 10.3 Tendons of the ankle and foot. The attachment of various tendons of the ankle and foot are depicted, as viewed from the dorsal aspect (**A**), lateral aspect (**B**), and medial aspect (**C**).

COMPOUND MOTION IN THE ANKLE AND FOOT

Supination

adduction (A–B) and inversion (Y) of forefoot

inversion (adduction) of heel

plantar flexion

Pronation

abduction (A–B) and eversion (X) of forefoot

eversion (abduction) of heel

dorsiflexion

Figure 10.4 Motion in the ankle and foot. Supination is a compound motion consisting of adduction and inversion of the forefoot, together with inversion of the heel and slight plantar flexion in the ankle joint. In pronation, the compound motion involves abduction and eversion of the forefoot with eversion of the heel and slight dorsiflexion in the ankle joint.

deformity. Occasionally, varus and valgus are used interchangeably with inversion and eversion to describe the applied stress.

Imaging of the Ankle and Foot

Ankle. The standard radiographic examination of the ankle, as a rule, includes the anteroposterior (including the mortise), lateral, and oblique projections. Stress views are also frequently obtained for evaluating ankle injuries. These may also need to be supplemented with special projections.

On the *anteroposterior* view, the distal tibia and fibula, including the medial and lateral malleoli, are well demonstrated (Fig. 10.5). On this projection, it is important to note that the fibular (lateral) malleolus is longer than the tibial (medial) malleolus. This anatomic feature, important for maintaining ankle stability, is crucial for reconstruction of the fractured ankle joint. Even minimal displacement or shortening of the lateral malleolus allows lateral talar shift to occur and may cause incongruity in the ankle joint, possibly leading to post-

traumatic arthritis. A variant of the anteroposterior projection, in which the ankle is internally rotated 10°, is called the mortise view because the ankle mortise is well demonstrated on it (Fig. 10.6).

The *lateral* view is used to evaluate the anterior aspect of the distal tibia and the posterior lip of this bone (the so-called third malleolus) (Fig. 10.7). Some fractures oriented in the coronal plane can be better visualized on this projection.

The *oblique* view of the ankle, best obtained with the foot internally rotated approximately 30° to 35°, is effective in demonstrating the tibiofibular syndesmosis and the talofibular joint (Fig. 10.8). An *external oblique* view may also be required to evaluate the lateral malleolus and the anterior tibial tubercle (Fig. 10.9).

Most ankle ligament injuries require stress radiography, ankle joint arthrography, computed tomography (CT), or magnetic resonance imaging (MRI) (see later) for demonstration and sufficient evaluation. Some, however, can be deduced from the site and extension of fractures on the standard radiographic examination. A thorough knowledge of the

Figure 10.5 Anteroposterior view. (A) For the anteroposterior view of the ankle, the patient is supine on the radiographic table with the heel resting on the film cassette. The foot is in neutral position, with the sole perpendicular to the leg and the cassette. The central beam is directed vertically to the ankle joint at the midpoint between both malleoli. **(B)** The radiograph in this projection demonstrates the distal tibia, particularly the medial malleolus, the body of the talus, and the tibiotalar joint. Note, however, the overlap of the distal fibula and the lateral aspect of the tibia. The tibiofibular syndesmosis is not clearly demonstrated.

Figure 10.6 Mortise view. (A) The mortise view, a variant of the anteroposterior projection obtained with 10° internal rotation of the ankle, eliminates the overlap of the medial aspect of the distal fibula and the lateral aspect of the talus, so the space between these bones is well demonstrated. **(B)** The ankle mortise, shown here on a tomographic cut through the ankle joint, is formed by the medial malleolus, the articular surface of the distal tibia (the ceiling or

Figure 10.7 Lateral view. (A) For the lateral projection of the ankle, the patient is placed on his or her side with the fibula resting on the film cassette and the foot in the neutral position. The central beam is directed vertically to the medial malleolus. (The lateral view can also be obtained by placing the medial side of the ankle against the cassette.) **(B)** On this view, the distal tibia, talus, and calcaneus are seen in profile, and the fibula overlaps the posterior aspect of the tibia and the posterior aspect of the talus. The tibiotalar and subtalar joints are well demonstrated. Note the posterior lip of the tibia, also known as the third malleolus.

Figure 10.8 Internal oblique view. (A) For the internal oblique view of the ankle, the patient is supine, and the leg and foot are rotated medially approximately 35° *(inset)*. The foot is in the neutral position, forming a 90° angle with the distal leg. The central beam is directed perpendicular to the lateral malleolus. **(B)** On the radiograph, the medial and lateral malleoli, the tibial plafond, the dome of the talus, the tibiotalar joint, and the tibiofibular syndesmosis are well demonstrated.

skeletal and soft-tissue topographic anatomy of the ankle, together with an understanding of the kinematics and mechanism of ankle injuries, will aid the radiologist in correctly diagnosing traumatic conditions and predicting ligament injuries. With such understanding, the radiologist can even determine the sequence of injury to the various structures.

Some ligament injuries may be diagnosed on the basis of disruption of the ankle mortise and displacement of the talus; others can be deduced from the appearance of fractured bones. For example, fibular fracture above the level of the ankle joint indicates that the distal anterior tibiofibular ligament is torn. Fracture of the fibula above its anterior tubercle strongly suggests that the tibiofibular syndesmosis is completely disrupted. Fracture of the fibula above the level of the ankle joint without accompanying fracture of the medial malleolus indicates rupture of the deltoid ligament. Transverse fracture of the medial malleolus indicates that the deltoid ligament is intact. High fracture of the fibula associated with a fracture of the medial malleolus or tear of the tibiofibular ligament, the so-called Maisonneuve fracture (see later), indicates rupture of the interosseous membrane up to the level of the fibular fracture.

When radiographs of the ankle are normal, however, stress views are extremely important in evaluating ligament injuries (see Fig. 4.3). Inversion (adduction) and anterior-draw stress films are most frequently obtained; only rarely is an eversion (abduction)-stress examination required.

On the *inversion-stress* film, obtained in the anteroposterior projection, the degree of talar tilt can be measured by the angle formed by lines drawn along the tibial plafond and the dome of the talus (Fig. 10.10). This angle helps diagnose tears of the lateral collateral ligament. However, the wide range of normal values for these measurements may make interpretation difficult, and thus comparison studies of the contralateral ankle should be obtained. Even this method is not always accurate; up to 25° of talar tilt has been reported in people with no history of injury, and occasionally there will be a patient whose ankles exhibit considerable variation in measurement. Many authorities advise that with forced inversion, tilt less than 5° is normal, 5° to 15° may be normal or abnormal, 15° to 25° strongly suggests ligament injury, and more than 25° is always abnormal. With forced eversion, talar tilting of more than 10° is probably pathologic.

The *anterior-draw* stress film, obtained in the lateral projection, provides a useful measurement for determining injury to the anterior talofibular ligament (Fig. 10.11). Values of up to 5 mm of separation

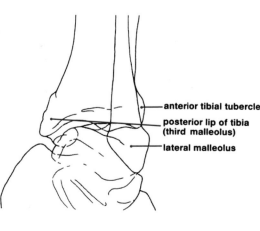

anterior tibial tubercle
posterior lip of tibia (third malleolus)
lateral malleolus

Figure 10.9 External oblique view. On the external oblique view, for which the patient is positioned as for the internal oblique view but with the limb rotated laterally approximately 40° to 45°; the lateral malleolus and the anterior tibial tubercle are well demonstrated.

Figure 10.10 Inversion stress view. (A) For inversion (adduction)-stress examination of the ankle, the foot is fixed in the device while the patient is supine. The pressure plate, positioned approximately 2 cm above the ankle joint, applies varus stress adducting the heel. (If the examination is painful, 5 to 10 mL of 1% Xylocaine or a similar local anesthetic is injected at the site of maximum pain.) **(B)** On the anteroposterior film, the degree of talar tilt is measured by the angle formed by lines drawn along the tibial plafond and the dome of the talus. The contralateral ankle is subjected to the same procedure for comparison.

Figure 10.11 Anterior-draw stress view. (A) For anterior-draw stress examination, the patient is placed on his or her side, with the foot in the device. The pressure plate, positioned anteriorly approximately 2 cm above the ankle, applies posterior stress on the heel. During the examination, the amount of pressure is monitored on a light-emitting diode digital reader. **(B)** On the lateral stress film, the amount of transposition of the talus in relation to the distal tibia can be determined.

between the talus and the distal tibia are considered normal; values between 5 and 10 mm may be normal or abnormal, and the opposite ankle should be stressed for comparison. Values above 10 mm always indicate abnormality.

Ancillary imaging techniques are essential to the diagnosis and evaluation of many ankle injuries. Tomography is useful in evaluating complex fractures of the distal tibia and fibula, and CT may be required to determine the position of comminuted fragments in complex fractures, for example, of the distal tibia, talus, and calcaneus.

Arthrography (Fig. 10.12) is occasionally used for assessing the integrity of the ligamentous structures in acute trauma, although recently it has been almost completely supplanted by MRI. It is still, however, an effective technique for evaluating the articular cartilage, and detecting and localizing loose osteocartilaginous bodies. In conjunction with tomography (arthrotomography), it is indispensable in the

Figure 10.12 **Arthrography of the ankle joint.** (A) For arthrographic examination of the ankle, the patient is supine on the table, with the foot in the neutral position (see Fig. 10.5A). Under fluoroscopic control, the injection site between the tendons of the tibialis anterior and the extensor hallucis longus is marked. Care should be taken to avoid puncturing the dorsalis pedis artery, which should be located by palpation and its site marked on the skin. The needle (preferably 21-gauge) is directed slightly cephalad to avoid the overhanging anterior margin of the tibia. After the joint is entered, approximatley 5 to 7 mL of 60% meglumine diatrizoate or a similar contrast agent is injected for a single-contrast arthrogram. For a double-contrast study, 1 to 2 mL of positive contrast agent and 6 to 8 mL of room air are injected. Films are then obtained in the standard anteroposterior, lateral, and oblique projections. (B) The normal anteroposterior view shows contrast agent outlining the ankle joint, coating the articular surface of the talus and extending into the syndesmotic recess, which normally should not exceed 2.5 cm. (C) On the lateral view, the anterior and posterior capsular recesses are outlined. Filling of the posterior facet of the subtalar joint represents a normal variant, occurring in approximately 10% of cases (see Fig. 10.60C). In approximately 20% of cases, the tendon sheaths of the flexor hallucis longus and flexor digitorum longus opacify on the medial aspect of the ankle. When this occurs, the full extension of the flexor hallucis longus should be noted as it passes proximal to the groove in the talar tubercle and into the groove beneath the sustentaculum tali. Under normal conditions, no tendon sheath opacification should occur on the lateral side of the ankle. (D) Oblique radiograph demonstrates the tibiofibular syndesmosis. No contrast agent should be seen in this area except for normal opacification of the syndesmotic recess.

evaluation of chondral and osteochondral fractures and osteochondritis dissecans, which usually affects the dome of the talus. A single-contrast study is usually performed to assess the integrity of the ankle ligaments. For evaluating the articular cartilage, a double-contrast study (combining a positive-contrast agent and air) is used in conjunction with tomography.

Ankle tenography is a useful procedure for evaluating tendon tears, particularly tears of the Achilles tendon, peroneus longus and brevis, tibialis posterior, flexor digitorum longus, and flexor hallucis longus. According to Bleichrodt and colleagues, tenography particularly has proved to be reliable in the diagnosis of injuries of the calcaneofibular ligament, with a sensitivity of 88% and specificity of 87% to 94%. In a procedure similar to that for ankle arthrography, a 22-gauge needle is inserted into the tendon sheath, with the needle tip directed distally, and 15 to 20 mL of contrast medium is injected under fluoroscopic guidance. Films are then obtained in the standard projections (Fig. 10.13). Tear is indicated by extravasation of contrast agent from the tendon sheath, abrupt termination of the contrast-filled tendon sheath, or leak of contrast into the adjoining articulations (Figs. 10.68B and 10.71). Recently, this technique has been completely replaced by MRI.

CT is an effective modality to evaluate various ligaments and tendons, because the soft-tissue contrast resolution of CT allows easy differentiation of these structures from surrounding fat. Specifically, tendon injuries including tendinitis, tenosynovitis, and rupture and dislocation of tendons can be effectively diagnosed. The major limitation in evaluating pathologic conditions of tendons with CT is the in-

ability to scan the tendons in the coronal and sagittal planes. Reformation images, while occasionally helpful, suffer from the lack of spatial resolution and require additional examination time.

For adequate CT of the ankle and foot, proper positioning of the leg in the gantry is essential. In addition, because nomenclature for imaging planes of the feet occasionally creates a problem, it is important to recognize that the coronal, sagittal, and axial planes of the ankle and foot are determined the same way as for the body (Fig. 10.14A). For coronal images, the knees are flexed and the feet are positioned flat against the gantry table. The coronal sections are obtained with the beam directed to the dorsum of the foot. More commonly modified coronal images are obtained by angling the gantry or by using a foot wedge (Fig. 10.14B). A lateral scanogram helps to establish the degree of necessary gantry tilt. Axial images are obtained with the feet perpendicular to the gantry table, great toes together, and the knees fully extended. The beam is directed parallel to the soles of the feet. Sagittal images are usually generated by using reformation technique, although direct sagittal sections can also be obtained by placing the patient in the lateral decubitus position. Images in all planes are usually acquired using 3- or 5-mm thin contiguous sections. For three-dimensional (3-D) reformation, 1.5- or 2-mm contiguous sections are required, although 5-mm sections with a 3-mm overlap can also be used.

MRI, with its direct multiplanar capabilities and excellent soft-tissue contrast resolution, has proved to be superior to CT for evaluation of ankle tendons and ligaments. The tendons show uniformly low signal intensity in all spin-echo pulse sequences, with the exception of

Figure 10.13 Ankle tenography. Tenograms in the oblique **(A)** and lateral **(B)** projections demonstrate the normal appearance of the tendon of the flexor hallucis longus. On the oblique view, note the distal direction of the needle tip at the beginning of the injection. Normally, the tendon of the flexor hallucis longus does not opacify beyond the limit of the Lisfranc joint. **(C)** On the normal tenogram of the peroneus longus and brevis, seen here on the lateral view, note the position of these tendons below the flexor hallucis longus. The tendon of the peroneus brevis is seen normally opacified; the tendon of the peroneus longus passes below it, crossing into the plantar aspect of the foot to its insertion at the base of the first metatarsal bone.

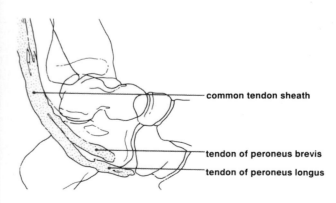

common tendon sheath

tendon of peroneus brevis

tendon of peroneus longus

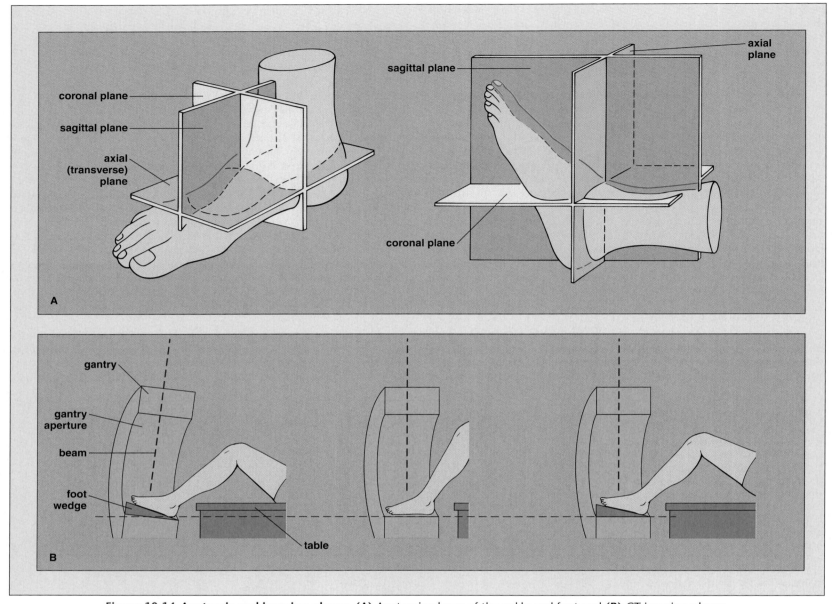

Figure 10.14 Anatomic and imaging planes. (A) Anatomic planes of the ankle and foot and **(B)** CT imaging planes.

the Achilles tendon and tibialis posterior tendon. These two tendons, on long TR sequences, occasionally show small foci of intermediate signal intensity within their substance, particularly near their insertions to the calcaneal tuberosity and the navicular bone, respectively. From a practical point of view, it is helpful to memorize the location and relationship of various tendons seen on axial MR image of the ankle by using the mnemonic phrase, "Tom, Dick, and Harry" for the medial aspect, and "TED" for the lateral aspect of the ankle (Fig. 10.15). The ankle ligaments, likewise, demonstrate low signal intensity on MR images, with the exception of the posterior talofibular ligaments, which often appears inhomogeneous, similar to the anterior cruciate ligament of the knee. The anterior and posterior talofibular ligaments can be visualized over their entire length on axial scans with the foot in neutral position (Fig. 10.16), because they are approximately in the same plane of section. The calcaneofibular ligament can be similarly visualized when the foot is in 40° plantar flexion. The anterior and posterior tibiofibular ligaments can be demonstrated on the axial images in more proximal sections (Fig. 10.17).

On the sections in the sagittal plane, the tibialis posterior, flexor digitorum longus, and flexor hallucis longus tendons are identified on the medial cuts. The peroneus longus and brevis tendons are seen on the lateral sections (Fig. 10.18). The Achilles tendon is best seen on midline sagittal section (Fig. 10.19). The coronal plane is also effective in visualization of various ligaments and tendons (Fig. 10.20).

The pathologic conditions of tendons and ligaments are demonstrated by discontinuity of the anatomic structure, the presence of high signal intensity within the tendon substance on T2-weighted images, and inflammatory changes within or around the tendons, which again can be demonstrated by a change in the normal signal intensity.

Foot. Most injuries to the foot can be sufficiently evaluated on the standard radiographic examination of the foot, which includes the anteroposterior, lateral, and oblique projections. Only occasionally are special tangential projections required.

The *anteroposterior* view of the foot adequately demonstrates the metatarsal bones and phalanges (Fig. 10.21) This view reveals an important anatomic feature known as the *first intermetatarsal angle,* which normally ranges from 5° to 10° (Fig. 10.21C). This angle is an important factor in the evaluation of forefoot deformities, because it represents a way to quantify the amount of metatarsus primus varus associated with hallux valgus. On the *lateral* projection, *Boehler angle,*

Figure 10.15 Schematic representation of ankle tendons on axial MRI. (Modified from Kaplan PA, et al., 2001)

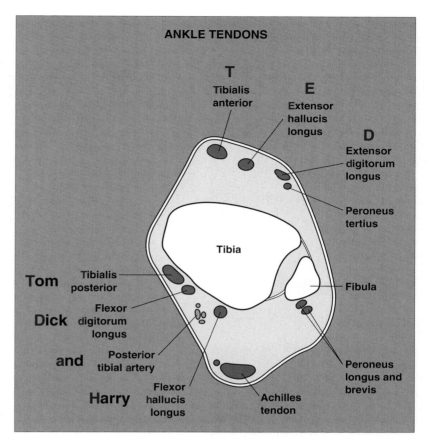

an important anatomic relation of the talus and the calcaneus, can be appreciated (Fig. 10.22). In fractures of the calcaneus, this angle, which normally ranges from 20° to 40°, is decreased because of compression of the superior aspect of the bone (Fig. 10.22A). This measurement also aids in evaluation of depression of the posterior facet of the subtalar joint. On the lateral view, calcaneal pitch can also be evaluated. This measurement is an indication of the height of the foot and normally ranges from 20° to 30° (Fig. 10.22D). Higher val-

ues indicate a cavus foot deformity. An *oblique* view of the foot is also obtained as part of the standard radiographic examination (Fig. 10.23). Injuries to the subtalar joint occasionally require special, tangential projections such as the posterior tangential *(Harris-Beath)* view (Fig. 10.24) or oblique tangential *(Broden)* view (Fig. 10.25). A tangential view of the sesamoid bones of the great toe (Fig. 10.26) may also be necessary.

Radiographic evaluation of foot injuries is complicated by the

Figure 10.16 MRI of the anterior talofibular ligament. Axial spin-echo MR image (SE; TR 2000/TE 20 msec) through the lateral malleolus and talus demonstrates normal anterior talofibular ligament. (From Beltran J, 1990, with permission.)

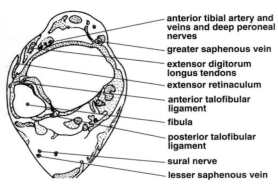

anterior tibial artery and
veins and deep peroneal
nerves

greater saphenous vein

extensor digitorum
longus tendons

extensor retinaculum

anterior talofibular
ligament

fibula

posterior talofibular
ligament

sural nerve

lesser saphenous vein

Figure 10.17 MRI of the anterior and posterior tibiofibular ligaments. Axial spin-echo MR image (SE; TR 2000/TE 20 msec) shows normal anterior and posterior tibiofibular ligaments. (From Beltran J, 1990, with permission.)

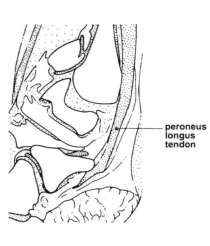

peroneus
longus
tendon

Figure 10.18 MRI of the peroneus longus tendon. Sagittal spin-echo MR image (SE; TR 800/TE 20 msec) through lateral malleolus shows normal appearance of peroneus longus as it curves around the lateral malleolus. (From Beltran J, 1990, with permission.)

extensor hallucis
longus tendon

tibia

Achilles tendon

talus

posterior subtalar joint

interosseous ligament

calcaneus

cuboid

plantaris fascia

Figure 10.19 MRI of the Achilles tendon. Midline sagittal spin-echo MR image (SE; TR 800/TE 20 msec) demonstrates normal Achilles tendon. Note the uniformly low signal intensity of the tendon contrasting with the high signal intensity of the anterior fat pad. (From Beltran J, 1990, with permission.)

Figure 10.20 MRI of the posterior talofibular and calcane-ofibular ligaments. Coronal spin-echo T1-weighted MR image of the ankle shows normal posterior talofibular and calcaneofibular ligaments. (From Beltran J, 1990, with permission.)

fibula
tibialis posterior tendon
posterior talofibular ligament
medial talocalcaneal ligament
calcaneofibular ligament
abductor hallucis muscle
peroneous longus tendon
calcaneus

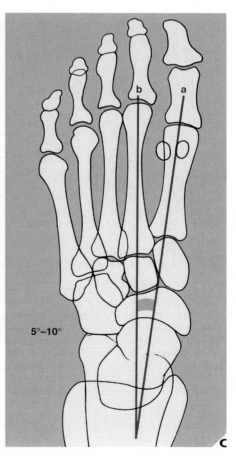

Figure 10.21 Anteroposterior view. (A) For the anteroposterior (dorsoplantar) view of the foot, the patient is supine, with the knee flexed and the sole placed firmly on the film cassette. The central beam is directed vertically to the base of the first metatarsal bone. **(B)** On the film in this projection, injury to the metatarsal bones and phalanges can be adequately assessed. Note that 75% of the talar head articulates with the navicular bone. (For identification of the bones of the foot, see Fig. 10.2.) **(C)** The first intermetatarsal angle is formed by the intersection of the lines bisecting the shafts of the first (*a*) and second (*b*) metatarsals.

5°–10°

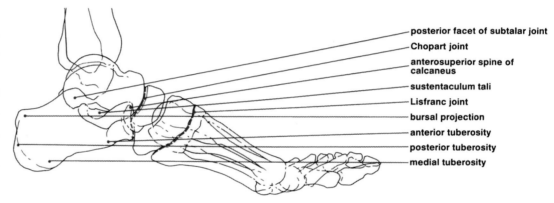

posterior facet of subtalar joint
Chopart joint
anterosuperior spine of calcaneus
sustentaculum tali
Lisfranc joint
bursal projection
anterior tuberosity
posterior tuberosity
medial tuberosity

Figure 10.22 Lateral view. (A) For the lateral view of the foot, the patient lies on his or her side with the knee slightly flexed and the lateral aspect of the foot against the film cassette. The central beam is directed vertically to the midtarsus. (B) The lateral radiograph demonstrates the bursal projection, the most prominent feature on the posterior aspect of the calcaneus; the posterior tuberosity where the Achilles tendon inserts; the medial tuberosity on the plantar surface where the plantar fascia inserts; the anterior tuberosity; the anterosuperior spine of the calcaneus; the posterior facet of the subtalar joint; the sustentaculum tali; and the talonavicular and calcaneocuboid articulations. The Chopart and Lisfranc joints are also well visualized. (C) The lateral view also allows evaluation of the angular relationship between the talus and the calcaneus—Boehler angle. This feature is determined by the intersection of a line (a) drawn from the posterosuperior margin of the calcaneal tuberosity (bursal projection) through the tip of the posterior facet of the subtalar joint, and a second line (b) drawn from the tip of the posterior facet through the superior margin of the anterior process of the calcaneus. Normally, this angle ranges between 20° and 40°. (D) Calcaneal pitch is described by the intersection of a line drawn tangentially to the inferior surface of the calcaneus and one drawn along the plantar surface of the foot.

Figure 10.23 Oblique view. (A) For the oblique view of the foot, the patient is supine on the table with the knee flexed. The lateral border of the foot is elevated about 40° to 45° *(inset)* so that the medial border of the foot is forced against the film cassette. The central beam is directed vertically to the base of the third metatarsal. **(B)** On the oblique film of the foot, the phalanges and metatarsals are well demonstrated, as are the anterior part of the subtalar joint and the talonavicular, naviculocuneiform, and calcaneocuboid joints.

Figure 10.24 Harris-Beath view. (A) For the posterior tangential (Harris-Beath) view of the foot, the patient is erect, with the sole of the foot flat on the film cassette. The central beam is usually angled 45° toward the midline of the heel, but 35° or 55° of angulation may also be used. **(B)** On the film in this projection, the middle facet of the subtalar joint is seen, oriented horizontally; the sustentaculum tali projects medially. The posterior facet projects laterally and is parallel to the middle facet. The body of the calcaneus is well demonstrated.

Figure 10.25 Broden view. (A) For the Broden view of the foot, the patient is supine, with the knee slightly flexed and supported by a small sandbag. The foot rests on the film cassette, dorsiflexed to 90°, and, together with the leg, rotated medially approximately 45° *(inset)*. The central beam is directed toward the lateral malleolus. Films may be obtained at 10°, 20°, 30°, and 40° of cephalad angulation of the tube. **(B)** A radiograph obtained at 30° cephalad angulation demonstrates the posterior facet of the subtalar joint. Note also the good demonstration of the sustentaculum tali and the excellent visualization of the talofibular joint and the tibiofibular syndesmosis.

Figure 10.26 Tangential view. (A) For a tangential view of the sesamoid bones, the patient is seated on the table, with the foot dorsiflexed on the cassette, holding the toes in a dorsiflexed position with a strip of gauze. The central beam is directed vertically to the head of the first metatarsal bone. **(B)** This sesamoid view demonstrates the metatarsal heads and the sesamoid bones of the first metatarsal.

1 talotibial ossicle (os talotibiale)
2 supratalar ossicle (os supratalare)
3 supranavicular ossicle (os supranaviculare)
4 intermetatarsal ossicle (os intermetatarsale)
5 secondary cuboid (cuboides secundarium)
6 secondary calcaneus (calcaneus secundarius)
7 external tibial ossicle (os tibiale externum)
8 trigone ossicle (os trigonum)
9 peroneal ossicle (os peronaeum)
10 vesalian ossicle (os vesalianum)
11 accessory talus (talus accessorius)
12 secondary talus (talus secundarius)

medial sesamoid
fracture line
lateral sesamoid

Figure 10.27 Accessory ossicles. (A), (B) The numerous accessory ossicles of the foot and ankle can complicate the evaluation of foot injuries by mimicking fracture. Fractures, however, may go undetected when misinterpreted as ossicles, as seen here on the anteroposterior **(C)** and sesamoid **(D)** views of the foot, which demonstrate a fracture of the lateral (fibular) sesamoid (compare with Fig. 10.26B).

Table 10.1 Standard and Special Radiographic Projections for Evaluating Injury to the Ankle and Foot

Projection	Demonstration	Projection	Demonstration
Anteroposterior (ankle)	Fractures of: Distal tibia Distal fibula Medial malleolus Lateral malleolus Pilon fractures (extension into tibiotalar joint)	*Lateral (continued)* (ankle and foot)	Talus (particularly neck) Calcaneus (particularly in coronal plane) Posterior facet of subtalar joint Sustentaculum tali Accessory ossicles Cuboid bone
(foot)	Fractures of: Distal portion of talus Navicular, cuboid, and cuneiform bones Metatarsals and phalanges (including stress fractures and accessory ossicles) Dislocations in: Subtalar joint Peritalar (anterior and posterior types) Total talar Tarsometatarsal (Lisfranc) joint	*Stress* (anterior-draw)	Dislocations in: Subtalar joint Peritalar (anterior and posterior types) Tarsometatarsal (Lisfranc) joint Tear of anterior talofibular ligament Ankle instability
With 10° internal ankle rotation (mortise view)	Same structures and abnormalities as anteroposterior but better demonstration of tibial plafond	*Oblique* Internal External	Fractures of: Medial malleolus Talus Tuberosity of calcaneus Metatarsals Phalanges
Stress (inversion, eversion)	Tear of lateral collateral ligament Ankle instability Boehler angle	*Posterior Tangential* (Harris-Beath)	Fractures involving: Middle and posterior facets of subtalar joint Calcaneus (in axial plane)
Lateral (ankle and foot)	Fractures of: Distal tibia Anterior aspect Posterior lip (third malleolus) Tibiotalar joint	*Oblique Tangential* (Broden)	Fractures involving: Posterior facet of subtalar joint Calcaneus Sustentaculum tali
		Axial (sesamoid view)	Fractures of sesamoid bones

presence of multiple accessory ossicles, which are considered secondary centers of ossification, and the sesamoid bones, which may mimic a fracture (Fig. 10.27A,B); conversely, a chip fracture can be misinterpreted as a mere ossicle (Fig. 10.27C,D). Thus, it is important to recognize these structures on conventional radiographs.

In addition to radiography, ancillary imaging techniques may need to be used in the evaluation of injury to the foot. Radionuclide imaging (bone scan) is a valuable means of detecting stress fractures, common foot injuries that are not always obvious on the standard radiographic examination. Likewise, tomographic examination may supply useful information about occult or subtle fractures and help with evaluation of fracture healing. CT is especially effective in assessing complex fractures, particularly of the calcaneus. Tenographic examination may also be required to evaluate injury to the tendons of the foot (see previous text and Fig. 10.13). MRI is now frequently used to evaluate trauma to the foot.

For a tabular summary of the preceding discussion, see Tables 10.1 and 10.2 and Figure 10.28.

Table 10.2 Ancillary Imaging Techniques For Evaluating Injury to the Ankle and Foot

Technique	Demonstration	Technique	Demonstration
Radionuclide Imaging (scintigraphy, bone scan)	Stress fractures Healing process	*Tenography*	Tears of: Achilles tendon Posterior tibialis tendon Peroneal tendons Digitorum longus tendon
Tomography	Position of fragments and extension of fracture lines in complex fractures Healing process and complications Nonunion Secondary infection	*Computed Tomography*	Complex fractures (particularly of os calcis) Intraarticular extension of fracture line Injuries to tendons (particularly peroneal, tibialis, and Achilles) and ligaments
Arthrography (single-contrast) (double-contrast usually combined with tomography or CT)	Tears of ligament structures of ankle joint Osteochondral fractures Osteochondritis dissecans of talus Osteochondral bodies in joint	*Magnetic Resonance Imaging*	Same as arthrography, tenography, and computed tomography

Figure 10.28 Spectrum of radiologic imaging techniques used to evaluate trauma to the ankle and foot.*
*The radiographic projections or radiologic techniques indicated throughout the diagram are only those that are the most effective in demonstrating the respective traumatic conditions.

Injury to the Ankle

All ankle injuries can be broadly classified, according to the mechanism of injury, as resulting from inversion (Fig. 10.29) or eversion (Fig. 10.30) stress forces. Inversion injuries are much more common, as O'Donoghue has pointed out, accounting for 85% of all traumatic conditions involving the ankle. These groupings apply to both fractures and injuries to the ligament complexes of the ankle. However, it is in the latter type of injuries that they are particularly helpful in determining and evaluating the specific type of ligament injury, especially in the presence of certain fractures about the ankle.

Fractures About the Ankle Joint

In addition to being classified by mechanism of injury, fractures about the ankle joint can also be classified by the anatomic structure involved (Fig. 10.31) and designated as:

1. *Unimalleolar,* when the fracture involves the medial (tibial) or lateral (fibular) malleolus (Fig. 10.32)

2. *Bimalleolar,* when both malleoli are fractured (Fig. 10.33)

3. *Trimalleolar,* when fractures involve the medial and lateral malleoli as well as the posterior lip (or tubercle) of the distal tibia (the third malleolus) (Fig. 10.34)

4. *Complex fractures,* known also as pilon fractures, when comminuted fractures of the distal tibia and fibula occur (Fig. 10.35).

These fractures, when viewed from the standpoint of pathomechanics, may be either inversion or eversion injuries or a combination of both. The various types of eversion fractures are best known by their eponyms, including the Pott, Maisonneuve, Dupuytren, and Tillaux fractures (see later).

All of the following ankle fractures involving the distal tibia and fibula can be diagnosed on the standard radiographic projections. However, CT may be useful in delineating the extent of the fracture line, and this modality is particularly effective in evaluating lateral displacement in the juvenile Tillaux fracture. To evaluate associated ligament injuries, MRI is the technique of choice.

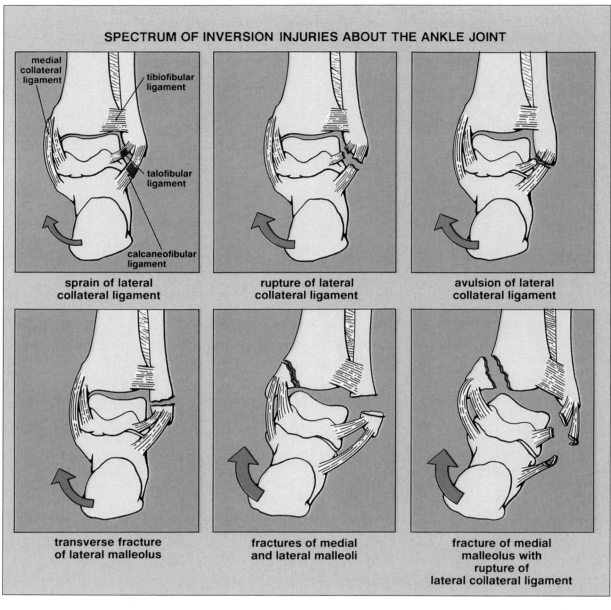

SPECTRUM OF INVERSION INJURIES ABOUT THE ANKLE JOINT

medial collateral ligament

tibiofibular ligament

talofibular ligament

calcaneofibular ligament

sprain of lateral collateral ligament

rupture of lateral collateral ligament

avulsion of lateral collateral ligament

transverse fracture of lateral malleolus

fractures of medial and lateral malleoli

fracture of medial malleolus with rupture of lateral collateral ligament

Figure 10.29 Inversion injuries. Depending on its severity, an inversion force delivered to the lateral structures of the ankle joint may manifest in a broad spectrum of injuries of the lateral collateral ligament complex, as well as the lateral and medial malleoli. Note, however, that inversion-stress forces do not affect the posterior tibiofibular or medial collateral ligaments. (Modified from Edeiken J, 1978, with permission.)

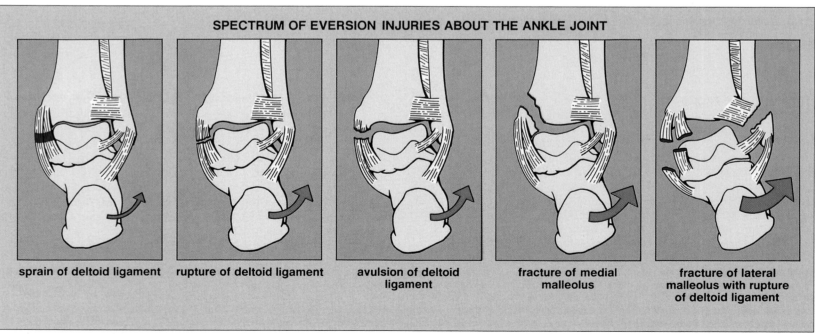

SPECTRUM OF EVERSION INJURIES ABOUT THE ANKLE JOINT

sprain of deltoid ligament

rupture of deltoid ligament

avulsion of deltoid ligament

fracture of medial malleolus

fracture of lateral malleolus with rupture of deltoid ligament

Figure 10.30 Eversion injuries. Depending on its severity, an eversion force delivered to the medial structures of the ankle joint may manifest in a broad spectrum of injuries of the medial collateral (deltoid) ligament complex, as well as the medial and lateral malleoli. Note, however, that eversion-stress forces do not affect the posterior tibiofibular or lateral collateral ligaments. (Modified from Edeiken J, 1978, with permission.)

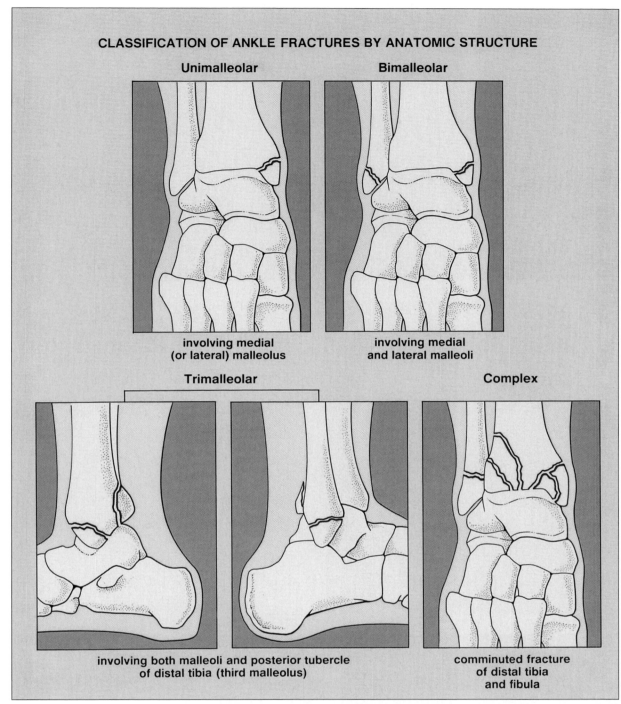

Figure 10.31 Classification of ankle fractures. Ankle fractures can be classified according to the anatomic structure as unimalleolar, bimalleolar, trimalleolar, or complex.

Figure 10.32 Unimalleolar fracture. Anteroposterior radiograph of the ankle (**A**) and coronal CT reformatted image (**B**) demonstrate the typical appearance of a unimalleolar fracture involving the medial malleolus.

Figure 10.33 Bimalleolar fracture. Oblique radiograph of the ankle shows a bimalleolar fracture involving the tibial and fibular malleoli.

Figure 10.34 Trimalleolar fracture. Oblique (**A**) and lateral (**B**) radiographs of the ankle show a trimalleolar fracture affecting both malleoli and the posterior lip of the distal tibia. The latter feature is better seen on the lateral view.

Figure 10.35 Pilon fracture. Anteroposterior **(A)** and lateral **(B)** films of the ankle demonstrate a complex, comminuted fracture of the distal tibia and fibula in a 30-year-old man who fell from a third-floor window. **(C)** Axial CT section through the tibial plafond shows typical appearance of pilon fracture.

Fractures of the Distal Tibia. *Pilon (Pylon) Fracture.* Fracture of the distal tibia is called a pilon (pylon) fracture when the comminuted fracture lines extend into the tibiotalar joint (Fig. 10.36; see also Fig. 10.35). These injuries comprise approximately 5% of all lower leg fractures. Most pilon fractures occur during fall from a height, motor vehicle accidents, snow or water skiing accidents, or are caused by a forward fall on a level surface with the foot entrapped. Although the pathomechanics of this injury may be complex, the predominant force is vertical compression. Not infrequently there is associated fracture of the distal fibula, talus, and subluxation in the ankle joint (Fig. 10.37), in addition to severe damage to the soft-tissue sleeve of the distal leg. Pilon fractures are a distinct clinical and radiologic entity and should not be confused with trimalleolar fractures. The following features distinguish pilon fractures from the trimalleolar fractures: the presence of profound comminution of the distal tibia; intraarticular extension of tibial fracture through the dome of the plafond; usual association of fracture of the talus; and usual preservation of tibiofibular syndesmosis. This fracture's significance comprises the intraarticular extension of the fracture line and its consequent potential to cause late complications of posttraumatic arthritis, as well as nonunion and malunion.

Müller's widely accepted classification of pilon fractures divides these injuries into three groups, depending on the displacement of the fragments and the incongruity of the joint (Fig. 10.38).

Tillaux Fracture. In 1872, Tillaux described an ankle fracture resulting from abduction and external-rotation injury and consisting of avulsion of the lateral margin of the distal tibia. The fracture line is vertical and extends from the distal articular surface of the tibia upward to the lateral cortex (Fig. 10.39). In children, a similar type of fracture, referred to as *juvenile Tillaux fracture,* is actually a Salter-Harris type III injury to the distal tibial growth plate (Fig. 10.40; see Fig. 4.28). This injury probably occurs because the growth plate fuses from medial to lateral, making the medial side stronger than the lateral.

The radiologic evaluation of a Tillaux fracture is critical for establishing whether surgery will be necessary. If the fracture fragment is laterally displaced more than 2 mm or if there is an irregularity of the articular surface of the distal tibia (a step-off), then surgical rather than conservative treatment is indicated. Conventional tomography and CT are the best methods for obtaining this information (Figs. 10.41, 10.42, and 10.43).

If, instead of avulsion of the lateral margin of the tibia, the medial portion of the fibula becomes detached and the anterior tibiofibular ligament remains intact, then the fracture is called a *Wagstaffe-LeFort fracture* (Fig. 10.44).

Triplanar (Marmor-Lynn) Fracture. Fractures involving the lateral aspect of the distal tibial epiphysis may be complicated by extension of the fracture line into two other planes, hence the term *triplanar fracture.* The mechanism of this type of injury is usually plantar flexion and external rotation. The three planes involved are the *sagittal plane,* in which there is a vertical fracture through the epiphysis; the *axial plane,* in which a horizontally oriented fracture extends through the lateral aspect of the growth plate; and the *coronal plane,* in which there is an oblique fracture through the metaphysis into the diaphysis, extending superiorly from the anterior aspect of the growth plate to the posterior cortex of the tibia (Fig. 10.45).

The epiphyseal component of this fracture is best seen on the anteroposterior view, the axial component on both the anteroposterior and lateral views, and the diaphyseal extension on the lateral view. The typical triplanar fracture thus consists of a combination of the juvenile Tillaux fracture and a Salter-Harris type II fracture (Figs. 10.46 and 10.47; see also Figs. 10.40 and 4.28) and should not be mistaken for a Salter-Harris type IV fracture (Fig. 10.48). Occasionally, metadiaphyseal component of the triplanar fracture may cross the growth plate and extend into the epiphysis, thus making the distinction from Salter-Harris type IV fracture more difficult (Fig. 10.49).

Figure 10.36 CT of pilon fracture. Coronal **(A)**, sagittal **(B)**, axial **(C)**, and three-dimensional **(D)** reformatted CT images show characteristic features of pilon fracture in a 30-year-old man who was injured in a motorcycle accident.

Figure 10.37 Pilon fracture. A 36-year-old man was injured in a motor vehicle accident and sustained a complex fracture of the distal tibia and fibula. **(A)** Conventional radiograph shows markedly comminuted intraarticular fracture of the distal tibia and segmental fracture of the distal fibula. Coronal **(B)** and sagittal **(C)** CT reformatted images demonstrate the number and direction of displaced fragments. **(D) and (E)** Three-dimensional CT images viewed from anterior and medial directions display spatial orientation of various fractured fragments, thus providing an orthopedic surgeon with a "road map" for successful open reduction and internal fixation of this complex fracture.

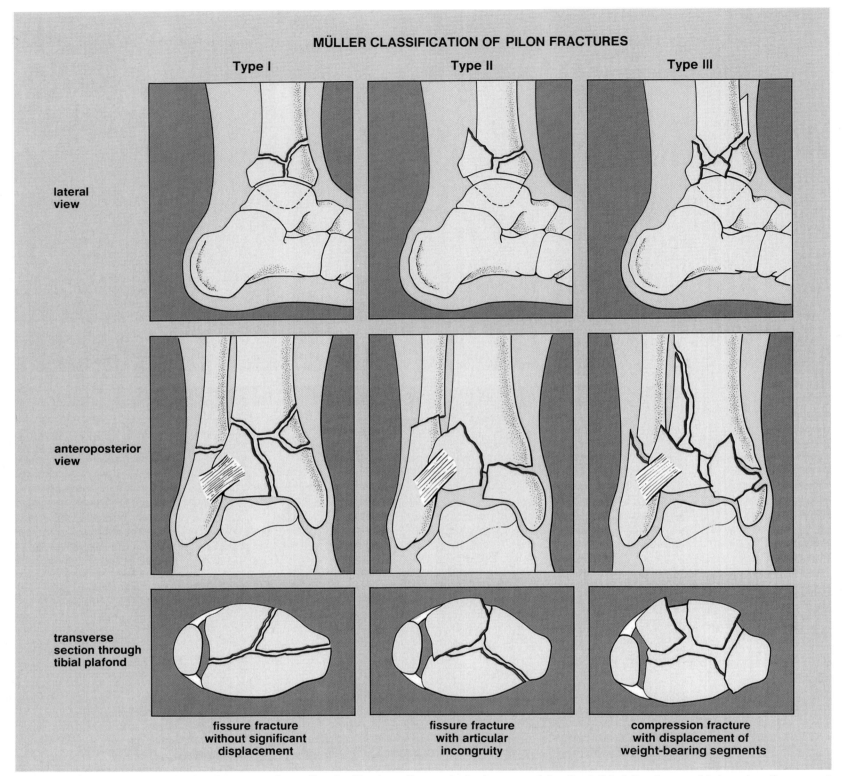

MÜLLER CLASSIFICATION OF PILON FRACTURES

Type I	Type II	Type III

lateral view

anteroposterior view

transverse section through tibial plafond

fissure fracture without significant displacement	fissure fracture with articular incongruity	compression fracture with displacement of weight-bearing segments

Figure 10.38 Classification of pilon fractures. The Müller classification of intraarticular fractures of the distal tibia (pilon fractures) is based on the amount of displacement of the fragments and the consequent degree of incongruity of the joint. (Modified from Müller ME, et al., 1979, with permission.)

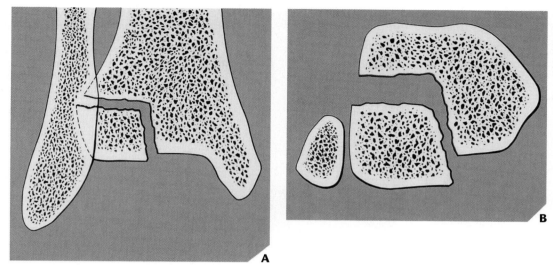

Figure 10.39 Tillaux fracture. In the classic Tillaux fracture, shown here schematically in coronal **(A)** and transverse **(B)** sections through the distal tibia, the fracture line extends from the distal articular surface of the tibia upward to the lateral cortex.

Figure 10.40 Juvenile Tillaux fracture. A 13-year-old girl injured her right ankle during a basketball game. Oblique view of the ankle **(A)** and tomographic sections in the oblique **(B)** and lateral **(C)** projections demonstrate a typical Salter-Harris type III injury to the growth plate, also called juvenile Tillaux fracture.

Figure 10.41 **CT of Tillaux fracture.** A 24-year-old woman twisted her ankle while ice-skating. Anteroposterior radiograph **(A)** and CT section **(B)** show a marginal fracture of the lateral aspect of the tibia, a characteristic Tillaux fracture. The minimal amount of displacement seen here would mandate only conservative treatment.

Figure 10.42 **CT of Tillaux fracture.** A 39-year-old man sustained a nondisplaced Tillaux fracture, demonstrated on **(A)** axial CT section and **(B)** coronal reformatted image.

Figure 10.43 **Tomography of Tillaux fracture.** A 45-year-old man twisted his right ankle in a basketball game. Anteroposterior radiograph **(A)** and frontal trispiral tomogram **(B)** show a displaced Tillaux fracture that requires surgical management.

Figure 10.44 Wagstaffe-LeFort fracture. In the Wagstaffe-LeFort fracture, seen here schematically on the anteroposterior view, the medial portion of the fibula is avulsed at the insertion of the anterior tibiofibular ligament. The ligament, however, remains intact.

Figure 10.45 Triplanar fracture. The Marmor-Lynn (or triplanar) fracture comprises a vertical fracture of the epiphysis in the sagittal plane, a horizontally oriented fracture in the axial plane through the lateral aspect of the growth plate, and an oblique fracture through the metaphysis into the diaphysis in the coronal plane, extending superiorly from the anterior aspect of the growth plate to the posterior cortex of the tibia.

Figure 10.46 Triplanar fracture. A 12-year-old girl fell on ice and sustained a typical triplanar fracture. **(A)** Anteroposterior view of the left ankle shows a vertical fracture of the epiphysis and horizontal extension through the lateral aspect of the growth plate. The metaphyseal and diaphyseal components of the fracture are barely seen. **(B)** Lateral view clearly demonstrates the posteriorly directed fracture line in the coronal plane, the third component of a triplanar fracture.

Figure 10.47 Triplanar fracture. A 13-year-old boy presented with a triplanar fracture. (A) Anteroposterior radiograph shows only horizontal and vertical components. (B) A trispiral lateral tomogram shows horizontal and oblique components.

Figure 10.48 Salter-Harris type IV fracture. Anteroposterior view of the ankle in an 8-year-old boy demonstrates that the fracture line traverses the epiphysis and metaphysis of the distal tibia, but there is no horizontal extension through the growth plate. Note the associated Salter-Harris type I fracture of the distal fibula (see also Fig. 4.28).

Figure 10.49 CT of triplanar fracture. (A) An anteroposterior radiograph shows horizontal (*arrow*) and vertical (*open arrow*) components of this injury. (B) Lateral radiograph shows the oblique component (*curved arrow*), but the distal extent of the fracture line is not well demonstrated. *(continued)*

Figure 10.49 CT of triplanar fracture. *Continued.* The coronal **(C)** and sagittal **(D)** CT reformatted images confirm the diagnosis of triplanar fracture. Note that the obliquely oriented fracture line extends into the epiphysis.

Fractures of the Fibula. *Pott Fracture.* After sustaining a fracture of his own leg, Sir Percivall Pott described in 1769 what he believed to be the most common type of ankle fracture, a fracture of the distal third of the fibula (Fig. 10.50). It is now recognized that this type of fracture usually occurs as a result of disruption of the tibiofibular syndesmosis. In fact, many authorities believe that the type of fracture Pott described does not exist as a primary fracture.

Dupuytren Fracture. Dupuytren fracture is the name given to a fracture of the fibula occurring 2 to 7 cm above the distal tibiofibular syndesmosis and including disruption of the medial collateral ligament (Fig. 10.51). The associated tear of the syndesmosis leads to ankle instability.

Maisonneuve Fracture. Like the Dupuytren fracture, the Maisonneuve fracture is an eversion-type injury of the fibula. The fracture, however, occurs in the proximal half of the bone, commonly at the junction of the proximal and middle thirds of the shaft (Fig. 10.52). The tibiofibular syndesmosis is disrupted, and either tear of the tibiofibular ligament or fracture of the medial malleolus is also present (Fig. 10.53). The more proximal the location of the fibular fracture, the more damage to the interosseous membrane between the tibia and the fibula, which is always disrupted up to the point of the fibular fracture.

Injury to the Soft Tissues About the Ankle Joint and Foot

As mentioned, all ankle injuries can be grossly classified as resulting from inversion- or eversion-stress forces (see Figs. 10.29 and 10.30). However, the forces delivered to the ankle are rarely pure inversion or pure eversion. A combination of forces is usually at work to produce ligament and tendon injuries that may occur secondary to fractures or

Figure 10.50 Pott fracture. In the Pott fracture, the fibula is fractured above the intact distal tibiofibular syndesmosis, the deltoid ligament is ruptured, and the talus is subluxed laterally.

Figure 10.51 **Dupuytren fracture.** (A) This fracture usually occurs 2 to 7 cm above the distal tibiofibular syndesmosis, with disruption of the medial collateral ligament and, typically, tear of the syndesmosis leading to ankle instability. (B) In the low variant, the fracture occurs more distally and the tibiofibular ligament remains intact.

as primary injuries. Several classifications have been developed to reflect the complexity of these forces. Lauge-Hansen classified ankle injuries based on the mechanism of injury by combining the position of the foot (supination or pronation) with the direction of the deforming force vector (external rotation, adduction, or abduction) (Table 10.3). He emphasized the close relationship between bone and ligament injuries, but the complexity of his classification diminishes its value in treatment.

From the practical orthopedic point of view, the Weber classification, based on the level of fibular fracture and therefore on the type of syndesmotic ligament injury, is much more useful (Fig. 10.54):

Stage A   The fibular fracture may be a transverse avulsion fracture at the level of or just distal to the ankle joint. There may be an associated fracture of the medial malleolus. Alternatively, the fibula is intact, but the lateral collateral ligament is disrupted. In either case, the tibiofibular syndesmosis, the interosseous membrane, and the deltoid ligament are intact.

Stage B   There is a spiral fracture of the distal fibula, beginning at the level of the tibiofibular syndesmosis, with partial disruption of mainly the posterior tibiofibular ligament. It may also be associated with an avulsion fracture of the medial malleolus below the level of the ankle joint (Fig. 10.55). Alternatively, the medial malleolus may be intact and the deltoid ligament may be disrupted.

Stage C   Fracture of the fibula occurs at a level higher than the ankle joint, with associated tear of the posterior tibiofibular ligament and resultant lateral talar instability. If the fibular fracture is high (Maisonneuve type), the interosseous membrane is torn to the level of the fracture. There is also an avulsion fracture of the medial malleolus, in which case the deltoid ligament is intact. Alternatively, the medial malleolus is intact, but the deltoid ligament is disrupted (Fig. 10.56).

The likelihood of injury to the distal tibiofibular syndesmosis can be inferred from the nature and level of the fibular fracture: The higher the fibular fracture, the more extensive the damage to the tibiofibular ligaments and, thus, the greater the risk of ankle instability. The greatest value of this classification lies in the fact that it emphasizes the lateral syndesmosis-malleolar complex as an important factor in congruence and stability in the ankle joint.

Tear of the Medial Collateral Ligament. Depending on the severity of the eversion force, injury to the medial collateral ligament

Figure 10.52 **Maisonneuve fracture.** The classic Maisonneuve fracture commonly occurs at the junction of the middle and distal thirds of the fibula. The tibiofibular syndesmosis is disrupted, and the interosseous membrane is torn up to the level of the fracture. The tibiotalar (medial) joint compartment is widened because of lateral subluxation of the talus.

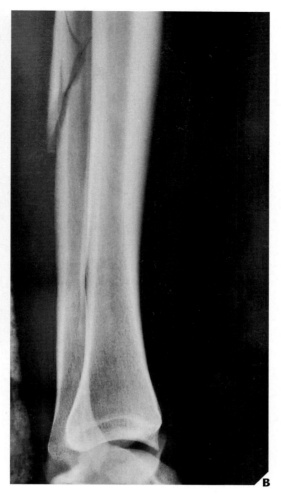

Figure 10.53 Maisonneuve fracture. A 22-year-old man injured his right ankle in a skiing accident. **(A)** Oblique view of the ankle shows a comminuted fracture of the medial malleolus, with extension into the anterior lip of the tibia. **(B)** On the lateral view, a comminuted fracture of the fibula is apparent. This is a characteristic of a Maisonneuve-type fracture.

ranges from sprain to complete rupture (Fig. 10.30). Tear may occur either in the body of the ligament or at its attachment to the medial malleolus. Rupture of the medial collateral ligament is typically associated with a tear of the tibiofibular ligament and lateral subluxation of the talus. On clinical examination, soft-tissue swelling is prominent distal to the tip of the medial malleolus. If the standard radiographic examination of the ankle reveals lateral shift of the talus in the ab-

sence of a spiral fracture of the fibula, one must assume that both the tibiofibular and the medial collateral ligaments are torn. Arthrographic examination shows leak of contrast agent beneath the medial malleolus (Fig. 10.57).

Although tears of the ligaments of the ankle can be demonstrated on CT examination, more commonly these injuries are evaluated by MRI. Acute tear of the medial collateral ligament appears as disrup-

Table 10.3 **Lauge-Hansen Classification of Ankle Injuries**

Pronation—Abduction Injuries		**Supination—Adduction Injuries**	
Stage I	Rupture of the deltoid ligament or transverse fracture of the medial malleolus	Stage I	Injury to the lateral collateral ligament or transverse fracture of the lateral malleolus below the level of the joint*
Stage II	Disruption of the distal anterior and posterior tibiofibular ligaments	Stage II	Steep oblique fracture of the medial malleolus
Stage III	Oblique fracture of the fibula at the level of the joint* (best seen on the anteroposterior projection)	**Supination—Lateral (External) Rotation Injuries**	
Pronation—Lateral (External) Rotation Injuries		Stage I	Disruption of the anterior tibiofibular ligament
		Stage II	Spiral fracture of the distal fibula near the joint* (best seen on the lateral projection)
Stage I	Rupture of the deltoid ligament or transverse fracture of the medial malleolus	Stage III	Rupture of the posterior tibiofibular ligament
Stage II	Disruption of the anterior tibiofibular ligament and interosseous membrane	Stage IV	Transverse fracture of the medial malleolus
Stage III	Fracture of the fibula usually 6 cm or more above the level of the joint*		
Stage IV	Chip fracture of the posterior tibia or rupture of the posterior tibiofibular ligament		

* The appearance of the fibular fracture is the key to determining the mechanism of injury. Modified from Lauge-Hansen N, 1950, with permission.

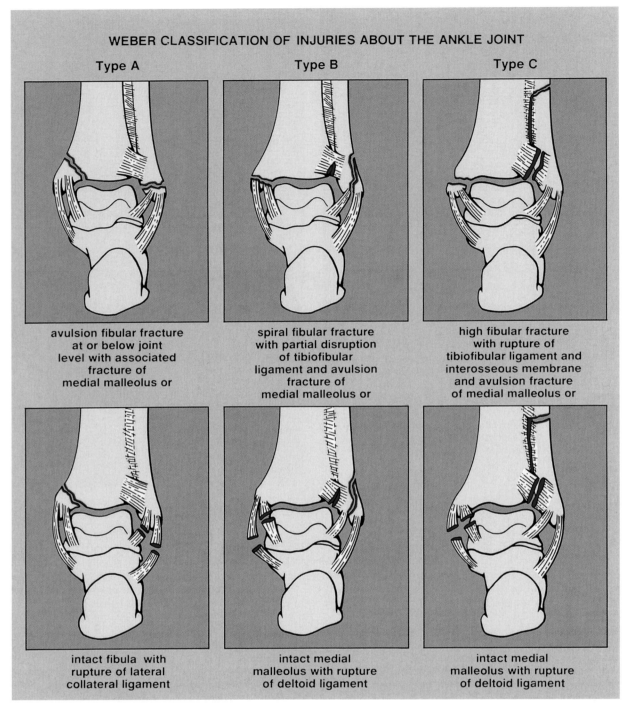

WEBER CLASSIFICATION OF INJURIES ABOUT THE ANKLE JOINT

Type A

avulsion fibular fracture
at or below joint
level with associated
fracture of
medial malleolus or

intact fibula with
rupture of lateral
collateral ligament

Type B

spiral fibular fracture
with partial disruption
of tibiofibular
ligament and avulsion
fracture of
medial malleolus or

intact medial
malleolus with rupture
of deltoid ligament

Type C

high fibular fracture
with rupture of
tibiofibular ligament and
interosseous membrane
and avulsion fracture
of medial malleolus or

intact medial
malleolus with rupture
of deltoid ligament

Figure 10.54 Weber classification. The Weber classification of injuries to the structures about the ankle joint is based on the level at which fibular fracture occurs, as well as the presence or absence of an associated fracture of the medial malleolus. Disruption of the medial and lateral ligament complexes can be deduced from the level of the fibular fracture, as well as that of the medial malleolar fracture. (Modified from Weber BG, 1972, with permission.)

tion of continuity or absence of the low-intensity ligamentous fibers surrounded by edema or hemorrhage (Fig. 10.58). Chronic or healed ligamentous disruption shows generalized thickening of the ligament.

Tear of the Lateral Collateral Ligament. Inversion-stress forces delivered to the lateral ankle structures may cause a spectrum of injuries to the lateral collateral ligament, ranging from sprain to complete rupture (Fig. 10.29). The body of the ligament or its attachment to the fibular malleolus may be the site of injury. In the absence of fracture of the fibular malleolus on the standard radiographic examination, disruption of the ligament complex can be recognized on the inversion-stress film of the ankle by an increase in talar tilt to 15° or more (Figs. 10.10B and 10.59A). Arthrographic examination, however, is always diagnostic.

The component ligaments of this complex may also be injured in-

dependently. The *anterior talofibular ligament* is the most frequently injured ankle ligament. It can be diagnosed on the inversion-stress film of the ankle (Fig. 10.10), but arthrographic examination may be required for confirmation (*Fig.* 10.59). Characteristically, contrast agent is seen to leak anteriorly to the lateral malleolus and laterally alongside it (*Fig.* 10.60); rupture of the *posterior talofibular ligament* is better appreciated on the lateral view. Rupture of the *calcaneofibular ligament* is invariably associated with tear of the anterior talofibular ligament (Fig. 10.61). The distinguishing arthrographic finding is opacification of the peroneal tendon sheath (Fig. 10.62).

MRI is equally effective evaluating injury to the lateral collateral ligament. The diagnosis of a tear is based on lack of visualization of the one or more components of this ligament. The tears of the calca-

Figure 10.55 Weber type B fracture. A 24-year-old woman injured her right ankle in a skiing accident. Anteroposterior view of the ankle demonstrates a spiral fracture of the fibula beginning at the level of the tibiofibular syndesmosis with consequent tear of the inferoposterior portion of the syndesmotic complex; the interosseous membrane is intact. The site of the fracture of the medial malleolus suggests that the deltoid ligament may be intact. According to the Weber classification, this is a type B fracture.

Figure 10.56 Weber type C fracture. A 32-year-old woman stepped into a pothole and injured her right ankle. Anteroposterior view of the ankle demonstrates a fracture of the fibula above the level of the ankle joint, indicating disruption of the interosseous membrane. The intact medial malleolus indicates a tear of the deltoid ligament. This type of fracture is classified as a Weber type C. The risk of ankle mortise instability due to disruption of the medial and lateral ligament complexes gives this type of injury a worse prognosis than type A or B.

Figure 10.57 Tear of the deltoid ligament. (A), (B). Tear of the deltoid ligament in the absence of fracture is characterized on the arthrogram, represented here schematically, by leak of contrast beneath the medial malleolus (compare with Fig. 10.12).

Figure 10.58 MRI of the tear of the deltoid ligament. (A) An axial T2-weighted image of the right ankle shows a partial tear of the deltoid ligament *(arrow)* with high-signal-intensity hemorrhage in the tibiotalar and tibiocalcaneal fibers. **(B)** An axial T2-weighted image of a normal deltoid ligament that demonstrates low signal intensity of its intact fibers *(arrow)* is shown for comparison.

Figure 10.59 Multiple tears of the ankle ligaments. A 28-year-old woman injured her ankle in a skiing accident. **(A)** Inversion-stress radiograph shows a talar tilt of 22°, suggesting tear of the lateral collateral ligament complex. Single-contrast arthrograms in the anteroposterior **(B)** and lateral **(C)** projections reveal tears of several ligaments: leakage around the tip of the fibula indicates a tear of the anterior talofibular ligament, filling of the peroneal tendon sheath indicates a tear of the calcaneofibular ligament, and leak of contrast into the tibiofibular syndesmosis indicates a tear of the distal anterior tibiofibular ligament. Filling of the posterior facet of the subtalar joint indicates a tear of the posterior talofibular ligament.

Figure 10.60 Tear of the anterior and posterior talofibular ligaments. (A), (B) On arthrography, leak of contrast around the tip of the lateral malleolus characterizes a tear of the anterior talofibular ligament. **(C)** Tear of the posterior talofibular ligament can be recognized on the lateral view by opacification of the posterior facet of the subtalar joint. In 10% of cases, however, this finding may represent a normal variant.

Figure 10.61 Tear of the calcaneofibular and anterior talofibular ligaments. A 27-year-old man twisted his ankle during a sports activity. Conventional radiographs were normal, and stress views were equivocal. Contrast arthrograms in the lateral **(A)** and oblique **(B)** projections of the ankle show opacification of the peroneal tendon sheath characteristic of tear of the calcaneofibular ligament. Leak of contrast agent along the fibular malleolus, seen on both views, indicates an associated tear of the anterior talofibular ligament.

Figure 10.62 Tear of the calcaneofibular ligament. (A), (B) The characteristic arthrographic finding in rupture of the calcaneofibular ligament is opacification of the peroneal tendon sheath.

neofibular ligament are best demonstrated in the coronal plane, while the tears of the anterior and posterior talofibular ligaments are best seen on the axial sections (Fig. 10.63).

Tear of the Distal Anterior Tibiofibular Ligament. Commonly associated with other ligament injuries, tear of the anterior tibiofibular ligament may also occur as an isolated injury (Fig. 10.64). Its arthrographic appearance is characterized by leak of contrast agent into the syndesmotic space (Fig. 10.65).

Tendon Ruptures. Most tendon ruptures can be diagnosed by history and clinical examination. For example, tear of the *Achilles tendon,* the most common injury to the soft tissues of the foot, is often indicated by severe tenderness at the tendon's insertion, together with limitation of plantar flexion. Avulsion of this tendon from its calcaneal insertion (Fig. 10.66) can be recognized on the lateral radiograph of the foot obtained with a low-kilovoltage/soft-tissue technique (Fig. 10.67), although tenography (Fig. 10.68) or MRI (Figs. 10.69 and

10.70; see also Fig. 10.19) is confirmatory. Tenography, although rarely performed at the present time, is also helpful in confirming rupture of the *posterior tibialis* (Fig. 10.71) and *peroneal tendons.*

Injury to the Foot

Fractures of the Foot

Fractures of the Calcaneus. Commonly sustained in falls from heights, fractures of the calcaneus are sometimes called "lover's fractures;" in 10% of cases, they are seen bilaterally. According to Cave,

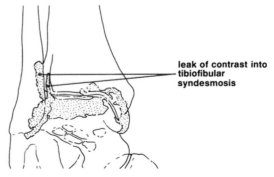

leak of contrast into tibiofibular syndesmosis

Figure 10.63 MRI of the tear of the anterior talofibular ligament. An axial T2-weighted MRI shows disruption of the anterior talofibular ligament resulting in its replacement by high-signal-intensity fluid *(straight arrow).* Note that the intact posterior talofibular ligament shows normal low signal intensity *(curved arrow).*

Figure 10.64 Tear of the distal anterior tibiofibular ligament. A 29-year-old man injured his ankle during a basketball game. Conventional radiograph and stress examination revealed no abnormalities. On arthrography, however, leak of contrast into the region of the tibiofibular syndesmosis indicates a tear of the distal anterior tibiofibular ligament (compare with Fig. 10.12B,D).

Figure 10.65 Tear of the distal anterior tibiofibular ligament. (A), (B) This injury can be recognized on arthrography by leak of contrast above the syndesmotic recess. Normally, opacification of the recess does not exceed 2.5 cm.

TYPES OF ACHILLES TENDON RUPTURE

| Normal | Avulsion | Rapture at musculotendinous interface | Incomplete rupture | Incomplete rupture | Complete rupture |

Figure 10.66 Achilles tendon injury. Schematic representation of various types of Achilles tendon injury.

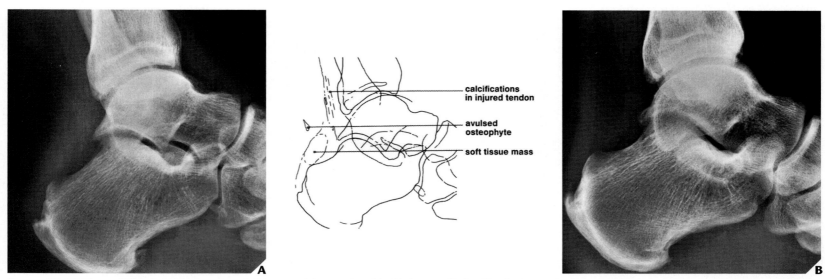

calcifications in injured tendon

avulsed osteophyte

soft tissue mass

Figure 10.67 Tear of the Achilles tendon. A 54-year-old man stumbled into a pothole. Physical examination revealed severe tenderness at the insertion of the Achilles tendon and marked limitation of plantar flexion. **(A)** Lateral view shows a lack of definition of the tendon, a lumpy soft-tissue mass, and an avulsion fracture of a small osteophyte from the posterior aspect of the calcaneus at the insertion of the ruptured tendon. **(B)** The other, normal foot is shown for comparison.

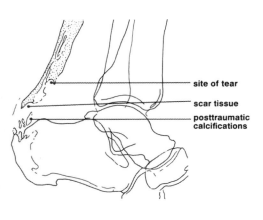

Figure 10.68 Tear of the Achilles tendon. (A) Lateral radiograph of the ankle shows a lack of definition of the Achilles tendon at its insertion on the posterior aspect of the os calcis and prominent soft-tissue swelling. Multiple calcifications are seen at the site of the tendon's insertion. **(B)** The tenogram demonstrates a tear of the tendon approximately 5 cm proximal to the insertion by the abrupt termination of contrast filling the tendon sheath.

fractures of the calcaneus account for 60% of all major tarsal injuries.

In the evaluation of such injuries, it is critical to determine whether the fracture line involves the subtalar joint and, if so, to assess the degree of depression of the posterior facet. Determination of the Boehler angle (see Fig. 10.22C) helps evaluate depression, but conventional tomography and CT are usually essential (Fig. 10.72). The CT examination should include coronal and axial sections. Sagittal and 3-D reformations may enhance depiction and characterization of calcaneal fractures (Figs. 10.73 and 10.74) and may be helpful in assessment of adequacy of postsurgical reduction. In all calcaneal fractures sustained in a fall from a height, a radiograph of the thoracolumbar spine is essential because of the commonly associated finding of compression fracture of one of the vertebral bodies (Fig. 10.75).

Essex-Lopresti classified calcaneal fractures into two main categories: those sparing the subtalar joint (25%) and those extending into it (75%), with the latter subdivided into joint-depression fractures and tongue-type fractures. Rowe and coworkers classified calcaneal fractures into five types (Fig. 10.76):

Stage I   Fractures of the tuberosity, sustentaculum tali, or anterior process (21%).

Stage II   Beak fractures and avulsion fractures of the Achilles tendon insertion (3.8%).

Stage III   Oblique fractures not extending into the subtalar joint (19.5%).

Stage IV   Fractures involving the subtalar joint (24.7%).

Stage V   Fractures with central depression and varying degrees of comminution (31%).

Stress fractures of the calcaneus occur in joggers and runners but do not spare the older population when bones are weakened by osteoporosis (Fig. 10.77). Like stress fractures in long bones, these fractures are not immediately evident but typically become obvious approximately 10 to 14 days after the precipitating incident. They can be recognized on radiographs by a band of sclerosis, representing formation of endosteal callus. The fracture line is usually oriented either vertically or parallel to the posterior contour of the bone. If stress fractures are suspected but radiographs are normal, a bone scan may validate the diagnosis.

Fractures of the Talus. Fractures of the talus are the second most common tarsal bone fractures, after the calcaneus. Fracture may involve the head, neck, body, or posterior process. The neck of the

Figure 10.69 MRI of the Achilles tendon tear. Sagittal STIR **(A)** and axial T2-weighted **(B)** MR images show a focus of high-signal intensity within the posterior part of the Achilles tendon *(arrows)*, indicating an acute partial tear. Edema is present within the fat pad and in the subcutaneous tissue.

Figure 10.70 MRI of the Achilles tendon tear. (A) A complete Achilles tendon tear with a large 3-cm gap *(arrows)* is seen on this sagittal STIR magnetic resonance image. There is massive edema and hemorrhage subcutaneously and deep to the Achilles tendon. (B) In another patient, a sagittal T1-weighted MRI shows a complete rupture of the Achilles tendon near the musculotendinous junction *(arrow)*.

Figure 10.71 Tenogram of the posterior tibialis muscle tendon tear. A 57-year-old man sustained an eversion injury to the left ankle while playing tennis. On clinical examination, he was diagnosed as having ruptured the tendon of the posterior tibialis muscle. Tenography confirms the clinical findings. Note the abnormal opacification of the subtalar, Chopart, and naviculocuneiform joints.

torn tendon of posterior tibialis

opacification of subtalar joint

opacification of Chopart's joint

opacification of naviculocuneiform joint

Figure 10.72 Fracture of the calcaneus. A 54-year-old man fell from a scaffold and sustained a fracture of the left calcaneus. **(A)** Lateral view shows a comminuted fracture of the calcaneus. There is a suggestion of extension of the fracture line into the subtalar joint. **(B)** Tomographic examination in the lateral projection confirms intraarticular extension of the fracture line. The amount of depression of the articular surface, however, cannot be definitely assessed. **(C)** CT section precisely demonstrates the position of the comminuted fragments and depression at the posterior facet of the subtalar joint. It also shows that the middle facet is intact, important information that the conventional and tomographic studies could not provide.

Figure 10.73 CT of the calcaneus fracture. A 34-year-old man sustained a comminuted fracture of the right calcaneus. **(A)** Coronal CT section shows extension of the fracture line to the subtalar joint. **(B)** Reformatted sagittal image shows in addition a fracture of the anterior process of the calcaneus with extension into the anterior facet of subtalar joint. **(C)** 3-D reformatted image shows the topography and complexity of the fracture.

Figure 10.74 CT of the calcaneus fracture. (A) Sagittal CT reformatted image and three-dimensional reconstractions viewed from the medial **(B)** and lateral **(C)** sides of the foot show a complex, intraarticular fracture of the calcaneus. The position of various fractured fragments is well depicted.

Figure 10.75 Fractures of the calcaneus and the thoracic vertebra. A 48-year-old man jumped from a second-floor window. **(A)** Lateral radiograph of the ankle demonstrates a comminuted fracture of the calcaneus. **(B), (C)** Coronal CT sections demonstrate the position of multiple, small, comminuted fragments and involvement of the sustentaculum tali. **(D)** Lateral radiograph of the thoracolumbar spine shows compression fracture of the T-12 vertebral body. *(continued)*

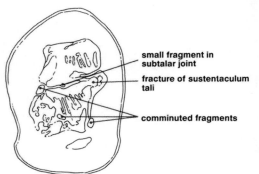

small fragment in subtalar joint

fracture of sustentaculum tali

comminuted fragments

Figure 10.75 Fractures of the calcaneus and the thoracic vertebra. *Continued.*

talus is the most vulnerable site, and the vertical fractures are most frequently encountered. Hawkins proposed three types of vertical fractures of the neck of the talus (Fig. 10.78). His classification, based on the damage to the blood supply of the talus, serves as a guide to prognosis for healing of the fracture, incidence of osteonecrosis, and indication for open reduction. Recently, Canale and Kelly modified this classification to include a fourth, rare type of a displaced fracture with subtalar or tibiotalar dislocation and subluxation or dislocation in the talonavicular joint.

Whether vertical or comminuted, fractures of the talus most often result from forced dorsiflexion of the foot, as may occur in automobile accidents. Accompanying dislocation in the subtalar and talonavicular joints is common. Talar fractures are usually obvious on the standard radiographic projections. MRI may be of value for detecting various complications (Fig. 10.79).

Osteochondritis Dissecans of the Talus. Osteochondritis dissecans should not be confused with osteochondral fracture of the dome of the talus resulting from inversion or eversion injury to the ankle. (The differential diagnosis of osteochondritis dissecans and osteochondral fracture is discussed in detail in Chapter 9.)

Osteochondritis dissecans results from chronic stress and is seen most commonly in athletes and ballet dancers. The best diagnostic procedures for demonstrating the lesion are arthrotomography (Fig. 10.80) and MRI (Fig. 10.81), as is also true for osteochondritis dissecans of the femoral condyles.

Navicular Fractures. Navicular fractures are rare and are usually sustained along with fractures of other bones of the foot. Occasionally, navicular fracture may be caused by a fall from a height. Sangeorzan and colleagues classified navicular fractures into three types based on the orientation of the fracture line and the degree of comminution. Type I fractures pass through the navicular bone in a coronal plane, without associated forefoot angulation. Type II fractures are associated with forefoot angulation and the fracture line runs from the dorsolateral to the plantar-medial aspect of the bone. Type III fractures

are comminuted and the forefoot is laterally displaced. Eichenholtz and Levine classified these fractures as cortical avulsion (47%), tuberosity avulsion (24%), and fractures of the body (29%).

Because navicular fractures can be missed on conventional radiography, CT including reformatted imaging is recommended when such fractures are suspected (Fig. 10.82).

Jones Fracture. This avulsion fracture of the base of the fifth metatarsal results from inversion stress placed on the peroneus brevis tendon, which is attached to the fifth metatarsal (Fig. 10.83; see also Fig. 4.29A). From a historical point of view, however, the term "Jones fracture" is used incorrectly, because the original fracture described by Robert Jones in 1902 was one sustained approximately three-fourths of 1 inch from the base of the fifth metatarsal (Fig. 10.84). The distinction between a "true" Jones fracture and an avulsion fracture of the base of the fifth metatarsal is also of prognostic value: Avulsion fractures generally heal quickly, while fractures through the proximal metatarsal shaft, because of poor blood supply, have a significant incidence of delayed union and fibrous union. In children, it is important not to confuse this fracture with the normal (and frequently present) secondary ossification center of the base of the fifth metatarsal (see Fig. 4.29B). The fracture line is transversely oriented, whereas the gap separating the ossification center from the fifth metatarsal is oblique.

Complications

The most common complications of ankle and foot fractures are nonunion and posttraumatic arthritis. Although conventional radiography can usually demonstrate the features of these complications, CT is the better technique for delineating their details.

Dislocations in the Foot

The most common dislocation in the foot occurs in the tarsometatarsal (Lisfranc) joint. In general, however, dislocations are less common than fractures of the ankle and foot. They are occasion-

ROWE CLASSIFICATION OF CALCANEAL FRACTURES

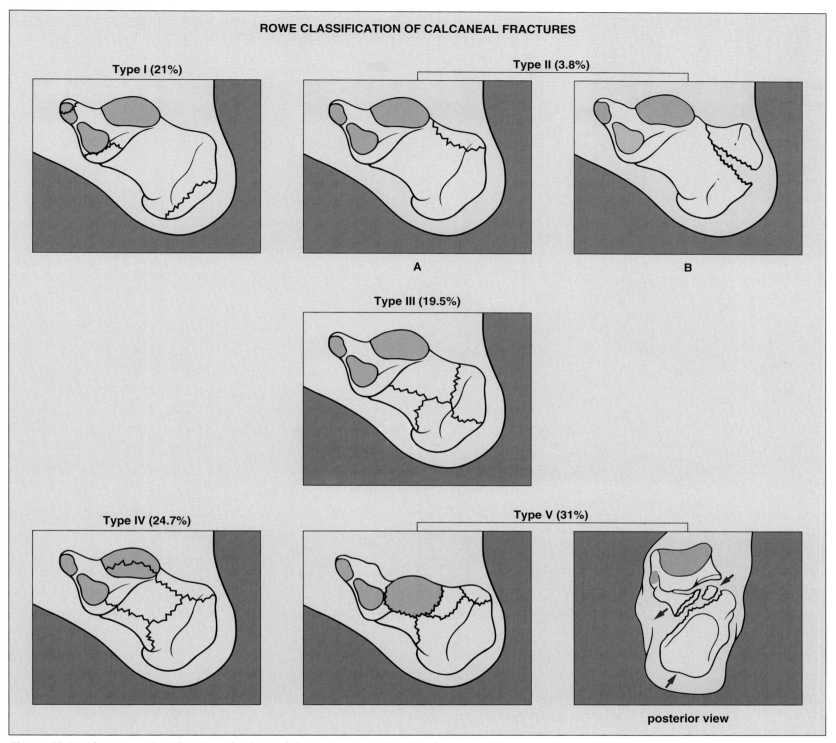

Figure 10.76 The Rowe classification of calcaneal fractures. Type I (21%)—fractures of the tuberosity, sustentaculum tali, or anterior process; type II (3.8%)—beak fractures **(A)** and avulsion fractures of the Achilles tendon insertion **(B)**; type III (19.5%)—oblique fractures not extending into the subtalar joint; type IV (24.7%)—fractures involving the subtalar joint; type V (31%)—fractures with central depression and varying degrees of comminution. (Modified from Rowe CR, et al., 1963, with permission.)

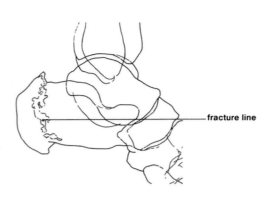

—fracture line

Figure 10.77 Stress fracture of the calcaneus. A 75-year-old woman reported pain in the left heel; she had no history of trauma. She walked about a mile to the super-market every day. Lateral radiograph of the right foot shows a typical stress fracture of the os calcis.

HAWKINS CLASSIFICATION OF TALAR NECK FRACTURES

Type I
(11%-21%)

Type II
(40%-42%)

Type III
(23%-47%)

Figure 10.78 The Hawkins classification of vertical talar neck fractures. Type I fracture shows no displacement of the talus in relation to the subtalar joint. Type II fracture exhibits subluxation or dislocation of the talus in the subtalar joint. Type III fracture is characterized by the displacement of the body of the talus, which is locked behind the sustentaculum tali, so that the fracture surface is pointing laterally.

Figure 10.79 Fracture of the talus. A 41-year-old woman injured her right foot in an automobile accident. **(A)** Lateral radiograph of the foot demonstrates a vertical fracture of the talus. T1-weighted **(B)** and T2-weighted **(C)** sagittal spin-echo MR images demonstrate lack of union and persistent joint effusion. The axial image **(D)** demonstrates segmental osteonecrosis of the posterolateral part of the talus.

ally seen as a result of motor vehicle or aircraft accidents, as in dislocation of the talus—the so-called aviator's astragalus. According to Shelton and Pedowitz, aircraft accidents account for 43% of all talar injuries.

Dislocations in the Subtalar Joint. The two major types of subtalar joint dislocations are peritalar dislocation of the foot and total dislocation of the talus.

Peritalar Dislocation. This type of abnormality involves simultaneous dislocations in the talocalcaneal and talonavicular joints with normal maintenance of the tibiotalar relationship. Often referred to as subtalar or subastragalar dislocation, peritalar dislocation, as Pennal has pointed out, accounts for approximately 15% of all talar injuries and approximately 1% of all dislocations. Patients vary in age

from 10 to older than 60 years, but three- to 10-times more men than women sustain these injuries.

Four subtypes of peritalar dislocation have been identified: medial, lateral, posterior, and anterior. *Medial dislocation* is the most common subtype, resulting from a violent inversion force acting as a fulcrum for the sustentaculum tali to cause initial dislocation of the talonavicular joint, together with rotary subluxation of the talocalcaneal joint. A greater force may cause complete dislocation. The dorsoplantar (anteroposterior) view of the foot is recommended to demonstrate this abnormality. The radiographs should be scrutinized carefully for associated fractures, particularly of both malleoli, the articular margin of the talus, and the navicular and fifth metatarsal bones.

Figure 10.80 Osteochondritis dissecans of the talus. A 29-year-old man, a professional ballet dancer, reported pain in the ankle over the preceding 8 months. Anteroposterior **(A)** and lateral **(B)** radiographs demonstrate a radiolucent defect in the medial aspect of the dome of the talus and a small osteochondral body within the defect, characteristic findings in osteochondritis dissecans. **(C)** Arthrotomography demonstrates the intact articular cartilage over the lesion, distinguishing it as an in situ lesion.

Figure 10.81 MRI of osteochondritis dissecans of the talus. (A) A sagittal T1-weighted image shows an area of low signal intensity at the talar dome *(arrows).* **(B)** A sagittal inversion recovery image shows high-signal-intensity lesion of osteochondritis dissecans *(arrows).*

Figure 10.82 CT of the navicular fracture. A sagittal **(A)** CT reformatted image and **(B)** three-dimensional CT show a fracture of the navicular bone (*arrow*).

Lateral dislocation is the next most common subtype, accounting for approximately 20% of all peritalar dislocations. At the time of injury, the foot is everted and, with the anterior calcaneal process acting as a fulcrum, the head of the talus is forced out of the talonavicular joint; the calcaneus is dislocated laterally. As in medial dislocation, the dorsoplantar view of the foot is diagnostic.

Posterior and anterior dislocations are the rarest subtypes, occurring as a result of a fall from a height onto the plantar-flexed foot (posterior dislocation) or the dorsiflexed foot (anterior dislocation). In either case, the lateral view of the foot and ankle is best for demonstrating the abnormality (Fig. 10.85).

Total Talar Dislocation. Characterized by complete disruption of both the ankle (tibiotalar) and the subtalar joints, total talar dislocation is the most serious of all talar injuries. It is frequently complicated by osteonecrosis of the astragalus.

Tarsometatarsal Dislocation. Also termed *Lisfranc fracture-dislocation*, this is the most common dislocation in the foot. It also frequently occurs in association with various types of fractures. Basically, this is a dorsal dislocation, often occurring as the result of a fall from a height

or down a flight of stairs or even of stepping off a curb. There are two basic forms of injury: *homolateral*—dislocation of the first to the fifth metatarsal, and *divergent*—lateral displacement of the second to the fifth metatarsals with medial or dorsal shift of the first metatarsal (Fig. 10.86). Associated fractures most often occur at the base of the second metatarsal bone; they may also be seen in the third metatarsal, first or second cuneiform, or navicular bones. The divergent form of tarsometatarsal dislocation is most frequently associated with such fractures. These injuries are well demonstrated on the standard views of the foot (Fig. 10.87). Ancillary imaging techniques are seldom required, although CT examination may demonstrate unsuspected associated fractures (Fig. 10.88). The most common complications of ankle and foot fractures are nonunion and posttraumatic arthritis. Although conventional radiography can usually demonstrate the features of these complications, CT is the better technique for delineating their details.

Tarsal Tunnel Syndrome

The tarsal tunnel is a fibro-osseous structure located in the medial side of the ankle and hindfoot, extending from the medial malleolus to the

Figure 10.83 Avulsion fracture. A 28-year-old man stumbled on uneven pavement and sustained an inversion injury of the right foot. **(A)** Oblique radiograph demonstrates a fracture of the base of the fifth metatarsal, frequently but incorrectly interpreted as the Jones fracture. **(B)** Inversion-stress forces on the peroneus brevis tendon cause avulsion fracture of the base of the fifth metatarsal.

tendon of peroneus brevis

inversion stress

fifth metatarsal

JONES FRACTURE

Figure 10.84 Jones fracture. (A) A "true" Jones fracture is located about an inch distally to the base of the fifth metatarsal. **(B)** A 43-year-old woman, while dancing, twisted her left foot and sustained a "true" Jones fracture of the fifth metatarsal.

Figure 10.85 Peritalar dislocation. A 25-year-old man fell from a ladder and landed on his plantar-flexed left foot. Lateral radiograph demonstrates posterior peritalar dislocation. Note that the talus articulates normally with the tibia, but there are simultaneous dislocations in the talocalcaneal and talonavicular joints. The entire foot (except for the talus) is posteriorly displaced. Associated fractures of the navicular and cuboid bones are evident.

Figure 10.86 Types of the Lisfranc fracture–dislocation. Tarsometatarsal dislocation (Lisfranc fracture-dislocation) may be seen in two variants. In the homolateral form, the first to the fifth metatarsals are dislocated laterally. In the divergent form, the first metatarsal is medially dislocated. Both types are often associated with fracture of the base of the second metatarsal bone.

navicular bone. The roof of the tunnel is formed by the flexor retinaculum, the lateral side is formed by the medial aspect of the talus and sustentaculum tali, and the medial side is bordered by the flexor retinaculum, abductor hallucis muscle, and the medial wall of the calcaneus. The tarsal tunnel contains the posterior tibial nerve, the posterior tibial artery and vein, the posterior tibial tendon, the flexor digitorum longus tendon, and the flexor hallucis longus tendon. The term "tarsal tunnel syndrome" was originally and independently coined by Keck and Lam in 1962. The syndrome is caused by compression of the posterior tibial nerve or its branches as they pass deep to the flexor retinaculum, either by extrinsic masses or posttraumatic fibrosis. The clinical symptoms include pain, a burning sensation, and paresthesias in the sole of the foot and the toes. MR imaging is very effective in demonstrating the cause of nerve impingement.

Sinus Tarsi Syndrome

The sinus tarsi (or tarsal sinus) is a cone-shaped space located in the lateral aspect of the foot between the neck of the talus and the anteroposterior surface of the calcaneus. The sinus tarsi contains fat, talocalcaneal ligaments, interosseous ligaments, portions of the joint capsule of the posterior subtalar joint, and neurovascular structures. The sinus tarsi syndrome is caused by abnormalities of one or more structures contained in the sinus and is characterized by pain in the lateral portion of the foot and a feeling of instability of the hindfoot. Pain relief can be achieved by injection of anesthetic agents into the tarsal sinus. In 70% of reported cases, the causing factor responsible

for the sinus tarsi syndrome was trauma, usually involving inversion injury to the foot. MR imaging may show obliteration of sinus tarsi fat, tear of calcaneofibular and anterior talofibular ligaments, and tear of the posterior tibial tendon.

fractures at base of 2d and 3d metatarsals

dislocation in metatarsocuneiform joint

lateral shift of 2d–5th metatarsals

Figure 10.87 Divergent Lisfranc fracture–dislocation. A 39-year-old man fell down a flight of stairs. Anteroposterior **(A)** and lateral **(B)** radiographs of the right foot show the divergent type of the Lisfranc fracture–dislocation. There is lateral shift of the second to fifth metatarsals, as well as dislocation and dorsal shift in the first metatarsocuneiform joint, which is better appreciated on the lateral film. Note the fractures at the base of the second and third metatarsals.

Figure 10.88 CT of the Lisfranc fracture-dislocation. A 54-year-old man fell down a flight of stairs and injured his left foot. **(A)** Dorsoplantar radiograph shows typical appearance of divergent Lisfranc fracture-dislocation. A small fractured fragment from the base of the second metatarsal is well-seen (*arrow*). CT reformatted image in axial (transverse) plane **(B)**, and three-dimensional CT **(C)** demonstrate an unsuspected fracture of the medial (*open arrow*) and lateral (*curved arrow*) cuneiform bones.

PRACTICAL POINTS TO REMEMBER

Ankle

[1] There are three principal sets of ligaments around the ankle joint:
- the medial collateral (deltoid) ligament
- the lateral collateral ligament
- the distal tibiofibular syndesmotic complex.

[2] Traumatic conditions of the ankle should be evaluated according to the mechanism that caused the injury, including:
- inversion-stress forces
- eversion-stress forces
- complex stresses combining supination or pronation with rotation, abduction, or adduction.

[3] Inversion-stress forces may manifest in a spectrum of injuries to the lateral collateral ligament, as well as in associated fractures of the distal tip of the fibula and occasionally the medial malleolus.

[4] Eversion-stress forces may manifest in a range of injuries to the medial collateral (deltoid) ligament, as well as fracture of the medial malleolus. Pott, Maisonneuve, and Dupuytren fractures are all eversion injuries.

[5] Pilon fracture is a comminuted fracture of the distal tibia with extension into the tibiotalar joint.

[6] Tillaux fracture consists of avulsion of the lateral margin of distal tibia resulting from abduction and external rotation injury.

[7] Juvenile Tillaux fracture is a Salter-Harris type III injury to the distal tibial growth plate.

[8] Triplanar Marmor-Lynn fracture consists of a vertical fracture through the distal tibial epiphysis (in the sagittal plane), horizontal fracture through the lateral aspect of the distal tibial growth plate (in the axial plane), and oblique fracture through the distal metaphysis extending into the diaphysis (in the coronal plane).

[9] Traumatic conditions of the structures about the ankle joint may not be obvious on the standard radiographic examination when only damage of soft-tissue structures is present. Correct management of such injuries may be much more important to a successful orthopedic outcome than correct management of a simple fracture. For this reason, stress views, arthrographic examination, and MRI are of paramount importance for full evaluation of the extent of damage to the complex structures about the joint.

[10] The ligament structure most important for congruence of the joint and ankle stability is the distal tibiofibular syndesmotic complex.

[11] Lauge-Hansen classification of ankle trauma is based on the mechanism of injury, combining the position of the foot with the direction of deforming force vector.

[12] The Weber classification of ankle fractures—based on the level of fibular fracture—is practical for assessing the risk of future ankle instability because of its emphasis on the lateral syndesmotic–malleolar complex as an important factor in ankle joint stability.

[13] On arthrographic examination of the ligament structures about the ankle and foot:
- leak of contrast around the tip of the fibular malleolus indicates a tear of the anterior talofibular ligament
- opacification of the peroneal tendon sheath suggests a tear of the calcaneofibular ligament
- leak of contrast more than 2.5 cm into the tibiofibular syndesmotic recess indicates a tear of the distal anterior tibiofibular ligament
- leak of contrast beneath the medial malleolus indicates a tear of the deltoid ligament.

[14] Tenography is a useful technique for evaluating tears of the tendons, such as the Achilles tendon, the posterior tibialis tendon, or the peroneal tendon.

[15] MRI is a noninvasive modality capable of demonstrating pathologic conditions of tendons and ligaments by displaying discontinuity of the anatomic structures, the presence of abnormal signal within them, and the presence of inflammatory changes.

Foot

[1] It is important to learn to recognize the multiple accessory ossicles of the foot:
- the normal appearance of these secondary ossification centers may mimic fractures
- conversely, an avulsion fracture may be misinterpreted as a normal ossicle.

[2] Harris-Beath and Broden views, tangential projections, are important techniques for evaluating injury to the subtalar joint.

[3] The Boehler angle demonstrates an important anatomic relation of the calcaneus and subtalar joint. It is useful for evaluating compression fracture of the calcaneus, particularly with extension into the subtalar joint.

[4] In fracture of the calcaneus (so-called lover's fracture), look for an associated compression fracture of the vertebral body in the thoracic or lumbar spine.

[5] Hawkins classification of talar neck fractures is based on the damage to the blood supply of the talus and serves as a prognostic guide for healing of the fracture, incidence of osteonecrosis, and indication for open reduction.

[6] In Lisfranc fracture–dislocation in the tarsometatarsal articulation, always look for an associated fracture either:
- at the base of the metatarsals
- or in the cuneiform bones.

SUGGESTED READINGS

Ala-Ketola L, Puranen J, Koivisto E, Puupera M. Arthrography in the diagnosis of ligament injuries and classification of ankle injuries. *Radiology* 1977;125:63–68.

Arimoto HK, Forrester DM. Classification of ankle fractures: An algorithm. *AJR Am J Roentgenol* 1980;135:1057–1063.

Baker K, Gilula L. The current role of tenography and bursography. *AJR Am J Roentgenol* 1990;154:129–133.

Beltran J. *MRI: musculoskeletal system.* Philadelphia: JB Lippincott; 1990.

Beltran J. MRI techniques and practical applications: magnetic resonance imaging of the ankle and foot. *Orthopedics* 1994;17:1075–1082.

Beltran J, Munchow AM, Khabiri H, Magee DG, McGhee RB, Grossman SB. Ligaments of the lateral aspect of the ankle and sinus tarsi: an MR imaging study. *Radiology* 1990;177:455–458.

Beltran J, Noto AM, Herman LJ, Lubbers LM. Tendons: high-field-strength, surface coil MR imaging. *Radiology* 1987;162:735–740.

Beltran J, Noto AM, Mosure JC, Shamam OM, Weiss KL, Zuelzer WA. Ankle: surface coil MR imaging at 1.5T. *Radiology* 1986;161:203–209.

Bencardino J, Rosenberg ZS. MR imaging and CT in the assessment of osseous abnormalities of the ankle and foot. *Magn Reson Imaging Clin North Am* 2001;9:567–577.

Berquist TM. Foot, ankle, and calf. In: Berquist TM, ed. *MRI of the musculoskeletal system.* New York: Raven Press, 1990:253–311.

Bleichrodt RP, Kingma LM, Binnendijk B, Klein J-P. Injuries of the lateral ankle ligaments: classification with tenography and arthrography. *Radiology* 1989;173:347–349.

Bone LB. Fractures of the tibial plafond. The pilon fracture. *Orthop Clin North Am* 1987;18:95–104.

Boruta PM, Bishop JO, Braly WG, Tullos HS. Acute lateral ankle ligament injuries: a literature review. *Foot Ankle Int* 1990;11:107–113.

Brostrom L, Liljedahl SO, Lindvall N. Sprained ankles. II. Arthrographic diagnosis of recent ligament ruptures. *Acta Chir Scand* 1965;129:485–499.

Brown KW Morrison WB, Schweitzer ME, Parellada JA, Nothnagel H. MRI findings associated with distal tibiofibular syndesmosis injury. *AJR Am J Roentgenol* 2004;182:131–136.

Bui-Mansfield LT, Kline M, Chew FS, Rogers LF, Lenchik L. Osteochondritis dissecans of the tibial plafond: imaging characteristics and a review of the literature. *AJR Am J Roentgenol* 2000;175:1305–1308.

Bureau NJ, Cardinal E, Hobden R, Aubin B. Posterior ankle impingement syndrome: MR imaging findings in seven patients. *Radiology* 2000;215:497–503.

Canale ST, Belding RH. Osteochondral lesions of the talus. *J Bone Joint Surg [Am]* 1980;62A:97–102.

Canale ST, Kelly FB. Fractures of the neck of the talus. *J Bone Joint Surg [Am]* 1978;60A:143–156.

Cetti R, Andersen I. Roentgenographic diagnoses of ruptured Achilles tendons. *Clin Orthop* 1993;286:215–221.

Chandnani VP, Bradley YC. Achilles tendon and miscellaneous tendon lesions. *Radiol Clin North Am* 1994;2:89–96.

Cheung Y, Rosenberg ZS, Magee T, Chinitz L. Normal anatomy and pathologic conditions of ankle tendons: current imaging techniques. *Radiographics* 1992;12:429–444.

Cone RO III, Nguyen V, Flournoy JG, Guerra J Jr. Triplane fracture of the distal tibial epiphysis: radiographic and CT studies. *Radiology* 1984;153:763–767.

Corbett M, Levy A, Abramowitz AJ, Whitelaw GP. A computer tomographic classification system for the displaced intraarticular fracture of the os calcis. *Orthopedics* 1995;18:705–710.

Daffner RH. Ankle trauma. *Radiol Clin North Am* 1990;28:395–421.

Daffner RH, Riemer BL, Lupetin AR, Dash N. Magnetic resonance imaging in acute tendon ruptures. *Skeletal Radiol* 1986;15:619–621.

De Smet AA, Fisher DR, Burnstein MI, Graf BK, Lange RH. Value of MR imaging in staging osteochondral lesions of the talus (osteochondritis dissecans): results in 14 patients. *AJR Am J Roentgenol* 1990;154:555–558.

De Smet AA, Reckling FW, McNamara GR. Radiographic classification of ankle injuries. *J Assoc Can Radiol* 1982;33:142–147.

DeLee JC. Fractures and dislocations of the foot. In: Mann RA, Coughlin MJ, eds. *Surgery of the foot and ankle*, 6th ed. St. Louis: CV Mosby; 1993:1550–1551.

Delfault EM, Demondion X, Biéganski A, Thiron M-C, Mestdagh H, Cotten A. Imaging of foot and ankle nerve entrapment syndromes: from well-demonstrated to unfamiliar sites. *Radiographics* 2003;23:613–623.

Dias LS, Giegerich CR. Fractures of the distal tibial epiphysis in adolescence. *J Bone Joint Surg [Am]* 1983;65A:438–444.

Dias LS, Tachdjian MO. Physeal injuries in the ankle in children. Classification. *Clin Orthop* 1978;136:230–233.

Donnelly EF. The Hawkins sign. *Radiology* 1999;210:195–196.

Edeiken J, Cotler JM. Ankle trauma. *Semin Roentgenol* 1978;13:145–155.

Edeiken J, Cotler JM. Ankle. In: Felson B, ed. *Fractures*. New York: Grune & Stratton; 1978.

Edeiken J, Cotler JM. Ankle. In: Felson B, ed. *Roentgenology of fractures and dislocations*. New York: Grune & Stratton; 1978:151.

Eichenholtz S, Levine DB. Fractures of the tarsal navicular bone. *Clin Orthop* 1964;34:142.

Erickson SJ, Quinn SF, Kneeland JB, et al. MR imaging of the tarsal tunnel and related spaces: normal and abnormal findings with anatomic correlation. *AJR Am J Roentgenol* 1990;155:323–328.

Erickson SJ, Rosengarten JL. MR imaging of the forefoot. Normal anatomic findings. *AJR Am J Roentgenol* 1993;169:567–571.

Erickson SJ, Smith JW, Ruiz ME, et al. MR imaging of the lateral collateral ligament of the ankle. *AJR Am J Roentgenol* 1991;156:131–136.

Essex-Lopresti P. The mechanism, reduction technique and results in fracture of the os calcis. *Br J Surg* 1982;39:395–419.

Evans GA, Frenyo SD. The stress-tenogram in the diagnosis of ruptures of the lateral ligament of the ankle. *J Bone Joint Surg [Br]* 1979;61B:347–351.

Faciszewski T, Burks RT, Manaster BJ. Subtle injuries of the Lisfranc joint. *J Bone Joint Surg [Am]* 1990;72A:1519–1522.

Farooki S, Yao L, Seeger LL. Anterolateral impingement of the ankle: effectiveness of MR imaging. *Radiology* 1998;207:357–360.

Feldman F, Singson RD, Rosenberg ZS, Berdon WE, Amodio J, Abramson SJ. Distal tibial triplane fractures: diagnosis with CT. *Radiology* 1987;164:429–435.

Finkel JE. Tarsal tunnel syndrome. *Radiol Clin North Am* 1994;2:67–78.

Fordyce AJW, Horn CV. Arthrography in recent injuries of the ligaments of the ankle. *J Bone Joint Surg [Br]* 1972;54B:116–121.

Fornage BD, Rifkin MD. Ultrasound examination of tendons. *Radiol Clin North Am* 1988;6:87–107.

Forrester DM, Kerr R. Trauma to the foot. *Radiol Clin North Am* 1990;28:423–433.

Freiberger RH. Introducing arthrography. In: Freiberger RH, Kaye JJ, eds. *Arthrography*. New York: Appleton-Century-Crofts; 1979:1–4.

Frost HM, Hanson CA. Technique for testing the drawer sign in the ankle. *Clin Orthop* 1977;123:49–51.

Gallo RA, Kolman BH, Daffner RH, Sciulli RL, Roberts CC, DeMeo PJ. MRI of tibialis anterior tendon rupture. *Skeletal Radiol* 2004;33:102–106.

Geissler WB, Tsao AK, Hughes JL. Fractures and injuries of the ankle. In: Rockwood CA, Green DP, Bucholz RW, Heckman JD, eds. *Rockwood and Green's fractures in adults*, 4th ed. Philadelphia: Lippincott-Raven Publishers; 1996:2236–2242.

Giannestras NJ. *Foot disorders. Medical and surgical management*, 2nd ed. Philadelphia, Lea & Febiger; 1973.

Giannestras NJ, Sammarco GL. Fractures and dislocations of the foot. In: Rockwood CA Jr, Green DP, eds. *Fractures*, vol. 2. Philadelphia: JB Lippincott; 1975.

Goldman AB. *Procedures in skeletal radiology*. New York: Grune & Stratton; 1984:181.

Gordon RB. Arthrography of the ankle joint. Experience in one hundred seven studies. *J Bone Joint Surg [Am]* 1970;52A:1623–1631.

Goss CM, Gray H, eds. *Anatomy of the human body*, 29th ed. Philadelphia; Lea & Febiger; 1973:355–359.

Greenspan A. Imaging of the foot and ankle. *Curr Opin Orthop* 1996;7:61–68.

Greenspan A, Anderson MW. Imaging of the foot and ankle. *Curr Opin Orthop* 1993;4:68–75.

Griffiths HJ. Trauma to the ankle and foot. *CRC Crit Rev Diagn Imaging* 1986;26:45–105.

Groshar D, Alperson M, Mendes DG, Barsky V, Liberson A. Bone scintigraphy findings in Lisfranc joint injury. *Foot Ankle Int* 1995;16:710–711.

Gross RH. Fractures and dislocations of the foot. In: Rockwood CA, Wilkins KE, Kuig RE, eds. *Fractures in children*, vol. 3. Philadelphia: JB Lippincott; 1984:1043–1103.

Hansen ST. Foot injuries. In: Browner BD, Jupiter JB, Levine AM, Trafton PG, eds. *Skele-*

tal trauma: fractures—dislocations—ligamentous injuries. Philadelphia: WB Saunders; 1992:1960–1961.

Haraguchi N, Kato F, Hayashi H. New radiographic projections for avulsion fractures of the lateral malleolus. *J Bone Joint Surg [Br]* 1998;80B:684–688.

Hauger O, Moinard M, Lasalarie JC, Chauveaux D, Diard F. Anterolateral compartment of the ankle in the lateral impingement syndrome: appearance on CT arthrography. *AJR Am J Roentgenol* 1999;173:685–690.

Hawkins LG. Fractures of the lateral process of the talus. *J Bone Joint Surg [Am]* 1965;47A:1170–1175.

Hawkins LG. Fractures of the neck of the talus. *J Bone Joint Surg [Am]* 1970;52A:991–1002.

Haygood TM. Magnetic resonance imaging of the musculoskeletal system. VII. The ankle. *Clin Orthop* 1997;336:318–336.

Heare MM, Gillespy T, Bittar ES. Direct coronal computed tomography arthrography of osteochondritis dissecans of the talus. *Skeletal Radiol* 1988;17:187–189.

Heckman JD. Fractures and dislocations of the foot. In: Rockwood CA Jr, Green DP, Bucholz RW, Heckman JD, eds. *Rockwood and Green's fractures in adults,* 4th ed. Philadelphia: Lippincott-Raven; 1996:2295–2308.

Helgason JW, Chandnani VP. MR arthrography of the ankle. *Radiol Clin North Am* 1998;36:729–738.

Herring C. Nomenclature for imaging planes of the feet [Letter]. *AJR Am J Roentgenol* 1997;168:277.

Jahss MH. *Disorders of the foot and ankle,* vol. 2, 2nd ed. Philadelphia: WB Saunders; 1991.

Janzen DL, Connell DG, Munk PL, Buckley RE, Meek RN, Schechter MT. Intraarticular fractures of the calcaneus: value of CT findings in determining prognosis. *AJR Am J Roentgenol* 1992;158:1271–1274.

Jones R. Fracture of the base of the fifth metatarsal by direct violence. *Ann Surg* 1902;35:697.

Kainberger FM, Engel A, Barton P, Huebsch P, Neuhold A, Salomonowitz E. Injury of the Achilles tendon: diagnosis with sonography. *AJR Am J Roentgenol* 1990;155:1031–1036.

Kaplan PA, Helms CA, Dussault R, Anderson MW, Major NM. *Musculoskeletal MRI.* Philadelphia: Saunders WB; 2001:393–437.

Kaye JJ. The ankle. In: Freiberger RH, Kaye JJ, eds. *Arthrography.* New York: Appleton-Century-Crofts; 1979:237–256.

Keck C. The tarsal-tunnel syndrome. *J Bone Joint Surg [Am]* 1962;44A:180–182.

Kerr R, Frey C. MR imaging in the tarsal tunnel syndrome. *J Comput Assist Tomogr* 1991;15:280–286.

Khoury NJ, El-Khoury GY, Saltzman CL, Brandser EA. Rupture of the anterior tibial tendon: diagnosis by MR imaging. *AJR Am J Roentgenol* 1996;167:351–354.

Khoury NJ, El-Khoury GY, Saltzman CL, Kathol MH. Peroneus longus and brevis tendon tears: MR imaging evaluation. *Radiology* 1996;200:833–841.

Kirch MD, Erickson SJ. Normal magnetic resonance imaging of the ankle and foot. *Radiol Clin North Am* 1994;2:1–22.

Kleiger B. A review of ankle fractures due to lateral strains. *Bull Hosp Joint Dis Orthop Inst* 1968;29:138–186.

Kleiger B. Mechanisms of ankle injury. *Orthop Clin North Am* 1974;5:127–146.

Kleiger B, Mankin HJ. A roentgenographic study of the development of the calcaneus by means of the posterior tangential view. *J Bone Joint Surg [Am]* 1961;43A:961–969.

Kleiger B, Mankin HJ. Fracture of the lateral portion of the distal tibial epiphysis. *J Bone Joint Surg [Am]* 1964;46A:25–32.

Klein MA, Spreitzer AM. MR imaging of the tarsal sinus and canal: normal anatomy, pathologic findings and features of the sinus tarsi syndrome. *Radiology* 1993;226:169–173.

Kneeland JB. Technical considerations for magnetic resonance imaging of the ankle and foot. *Radiol Clin North Am* 1994;2:23–28.

Kneeland JB, Dalinka MK. Magnetic resonance imaging of the foot and ankle. *Magn Reson Q* 1992;8:97–115.

Kneeland JB, Macrandar S, Middleton WD, Cates JD, Jesmanowicz A, Hyde JS. MR imaging of the normal ankle: correlation with anatomic sections. *AJR Am J Roentgenol* 1988;151:117–123.

Lam SJS. A tarsal-tunnel syndrome. *Lancet* 1962;2:1354–1355.

Lau JTC, Daniels TR. Tarsal tunnel syndrome: a review of the literature. *Foot Ankle Int* 1999;20:201–209.

Lauge-Hansen N. Fractures of the ankle. Analytical survey as the basis of new experimental, roentgenological, and clinical investigations. *Arch Surg* 1948;56:259–317.

Lauge-Hansen N. Fractures of the ankle. II. Combined experimental-surgical and experimental-roentgenologic investigations. *Arch Surg* 1950;60:957–985.

Lauge-Hansen N. "Ligamentous" ankle fractures: diagnosis and treatment. *Acta Chir Scand* 1949;97:544–550.

Lee SH, Jacobson J, Trudell D, Resnick D. Ligaments of the ankle: normal anatomy with MR arthrography. *J Comput Assist Tomogr* 1998;22:807–813.

Leitch JM, Cundy PJ, Paterson DC. Three-dimensional imaging of a juvenile Tillaux fracture. *J Pediatr Orthop* 1989;9:602–603.

Lektrakul N, Chung CB, Theodorou DJ, Yu J, Haghighi P, Trudell D, Resnick D. Tarsal sinus: arthrographic, MR imaging, MR arthrographic, and pathologic findings in cadavers and retrospective study data in patients with sinus tarsi syndrome. *Radiology* 2001;219:802–810.

Lindsjo U. Classification of ankle fractures: the Lauge-Hansen or AO system? *Clin Orthop* 1985;199:12–16.

Lowery RBW. Fractures of the talus and os calcis. *Curr Opin Orthop* 1995;6:25–34.

Lowrie IG, Finlay BB, Brenke IJ, Gregg PJ. Computed tomographic assessment of the subtalar joint in calcaneal fractures. *J Bone Joint Surg [Br]* 1988;70B:247–250.

Ly JQ, Bui-Mansfield LT. Anatomy of the abnormalities associated with Kager's fat pad. *AJR Am J Roentgenol* 2004;182:147–154.

Lynn MD. The triplane distal tibial epiphyseal fracture. *Clin Orthop* 1972;86:187–190.

Magee TH, Hinson GW. Usefulness of MR imaging in the detection of talar dome injuries. *AJR Am J Roentgenol* 1998;170:1227–1230.

Magid D, Michelson JD, Ney DR, Fishman EK. Adult ankle fractures: comparison of plain films and interactive two- and three-dimensional CT scans. *AJR Am J Roentgenol* 1990;154:1017–1023.

Mainwaring BL, Daffner RH, Riemer BL. Pylon fractures of the ankle: a distinct clinical and radiologic entity. *Radiology* 1988;168:215–218.

Marmor L. An unusual fracture of the tibial epiphysis. *Clin Orthop* 1970;73:132–135.

Mast J. Pilon fractures of the tibia. In: Chapman MW, ed. *Operative orthopaedics,* 2nd ed. Philadelphia: JB Lippincott; 1993:711–729.

Meschan I. *Synopsis of roentgen signs.* Philadelphia: WB Saunders; 1962.

Mesgarzadeh M, Schneck CD, Tehranzadeh J, Chandnani VP, Bonakdarpour A. Magnetic resonance imaging of ankle ligaments. Emphasis on anatomy and injuries to lateral collateral ligaments. *Radiol Clin North Am* 1994;2:39–58.

Michelson JD. Current concepts review: fractures about the ankle. *J Bone Joint Surg [Am]* 1995;77A:142–152.

Mink JH. Tendons. In: Deutsch AL, Mink JH, Kerr R, eds. *MRI of the foot and ankle.* Philadelphia: Lippincott-Raven Publishers; 1992:135–172.

Morrey BF, Cass JR, Johnson KA, Berquist TH. Foot and ankle. In: Berquist TH, ed. *Imaging of orthopedic trauma and surgery.* Philadelphia: WB Saunders; 1986:407–498.

Muhle C, Frank LR, Rand T, et al. Collateral ligaments of the ankle: high-resolution MR imaging with a local gradient coil and anatomic correlation in cadavers. *Radiographics* 1999;19:673–683.

Müller ME, Allgower M, Schneider R, Willenegger H. *Manual of internal fixation techniques recommended by AO Group,* 2nd ed. New York: Springer-Verlag; 1979.

Müller ME, Nazarian S, Koch P. *The AO classification of fractures.* New York: Springer-Verlag; 1979.

Newburg AH. Osteochondral fractures of the dome of the talus. *Br J Radiol* 1979;52:105–109.

Nielson JO, Dons-Jensen H, Sorensen HT. Lauge-Hansen classification of malleolar fractures: an assessment of the reproducibility in 118 cases. *Acta Orthop Scand* 1990;61:385–387.

Norman A, Kleiger B, Greenspan A, Finkel JE. Roentgenographic examination of the normal foot and ankle. In: Jahss MM, ed. *Disorders of the foot and ankle. Medical and surgical management,* vol. 1, 2nd ed. Philadelphia: WB Saunders; 1991:64–90.

Oae K, Takao M, Naito K, Uchio Y, Kono T, Ishida J, Ochi M. Injury of the tibiofibular syndesmosis: value of MR imaging for diagnosis. *Radiology* 2003;227:155–161.

Ohashi K, El-Khoury GY, Bennett DL. MDCT of tendon abnormalities using volume-rendered images. *AJR Am J Roentgenol* 2004;182:161–165.

Ouzounian TJ, Anderson R. Anterior tibial tendon rupture. *Foot Ankle Int* 1995;16:406–410.

Pankovich AM. Fractures of the fibula proximal to the distal tibiofibular syndesmosis. *J Bone Joint Surg [Am]* 1978;60A:221–229.

Pavlov H. Talo-calcaneonavicular arthrography. In: Freiberger RH, Kaye JJ, eds. *Arthrography.* New York: Appleton-Century-Crofts; 1979:257–260.

Peltier LF. Eponymic fractures: Robert Jones and Jones' fracture. *Surgery* 1972;71:522–526.

Peltier LF. Guillaume Dupuytren and Dupuytren's fracture. *Surgery* 1958;43:868–874.

Peltier LF. Percival Pott and Pott's fracture. *Surgery* 1962;51:280–286.

Pennal GF. Fractures of the talus. *Clin Orthop* 1963;30:53–63.

Prokuski LJ, Saltzman CL. Challenging fractures of the foot and ankle. *Radiol Clin North Am* 1997;35:655–670.

Protas JM, Kornblatt BA. Fractures of the lateral margin of the distal tibia. The Tillaux fracture. *Radiology* 1981;138:55–57.

Raatikainen T, Putkonen M, Puranen J. Arthrography, clinical examination, and stress radiograph in the diagnosis of acute injury to the lateral ligaments of the ankle. *Am J Sports Med* 1992;20:2–6.

Rasmussen S, Madsen PV, Bennicke K. Observer variation in the Lauge-Hansen classification of ankle fractures: precision improved by instruction. *Acta Orthop Scand* 1993;74:693–694.

Rijke AM, Jones B, Vierhovt PAM. Stress examination of traumatized lateral ligaments of the ankle. *Clin Orthop* 1986;210:143–151.

Robbins MI, Wilson MG, Sella EJ. MR imaging of the anterior calcaneal process fractures. *AJR Am J Roentgenol* 1999;172:475–479.

Robinson P, White LM, Salonen DC, Daniels TR, Ogilvie-Harris D. Anterolateral ankle impingement: MR arthrographic assessment of the anterolateral recess. *Radiology* 2001;221:186–190.

Robinson P, White LM, Salonen DC, Ogilvie-Harris D. Anteromedial impingement of the ankle: using MR arthrography to assess the anteromedial recess. *AJR Am J Roentgenol* 2002;178:601–604.

Robinson P, White LM. Soft-tissue and osseous impingement syndromes of the ankle: role of imaging in diagnosis and management. *Radiographics* 2002;22:1457–1471.

Rogers LF. *Radiology of skeletal trauma.* New York: Churchill Livingstone, 1992:1319–1385.

Rosenberg ZS. Chronic rupture of the posterior tibial tendon. *Radiol Clin North Am* 1994;2:79–87.

Rosenberg ZS. Normal anatomy of ankle tendons and ligaments: computed tomography and magnetic resonance imaging. In: Taveras JM, Ferrucci JT, eds. *Radiology,* vol. 5. Hagerstown, MD: JB Lippincott; 1989:1–6.

Rosenberg ZS, Cheung Y, Jahss MH. Computed tomography scan and magnetic resonance imaging of ankle tendons: an overview. *Foot Ankle* 1988;8:297–307.

Rosenberg ZS, Feldman F, Singson RD. Peroneal tendon injuries: CT analysis. *Radiology* 1986;161:743–748.

Rosenberg ZS, Feldman F, Singson RD, Kane R. Ankle tendons: evaluation with CT. *Radiology* 1988;166:221–226.

Rosenberg ZS, Feldman F, Singson RD, Price GJ. Peroneal tendon injury associated with calcaneal fractures: CT findings. *AJR Am J Roentgenol* 1987;149:125–129.

Rowe CR, Sakellarides HT, Freeman PA, Sorbie C. Fracture of the os calcis: a long-term follow-up study of 146 patients. *JAMA* 1963;184:920.

Rubin DA, Towers JD, Britton CA. MR imaging of the foot: utility of complex oblique imaging planes. *AJR Am J Roentgenol* 1996;166:1079–1084.

Sammarco GJ. Peroneal tendon injuries. *Orthop Clin North Am* 1994;25:135–145.

Sangeorzan BJ, Benirschke SK, Mosca V, et al. Displaced intra-articular fractures of the tarsal navicular. *J Bone Joint Surg [Am]* 1989;71A:1504–1510.

Sarrafian S. *Anatomy of the foot and ankle,* 2nd ed. Philadelphia: JB Lippincott; 1993.

Sartoris DJ, Mink JH, Kerr R. The foot and ankle. In: Mink JH, Deutsch AL, eds. *MRI of the musculoskeletal system: a teaching file.* New York: Raven Press; 1990:389–450.

Schneck CD, Mesgarzadeh M, Bonakdarpour A. MR imaging of the most commonly injured ankle ligaments. Part II. Ligament injuries. *Radiology* 1992;184:507–512.

Schneck CD, Mesgarzadeh M, Bonakdarpour A, Ross GJ. MR imaging of the most commonly injured ankle ligaments. Part I. Normal anatomy. *Radiology* 1992;184:499–506.

Schreibman KL, Gilula LA. Ankle tenography. A therapeutic imaging modality. *Radiol Clin North Am* 1998;36:739–756.

Schweitzer ME, Karasick D. MR imaging of disorders of the Achilles tendon. *AJR Am J Roentgenol* 2000;175:613–625.

Shereff MJ, Johnson KA. Radiographic anatomy of the hindfoot. *Clin Orthop* 1983;117:16.

Smith RW. Computerized sectional imaging: computed tomography and magnetic resonance imaging of the foot and ankle. In: Jahss MH, ed. *Disorders of the foot and ankle. Medical and surgical management,* vol. 1. 2nd ed. Philadelphia, WB Saunders; 1991:155–204.

Spiegel PK, Staples OS. Arthrography of the ankle joint: problems in diagnosis of acute lateral ligament injuries. *Radiology* 1975;114:587–590.

Staples OS. Ligamentous injuries of the ankle joint. *Clin Orthop* 1965;42:21–35.

Stewart I. Jones' fracture: fracture of the base of the fifth metatarsal. *Clin Orthop* 1960;16:190–198.

Swanson TV. Fractures and dislocations of the talus. In: Chapman MW, ed. *Operative orthopaedics,* 2nd ed. Philadelphia: JB Lippincott; 1993:2143–2145.

Tehranzadeh J, Stuffman E, Ross SDK. Partial Hawkins sign in fractures of the talus: a report of three cases. *AJR Am J Roentgenol* 2003;181:1559–1563.

Teng MMH, Destovet JM, Gilula LA, Resnick D, Hembree JL, Oloff LM. Ankle tenography: a key to unexplained symptomatology. Part I: Normal tenographic anatomy. *Radiology* 1984;151:575–580.

Theodorou DJ, Theodorou SJ, Kakitsubata Y, Botte MJ, Resnick D. Fractures of proximal portion of fifth metatarsal bone: anatomic and imaging evidence of a pathogenesis of avulsion of the plantar aponeurosis and the short peroneal muscle tendon. *Radiology* 2003;226:857–865.

Theodorou DJ, Theodorou SJ, Resnick D. Proximal fifth metatarsal bone: not everything is a Jones' fracture (abstr). *Radiology* 2001;221(P):667.

Trafton PG, Bray TJ, Simpson LA. Fractures and soft tissue injuries of the ankle. In: Browner BD, Jupiter JB, Levine AM, Trafton PG, eds. *Skeletal trauma: fractures—dislocations—ligamentous injuries.* Philadelphia: WB Saunders; 1992:1871–1957.

Urman M, Ammann W, Sisler J, et al. The role of bone scintigraphy in the evaluation of talar dome fractures. *J Nucl Med* 1991;32:2241–2244.

Vogl TJ, Hochmut K, Diebold T, et al. Magnetic resonance imaging in the diagnosis of acute injured distal tibiofibular syndesmosis. *Invest Radiol* 1997;32:401–409.

Vuori JP, Aro HT. Lisfranc joint injuries: trauma mechanisms and associated injuries. *J Trauma* 1993;35:40–45.

Watson-Jones R. *Fractures and joint injuries,* vols. I, II. St. Louis: Mosby; 1952,1955.

Weber BG. *Die Verletzungen des Oberen Sprunggelenkes.* Stuttgart: Verlag Hans Huber; 1972.

Weber MJ. Ankle fractures and dislocations. In: Chapman MW, ed. *Operative Orthopaedics,* 2nd ed. Philadelphia: JB Lippincott; 1993:731–745.

Wechsler RJ, Schweitzer ME, Karasick D, Deely DM, Glaser JB. Helical CT of talar fractures. *Skeletal Radiol* 1997;26:137–142.

Wetzel LH, Murphey MD. Magnetic resonance imaging and computed tomography of the foot and ankle. In: Bloem JL, Sartoris DJ, eds. *MRI and CT of the musculoskeletal system. A text-atlas.* Baltimore: Williams & Wilkins; 1992:498–524.

Yulish BS, Mulopulos GP, Goodfellow DB, Bryan PJ, Modic MT, Dollinger BM. MR imaging of osteochondral lesions of talus. *J Comput Assist Tomogr* 1987;11:296–301.

SPINE

Fractures of the vertebral column are important not only because of the structures involved but also because of the complications that may arise affecting the spinal cord. Constituting approximately 3% to 6% of all skeletal injuries, fractures of the vertebral column are most commonly encountered in people between the ages of 20 and 50 years, with the majority of cases (80%) being seen in males. Most spinal fractures occur at the thoracic and lumbar levels, but injury to the cervical area has a greater potential risk for spinal cord damage. Automobile accidents, sports-related activities (e.g., diving, skiing), and falls from heights are usually the circumstances in which spinal injuries are sustained.

The spine is composed of 33 vertebrae: 7 cervical, 12 thoracic, 5 lumbar, a sacrum of 5 fused segments, and a coccyx of 4 fused segments. With the exception of the first and second cervical vertebrae (C-1 and C-2), the vertebral bodies are separated from each other by intervertebral disks.

Cervical Spine

Anatomic–Radiologic Considerations

Structurally, the first and second cervical vertebrae possess anatomic features distinct from those of the remaining five cervical vertebrae (Fig. 11.1). The first cervical vertebra, C-1 or atlas, is a bony ring consisting of anterior and posterior arches connected by two lateral masses. The atlas has no body; its main structures are the lateral masses, also called "articular pillars." The second vertebra, C-2 or axis, is a more complex structure whose distinguishing feature is the odon-toid process, also known as the "dens" (tooth), projecting cephalad from the anterior surface of the body. The space between the odontoid process and the anterior arch of the atlas, called the "atlantal–dens interval," should not exceed 3 mm in adults, whether the head is flexed or extended. In children younger than age 8 years, this distance has been reported to be as much as 4 mm, particularly in flexion, secondary to greater ligamentous laxity.

The vertebrae C3-7 exhibit identical anatomic features and are more uniform in appearance, consisting of a vertebral body and a posterior neural arch, including the right and left pedicles and laminae, which together with the posterior aspect of the body enclose the spinal canal (Fig. 11.2). Extending caudad and cephalad from the junction of the pedicle and lamina on each side are superior and inferior articular processes, which form the apophyseal joints between the successive vertebrae. Extending laterally from the pedicle on each side is a transverse process and, in the posterior portion, a spinous process extends from the junction of the laminae in the midline. The vertebra C-7, in addition, is distinguished by its long spinous process and large transverse processes.

Radiographic examination of a patient with cervical spine trauma may be difficult and is usually limited to one or two projections; because frequently the patient is unconscious, there are associated injuries, and unnecessary movement risks damage to the cervical cord. The single most valuable projection in these instances is the lateral view, which may be obtained in the standard fashion or with the patient supine, depending on the condition (Fig. 11.3). This projection suffices to demonstrate most traumatic conditions of the cervical spine, including injuries involving the anterior and posterior arches of C-1; the odontoid process, which is seen in profile; and the anterior at-

TOPOGRAPHIC ANATOMY OF THE C-1 AND C-2 VERTEBRAE

anteroposterior view

lateral view

axial view (superior)

▭▭ atlantoaxial joint
▮ atlantal–dens interval

1 odontoid process of axis (dens)
2 lateral masses of atlas
3 body of axis
4 superior articular facet
5 transverse process
6 inferior articular facet

7 pedicle
8 lamina
9 spinous process
10 transverse foramen
11 anterior arch of atlas
12 posterior arch of atlas

Figure 11.1 Topographic anatomy of the C-1 and C-2 vertebrae.

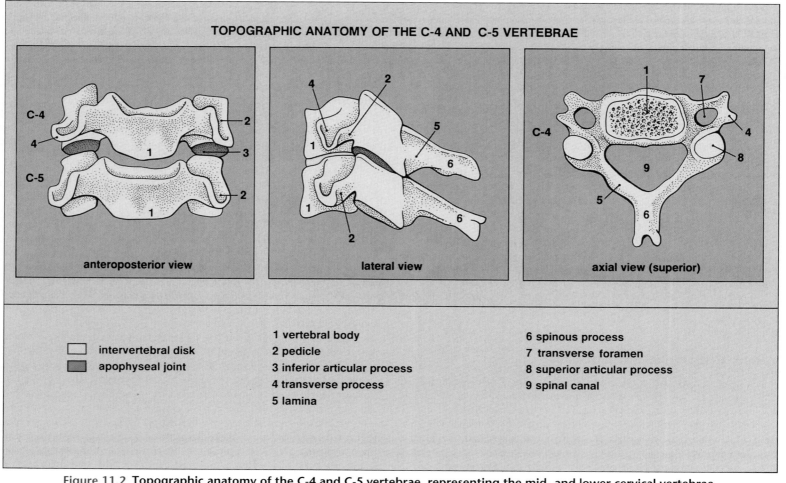

TOPOGRAPHIC ANATOMY OF THE C-4 AND C-5 VERTEBRAE

anteroposterior view

lateral view

axial view (superior)

▯ intervertebral disk
▮ apophyseal joint

1 vertebral body
2 pedicle
3 inferior articular process
4 transverse process
5 lamina

6 spinous process
7 transverse foramen
8 superior articular process
9 spinal canal

Figure 11.2 Topographic anatomy of the C-4 and C-5 vertebrae, representing the mid- and lower cervical vertebrae.

Figure 11.3 Lateral view. (A) For the erect lateral view of the cervical spine, the patient is standing or seated, with the head straight in the neutral position. The central beam is directed horizontally to the center of the C-4 vertebra (at the level of the chin). **(B)** For the cross-table lateral view, the patient is supine on the radiographic table. The radiographic cassette (a grid cassette to obtain a clearer image) is adjusted to the side of the neck, and the central beam is directed horizontally to a point *(red dot)* approximately 2.5 to 3 cm caudal to the mastoid tip. **(C)** The film in this projection clearly shows the vertebral bodies, apophyseal joints, spinous processes, and intervertebral disk spaces. It is mandatory to demonstrate the C-7 vertebra. *(continued)*

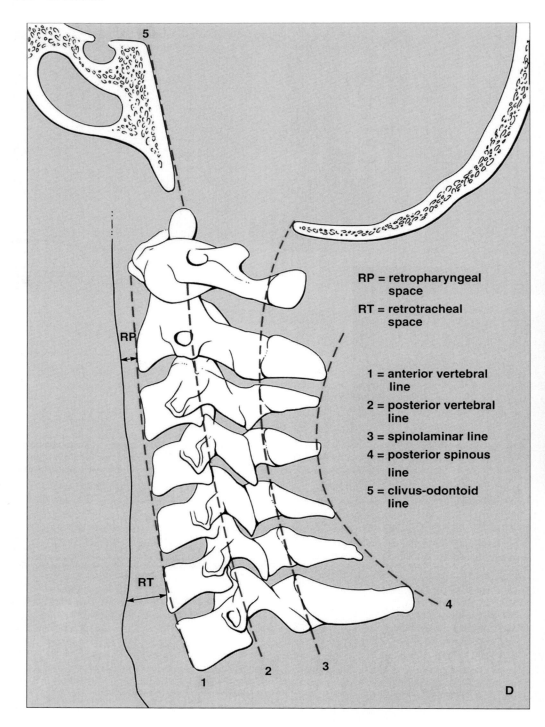

RP = retropharyngeal
        space

RT = retrotracheal
        space

1 = anterior vertebral
        line

2 = posterior vertebral
        line

3 = spinolaminar line

4 = posterior spinous
        line

5 = clivus-odontoid
        line

Figure 11.3 Lateral view. *Continued.* **(D)** With this view, the five contour lines of the normal cervical spine can be demonstrated: anterior vertebral line drawn along anterior margins of the vertebral bodies; posterior vertebral line (outlines anterior margin of spinal canal), drawn along posterior margins of the vertebral bodies; spinolaminar line (outlines posterior margin of the spinal canal), drawn along the anterior margins of the bases of the spinous processes at the junction with lamina; posterior spinous line drawn along the tips of the spinous processes from C2-7, which should be running smoothly, without angulation or interruption; and the clivus-odontoid line, drawn from the dorsum sellae along the clivus to the anterior margin of the foramen magnum should point to the tip of the odontoid process at the junction of the anterior and middle thirds. The retropharyngeal space (distance from the posterior pharyngeal wall to the anteroinferior aspect of C-2) should measure 7 mm or less; the retrotracheal space (distance from the posterior wall of the trachea to the anteroinferior aspect of C-6) should measure no more than 22 mm in adults and 14 mm in children. **(E)** Low-kilovoltage technique demonstrates prevertebral soft tissues to better advantage.

lantal–dens interval. The bodies and spinous processes of C2-7 are fully visualized, and the intervertebral disk spaces and prevertebral soft tissues can be adequately evaluated. The lateral radiograph may also be obtained in flexion of the neck, which is particularly effective in demonstrating suspected instability at C1-2 by allowing evaluation of the atlanto–odontoid distance; an increase in this distance to more than 3 mm indicates atlantoaxial subluxation. It is of the utmost importance on the lateral projection of the cervical spine that the C-7 vertebra be visualized, because this is the most commonly overlooked site of injuries.

The lateral view of the cervical spine, including the lower part of the skull, is extremely important to evaluate the vertical subluxation involving the atlantoaxial articulation and the migration of the odontoid process into the foramen magnum. Several measurements are helpful to determine atlantoaxial impaction or cranial settling resulting in superior migration of the odontoid process (Figs. 11.4–11.7).

On the anteroposterior view of the cervical spine (Fig. 11.8), the bodies of the C3-7 vertebrae (and occasionally in young persons, even the C-1 and C-2 vertebrae) are well demonstrated, as are the uncovertebral (Luschka) joints and the intervertebral disk spaces. The

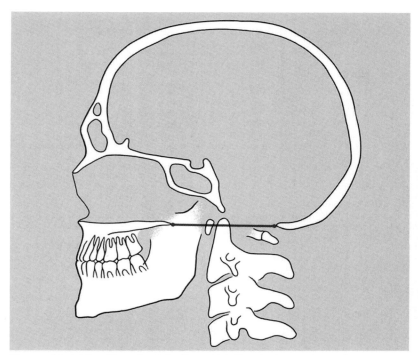

Figure 11.4 The Chamberlain line. This line is drawn from the posterior margin of the foramen magnum (opisthion) to the dorsal (posterior) margin of the hard palate. The odontoid process should not project above this line more than 3 mm; a projection of 6.6 mm (±2 SD) above this line strongly indicates cranial settling.

Figure 11.5 The McRae line. This line defines the opening of the foramen magnum and connects the anterior margin (basion) with posterior margin (opisthion) of the foramen magnum. The odontoid process should be just below this line or the line may intersect only at the tip of the odontoid process. In addition, a perpendicular line drawn from the apex of the odontoid to this line should intersect it in its ventral quarter.

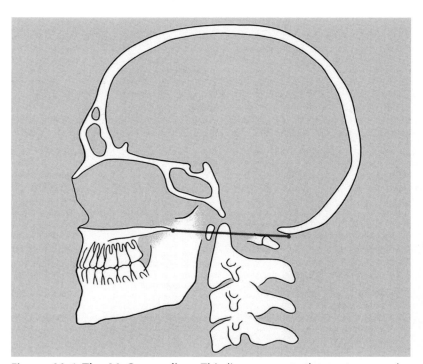

Figure 11.6 The McGregor line. This line connects the posterosuperior margin of the hard palate to the most caudal part of the occipital curve of the skull. The tip of the odontoid normally does not extend more than 4.5 mm above the line.

Figure 11.7 Ranawat method. Ranawat and associates developed a method for determining the extent of the superior margin of the odontoid process, since the hard palate often is not identifiable on radiographs of the cervical spine. The coronal axis of C-1 is determined by connecting the center of the anterior arch of the first cervical vertebra with its posterior ring. The center of the sclerotic ring in C-2, representing the pedicles, is marked. The line is drawn along the axis of the odontoid process to the first line. The normal distance between C-1 and C-2 in men averages 17 mm (±2 mm SD), and in women, 15 mm (± 2 mm SD). A decrease in this distance indicates cephalad migration of C-2.

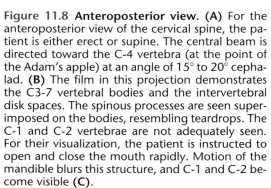

Figure 11.8 Anteroposterior view. (A) For the anteroposterior view of the cervical spine, the patient is either erect or supine. The central beam is directed toward the C-4 vertebra (at the point of the Adam's apple) at an angle of 15° to 20° cephalad. **(B)** The film in this projection demonstrates the C3-7 vertebral bodies and the intervertebral disk spaces. The spinous processes are seen superimposed on the bodies, resembling teardrops. The C-1 and C-2 vertebrae are not adequately seen. For their visualization, the patient is instructed to open and close the mouth rapidly. Motion of the mandible blurs this structure, and C-1 and C-2 become visible **(C)**.

Figure 11.9 Open-mouth view. For the open-mouth view, the patient is positioned in the same manner as for the supine anteroposterior projection; the head is straight, in the neutral position. With the patient's mouth open as widely as possible, the central beam is directed perpendicular to the midpoint of the open mouth. During the exposure, the patient should softly phonate "ah" to affix the tongue to the floor of the mouth so that its shadow is not projected over C-1 and C-2. On the radiograph, the odontoid process, the body of C-2, and the lateral masses of the atlas are well demonstrated; the atlantoaxial joints are seen to best advantage.

spinous processes are seen almost on end, casting oval shadows resembling teardrops. A variant of the anteroposterior projection known as the open-mouth view (Fig. 11.9) may also be obtained as part of the standard examination. This view provides effective visualization of the structures of the first two cervical vertebrae. The body of C-2 is clearly imaged, as are the atlantoaxial joints, the odontoid process, and the lateral spaces between the odontoid process and the articular pillars of C-1. If the open-mouth view is difficult to obtain or the odontoid process is not clearly visualized, particularly its upper half, then the Fuchs view may be helpful (Fig. 11.10). Oblique projections of the cervical spine (Fig. 11.11) are not routinely obtained, although at times they help visualize obscure fractures of the neural

arch and abnormalities of the neural foramina and apophyseal joints. Special projections may occasionally be required for sufficient evaluation of the structures of the cervical spine. The pillar view (Fig. 11.12), which may be obtained in the anteroposterior or oblique projection, serves to demonstrate the lateral masses of the cervical vertebrae, and the swimmer's view (Fig. 11.13) may be used for better demonstration of the C-7, T-1, and T-2 vertebrae, which on the standard lateral or oblique projection are obscured by the overlapping clavicle and soft tissues of the shoulder girdle. Fluoroscopy and videotaping are usually of little help in acute injuries because pain may prevent the necessary movement for positioning.

Ancillary imaging techniques play an important role in the eval-

Figure 11.10 Fuchs view. (A) For the Fuchs views of the odontoid process, the patient is supine on the table, with the neck hyperextended. The central beam is directed vertically to the neck just below the tip of the chin. **(B)** On the radiograph obtained in this projection, the odontoid, especially its upper half, is clearly visualized.

Figure 11.11 Oblique view. (A) An oblique view of the cervical spine may be obtained in the anteroposterior (as shown here) or posteroanterior projection. The patient may be erect or recumbent, but the erect position (seated or standing) is more comfortable. The patient is rotated 45° to one side—to the left, as shown here, to demonstrate the right-sided neural foramina and to the right to demonstrate the left-sided neural foramina. The central beam is directed to the C-4 vertebra with 15° to 20° cephalad angulation. **(B)** The film in this projection is effective primarily for demonstrating the intervertebral neural foramina.

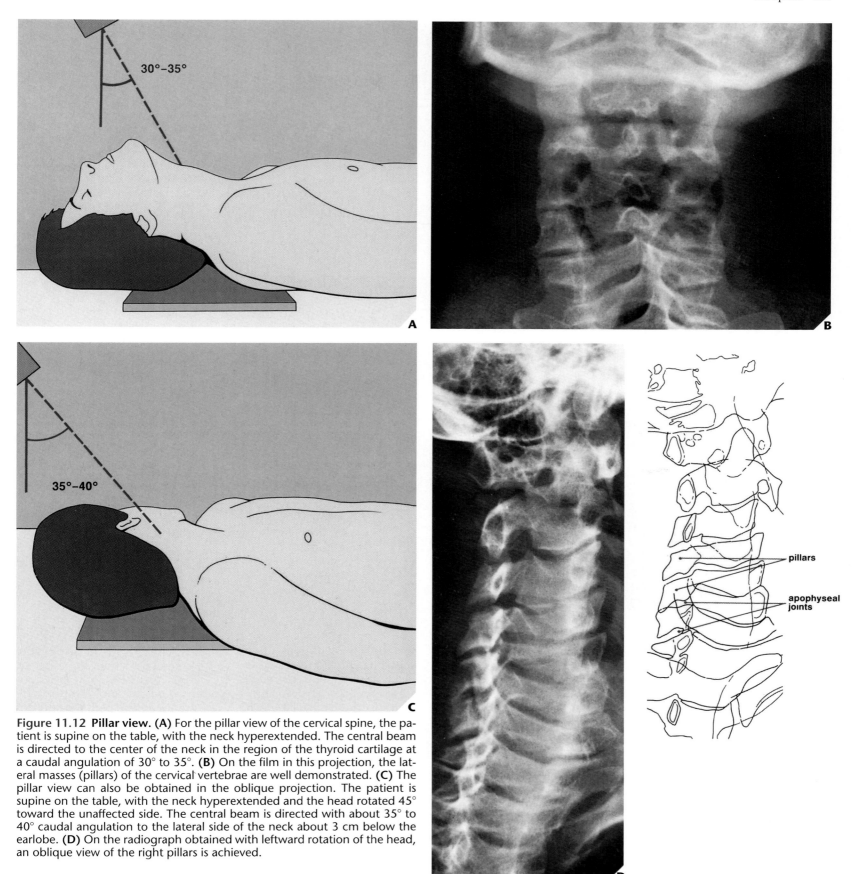

Figure 11.12 Pillar view. (A) For the pillar view of the cervical spine, the patient is supine on the table, with the neck hyperextended. The central beam is directed to the center of the neck in the region of the thyroid cartilage at a caudal angulation of 30° to 35°. **(B)** On the film in this projection, the lateral masses (pillars) of the cervical vertebrae are well demonstrated. **(C)** The pillar view can also be obtained in the oblique projection. The patient is supine on the table, with the neck hyperextended and the head rotated 45° toward the unaffected side. The central beam is directed with about 35° to 40° caudal angulation to the lateral side of the neck about 3 cm below the earlobe. **(D)** On the radiograph obtained with leftward rotation of the head, an oblique view of the right pillars is achieved.

Figure 11.13 Swimmer's view. (A) For the swimmer's view of the cervical spine, the patient is placed prone on the table with the left arm abducted 180° and the right arm by the side, as if swimming the crawl. The central beam is directed horizontally toward the left axilla. The radiographic cassette is against the right side of the neck, as for the standard cross-table lateral view. **(B)** The film in this projection provides adequate visualization of the C-7, T-1, and T-2 vertebrae, which would otherwise be obscured by the shoulders.

uation of suspected spinal trauma. Conventional tomography and computed tomography (CT) are commonly used techniques. In the evaluation of fractures of the odontoid process, for example, conventional tomography is particularly helpful; in determining the extent of cervical spine injuries in general, including soft-tissue trauma, CT (Fig. 11.14) provides valuable information regarding the integrity of the spinal canal and the localization of fracture fragments within the canal.

In the past decade, magnetic resonance imaging (MRI) has become the most effective modality to evaluate vertebral trauma because of the impressive quality of its images and its multiplanar capabilities, which allow examination of acutely traumatized patients without moving them. In evaluating fractures, MRI is useful not only to determine the relationship of bony fragments that may be displaced in the vertebral canal but also to demonstrate the full extent of injury, especially to the soft tissues and the spinal cord. The effect of the trauma on the spinal cord can be directly imaged, and spinal cord compression can be diagnosed. The superior soft-tissue contrast resolution of MRI can reveal minimal edema and small quantities of hemorrhage within the spinal cord. Injury to ligamentous structures and extradural pathology also may be readily identified. In the cervical spine, 3-mm-thick sagittal sections and 5-mm-thick axial sections are routinely obtained. The most effective are spin-echo T1- and T2- or T2*-weighted images obtained in the sagittal plane. Sagittal MR images permit evaluation of

vertebral body alignment and integrity, along with the size of the spinal canal (Fig. 11.15A). On the parasagittal section, the articular facets are well demonstrated (Fig. 11.15B). More recently, fast scans (fast spin-echo [FSE]) have been advocated for demonstrating injuries in the axial plane. These fast gradient-echo pulse sequences have become a popular addition to, or a replacement for, spin-echo T2-weighted sequences. Gradient-echo sequences have short acquisition times and adequate resolution and show a satisfactory "myelographic effect" between cerebrospinal fluid and adjacent structures (Fig. 11.15C,D).

On T1-weighted sagittal images of the cervical spine, the vertebral bodies that contain yellow (or fatty) marrow are imaged as high-signal-intensity structures (Fig. 11.15A). The intervertebral disks and the cord demonstrate intermediate signal intensity, while cerebrospinal fluid demonstrates low signal intensity.

On T2-weighted sagittal images, the vertebral bodies are imaged with low signal intensity, the intervertebral disks and cerebrospinal fluid demonstrate high signal intensity, and the cord demonstrates intermediate-to-low signal intensity.

On the axial images obtained in T1 weighting, the disk demonstrates intermediate signal intensity, the spinal fluid has low signal intensity, and the cord has high-to-intermediate signal intensity.

On the axial images obtained in T2* weighting, multiplanar gradient recalled (MPGR), the disk is of high signal intensity and the

Figure 11.14 **CT of the cervical spine.** CT sections through the body of C-6 **(A)**, C-7 **(B)**, and the C6-7 intervertebral space **(C)** show the normal appearance of these structures.

Figure 11.15 **MRI of normal cervical spine. (A)** T1-weighted (TR 800/TE 20 msec) spin-echo sagittal midline section demonstrates anatomic details of the bones and soft tissues. The craniocervical junction is well outlined. The foramen magnum is defined by the fat within the occipital bone and clivus. The anterior and posterior arches of C-1 appear as small oval marrow-containing structures at the upper cervical spine. The spinal cord is of an intermediate signal intensity outlined by lower signal of CSF. The intervertebral disks are imaged with low signal intensity. **(B)** Parasagittal section demonstrates the apophyseal joints. *(continued)*

Figure 11.15 MRI of normal cervical spine. *Continued.* (C) T2*-weighted multiplanar gradient-recalled sagittal image shows vertebral bodies and spinous processes to be of low signal intensity. The high water content of the intervertebral disks produces a very high signal similar to that of cerebrospinal fluid. The cord is imaged as an intermediate signal intensity structure. **(D)** Axial section demonstrates neural foramina and nerve roots. The cervical cord is faintly outlined. (From Beltran J, 1990, with permission.)

spinal fluid is also of high signal intensity, in contrast to the spinal cord, which images as an intermediate-signal-intensity structure. The bone demonstrates low signal intensity (Fig. 11.15C,D).

In addition to its imaging capabilities, MR also has, according to some investigators, a prognostic value when attempting to predict the degree of neurologic recovery following trauma.

It has to be stressed, however, that CT alone or combined with

myelography remains the better choice for evaluating vertebral fractures, especially when they are nondisplaced or involve the posterior elements (lateral masses, facets, laminae, spinous processes), largely because of the limitations of spatial resolution of MRI. In addition, imaging the acutely injured patient is difficult. The patient may be unstable or immobilized with either a halo or traction device unsuitable for the magnetic environment. For this reason, radiographs, CT, and myelography continue to play a significant role in the evaluation of the acutely traumatized spine. However, as Hyman and Gorey noted, chronic injury to the spinal cord is most accurately evaluated with MRI.

Since the advent of CT and MRI, myelography alone (Fig. 11.16) is now rarely indicated in the evaluation of cervical injuries; if needed, this examination is usually performed in conjunction with CT (Fig. 11.16D).

For a summary of the preceding discussion in tabular form, see Tables 11.1, 11.2, and 11.3.

Injury to the Cervical Spine

Traumatic conditions involving the cervical spine are almost always the result of indirect stress forces acting on the head and neck, the position of which at the time of impact determines the site and type of damage. As Daffner stressed, vertebral fractures occur in predictable and reproducible patterns that are related to the type of force applied to the vertebral column. The same force applied to the cervical, thoracic, or lumbar spine will result in injuries that appear quite similar, producing a pattern of recognizable signs that span the spectrum from mild soft-tissue damage to severe skeletal and ligamentous disruption. These patterns Daffner termed "fingerprints" of spinal injury; they depend on the mechanism of injury, which may be an excessive movement in any direction: flexion, extension, rotation, vertical compression, shearing, distraction—or a combination of these.

Of the greatest initial importance in suspected cervical injuries, however, is the question of stability of a fracture or dislocation (Table 11.4). Stability of the vertebral column depends on the integrity of the major skeletal components, the intervertebral disks, the apophyseal joints, and the ligamentous structures. One of the most important factors is the integrity of the ligaments of the spine: the supraspinous and interspinous ligaments, the posterior longitudinal ligament, and the ligamenta flava, which together with the capsule of the apophyseal joints constitute the so-called posterior ligament complex of Holdsworth (Fig. 11.17). Injuries are stable by virtue of intact ligamentous structures; the more severe the damage to these structures, the more liable they are to further displacement, with greater risk of sequelae involving the spinal cord. Radiographic findings that indicate instability, according to Daffner, are: displacement of vertebrae, widening of the interspinous or interlaminar spaces, widening of the apophyseal joints, widening and elongation of the vertebral canal manifesting as widening of the interpedicular distance in transverse and vertical planes, and disruption of the posterior vertebral body line. Only one of these features needs to be present to make a radiographic assumption of an unstable injury. These remarks on stability also apply to injuries of the thoracic and lumbar segments.

Recently, Daffner and colleagues modified the classification of cervical vertebral injuries on the basis of CT findings, introducing "major" injuries and "minor" injuries. The former are defined as having either radiographic or CT evidence of instability, with or without associated localized or central neurologic findings. The latter injuries have no radiographic or CT evidence of instability and do not produce or have no potential to cause neurologic findings. According to these authors, cervical injury should be classified as "major" if the following radiographic and CT criteria are present: displacement of more than 2 mm in any plane, widening of the vertebral body in any plane, widening of the interspinous or interlaminar space, widening of the facet joints, disruption of the posterior vertebral body line, widening of the disk space, vertebral burst, locked or perched facets

Figure 11.16 Myelography of the cervical spine. For myelographic examination of the cervical spine, the patient is recumbent on the table, lying on the left side. Using fluoroscopy, the point of entrance of the needle is marked at the C1-2 level, and a 22-gauge needle is inserted vertically, the tip being directed to the dorsal aspect of the subarachnoid space, above the lamina of C-2. Free flow of spinal fluid indicates the correct position of the needle. **(A)** Approximately 10 mL of iohexol or iopamidol, water-soluble nonionic iodinated contrast agents, at a concentration of 240 mg iodine/mL, is slowly injected. Films are obtained in the posteroanterior **(B)**, cross-table lateral **(C)**, and oblique projections. (Oblique projections, however, are obtained not by rotating the patient but by angling the radiographic tube 45°.) If the lower segment of the cervical spine is not satisfactorily demonstrated or if the upper thoracic segment needs to be visualized, a film may also be obtained in the swimmer's position. Myelography demonstrates the thecal sac filled with contrast and the outline of the normal nerve roots and nerve root sleeves. **(D)** CT section at the level C3-4 obtained following myelography demonstrates the normal appearance of contrast in the subarachnoid space.

A

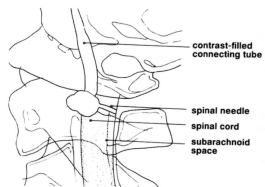

contrast-filled
connecting tube

spinal needle
spinal cord
subarachnoid
space

B

C

spinal cord

subarachnoid
space

D

nerve exit
contrast in
subarachnoid
space
cervical cord

Table 11.1 **Tissue MRI Signal Characteristics**

Signal Intensity	T1 Weighting	T2 Weighting	Gradient Echo (T2*)
Low signal	Cortical bone Vertebral end plates Degenerated disks Osteophytes Spinal vessels Cerebrospinal fluid	Cortical bone Vertebral end plates Ligaments Degenerated disks Osteophytes Spinal vessels Nerve roots	Bone marrow Vertebral bodies Vertebral end plates Ligaments Osteophytes
Intermediate signal	Spinal cord Paraspinal soft tissue Intervertebral disks Nerve roots Osteophytes	Paraspinal soft tissue Osteophytes Spinal cord Facet cartilage Bone marrow Vertebral bodies	Annulus fibrosus Spinal cord Nerve roots

High signal	Epidural venous
	  plexus
	Hyaline cartilage
	Epidural and
	  paraspinal fat
	Bone marrow
	Vertebral bodies
		Intervertebral disks
		Cerebrospinal fluid
			Intervertebral disk
			Cerebrospinal fluid
			Facet cartilage
			Epidural venoas
			  plexus
			Arteries

Modified from Kaiser MC, Ramos L, 1990, with permission.

Table 11.2 **Standard and Special Radiographic Projections for Evaluating Injury to the Cervical Spine**

Projection	Demonstration

Anteroposterior	Fractures of the bodies of C3–7
	Abnormalities of the
	  Intervertebral disk spaces
	  Uncovertebral (Luschka) joints

Open-mouth	Fractures of:
	  Lateral masses of C-1
	  Odontoid process
	  Body of C-2
	Jefferson fracture
	Abnormalities of atlantoaxial joints

Fuchs	Fractures of odontoid process

Lateral	Occipito-cervical dislocation
	Fractures of:
	  Anterior and posterior arches of
	  C-1
	  Odontoid process
	  Bodies of C2–7
	  Spinous processes
	Hangman's fracture
	Burst fracture
	Teardrop fracture
	Clay-shoveler's fracture
	Simple wedge (compression) fracture
	Unilateral and bilateral locked facets
	Abnormalities of:
	  Intervertebral disk spaces
	  Prevertebral soft tissues
	  Atlanto-odontoid space

In flexion	Atlantoaxial subluxation

Oblique	Abnormalities of:
	  Intervertebral (neural) foramina
	  Apophyseal joints

Pillar (anteroposterior or oblique)	Fractures of lateral masses (pillars)
Swimmer's	Fractures of C-7, T-1, and T-2

Table 11.3 **Ancillary Imaging Techniques for Evaluating Injury to the Cervical, Thoracic, and Lumbar Spine**

Technique	Demonstration

Tomography	Fractures, particularly of the odontoid
	  process
	Localization of displaced fracture
	  fragments
	Progress of treatment
	  Fracture healing
	  Status of spinal fusion

Myelography	Obstruction or compression of the
	  dural (thecal) sac
	Displacement or compression of the
	  spinal cord
	Abnormalities of:
	  Spinal nerve root sleeves (sheaths)
	  Subarachnoid space
	  Herniated disk

Diskography	Limbus vertebra Schmorl node Herniated disk

Computed Tomography (alone or combined with myelography) (and/or diskography)	Fractures of the occipital condyles
	Abnormalites of:
	  Lateral recesses and neural
	    foramina
	  Spinal cord
	Complex fractures of the vertebrae
	Localization of displaced fracture
	  fragments in spinal canal
	Spondylolysis
	Disk herniation
	Paraspinal soft tissue injury (e.g.,
	  hematoma)
	Progress of treatment
	  Fracture healing
	  Status of spinal fusion

Radionuclide Imaging (scintigraphy, bone scan)	Subtle or obscure fractures Recent versus old fractures Fracture healing
Magnetic Resonance Imaging	Same as myelography and computed tomography combined Annular tears

Table 11.4 Classification of Injuries to the Cervical Spine by Mechanism of Injury and Stability

Condition	Stability
Flexion Injuries	
Occipitocervical dislocation	Unstable
Subluxation	Stable
Dislocation in facet joints (locked facets)	
Unilateral	Stable
Bilateral	Unstable
Odontoid fractures	
Type I	Stable
Type II	Unstable
Type III	Stable
Wedge (compression) fracture	Stable
Clay-shoveler's fracture	Stable
Teardrop fracture	Unstable
Burst fracture	Stable or unstable
Extension Injuries	
Occipitocervical dislocation	Unstable
Fracture of posterior arch of C-1	Stable
Hangman's fracture	Unstable
'Extension teardrop' fracture	Stable
Hyperextension fracture—dislocation	Unstable
Compression Injuries	
Occipital condyle fracture (types I, II)	Stable
Jefferson fracture	Unstable
Burst fracture	Stable or unstable
Laminar fracture	Stable
Compression fracture	Stable
Shearing Injuries	
Lateral vertebral compression	Stable
Lateral dislocation	Unstable
Transverse process fracture	Stable
Lateral mass fracture	Stable
Rotation Injuries	
Occipital condyle fracture (type III)	Unstable
Rotary subluxation C1–2	Stable
Fracture-dislocation	Unstable
Facet and pillar fractures	Stable or unstable
Transverse process fracture	Stable
Distraction Injuries	
Occipito-cervical dislocation	Unstable
Hangman's fracture	Unstable
Atlantoaxial subluxation	Stable or unstable

either unilateral or bilateral, "hanged man" fracture of C2, fracture of the odontoid process, and type III occipital condyle fracture. All other types of fractures are considered to be "minor."

Fractures of the Occipital Condyles

Fractures of the occipital condyles are rare. This injury is often overlooked and is not obvious on the conventional radiography. Instead, the diagnosis requires a high index of suspicion, after which confirmation can easily be obtained by either CT with coronal reformation or conventional tomography. A classification system of occipital condyle fractures was devised by Anderson and Montesano in 1988 based on fracture morphology, pertinent anatomy, and biomechanics (Fig. 11.18).

Type I is an impacted occipital condyle fracture occurring as the result of axial loading force on the skull, similar to the mechanism for a Jefferson fracture. CT shows comminution of the occipital condyle with minimal or no displacement of fragments into the foramen magnum (Fig. 11.19). Although the ipsilateral alar ligament may be functionally inadequate, spinal stability is ensured by the intact tectorial membrane and contralateral alar ligament.

Type II occipital condyle fracture occurs as a component of a basilar skull fracture. On axial CT sections of the base of the skull, a fracture line can be seen exiting the occipital condyle and entering the foramen magnum. The mechanism of injury is a direct blow to the skull. Stability is maintained by intact alar ligaments and tectorial membrane.

Type III is an avulsion fracture of the medial aspect of occipital condyle by the alar ligament: a small fragment of the condyle is displaced toward the tip of odontoid process (Fig. 11.20). The alar ligaments are primary restraints of occipitocervical rotation and lateral bending. Therefore, the mechanism of injury in this type is rotation, lateral bending, or a combination of the two. After avulsion of the occipital condyle, the contralateral alar ligament and tectorial membrane are loaded. Therefore, this type of occipital condyle fracture is a potentially unstable injury.

Occipitocervical Dislocations

Traumatic occipitocervical dislocations are usually fatal and therefore rarely present a clinical problem. With the improvement in trauma care, which now includes on-site-intubation and immediate resuscitation as well as early hospital transport, more and more victims of this injury are presenting for definitive care. The radiographic diagnosis, however, still remains somewhat difficult because of the overlapping shadows of the base of the cranium and the mastoid processes. Traynelis and colleagues have classified occipital cervical dislocations according to the direction of displacement of the occiput: anterior, vertical, or posterior. Anderson and Montesano have modified this classification as follows.

Type I injuries are characterized by anterior translation of both occipital condyles on their corresponding atlantal facets (Fig. 11.21A). Biomechanical studies have demonstrated that for this injury to occur, all major structures (alar ligaments, tectorial membrane, and occipital atlantal facet joint capsules) crossing the occipitocervical junction must be ruptured. This type of injury is seen more commonly in patients who survive transport to the hospital.

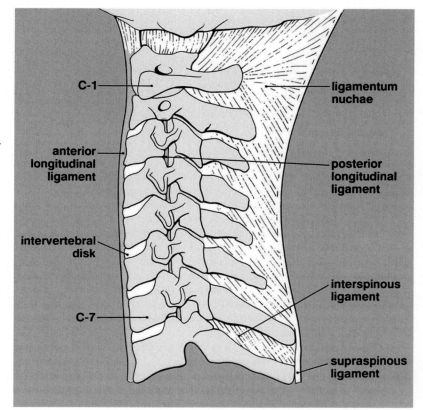

Figure 11.17 Anatomy of the principal ligaments of the cervical spine.

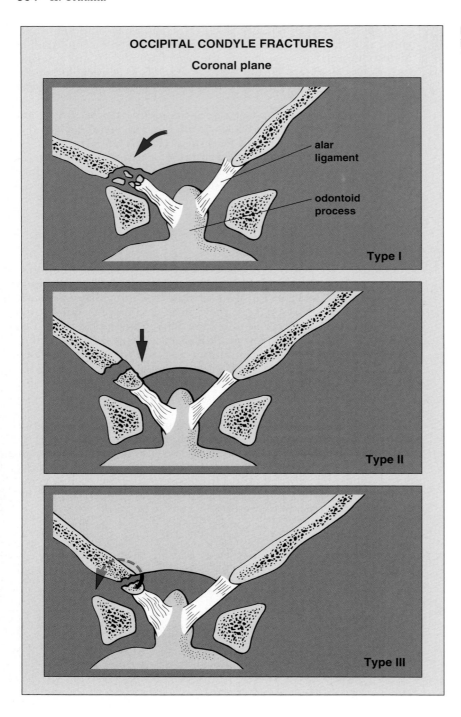

OCCIPITAL CONDYLE FRACTURES

Coronal plane

alar ligament

odontoid process

Type I

Type II

Type III

Figure 11.18 **Anderson and Montesano classification of the occipital condyle fractures.** (Modified from Anderson PA, Montesano PX, 1988, with permission.)

Type II injuries are associated with a vertical translation of the occiput on the cervical spine, secondary to the rupture of all occipitocervical ligaments. In type IIA, there is distraction between the occiput and C1, and vertical translation of the occiput on C1 is usually less than 2 mm. Vertical displacement greater than this represents failure of the tectorial membrane, alar ligaments, and occipitoatlantal facet joint capsules (Fig. 11.21B). If, conversely, the occipitoatlantal facet joint capsules remain intact and failure occurs at a more distal level of the tectorial membrane (i.e., at the level of the atlantoaxial facet joint ligaments), a type IIB injury results. In this type, there is also a vertical displacement of the spine, which occurs, however, between C1 and C2 rather than at the atlantooccipital level.

Type III injuries consist of posterior displacement of the occiput that is translated posteriorly to the atlas.

In all types of occipitocervical instability, associated injury to the transverse ligament and C1–2 instability should be suspected. Radiologic examination should include a standard lateral radiograph of the cervical spine that demonstrates the region from the occiput to the cervicothoracic junction. The articulations between occipital condyles and the atlanto-lateral masses must always be included and the clivus clearly visualized. In type III injuries, the clivus-odontoid line, which normally points into the tip of the odontoid process (Fig. 11.3D), points posteriorly to the odontoid. Other suggestive findings on the lateral radiograph of the cervical spine are the absence of the projection of the mastoid processes over the odontoid and retropharyngeal soft-tissue swelling. CT is more effective for evaluating the occipitocervical junction. Using 1-mm thin contiguous sections with multiplanar reformation, the alignment of the occiput-C1 and C1–2 articulations can be readily discerned.

Fractures of the C-1 and C-2 Vertebrae

Jefferson Fracture. This fracture results from a blow to the vertex of the head. The axial forces transmitted symmetrically through the cranium and occipital condyles into the superior surfaces of the lateral masses of the atlas drive the lateral masses outward, resulting in bilateral, symmetrical fractures of the anterior and posterior arches of

Figure 11.19 Fracture of the occipital condyle. A 23-year-old woman was injured in a motorcycle accident. **(A)** Coronal reformatted CT image shows a comminuted fracture of the right occipital condyle (*arrows*) and a fracture of the right lateral mass of the atlas (*curved arrow*). **(B)** Three-dimensional CT (bird's eye view) shows no displacement of the fractured fragments (*arrows*) into the foramen magnum, classifying this injury as a type I.

C-1, which are invariably associated with disruption of the transverse ligaments (Fig. 11.22). Neck pain and unilateral occipital headache are characteristic clinical features of Jefferson fracture.

The best radiographic projection for demonstrating this injury is the open-mouth anteroposterior view (Fig. 11.23A); trispiral tomography in the lateral projection using 1-mm thin cuts, as well as CT, may also be required in the evaluation of complex fractures (Fig. 11.23C,D).

Fractures of the Odontoid Process. Fractures of the dens belong to the group of flexion injuries, although at times forces causing hyperextension of the cervical spine may also result in damage to the dens. In hyperflexion injuries, the odontoid process is usually displaced anteriorly, and there may be associated forward subluxation of C-1 or C-2. Hyperextension injuries, however, usually cause the odon-

toid to be displaced posteriorly, with posterior subluxation of C-1 or C-2.

Several classifications of odontoid fractures have been proposed, based on the site and amount of displacement of a fracture. The system suggested by Anderson and D'Alonzo, however, is practical and has gained wide acceptance because of its emphasis on the most important feature of such fractures—their stability (Fig. 11.24):

Stage I   Fractures of the body of the dens distal (cephalad) to the base. They are usually obliquely oriented and are considered stable injuries. Conservative treatment usually suffices for healing. Some authorities do not recognize type I fractures, postulating that these "injuries" in fact represent a nonunited secondary ossification center (ossiculum terminale of Bergman) or os odontoideum.

Figure 11.20 Fracture of the occipital condyle. A 16-year-old girl was assaulted and sustained a blow injury to the head. Conventional radiographs of the skull and upper cervical spine were interpreted as normal. **(A)** Axial CT section through the base of the skull shows a type III fracture of the occipital condyle *(arrow)*. **(B)** Coronal reformatted CT image confirms the presence of an evulsion fracture *(arrow)*.

Figure 11.21 Occipito-cervical dislocation. (A) Lateral radiograph of the cervical spine in a 24-year-old man, who injured his head and neck in a motorcycle accident that resulted in complete quadriplegia, shows type I of occipitocervical dislocation: the occipital condyles are anteriorly displaced in relation to C-1 vertebra. (From Greenspan A, Montesano PX, 1993, with permission.) **(B)** In another patient, lateral radiograph demonstrates a type IIA vertical occipito-cervical dislocation. (From Chapman MW, 1993, with permission.)

Figure 11.22 Jefferson fracture. The classic Jefferson fracture, seen here schematically on the anteroposterior (**A**) and axial (**B**) views, exhibits a characteristic symmetric overhang of the lateral masses of C-1 over those of C-2. Lateral displacement of the articular pillars results in disruption of the transverse ligaments. (**C**) On occasion, only unilateral lateral displacement of an articular pillar may be present.

Figure 11.23 Jefferson fracture. A 19-year-old man sustained a neck injury while being mugged. (**A**) Open-mouth anteroposterior view of the cervical spine shows lateral displacement of the lateral masses of the atlas, suggesting a ring fracture of C-1. (**B**) Lateral view demonstrates fracture lines of the posterior and anterior arch of C-1. *(continued)*

Figure 11.23 Jefferson fracture. *Continued.* (C) CT section demonstrates two fracture lines of the posterior arch and a fracture of the anterior arch. **(D)** CT coronal reformation confirms lateral displacement of the lateral masses.

fracture of anterior arch

odontoid

fractures of posterior arch

displaced lateral masses of C-1

odontoid process

atlantoaxial joints

Stage II Transverse fractures through the base of the odontoid are unstable injuries (Fig. 11.26). Conservative treatment has been complicated by nonunion in approximately 35% of cases; therefore, surgical fusion is the usual method of treatment.

Stage III Fractures through the base of the odontoid extending into the body of the axis are stable injuries (Fig. 11.25). Conservative treatment is usually sufficient.

The best techniques for demonstrating fractures of the dens are the anteroposterior view, including the open-mouth variant, or Fuchs projection, and the lateral projection; thin-section trispiral tomography may also prove effective in delineating ambiguous or subtle features (Fig. 11.26).

CT detection of the dens fractures, particularly type II, may be difficult if the axial sections are obtained parallel to the usually horizontally oriented fracture line. For this reason, it is essential to obtain routinely reformatted images in coronal and sagittal planes (Fig. 11.27).

Hangman's Fracture. In 1912, Wood-Jones described the pathomechanism associated with execution by hanging. He found that hyperextension and distraction resulted in bilateral fractures through the pedicles of the axis, with anterior dislocation of the body and subsequent tearing of the spinal cord. A similar fracture, which in fact constitutes traumatic spondylolisthesis of C-2, is common in automobile accidents, when the face strikes the windshield before the vertex of the head, forcing the neck into hyperextension. This injury, which accounts for 4% to 7% of all cervical spine fractures and dislocations, may present as simple, nondisplaced fractures through the pedicles of the axis or as fractures through the arches with anterior subluxation and angulation of C-2 onto C-3 (Fig. 11.28). The fracture line usually lies anterior to the inferior articular facet of C-2 in both variants, but displaced fractures are more often associated with ligament disruption and intervertebral disk injuries. The best projection for demonstrating this injury is the lateral view (Fig. 11.29).

Hangman's fractures (which probably should be correctly called "hanged man" fractures) have been classified into three types (Fig. 11.30). Type I injury is characterized by the fracture through the pedicle of C2 extending between the superior and inferior facets. Type II injury constitutes a type I fracture with concomitant disruption of intervertebral disk C2-3. Type III injury consists of a type II fracture associated with a C2-3 facet dislocation.

Fractures of the Mid and Lower Cervical Spine

Burst Fracture. The mechanism of this fracture is identical to that of Jefferson fractures involving C-1, but burst fractures are seen in the lower cervical vertebrae (C3-7). When the nucleus pulposus, which is normally contained within the intervertebral disk, is driven through the fractured vertebral end plate into the vertebral body, the body explodes from within, resulting in a comminuted fracture. Typically, the posterior fragment is posteriorly displaced and may cause injury to the spinal cord. If the posterior ligament complex is not disrupted, a burst fracture is stable. Occasionally, with ligamentous disruption, a burst fracture becomes unstable. Radiographically, it is characterized by a vertical split in the vertebral body, as seen on the anteroposterior view, but the lateral projection or lateral tomography better demonstrates the extent of comminution and posterior displacement (Fig. 11.31A). The most revealing modality in the case of burst fracture is CT since it demonstrates the details of fracture of the posterior part of the vertebral body in the axial plane (Fig. 11.31B).

Teardrop Fracture. The most severe and most unstable of injuries of the cervical spine, teardrop fracture is characterized by posterior displacement of the involved vertebra into the spinal canal, fracture of its posterior elements, and disruption of the soft tissues, including the ligamentum flavum and the spinal cord, at the level of injury. In addition, stress applied to the anterior longitudinal ligament causes it either to rupture or to avulse from the vertebral body, taking along a piece of the anterior surface of the body. This small, triangular or teardrop-shaped fragment is usually anteriorly and inferiorly displaced (Fig. 11.32). Associated spinal cord injury results in the acute anterior cervical cord syndrome, consisting of abrupt quadriplegia and loss of pain and temperature distinction; however, posterior column senses—position, vibration, and motion—are usually preserved.

The lateral view is the best radiographic projection for demonstrating this injury; lateral tomography may also be necessary, as well as CT (Figs. 11.33 and 11.34). The evaluation of spinal cord compression requires MRI (Fig. 11.35).

It should be kept in mind in the evaluation of this fracture that occasionally a triangular fragment of bone similar in shape and location to that seen in the classic teardrop fracture may be noted in an extension type of injury. This "extension teardrop" fracture, however, is completely different; it is a stable fracture without the potentially

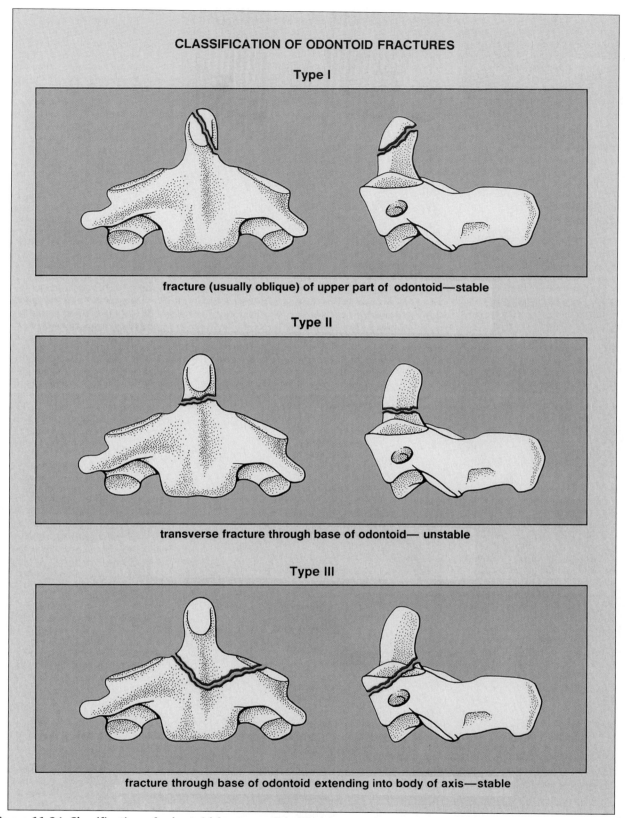

CLASSIFICATION OF ODONTOID FRACTURES

Type I

fracture (usually oblique) of upper part of odontoid—stable

Type II

transverse fracture through base of odontoid— unstable

Type III

fracture through base of odontoid extending into body of axis—stable

Figure 11.24 Classification of odontoid fractures. (Modified from Anderson LD, D'Alonzo RT, 1974, with permission.)

fracture line
extending into
vertebral body

fracture line

Figure 11.25 Fracture of the odontoid process. A 24-year-old man fell on his head in a skiing accident. Open-mouth anteroposterior (**A**) and lateral (**B**) views of the cervical spine demonstrate a fracture of the odontoid process extending into the body of C-2—a type III stable fracture. The diagnosis was confirmed by trispiral tomography in the anteroposterior projection (**C**).

Figure 11.26 Fracture of the odontoid process. A 62-year-old man sustained a flexion injury of the cervical spine in an automobile accident. Open-mouth anteroposterior (**A**) and lateral (**B**) views demonstrate a fracture line at the base of the odontoid process, but the details of this injury cannot be well appreciated. Thin-section trispiral tomographic sections in the anteroposterior (**C**) and lateral (**D**) projections confirm the fracture at the base of the dens. This is a type II (unstable) fracture.

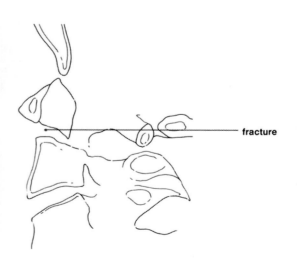

fracture

Figure 11.27 Fracture of the odontoid process. A 50-year-old man sustained a flexion neck injury during a motorcycle accident. The conventional radiographs of the cervical spine suggested odontoid fracture but were not conclusive. Coronal (**A**) and sagittal (**B**) reformatted CT images clearly demonstrate a type II odontoid fracture.

1 odontoid process   4 lamina
2 superior articular facet of C-2   5 spinous process
3 inferior articular facet of C-2

Figure 11.28 Hangman's fracture. This injury may present as nondisplaced fractures through the arches of C-2, as seen here schematically on the lateral (**A**) and axial (**B**) views, or as displaced fractures with anterior angulation (**C**) and (**D**) associated with disruption of ligaments, the intervertebral disk, or articular facets.

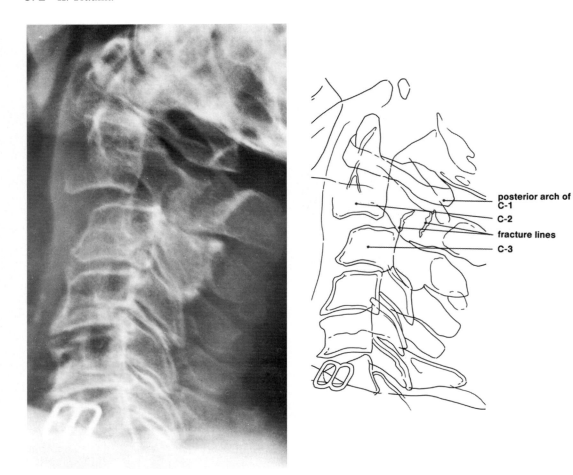

posterior arch of
C-1
C-2
fracture lines
C-3

Figure 11.29 Hangman's fracture. A 62-year-old man sustained a severe hyperextension injury to the cervical spine in an automobile accident. Lateral film shows a fracture through the pedicles of C-2 associated with C2-3 subluxation, a typical finding in hangman's fracture.

CLASSIFICATION OF HANGMAN'S FRACTURES

Type I   Type II   Type III

Figure 11.30 Classification of hangman's fractures. (Modified from Levine AM, Edwards CC, 1985, with permission.)

Figure 11.31 Burst fracture. A 40-year-old man was ejected from a motorcycle and hit the pavement with the vertex of his head. **(A)** Lateral radiograph of the cervical spine demonstrates a comminuted fracture of the body of C-7, involving the anterior and middle columns. **(B)** A CT section confirms the burst fracture. The posterior part of the vertebral body is displaced into the spinal canal.

Figure 11.32 Teardrop fracture. Teardrop fracture, seen here schematically in a sagittal section of the lower cervical spine, is the most serious and unstable of cervical spine injuries. Disruption of the anterior longitudinal ligament may cause avulsion of a teardrop-shaped fragment of the anterior surface of the body of C-5. This fracture is also typified by posterior displacement of the involved vertebra and fracture of its posterior elements. Depending on the severity of the injury, varying degrees of spinal cord damage may result.

Figure 11.33 Teardrop fracture. A 38-year-old man sustained an injury of the neck in a motorcycle accident. **(A)** Lateral view of the cervical spine demonstrates an avulsion fracture of the anteroinferior aspect of the body of C-5 and a fracture of its spinous process. The lamina of C-4 is fractured as well. There is disruption of the facets at the level of C5-6 with marked widening. There is posterior displacement of all vertebrae including and above C-5. **(B)** CT section demonstrates in addition a markedly comminuted fracture of the body of C-5.

Figure 11.34 Teardrop fracture. A 36-year-old man sustained a neck injury in a motorcycle accident. **(A)** A lateral radiograph of the cervical spine shows a typical teardrop fracture of C-5 associated with C5-6 subluxation. CT axial section **(B)** and sagittal reformation **(C)** demonstrate the details of this injury. **(D)** CT coronal reformation shows the vertical fracture of the body of C-5 oriented in the sagittal plane.

Figure 11.35 **Teardrop fracture.** A 38-year-old man, an unrestrained passenger, was injured in a car accident. **(A)** A lateral radiograph of the cervical spine shows a teardrop fracture of C-4. **(B)** A sagittal gradient-echo (multiplanar gradient-recalled) MR image shows posterior displacement of the C-4 vertebral body compromising the spinal canal and almost complete transection of the cervical cord. Extensive high-signal soft-tissue edema and hemorrhage is evident.

dangerous complications of the flexion type of injury, and usually occurs at the level of C-2 or C-3 (Fig. 11.36).

Clay-Shoveler's Fracture. This oblique or vertical fracture of the spinous process of C-6 or C-7 is caused by an acute powerful flexion, such as that produced by shoveling. Deriving its name from its common occurrence in Australian clay miners in the 1930s, clay-shoveler's fracture was simultaneously labeled with the same name in Germany, where it was seen among workers building the Autobahn. A direct blow to the cervical spine or indirect trauma to the neck in automobile accidents can result in similar injury.

Clay-shoveler's fracture is a stable fracture, the posterior ligament complex remaining intact, and is thus not associated with neurologic damage. The best radiographic projection for demonstrating this in-

jury is the lateral view of the cervical spine (Fig. 11.37A). If C-7 cannot be visualized despite good positioning and technique, for example, because of a short, thick neck or wide shoulders, then the swimmer's view should be obtained. This fracture can also be identified on the anteroposterior view by the so-called ghost sign (Fig. 11.37B) produced by displacement of the fractured spinous process.

Simple Wedge (Compression) Fracture. Resulting from hyperflexion of the cervical spine, a simple wedge fracture generally occurs in the mid-cervical or lower cervical segment. There is anterior compression (wedging) of the vertebral body, and although the posterior ligament complex is stretched, it remains intact, making this a stable fracture. The lateral projection of the cervical spine adequately demonstrates this injury (Fig. 11.38).

Figure 11.36 **Extension teardrop fracture.** A 37-year-old man sustained an extension injury to the cervical spine in a fall. Lateral view of the spine demonstrates an extension teardrop fracture of the vertebral body of C-3. Note that, in contrast to a flexion-type injury, there is no subluxation, and the posterior vertebral and spinolaminar lines are not disrupted.

normal spinous
process of C-6

double outline
of C-7 spinous
process

normal spinous
process of T-1

Figure 11.37 Clay-shoveler's fracture. A 22-year-old man sustained a neck injury in an automobile accident. **(A)** Lateral view of the cervical spine shows a fracture of the spinous process of C-7, identifying this injury as a clay-shoveler's fracture. **(B)** On the anteroposterior view, clay-shoveler's fracture can be identified by the appearance of a double spinous process for C-7. This ghost sign is secondary to slight caudal displacement of the fractured tip of the spinous process.

Figure 11.38 Compression (wedge) fracture. A 30-year-old woman sustained a neck injury in an automobile accident. Lateral radiograph of the cervical spine demonstrates a simple wedge fracture of C-5.

Locked Facets

Unilateral Locked Facets. This type of injury is secondary to the flexion-rotation force with subsequent tearing of the joint capsule of one facet and posterior ligamentous complex. In the absence of disk space widening or subluxation, unilateral facet locking is a relatively stable injury. Frequently, however, there is approximately 25% anterior subluxation. These patients are at risk of sustaining nerve root injury or, rarely, a Brown-Sequard type spinal cord injury.

Bilateral Perched Facets. This type of vertebral subluxation occurs as a result of a flexion injury. There is disruption of the posterior ligamentous complex, and the inferior and superior articular processes of the involved vertebrae are in apposition. The shingled appearance of the facet joints is changed to a configuration in which the laminar cortices intersect at one point (Figs. 11.39 and 11.40A). This injury is best diagnosed on the lateral and oblique projections of the cervical spine, or CT with sagittal and oblique reformation.

Bilateral Locked Facets. Bilateral dislocation of the cervical

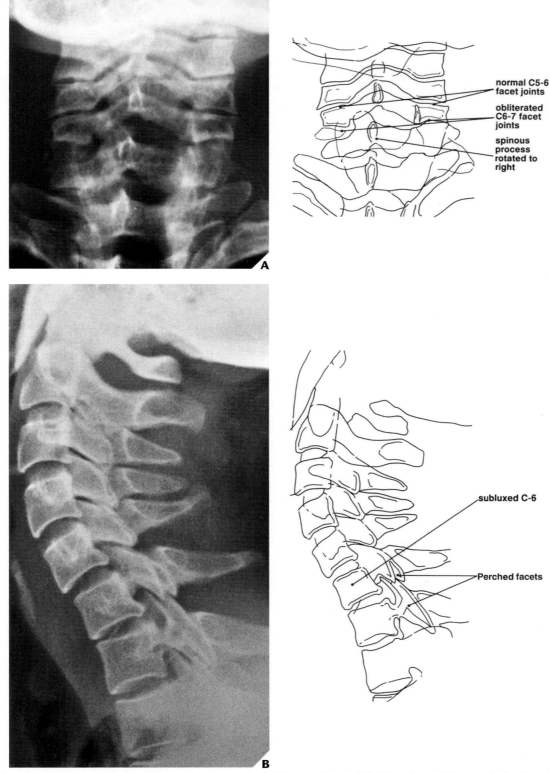

Figure 11.39 Perched facets. A 34-year-old woman injured her neck in a skiing accident. **(A)** Pillar view of the cervical spine demonstrates bilateral obliteration of the facet joints at the C6-7 level. The joints above appear normal. Displacement of the spinous process to the right is the result of rotation. **(B)** Lateral view shows perched facets of vertebrae C-6 and C-7.

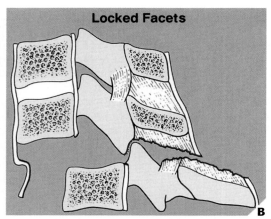

Figure 11.40 **Locked facets.** (A), (B) Bilateral locked facets is a hyperflexion injury characterized by complete anterior dislocation of the affected vertebra. It is always associated with extensive ligament disruption and carries a great risk of cervical spinal cord damage. (C) A 36-year-old man injured his neck in a motor vehicle accident that resulted in quadriplegia. Lateral radiograph of the cervical spine shows bilateral locked facets at the C5-6 level.

spine in the facet joints is the result of extreme flexion of the head and neck; it is an unstable condition caused by extensive disruption of the posterior ligament complex. Interlocking of the articular facets is initiated by the forward movement of the inferior articular facet of the upper vertebra over the superior articular facet of the underlying vertebra (Fig. 11.40). This causes the lamina and spinous process of the two adjacent vertebrae to spread apart and the vertebral bodies to sublux. In the later stage of dislocation, the inferior articular facet of the upper vertebra locks in front of the superior articular facet of the lower vertebra, which results in complete anterior dislocation. The configuration of this injury leads to complete disruption of the posterior ligament complex, the posterior longitudinal ligament, the annulus fibrosus, and frequently the anterior longitudinal ligament. It is also associated with a high incidence of cervical spinal cord damage.

The lateral projection of the cervical spine, preferably a cross-table lateral, is sufficient to demonstrate bilaterally locked facets. The key to the correct diagnosis is the presence of malalignment of the affected vertebrae associated with disruption of all lateral cervical spine landmarks (Fig. 11.3D) and position of the dislocated facets posteriorly and cephalad in relation to the facets of the vertebra above (Fig. 11.40C).

Thoracolumbar Spine

Anatomic–Radiologic Considerations

The standard radiographic projections for evaluating an injury to the *thoracic spine* are the anteroposterior (Fig. 11.41) and lateral (Fig. 11.42) views. The lateral projection is obtained using a technique called autotomography, which requires shallow breathing by the patient to blur the structures involved in respiratory motion and give a clear view of the thoracic vertebral column.

As in cervical spine injuries, conventional tomography, CT, and MRI play leading roles in the evaluation of fractures of the thoracic spine, particularly in defining the extent of injury. Conventional tomography offers the possibility of obtaining direct coronal and sagittal sections of the spine, but it has the disadvantages of not being able to obtain axial sections and exposing the patient to a relatively high dose of radiation. Axial images can be obtained on CT, which provides in addition an excellent means of evaluating soft-tissue injuries and exposes the patient to a relatively low dose of radiation. Unless reformation images are obtained, however, axially oriented fracture lines can be missed on axial CT sections. MR images are ideal for evaluating concomitant soft-tissue injury, particularly to the spinal cord and thecal sac.

The standard radiographic examination for evaluating injuries of the *lumbar spine* includes the anteroposterior, lateral, and oblique projections, supplemented by coned-down lateral spot films of the lumbosacral junction (L5-S1). The anteroposterior view is usually sufficient for evaluating traumatic conditions involving the vertebral bodies and transverse processes; the intervertebral disk spaces are also well demonstrated, except for the lowest (L5-S1) (Fig. 11.43). The spinous processes, seen as teardrops, and the articular facets, however, are not well demonstrated on this projection. A characteristic configuration of the end plates of the L3-5 vertebral bodies can be observed on the anteroposterior projection. Normally, the inferior aspects of these vertebrae form what is called a "Cupid's bow" contour (Fig. 11.44), which is lost in cases of compression fractures affecting this part of the column.

normal paraspinal line

T-12

L-1

Figure 11.41 Anteroposterior view of the thoracic spine. (A) For the anteroposterior view of the thoracic spine, the patient is supine on the table, with the knees flexed to correct the normal thoracic kyphosis. The central beam is directed vertically about 3 cm above the xiphoid process. **(B)** On the film in this projection, the vertebral end plates and pedicles and the intervertebral disk spaces are seen. The height of the vertebrae can be determined, and changes in the paraspinal line can be evaluated.

Figure 11.42 Lateral view of the thoracic spine. For the lateral view of the thoracic spine, the patient is erect with the arms elevated. To eliminate structures that would obscure the bony elements of the thoracic spine, the patient is instructed to breathe shallowly during the exposure. The central beam is directed horizontally to the level of the T-6 vertebra with about 10° cephalad angulation. The film in this projection demonstrates a lateral image of the vertebral bodies and intervertebral disk spaces.

Figure 11.43 Anteroposterior view of the lumbar spine. (A) For the anteroposterior projection of the lumbar spine, the patient is supine on the table, with the knees flexed to eliminate the normal physiologic lumbar lordosis. The central beam is directed vertically to the center of the abdomen at the level of the iliac crests. **(B)** The radiograph in this projection demonstrates the vertebral bodies, the vertebral end plates, and the transverse processes; the intervertebral disk spaces are also well delineated. The spinous processes are seen en face, appearing as teardrops; the pedicles, also visualized en face, project as oval densities on either side of the bodies.

Figure 11.44 Cupid's bow sign. Anteroposterior coned-down view of the lumbar spine demonstrates a characteristic configuration of the lower aspects of L-3 and L-4. This "Cupid's bow" contour is lost in cases of compression fracture.

Figure 11.45 Lateral view of the lumbar spine. (A) For the lateral projection of the lumbar spine, the patient is recumbent on the radiographic table on either the left or right side; the knees and hips are flexed to eliminate the lordotic curve. The central beam is directed vertically to the center of the body of L-3, at the level of the patient's waist. **(B)** The lateral film of the lumbar spine allows adequate demonstration of the vertebral bodies, pedicles, and spinous processes, as well as the intervertebral foramina and disk spaces.

ear—superior
articular process

nose—transverse
process

eye—pedicle

neck—pars
interarticularis
(isthmus)

foreleg—inferior
articular
process

tail—superior
articular
process
of opposite side

body—lamina
and spinous
process

hindleg—inferior
articular
process
of opposite side

Figure 11.46 Oblique view of the lumbar spine.
(A) For the posteroanterior oblique projection of the lumbar spine, the patient is recumbent on the table, with the right side rotated 45° to demonstrate the right-sided articular facets. (Elevation of the left side allows demonstration of the left-sided articular facets.) The central beam is directed vertically toward the center of L-3. **(B)** The posteroanterior oblique film demonstrates the facet joints, the superior and inferior articular process, the pedicles, and the pars interarticularis. **(C), (D)** The oblique film also demonstrates a characteristic configuration of the elements of adjacent lumbar vertebrae known as the "Scotty dog."

On the lateral projection of the lumbar spine, the vertebral bodies are seen in profile, and the superior and inferior end plates are well demonstrated (Fig. 11.45). Fractures of the spinous processes can be adequately evaluated on this projection, as can abnormalities involving the intervertebral disk spaces, including L5-S1. As in the cervical spine, an oblique projection of the lumbar spine can be obtained from the patient's anterior or posterior aspect, although the posteroanterior oblique projection is preferable (Fig. 11.46). This view is particularly effective in demonstrating the facet joints (articular facets) and reveals a configuration of the elements of adjoining vertebrae, known as the "Scotty dog" formation (Fig. 11.46C,D), which was first identified by Lachapele.

Ancillary imaging techniques are frequently used in the evaluation of traumatic conditions of the lumbar spine. As in cervical and thoracic injuries, conventional tomography and CT provide useful information; CT is frequently used to assess the extent of damage in vertebral body fractures and abnormalities involving the intervertebral disks (Fig. 11.47). Moreover, myelography (Fig. 11.48) and diskography (Fig. 11.49) are often required, and they are frequently performed in conjunction with CT examination (Fig. 11.50).

MRI is now frequently used in the evaluation of injury to the thoracic and lumbar spine. In general, the images are obtained using a planar surface coil with its long axis oriented parallel to the spine. The slice thickness used to image the thoracic and lumbar spine in both sagittal and axial planes is usually 5 mm, with a 1-mm gap between slices to reduce the artifactual signal from adjacent slices. Sagittal images of the thoracic and lumbar spine are obtained with T1 and T2 weighting. In the axial plane, T1- and T2*-gradient-recalled echo pulse sequences (MPGR or GRASS) are usually obtained. Similarly to the imaging of the cervical spine, cerebrospinal fluid is visualized with low signal intensity on the sagittal images in T1 weighting, in contrast to the intermediate signal intensity of the spinal cord. The marrow within the vertebral bodies is seen as a high signal intensity, in contrast to the intermediate signal intensity of the intervertebral disks (Fig. 11.51A).

On T2-weighted images, the thoracic cord is visualized as low-to-intermediate signal intensity, in contrast to the high signal intensity of the cerebrospinal fluid. The intervertebral disks demonstrate high signal intensity on both T2- and T2*-(MPGR) weighted images. The vertebral body marrow is imaged as intermediate signal intensity on T2-weighted images and low signal intensity on T2*-weighted MPGR and GRASS images (Fig. 11.51B).

The axial images effectively demonstrate the relation of the intervertebral disk spaces to the thecal sac. On axial T1-weighted images, the vertebral body, pedicles, laminae, transverse, and spinous processes demonstrate high signal intensity, whereas the nucleus pulposus yields intermediate signal intensity, in contrast to the low signal intensity peripherally of the annulus fibrosus. The nerve roots demonstrate low-to-intermediate signal intensity and are in contrast with the high signal intensity of the surrounding fat (Fig. 11.51C). On T2-

Figure 11.47 CT of the lumbar spine. (A) CT section through the L4-5 disk space demonstrates the facet joints in full view, as well as the spinous process and laminae of L-4. Note the appearance of the ligamentum flavum. **(B)** CT section through upper third of the body of L-5 demonstrates an axial view of the pedicles, transverse processes, and laminae, as well as a cross section of the thecal sac and the superior part of the spinous process. **(C)** In a section through the lower third of the body of L-5 intervertebral foramina, the caudal part of the body, and the spinous process are seen. Note the L5-S1 facet joints.

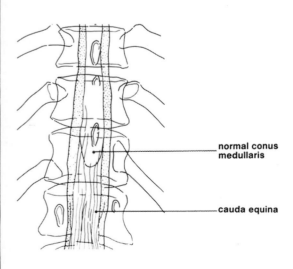

Figure 11.48 Myelography of the lumbar spine. For myelographic examination of the lumbar spine, the patient is prone on the table. The puncture site, usually at the L3-4 or L2-3 level, is marked under fluoroscopic control. A 22-gauge needle is inserted into the subarachnoid space, and free flow of spinal fluid indicates proper placement. Iohexol or iopamidol (15 mL), in a concentration of 180 mg iodine/mL is slowly injected, and films are obtained in the posteroanterior (**A**), left and right oblique (**B**), and cross-table lateral (**C**) projections. In these normal studies, contrast is seen outlining the subarachnoid spaces of the thecal sac, as well as the cul-de-sac or most caudal part of the subarachnoid space. The nerve roots appear symmetric on both sides of the contrast column. A linear filling defect represents a nerve root in its contrast-filled sleeve. The length of the root pocket may vary from one patient to another, but in each patient, all roots are approximately equal in length. It is imperative during myelographic examination of the lumbar segment to obtain one spot film of the thoracic segment at the level T10-12 (**D**), because tumors localized in the conus medullaris may mimic the clinical symptoms of a herniated lumbar disk.

Figure 11.49 Diskography of the lumbar spine.
For diskographic examination of the lumbar spine, the patient is prone on the table, and the level of the injection, depending on the indication, is marked. The needle is inserted into the center of the nucleus pulposus, and about 2 to 3 mL of metrizamide is injected. **(A)** Lateral view of a normal diskogram shows a concentration of contrast medium in the nucleus pulposus outlining the disk; there should be no leak of contrast while the needle is in place. **(B)** CT section through the L3-4 disk space after diskography shows the normal appearance of this structure.

contrast outlining normal disk

thecal sac

weighted images, the nucleus pulposus demonstrates high signal intensity, in contrast to the low signal intensity of the annulus fibrosus. The nerve roots are imaged as low-signal-intensity structures (Fig. 11.51D).

For a summary of the preceding discussion in tabular form, see Tables 11.1, 11.3, 11.5 and Fig. 11.52.

Injury to the Thoracolumbar Spine

Fractures of the Thoracolumbar Spine

Classification. Fractures of the thoracolumbar segment of the spine may involve the vertebral body and arch, as well as the transverse, spinous, and articular processes. They can generally be grouped by mechanism of injury as compression fractures, burst fractures, distraction fractures (Chance and other seat-belt injuries), and fracture–dislocations.

Because different classifications of thoracolumbar spine fractures have been used in the past by numerous authors, reports concerning the stability or lack of stability of a particular fracture pattern have varied. In 1983, Denis introduced the concept of the three-column spine classification of acute injuries to the thoracic and lumbar segments (Fig. 11.53). The significance of this system is its usefulness in determining the stability of various fractures, based on the site of injury in one or more of the spinal columns or elements:

The *anterior column* comprises the anterior two-thirds of the annulus fibrosus and vertebral body, and the anterior longitudinal ligament. The *middle column* includes the posterior longitudinal ligament, and the posterior third of the vertebral body and annulus fibrosus. The *posterior column* consists of the posterior ligament complex, which has been defined by Holdsworth to include the supraspinous and infraspinous ligaments, the capsule of the intervertebral joints, and the ligamentum flavum (or interlaminar ligament), as well as the posterior portion of the neural arch. Generally, one-column fractures are

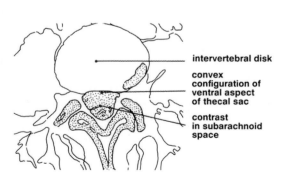

intervertebral disk

convex configuration of ventral aspect of thecal sac

contrast in subarachnoid space

Figure 11.50 CT–myelography of the lumbar spine. CT section obtained after myelography shows the normal appearance of contrast medium in the subarachnoid space. Note that the disk does not encroach on the ventral aspect of the thecal sac.

Figure 11.51 MRI appearance of a normal lumbar spine. (A) On this spin-echo T1-weighted sagittal midline section (TR 800/TE 20 msec) the tip of the conus medullaris is identified at the T12-L1 level, surrounded by low-signal-intensity cerebrospinal fluid. Epidural fat is of a very high signal intensity. It is most clearly seen posteriorly but also some fat is present anteriorly at the lumbosacral junction. Intervertebral disks are of an intermediate signal intensity because of their high water content. The low-signal-intensity lines along the ventral and dorsal aspects of the vertebral body are related to the anterior and posterior longitudinal ligaments and cortical bone of the vertebral bodies. These ligaments also span and cover the anterior and posterior portions of the disks. The thin black line along the inferior end plate and the bright line at the superior portion of each vertebral body are due to a chemical shift artifact. **(B)** Gradient-echo T2-weighted sagittal midline section (MPGR; TR 1000/TE 12 msec, flip angle 22.5°) provides an image with a similar appearance to that of the myelographic technique, because of its very high gray-scale contrast. There is clear delineation of the thecal sac filled with high-signal-intensity cerebrospinal fluid. The posterior longitudinal ligament and dura are silhouetted against the high water signal of the cerebrospinal fluid and the intervertebral disks. The epidural fat is of intermediate-to-low signal intensity and the vertebral bodies are of a very low signal intensity. A high signal intensity of the mid posterior cleft in the vertebral bodies is related to the basivertebral veins. **(C)** On the spin-echo T1-weighted axial section (SE; TR 800/TE 20 msec), the nerve roots are surrounded by high-signal-intensity fat in the neural foramen. The ventral margin of the thecal sac at the disk level is convex outward and the canal is ample in size. The facet joints are well seen as the two low-signal-intensity arcs of the cortical bone. **(D)** Gradient-echo T2-weighted axial section (MPGR; TR 1000/TE 12 msec, flip angle 22.5°) demonstrates low-signal nerve roots of the cauda equina surrounded by high-signal-intensity cerebrospinal fluid. The anterior margin of the thecal sac is well delineated. The individual nerve-root sheaths in the foramen also appear at a somewhat higher signal intensity. Some signal is visible from the disk interspace.

Table 11.5 **Standard and Special Radiographic Projections for Evaluating Injury to the Thoracic and Lumbar Spine***

Projection	Demonstration	Projection	Demonstration

Anteroposterior	Fractures of:
	    Vertebral bodies
	    Vertebral end plates
	    Pedicles
	    Transverse processes
	Fracture—dislocations
	Abnormalities of intervertebral
	    disk spaces
	Paraspinal bulge
	Inverted Napoleon's-hat sign
		Lateral
		(continued)
		
		Oblique
			Chance fracture (seat-belt frac-
			    tures)
			Abnormalities of:
			    Intervertebral foramina
			    Intervertebral disk spaces
			Limbus vertebra
			Schmorl node
			Spondylolisthesis
			Spinous-process sign
			Abnormalities of:

Lateral	Fractures of:
	    Vertebral bodies
	    Vertebral end plates
	    Pedicles
	    Spinous processes
			Articular facets
			    Pars interarticularis
			Spondylolysis
			"Scotty dog" configuration

* For the ancillary imaging techniques, see Table 11.3.

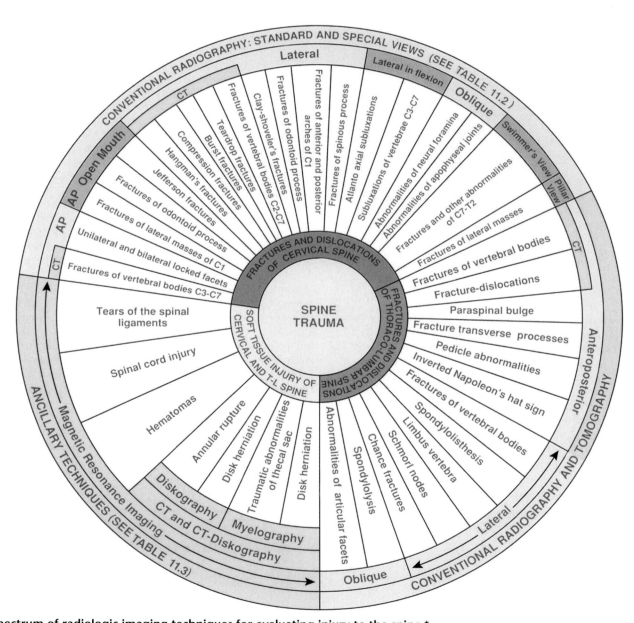

Figure 11.52 Spectrum of radiologic imaging techniques for evaluating injury to the spine.*
  The radiographic projections or radiologic techniques indicated throughout the diagram are only those that are the most effective in demonstrating the respective traumatic conditions.

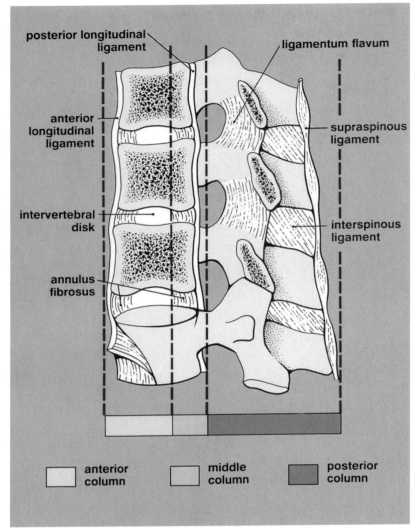

Figure 11.53 Division of the spine into three columns. The three-column concept in viewing the thoracolumbar spine is helpful in determining the stability of various injuries. Fractures involving all three columns are unstable and those affecting one column are stable. (Modified from Denis F, 1983, with permission.)

11.56). The anteroposterior radiograph reveals buckling of the lateral cortices of the vertebral body close to the involved end plate, together with a decrease in the height of the body. In lateral-flexion injuries, compression forces may result in a wedge-shaped deformity of the vertebral body. In subtle cases, a clue to the diagnosis may be seen in a localized bulge of the paraspinal line secondary to hemorrhage and edema. However, it should be kept in mind that this finding may also be seen in pathologic fractures secondary to skeletal metastases to the spine. On the lateral projection, a simple vertebral compression fracture can be identified by a decrease in the height of the anterior part of the body, while the height of the posterior part and posterior cortex is maintained.

Burst Fractures. A burst fracture results from a failure of the anterior and middle columns secondary to axial-compression forces or a combination of axial compression with rotation or anterior or lateral flexion. The anteroposterior and lateral projections of the thoracic and lumbar spine are usually adequate to demonstrate these fractures. The anteroposterior radiograph characteristically reveals a vertical fracture of the lamina, together with an increase in the interpedicular distance and splaying of the posterior facet joints. On the lateral radiograph, fracture of the posterior part of the vertebral body results in a decrease in the height of this portion of the bone. Comminution is often present, and fragments are retropulsed into the spinal canal, leading to compression of the thecal sac. For this reason, CT is an essential technique in the evaluation of burst fractures (Fig. 11.57A–C), and MRI (Fig. 11.57D,E) or myelography (Fig. 11.58) may be required to localize the site and demonstrate the degree of compression on the thecal sac.

Chance Fractures. Originally described by G. Q. Chance, this type of distraction injury of the lumbar spine has also come to be called a "seat-belt" fracture, because of the frequency of its occurrence in automobile accidents in individuals wearing only lap seat-belts. Acute forward flexion of the spine across a restraining lap seat-belt during sudden deceleration causes the spine above the belt to be pushed forward and distracted from the lower, fixed part of the spine. The classic Chance fracture involves a horizontal splitting of the vertebra, beginning in the spinous process or lamina and extending through the pedicles and the vertebral body without damage to ligament structures. Its constant feature is a transverse fracture without dislocation or subluxation (Figs. 11.59 and 11.60). The transverse process may be horizontally fractured as well, and at times there is compression of the anterior aspect of the vertebral body. Chance fracture tends to be stable, because the upper half of the neural arch remains firmly attached to the vertebra above and the lower half to the vertebra below. Since the original description of this fracture, three more types of seat-belt fractures have been reported, which involve varying degrees of ligament and intervertebral disk disruption (Figs. 11.61, 11.62). According to the Denis three-column concept of thoracolumbar spine injuries, these latter types of fractures are essentially the result of failure of the posterior and middle columns, with the intact anterior element acting as a hinge. These injuries may be stable or unstable, depending on their extent and severity.

Fracture–Dislocations

Resulting from various forces—flexion, rotation, distraction, or anteroposterior or posteroanterior shear—acting on the thoracolumbar

stable, and three-column unstable; two-column fractures may be stable or unstable, depending on the extent of injury (Table 11.6).

Compression Fractures. Usually resulting from anterior or lateral flexion, compression fracture is a failure of the anterior column under compression forces; the middle column remains intact, acting as a hinge, even in severe cases in which there may also be partial failure of the posterior column. The standard radiographic examination of the thoracic and lumbar segments is usually sufficient to demonstrate this injury (Fig. 11.54), although CT or MRI may be required to delineate the extent of the fracture or demonstrate obscure features (Figs. 11.55 and

Table 11.6 **Basic Types of Spinal Fractures and the Columns Involved in Each**

Type of Fracture	Column Involvement		
	Anterior	*Middle*	*Posterior*
Compression	Compression	None	None or distraction (in severe fractures)
Burst	Compression	Compression	None or distraction
Seat-belt	None or compression	Distraction	Distraction
Fracture-dislocation	Compression and/or rotation, shear	Distraction and/or rotation, shear	Distraction and/or rotation, shear

(From Montesano PX, Benson DR, 1991, with permission).

Figure 11.54 Compression fracture. A 48-year-old woman fell from a ladder and hurt her back. **(A)** Anteroposterior radiograph of the thoracic spine demonstrates a decrease in the height of the vertebral body of T-8, secondary to compression fracture. Note the localized widening of the paraspinal line secondary to hemorrhage and edema. **(B)** The lateral radiograph demonstrates anterior wedging. Note the intact posterior vertebral body line. These are the features of simple compression fracture affecting only the anterior column.

Figure 11.55 CT of the compression fracture. (A) Lateral radiograph of the lumbar spine shows compression of the anterior part of the vertebral body of L-3, although the posterior part is not well demonstrated. **(B)** Sagittal CT reformatted image clearly shows intact middle column, confirming the presence of the compression and not the burst fracture.

Figure 11.56 MRI of the compression fracture. (A) Lateral radiograph of the lumbar spine shows compression of the anterosuperior part of the vertebral body of L-1. **(B)** Sagittal proton-density MRI demonstrates a fracture involving only the anterior column, confirming the diagnosis of compression fracture.

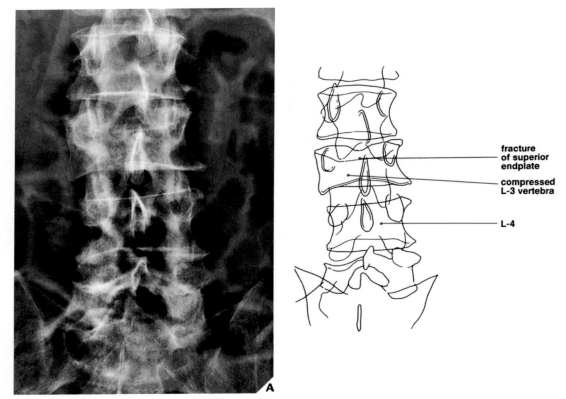

Figure 11.57 Burst fracture. A 56-year-old merchant seaman fell from a 60-foot-high ladder on a ship. Anteroposterior **(A)** and lateral **(B)** films of the lumbar spine show a burst fracture of the body of L-3. Note widening of the interpediculate distance on the anteroposterior radiograph, the hallmark of burst fracture. The severity of the injury, however, is better appreciated on a CT section **(C)** through the body of L-3. There is comminution of the vertebral fracture and displacement of two bony fragments into the spinal canal, with compression of the thecal sac, indicating involvement of anterior and middle columns. **(D)** In another patient, a 26-year-old man with a burst fracture of L-3, sagittal T1-weighted MR image (SE; TR 800/TE 20 msec) demonstrates posterior displacement of the middle column with compression of the thecal sac. **(E)** Sagittal T2-weighted MR image of a 58-year-old man who fell from the roof of a three-story building shows a typical appearance of a burst fracture of T-11. Note compression of the thecal sac. *(continued)*

Figure 11.57 **Burst fracture.** *Continued.*

Figure 11.58 Myelography of the burst fracture. A 28-year-old woman made a parachute jump and landed on her back. Hemiplegia and incontinence developed thereafter. **(A)** Anteroposterior radiograph of the lumbar spine shows a burst fracture of L-1. **(B)** Lateral view as part of a myelogram shows complete obstruction of the flow of contrast medium at the level of fracture caused by a small bony fragment impinging on the thecal sac.

Figure 11.59 Chance fracture. A 30-year-old woman sustained an injury to the lower back in a car collision; she had been wearing a lap seat belt. Anteroposterior **(A)** and lateral **(B)** tomograms of the lumbar spine show a fracture of the vertebral body of L-1 extending into the lamina and spinous process. Coronal **(C)** and sagittal **(D)** CT reformation images confirm the conventional tomographic findings. (Courtesy of Dr. D. Faegenburg, Mineola, NY.)

Figure 11.60 CT of the Chance fracture. A 36-year-old woman was injured in a car accident. She had been wearing a lap seat belt but not a restraining shoulder belt. Reformatted CT images in coronal (**A**) and sagittal (**B**) planes show a typical one-level Chance fracture through the L-2 vertebra.

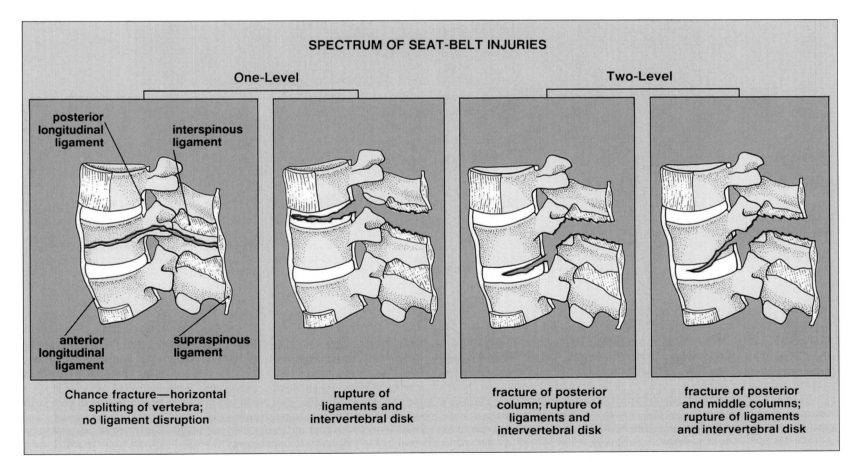

Figure 11.61 **The spectrum of seat-belt injuries involving the lumbar spine.**

Figure 11.62 Two-level seat-belt injury. A 21-year-old woman sustained an injury to the lower back in a car accident. **(A)** Anteroposterior view of the lumbar spine demonstrates a horizontal cleft in the L-2 vertebral body. Note increased distance between the pedicles of L-2 and L-3 and fractures of several transverse processes. **(B)** Lateral view shows posterior angulation at the L2-3 level and an oblique fracture extending from the inferoposterior part of the L-2 vertebral body to the lamina and posterior elements. **(C)** Sagittal CT reformation demonstrates the fracture of posterior elements to better advantage. **(D)** Parasagittal MR image demonstrates disruption of the posterior ligaments and a large soft-tissue hematoma. The findings are typical of a two-level seat-belt injury.

segment either alone or in combination, fracture–dislocations result in failure of all three columns of the spine (Fig. 11.63); hence, such injuries are unstable and are usually associated with severe neurologic complications.

In the *flexion-rotation type* of injury, the posterior and middle columns are completely disrupted, and the anterior column may show on the lateral radiograph anterior wedging of the vertebral body. The lateral film also demonstrates subluxation or dislocation, together with an increase in the interspinous distance (Fig. 11.64). The posterior wall of the vertebral body may be intact if the dislocation occurs at the level of the intervertebral disk. The anteroposterior projection may not be diagnostic, but it occasionally reveals a displaced fracture of the superior articular process on one side, representing failure of the posterior column secondary to rotational forces.

In the *shear types* of fracture–dislocation, all three columns are dis-

rupted, including the anterior longitudinal ligament. The *posteroanterior shear variant* is characterized by forward displacement of the spinal segment onto the vertebra below at the point of shear; the vertebral bodies are intact without any decrease in their anterior or posterior height. However, the posterior elements of the dislocated vertebral segment, including the laminae, articular facets, and spinous processes, are usually fractured at several levels (Fig. 11.65). In *anteroposterior shear*, the spinal segment above the point of shear is dislocated posterior to the segment below (Fig. 11.66). It may be accompanied by a fracture of the spinous process.

Fracture–dislocation of the *flexion-distraction type* resembles seat-belt injuries involving failure of the posterior and middle columns (Fig. 11.67; Fig. 11.61). However, unlike seat-belt injuries, the entire annulus fibrosus is torn, which allows the vertebra above to dislocate or sublux onto the vertebra below.

FRACTURE-DISLOCATIONS

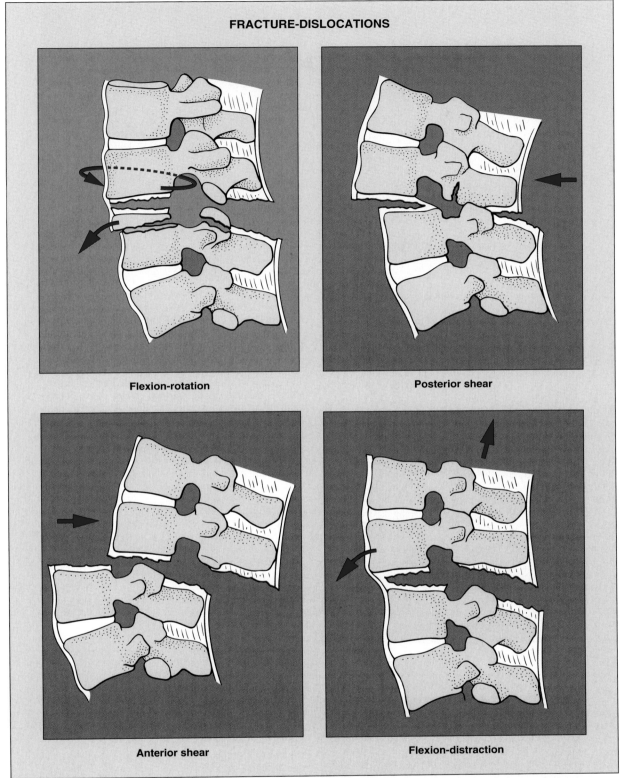

Flexion-rotation

Posterior shear

Anterior shear

Flexion-distraction

Figure 11.63 Types of fracture–dislocations. Schematic representation of various types of fracture–dislocation of the thoracolumbar spine.

Figure 11.64 Fracture–dislocation. A 27-year-old man was injured in a motorcycle accident and sustained a flexion-rotation type of fracture-dislocation at the T12-L1 level. **(A)** Lateral radiograph shows anterior wedging of the body of L-1 and disruption of the middle column. There is also slight anterior displacement of vertebra T-12. **(B)** CT section through the vertebra L-1 shows fracture of the middle column associated with retropulsion of the fractured fragment into the spinal canal, similar to that in the burst fracture. **(C)** Sagittal T2-weighted MR image shows in addition disruption of the posterior column and compression of the thecal sac.

Figure 11.65 Fracture–dislocation. Lateral radiograph of the lumbar spine demonstrates a posteroanterior shear-type fracture–dislocation at the L4-5 level. The vertebral bodies are intact, but there are fractures of the posterior elements of the affected vertebrae.

Figure 11.66 Fracture–dislocation. Sagittal T2-weighted MR image demonstrates an anteroposterior shear-type fracture–dislocation at the lower thoracic level.

Spondylolysis and Spondylolisthesis

Spondylolysis, a defect in the pars interarticularis (neck of the "Scotty dog") of a vertebra, may be an acquired abnormality, secondary to an acute fracture, or, as is more commonly the case, it may result from chronic stress (stress fracture). Rarely is it seen as a result of a congenital defect in the isthmus. Spondylolisthesis, a term introduced by Killian in 1854, is defined as ventral slipping or gliding of all or part of one vertebra on a stationary vertebra beneath it. These abnormalities are seen predominantly in the lumbar spine (90% of cases) and most commonly at the L4-5 and L5-S1 levels.

It is important to distinguish spondylolisthesis associated with spondylolysis from spondylolisthesis occurring without an associated defect in the pars interarticularis (Fig. 11.68). As a rule, this latter form, designated "pseudospondylolisthesis" by Junghanns in 1931, is associated with degenerative disk disease and degeneration and subluxation in the apophyseal joints, and it is often referred to as degenerative spondylolisthesis (see Chapter 13). Although the defect in the pars interarticularis cannot always be demonstrated on conventional radiographs, true spondylolisthesis can be differentiated from pseudospondylolisthesis by the spinous-process sign introduced by Bryk and Rosenkranz (Fig. 11.69). The sign is a logical outgrowth of the different processes at work in the two conditions. In true spondylolisthesis, a bilateral defect in the pars interarticularis leads to forward (ventral) slippage of the body, pedicles, and superior articular process of the involved vertebra, while the spinous process, laminae, and inferior articular process remain in normal position. Therefore, study of the most dorsal aspects of the spinous processes reveals a step-off at the interspace above the level of the slip (Fig. 11.70A). In pseudospondylolisthesis, however, the entire vertebra, including the spinous process, moves forward; in this situation, the most dorsal aspects of the spinous processes exhibit a step-off at the interspace below the level of the slipped vertebra (Fig. 11.70B). Application of this sign allows a correct diagnosis to be made on a single lateral film; oblique projections are not necessary. In obtaining the films, however, it is important to avoid overexposure, which may obscure the posterior margins of the spinous processes.

The defect in the pars interarticularis precipitating spondylolisthesis can be demonstrated on the standard oblique projection of the lumbar spine, which may need to be supplemented by conventional tomography or CT (Fig. 11.71 A–C); myelography on the lateral view may show an extradural defect on the ventral aspect of the thecal sac, similar to that created by disk herniation (Fig. 11.71D). A severe degree of spondylolisthesis at the L5-S1 level can be identified on the anteroposterior view by the ventrocaudal displacement of L-5 over the sacrum. This configuration creates curvilinear densities forming what is called the "inverted Napoleon's hat" sign (Fig. 11.72). The simple grading of spondylolisthesis proposed by Meyerding is based on the amount of forward slipping (Fig. 11.73).

Injury to the Diskovertebral Junction

One of the most frequent conditions affecting the diskovertebral junction is herniation of an intervertebral disk. The chief structural unit between adjacent vertebral bodies, the intervertebral disk, comprises a soft central portion, the nucleus pulposus, composed of collagen fibrils and mucoprotein gel, lying eccentrically and somewhat posteriorly, and a firm fibrocartilaginous ring, the annulus fibrosus, surrounding the nucleus pulposus and reinforced by the anterior and

Figure 11.67 Fracture–dislocation. Lateral radiograph of the thoracolumbar spine **(A)** and sagittal reformatted CT image **(B)** demonstrate characteristic features of a flexion-distraction type of fracture–dislocation.

Figure 11.68 Types of spondylolisthesis. Spondylolisthesis may occur in association with spondylolysis resulting from a defect in the pars interarticularis, or secondary to degenerative disk disease and degeneration and subluxation of the apophyseal joints (pseudospondylolisthesis).

Figure 11.69 The spinous-process sign. The spinous-process sign can help differentiate true spondylolisthesis from pseudospondylolisthesis by the appearance of a step-off in the spinous processes above the level of vertebral slip in the former and below that level in the latter.

Figure 11.70 Spondylolisthesis and "pseudospondylolisthesis." (A) Lateral view of the lumbar spine demonstrates the typical appearance of spondylolisthesis secondary to a defect in the pars interarticularis. Note that the most dorsal aspect of the spinous process of L-5 forms a step with that of L-4 above the level of slippage of L-5. **(B)** In spondylolisthesis without spondylolysis (degenerative spondylolisthesis), a step-off in the spinous processes below the level of vertebral slippage is an identifying feature.

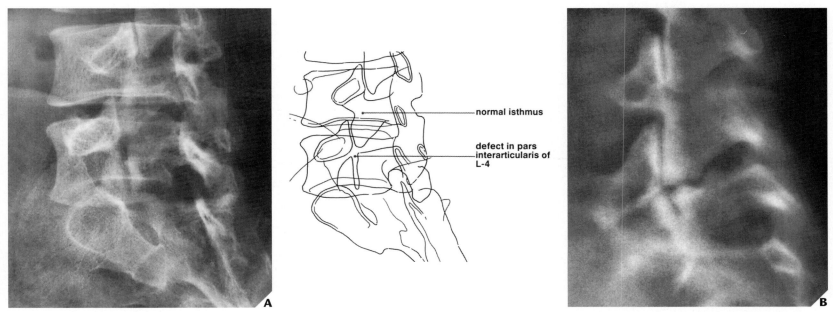

Figure 11.71 Spondylolysis and spondylolisthesis. Oblique radiograph **(A)** and trispiral tomogram **(B)** of the lumbar spine in a 28-year-old man show a defect in the pars interarticularis (neck of the "Scotty dog") of L-4 typical of spondylolysis. *(continued)*

Figure 11.71 Spondylolysis and spondylolisthesis. *Continued.* **(C)** CT section through the body clearly demonstrates defects in the left and right pars interarticularis. **(D)** Lateral spot film obtained during myelography shows an extradural defect, similar to that of disk herniation, on the ventral aspect of the thecal sac caused by grade 2 spondylolisthesis at L4-5. The defect in the pars interarticularis is also clearly seen.

Figure 11.72 Inverted Napoleon's hat sign. (A) Anteroposterior view of the lumbosacral spine in a 21-year-old man with severe (grade 4) spondylolisthesis shows curvilinear densities in the sacral area forming an inverted Napoleon's hat. This configuration is caused by a severe degree of slip at the L5-S1 level, as seen on the lateral projection **(B)**. **(C)** The sign is created by imaging the vertebral body in the axial projection, similar to that seen on a CT section of a normal vertebra. *(continued)*

Figure 11.72 Inverted Napoleon's hat sign. *Continued.*

L-5

S-1

Grade 1 Grade 2 Grade 3 Grade 4

Figure 11.73 **Grades of spondylolisthesis.** The grading of spondylolisthesis, as proposed by Meyerding, is based on the amount of forward displacement of L-5 on S-1.

posterior longitudinal ligaments. Injury to the intervertebral disk and the disko-vertebral junction can result from acute trauma or from subtle subclinical, often endogenous injury. Depending on the direction of herniation of disk material, a spectrum of injuries of the intervertebral disk and adjacent vertebrae may be seen (Fig. 11.74).

Anterior Disk Herniation. When the normal attachments of the annulus fibrosus to the vertebral rim by Sharpey fibers and to the anterior longitudinal ligament loosen, disk material (nucleus pulposus) herniates anteriorly. Elevation of the anterior longitudinal ligament by herniating material stimulates the formation of peripheral osteophytes, leading to a degenerative condition known as spondylosis deformans (see Chapter 13 on arthritides), which can be demonstrated on the lateral view of the lumbar spine (Fig 11.75A; see also Fig.

13.29). Anterior herniation can also be demonstrated on diskography (Fig. 11.75B) and MRI.

Intravertebral Disk Herniation. Ventrocaudal disk herniation, as well as ventrocephalad herniation, which is much less commonly seen, produces an abnormality known as limbus vertebra. Herniation of disk material into a vertebral body at the site of attachment of the annulus fibrosus to the body's rim separates a small, triangular fragment of bone, which is commonly mistaken for an acute fracture or infectious spondylitis. Reactive bone sclerosis adjacent to the defect, however, indicates a chronic process. The adjacent disk space is invariably narrowed, and a radiolucent cleft known as the vacuum phenomenon may be seen in the disk space, representing degeneration of the disk (Fig. 11.76). This abnormality is invariably asymptomatic it

Figure 11.74 **The spectrum of intervertebral disk herniation.**

SPECTRUM OF INTERVERTEBRAL DISK HERNIATION

Normal

Anterior Herniation

ventrad extrusion leading to elevation of anterior longitudinal ligament; osteophyte formation—spondylosis deformans

Intravertebral Herniation

anterocaudad extrusion separating a triangular fragment from adjacent vertebra—limbus vertebra

cephalad or caudad extrusion through end plate into adjacent vertebra—Schmorl node

Intraspinal Herniation

posterior or posterolateral extrusion into spinal canal—"herniated disk"

Figure 11.75 Spondylosis deformans and anterior disk herniation. (A) Lateral radiograph of the lumbar spine shows a late stage of spondylosis deformans at the L2-3, L3-4, and L4-5 levels characterized by large osteophytes on the anterior aspects of adjacent vertebral bodies as a result of anterior disk herniation. (B) Anterior disk herniation can also be identified on diskography by contrast medium outlining the extruded material, as seen here at the L5-S1 level.

contrast outlining
anterior disk
herniation

spinal needle
in intervertebral
disk

is the product of chronic, endogenous trauma. The characteristic radiographic changes are best seen on the lateral projection of the lumbar spine (Fig. 11.76); only rarely is conventional tomography or CT indicated to exclude a true vertebral fracture (Fig. 11.77). MRI may be performed to confirm or exclude the concomitant posterior disk herniation (Fig. 11.78, see also Fig. 11.89). Occasionally, more than one vertebra is affected and although limbus vertebra is usually seen in the lumbar spine, it may also be present in a thoracic vertebra.

Limbus vertebra should not be confused with the secondary ossification centers of the vertebral ring apophysis, which are commonly seen in the growing skeleton (Fig. 11.79); at skeletal maturity, these centers become fully united with the vertebral body.

Intravertebral disk herniation may also occur when the nucleus pulposus breaks through the vertebral end plate, extruding into a vertebra. This abnormality may be the result of acute trauma, as in a burst fracture, but it is much more commonly encountered secondary to

Figure 11.76 Limbus vertebra. Lateral radiograph of the lumbar spine in a 55-year-old woman with breast cancer who underwent radiographic examination to exclude bone metastases shows anterior intravertebral disk herniation into the body of L-2 (limbus vertebra). Note the vacuum phenomenon, indicating disk degeneration.

vacuum
phenomenon

anterior disk
herniation into
vertebral body

Figure 11.77 Limbus vertebra. An 18-year-old man injured his lumbar spine in an automobile accident. The standard radiographic examination was equivocal regarding fracture. **(A)** Lateral tomogram shows the typical appearance of a limbus vertebra secondary to anterior herniation of the nucleus pulposus. The small triangular segment is separated from the body of L-4 by a rim of reactive sclerosis, indicating a chronic process. Note the characteristic disk space narrowing. **(B)** CT examination was performed to investigate the possibility of concomitant posterior disk herniation into the spinal canal. The examination was negative for posterior herniation but confirmed the anterior herniation into the vertebral body, as seen in this more proximal section.

Figure 11.78 MRI of anterior intravertebral disk herniation (limbus vertebra). A 39-year-old woman presented with radicular pain after lifting a heavy object. **(A)** Lateral radiograph of the lumbar spine shows a typical appearance of limbus vertebra. Axial **(B)** and sagittal **(C)** MR images demonstrate anterior intravertebral disk herniation (*open arrows*), but there is no evidence of posterior disk herniation.

Figure 11.79 Secondary ossification centers. The secondary ossification centers of the vertebral ring apophysis in the growing skeleton, as seen here in a 5-year-old girl, should not be mistaken for limbus vertebrae.

weakening of the vertebral body, as in osteoporosis. In the latter condition, the lesion is known as a Schmorl node. It may be small and localized, or large and diffuse, in which case it is often referred to as "ballooned disk" (Fig. 11.80).

Scheuermann Disease. Also known as juvenile thoracic kyphosis, Scheuermann disease was first described by Scheuermann in 1921. The underlying abnormality is characterized by intravertebral herniation of disk material (Schmorl nodes), associated with anterior wedging (of 5° or more) of at least three contiguous vertebral bodies. There is a wavy appearance of vertebral endplates and narrowing of the intervertebral disk spaces. Thoracic kyphosis is often present (Fig. 11.81). This condition usually affects adolescent boys and young adults. The clinical manifestations are variable. Some patients are completely asymptomatic, whereas others may experience fatigue and thoracic pain aggravated by physical exertion. Neurologic findings are rare. Although the thoracic spine is predominantly affected, involvement of the lumbar spine has also been reported. This condition is called Scheuermann disease type II (in contrast to type I, which involves the upper thoracic spine), although some investigators prefer the term "juvenile lumbar osteochondrosis." Imaging studies demonstrate changes almost identical to those seen in Scheuermann disease type I, including prominent Schmorl nodes, irregularity of the endplates, and narrowing of the disk spaces (Fig. 11.82). However, anterior vertebral wedging is not a constant feature of this variant.

Posterior and Posterolateral Disk Herniation. Intraspinal herniation or "herniated disk" is the most serious of the three variants of diskovertebral junction injury. It is most commonly seen in the lumbar spine, particularly L4-5 and L5-S1, although it may be seen in the cervical region. It is commonly associated with clinical symptoms such as sciatic pain and weakening of the lower extremity, especially when herniation in the lumbar segment causes compression on an exiting nerve root or the thecal sac. A predisposing factor in some patients may be the loss of elasticity of the annulus fibrosus caused by degen-

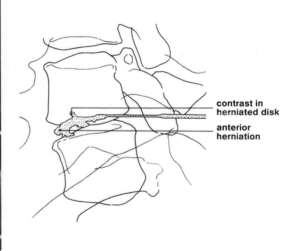

contrast in herniated disk

anterior herniation

Figure 11.80 Schmorl nodes. (A) Lateral radiograph of the lumbar spine in an asymptomatic 77-year-old woman with osteoporosis of the spine shows multiple indentations particularly of the inferior end plates, representing the Schmorl nodes, secondary to intravertebral disk herniation caused by weakening of the vertebral end plates. **(B)** In another patient, a small Schmorl node is demonstrated on diskography by opacification of extruded disk material in the body of L-4. Some anterior herniation is also evident.

Figure 11.81 Scheuermann disease. Lateral tomogram of the thoracic spine in a 23-year-old man demonstrates several Schmorl nodes in T5-8 and slight anterior wedging of the vertebral bodies. Note the wavy outline of the superior and inferior end plates and the mild kyphotic curve of the thoracic spine in this patient, an abnormality also called juvenile thoracic kyphosis.

Radicular symptoms represents one of the most common reasons why patients are referred for MRI of the spine. MRI is particularly sensitive and is used to detect and characterize disk herniation because it allows for direct evaluation of the internal morphology of the disk. The sagittal imaging plane is more sensitive for defining disk impingement on the thecal sac, or for demonstrating extruded fragments and showing the relationship to the vertebral bodies and intervertebral disk spaces (Fig. 11.89A). The axial imaging plane can demonstrate the effect of the herniated disk on the exiting nerve roots and thecal sac (Fig. 11.89B). Axial images are also important in evaluating neural foramina and nerve root effacement in cases of lateral and posterolateral disk herniation. Free disk fragments can be easily identified.

The use of T1-weighted images in the axial plane provides excellent contrast between high-signal fat and low-signal thecal sac, nerve roots, and disk fragments. Fast-scan techniques provide increased cerebrospinal fluid signal and allow enhanced contrast between herniated fragments and cerebrospinal fluid. Some advantages of MRI in comparison with myelography and CT of lumbar disk disease are evident. MRI is sensitive to the water content of the nucleus pulposus. As the water content of this structure decreases with aging or degeneration, decreased signal appears, particularly on T2-weighted images. In addition, the myelographic effect provided with heavily T2-weighted

erative changes, with subsequent rupture of the annulus or even the posterior longitudinal ligament and retropulsion of the nucleus pulposus into the spinal canal. Typically, the patient, usually a young adult man, gives a history of straining his back by lifting a heavy object. The subsequent pain in the lumbar region radiates to the posterior aspect of the thigh and buttock and the lateral aspect of the leg, and is aggravated by coughing and sneezing; sometimes, there is associated paresthesia or numbness in the foot. Physical examination reveals muscular spasm, limitation of forward bending, and restriction of straight-leg raising on the affected side. Various other symptoms and physical findings may be present depending on the level and degree of injury.

The standard radiographic examination in herniated disks is usually normal, and ancillary radiologic techniques including myelography and CT, either alone or in conjunction with one another, as well as diskography, and now MRI, are required to make a diagnosis. The myelographic findings in disk herniation may be very subtle, such as absent opacification of a nerve sheath (Fig. 11.83), or more obvious, such as an extradural pressure defect in the contrast-filled thecal sac (Fig. 11.84). Disk herniation can also be diagnosed on plain CT examination (Fig. 11.85) or on CT sections obtained after myelography (Figs. 11.86 and 11.87) or diskography (Fig. 11.88). The most effective technique, however, is MRI (Fig. 11.89).

The latter imaging modality is being used increasingly for the diagnosis of conditions causing acute low back pain and sciatica. The sensitivity of MRI for the diagnosis of herniated disk and spinal stenosis is equivalent to or better than that of computed tomography, even in combination with myelography and diskography.

Figure 11.82 MRI of Scheuermann disease. A 28-year-old man presented with low back pain lasting several months. Sagittal MRI of the lumbar spine demonstrates characteristic features of Scheuermann disease, type II. Note prominent Schmorl nodes involving all five vertebral bodies, decreased height of the vertebral bodies, and narrowing of the intervertebral disk spaces.

Figure 11.83 Lateral disk herniation. In lifting a heavy object, a 27-year-old man felt sudden, sharp pain in the lower back radiating to the left lower extremity. The standard radiographs of the lumbosacral spine were normal. Anteroposterior view of a myelogram demonstrates a subtle lack of filling of the left L-5 nerve sheath, which at surgery was found to be compressed by a lateral herniation of the L4-5 disk.

lack of filling of L-5 nerve sheath

normal nerve root

Figure 11.84 Myelography of herniated disk. Lateral spot film obtained during myelography in a 38-year-old man demonstrates a large posterior herniation of the intervertebral disk at L4-5.

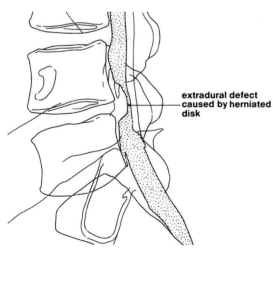

extradural defect caused by herniated disk

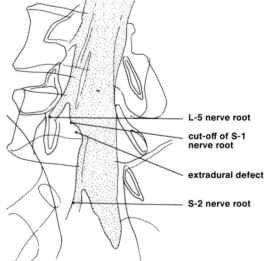

Figure 11.85 CT of herniated disk. Axial CT section of the lumbar spine at the L5-S1 level demonstrates a large centrolateral disk herniation encroaching on the left intervertebral foramen.

Figure 11.86 CT–myelography of herniated disk. A 47-year-old man presented with severe back pain radiating to the right buttock and leg. **(A)** Spot film in the oblique projection obtained during myelography shows an extradural defect on the right side of the thecal sac at the L5-S1 disk space involving the right S-1 nerve root. The L-5 and S-2 nerve roots are normally outlined. CT sections **(B)**, **(C)** also obtained during myelography, demonstrate the lack of opacification of the S-1 nerve root on the right side and a large herniation of the L5-S1 disk compressing the thecal sac from the right.

Figure 11.87 Three-dimensional CT–myelography of herniated disk. A three-dimensional CT of the lower thoracic spine was obtained after contrast agent was injected into the thecal sac (CT–myelography). There is disk herniation at the level of T7-T8 (*arrow*) associated with complete obstruction of contrast flow (*open arrows*). The curved arrow points to the spinal cord.

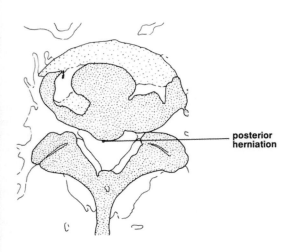

Figure 11.88 CT-diskography of herniated disk. A 30-year-old male construction worker strained his lower back at work and was admitted to the hospital with severe sciatica. (A) Lateral radiograph of the lumbar spine during myelographic examination reveals a slight separation of the ventral aspect of the dural sac from the dorsal aspect of L-5 due to grade 1 spondylolisthesis. In addition, there is an extradural pressure defect on the ventral aspect of the dural sac at the L4-5 level and a much smaller defect at the L3-4 disk space. (B) A diskogram using metrizamide was performed at the L3-4 and L4-5 levels, the latter demonstrating posterior herniation. (C) CT at the L4-5 level following diskography shows posterior protrusion of the opacified disk material.

Figure 11.89 MRI of herniated disk. A 44-year-old man presented with sciatic pain radiating to the right buttock and thigh. **(A)** Sagittal MRI (SE; TR 1500/TE 20 msec) demonstrates a posterior herniation of disk L4-5 and a bulging disk at L5-S1. **(B)** Axial MRI (SE; TR 1500/TE 30 msec) clearly shows posterolateral disk herniation with marked compression of the thecal sac. **(C)** The levels of the several axial sections obtained at the L4-5 disk space are indicated.

images and fast-scan techniques allows the visualization of nerve roots within the thecal sac. Anomalies such as conjoint nerve roots, which may simulate a herniated nucleus pulposus on CT studies, can be visualized directly with MRI. It has to be stressed, however, that evaluating patients with radiculopathy and herniated disk is an area in which both MRI and CT can be complementary. When an extradural defect is identified with MRI, it may be difficult to ascertain whether the lesion represents a herniated nucleus pulposus or an osteophyte; in these situations, CT can make the distinction easily, by identifying the increased mineralization within the osteophyte. When the herniated fragment is clearly in continuity with the intervertebral disk and is of the same signal intensity, the diagnosis is suggested by MRI alone.

Annular Tears. Tears or fissures of the annulus fibrosus of lumbar intervertebral disks may occur secondary to trauma and may also be caused by degenerative changes of the disk related to normal aging. According to Munter and associates these tears represent separations between annular fibers, separations of annular fibers from their vertebral insertions, or breaks through these fibers in any orientation, involving one or more layers of the annular lamellae. Annular tears are found in both symptomatic and asymptomatic individuals. In a cadaver study, Yu and colleagues identified three types of annular tears. Type I is a concentric tear that is characterized by rupture of the transverse fibers connecting adjacent lamellae in the annulus, without disruption of the longitudinal fibers. Type II is a radial tear that represents fissures extending from the periphery of the annulus to the nucleus pulposus associated with disruption of the longitudinal fibers. Type III is a transverse tear caused by disruption of Sharpey fibers at the periphery of the annulus fibrosus. Type II and III tears can be seen on T2-weighted MRI as hyperintense foci within the annulus. These tears can also be occasionally demonstrated by CT diskography.

PRACTICAL POINTS TO REMEMBER

Cervical Spine

[1] The single most important projection in the radiographic examination of the cervical spine is the lateral view—either the erect or cross-table lateral.

[2] In the evaluation of injury to the cervical spine, it is mandatory to visualize the C-7 vertebra, the site of the most commonly missed fractures. If this cannot be accomplished on the lateral projection, the swimmer's view should be attempted.

[3] CT examination and MRI are useful techniques for evaluating vertebral-column trauma and associated soft-tissue and spinal cord injuries.

[4] Stability of a cervical spine fracture is the most important practical factor in evaluation of injuries to this region.

[5] Fractures of the occipital condyles are best demonstrated on CT with coronal reformation.

[6] A classification system of three types of occipital condyle fractures devised by Anderson and Montesano is based on fracture morphology, pertinent anatomy, and biomechanics.

[7] Occipitocervical dislocation is effectively demonstrated on the lateral radiographs supplemented with CT reformatted images.

[8] Jefferson fracture—a symmetrical fracture of the anterior and posterior arches of C-1—can be diagnosed on the anteroposterior open-mouth view by the lateral displacement of the lateral masses.

[9] In the evaluation of fractures of the odontoid process (dens), note that:
  • type I (an oblique fracture distal [cephalad] to the base) and type III (a fracture through the base extending into the body) are stable

- type II (a transverse fracture through the base) is unstable.
[10] Teardrop fracture, a flexion injury representing a variant of a burst fracture, is the most severe and unstable of cervical spine fractures; it is frequently associated with spinal cord damage.
[11] Extension teardrop fracture, which usually occurs at the level of C-2 or C-3, is a stable injury without the potentially dangerous compliations of the flexion teardrop fracture.
[12] Clay-shoveler's fracture, involving the spinous processes of C-6 or C-7, can be recognized on the anteroposterior projection of the cervical spine by the ghost sign produced by caudal displacement of the fractured spinous process.
[13] In the radiographic evaluation of locked facets, a bow-tie or bat-wing appearance of the dislocated articular pillars on the lateral projection is characteristic.

Thoracolumbar Spine

[1] The three-column spine classification of acute injuries to the thoracic and lumbar segments is a practical approach to defining the stability of various fractures.
[2] Subtle fractures of the thoracic vertebrae can be recognized by a localized bulge in the paraspinal line secondary to edema and hemorrhage.
[3] Chance fracture, known also as a seat-belt fracture, is a horizontal fracture through a lumbar vertebral body with extension into the lamina and spinous process.
[4] Fracture-dislocations of thoracic and lumbar spine, which are unstable injuries, are classified into four types:
  - flexion-rotation injury
  - posteroanterior shear injury
  - anteroposterior shear injury
  - flexion-distraction injury
[5] Spondylolysis, a defect in the pars interarticularis (neck of the "Scotty dog"), leads to ventral slipping of one vertebra on the vertebra beneath it—spondylolisthesis.
[6] Spondylolisthesis
  - may be associated with a defect in the pars interarticularis, so-called true spondylolisthesis
  - or exist without an isthmic defect, so-called pseudospondylolisthesis or degenerative spondylolisthesis (associated with degenerative changes in the intervertebral disk and apophyseal joints).
[7] A simple test to distinguish between the two types of spondylolisthesis is the spinous-process sign.
[8] A severe degree of spondylolisthesis at the L5-S1 level can be recognized on the anteroposterior projection by the phenomenon known as the "inverted Napoleon's hat" sign.
[9] An intervertebral disk can herniate anteriorly or anterolaterally, as well as posteriorly, or posterolaterally. Intraosseous herniation into a vertebral body may occur caudad or ventrocaudad, cephalad, or ventrocephalad.
[10] Intravertebral ventrocaudad or ventrocephalad herniation results in separation of a small, triangular segment of a vertebra. This limbus vertebra should not be mistaken for a fracture.
[11] Posterior disk herniation can be documented by:
  - CT
  - myelography
  - diskography
  - MRI
  - or a combination of these
[12] As a rule, diskography is performed if the results of CT, myelography, and MRI are equivocal.

SUGGESTED READINGS

Amundsen P, Skalpe IO. Cervical myelography with a watersoluble contrast medium (metrizamide). *Neuroradiology* 1975;8:209–212.

Anand AK, Lee BCP. Plain and metrizamide CT of lumbar disk disease: comparison with myelography. *AJNR* 1982;3:567–571.

Anderson LD, D'Alonzo RT. Fractures of the odontoid process of the axis. *J Bone Joint Surg [Am]* 1974;56A:1663–1674.

Anderson PA, Montesano PX. Injuries to the occipitocervical articulation. In: Chapman MW, ed. *Operative orthopaedics*, vol. 4, 2nd ed. Philadelphia; JB Lippincott; 1993:2631–2640.

Anderson PA, Montesano PX. Morphology and treatment of occipital condyle fractures. *Spine* 1988;13:731–736.

Anderson PA, Montesano PX. Treatment of sacral fractures and lumbosacral injuries. In: Chapman MW, ed. *Operative orthopaedics*, vol. 4, 2nd ed. Philadelphia: JB Lippincott; 1993:2699–2710.

Beltran J. *MRI: musculoskeletal system.* Philadelphia: JB Lippincott; 1990.

Blackmore CC, Deyo RA. Specificity of cervical spine radiography. Importance of clinical scenario. *Emerg Radiol* 1997;4:283–286.

Blacksin MF, Lee HJ. Frequency and significance of fractures of the upper cervical spine detected by CT in patients with severe neck trauma. *AJR Am J Roentgenol* 1995;165:1201–1204.

Boden SD, Davis DO, Dina TS, Patronas NJ, Wiesel SW. Abnormal magnetic-resonance scans of the lumbar spine in asymptomatic subjects. *J Bone Joint Surg [Am]* 1990;72A:403–408.

Boyd WR, Gardiner GA Jr. Metrizamide myelography. *AJR Am J Roentgenol* 1977;129:481–484.

Brandser EA, El-Khoury GY. Thoracic and lumbar spine trauma. *Radiol Clin North Am* 1997;35:533–557.

Brashear R Jr, Venters GC, Preston ET. Fractures of the neural arch of the axis: a report of twenty-nine cases. *J Bone Joint Surg [Am]* 1975;57A:879–887.

Brodsky AE, Binder WF. Lumbar discography. Its value in diagnosis and treatment of lumbar disc lesions. *Spine* 1979;4:110–120.

Brown RC Evans ET. What causes the "eye in the Scotty dog" in the oblique projection of the lumbar spine? *AJR Am J Roentgenol* 1973;118:435–437.

Bryk D, Rosenkranz W. True spondylolisthesis and pseudospondylolisthesis—the spinous process sign. *J Can Assoc Radiol* 1969;20:53–56.

Bucholz RW. Unstble hangman's fractures. *Clin Orthop* 1981;154:119–124.

Bucholz RW, Burkhead WZ. The pathologic anatomy of fatal atlanto-occipital dislocations. *J Bone Joint Surg [Am]* 1979;61A:248–250.

Burke JT, Harris JH. Acute injuries of the axis vertebra. *Skeletal Radiol* 1989;18:335–346.

Cancelmo JJ Jr. Clay shoveler's fracture: a helpful diagnostic sign. *AJR Am J Roentgenol* 1972;115:540–543.

Chance CQ. Note on a type of flexion fracture of the spine. *Br J Radiol* 1948;21:452–453.

Christenson PC. The radiologic study of the normal spine: cervical, thoracic, lumbar, and sacral. *Radiol Clin North Am* 1977;15:133–154.

Clark WM, Gehweiler JA Jr, Laib R. Twelve significant signs of cervical spine trauma. *Skeletal Radiol* 1979;3:201–205.

Collis JS Jr, Gardner WJ. Lumbar discography. An analysis of one thousand cases. *J Neurosurg* 1962;19:452–461.

Daffner RH. Helical CT of the cervical spine for trauma patients: a time study. *AJR Am J Roentgenol* 2001;177:677–679.

Daffner RH. *Imaging of vertebral trauma,* 2nd ed. Philadelphia: Lippincott-Raven; 1996.

Daffner RH. Injuries of the thoracolumbar vertebral column. In: Dalinka MK, Kaye JJ, eds. *Radiology in emergency room medicine.* New York: Churchill Livingstone; 1984:317–341.

Daffner RH, Brown RR, Goldberg AL. A new classification of cervical vertebral injuries: influence of CT. *Skeletal Radiol* 2000;29:125–132.

Daffner RH, Deeb ZL, Rothfus WE. "Fingerprints" of vertebral trauma—a unifying concept based on mechanisms. *Skeletal Radiol* 1986;15:518–525.

Denis F. Spinal instability as defined by the three-column spine concept in acute spinal trauma. *Clin Orthop* 1984;189:65–76.

Denis F. Three column spine and its significance in the classification of acute thoracolumbar spinal injuries. *Spine* 1983;8:817–831.

Dietz GW, Christensen EE. Normal "Cupid's bow" contour of the lower lumbar vertebrae. *Radiology* 1976;121:577–579.

Dortwart RH, DeGroot J, Sauerland EK, Helms CA, Vogler JB. Computed tomography of the lumbosacral spine: normal anatomy, anatomic variants and pathologic anatomy. *Radiographics* 1982;2:459–499.

Dublin AB, McGahan JP, Reid MH. The value of computed tomographic metrizamide myelography in the neuroradiological evaluation of the spine. *Radiology* 1983;146:79–86.

Dullerud R, Johansen JG. CT-diskography in patients with sciatica. Comparison with plain CT and MR imaging. *Acta Radiol* 1995;36:497–504.

Ellis JH, Martel W, Lillie JH, Aisen AM. Magnetic resonance imaging of the normal craniovertebral junction. *Spine* 1991;16:105–111.

Epstein BS, Epstein JA, Jones MD. Lumbar spondylolisthesis with isthmic defects. *Radiol Clin North Am* 1977;15:261–273.

Ferguson RL, Allen BL Jr. A mechanistic classification of thoracolumbar spine fractures. *Clin Orthop* 1984;189:77–88.

Firooznia H, Benjamin V, Kricheff II, Rafii M, Golimbu C. CT of lumbar spine disc herniation: correlation with surgical findings. *AJR Am J Roentgenol* 1984;142:587–592.

Freyschmidt J, Brossmann J, Wiens J, Sternberg A. *Freyschmidt's "Koehler/Zimmer" Borderlands of Normal and Early Pathological Findings in Skeletal Radiography.* 5th ed, Thieme, Stuttgart-New York; 2003:671–730.

Fuchs AW. Cervical vertebrae (Part I). *Radiogr Clin Photogr* 1940;16:2–17.

Gabrielsen TO, Maxwell JA. Traumatic atlanto-occipital dislocation. *AJR Am J Roentgenol* 1966;97:624–629.

Gehweiler JA Jr, Osborn RL, Becker RF. *The radiology of vertebral trauma.* Philadelphia: WB Saunders; 1980.

Gerlock AJ Jr, Kirchner SG, Heller RM, Kaye JJ. *The cervical spine in trauma.* Philadelphia: WB Saunders; 1978.

Gerlock AJ Jr, Mirfakhraee M. Computed tomography and hangman's fractures. *South Med J* 1983;76:727–728.

Glickstein MF, Burke DL, Kressel HY. Magnetic resonance demonstration of hyperintense herniated discs and extruded disc fragments. *Skeletal Radiol* 1989;18:527–530.

Greenspan A. CT-discography vs. MRI in intervertebral disk herniation. *Appl Radiol* 1993;22:34–40.

Greenspan A, Amparo EG, Gorczyca D, Montesano PX. Is there a role for diskography in the era of magnetic resonance imaging? Prospective correlation and quantitative analysis of computed tomography-diskography, magnetic resonance imaging, and surgical findings. *J Spinal Disord* 1992;5:26–31.

Guerra J Jr, Garfin SR, Resnick D. Vertebral burst fractures: CT analysis of the retropulsed fragment. *Radiology* 1984;153:769–772.

Gumley G, Taylor TK, Ryan MD. Distraction fractures of the lumbar spine. *J Bone Joint Surg [Br]* 1982;64B:520–525.

Han SY, Witten DM, Mussleman JP. Jefferson fracture of the atlas. Report of six cases. *J Neurosurg* 1976;44:368–371.

Harrington PR, Tullos HS. Spondylolisthesis in children: observations and surgical treatment. *Clin Orthop* 1971;79:75–84.

Harris Jr JH. The cervicocranium: its radiographic assessment. *Radiology* 2001;218:337–351.

Haughton VM. MR imaging of the spine. *Radiology* 1988;166:297–301.

Haughton VM, Eldevik OP, Magnaes B, Amundsen P. A prospective comparison of computed tomography and myelography in the diagnosis of herniated lumbar disks. *Radiology* 1982;142:103–110.

Hayes CW, Conway WF, Walsh JW, Coppage L, Gervin AS. Seat belt injuries: radiologic findings and clinical correlation. *Radiographics* 1991;11:23–36.

Hecht ST, Greenspan A. Digital subtraction lumbar diskography: technical note. *J Spinal Disord* 1993;6:68–70.

Holdsworth F, Chir M. Fractures, dislocations and fracture-dislocations of the spine. *J Bone Joint Surg [Am]* 1970;52A:1534–1551.

Holt EP Jr. The question of lumbar discography. *J Bone Joint Surg [Am]* 1968;50A:720–726.

Hyman RA, Gorey MT. Imaging strategies for MR of the spine. *Radiol Clin North Am* 1988;26:505–533.

Jefferson G. Fractures of the atlas vertebra. Report of four cases, and a review of those previously recorded. *Br J Surg* 1920;7:407–422.

Johansen JG, Orrison WW, Amundsen P. Lateral C1-2 puncture for cervical myelography. Part I: Report of a complication. *Radiology* 1983;146:391–393.

Kaiser MC, Ramos L. *MRI of the spine. A guide to clinical applications.* Stuttgart: Thieme Verlag; 1990.

Kathol MH. Cervical spine trauma. What is new? *Radiol Clin North Am* 1997;35:507–532.

Kim KS, Chen HH, Russell EJ, Rogers LF. Flexion teardrop fracture of the cervical spine: radiographic characteristics. *AJR Am J Roentgenol* 1989;152:319–326.

Kornberg M. Discography and magnetic resonance imaging in the diagnosis of lumbar disc disruption. *Spine* 1989;14:1368–1372.

Kricun R, Kricun ME, Dalinka MK. Advances in spinal imaging. *Radiol Clin North Am* 1990;28:321–339.

Lee C, Woodring JH. Unstable Jefferson variant atlas fractures: an unrecognized cervical injury. *AJR Am J Roentgenol* 1992;158:113–118.

Lustrin ES, Karakas SP, Ortiz AO, et al. Pediatric cervical spine: normal anatomy, variants, and trauma. *Radiographics* 2003;23:539–560.

MacDonald RL, Schwartz ML, Mirich D, Sharkey PW, Nelson WR. Diagnosis of cervical spine injury in motor vehicle crash victims: how many X-rays are enough? *J Trauma* 1990;30:392–397.

Mirvis SE, Geisler FH, Jelinek JJ, Joslyn JN, Gellad F. Acute cervical spine trauma: evaluation with 1.5T MR imaging. *Radiology* 1988;166:807–816.

Mirvis SE, Young JW, Lim C, Greenberg J. Hangman's fracture: radiologic assessment in 27 cases. *Radiology* 1987;163:713–717.

Modic MT. Degenerative disorders of the spine. In: Modic MT, Masaryk TJ, Ross JS, eds. *Magnetic resonance imaging of the spine.* Chicago: Year Book Medical Publishers; 1989.

Modic MT. Magnetic resonance imaging of the spine. In: Modic MT, Masaryk TJ, Ross JS, eds. *Magnetic resonance imaging of the spine.* Chicago, Year Book Medical Publishers; 1989.

Montesano PX, Benson DR. The thoracolumbar spine. In: Rockwood CA, Green DP, Bucholz RW, eds. *Rockwood and Green's fractures in adults,* 3rd ed. Philadelphia: JB Lippincott; 1991:1359–1397.

Montesano PX, Benson DR. Thoracolumbar spine fractures. In: Chapman MW, ed. *Operative orthopaedics,* vol. 4, 2nd ed. Philadelphia: JB Lippincott; 1993:2665–2697.

Munter FM, Wasserman BA, Wu H-M, Yousem DM. Serial MR imaging of annular tears in lumbar intervertebral disks. *AJNR Am J Neuroradiol* 2002;23:1105–1109.

Murphey MD. Trauma oblique cervical spine radiographs. *Ann Emerg Med* 1993;22:728–730.

Myerding HW. Spondylolisthesis. *Surg Gynecol Obstet* 1932;34:371–377.

Newman PH. The etiology of spondylolisthesis. *J Bone Joint Surg [Br]* 1963;45B:39–59.

Nuñez DB Jr, Quencer RM. The role of helical CT in the assessment of cervical spine injuries. *AJR Am J Roentgenol* 1998;171:951–957.

Nuñez DB Jr, Zuluaga A, Fuentes-Bernardo DA, Rivas LA, Becerra JL. Cervical spine trauma: how much more do we learn by routinely using helical CT? *Radiographics* 1996;16:1307–1318.

Orrison WW, Eldevik OP, Sackett JF. Lateral C1-2 puncture for cervical myelography. Part III: Historical, anatomic and technical considerations. *Radiology* 1983;146:401–408.

Raila FA, Aitken AT, Vickers GN. Computed tomography and three-dimensional reconstruction in the evaluation of occipital condyle fracture. *Skeletal Radiol* 1993;22:269–271.

Rogers LF. The roentgenographic appearance of transverse or Chance fractures of the spine: the seat belt fracture. *AJR Am J Roentgenol* 1971;111:844–849.

Rogers LF, Lee C. Cervical spine trauma. In: Dalinka MK, Kaye JJ, eds. *Radiology in emergency room medicine.* New York: Churchill Livingstone; 1984.

Scher AT. "Tear-drop" fractures of the cervical spine—radiologic features. *S Afr Med J* 1982;61:355–356.

Scher AT. Unilateral locked facet in cervical spine injuries. *AJR Am J Roentgenol* 1977;129:45–48.

Schneider RC, Livingston KE, Cave AJE, Hamilton G. "Hangman's fracture" of the cervical spine. *J Neurosurg* 1965;22:141–154.

Shipley JA, Beukes CA. The nature of the spondylolytic defect. Demonstration of a communicating synovial pseudoarthrosis in the pars interarticularis. *J Bone Joint Surg [Br]* 1998;80B:662—664.

Slone RM, MacMillan M, Montgomery WJ. Spinal fixation. Part 1. Principles, basic hardware, and fixation techniques for the cervical spine. *Radiographics* 1993;13:341—356.

Slone RM, MacMillan M, Montgomery WJ, Heare M. Spinal fixation. Part 2. Fixation techniques and hardware for the thoracic and lumbosacral spine. *Radiographics* 1993;13:521–543.

Smith GR, Northrop CH, Loop JW. Jumper's fractures: patterns of thoracolumbar spine injuries associated with vertical plunges. A review of 38 cases. *Radiology* 1977;122:657–663.

Spencer JA, Yeakley JW, Kaufman HH. Fracture of the occipitale condyle. *Neurosurgery* 1984;15:101–103.

Spengler DM. Lumbar disc herniation. In: Chapman MW, ed. *Operative orthopaedics,* vol. 4, 2nd ed. Philadelphia: JB Lippincott; 1993:2735–2744.

Taber KH, Herrick RC, Weathers SW, Kumar AJ, Schomer DF, Hayman LA. Pitfalls and artifacts encountered in clinical MR imaging of the spine. *Radiographics* 1998;18:1499–1521.

Tehranzadeh J. Discography 2000. *Radiol Clin North Am* 1998;36:463–495.

Thomas HM. Atlantoaxial injuries. *Semin Orthop* 1987;2:110–118.

Turetsky DB, Vines FS, Clayman DA, Northrup HM. Technique and use of supine oblique views in acute cervical spine trauma. *Ann Emerg Med* 1993;22:685–689.

Wiltse LL. Spondylolisthesis: classification and etiology. In: *AAOS Symposium on the Spine.* American Academy of Orthopedic Surgeons. St. Louis: Mosby; 1969:143–167.

Wiltse LL, Winter RB. Terminology and measurement of spondylolisthesis. *J Bone Joint Surg [Am]* 1983;65A:768–772.

Whitley JE, Forsyth HF. Classification of cervical spine injuries. *AJR Am J Roentgenol* 1958;83:633–644.

Wintermark M, Mouhsine E, Theumann N, Mordasini P, van Melle G, Leyvraz P, Schnyder P. Thoracolumbar spine fractures in patients who have sustained severe trauma: depiction with multi-detector row CT. *Radiology* 2003;227:681–689.

Woodring JF, Lee C. Limitations of cervical radiography in the evaluation of acute cervical trauma. *J Trauma* 1993;34:32–39.

Yu S, Sether IA, Ho PS, Wagner M, Haughton VM. Tears of the annulus fibrosus: correlation between MR and pathologic findings in cadavers. *AJNR* 1988;9:367–370.

Zanca P, Lodmell EA. Fracture of spinous processes: new sign for the recognition of fractures of cervical and upper dorsal spinous processes. *Radiology* 1951;56:427–429.

PART

III

ARTHRITIDES

RADIOLOGIC EVALUATION OF THE ARTHRITIDES

In its general meaning, the term *arthritis* indicates an abnormality of the joint as the result of a degenerative, inflammatory, infectious, or metabolic process (Fig. 12.1). Also included among the arthritides are connective tissue arthropathies, such as those associated with systemic lupus erythematosus (SLE) and scleroderma.

Radiologic Imaging Modalities

Conventional Radiography

The radiologic modalities used to evaluate arthritis are very similar to those used in traumatic conditions involving the bones and joints (see Chapter 4), although there are some modifications. The most important modality for the evaluation of arthritis is conventional radiography. As in the radiographic examination of traumatic conditions, standard films of the involved joint should be obtained in at least two projections at 90° to each other (Fig. 12.2; see also Fig. 4.1). A weight-bearing view may be of value, particularly for a dynamic evaluation of any decrement in the joint space under the weight of the body (Fig. 12.3). Special projections may at times be required to demonstrate destructive changes in the joint to better advantages.

The radial head–capitellum view (see Chapter 6), by eliminating overlap of the radial head and coronoid process and by more clearly demonstrating the humeroradial and humeroulnar joints, shows the inflammatory changes in the elbow joint to better advantage (Fig. 12.4). The semisupinated oblique view of the hand and wrist (the so-called Allstate or ball-catcher's view), introduced by Norgaard in 1965, effectively demonstrates the radial aspects of the metacarpal heads and of the base of the proximal phalanges in the hand and the triquetrum and pisiform in the wrist (Fig. 12.5). Because the earliest erosive changes of some inflammatory arthritides begin in these areas, the Norgaard view may provide important information at the early stages of arthritides (Fig. 12.6). It may also demonstrate subtle subluxations in metacarpophalangeal joints frequently seen in SLE.

Magnification Radiography

This technique is used to diagnose the very early articular changes of arthritis, which are not well appreciated on standard projections (Fig. 12.7). The method involves a special screen-film system and geometric enlargement that yields magnified images of the bones and joints with greater sharpness and bony detail.

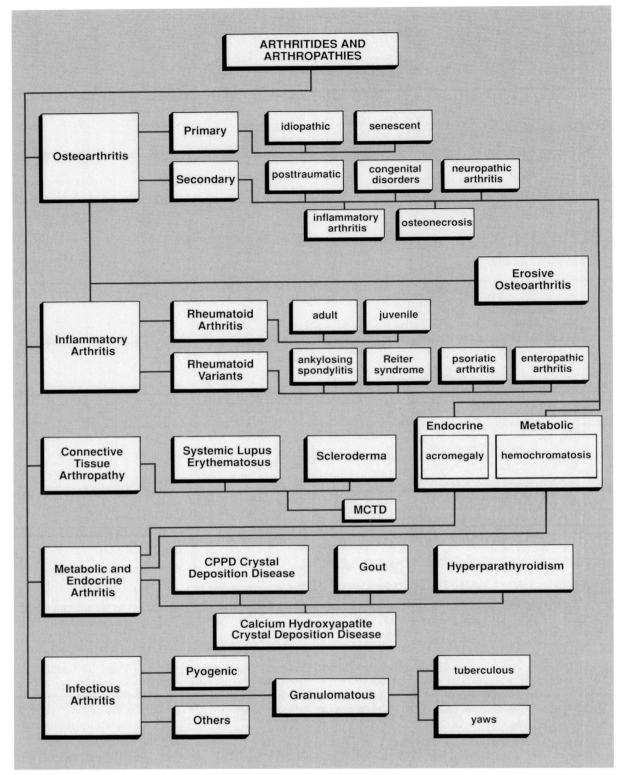

Figure 12.1 Classification of the arthritides.

Figure 12.2 Osteoarthritis. A 58-year-old woman presented with a history of pain in the left knee. **(A)** Anteroposterior radiograph demonstrates narrowing of the medial femorotibial joint compartment and marginal osteophytes arising from both the medial and lateral femoral condyles—findings typical of osteoarthritis (degenerative joint disease). **(B)** Lateral radiograph demonstrates, in addition, osteophytes at the anterior and posterior aspects of the articular end of the tibia, which are not appreciated on the anteroposterior projection. Involvement of the femoropatellar joint compartment and the presence of synovitis, represented by suprapatellar joint effusion, are also well demonstrated.

Figure 12.3 Osteoarthritis. Weight-bearing anteroposterior film of the left knee of the same patient shown in Figure 12.2 demonstrates collapse of the medial femorotibial compartment under the weight of the body, with a resulting varus configuration of the knee.

Figure 12.4 Rheumatoid arthritis. (A) Standard lateral view of the elbow of a 48-year-old woman with known rheumatoid arthritis of several years' duration shows destructive changes typical of inflammatory arthritis. **(B)** A special projection known as the radial head-capitellum view (see Fig. 6.12) demonstrates to better advantage the details of the arthritic process involving the humeroradial and humeroulnar joints. (From Greenspan A, Norman A, 1983 with permission.)

Figure 12.5 Ball-catcher's view. (A) For the "Allstate" Norgaard view of the hands and wrists, the patient's arm is fully extended and resting on its ulnar side. Fingers are extended. The hands are in slight pronation, as when catching a ball. The central beam is directed toward the metacarpal heads. **(B)** On the film in this projection, the radial aspects of the base of the proximal phalanges, the triquetrum, and pisiform bones are well demonstrated.

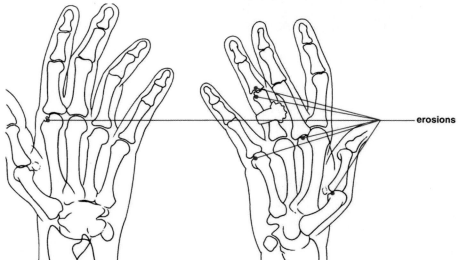

Figure 12.6 Rheumatoid arthritis. The "Allstate" view of the hands and the wrists of this 62-year-old woman with rheumatoid arthritis demonstrates erosions in the radiocarpal and intercarpal articulations as well as the carpometacarpal joint, bilaterally. Note, in addition, subtle erosions of the head of the first, third, fourth, and fifth metacarpals of the left hand and of the head of the second metacarpal of the right hand. A small erosion at the base of the middle phalanx of the ring finger of the left hand is also well seen.

periarticular soft
tissue swelling

juxtaarticular
osteoporosis

subtle erosions

Figure 12.7 Magnification radiography of early rheumatoid arthritis. Dorsovolar view of the fingers obtained with the magnification technique demonstrates the early changes of rheumatoid arthritis: juxta-articular osteoporosis, periarticular soft-tissue swelling representing intracapsular fluid, and subtle erosions at the bases of the proximal phalanges and heads of the metacarpals—a finding not appreciated on the standard radiographs of this patient.

Tomography, Computed Tomography, and Arthrography

Among the ancillary imaging techniques used to evaluate the arthritides, conventional tomography is rarely used for the purpose of making a specific diagnosis, its major purpose being demonstration to better advantage of the degree of joint destruction (Fig. 12.8). Computed tomography (CT) is effective in evaluating degenerative and inflammatory changes of various joints (Fig. 12.9A-C), and in the spine to document spinal stenosis (Fig. 12.9D). In the assessment of spinal stenosis secondary to degenerative changes, CT examination may also be performed after myelography (Fig. 12.10), although myelography

Figure 12.8 Tomography of secondary osteoarthritis in Paget disease. A 74-year-old woman with Paget disease and secondary degenerative changes in the hip joint was evaluated for a possible total hip arthroplasty. **(A)** Standard anteroposterior view of the right hip shows extensive Paget disease evident in the thickening of the cortex of the pelvic bones, particularly the ischium, and a coarse trabecular pattern. Note the narrowing of the radiographic joint space indicative of osteoarthritis of the hip joint. Conventional tomograms show predominant involvement of the acetabulum **(B)** with preservation of the femoral head **(C)**.

Figure 12.9 Evaluation of arthritides with CT. (A) Axial CT section through the hip joints of a 55-year-old man with hip osteoarthritis shows narrowing of the joint spaces, subchondral sclerosis, and osteophytes (*arrows*). The intraarticular osteochondral body (*open arrow*) was not clearly demonstrated on conventional radiographs. **(B)** Axial CT section through the sacroiliac joints of a 49-year-old man with psoriatic arthritis show diffuse narrowing of the joints and articular erosions (*arrows*). **(C)** Coronal CT section through the ankle and foot of a 52-year-old woman with rheumatoid arthritis shows erosions of the tibiotalar and subtalar joints. **(D)** CT scan of the lumbar spine in a 66-year-old patient with advanced osteoarthritis of the facet joints shows marked narrowing of the spinal canal secondary to degenerative changes. At 8 mm, the transverse diameter is well below normal.

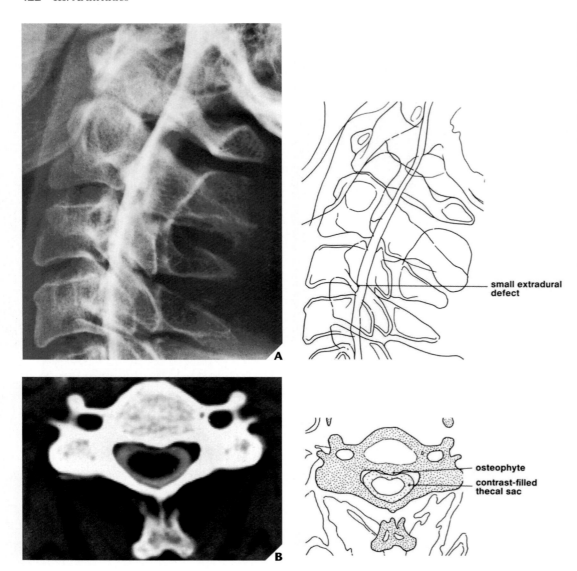

Figure 12.10 CT-myelography of impingement of the thecal sac. A 56-year-old man reported constant pain in the neck radiating to the left arm; there was also associated weakness and numbness in the left hand. **(A)** Cervical myelogram in the lateral projection shows a small extradural defect on the ventral aspect of the thecal sac at C3-4. **(B)** CT section obtained after myelography shows impingement of a posterior osteophyte on the thecal sac at the corresponding level.

alone is often sufficient (Fig. 12.11). Arthrography has some limited application in the evaluation of degenerative (Fig. 12.12), inflammatory, and infectious (see Fig. 25.16B) conditions of the joint.

Scintigraphy

Radionuclide bone scan is much more commonly used than these other techniques, mainly for evaluating the distribution of arthritis in different joints (see Chapter 2). The radiopharmaceuticals currently in use in bone scan include organic diphosphonates—ethylene diphosphonate (HEPD) and methylene diphosphonate (MDP)—labeled with technetium (Tc) 99m, a gamma emitter with a 6-hour half-life; MDP is more commonly used, typically in a dose that provides 15 mCi (555 MBq) of ^{99m}Tc. After intravenous injection of the radiopharmaceutical, approximately 50% of the dose localizes in bone, with the remainder circulating freely in the body and eventually excreted by the kidneys. A gamma camera can then be used in a procedure known as a three-phase radionuclide bone scan. Scintigraphy can determine the distribution of arthritic changes in large and small joints (Fig. 12.13). It can also distinguish an infected joint from infected periarticular soft tissues (see Fig. 24.9). To distinguish infectious arthritis from other forms of arthritides, indium (In) 111-labeled leukocytes and gallium (Ga) 57 scans have recently been used (see Chapter 2, section on Scintigraphy).

Serial examinations with bone scintigraphy, as Brower and Flem-

ming have pointed out, have also been helpful in evaluating the activity of given arthritis at a particular point in time. Such examinations may differentiate active disease from arthritis in remission.

Ultrasound

Ultrasound is rarely used in evaluation of joint abnormalities. Occasionally, it helps to differentiate popliteal fossa masses in patients with rheumatoid arthritis, in whom complications of an arthritic process (such as popliteal cyst or hypertrophied synovium) may be distinguished from conditions not related to arthritis (such as popliteal artery aneurysm). It may also effectively diagnose deep vein thrombosis, occasionally seen in patients with rheumatoid arthritis.

Magnetic Resonance Imaging

Magnetic resonance imaging (MRI) of the joints provides excellent contrast between soft tissues and bone. Articular cartilage, fibrocartilage, cortex, and spongy bone can be distinguished from each other by their specific signal intensities. It is an excellent modality for demonstrating the rheumatoid nodules and synovial abnormalities in patients with rheumatoid arthritis. MRI's ability to contrast the synovium-covered joint from other soft-tissue structures allows for noninvasive delineation of the degree of synovial hypertrophy that accompanies synovitis, previously demonstrable only by means

intact articular
cartilage

loss of articular
cartilage

Figure 12.11 Myelography of spinal stenosis. Lateral radiograph of the lumbosacral spine obtained after injection of metrizamide into the subarachnoid space shows an "hourglass" configuration of the contrast medium in the thecal sac, a feature characteristic of spinal stenosis. This appearance results from concomitant hypertrophy of the facet joints and posterior bulging of the intervertebral disks.

Figure 12.12 Arthrography of osteoarthritis. Double-contrast arthrogram in a 62-year-old man with progressive pain localized to the medial femorotibial joint compartment demonstrates destruction of the articular cartilage, consistent with osteoarthritis.

Figure 12.13 Scintigraphy of psoriatic arthritis. Radionuclide bone scan **(A)** obtained 2 hours after the intravenous injection of 15 mCi (555 MBq) of technetium 99m-labeled methylene diphosphonate shows an increased uptake of radiopharmaceutical in several joints of the hand and wrist. A conventional radiograph **(B)** of the same patient shows advanced psoriatic arthritis.

Figure 12.14 MRI of rheumatoid arthritis. Conventional radiograph was normal in this patient with known rheumatoid arthritis of the wrist. MRI in the coronal plane using **(A)** spin-echo sequence and **(B)** gradient echo technique demonstrates marginal scaphoid erosions with adjacent fluid and inflammatory panus. Inflammatory fluid is also seen in the radioulnar, midcarpal, radiocarpal, and carpometacarpal joints.

of arthrography or arthroscopy. Because synovitis is often accompanied by joint effusion, this too can be effectively demonstrated by MRI (Fig. 12.14). Joint fluid normally gives an intermediate signal intensity on T1-weighted images and a high signal intensity on T2-weighted images. This has proved to be helpful in diagnosing Baker cysts (Fig. 12.15). Although MRI is quite sensitive in detecting joint effusion, it cannot yet distinguish between inflammatory and noninflammatory fluid. Occasionally, MRI may provide some additional information in osteoarthritis (Fig. 12.16) and hemophilic arthropathy (Fig. 12.17). With the development of more sophisticated orthopedic methods for cartilage repair in osteoarthritis, such as new articular cartilage replacement techniques, including chondrocyte transplantation, osteochondral transplantation, and cartilage growth-stimulating factors, optimized MR imaging of these interventions for diagnosis and treatment planning in osteoarthritis is essential.

The most promising role of MRI, however, is in the evaluation of the spine. MR images in the sagittal plane are useful for demonstrating hypertrophy of the ligamentum flavum or the vertebral facets, grading the degree of foramina stenosis, and measuring the sagittal diameter of the spinal cord. MR images in the axial plane facilitate detailed analysis of the facet joints and more accurate measurement of the thickness of the ligamentum flavum and the diameter of the spinal canal. The quality of evaluation of spinal cord abnormalities by MRI in the cervical area in patients with rheumatoid arthritis and of spinal stenosis in patients with advanced degenerative changes of the spine surpasses that obtained with other modalities. MRI is particularly useful in examination of patients with pain related to disk disease because it can differentiate normal, degenerated, and herniated disks noninvasively (see Chapter 11). In fact, the changes of disk degeneration can be identified by MRI long before they can be detected by conventional radiography or CT.

Figure 12.15 MRI of the Baker cyst. A 68-year-old woman with rheumatoid arthritis reported pain in the region of the popliteal fossa. The presumptive diagnosis of thrombophlebitis was made. **(A)** Sagittal MRI (SE; TR 900/TE 20 msec) demonstrates an oval structure in the popliteal fossa displaying intermediate signal intensity. Also note a small subchondral erosion of the anterior aspect of the medial femoral condyle. **(B)** Coronal MRI (SE; TR 1800/TE 80 msec) at the level of the popliteal fossa demonstrates a large Baker cyst that displays a high signal intensity caused by fluid content.

Figure 12.16 MRI of osteoarthritis. (A) Sagittal proton density MRI of a 62-year-old woman with osteoarthritis of the right knee shows involvement of the femoropatellar compartment. Note joint space narrowing, subchondral cyst (*arrow*), and osteophytes (*open arrows*). **(B)** Coronal T2-weighted fat-suppressed MR image shows complete destruction of articular cartilage of the lateral joint compartment (*arrows*), subchondral edema (*open arrows*), and tear of the lateral meniscus (*curved arrow*). **(C)** Sagittal T2-weighted fat-suppressed MRI in another patient shows osteoarthritis of the knee complicated by multiple osteochondral bodies (*arrows*).

Figure 12.17 MRI of hemophilic arthropathy. A 29-year-old man with hemophilia and multiple episodes of intraarticular bleeding. **(A)**, **(B)** Anteroposterior and lateral radiographs of the knee demonstrate an advanced stage of hemophilia. Abnormalities include periarticular osteoporosis, irregularity of subchondral bone at the tibial plateau and femoral condyles, narrowing of the radiographic joint space, and erosion of the subchondral bone. **(C)** Coronal MRI (SE; TR 1900/TE 20 msec) demonstrates, in addition, complete destruction of articular cartilage at the medial joint compartment, and a large, subchondral cyst in the proximal tibia, not well appreciated on the radiographic films. **(D)** Sagittal MRI (SE; TR 800/TE 20 msec) demonstrates to better advantage the intraarticular blood in the suprapatellar and infrapatellar bursae, displaying intermediate signal intensity. **(E)** Axial MRI (TR 400/TE 20 msec) shows erosive changes of the articular cartilage of the femoral condyles.

The Arthritides

Diagnosis

Clinical Information

The clinical manifestations and laboratory data, in conjunction with the radiographic findings, are of significant help in making the diagnosis of a specific arthritic process. The various arthritides, for example, have different frequencies of occurrence between the sexes. Rheumatoid arthritis is much more common in females, and erosive osteoarthritis is seen almost exclusively in middle-aged women. Psoriatic arthritis, Reiter syndrome, and gouty arthritis, however, are more common in males. Clinical symptoms are of further assistance. Patients with Reiter syndrome, for example, usually present with urethritis, conjunctivitis, and mucocutaneous lesions, and those with psoriatic arthritis may present with swelling of a single finger, the so-called sausage digit, as well as changes in the skin and fingernails. Patients with gouty arthritis may exhibit soft-tissue masses, representing chronic tophi, on the dorsal aspect of the hands or feet.

Laboratory data are also essential. Gouty arthritis, for instance, is associated with elevated serum uric acid concentrations, and a synovial fluid examination reveals monosodium urate crystals in leukocytes in the fluid. The synovial fluid of patients with pseudogout, however, contains calcium pyrophosphate crystals. The detection of autoantibodies is another important aid in the diagnostic work-up. Rheumatoid factor (RF) is a typical finding in rheumatoid arthritis. Patients lacking the specific antibodies represented by RF are said to have "seronegative" arthritis. Patients with lupus arthritis have a positive lupus erythematosus cell test. Lastly, identification of the antigens of the major histocompatibility complex, particularly human leukocyte-associated antigens HLA-B27 and HLA-DR4, has in recent years become a crucial test in the diagnosis of arthritic disease. It has been reported that 95% of patients with ankylosing spondylitis, 86% of patients with Reiter syndrome, and 60% of patients with psoriatic arthropathy test positively for antigen HLA-B27, whereas a majority of those with rheumatoid arthritis exhibit the HLA-DR4 antigen. This is helpful in differentiating certain types of arthritides, as well as distinguishing psoriatic arthritis from rheumatoid arthritis in cases in which the radiographic presentation of these conditions may be very similar.

Figure 12.18 The constituent structures of a true or diarthrodial joint.

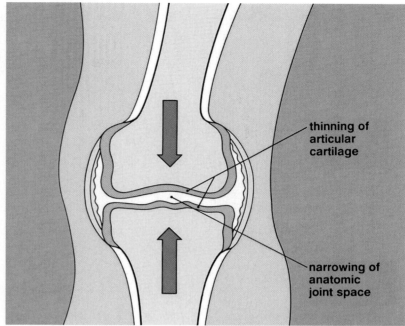

Figure 12.19 Narrowing of the joint space. The cardinal sign of an arthritic process is narrowing of the radiographic joint space. Thinning of the articular cartilage reduces the space mechanically.

Radiographic Features

The true or diarthrodial joint consists of cartilage covering the articular ends of the bones forming the joint; the articular capsule, which is reinforced by ligamentous structures; and the joint space, which is lined with synovial membrane and filled with synovial fluid (Fig. 12.18). Because of its physicochemical constitution, articular cartilage absorbs only a minimal amount of x-rays, thus appearing radiolucent on a radiographic film. The radiolucent articular cartilage, together with the joint cavity filled with synovial fluid, creates the so-called radiographic joint space.

The abnormality of the joint in arthritis usually consists of destruction of the articular cartilage, which appears on a film as a narrowing of the radiographic joint space, usually accompanied by subchondral erosion; narrowing of the joint is the cardinal sign of arthritis (Fig. 12.19). It should be kept in mind, however, that in some

arthritic processes the joint space may not become narrow, appearing instead slightly expanded. This happens, for example, in the early stages of some arthritides, when joint effusion and ligamentous laxity cause distention of the joint with fluid, but the articular cartilage has not yet been destroyed. It may also be seen in rare instances when granulation pannus erodes the subchondral bone without destroying the articular cartilage (Fig. 12.20).

Other radiographic signs specific to different types of arthritis include periarticular soft-tissue swelling, periarticular osteoporosis, and, in the more advanced stages of some arthritides, complete destruction of the joint with subluxation or dislocation and ankylosis (joint fusion) (Fig. 12.21).

The radiographic presentation of arthritis depends on the type and stage of the disease, as well as the site of the original insult characteristic for the various forms of arthritis (Fig. 12.22)—whether it is

Figure 12.20 Variations in the width of the joint space. In the early stage of some arthritides, widening rather than narrowing of the joint space may be seen radiographically. This may be caused by distention of the joint with fluid **(A)** or erosion of the subchondral bone by granulation pannus with some preservation of the articular cartilage **(B)**.

Figure 12.21 **Radiographic features of arthritides.** Summary representation of radiographic features seen in the arthritides. Not all of these features are seen in every type of arthritis.

Figure 12.22 **Target sites of various arthritides in a joint.**

the articular cartilage, as in osteoarthritis (see Figs. 12.2 and 12.26); the synovial membrane, as in inflammatory arthritis (Fig. 12.23A); the synovial membrane, subchondral bone, and periarticular soft tissues, as in infectious arthritis (see Fig. 25.15); or the synovial membrane, articular cartilage, subchondral bone, and periarticular soft tissues as in some metabolic arthritides (Fig. 12.23B,C).

The radiographic diagnosis of arthritis, as Resnick observed, is based on the evaluation of two fundamental parameters: the *morphology* of the articular lesion and its *distribution* in the skeleton. If these findings are combined with the history, physical examination, and relevant laboratory data in a given case, then the accuracy of the diagnosis is markedly improved.

Morphology of the Articular Lesion. The various arthritides exhibit morphologically distinct features, as observed radiographically

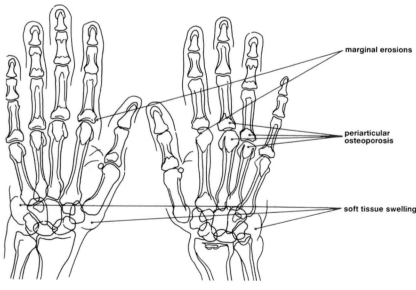

Figure 12.23 **Radiographic features of various arthritides. (A)** Early changes of rheumatoid arthritis, as seen in the hands of a 40-year-old woman, present as marginal erosions in so-called bare areas at the locus of attachment of the capsular synovial lining. Also note the periarticular osteoporosis and soft-tissue swelling, particularly in both wrists. **(B)** The asymmetric marginal erosions affecting various articulations in the hand of a 38-year-old man with tophaceous gout are characteristic of a metabolic process involving the subchondral bone. Note the preservation of part of the joint and the location of several erosions at some distance from the joint space. **(C)** In calcium pyrophosphate dihydrate (CPPD) crystal deposition arthropathy, seen here in the knee of a 70-year-old woman, there is calcification of the fibrocartilage (semilunar cartilage or menisci) and hyaline cartilage (articular cartilage) in association with narrowing of the medial femorotibial joint compartment. Aspirated fluid from the knee joint yielded CPPD crystals.

Figure 12.23 Radiographic features of various arthritides. *Continued.*

in the large (Fig. 12.24) and small (Fig. 12.25) joints. In the degenerative form of the disease known as osteoarthritis, thinning of the articular cartilage results in localized narrowing of the joint space; there is also subchondral sclerosis and osteophyte and cyst formation, but generally osteoporosis is absent (Fig. 12.26). Inflammatory arthritides, such as rheumatoid arthritis, are characterized by a diffuse, usually multi-compartmental narrowing of the joint space associated with marginal or central erosions, periarticular osteoporosis, and symmetric periarticular soft-tissue swelling; subchondral sclerosis is minimal or absent, and formation of osteophytes is lacking (Fig. 12.27). In a metabolic arthritis such as gout, well-defined bony erosions displaying a so-called overhanging edge are usually associated with preservation of part of the joint space and a localized, asymmetric soft-tissue mass; osteophyte formation and osteoporosis are absent (Fig. 12.28).

RADIOGRAPHIC MORPHOLOGY OF ARTHRITIDES IN A LARGE JOINT

Osteoarthritis

1 localized joint-space narrowing

2 subchondral sclerosis

3 osteophytes

4 cyst or pseudocyst

Inflammatory Arthritis (Rheumatoid Arthritis)

1 diffuse joint-space narrowing

2 marginal or central erosions

3 absent or minimal subchondral sclerosis

4 lack of osteophytes

5 cystic lesions

6 osteoporosis

7 periarticular soft tissue swelling (symmetric, usually fusiform)

Metabolic Arthritis (Gout)

1 marginal erosion with overhanging edge

2 partial preservation of joint space

3 lack of osteoporosis

4 lobulated, asymmetric soft tissue mass

Infectious Arthritis

1 destruction of joint space

2 joint effusion

3 soft tissue swelling

4 osteoporosis

Neuropathic Joint

1 destruction of joint with gross disorganization

2 bony debris

3 joint instability

4 joint effusion

5 (usual) lack of osteoporosis

Figure 12.24 Morphologic features distinguishing the various arthritides in a large joint.

RADIOGRAPHIC MORPHOLOGY OF ARTHRITIDES IN THE HAND

Osteoarthritis

1 Heberden nodes
2 Bouchard nodes
3 joint space narrowing
4 subchondral sclerosis

Erosive Osteoarthritis

1 gull-wing erosion
2 Heberden nodes (occasionally)
3 interphalangeal ankylosis

Rheumatoid Arthritis

1 periarticular osteoporosis
2 joint space narrowing
3 marginal erosions
4 boutonniére deformity
5 swan-neck deformity
6 subluxations and dislocations
7 soft tissue swelling (symmetric, fusiform)

Gouty Arthritis

1 asymmetric erosion with
   overhanging edge
2 partial preservation of joint space
3 asymmetric soft tissue swelling with
   or without calcifications (tophus)
   (usually at dorsal aspect)

Psoriatic Arthritis

1 joint space narrowing
2 fluffy periostitis
3 "sausage digit" (soft tissue
   swelling of single digit)
4 erosion of terminal tufts
5 "mouse-ear" type of articular erosion
6 interphalangeal ankylosis
7 soft tissue swelling

Lupus Arthritis

1 hitchhiker's thumb deformity
2 flexible deformities
   (subluxations)

Figure 12.25 Morphologic features distinguishing the various arthritides in the small joints of the hand.

Figure 12.26 Osteoarthritis. Conventional radiograph of the hip demonstrates the typical morphologic changes seen in degenerative joint disease (osteoarthritis): focal narrowing of the joint space (here at the weight-bearing segment), subchondral sclerosis, cyst-like lesions, and marginal osteophytes. Note the lack of osteoporosis.

Infectious arthritis is characterized by the complete destruction of both articular ends of the bones forming the joint; all communicating joint compartments are invariably involved, with diffuse osteoporosis, joint effusion, and periarticular soft-tissue swelling (see Fig. 25.16A). Neuropathic arthritis is marked by destruction of the articular surfaces, which leaves bony debris, and a substantial joint effusion; osteoporosis is usually lacking. Depending on the amount of destruction, varying degrees of joint instability are present (Fig. 12.29).

Analysis of the morphologic features of an arthritic lesion at certain sites other than the diarthrodial joints may be of further assistance in differentiating the various arthritides and reaching a correct diagnosis. Two such sites that are frequently affected are the heel (Fig. 12.30) and the spine (see Fig. 12.32). In the heel, degenerative changes are usually manifested by a traction osteophyte at the posterior and plantar aspects of the os calcis (Fig. 12.31A). Rheumatoid

Figure 12.27 Rheumatoid arthritis. Inflammatory arthritis, seen here in the hip, is marked by diffuse, uniform narrowing of the joint space, axial migration of the femoral head, marginal and central subchondral erosions, and severe periarticular osteoporosis. Note the almost total absence of reactive subchondral sclerosis and the lack of osteophyte formation.

Figure 12.28 Gouty arthritis. Asymmetric periarticular erosions that spare part of the joint are typical of gouty arthritis, seen here involving the first metatarsophalangeal joint of the right foot. Note the characteristic overhanging edge at the site of erosion and the soft-tissue mass representing a tophus; osteophytes and osteoporosis are absent, and the joint is partially preserved.

Figure 12.29 Neuropathic joint. The neuropathic joint is morphologically identified by gross articular disorganization, multiple bony debris, and joint effusion, as seen here in the knee. Note the lack of osteoporosis. The amount of destruction evident in this case results in severe joint instability.

RADIOGRAPHIC MORPHOLOGY OF ARTHRITIDES IN THE HEEL

Degenerative Arthritis

Rheumatoid Arthritis

Psoriatic Arthritis, Ankylosing Spondylitis, and Reiter Syndrome

traction osteophytes at
1 posterior aspect of os calcis (insertion of Achilles tendon) and
2 plantar aspect of os calcis (insertion of fascia plantaris)
3 osteophytes at the posterior facet of subtalar joint

1 erosion at posterosuperior aspect of os calcis (secondary to retrocalcaneal bursitis)
2 thickening of Achilles tendon
3 focal osteoporosis

1 fluffy periostitis
2 erosions at posterior aspect of os calcis above attachment of Achilles tendon, at attachment of plantar fascia, and at plantar surface of os calcis anterior to aponeurotic attachment
3 broad-based osteophyte

Figure 12.30 Arthritic changes in the heel. Morphologic features distinguishing the various arthritides as manifest in arthritic lesions at the heel.

Figure 12.31 Arthritic changes in the heel. The morphology of arthritic lesions in the heel can be helpful in differentiating the various arthritides. **(A)** In the degenerative variant, traction osteophytes are evident at the insertions of the Achilles tendon and fascia plantaris on the posterior and plantar aspects of the os calcis. **(B)** Rheumatoid arthritis typically exhibits retrocalcaneal bursitis and erosion of the posterosuperior aspect of the os calcis at the site of the bursa. Note the fluid-filled retrocalcaneal bursa projecting into the triangular-shaped fat pad anterior to the Achilles tendon. **(C)** The calcaneus in psoriatic arthritis characteristically shows a coarse, broad-based osteophyte arising from the plantar aspect of the bone at the insertion of the fascia plantaris. Note the "fluffy" outline and bone proliferation along the plantar aspect of the os calcis. **(D)** In this case of Reiter syndrome, there is erosion of the posterior aspect of the os calcis, bone sclerosis, and a "fluffy" periostitis along its plantar aspect.

arthritis produces erosive changes in the area of the retrocalcaneal bursa secondary to inflammatory rheumatoid bursitis (Fig. 12.31B). Psoriatic arthritis (Fig. 12.31C), Reiter syndrome (Fig. 12.31D), and ankylosing spondylitis all produce a characteristic "fluffy" periostitis that results in a broad-based osteophyte at the site of attachment of the fascia plantaris on the plantar aspect of the os calcis, associated with erosions of the plantar surface and the posterior aspect of the calcaneus.

Similarly, the morphology of arthritic lesions in the spine offers important indications of the disease process at work (Fig. 12.32).

Among the inflammatory arthritides, for instance, rheumatoid arthritis causes a characteristic erosion of the odontoid process (Fig. 12.33). Moreover, as a result of inflammatory pannus and erosion of the transverse ligament between the anterior arch of the atlas and C-2, there may be subluxation in the atlantoaxial joint. This is usually manifested by an increase to more than 3 mm in the distance between the arch of the atlas and the dens, as demonstrated on a lateral view of the cervical spine in flexion (Fig. 12.34). Erosion of the apophyseal joints of the cervical spine, sometimes leading to fusion, is frequently seen in juvenile rheumatoid arthritis (Fig. 12.35).

RADIOGRAPHIC MORPHOLOGY OF ARTHRITIDES IN THE SPINE

Rheumatoid Arthritis

1 erosion of anterior aspect of odontoid
2 atlantoaxial subluxation with cephalad migration of C-2
3 erosion and fusion of apophyseal joints

4 erosion and whittling of spinous processes
5 destruction of intervertebral disks
6 erosion of vertebral bodies

Degenerative Spine Disease

1 disk-space narrowing
2 osteophytes
3 stenosis of the neural foramina

4 facet narrowing and eburnation
5 stenosis of the spinal canal

Ankylosing Spondylitis

1 squaring of vertebral bodies
2 thin syndesmophytes
3 preservation of disk space

4 fusion of apophyseal joints
5 ossifications of paravertebral ligaments
6 "bamboo" spine

Psoriatic Arthritis and Reiter Syndrome

1 single broad-based, coarse syndesmophyte
2 paraspinal ossifications

Figure 12.32 Arthritides of the spine. Morphologic features distinguishing the various arthritides as manifested in the spine.

Figure 12.33 Rheumatoid arthritis. Antero-posterior **(A)** and lateral **(B)** trispiral tomograms of the cervical spine in a 55-year-old woman with a 15-year history of rheumatoid arthritis show erosion of the odontoid process typical for this condition.

increased
distance
between
anterior
arch of atlas
and odontoid

Figure 12.34 Rheumatoid arthritis. (A) Lateral film of the cervical spine in flexion in a 68-year-old woman with a long history of rheumatoid arthritis shows a marked increase in the distance between the anterior arch of the atlas and the odontoid process, measuring 12 mm; normally, it should not exceed 3 mm. **(B)** Trispiral tomogram demonstrates the atlantoaxial subluxation in detail.

Figure 12.35 Juvenile rheumatoid arthritis. Lateral view of the cervical spine in a 34-year-old woman with juvenile rheumatoid arthritis since age 20 shows the typical involvement of the apophyseal joints. In this case, there is complete fusion of the joints.

Arthritic lesions involving other segments of the spine also exhibit distinguishing features that help in differentiating the disease process. Degenerative changes may manifest in the cervical, thoracic, or lumbar (Fig. 12.36) spine by the appearance of marginal osteophytes, narrowing and sclerosis of the apophyseal joints, and narrowing of the disk spaces. In ankylosing spondylitis, there is a characteristic "squaring" of the vertebral bodies, with the formation of delicate syndesmophytes, which differ morphologically from degenerative osteophytes, arising from the anterior aspects of the vertebral bodies. In the later stages of this condition, inflammation and fusion of the apophyseal joints lead to the appearance of what has been called "bamboo" spine; the sacroiliac joints are also invariably affected (Fig. 12.37). In psoriasis and Reiter syndrome, one can occasionally see a single, coarse osteophyte in the lumbar spine, frequently bridging adjacent vertebral bodies, as well as paravertebral ossifications; there are also associated inflammatory changes in the sacroiliac joints (Fig. 12.38).

Distribution of the Articular Lesion. Osteoarthritis tends to have a characteristic distribution in the skeletal system. Typically, the large joints such as the hip and knee and the small joints of the hand and wrist are involved, whereas the shoulder, elbow, and ankle are spared (Fig. 12.39). Inflammatory arthritides, however, have different sites of predilection in the skeleton, depending on the specific variant of the disease. Rheumatoid arthritis, for example, involves most of the large joints such as the hip, knee, elbows, and shoulders. In the hand, it has a characteristic distribution that spares the distal interphalangeal joints (see Fig. 12.39); in the cervical spine, the C1-2 articulation and the apophyseal joints are frequently affected. Juvenile rheumatoid arthritis has a similar pattern of distribution, except that the distal interphalangeal joints of the hand may also be affected. Psoriatic arthritis, in contrast to rheumatoid arthritis, has a predilection for the distal interphalangeal joints, as well as the sacroiliac joints, resembling Reiter syndrome in this respect (see Fig. 12.39). Erosive osteoarthritis, which some investiga-

tors consider a variant of osteoarthritis, others a variant of rheumatoid arthritis, and still others a distinct form of arthritis, has a tendency to affect the proximal and distal interphalangeal joints of the hand (see Fig. 12.25).

Management

Monitoring the Results of Treatment

Similar modalities are used for monitoring the results of medical and surgical treatment of arthritis. Because the most effective treatment, particularly when large joints are involved, entails corrective and reconstructive procedures such as femoral or tibial osteotomy or total joint replacement of the hip or knee, the surgeon follows the postsurgical progress of the patient with sequential radiographic examinations. In osteoarthritis of the hip, the corrective procedures most often performed are varus or valgus osteotomies of the proximal femur to improve the congruence of the articular surfaces and redistribute the stress forces over different areas of the joint. Similarly, a high tibial osteotomy is performed to correct severe varus or valgus deformities in osteoarthritis of the knee, particularly in cases of unicompartmental involvement. The radiographic techniques used in monitoring the outcome of these procedures, which in fact represent iatrogenic surgical fractures, are similar to those used in evaluating traumatic fractures. As in traumatic fractures, the radiologist also pays attention to similar features, such as bone union, nonunion, or delayed union (see Chapter 4). In patients in whom total hip arthroplasties are performed, radiographic scrutiny is also essential. At present, three basic types of hip arthroplasty are used in orthopedic practice: unipolar hip hemiarthroplasty, bipolar hip hemiarthroplasty, and total hip arthroplasty. The first two of these are used mainly for patients with fracture of the femoral head and neck, and those with advanced femoral head osteonecrosis. Total hip arthro-

Figure 12.36 Degenerative spine disease. Oblique view of the lumbar spine in a 72-year-old woman shows narrowing and eburnation of the articular margins of the facet joints, osteophytosis, and narrowing of the intervertebral disk spaces—a combination of the effects of true facet joint arthritis, spondylosis deformans, and degenerative disk disease.

Figure 12.37 Ankylosing spondylitis. Anteroposterior **(A)** and lateral **(B)** radiographs of the lumbar spine in a 31-year-old man with advanced ankylosing spondylitis demonstrate the typical appearance of "bamboo spine" secondary to inflammation, ossification, and fusion of the apophyseal joints associated with ossification of the anterior and posterior longitudinal ligaments, as well as the supraspinous and interspinous ligaments. Note also the fusion of the sacroiliac joints.

Figure 12.38 Reiter syndrome. Lateral radiograph **(A)** of the lumbar spine in a 27-year-old man with Reiter syndrome shows a single, coarse osteophyte bridging the bodies of L-1 and L-2. Anteroposterior radiograph **(B)** of the lumbosacral segment shows the effects of the inflammatory process on the sacroiliac joints.

Figure 12.39 Distribution of arthritic lesions in the skeleton in various arthritides.

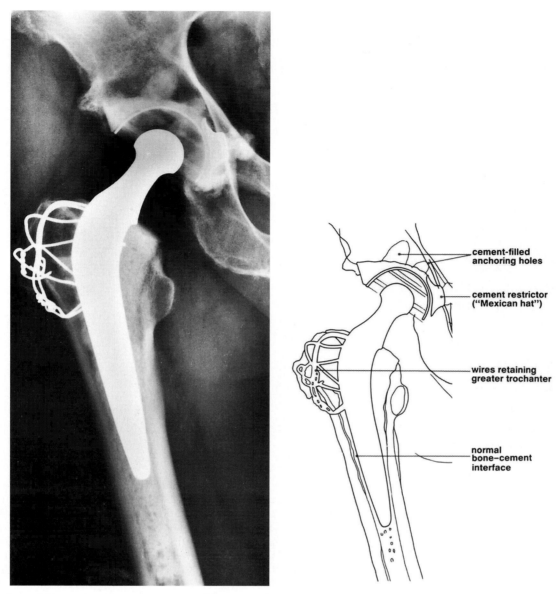

Figure 12.40 Cemented total hip arthroplasty. A 69-year-old man underwent total hip replacement because of advanced degenerative joint disease; a Charnley low-friction arthroplasty was performed. On the anteroposterior radiograph of the right hip, one can evaluate all the parts of the prosthesis. Note that the acetabular component is oriented approximately 45° to the horizontal plane and is cemented to the bone with methylmethacrylate previously impregnated with barium sulfate to make it visible radiographically. A wire-mesh cement restrictor ("Mexican hat") prevents significant leakage of methylmethacrylate into the pelvis. The stem of the prosthesis is in the neutral position in the medullary canal of the femur. Note the extent of cement below the distal end of the prosthesis, for secure anchoring. The greater trochanter, which was osteotomized to facilitate exposure of the joint, has been reattached by metallic wires slightly distal and lateral for improved stability. Note the normal appearance of the bone–cement interface.

plasty is commonly used in patients with advanced arthritis of the hip joint. The prosthetic components are usually cemented to the bone with methylmethacrylate, although cementless fixation is now gaining popularity. The latter technique is based on the use of a rough or porous surface on the prosthetic parts that enables ingrowth of the bone. A bioactive coating (i.e., hydroxyapatite) can also be used for the same purpose. Acetabular components usually have a porous coating over the entire surface of the cup, whereas femoral components can be either partially or fully coated. Cementless acetabular components are sometimes reinforced with screws. Occasionally, so-called hybrid arthroplasties are performed with cementless acetabular and cemented femoral components. After total hip replacement using cemented components it is important to evaluate the position of the prosthesis, with particular reference to the degree of inclina-

tion of the acetabular component, the position of the stem of the prosthesis (whether it is in valgus, varus, or the neutral position), and the status of the separated and rejoined greater trochanter, among other features (Fig. 12.40). Equally important is evaluation of cement-bone interface to detect the radiolucent area suggestive of prosthesis loosening (see Fig. 12.43). After total hip arthroplasty using noncemented components (Fig. 12.41), radiologic evaluation should focus on the interface between the prosthesis and bone to detect areas of bone resorption (focal osteolysis) that may indicate loosening of the prosthesis. After a total knee arthroplasty with a condylar type of prothesis, it is important to evaluate the position of the tibial component relative to the tibial shaft, as well as the axial alignment and the status of the methylmethacrylate fixation of the components (Fig. 12.42).

Figure 12.41 **Cementless total hip arthroplasty.** A 48-year-old woman underwent total hip arthroplasty because of advanced osteoarthritis. Note porous-coated acetabular component and partially coated femoral stem. The prosthetic components are in anatomic alignment, the femoral stem is in neutral position, the endocortex is intact, and there are no signs of loosening.

Complications of Surgical Treatment

As important as evaluating the outcome of the surgical treatment of arthritic disease is monitoring the complications that may arise from such treatment, especially those after osteotomies and joint-replacement procedures. These complications include thrombophlebitis, hematomas, heterotopic bone formation, the intrapelvic leakage of acrylic cement, infection, loosening, subluxation or dislocation of a prosthesis, and fracture of a prosthesis.

Thrombophlebitis. A rather frequent complication in the immediate postoperative period, particularly in patients with previous circulatory problems, thrombophlebitis is related to venous stasis and the lack of movement of the surgically treated extremity; sudden pain and swelling of the leg are common clinical findings. The venous soleal plexus in the calf is the most common site of thrombus formation. Radiologically, this complication can be detected by venography, radionuclide scanning, or ultrasound. On radionuclide

Figure 12.42 **Cemented total knee arthroplasty.** A 62-year-old woman underwent total knee arthroplasty using a nonconstrained three-part cemented condylar prosthesis. **(A)** Anteroposterior radiograph demonstrates that the tibial component is aligned with the surface of the bone, forming a 90° angle with the long axis of the tibia. There is no evidence of a radiolucent line at the cement–bone interface. The slight valgus configuration at the knee (approximately 7°) is acceptable. On the lateral projection **(B)**, note the tight adherence of the femoral component of the prosthesis to the bone.

scan, an increased gamma-count rate in an area of the lower extremities following intravenous administration of ^{125}I-labeled fibrinogen suggests adherence of the tracer to a developing clot. Ultrasound can detect venous thrombosis using compression technique. Lack of compressibility of a vein is thought to be the single most reliable finding in differentiating between thrombosed and normal veins. Other criteria useful in detection of vein thrombosis are the presence of echogenic intraluminal material and enlargement of the vein.

Hematoma. The formation of a hematoma is a common complication of surgery for arthritic disease. However, it usually subsides within a short time, unless it is associated with infection. This complication can be easily detected with MRI.

Leakage of Acrylic Cement. Intrapelvic leakage of methylmethacrylate may lead to vascular and neurologic damage, visceral necrosis, and urinary tract disorders, as a result of the heat of polymerization of the acrylic cement. To prevent an accidental leak, a wire mesh restrictor ("Mexican hat") is applied around the acetabular anchoring holes of the prosthesis (see Fig. 12.40).

Heterotopic Bone Formation. This is a relatively frequent complication of surgery for arthritic disease in the hip. The amount of new bone that forms in the adjacent soft tissues varies: if extensive, it may interfere with function of the hip joint. Conventional radiography and occasionally CT are sufficient to evaluate this complication.

Infection. Although infection may occur at any time postoperatively, it is usually observed shortly after the joint-replacement procedure. Clinically, it is manifested by pain, elevation of temperature, and discharge from the wound. The radiographic findings in cases of infection include soft-tissue swelling, rarefaction of bone, and, occasionally, a periosteal reaction. Scintigraphy using ^{111}In-oxine–labeled white blood cells has been reported to be very useful in these circumstances.

Loosening of a Prosthesis. Infection after a joint-replacement procedure may result in loosening of a prosthesis, but loosening may also be seen as a late complication resulting from mechanical factors. The standard radiographic projections are usually sufficient to reveal this development (Fig. 12.43). The most effective technique for demonstrating loosening of a prosthesis, however, is arthrography. The subtraction technique is commonly used to demonstrate the cardinal sign of loosening—the extension of contrast medium into the gap that develops at the interface of the bone and acrylic cement (Fig. 12.44). At times, when even arthrography is inconclusive, traction applied on the examined hip by pulling on the leg can be helpful in demonstrating occult loosening of a prosthesis. A radionuclide bone scan may occasionally be helpful in differentiating mechanical loosening from infectious loosening. Foci of increased activity, representing accumulation of radioisotope, are consistent with mechanical loosening, while diffuse increased activity indicates infection.

Figure 12.43 Failure of cemented total hip arthroplasty. Anteroposterior radiograph of the right hip of a 69-year-old woman shows a wide radiolucent zone at the bone–cement interface characteristic of loosening of a Charnley prosthesis. Note the fracture through the acrylic cement at the distal segment of the prosthetic stem.

radiolucent zone at bone–cement interface

fracture through acrylic cement

Figure 12.44 Failure of cemented total hip arthroplasty. An 80-year-old man had his right hip replaced 8 years before this radiographic examination. **(A)** Anteroposterior radiograph shows nonunion of the greater trochanter, broken wire sutures, and the suggestion of a radiolucent zone at the interface of the acrylic cement and bone in the acetabular component of the Charnley-Müller prosthesis. On a subsequent arthrogram **(B)** and a subtraction-enhanced film **(C)**, loosening of the prosthesis is clearly evident from the contrast medium seen entering the bone–cement gap and leaking medial and lateral to the neck of the prosthesis; the gap between the femur and separated greater trochanter is also opacified.

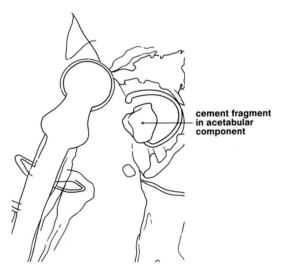

cement fragment in acetabular component

Figure 12.45 Complication of cemented total hip arthroplasty. A 77-year-old man had a Charnley low-friction arthroplasty 10 years previously for osteoarthritis of the right hip. Recently, he fell and dislocated the prosthesis, as shown on this anteroposterior radiograph **(A)**. Several attempts to reduce the dislocation, even under anesthesia, failed. **(B)** Tomographic cut demonstrates a small fragment of cement in the acetabular component of the prosthesis, which blocked reduction of the dislocation.

Dislocation of a Prosthesis. This complication is easily diagnosed on the lateral view of the knee or anteroposterior view of the hip. Tomography may occasionally be required, particularly if there are difficulties in reducing a dislocation (Fig. 12.45).

PRACTICAL POINTS TO REMEMBER

[1] The radiographic hallmarks of an arthritic process regardless of cause are:
  • narrowing of the joint space
  • bony erosion of various forms depending on the specific type of arthritis.

[2] The most effective radiologic imaging modality for evaluating arthritis is conventional radiography. Ancillary techniques, in order of their frequency of use, include:
  • radionuclide bone scan
  • magnification radiography
  • magnetic resonance imaging
  • arthrography
  • computed tomography.

[3] Radionuclide imaging is an effective technique for:
  • determining the skeletal distribution of arthritic changes
  • differentiating arthritis from periarticular soft-tissue infection
  • narrowing the differential diagnosis between infectious arthritis and other arthritides
  • monitoring the various complications of joint-replacement surgery.

[4] CT is effective in demonstrating complications of degenerative spine disease, such as spinal stenosis.

[5] MRI is effective in demonstrating abnormalities of the articular cartilage, synovial abnormalities, inflammatory panus, joint effusion, rheumatoid nodules, early subchondral erosions, and bone marrow edema.

[6] The radiographic diagnosis of arthritis is based on:
  • the morphology of an articular lesion
  • its distribution in the skeleton.

[7] The morphologic changes characteristic of different arthritides can be effectively analyzed in several important anatomic sites, including the hand, heel, and spine. These changes, together with the characteristic distribution of lesions in the skeleton and the clinical and laboratory data in a given case, facilitate a specific diagnosis.

[8] In the hand, the various arthritides have predilections for specific sites:
  • in osteoarthritis and erosive osteoarthritis—the proximal and distal interphalangeal joints
  • in psoriatic arthritis—the distal interphalangeal joints
  • in rheumatoid arthritis—the metacarpophalangeal and proximal interphalangeal joints
  • in multicentric reticulohistiocytosis—distal and proximal interphalangeal joints
  • in gouty arthritis—metacarpophalangeal and interphalangeal joints
  • in hyperparathyroid arthropathy—distal and proximal interphalangeal joints and metacarpophalangeal joints
  • in calcium pyrophosphate dihydrate crystal deposition disease—metacarpophalangeal joints
  • in scleroderma—distal interphalangeal joints.

[9] Patterns of migration of the femoral head within the acetabulum may suggest the etiology of hip arthritis:
  • osteoarthritis: superior, superoloteral, superomedial, and medial migrations
  • inflammatory arthritides: axial migration.

[10] In the spine, the various arthritides exhibit characteristic morphologic features in:
  • degenerative disease—marginal osteophytes and narrowing of the apophyseal joints and disk spaces

  • rheumatoid arthritis—atlantoaxial subluxation and erosion of the odontoid process
  • juvenile rheumatoid arthritis—fusion of the apophyseal joints of the cervical spine
  • psoriatic arthritis and Reiter syndrome—coarse, asymmetric paraspinal ossifications
  • ankylosing spondylitis—delicate syndesmophytes.

[11] Certain arthritides show lack of periarticular osteoporosis-osteoarthritis, gouty arthritis, calcium pyrophosphate dihydrate crystal deposition disease, and multicentric reticulohistiocytosis.

[12] Sacroiliitis is commonly seen in ankylosing spondylitis (in which it is bilateral and symmetrical) and in psoriatic arthritis and Reiter syndrome (in which it is either unilateral or bilateral but asymmetric in terms of degree of involvement).

[13] Monitoring the results of treatment of the arthritides involves detecting possible complications of various osteotomies and joint-replacement procedures. These complications include:
  • thrombophlebitis
  • intrapelvic leakage of methylmethacrylate cement
  • heterotopic bone formation
  • infection
  • loosening, dislocation, and fracture of a prosthesis.

[14] Contrast arthrography utilizing the subtraction technique is useful in detecting loosening of a prosthesis.

SUGGESTED READINGS

Aisen AM, Martel W, Ellis JE, McCune WJ. Cervical spine involvement in rheumatoid arthritis: MR imaging. *Radiology* 1987;165:159–163.

Alazraki NP, Fierer J, Resnick D. The role of gallium and bone scanning in monitoring response to therapy in chronic osteomyelitis. *J Nucl Med* 1978;19:696–697.

Allen AM, Ward WG, Pope Jr, TL. Imaging of the total knee arthroplasty. *Radiol Clin North Am* 1995;33:289–303.

Anderson LS, Staple TW. Arthrography of total hip replacement using substraction technique. *Radiology* 1973;109:470–472.

Beabout JW. Radiology of total hip arthroplasty. *Radiol Clin North Am* 1975;13:3–19.

Beltran J. *MRI: musculoskeletal system.* Philadelphia: JB Lippincott; 1990.

Beltran J, Caudill JL, Herman LA, et al. Rheumatoid arthritis: MR imaging manifestations. *Radiology* 1987;165:153–157.

Bianchi S, Martinoli C, Abdelwahab, IF. High-frequency ultrasound examination of the wrist and hand. *Skeletal Radiol* 1999;28:121–129.

Breedveld FC, Algra PR, Vielvoye CJ, Cats A. Magnetic resonance imaging in the evaluation of patients with rheumatoid arthritis and subluxations of the cervical spine. *Arthritis Rheum* 1987;30:624–629.

Brower AC, Flemming DJ. *Arthritis in black and white.* 2nd ed. Philadelphia: WB Saunders; 1997.

Charkes MD. Skeletal blood flow: implication for bone-scan interpretation. *J Nucl Med* 1980;21:91–98.

Datz FL, Morton KA. New radiopharmaceuticals for detecting infection. *Invest Radiol* 1993;28:356–365.

Erickson SJ. High-resolution imaging of the musculoskeletal system. *Radiology* 1997; 205:593–618.

Forrester DM. Imaging of the sacroiliac joints. *Radiol Clin North Am* 1990;28:1055–1072.

Forrester DM, Brown JC. *The radiology of joint disease,* 3rd ed. Philadelphia: WB Saunders; 1987.

Freiberger RH. Evaluation of hip prostheses by imaging methods. *Semin Roentgenol* 1986;21:20–28.

Gee R, Munk PL, Keogh C, et al. Radiography of the PROSTALAC (prosthesis with antibiotic-loaded acrylic cement) orthopedic implant. *AJR Am J Roentgenol* 2003;180:1701–1706.

Gelman MI, Coleman RE, Stevens PM, Davey BW. Radiography, radionuclide imaging, and arthrography in the evaluation of total hip and knee replacement. *Radiology* 1978;128:677–682.

Genant HK, Doi K, Mall JC, Sickles EA. Direct radiographic magnification for skeletal radiology. *Radiology* 1977;123:47–55.

Greenspan A, Norman A. Gross hematuria: a complication of intrapelvic cement intrusion in total hip replacement. *AJR Am J Roentgenol* 1978; 130: 327–329.

Greenspan A, Norman A. Radial head-capitellum view in elbow trauma [Letter]. *AJR Am J Roentgenol* 1983;140:1273–1275.

Greenspan A, Norman A. Radial head-capitellum view: an expanded imaging approach to elbow injury. *Radiology* 1987;164:272–274.

Griffiths HJ, Priest D, Kushner D. Total hip replacement and other orthopedic hip procedures. *Radiol Clin North Am* 1995;33:267–287.

Gristina AG, Kolkin J. Current concepts review. Total joint replacement and sepsis. *J Bone Joint Surg [Am]* 1983;65A:128–134.

Habermann ET. Total joint replacement: an overview. *Semin Roentgenol* 1986;21:7–19.

Hendrix RW, Wixson RL, Rana NA, Rogers LF. Arthrography after total hip arthroplasty: a modified technique used in the diagnosis of pain. *Radiology* 1983;148:647–652.

Insall J, Tria AJ, Scott WN. The total condylar knee prosthesis: the first 5 years. *Clin Orthop* 1979;145:68–77.

Jones MM, Moore WH, Brewer EJ, Sonnemaker RE, Long SE. Radionuclide bone/joint imaging in children with rheumatic complaints. *Skeletal Radiol* 1988;17:1–7.

Kattan KR, Marsch JT. Some extra-articular manifestations of arthritis and complications of therapy. A pictorial essay. *Radiol Clin North Am* 1988;26:1277–1293.

Kim S-H, Chung S-K, Bahk Y-W, Park Y-H, Lee S-Y, Son H-S. Whole-body and pinhole bone scintigraphic manifestations of Reiter's syndrome: distribution patterns and early and characteristic signs. *Eur J Nucl Med* 1999;26:163–170.

Kramer J, Recht MP, Imhof H, Stiglbauer R, Engel A. Postcontrast MR arthrography in assessment of cartilage lesions. *J Comput Assist Tomogr* 1994;18:218–224.

Kursunoglu-Brahme S, Riccio T, Weissman MH, et al. Rheumatoid knee: role of gadopentetate-enhanced MR imaging. *Radiology* 1990;176:831–835.

Larsson EM, Holtas S, Zygmunt S. Pre- and postoperative MR imaging of the craniocervical junction in rheumatoid arthritis. *AJR Am J Roentgenol* 1989;152:561–566.

Lund PJ, Heikal A, Maricic MJ, Krupinski EA, Williams CS. Ultrasonographic imaging of the hand and wrist in rheumatoid arthritis. *Skeletal Radiol* 1995;24:591–596.

Manaster BJ. Total hip arthroplasty: radiographic evaluation. *Radiographics* 1996;16:645–660.

McAfee JG. Update on radiopharmaceuticals for medical imaging. *Radiology* 1989;171:593–601.

McCauley TR, Disler DG. State of the art. MR imaging of articular cartilage. *Radiology* 1998;209:629–640.

Oudjhane K, Azouz EM, Hughes S, Paquin JD. Computed tomography of the sacroiliac joints in children. *Can Assoc Radiol J* 1993;44:313–314.

Perri JA, Rodman P, Mankin HJ. Giant synovial cysts of the calf in patients with rheumatoid arthritis. *J Bone Joint Surg [Am]* 1968;50A:709–719.

Peterfy CG, Genant HK. Emerging applications of magnetic resonance imaging in the evaluation of articular cartilage. *Radiol Clin North Am* 1996;34:195–213.

Peterfy CG, Majumdar S, Lang P, van Dijke CF, Sack K, Genant HK. MR imaging of the arthritic knee: improved discrimination of cartilage, synovia, and effusion with pulsed saturation transfer and fat-suppressed T1-weighted sequences. *Radiology* 1994;191:413–419.

Recht MP, Resnick D. MR imaging of articular cartilage: current status and future directions. *AJR Am J Roentgenol* 1994;163:283–290.

Rupani HD, Holder LE, Espinola DA, Engin SI. Three-phase radionuclide bone imaging in sports medicine. *Radiology* 1985;156:187–196.

Salvati EA, Ghelman B, McLaren T, Wilson PD Jr. Subtraction technique in arthrography for loosening of total hip replacement fixed with radiopaque cement. *Clin Orthop* 1974;101:105–109.

Schneider R, Abenavoli AM, Soundry M, Insall J. Failure of total condylar knee replacement. *Radiology* 1984;152:309–315.

Schneider R, Goldman AB, Insall JN. Knee prosthesis. *Semin Roentgenol* 1986;21:29–46.

Schneider R, Hood RW, Ranawat CS. Radiologic evaluation of knee arthroplasty. *Orthop Clin North Am* 1982;13:225–244.

Schumacher TM, Genant HK, Kellet MJ, Mall JC, Fye KM. HLA-B27 associated arthropathies. *Radiology* 1978;126:289–297.

Sebes JI, Nasrallah NS, Rabinowitz JG, Masi AT. The relationship between HLA-B27 positive peripheral arthritis and sacroillitis. *Radiology* 1978;126:299–302.

Seltzer SE, Weissman BN, Finberg HJ. Improved diagnostic imaging in joint diseases. *Semin Arthritis Rheum* 1982;11:315–330.

Steinbach L, Hellman D, Petri M, Sims R, Gillespy T, Genant H. Magnetic resonance imaging: a review of rheumatologic applications. *Semin Arthritis Rheum* 1986;16:79–91.

Subramanian G, McAfee JG. A new complex of 99m-Tc for skeletal imaging. *Radiology* 1971;99:192–196.

Subramanian G, McAfee JG, Blair RJ, Kallfelz FA, Thomas FD. Technetium-99m methylene diphosphonate—a superior agent for skeletal imaging. Comparison with other technetium complexes. *J Nucl Med* 1975;16:744–755.

Sugimoto H, Hirose I, Miyaoka E, Fujita A, Kinebuchi Y, Yamamoto W, Itoh Y-i. Low-field-strength MR imaging of failed hip arthroplasty: association of femoral periprosthetic signal intensity with radiographic, surgical, and pathologic findings. *Radiology* 2003;229:718–723.

Taljanovic MS, Jones MD, Hunter TB, Benjamin JB, Ruth JT, Brown AW, Sheppard JE. Joint arthroplasties and prostheses. *Radiographics* 2003;23:1295–1314.

Waldschmidt JG, Rilling RJ, Kajdacsy-Balla AA, Boynton MD, Erickson SJ. In vitro and in vivo MR imaging of hyaline cartilage: zonal anatomy, imaging pitfalls, and pathologic conditions. *Radiographics* 1997;17:1387–1402.

Weissman BN. Spondyloarthropathies. *Radiol Clin North Am* 1987;25:1235–1262.

Winalski CS, Palmer WE, Rosenthal DI, Weissman BN. Magnetic resonance imaging of rheumatoid arthritis. *Radiol Clin North Am* 1996;34:243–258.

CHAPTER 13

DEGENERATIVE JOINT DISEASE

Osteoarthritis

Degenerative joint disease (osteoarthritis, osteoarthrosis) is the most common form of arthritis. In its primary (idiopathic) form, it affects individuals age 50 and older; in its secondary form, however, osteoarthritis may be seen in a much younger age group. Patients in the latter group have clearly defined underlying conditions leading to the development of degenerative joint disease (see Fig. 12.1).

Some authorities postulate that there are two types of primary degenerative joint disease. The first form is apparently closely related to the aging process ("wear and tear") and represents not a true arthritis but a senescent process of the joint. It characteristically shows limited destruction of the cartilage, slow progression, lack of significant joint deformity, and no restriction of joint function. This process is not affected by gender or race. The second type, a true osteoarthritis, is unrelated to the aging process, although it shows an increased prevalence with age. Marked by progressive destruction of the articular cartilage and reparative processes such as osteophyte formation and subchondral sclerosis, true osteoarthritis progresses rapidly, leading to significant joint deformity. This form may be related to genetic factors, as well as to gender, race, and obesity. It has been shown that osteoarthritis tends to affect women more commonly than men, particularly in the proximal and distal interphalangeal joints and the first carpometacarpal joints. In the population older than age 65, osteoarthritis affects whites more frequently than blacks. Obesity is associated with a higher incidence of osteoarthritis in the knees, which may be related to an excessive weight-bearing load on these joints.

Generally, in osteoarthritis the large diarthrodial joints such as the hip or knee and the small joints such as the interphalangeal joints of the hand are most often affected; the spine, however, is just as frequently involved in the degenerative process (Fig. 13.1). The shoulder, elbow, wrist, and ankle are unusual sites for primary osteoarthritis, and if degenerative changes are encountered in these locations, secondary arthritis should be considered. It should be kept in mind, however, that evidence exists for an association between degenerative arthritis in unusual sites and certain occupations. Even primary osteoarthritic changes may develop more rapidly, for example, in the lumbar spine, knees, and elbows of coal miners and in the wrists, elbows, and shoulders of pneumatic drill operators. Degenerative changes are also commonly seen in the ankles and feet of ballet dancers and in the femoropatellar joints of bicyclists.

An overview of the clinical and radiographic hallmarks of degenerative joint disease is presented in Table 13.1.

Osteoarthritis of the Large Joints

The hip and knee joints are the most common sites of osteoarthritis. The severity of radiographic changes does not always correlate with

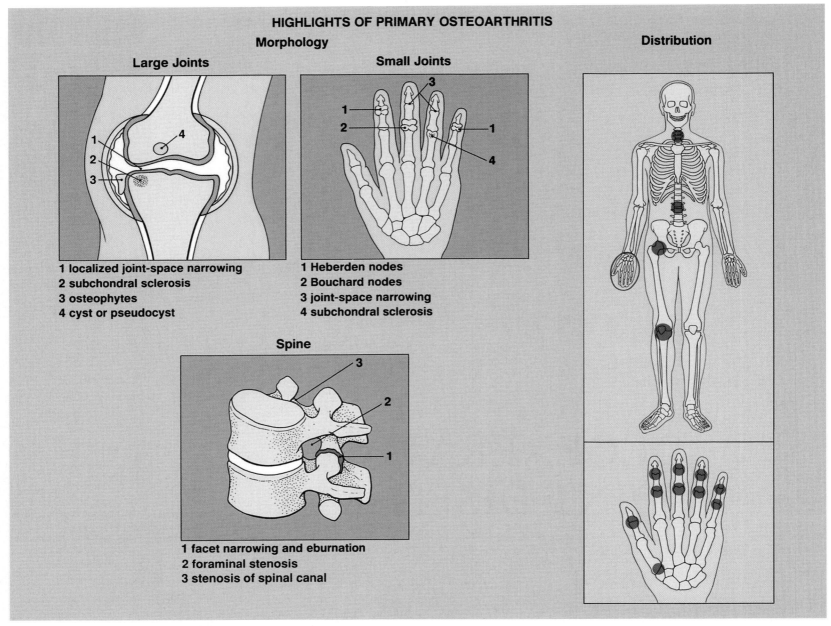

HIGHLIGHTS OF PRIMARY OSTEOARTHRITIS

Morphology

Large Joints

1 localized joint-space narrowing
2 subchondral sclerosis
3 osteophytes
4 cyst or pseudocyst

Small Joints

1 Heberden nodes
2 Bouchard nodes
3 joint-space narrowing
4 subchondral sclerosis

Spine

1 facet narrowing and eburnation
2 foraminal stenosis
3 stenosis of spinal canal

Distribution

Figure 13.1 Highlights of the morphology and distribution of arthritic lesions in primary osteoarthritis.

the clinical symptoms, which may vary from stiffness and pain to severe deformities and limitation of joint function.

Osteoarthritis of the Hip

There are four cardinal radiographic features of degenerative joint disease in the hip:

1. Narrowing of the joint space as a result of thinning of the articular cartilage
2. Subchondral sclerosis (eburnation) caused by reparative processes (remodeling)
3. Osteophyte formation (osteophytosis) as a result of reparative processes in sites not subjected to stress (so-called low-stress areas), which are usually marginal (peripheral) in distribution
4. Cyst or pseudocyst formation resulting from bone contusions that lead to microfractures and intrusion of synovial fluid into

the altered spongy bone; in the acetabulum, these subchondral cyst-like lesions are referred to as *Eggers cysts*.

These hallmarks of degenerative joint disease can be readily demonstrated on the standard projections of the hip (Fig. 13.2). Occasionally, tomography is used to demonstrate the details of the degenerative process; however, it is not used to make a specific diagnosis but rather to confirm or exclude possible complications (see Fig. 12.8). CT scanning may further delineate the characteristic features of osteoarthritis (Fig. 13.3).

As articular cartilage is destroyed and reparative changes develop, evidence emerges of a change in the relation of the femoral head with respect to the acetabulum, known as "migration." Generally, three patterns of femoral head migration can be observed: superior, which may be either superolateral or superomedial; medial; and axial (Fig. 13.4). The most common pattern is superolateral migration; the medial pattern is less common, whereas axial migration is

Table 13.1 **Clinical and Radiographic Hallmarks of Degenerative Joint Disease**

Type of Arthritis	Site	Crucial Abnormalities	Technique*/Projection

Primary osteoarthritis (F> M; >50 years)	Hand	Degenerative changes in:
		  Proximal interphalangeal joints
		    (Bouchard nodes)
		  Distal interphalangeal joints
		    (Heberden nodes)
			Dorsovolar view

	Hip	Narrowing of joint space Subchondral sclerosis Marginal osteophytes Cysts and pseudocysts Superolateral subluxation	Anteroposterior view

	Knee	Same changes as in hip
		Varus or valgus deformity
		Degenerative changes in:
		  Femoropatellar compartment
		  Patella (tooth sign)
			Anteroposterior view
			Weight-bearing anteroposterior view
			Lateral view
			Axial view of patella

	Spine	Degenerative disk disease:
		  Narrowing of disk space
		  Degenerative spondylolisthesis
		  Osteophytosis
		Spondylosis deformans
		Degenerative changes in apophyseal joints
		Foraminal stenosis
		Spinal stenosis
			Lateral view
			Lateral flexion/extension views
			Anteroposterior and lateral views
			Anteroposterior and lateral views
			Oblique views (cervical, lumbar)
			
			CT, myelogram, MRI

Secondary osteoarthritis Posttraumatic	Hip Knee Shoulder, elbow, wrist, ankle (unusual sites)	Similar changes to those in primary osteoarthritis History of previous trauma Younger age	Standard views Tomography
Slipped capital femoral epiphysis	Hips	Herndon hump Narrowing of joint space Osteophytosis	Anteroposterior and frog-lateral views
Congenital hip dislocation (F>M)	Hips	Signs of acetabular hypoplasia	Anteroposterior and frog-lateral views
Perthes disease (M>F)	Hip	Unilateral or bilateral Osteonecrosis of femoral head Coxa magna Lateral subluxation	Anteroposterior and frog-lateral views
Inflammatory arthritis	Hip Knee	Medial and axial migration of femoral head Periarticular osteoporosis Limited osteophytosis	Standard views
Osteonecrosis	Hip Shoulder	Increased bone density Joint space usually preserved or only slightly narrowed Crescent sign	Anteroposterior views (hip, shoulder) Grashey view (shoulder) Frog-lateral view (hip)
Paget disease (>40 years)	Hips, knees, shoulders	Coarse trabeculations Thickening of cortex	Standard views of affected joints Radionuclide bone scan
Multiple epiphyseal dysplasia	Epiphyses of long bones	Dysplastic changes Narrowing of joint space Osteophytes	Standard views of affected joints
Hemochromatosis	Hands	Degenerative changes in second and third metacarpophalangeal joints with beak-like osteophytes Chondrocalcinosis	Dorsovolar view
Acromegaly	Large joints	Joint spaces widened or only slightly narrowed	Standard views of affected joint
	Hands	Enlargement of terminal tufts Beak-like osteophytes in heads of metacarpals	Dorsovolar view

*Radionuclide bone scan is used to determine the distribution of arthritic lesions in the skeleton.

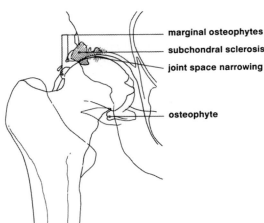

marginal osteophytes
subchondral sclerosis
joint space narrowing

osteophyte

Figure 13.2 Osteoarthritis of the hip joint. A 51-year-old woman presented with a history of right hip pain for the past 10 years and no previous history suggesting predisposing factors for osteoarthritis. Anteroposterior radiograph of the hip demonstrates the radiographic hallmarks of osteoarthritis: narrowing of the joint space, particularly at the weight-bearing segment; formation of marginal osteophytes; and subchondral sclerosis. Note the lack of osteoporosis.

only exceptionally seen. It should be kept in mind, however, that in inflammatory arthritis of the hip, such as rheumatoid arthritis, in which a previous axial migration of the femoral head is commonly associated with acetabular protrusio, degenerative changes might develop as a complication of the inflammatory process. Thus, one may see secondary osteoarthritis with axial migration (Fig. 13.5).

Occasionally, the degenerative process in the hip may run a more rapid course. This destructive arthrosis of the hip joint is known as *Postel coxarthropathy*, a condition characterized by rapid chondrolysis that may quickly lead to complete destruction of the hip joint. Originally described by Lequesne, and also by Postel and Kerboull in 1970, this unique hip disorder occurs predominantly in women, with age of onset at 60 to 70 years. In all cases, a rapid clinical course of hip pain is the consistent common symptom. The histologic findings are those of conventional osteoarthritis with severe

degenerative changes in the articular cartilage. However, osteophyte formation is absent or minimal. Hypervascularity in the subchondral bone is a common finding. The bone trabeculae are either abnormally thickened or abnormally thinned. Occasionally, one can observe foci of fibrosis, interstitial edema and hemorrhage in the marrow spaces, focal marrow fat fibrosis, and focal areas of bone resorption. The precise pathogenesis of this condition remains unclear, although direct drug toxicity and the analgesic effects of nonsteroidal anti-inflammatory drugs have been implicated. Some investigators have suggested that intraarticular deposition of hydroxyapatite crystals might lead to joint destruction. Others have proposed subchondral insufficiency fracture of the femoral head as a cause of this arthritis. Because of the rapidity of the process, the radiographic presentation of this condition is marked by very little, if any, reparative changes, mimicking infectious or neuropathic arthritis (Charcot joint) (Fig. 13.6). More recently, Boutry and colleagues reported MRI findings of this form of osteoarthritis. These included joint effusion, a bone marrow edema-like pattern in the femoral head, neck, and acetabulum, femoral head flattening, and cyst-like subchondral defects (Fig. 13.7).

Secondary osteoarthritis is often seen in the hip joint in patients with predisposing conditions such as previous trauma (Fig. 13.8), slipped capital femoral epiphysis, congenital hip dislocation, Perthes disease, osteonecrosis, Paget disease, and inflammatory arthritides. The radiographic findings are the same as those described for primary osteoarthritis, but the features of the underlying process also can often be detected. Although the standard radiographic views are usually sufficient for demonstrating these changes, computed tomography, arthrography, or magnetic resonance imaging may at times be needed for a more accurate assessment of the status of the articular cartilage.

Treatment. Advanced osteoarthritis, whether primary or secondary, is usually treated surgically by total hip arthroplasty using, among the various types available, either a cemented or a noncemented prosthesis. The reader is referred to Chapter 12 for further discussion of management.

Figure 13.3 CT of osteoarthritis of the hip. Coronal reformatted image shows diminution of the joint space, osteophytes, and subchondral cysts in the femoral head.

Figure 13.4 **Migration of the femoral head.**
(A) Anteroposterior radiograph of the right hip of a 65-year-old woman with long-standing degenerative joint disease in both hips demonstrates superolateral migration of the femoral head, the most common pattern seen in osteoarthritis of the hip joint. Note the typical Eggers cyst in the acetabulum. **(B)** Medial migration of the femoral head is apparent in this 48-year-old woman with osteoarthritis of the right hip. **(C)** Axial migration of the femoral head is evident in this 57-year-old woman who was suspected of having inflammatory arthritis. Clinical and laboratory investigations, however, led to a diagnosis of idiopathic osteoarthritis, which was confirmed on histopathologic examination after total hip replacement.

Eggers' cyst

Figure 13.5 **Rheumatoid arthritis with superimposed osteoarthritis.** Anteroposterior radiograph of the right hip of a 42-year-old woman with a known history of long-standing rheumatoid arthritis shows the typical changes of inflammatory arthritis, including axial migration of the femoral head and acetabular protrusio. Superimposition of secondary osteoarthritis is evident in subchondral sclerosis and marginal osteophytes.

Figure 13.6 **Postel coxarthropathy.** Anteroposterior radiograph of the right hip of a 72-year-old man who had pain in the hip for 4 months shows the typical appearance of Postel coxarthropathy, which often mimics Charcot joint or infectious arthritis. Note the destruction of the articular portion of the femoral head, which is laterally subluxed. The same destructive process has led to widening of the acetabulum.

Osteoarthritis of the Knee

The knee is a complex joint comprising three major compartments—the medial femorotibial, the lateral femorotibial, and the femoropatellar—and each of which may be affected by degenerative changes. The radiographic features of these changes are similar to those seen in osteoarthritis of the hip, including narrowing of the joint space (usually one or two compartments), subchondral sclerosis, osteophytosis, and subchondral cyst (or pseudocyst) formation. The standard anteroposterior and lateral projections of the knee are sufficient to demonstrate these processes (Fig. 13.9). If the medial joint compartment is affected, the knee may assume a varus configuration, which is best demonstrated on the weight-bearing anteroposterior view (Fig. 13.10A); involvement of the lateral compartment may lead to a valgus configuration (Fig. 13.10B). A frequent complication of osteoarthritis of the knee is the formation of osteochondral bodies, which can be demonstrated on the standard projections of the knee

(Fig. 13.11) but may occasionally require arthrography. MRI may also be effective in this respect (Figs. 13.12 and 13.13). The femoropatellar joint compartment is also commonly involved in primary osteoarthritis. The lateral radiograph of the knee and axial view of the patella are the most effective means of visualizing degenerative changes of the femoropatellar compartment (Fig. 13.14).

Often, particularly in individuals past their fifth decade of life, degenerative changes unrelated to femoropatellar osteoarthritis are seen at the insertion of the quadriceps tendon into the base of the patella. These changes are manifest as vertical ridges resembling teeth on an axial view of the patella and have been designated by Greenspan and colleagues as the "tooth" sign (Fig. 13.15A). The dentate structures represent an enthesopathy probably related to stress at the attachment of the quadriceps apparatus, and their nature is clearly demonstrated on the lateral projection (Fig. 13.15B). At times they can be recognized on the anteroposterior view as well (Fig. 13.15C). MR imaging effectively demonstrates these changes (Fig. 13.16).

Figure 13.7 Postel coxarthropathy. (A) Anteroposterior radiograph of the right hip of a 44-year-old man shows destructive changes of the femoral head and acetabulum. **(B)** Aspiration arthrogram, that was performed to rule out infection, shows hypertrophic synovitis. **(C)** A gradient-echo T2*-weighted MRI shows joint effusion, hypertrophied synovium, and subchondral cysts in the acetabulum and femoral head.

Figure 13.8 Posttraumatic osteoarthritis. A 64-year-old man, who in the past sustained complex right acetabular and femoral fractures, developed secondary osteoarthritis. **(A)** A preliminary scout CT image shows posttraumatic deformity of the acetabulum and femoral head associated with acetabular protrusio. **(B)** Axial CT section through both hips shows osteoarthritic changes of the right femoral head and ununited fracture of the anterior column (*arrow*). **(C)** Coronal reformatted image demonstrates significant narrowing of the joint space, deformity of the femoral head, and periarticular sclerosis. **(D)** 3-D reformation shows almost complete obliteration of the hip joint, acetabular protrusio, and osteophyte formation. All CT findings are consistent with posttraumatic osteoarthritis.

Figure 13.9 Osteoarthritis. Anteroposterior **(A)** and lateral **(B)** projections of the knee of a 57-year-old woman demonstrate narrowing of the medial femorotibial and femoropatellar compartments, subchondral sclerosis, and osteophytosis, which are the typical features of osteoarthritis. Note that osteophytes that were not obvious on the frontal projection are much better-demonstrated on the lateral radiograph.

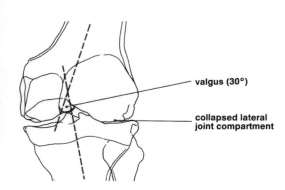

valgus (30°)

collapsed lateral
joint compartment

Figure 13.10 Osteoarthritis. (A) Weight-bearing anteroposterior radiograph of the knee of a 58-year-old woman demonstrates advanced osteoarthritis of the medial femorotibial joint compartment, which has led to a varus configuration of the joint. **(B)** Involvement of the lateral femorotibial joint compartment in advanced osteoarthritis as seen on this weight-bearing anteroposterior radiograph of another patient has resulted in a valgus configuration.

osteochondral bodies

arthritic changes
in medial joint
compartment

osteochondral bodies

arthritic changes in
femoropatellar compartment

Figure 13.11 Osteoarthritis with osteochondral bodies. Anteroposterior **(A)** and lateral **(B)** radiographs of the knee of a 66-year-old man with advanced osteoarthritis demonstrate predominant involvement of the medial femorotibial and femoropatellar joint compartments, with formation of two large osteochondral bodies.

Figure 13.12 MRI of osteochondral body. A low-signal-intensity osteocartilaginous loose body in suprapatellar bursa (*arrow*) is revealed on T1-weighted **(A)** and T2*-weighted **(B)** sagittal MR images.

Figure 13.13 Baker cyst with osteochondral bodies. Sagittal T1-weighted **(A)** and T2*-weighted **(B)** MR images show multiple osteochondral loose bodies (*arrows*) in a popliteal (Baker) cyst adjacent to the medial head of gastrocnemius muscle.

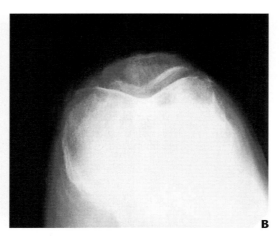

Figure 13.14 **Femoropatellar osteoarthritis.** Lateral radiograph of the knee (**A**) and axial radiograph of the patella (**B**) of a 72-year-old woman demonstrate narrowing of the medial femoropatellar joint compartment and osteophyte formation on the medial aspect of the joint.

Figure 13.15 **Patellar enthesopathy.** (**A**) Axial view of the patella demonstrates dentate structures (the "tooth" sign), which represent degenerative ossifications (enthesopathy) at the insertion of the quadriceps tendon into the base of patella, as seen on the lateral view (**B**) in this 55-year-old man. (**C**) Occasionally, the tooth sign can also be demonstrated on the anteroposterior projection of the knee, seen here in a 54-year-old woman. (**A** and **B** from Greenspan A, et al., 1977, with permission.)

Figure 13.16 **MRI of patellar enthesopathy.** Coronal T1-weighted (**A**) and axial T2-weighted (**B**) MR images show "tooth sign" of the patella.

Figure 13.17 Osteoarthritis. Anteroposterior radiograph of the right shoulder of a 58-year-old man shows the typical features of osteoarthritis; both shoulders were affected. The patient had no history of trauma or other underlying condition to suggest the possibility of secondary arthritis.

As in the hip joint, one may encounter secondary osteoarthritis in the knee. One of the most common predisposing factors is previous trauma or surgery.

Osteoarthritis of Other Large Joints

Other large joints such as the shoulder and ankle can be affected by osteoarthritis (Fig. 13.17), but involvement of these sites in the idiopathic form of the disease is much less common than involvement of the hip or knee. In fact, with evidence of degenerative changes in such sites, one must consider the possibility of secondary rather than idiopathic arthritis (see Table 13.1).

Osteoarthritis of the Small Joints

Primary Osteoarthritis of the Hand

The most commonly affected small joints are those of the hand, particularly the proximal and distal interphalangeal and the first carpometacarpal articulations (see Figs. 12.24 and 13.1). In the distal interphalangeal joints, if hypertrophic phenomena supervene and osteophytes are prominent, degenerative changes are accompanied by *Heberden nodes*. Similar deformities in the proximal interphalangeal joints are called *Bouchard nodes* (Fig. 13.18). If the degenerative changes involve the first carpometacarpal joint, they may result in an odd deformation of the thumb (Fig. 13.19). The midcarpal articulations may also be affected, particularly the scaphotrapeziotrapezoid joint.

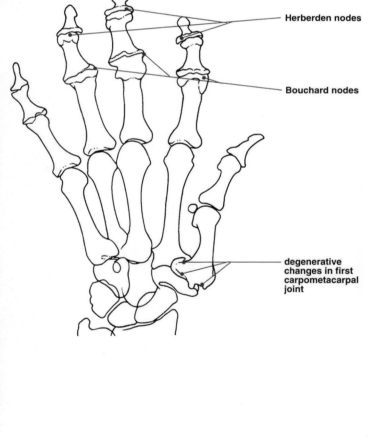

Figure 13.18 Interphalangeal osteoarthritis. Dorsovolar radiograph of right hand of a 74-year-old woman shows degenerative changes in the distal interphalangeal joints, manifested by Heberden nodes, and in the proximal interphalangeal joints, manifested by Bouchard nodes. Note also degenerative changes in the first carpometacarpal joint.

Figure 13.19 **Interphalangeal and carpometacarpal osteoarthritis.** Dorsovolar radiograph of both hands of a 52-year-old woman with osteoarthritis in addition to the typical Heberden and Bouchard nodes shows deformative changes at the first carpometacarpal articulations, resulting in an odd configuration of both thumbs.

Figure 13.20 **Acromegalic osteoarthritis.** Dorsovolar radiograph of both hands of a 42-year-old man with acromegaly shows widening of some and narrowing of other joint spaces, enlargement of the distal tufts and the bases of terminal phalanges, and beak-like osteophytes affecting particularly the heads of the metacarpals. Note the soft tissue prominence and the large sesamoid bones at the first metacarpophalangeal joints. The sesamoid index (derived by multiplying the vertical and horizontal diameters of the sesamoid bone) is 48 in this patient; normally, it should not exceed 20 to 25.

Figure 13.21 Hemochromatosis arthropathy. Oblique radiographs of both hands of a 53-year-old woman with hemochromatosis show beak-like osteophytes arising from the heads of the second and third metacarpals on the radial aspect. The interphalangeal, metacarpophalangeal, and carpal articulations are also affected.

Secondary Osteoarthritis of the Hand

Acromegaly. The most characteristic secondary osteoarthritic changes in the small joints may be observed in acromegalic patients. Although the degenerative process in acromegaly also affects large joints such as the hip, knee, shoulder, and the spine, the hand displays the most typical features of this condition. These include soft-tissue prominence and enlargement of the terminal tufts and the bases of the terminal phalanges; there may also be widening of some articular spaces and narrowing of others; beak-like osteophytes at the heads of the metacarpals are a prominent feature (Fig. 13.20). Degenerative changes in acromegaly are the result of hypertrophy of articular cartilage, which is not properly nourished by synovial fluid because of its abnormal thickness. (The reader is also referred to the discussion of acromegaly in Chapters 15 and 30.)

Hemochromatosis. Commonly associated with the development of secondary osteoarthritis in the small joints, hemochromatosis (iron storage disease) is a rare disorder characterized by iron deposition in internal organs, articular cartilage, and synovium. Some investigators believe that the arthropathy seen in this condition differs from typical degenerative joint disease and warrants classification in the group of metabolic arthritides (see Chapter 15).

In the hand, the second and third metacarpophalangeal joints are characteristically affected (Fig. 13.21), although other small joints such as the interphalangeal and carpal articulations may be involved. Degenerative changes may also be seen at the shoulders, knees, hips, and ankles. Loss of the articular space, eburnation, subchondral cyst formation, and osteophytosis are the most prominent radiographic features of hemochromatosis. The changes may occasionally mimic those seen in calcium pyrophosphate dihydrate deposition disease and rheumatoid arthritis.

Osteoarthritis of the Foot

In the foot, the most commonly affected articulation is the metatarsophalangeal joint of the great toe. This condition is known as *hallux rigidus* or *hallux limitus* (Fig. 13.22).

Degenerative Diseases of the Spine

Degenerative changes may involve the spine at the following sites:
1. The synovial joints—atlantoaxial, apophyseal, costovertebral, and sacroiliac—leading to *osteoarthritis* of these structures
2. The intervertebral disks, leading to the condition known as *degenerative disk disease*
3. The vertebral bodies and annulus fibrosus, leading to the condition known as *spondylosis deformans*
4. The fibrous articulations, ligaments, or sites of ligament attachment to the bone (entheses), leading to the condition known as *diffuse idiopathic skeletal hyperostosis* (DISH).

Frequently, all four conditions coexist in the same patient.

Osteoarthritis of the Synovial Joints

Degenerative changes of the vertebral facet joints are very common, particularly in the mid and lower cervical and the lower lumbar segments. As in the other synovial joints, the characteristic radiographic features include diminution of the joint space, eburnation of subchondral bone, and osteophyte formation, all of which are most easily demonstrated on the oblique projection of the spine (Fig. 13.23). In the cervical spine, osteophytes on the posterior aspect of a vertebral body may encroach on the neural foramina or the thecal sac,

Figure 13.22 Hallux rigidus. Dorsoplantar radiograph of the great and second toes of the feet of a 33-year-old man shows osteoarthritis of the first metatarsophalangeal joints, which are known as hallux rigidus (hallux limitus). Note the narrowing of the joint space, subchondral sclerosis, and marginal osteophytes.

subchondral sclerosis

narrowing of facet joints

Figure 13.23 Osteoarthritis of the facet joints. Oblique radiograph of the lumbar spine in a 68-year-old man demonstrates advanced osteoarthritis of the facet joints. Narrowing of the joint spaces, eburnation of the articular margins, and small osteophytes are similar to the changes seen in osteoarthritis of the large synovial joints.

causing various neurologic symptoms. In addition to the standard oblique views (Fig. 13.24), conventional tomography or computed tomography (CT) is usually required to demonstrate these changes (Fig. 13.25). Anterior osteophytes, however, are as a rule asymptomatic unless they are unusually prominent. Involvement of the apophyseal joints may exhibit a "vacuum phenomenon" (Fig. 13.26), which in fact represents gas in the joint. This finding is almost pathognomonic for a degenerative process.

As in other diarthrodial joints, degenerative changes of the sacroiliac joints are manifested by narrowing of the joint space, subchondral sclerosis, and osteophytosis (Fig. 13.27). It is important to note in the evaluation of the sacroiliac joints that only the lower half of the radiographic sacroiliac joint space is lined by synovium; the upper portion is a syndesmotic joint (Fig. 13.28).

Degenerative Disk Disease

In degenerative disk disease, the vacuum phenomenon in the disk space is common. These radiolucent collections of gas, principally nitrogen, are related to the negative pressure created by abnormally altered joint or disk spaces.

Other radiographic findings of degenerative disk disease include disk space narrowing and osteophytosis at the marginal borders of the adjacent vertebral bodies (Fig. 13.29). Degenerative disk disease, in combination with degenerative changes in the apophyseal joints, may lead to degenerative spondylolisthesis (see Figs. 11.68, 11.70, and 13.29).

Magnetic resonance imaging is highly effective in demonstrating changes of disk degeneration. Decrease in the water content results in a decreased signal intensity of the nucleus pulposus on T2-weighted images (Fig. 13.30). Frequently, additional characteristic alterations are seen in the end-plates of the vertebral bodies adjacent to the degenerative disk. These abnormalities consist of a focal decreased signal intensity of the marrow on T1-weighted images and increased signal on T2- or T2*-weighted images (Fig. 13.31). According to Modic, these alterations represent subchondral vascularized fibrous tissue associated with end-plate fissuring and disruption (type I). These changes may progress to fatty marrow end-plate conversion (type II) (Fig. 13.32), and later to sclerosis (type III).

Spondylosis Deformans

Spondylosis deformans is a degenerative condition marked by the formation of anterior and lateral osteophytes as a result of anterior and anterolateral disk herniation (see Figs. 11.74 and 11.75). As Schmorl and other investigators have pointed out, the initiating factors in the development of this condition are abnormalities in the peripheral fibers of the annulus fibrosus that result in weakening of the anchor-

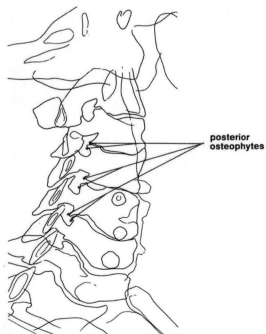

posterior osteophytes

Figure 13.24 Encroachment of the neural foramina. Oblique radiograph of the cervical spine in a 72-year-old woman who reported neck pain radiating to both shoulders reveals multiple posterior osteophytes encroaching on numerous neural foramina.

Figure 13.25 Encroachment of the neural foramina and the thecal sac. (A) Conventional lateral tomogram of the cervical spine in a 56-year-old man demonstrates encroachment of the neural foramina by posterior osteophytes. **(B)** CT section at the level of C-3 obtained during myelography demonstrates a large posterior osteophyte impinging on the thecal sac and compressing the subarachnoid space filled with contrast medium.

Figure 13.26 Osteoarthritis of the apophyseal joints. A 56-year-old man with osteoarthritis affecting the apophyseal joints of the lumbar spine. **(A)** Oblique radiograph of the lumbosacral spine demonstrates a vacuum phenomenon of the facet joint L5-S1 and eburnation of the subarticular bone. **(B)** CT section through both facets clearly demonstrates the presence of gas, as confirmed by the Hounsfield values. These units are related to the attenuation coefficient for various tissues in the body and represent absorption values directly related to tissue density. Note also the hypertrophic spur arising from the right facet and encroaching on the spinal canal.

eburnation of
subarticular bone

vacuum phenomenon

Figure 13.27 Osteoarthritis of the sacroiliac joints. (A) Degenerative changes in the sacroiliac joints, seen here affecting predominantly the right sacroiliac joint in an 82-year-old woman, are manifested by narrowing of the joint space and osteophytosis. **(B)** In another patient, a 68-year-old man, osteoarthritis of both sacroiliac joints is demonstrated on axial CT image.

Figure 13.28 Sacroiliac joints. The true diarthrodial portion of the sacroiliac joint comprises only approximately 50% of the radiographic joint space. The upper part is a syndesmotic joint.

Figure 13.29 Degenerative disk disease. Lateral radiograph of the lumbosacral spine in a 66-year-old woman demonstrates advanced degenerative disk disease at multiple levels. Note the radiolucent collections of gas in several disks (the vacuum phenomenon) as well as the narrowing of the disk spaces and marginal osteophytes. Grade 1 degenerative spondylolisthesis is seen at the L4-5 level.

Figure 13.30 MRI of degenerative disk disease. Sagittal T2-weighted MR image shows early degenerative changes in the T12-L1, L1-2, and L2-3 intervertebral disks (*arrows*), more advanced process in the L3-4 disk, and severe degenerative disk disease at L4-5 and L5-S1. At the latter levels, markedly decreased intervertebral spaces and low signal intensity of degenerated disks are seen.

age of the intervertebral disk to the vertebral body at the site where Sharpey fibers attach to the vertebral rim. Unlike degenerative disk disease, the intervertebral spaces in spondylosis deformans are relatively well-preserved, with the primary radiographic feature being extensive osteophytosis (Fig. 13.33). These osteophytes must be differentiated from the delicate syndesmophytes of ankylosing spondylitis, from the large characteristically asymmetric bone excrescences that are seen in psoriatic arthritis and Reiter syndrome involving the lateral aspect of vertebral bodies, and from the flowing, usually anterior, hyperostosis of the DISH syndrome.

Diffuse Idiopathic Skeletal Hyperostosis

Diffuse idiopathic skeletal hyperostosis (DISH), originally described by Forestier and popularized by Resnick, is characterized by flowing ossification along the anterior aspect of the vertebral bodies extending across the disk spaces. It is also associated with hyperostosis at the sites of tendon and ligament attachments to the bone, ligament ossification, and osteophytosis involving the axial and appendicular skeleton. A lateral radiograph of the spine best demonstrates these changes. As in spondylosis deformans, the disk spaces are usually well-preserved (Fig. 13.34). It is important to distinguish this condition from the apparently similar "bamboo spine" seen in ankylosing spondylitis (see Fig. 14.31).

Figure 13.31 MRI of degenerative disk disease. A type I vertebral end-plate change (*arrows*) demonstrates a focus of low signal intensity in subchondral marrow on a T1-weighted sagittal MRI **(A)** and a high signal intensity on T2* weighting **(B)**.

A   **B**

Figure 13.32 MRI of degenerative disk disease. Type II end-plate changes in degenerative disk disease consisting of focal areas of yellow marrow conversion (*arrows*) are seen on a sagittal T1-weighted MR image.

Figure 13.33 Spondylosis deformans. Anteroposterior projection of the lumbosacral spine in a 68-year-old woman exhibits the typical changes of spondylosis deformans. Note the extensive osteophytosis and relatively well-preserved intervertebral disk spaces.

Figure 13.34 Diffuse idiopathic skeletal hyperostosis. Lateral radiographs of the cervical (**A**), thoracic (**B**), and lumbar (**C**) spine in a 72-year-old man with Forestier disease (DISH) show the characteristic flowing hyperostosis extending across the vertebral disk spaces, which are relatively well-preserved.

Complications of Degenerative Disease of the Spine

Degenerative Spondylolisthesis

One of the most common complications of degenerative disease of the spine, degenerative spondylolisthesis, results from degenerative changes in the disk and apophyseal joints. In this condition, there is anterior displacement of a vertebra onto the one below, which usually is easily recognized on the lateral view of the spine by the spinous-process sign (Fig. 13.35; see also Fig. 11.69). However, on occasion, the displacement may not be obvious on the standard lateral film, and radiographs must be obtained while the patient maximally extends and flexes the spine (Fig. 13.36). As Milgram pointed out, the stress applied by forward and backward motion of the spine discloses instability (spondylolisthesis), which may be overlooked on other projections.

Degenerative spondylolisthesis occurs in approximately 4% of patients with degenerative disk disease and affects women more frequently than men. It has a predilection for the L4-5 spinal level. This predilection has been attributed to developmental or acquired alterations in the neural arch that lead to instability and abnormal stress. The stress applied to the vertebra may result in decompensation of the

ligaments, hypermobility, instability, and osteoarthritis of adjacent apophyseal joints.

Clinical symptoms associated with degenerative spondylolisthesis include low back pain with or without radiation into the leg, sciatic pain with signs of nerve root compression, and intermittent claudication of the cauda equina. It should be noted, however, that many patients with degenerative spondylolisthesis are asymptomatic.

Radiographic findings of degenerative spondylolisthesis include osteoarthritic changes of the facet joints (joint narrowing, marginal eburnation, and osteophyte formation), anterior slippage of the superior vertebra on the inferior vertebra, and, in many instances, intervertebral vacuum phenomenon (see Fig. 13.29). Invariably, the affected intervertebral disk space is narrowed. CT may also effectively demonstrate this complication (Fig. 13.37).

The intervertebral vacuum phenomenon associated with degenerative disk disease should not be confused with the intravertebral vacuum cleft sign. This sign appears on radiographs as a transverse, linear, or semilunar radiolucency located within the vertebral body. According to recent reports, this sign represents gas (principally nitrogen) in the fracture line of the vertebral body. Although the pathogenesis of this process is not completely clear, the sign is most sugges-

Figure 13.35 Degenerative spondylolisthesis. A 55-year-old woman with degenerative disk disease at L4-5 and degenerative facet arthritis developed spondylolisthesis, a common complication of this condition. Lateral radiograph of the lumbosacral spine is sufficient to differentiate this condition from spondylolisthesis associated with spondylolysis by the appearance of a step-off of the spinous process at the vertebra below the involved intervertebral space (see Fig. 11.69).

Figure 13.36 Degenerative spondylolisthesis. A 50-year-old man presented with chronic low back pain. **(A)** Standard lateral view of the lumbosacral spine in the neutral position shows narrowing of the L4-5 disk space, indicating degenerative disk disease. There is no evidence of vertebral list. **(B)** Lateral radiograph in flexion, however, demonstrates grade 1 spondylolisthesis at L4-5.

Figure 13.37 Degenerative spondylolisthesis and spinal stenosis. (A) Axial CT of a 70-year-old woman with chronic low back pain shows the vacuum phenomenon at the disk level L5-S1. **(B)** Sagittal reformatted image demonstrates degenerative disk disease at L5-S1 associated with a vacuum phenomenon and spondylolisthesis. There is also evidence of spinal stenosis at the S-1 level.

tive of ischemic necrosis of bone. This phenomenon has been also reported in association with Kümmell disease, a delayed posttraumatic collapse of the vertebral body (Fig. 13.38).

Spinal Stenosis

Spinal stenosis is a much more severe complication of degenerative disease of the spine. In its acquired form, it results from hypertrophy of the structures surrounding the spinal canal, such as the pedicles, laminae, articular processes, and posterior aspect of the vertebral bodies, as well as the ligamentum flavum. These alternations usually are apparent on plain film radiography; however, spinal stenosis can be better demonstrated by ancillary techniques. Spinal stenosis can be demonstrated by myelography, which can show the impingement of

the thecal sac by hypertrophic changes of the posterior parts of the vertebral body and bulging disks, but CT best delineates its details (Fig. 13.39). Magnetic resonance imaging is also an effective modality in this respect (Fig. 13.40).

Spinal stenosis in the lumbar segment can be divided into three groups on the basis of its anatomic location: stenosis of the spinal canal, stenosis of the subarticular or lateral recesses, and stenosis of the neural foramina.

The causes of stenosis of the central canal are related to hypertrophic changes of osteoarthritis of the apophyseal joints, thickening of the ligamentum flavum, and osteophytes arising from the vertebral bodies. Bone hypertrophy at the site of the facet joints is a major cause of stenosis of the subarticular or lateral recesses, leading to encroachment on the neural elements in this region. Clinical manifestations of lateral recess syndrome include unilateral or bilateral leg pain, which is initiated or aggravated by long periods of standing or walking. These symptoms are usually relieved entirely by sitting or squatting.

The stenosis of the neural foramina is caused by hypertrophic changes and osteophytosis involving the vertebral body and articular process. Moreover, degenerative spondylolisthesis may be associated with distortion of the intervertebral foramen and may lead to compromise of the exiting nerve.

Neuropathic Arthropathy

This acute or chronic destructive arthritis, also known as Charcot joint, is grouped with other degenerative joint diseases because it exhibits manifestations similar to those seen in other forms of osteoarthritis—destruction of articular cartilage, subchondral sclerosis, and marginal osteophytosis—but in their most severe form. Neuropathic arthropathy comprises a spectrum of destructive processes in the joint associated with neurosensory deficit. Pathognomonic for neuropathic joints are fragmentation of the bone and cartilage, which are discharged as debris into the joint; chronic synovitis with accumulation of varying amounts of fluid in the joint; and joint instability manifested by subluxation and dislocation (Fig. 13.41). Underlying conditions leading to neuropathic joint include, among others, diabetes mellitus, syphilis, leprosy, syringomyelia, congenital indifference to pain, and spina bifida with meningomyelocele (Table 13.2). In diabetic patients, the condition has a greater predilection for the joints of the foot and ankle (Fig. 13.42); in pa-

Figure 13.38 Kümmell disease. Lateral radiograph of the lumbar spine shows posttraumatic collapse of the vertebral body of L-4 associated with intravertebral vacuum cleft sign (*arrow*).

Figure 13.39 Spinal stenosis. A 71-year-old woman was evaluated for severe low back pain. **(A)** Standard lateral radiograph of the lumbar spine shows degenerative spondylolisthesis at the L4-5 interspace. Note the short appearance of the pedicles. **(B)** Myelogram in the antero-posterior projection also discloses segmental narrowing of the thecal sac; the upper defect is related to spondylolisthesis, the lower to spinal stenosis. CT sections **(C, D)** demonstrate the details of the abnormalities—severe spinal and foraminal stenosis, hypertrophy of the ligamenta flava, and posterior bulging of the intervertebral disk. Note the cloverleaf configuration of the spinal canal secondary to marked hypertrophy of the facet joints. The vacuum phenomenon in the apophyseal joints is well demonstrated.

Figure 13.40 MRI of spinal stenosis. Degenerative changes of the facet joints and disk bulging contributed to central canal stenosis at the L4-5 disk level, as demonstrated here on T2*-weighted axial MR images.

Table 13.2 **Causes of Neuropathic Arthropathy**

Alcoholism	Multiple sclerosis
Amyloidosis	Peripheral nerve tumors
Charcot-Marie-Tooth disease	Pernicious anemia
Congential indifference to pain	Poliomyelitis
Diabetes mellitus	Spinal cord tumors
Extrinsic compression of	Steroids (systemic or
the spinal cord	intraarticular)
Familial dysautonomia	Syringomyelia
(Riley-Day syndrome)	Tabes dorsalis (syphilis)
Leprosy	Uremia
Meningomyelocele	

(Modified from Jones E.A. et al., 2000 with permission.)

Figure 13.42 Neuropathic joint. A 59-year-old woman with long-standing diabetes mellitus presented with neuropathic changes of left ankle joint, demonstrated here on the anteroposterior (**A**) and lateral (**B**) radiographs.

Figure 13.41 Neuropathic joint. Anteroposterior radiograph of the right hip of a 57-year-old woman with neurosyphilis (tabes dorsalis) shows the typical features of neuropathic (Charcot) joint. There is complete disorganization of the joint, fragmentation, and subluxation. The absence of osteoporosis is a characteristic feature of the neuropathic joint. This condition represents the most severe manifestation of degenerative joint disease.

Figure 13.43 Neuropathic joint. A 59-year-old woman with syringomyelia developed a neuropathic shoulder joint. Anteroposterior radiograph shows destruction of the joint, bony debris, and subluxation of the humeral head.

tients with syringomyelia, joints of the upper extremities are more commonly affected (Fig. 13.43). The eponym *Charcot joint* was originally reserved for neuropathic joint in syphilitic patients with tabes dorsalis (Fig. 13.44). Currently, this term applies to any joint displaying features of neuropathic arthropathy, regardless of the causative factor.

Figure 13.44 Neuropathic joint. A 62-year-old man with syphilis presented with a typical neuropathic (Charcot) knee joint.

PRACTICAL POINTS TO REMEMBER

Osteoarthritis
[1] Degenerative joint disease (osteoarthritis, osteoarthrosis, degenerative arthritis) is classified as primary (idiopathic) or secondary; in the latter, there is an underlying predisposing disorder.
[2] The radiographic hallmarks of osteoarthritis are:
  • diminution (narrowing) of the joint space
  • subchondral sclerosis
  • osteophytosis
  • cyst or pseudocyst formation
  • lack of pronounced osteoporosis.

Osteoarthritis of the Large Joints
[1] In the hip joint, the degenerative process results in migration of the femoral head, most commonly in a superolateral direction.
[2] Postel coxarthropathy is a rapidly destructive arthrosis of the hip joint, which radiographically can mimic infection or neuropathic joint.
[3] The medial femorotibial and femoropatteller compartments of the knee joint are commonly involved in osteoarthritis. Weight-bearing examination may reveal a varus configuration of the knee.
[4] The "tooth" sign of the patella, recognized on an axial view by vertical ridges at the insertion of the quadriceps tendon into the base of the patella, represents a type of degenerative change (enthesopathy) unrelated to femoropatellar osteoarthritis. It is commonly seen after the fifth decade of life.
[5] If the shoulder, elbow, or ankle joints are affected by degenerative joint disease, a diagnosis of secondary rather than primary osteoarthritis should be considered.

Osteoarthritis of the Small Joints
[1] In the hand, the hallmarks of primary degenerative joint disease are:
  • Heberden nodes affecting the distal interphalangeal joints
  • Bouchard nodes affecting the proximal interphalangeal joints.
[2] The first carpometacarpal articulation is frequently involved in primary degenerative joint disease.

Degenerative Disease of the Spine
[1] In the spine, degenerative changes may be present in four major forms:
  • as osteoarthritis of the synovial joints, including the atlantoaxial, apophyseal, costovertebral, and sacroiliac
  • as spondylosis deformans, a condition manifested by formation of anterior and lateral marginal osteophytes with preservation of the disk spaces (at least in the early stages)
  • as degenerative disk disease, a condition primarily involving the intervertebral disks and manifested by destruction of these structures, the vacuum phenomenon, and narrowing of the disk spaces
  • as diffuse idiopathic skeletal hyperostosis (DISH syndrome or Forestier disease), characterized by flowing ossifications along the anterior aspects of vertebral bodies extending across the disk spaces, relative preservation of the intervertebral disks, and hyperostosis at the sites of tendon and ligament attachment to the bone (enthesopathy).
[2] Two common conditions can complicate degenerative spine disease:
  • degenerative spondylolisthesis
  • spinal stenosis.
[3] Degenerative spondylolisthesis is marked by anterior (ventral) displacement of a vertebra onto the one below and recognized on the lateral view of the spine by the spinous-process sign.
[4] Spinal stenosis can readily be diagnosed using computed tomography or magnetic resonance imaging.

Neuropathic Arthropathy
[1] Neuropathic (Charcot) joint manifests with the same degenerative changes as osteoarthritis, but they are seen in their most severe form. This condition is also marked by:
  • fragmentation of the bone and cartilage, filling the joint with debris

- chronic synovitis with joint effusion
- joint instability with subluxation or dislocation.

[2] The underlying conditions leading to neuropathic joint include diabetes mellitus, syphilis, leprosy, syringomyelia, and congenital indifference to pain.

SUGGESTED READINGS

Adamson TC 3rd, Resnik CS, Guerra Jr J, Vint VC, Weisman MH, Resnick D. Hand and wrist arthropathies of hemochromatosis and calcium pyrophosphate deposition disease: distinct radiographic features. *Radiology* 1983;147:377–381.

Bennett GL, Leeson MC, Michael A. Extensive hemosiderin deposition in the medial meniscus of a knee. Its possible relationship to degenerative joint disease. *Clin Orthop* 1988;230:182–185.

Bhalla S, Reinus WR. The linear intravertebral vacuum: a sign of benign vertebral collapse. *AJR Am J Roentgenol* 1998;170:1563–1569.

Blackburn WD Jr, Chivers S, Bernreuter W. Cartilage imaging in osteoarthritis. *Semin Arthritis Rheum* 1996;25:273–281.

Bloem JL, Sartoris DJ, eds. *MRI and CT of the musculoskeletal system. A text-atlas.* Baltimore: Williams & Wilkins; 1992.

Bock GW, Garcia A, Weisman MH, et al. Rapidly destructive hip disease: clinical and imaging abnormalities. *Radiology* 1993;186:461–466.

Bora FW Jr, Miller G. Joint physiology, cartilage metabolism, and the etiology of osteoarthritis. *Hand Clin* 1987;3:325–336.

Boutry N, Paul C, Leroy X, Fredoux D, Migaud H, Cotten A. Rapidly destructive osteoarthritis of the hip: MR imaging findings. *AJR Am J Roentgenol* 2002;179:657–663.

Brandt KD. Osteoarthritis. *Clin Geriatr Med* 1988;4:279–293.

Braunstein EM, Brandt KD, Albrecht M. MRI demonstration of hypertrophic articular cartilage repair in osteoarthritis. *Skeletal Radiol* 1990;19:335–339.

Broderick LS, Turner DA, Renfrew DL, Schnitzer TJ, Huff JP, Harris C. Severity of articular cartilage abnormality in patients with osteoarthritis: evaluation with fast spin-echo MR vs arthroscopy. *AJR Am J Roentgenol* 1994;162:99–103.

Brower AC, Downey EF. Kümmell disease: report of a case with serial radiographs. *Radiology* 1981;141:363–364.

Buckwalter JA, Mankin HG. Articular cartilage. II. Degeneration and osteoarthritis, repair, regeneration, and transplantation. *J Bone Joint Surg [Am]* 1997;79A:612–632.

Buckwalter JA, Mow VC. Cartilage repair in osteoarthritis. In: Moskowitz RW, Howell DS, Goldberg VM, Mankin HJ, eds. *Osteoarthritis,* 2nd ed. Philadelphia: WB Saunders; 1992:71–107.

Bullough PG. The pathology of osteoarthritis. In: Moskowitz RW, Howell DS, Goldberg VM, Mankin HJ, eds. *Osteoarthritis,* 2nd ed. Philadelphia: WB Saunders; 1992:39–69.

Bullough PG, Bansal M. The differential diagnosis of geodes. *Radiol Clin North Am* 1988;26:1165–1184.

Chan WP, Lang P, Stevens MP, et al. Osteoarthritis of the knee: comparison of radiography, CT, and MR imaging to assess extent and severity. *AJR Am J Roentgenol* 1991;157:799–806.

Charcot JM. Sur quelques arthropathies qui paraissent dépendre d'une lesion du cerveau ou de la moëlle épindère. *Arch Physiol Norm Pathol* 1868;1:161–178.

Chou L, Knight R. Idiopathic avascular necrosis of a vertebral body: a case report and literature review. *Spine* 1997;22:1928–1932.

Cohn EL, Maurer EJ, Keats TE, Dussault RG, Kaplan PA. Plain film evaluation of degenerative disk disease at the lumbosacral junction. *Skeletal Radiol* 1997;26:161–166.

Cone RO, Resnick D. Degenerative disease of the shoulder. *Australas Radiol* 1984;28:232–239.

Danielsson L. Incidence and osteoarthritis of the hip (coxarthrosis). *Clin Orthop* 1966;45:67–72.

Davis MA. Epidemiology of osteoarthritis. *Clin Geriatr Med* 1988;4:241–255.

Della Torre P, Picuti G, Di Filippo P. Rapidly progressive osteoarthritis of the hip. *Ital J Orthop Traumatol* 1987;13:187–200.

Dieppe P, Cushnaghan J. The natural course and prognosis of osteoarthritis. In: Moskowitz RW, Howell DS, Goldberg VM, Mankin HJ, eds. *Osteoarthritis,* 2nd ed. Philadelphia: WB Saunders; 1992:399–412.

Epstein BS, Epstein JA, Jones MD. Lumbar spinal stenosis. *Radiol Clin North Am* 1977;15:227–239.

Erkintalo MO, Salminen JJ, Alanen AM, Paajanen HEK, Kormano MJ. Development of degenerative changes in the lumbar intervertebral disk: results of a prospective MR imaging study in adolescents with and without low-back pain. *Radiology* 1995;196:529–533.

Fairbank TJ. Knee joint changes after menisectomy. *J Bone Joint Surg [Br]* 1948;30B:664–670.

Felson DT. The course of osteoarthritis and factors that affect it. *Rheum Dis Clin North Am* 1993;19:607–615.

Forestier J, Rotes Querol J. Senile ankylosing hyperostosis of the spine. *Ann Rheum Dis* 1950;9:321–330.

Freeman MAR. Total replacement of the knee. *Orthop Rev* 1974;3:21–29.

Gibson MJ, Buckley J, Mawhinney RC, Mulholland RC, Worthington BS. Magnetic resonance imaging and discography in the diagnosis of disc degeneration. *J Bone Joint Surg [Br]* 1986;68B:369–373.

Golimbu C, Firooznia H, Rafii M. The intravertebral vacuum sign. *Spine* 1986;11:1040–1043.

Greenspan A, Norman A, Tchang FKM. "Tooth" sign in patellar degenerative disease. *J Bone Joint Surg [Am]* 1977;59A:483–485.

Grenier N, Grossman RI, Schiebler ML, Yeager BA, Goldberg HI, Kressel HY. Degenerative lumbar disk disease: pitfalls and usefulness of MR imaging in detection of vacuum phenomenon. *Radiology* 1987;164:861–865.

Harrison MH, Schajowicz F, Trueta J. Osteoarthritis of the hip: a study of the nature and evolution of the disease. *J Bone Joint Surg [Br]* 1953;35B:598–629.

Hayward I, Bjorkengren AG, Pathria MN, Zlatkin MB, Sartoris DJ, Resnick D. Patterns of femoral head migration in osteoarthritis of the hip: A reappraisal with CT and pathologic correlation. *Radiology* 1988;166:857–860.

Hill CL, Gale DG, Chaisson CE, et al. Knee effusions, popliteal cysts, and synovial thickening: association with knee pain in osteoarthritis. *J Rheumatol* 2001;28:1330–1337.

Howell DS, Altman RD. Cartilage repair and conservation in osteoarthritis. *Rheum Dis Clin North Am* 1993;19:713–724.

Jones EA, Manaster BJ, May DA, Disler DG. Neuropathic osteoarthropathy: diagnostic dilemmas and differential diagnosis. *Radiographics* 2000;20:S279–S293.

Karvonen RL, Negendank WG, Teitge RA, Reed AH, Miller PR, Fernandez-Madrid F. Factors affecting articular cartilage thickness in osteoarthritis. *J Rheumatol* 1994;21:1310–1318.

Kellgren JH, Moore R. Generalized osteoarthritis and Heberden's nodes. *BMJ* 1952;1:181–187.

Kerr R, Resnick D, Pineda C, Haghighi P. Osteoarthritis of the glenohumeral joint: a radiologic-pathologic study. *AJR Am J Roentgenol* 1985;144:967–972.

Kirkaldy-Willis WH, Farfan HF. Instability of the lumbar spine. *Clin Orthop* 1982;165:110–123.

Knutsson F. The vacuum phenomenon in the intervertebral discs. *Acta Radiol* 1942;23:173–175.

Kumpan W, Salomonowitz E, Seidl G, Wittich GR. The intervertebral vacuum phenomenon. *Skeletal Radiol* 1986;15:444–447.

Lawrance JAL, Athanasou NA. Rapidly destructive hip disease. *Skeletal Radiol* 1995;24:639–641.

Leach RE, Gregg T, Siber FJ. Weight-bearing radiography in osteoarthritis of the knee. *Radiology* 1970;97:265–268.

Lee SH, Coleman PE, Hahn FJ. Magnetic resonance imaging of degenerative disk disease of the spine. *Radiol Clin North Am* 1988;26:949–964.

Lefkowitz DM, Quencer RM. Vacuum facet phenomenon: a computed tomographic sign of degenerative spondylolisthesis. *Radiology* 1982;144:562.

Lequesne M. La coxarthrose destructrice rapide. *Rhumatologie* 1970;22:51–63.

Lequesne MG, Laredo J-D. The faux profil (oblique view) of the hip in the standing position. Contribution to the evaluation of osteoarthritis of the adult hip. *Ann Rheum Dis* 1998;57:676–681.

Link TM, Steinbach LS, Ghosh S, Ries M, Lu Y, Lane N, Majumdar S. Osteoarthritis: MR imaging findings in different stages of disease and correlation with clinical findings. *Radiology* 2003;226:373–381.

Maldague BE, Noel HM, Malghem JJ. The intravertebral vacuum cleft: a sign of ischemic vertebral collapse. *Radiology* 1978;129:23–29.

Mankin HJ, Brandt KD. Biochemistry and metabolism of articular cartilage in osteoarthritis. In: Moskowitz RW, Howell DS, Goldberg VM. Mankin HJ, eds. *Osteoarthritis,* 2nd ed. Philadelphia: WB Saunders; 1992:109–154.

Martel W, Snarr JW, Horn JR. The metacarpophalangeal joints in interphalangeal osteoarthritis. *Radiology* 1973;108:1–7.

McAfee PC, Ullrich CG, Yuan HA, Cacayorill ED, Lockwood RC. Computed tomography in degenerative lumbar spinal stenosis: the value of multiplanar reconstruction. *Radiographics* 1982;2:529–537.

McCauley TR, Disler DG. Magnetic resonance imaging of articular cartilage of the knee. *J Am Acad Orthop Surg* 2001;9:2–8.

Milgram JE. Recurrent articular spondylolisthesis: common cause of vertebral instabilities, root pain, sciatica, and ultimately spinal stenosis. Early detection and blocking of specific dislocations. *Bull Hosp Joint Dis Orthop Inst* 1986;46:47–51.

Modic MT, Masaryk TJ, Ross JS, Carter JR. Imaging of degenerative disk disease. *Radiology* 1988;168:177–186.

Modic MT, Steinberg PM, Ross JS, Masaryk TJ, Carter JR. Degenerative disk disease: assessment of changes in vertebral body marrow with MR imaging. *Radiology* 1988;166:193–199.

Norman A, Robbins H, Milgram JE. The acute neuropathic arthropathy—a rapid severely disorganizing form of arthritis. *Radiology* 1968;90:1159–1164.

Pathria M, Sartoris DJ, Resnick D. Osteoarthritis of the facet joints: accuracy of oblique radiographic assessment. *Radiology* 1987;164:227–230.

Pepper HW, Noonan CD. Radiographic evaluation of total hip arthroplasty. *Radiology* 1973;108:23–29.

Peyron JG. Epidemiologic and etiologic approach of osteoarthritis. *Semin Arthritis Rheum* 1979;8:288–306.

Peyron JG, Altman RD. The epidemiology of osteoarthritis. In: Moskowitz RW, Howell DS, Goldberg VM, Mankin HJ, eds. *Osteoarthritis,* 2nd ed. Philadelphia: WB Saunders; 1992:15–37.

Postel M, Kerboull M. Total prosthetic replacement in rapidly destructive arthrosis of the hip joint. *Clin Orthop* 1970;72:138–144.

Pritzker KP. Aging and degeneration in the lumbar intervertebral disc. *Orthop Clin North Am* 1977;8:66–77.

Resnick D. Degenerative diseases of the vertebral column. *Radiology* 1985;156:3–14.

Resnick D. Patterns of migration of the femoral head in osteoarthritis of the hip. Roentgenographic-pathologic correlation and comparison with rheumatoid arthritis. *AJR Am J Roentgenol* 1975;124:62–74.

Resnick D, Niwayama G. Degenerative disease of extraspinal locations. In: Resnick D, ed. *Diagnosis of bone and joint disorders,* 3rd ed. Philadelphia: WB Saunders; 1995:1263–1371.

Resnick D, Niwayama G. Entheses and enthesopathy. Anatomical, pathological and radiological correlation. *Radiology* 1983;146:1–9.

Resnick D, Niwayama G. Diffuse idiopathic skeletal hyperostosis (DISH): ankylosing hyperostosis of Forestier and Rotes-Querol. In: Resnick D, ed. *Diagnosis of bone and joint disorders,* 3rd ed. Philadelphia: WB Saunders; 1995:1463–1495.

Resnick D, Niwayama G, Coutts RD. Subchondral cysts (geodes) in arthritic disorders: pathologic and radiographic appearance of the hip joint. *AJR Am J Roentgenol* 1977; 128:799–806.

Resnick D, Niwayama G, Goergen TG. Degenerative disease of the sacroiliac joint. *Invest Radiol* 1975;10:608–621.

Resnick D, Shaul SR, Robins JM. Diffuse idiopathic skeletal hyperostosis (DISH). Forestier's disease with extraspinal manifestations. *Radiology* 1975;115:513–524.

Rosenberg ZS, Shankman S, Steiner GC, Kastenbaum DK, Norman A, Lazansky MG. Rapid destructive osteoarthritis: clinical, radiographic, and pathologic features. *Radiology* 1992;182:213–216.

Ross JS, Modic MT, Masaryk TJ, Carter J, Marcus RE, Bohlman H. Assessment of extradural degenerative disease with Gd DTPA-enhanced MR imaging: correlation with surgical and pathologic findings. *AJNR* 1989;10:1243–1249.

Rubenstein JD, Li JG, Majumdar S, Henkelman RM. Image resolution and signal-to-noise ratio requirements for MR imaging of degenerative cartilage. *AJR Am J Roentgenol* 1997;169:1089–1096.

Schiebler ML, Grenier N, Fallon M, Camerino V, Zlatkin M, Kressel HY. Normal and degenerated intervertebral disk: in vivo and in vitro MR imaging with histopathologic correlation. *AJR Am J Roentgenol* 1991;157:93–97.

Schmorl G, Junghanns H. *The human spine in health and disease,* 2nd ed. New York: Grune & Stratton; 1971.

Schumacher HR. Articular cartilage in the degenerative arthropathy of hemochromatosis. *Arthritis Rheum* 1982;25:1460–1468.

Sokoloff L. Pathology and pathogenesis of osteoarthritis. In: Hollander JL, McCarty DJ, eds. *Arthritis and allied conditions,* 8th ed. Philadelphia: Lea & Febiger; 1972:1009–1031.

Stoller DW, Cannon WD Jr, Anderson LJ. The knee. In: *Magnetic resonance imaging in orthopaedics & sports medicine.* Philadelphia: JB Lippincott; 1993:139–372.

Theodorou DJ. The intravertebral vacuum cleft sign. *Radiology* 2001;221:787–788.

Waldschmidt JG, Braunstein EM, Buckwalter KA. Magnetic resonance imaging of osteoarthritis. *Rheum Dis Clin North Am* 1999;25:451–465.

Watt I, Dieppe P. Osteoarthritis revisited. *Skeletal Radiol* 1990;19:1–3.

Weber BG. Total hip replacement: rotating versus fixed and metal versus ceramic heads. In: Salvati EA, ed. *The hip. Proceedings of the Ninth Open Scientific Meeting of the Hip Society, 1981.* St. Louis: CV Mosby; 1981:264–275.

Weisz GM. Value of computerised tomography in diagnosis of diseases of the lumbar spine. *Med J Aust* 1982;1:216–219.

Weisz GM, Lee P. Spinal reserve capacity. A radiologic concept of lumbar canal stenosis. *Orthop Rev* 1984;13:579–582.

Weisz GM, Lee P. Spinal canal stenosis. *Clin Orthop* 1983;179:134–140.

Yazici H, Saville PD, Salvati EA, Bohne WH, Wilson PD Jr. Primary osteoarthritis of the knee or hip. Prevalence of Heberden nodes in relation to age and sex. *JAMA* 1975;231:1256–1260.

Yu SW, Haughton VM, Ho PS, Sether LA, Wagner M, Ho KC. Progressive and regressive changes in the nucleus pulposus. *Radiology* 1988;169:93–97.

Yu SW, Haughton VM, Lynch KL, Ho KC, Sether LA. Fibrous structure in the intervertebral disk correlation of MR appearance with anatomic sections. *AJNR* 1989;10:1105–1110.

INFLAMMATORY ARTHRITIDES

The inflammatory arthritides comprise a group of different and for the most part systemic disorders (see Fig. 12.1) that have in common one important feature: inflammatory pannus eroding articular cartilage and bone (Fig. 14.1). An overview of the clinical and radiographic hallmarks of the various inflammatory arthritides is shown in Table 14.1.

Erosive Osteoarthritis

Erosive osteoarthritis was first described by Kellgren and Moore in 1952 and reintroduced in 1961 by Crain, who called it *interphalangeal osteoarthritis*. He defined this disorder as a localized variant of osteoarthritis involving the finger joints, characterized by degenerative changes with intermittent inflammatory episodes leading to deformities and ankylosis. In 1966, Peter and Pearson coined the term *erosive osteoarthritis,* and Ehrlich in 1972 described it as *inflammatory osteoarthritis*. It can be defined as a progressive disorder of the interphalangeal joints with severe synovitis, superimposed on the changes of

degenerative joint disease. Although the cause is still unclear, several investigators have suggested hormonal influences, metabolic background, autoimmunity, and heredity as being involved.

Erosive osteoarthritis is a progressive inflammatory arthritis seen predominantly in middle-aged women. Only rarely are men affected, with an estimated female-to-male ratio of 12:1. Patients' ages range from 36 to 83 years, and mean age of onset is 50.5 years. This condition combines certain clinical manifestations of rheumatoid arthritis with certain radiographic features of degenerative joint disease. Involvement is limited to the hands, with the proximal and distal interphalangeal joints being the most frequently affected. Large joints, such as the hip or shoulder, are only rarely involved. The arthritis usually begins abruptly and is characterized by pain, swelling, and tenderness of the small joints of the hands. Also described are throbbing paresthesias of the fingertips and morning stiffness.

In the early stage of the disease, the main feature is symmetric synovitis of the interphalangeal joints. Later, this is followed by articular erosions, which exhibit a characteristic radiographic feature named the "gull-wing" deformity by Martel. This configuration is seen

Figure 14.1 Inflammatory arthritides. Highlights of the morphology and distribution of arthritic lesions in the inflammatory arthritides.

as a result of central erosion and marginal proliferation of bone (Fig. 14.2); Heberden nodes may also be present. Periosteal reaction taking the form of linear or fluffy bone apposition over the cortex near the affected joints is occasionally observed. Swelling of soft tissue, usually fusiform, may be present around involved articulations (Fig. 14.2 B and C); however, periarticular osteoporosis is rarely present. Later in the disease process, bone ankylosis of the phalanges may develop. Approximately 15% of patients with erosive osteoarthritis may have clinical, laboratory, and radiographic manifestations of rheumatoid arthritis (Fig. 14.3). The exact relationship between these two conditions is still unclear. Some investigators believe that erosive osteoarthritis is actually rheumatoid arthritis originating in unusual sites but subsequently progressing to the articulations that are more typically involved. Others suggest that each is a distinct entity, citing as evidence the fact that the synovial fluid of patients with rheumatoid arthritis does not resemble that of patients with erosive osteoarthritis, that the immunologic abnormalities commonly seen in rheumatoid arthritis are absent in the latter condition, and that the serologic test for rheumatoid factor is negative.

Occasionally, a variant of erosive osteoarthritis may be seen as one of the features of Cronkhite-Canada syndrome. This rare systemic disorder also manifests with generalized gastrointestinal polyposis, hyperpigmentation of the skin, and nail atrophy.

Treatment

The main objective of therapy in patients with inflammatory erosive osteoarthritis is relief of pain and restoration of joint function. Nonpharmacologic therapy includes physical and occupational therapy. Range-of-motion exercises and moist heat, in the form of a paraffin bath, are helpful. Pharmacologic methods include analgesics, nonsteroidal antiinflammatory drugs, and corticosteroids. Selected cases

have also been treated with methotrexate and oral gold salts. Surgical intervention is often necessary for the relief of persistent pain and the correction of severe deformities. One of the most effective procedures is joint replacement by means of silicone–rubber arthroplasties (Fig. 14.3B). The indications for this type of surgery are loss of the joint space, synovial proliferation with joint destruction, loss of normal alignment, and uncontrollable pain.

Rheumatoid Arthritis

Adult Rheumatoid Arthritis

Rheumatoid arthritis is a progressive, chronic, systemic inflammatory disease affecting primarily the synovial joints; women are affected three-times more often than men. The course of the disease varies from patient to patient, and there is a striking tendency toward spontaneous remissions and exacerbations. The detection of rheumatoid factor, representing specific antibodies in the patient's serum, is an important diagnostic finding. Although it is still debatable, some investigators also include under this rubric a condition called *seronegative rheumatoid arthritis* (see later), in which patients present without rheumatoid factor but with the clinical and radiographic picture of rheumatoid arthritis.

Rheumatoid Factors

Rheumatoid factors, so widely used by clinicians, are anti-gamma-globulin antibodies that are elaborated in part by rheumatoid synovium. Rheumatoid factors in synovial fluid are either of the IgG or of the IgM variety. They combine with their antigens (immunoglobulin G [IgG]) to form immune complexes. These complexes activate the complement system, which releases mediators responsive for produc-

Table 14.1 **Clinical and Radiographic Hallmarks of Inflammatory Arthritides**

Type of Arthritis	Site	Crucial Abnormalities	Technique*/Projection

Erosive osteoarthritis (F; middle age)	Hands	Involvement of:
		    Proximal interphalangeal joints
		    Distal interphalangeal joints
		Gull-wing deformities associated with erosions
		Heberden nodes
		Joint ankylosis
			Dorsovolar view

Rheumatoid arthritis (F>M; presence of rheumatoid factor and DRW4)	Hands and wrists	Involvement of:
		    Metacarpophalangeal joints
		    Proximal interphalangeal joints
		Central and marginal erosions
		Periarticular osteoporosis
			Dorsovolar view

		Joint deformities: swan-neck, boutonnière, main-en-lorgnette, hitchhiker's thumb	Dorsovolar and lateral views
	Hip	Narrowing of joint space Erosions Acetabular protrusio	Anteroposterior and lateral views
	Knee	Narrowing of joint space Synovial cysts Erosions	Anteroposterior and lateral views
	Ankle and foot	Involvement of subtalar joint	Anteroposterior and lateral views Lateral and Broden views
		Erosions of calcaneus	Lateral view (heel)
Juvenile rheumatoid arthritis	Hands	Joint ankylosis Periosteal reaction Growth abnormalities	Dorsovolar view (wrist and hand)
	Knees	Growth abnormalities	Anteroposterior and lateral views
	Cervical spine	Fusion of apophyseal joints	Anteroposterior, lateral, and oblique views
Rheumatoid variants		C1–2 subluxation	Lateral view in flexion
Ankylosing spondylitis (M>F; young adult; 95% positive for HLA-B27)	Spine	Squaring of vertebral bodies Syndesmophytes "Bamboo" spine Paravertebral ossifications	Anteroposterior and lateral views
	Sacroiliac joints	Inflammatory changes Fusion	Posteroanterior and Ferguson views
	Pelvis	Whiskering of iliac crests and ischial tuberosity	Anteroposterior view
Reiter syndrome (M > F)	Foot	Involvement of great toe articulations Erosions of calcaneus	Anteroposterior and lateral views
	Spine	Single, coarse syndesmophyte	Anteroposterior and lateral views
	Sacroiliac joints	Unilateral or bilateral but asymmetric involvement	Posteroanterior and Ferguson views
Psoriatic arthritis (M ≥ F; skin changes; HLA-B27 positive)	Hands	Involvement of distal interphalangeal joints Erosion of terminal tufts Mouse-ear erosions Pencil-in-cup deformities Sausage digit Joint ankylosis Fluffy periosteal reaction	Dorsovolar view
	Foot	Involvement of distal interphalangeal joints Erosions of terminal tufts and calcaneus	Anteroposterior and lateral views (ankle and foot)
	Spine	Single, coarse syndesmophyte	Anteroposterior and lateral views
	Sacroiliac joints	Unilateral or bilateral but asymmetric involvement	Posteroanterior and Ferguson views
Enteropathic Arthropathies	Sacroiliac joints	Symmetric involvement	Posteroanterior and Ferguson views Computed tomography

*Radionuclide bone scan is used to determine the distribution of arthritic lesions in the skeleton.

ing inflammation within the joint structures. Because rheumatoid factors can be found in the joint fluids of patients with nonrheumatoid disorders, their presence alone is not diagnostic of rheumatoid arthritis. However, finding high titers of these factors in a joint effusion strongly suggests the diagnosis of rheumatoid arthritis. Early in the course of disease, rheumatoid factors may be demonstrated in the synovial fluid before they are positive in the serum, allowing early diagnosis.

Rheumatoid factors participate in the pathogenesis of rheumatoid arthritis through the formation of local and circulating antigen–antibody complexes. In synovial fluid, IgM and IgG rheumatoid factors can combine with antigen (IgG) to form immune complexes. The complement system is activated, resulting in the attraction of polymorphonuclear leukocytes into the joint space. Discharge of their hydrolytic enzymes causes destruction of joint tissues. The process initiating these events is as yet unknown.

Rheumatoid factors are not, however, absolutely diagnostic of rheumatoid arthritis and are found in the synovial fluid and serum in approximately 70% to 80% of patients with a clinical diagnosis of rheumatoid arthritis. In rheumatoid arthritis of recent onset, the test for rheumatoid factors initially may be negative in serum or synovial fluid, but later may become positive. Patients who are seropositive at

Figure 14.2 Erosive osteoarthritis. (A) Dorsovolar film of the left hand of a 48-year-old woman with erosive osteoarthritis shows the typical involvement of the proximal and distal interphalangeal joints. Note the "gull-wing" pattern of articular erosion, a configuration resulting from peripheral bone erosion in the distal side of the joint and central erosion in the proximal side of the joint associated with marginal bone proliferation. **(B)** Dorsovolar radiograph of the left thumb of a 51-year-old woman shows characteristic "gull-wing" erosion of the interphalangeal joint. Note adjacent fusiform soft tissue swelling and lack of periarticular osteoporosis. **(C)** In another patient, a 50-year-old woman, "gull-wing" erosion is accompanied by periosteal reaction and fusiform soft tissue swelling.

the onset of their disease will often sustain persistent disease activity and disability. Patients with rheumatoid arthritis with subcutaneous nodules almost always will have positive agglutination tests, generally in high titer.

Radiographic Features

Rheumatoid arthritis is characterized by a diffuse, usually multicompartmental, symmetric narrowing of the joint space associated with marginal or central erosions, periarticular osteoporosis, and periarticular soft-tissue swelling; subchondral sclerosis is minimal or absent and formation of osteophytes is lacking.

Large Joint Involvement

Any of the large weight-bearing and non-weight-bearing joints can be affected by rheumatoid arthritis. Regardless of the size of the joint and the site of involvement, certain radiographic features can be identified that are characteristic of this inflammatory process.

Osteoporosis. In rheumatoid arthritis, unlike osteoarthritis, osteoporosis is a striking feature. In the early stage of the disease, osteoporosis is localized to periarticular areas, but with progression of the condition a generalized osteoporosis can be observed.

Joint Space Narrowing. This is usually a symmetric process with concentric narrowing of the joint. In the knee, all three joint com-

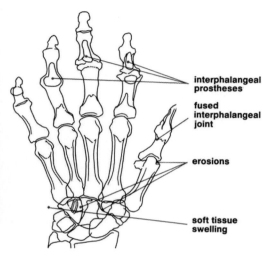

Figure 14.3 Progression of erosive osteoarthritis into rheumatoid arthritis. (A) Dorsovolar radiograph of the hand of a 58-year-old woman demonstrates the gull-wing configuration of erosive changes in the proximal interphalangeal joints and the distal interphalangeal joint of the small finger. Because of protracted pain and lack of response to conservative treatment, she underwent joint resection followed by implantation of silicone–rubber prostheses in the proximal interphalangeal joints of the index, middle, and ring fingers, together with fusion of the interphalangeal joint of the thumb and the distal interphalangeal joint of the small finger. Five years after surgery, the classic radiographic features of rheumatoid arthritis developed, involving the wrists **(B)**, elbows, shoulders, hips, and cervical spine. Note the surgical fusion of interphalangeal joints of the thumb and fifth finger, as well as the spontaneous fusion of the distal interphalangeal joints of the index and ring fingers.

partments are involved (Fig. 14.4). Concentric narrowing in the hip joint leads to axial migration of the femoral head, which in more advanced stages may result in acetabular protrusio (Fig. 14.5). Cephalad migration of the humeral head may also be seen secondary to destructive changes in the shoulder joint and rupture of the rotator cuff (Fig. 14.6); resorption of the distal end of the clavicle, which assumes a pencil-like appearance, may also be observed. Tear of the rotator cuff in this condition must be differentiated from the chronic traumatic form of this abnormality (see Fig. 5.52).

Articular Erosions. Erosive destruction of a joint may be central or peripheral in location. As a rule, reparative processes are absent or very minimal; thus, there is no evidence of subchondral sclerosis or osteophytosis (Fig. 14.7), which may be present only if secondary degenerative changes are superimposed on the underlying inflammatory process (see Fig. 13.5).

Synovial Cysts and Pseudocysts. These radiolucent defects are usually seen in close proximity to the joint (Fig. 14.8). They may or may not communicate with the joint space.

Joint Effusion. Fluid can be best demonstrated in the knee joint on the lateral projection (see Fig. 14.4B). Fluid in the other large joints such as the shoulder, elbow, and hip can be best demonstrated by magnetic resonance imaging.

Figure 14.4 Rheumatoid arthritis. Anteroposterior **(A)** and lateral **(B)** radiographs of the knee of a 52-year-old woman with rheumatoid arthritis affecting several joints show tricompartmental involvement. Note the periarticular osteoporosis, joint effusion, and lack of osteophytosis.

Figure 14.5 Rheumatoid arthritis. (A) Anteroposterior radiograph of the right hip of a 60-year-old woman with advanced rheumatoid arthritis shows concentric joint space narrowing, with axial migration of the femoral head leading to acetabular protrusion. **(B)** Anteroposterior radiograph of the left hip of a 64-year-old woman shows erosions of the femoral head and acetabulum, concentric narrowing of the hip joint, and acetabular protrusion.

Figure 14.6 Rheumatoid arthritis. Anteroposterior view of the right shoulder of a 72-year-old man with advanced rheumatoid arthritis shows upward migration of the humeral head secondary to rotator cuff tear, a common complication of rheumatoid changes in the shoulder joint. Note the characteristic tapered erosion of the distal end of the clavicle, erosions of the humeral head, and the substantial degree of periarticular osteoporosis.

Figure 14.7 Rheumatoid arthritis. Anteroposterior view of the left hip of a 59-year-old woman with advanced rheumatoid polyarthritis demonstrates the typical erosions of the femoral head and acetabulum. Note the lack of osteophytosis and the only very minimal reactive sclerosis.

Figure 14.8 Rheumatoid cyst. Anteroposterior radiograph of the left knee of a 35-year-old woman with rheumatoid arthritis shows a large synovial cyst in the proximal tibia. Note also articular erosions and periarticular osteoporosis.

Small Joint Involvement

Rheumatoid arthritis characteristically affects the small joints of the wrist, as well as the metacarpophalangeal and proximal interphalangeal joints of the hands and feet (Fig. 14.9). As a rule, the distal interphalangeal joints in the hand are spared, although in advanced stages of the disease even these may be affected. This latter point, however, is controversial, because some investigators believe that if the distal interphalangeal joints are involved, the condition may represent juvenile rheumatoid arthritis or another form of polyarthritis, not classic rheumatoid arthritis.

In addition to the characteristic changes exhibited in large joint involvement, the small joints may also show radiographic features specific for these sites.

Soft-Tissue Swelling. This earliest sign of rheumatoid arthritis usually has a fusiform, symmetric shape. It is periarticular in location and represents a combination of joint effusion, edema, and tenosynovitis.

Marginal Erosions. The earliest articular changes manifest as marginal erosions at so-called bare areas. These are the sites within the small joints that are not covered by articular cartilage. The most common locations for these erosions are the radial aspects of the second

Figure 14.9 Rheumatoid arthritis of the small joints. Radiographs of the hand **(A)** and foot **(B)** of a 51-year-old woman with rheumatoid arthritis show typical erosions of the small joints.

Figure 14.10 **Rheumatoid arthritis.** Typical erosions in the bare areas are seen in this 55-year-old woman with rheumatoid arthritis. Note also periarticular osteoporosis and soft-tissue swelling.

and third metacarpal heads and the radial and ulnar aspects of the bases of the proximal phalanges (Fig. 14.10). Synovial inflammation in the prestyloid recess, a diverticulum of the radiocarpal joint that is intimate with the styloid process of ulna, as Resnick pointed out, produces marginal erosion of the styloid tip.

Joint Deformities. Although not pathognomonic for rheumatoid arthritis, certain deformations such as the *swan-neck deformity* and the *boutonnière deformity* are more often seen in this form of arthritis than in other inflammatory arthritides. The first of these represents hyperextension in the proximal interphalangeal joint and flexion in the distal interphalangeal joint, a configuration resembling a swan's neck (Fig. 14.11). In the boutonnière deformity,

the configuration is just the opposite, with flexion in the proximal joint and extension in the distal interphalangeal joint (Fig. 14.12). The word *boutonnière* is French for "buttonhole," the term for this deformity deriving from the configuration of the finger while securing a flower to a lapel. A similar deformation of the thumb is called *hitchhiker's thumb.*

Moreover, subluxations and dislocations with malalignment of the fingers are common findings in advanced stages of rheumatoid arthritis. Particularly characteristic are ulnar deviation of the fingers in the metacarpophalangeal joints and radial deviation of the wrist in the radiocarpal articulation (Fig. 14.13). In far-advanced stages of rheumatoid arthritis, shortening of several phalanges may be en-

Figure 14.11 **Rheumatoid arthritis.** Oblique radiograph of the hand of a 59-year-old woman shows the swan-neck deformity of the second through fifth fingers. Note the flexion in the distal interphalangeal joints and the extension in the proximal interphalangeal joints, the hallmarks of this abnormality.

Figure 14.12 Rheumatoid arthritis. Dorsovolar radiograph of the hands of a 48-year-old woman with rheumatoid arthritis demonstrates the boutonnière deformity in the small and ring fingers of the right hand and in the ring finger of the left hand.

Figure 14.13 Rheumatoid arthritis. Dorsovolar projection of both hands of a 51-year-old woman shows subluxation in the metacarpophalangeal joints resulting in ulnar deviation of the fingers and radial deviation in the radiocarpal articulations. Note also ankylosis of the midcarpal articulations of the right hand.

Figure 14.14 Rheumatoid arthritis. Dorsovolar view of the right hand of a 54-year-old woman with long-standing advanced rheumatoid arthritis demonstrates the *main-en-lorgnette* deformity. Note the telescoping of the fingers secondary to destructive joint changes and dislocations in the metacarpophalangeal joints. There is also ankylosis of the radiocarpal and intercarpal articulations and "penciling" of the distal ulna.

Figure 14.15 Rheumatoid arthritis. Dorsovolar view of the hand of a 60-year-old woman shows a gap between the scaphoid and lunate, indicating destruction of the scapholunate ligament. Note also the subluxation in the metacarpophalangeal joints resulting in ulnar deviation of the fingers.

countered secondary to destructive changes in the joints associated with dislocations in the metacarpophalangeal joints. This deformity appears as a "telescoping" of the fingers, hence its name, *main-en-lorgnette,* from the French name for the telescoping type of opera glass (Fig. 14.14). An abnormally wide space between the lunate and scaphoid may also be encountered in advanced stages of the disease secondary to erosion and rupture of the scapholunate ligament (Fig. 14.15); this phenomenon resembles the Terry-Thomas sign seen secondary to trauma (see Fig. 7.68). Joint deformities are also often seen in the foot; the subtalar joint is frequently affected, and subluxation in the metatarsophalangeal joints often leads to deformities such as hallux valgus and hammertoes.

Joint Ankylosis. A rare finding that may be observed in advanced stages of rheumatoid arthritis is joint ankylosis, which is most commonly encountered in the midcarpal articulations (see Figs. 14.13 and 14.14). Ankylotic changes in the wrist are more common in patients with juvenile rheumatoid arthritis and with so-called seronegative rheumatoid arthritis.

Involvement of the Spine

The thoracic and lumbar segments are affected by rheumatoid arthritis only on rare occasions. The cervical spine, however, is involved in approximately 50% of individuals with this condition (Table 14.2). The most characteristic radiographic features of rheumatoid arthritis in the cervical spine can be observed in the odontoid process, the atlantoaxial joints, and the apophyseal joints. Erosive changes may be encountered in the odontoid process (see Fig. 12.33) and apophyseal joints (Fig. 14.16), whereas subluxation is a common finding in the at-

lantoaxial joint (see Fig. 12.34), frequently accompanied by vertical translocation of the odontoid process (also known as cranial settling or atlantoaxial impaction) (Fig. 14.17 and Fig. 14.19). The most frequent abnormality is laxity of the transverse ligament connecting the odontoid to the atlas. This laxity becomes apparent on the radiograph obtained in the lateral view of the flexed cervical spine, is expressed by subluxation in the atlantoaxial joint (Fig. 14.18), and is frequently accompanied by superior migration of the odontoid process. This complication often requires surgical intervention, and the most common procedure to correct this is posterior fusion.

Table 14.2 **Abnormalities of the Cervical Spine in Rheumatoid Arthritis**

Osteoporosis
Erosion of the odontoid process
Atlantoaxial (C1–2) subluxation
Vertical translation of the odontoid (cranial settling)
Erosions of the apophyseal joints
Fusion of the apophyseal joints
Erosions of the Luschka joints
Disk space narrowing
Erosions and sclerosis of the vertebral body margins
Erosions (whittling) of the spinous processes
Subluxations of the vertebral bodies ("stepladder" or "doorstep" appearance on lateral radiographs)

Modified from Resnick D, Niwayama G, 1995, with permission.

Figure 14.16 Rheumatoid arthritis of the cervical spine. Lateral radiograph of the cervical spine of a 52-year-old woman with advanced rheumatoid arthritis shows erosive changes of the apophyseal joints. In addition, note osteoporosis, erosion of the odontoid, erosions at the diskovertebral junctions, and whittling of the spinous processes.

Severe involvement of the apophyseal joints leads to subluxations. In extremely rare cases, in a manner similar to that in juvenile rheumatoid arthritis, the apophyseal joints may ankylose. The other structures occasionally affected by rheumatoid process are the intervertebral disks and adjacent vertebral bodies, which become involved as a result of synovitis extending from the joints of Luschka. Only a small percentage of patients with cervical disease may have cervical myelopathy. Magnetic resonance imaging is an ideal modality to evaluate spinal cord involvement in these patients (Fig. 14.19).

Figure 14.17 Rheumatoid arthritis of the cervical spine. Lateral radiograph of the cervical spine of a 41-year-old woman with rheumatoid arthritis shows a vertical translocation of the odontoid process (cranial settling). Note also erosive changes at the diskovertebral junctions, erosions of the apophyseal joints, and whittling of the spinous processes.

Figure 14.18 **Rheumatoid arthritis—C1-C2 instability.** Flexion (**A**) and extension (**B**) lateral radiographs demonstrate C1-2 subluxation in a 66-year-old woman with rheumatoid arthritis.

Complications of Rheumatoid Arthritis

The complications of rheumatoid arthritis are related not only to the inflammatory process itself but also to the sequelae of treatment (see the discussion on the complications of treatment in Chapter 12). The large doses of steroids that are commonly prescribed in therapy often lead to the development of generalized osteoporosis. Severe osteoporosis and large bony erosions may in turn precipitate pathologic fracture, a frequent complication. Tear of the rotator cuff may also occur because of erosion by inflammatory pannus in the shoulder joint (see Fig. 14.6). In the knee, a large popliteal (Baker) cyst may complicate rheumatoid arthritic changes (Figs. 14.20 and 14.21); this condition may be misdiagnosed as thrombophlebitis.

Rheumatoid Nodulosis

A variant of rheumatoid arthritis is rheumatoid nodulosis, which occurs predominantly in men. It is a nonsystemic disorder characterized by the presence of multiple subcutaneous nodules (Fig. 14.22) and a very high rheumatoid factor titer; as a rule, there are no joint abnormalities. Occasionally, small cystic lesions may be present in various bones. Nodules are usually different in size and consistency, and distribution is over the elbows, extensor surfaces of hands and feet, and other pressure points. The most striking feature is lack of systemic manifestations of rheumatoid arthritis.

On histologic examination, the nodules show typical rheumatoid changes, including central necrosis surrounded by palisading histiocytes and fibroblasts, with an outer layer of connective tissue and chronic inflammatory cells. Only occasionally will the histologic appearance be atypical. In these cases, the nodule may contain abundant cholesterol clefts and lipid-loaded macrophages, suggestive of xanthoma or even multicentric reticulohistiocytosis.

Figure 14.19 **MRI of rheumatoid arthritis of the cervical spine.** A 52-year-old woman with advanced rheumatoid arthritis presented with chronic neck pain, weakness of the upper limbs, numbness in both hands, and occasional dyspnea and cardiac arrhythmia. A sagittal spin-echo T1-weighted MR image shows inflammatory pannus eroding odontoid (*arrow*), and cranial settling with cephalad migration of C-2 impinging on the medulla oblongata (*open arrow*).

Figure 14.20 **Rheumatoid arthritis complicated by a Baker cyst.** A 31-year-old woman with a 2-year history of seropositive rheumatoid arthritis developed swelling of the upper calf and tenderness in the popliteal fossa. A presumptive diagnosis of thrombophlebitis was made, but a venogram failed to corroborate this. This lateral view of a knee arthrogram shows a large popliteal (Baker) cyst dissecting into the medial aspect of the calf. This condition is a well-documented complication in patients with rheumatoid arthritis. (From Greenspan A, et al., 1983, with permission.)

Figure 14.21 Rheumatoid arthritis complicated by a Baker cyst. A 60-year-old woman with rheumatoid arthritis developed a popliteal cyst. Sagittal (**A**) and axial (**B**) T2-weighted fat-suppressed MR images demonstrate a large Baker cyst (*arrows*). Open arrows point to erosive changes of the articular cartilage, curved arrow indicates joint effusion.

Therapy is usually limited to the occasional use of nonsteroidal antiinflammatory drugs. Nodules that cause local pain because of nerve compression can be surgically removed. Some investigators have reported a decrease in nodule size after the use of penicillamine. These reports are controversial, however, because the regression and even disappearance of rheumatoid nodules may occur without any treatment at all.

In classic rheumatoid arthritis, small-vessel vasculitis is a primary factor in nodule development, and circulating immune complexes used by rheumatoid synovium are responsible for such extraarticular manifestations as vasculitis, polyserositis, and nodules. In rheumatoid nodulosis, however, nodules develop in the absence of active joint disease. Thus, the pathogenesis of rheumatoid nodulosis remains unclear.

A positive family history of rheumatoid arthritis in some patients with rheumatoid nodulosis and the occurrence of familial nodulosis suggest the involvement of hereditary factors. Investigations into tissue typing, particularly the search for DW4/DRW4 antigens, may illustrate the pathogenesis of this rheumatoid variant. The strong male preponderance suggests that androgens may modify disease expression in genetically predisposed individuals. Rheumatoid nodulosis is often misdiagnosed as gout or xanthomatosis. Moreover, it should be kept in mind when evaluating this condition that approximately 20% of patients with classic rheumatoid arthritis have rheumatoid nodules, which are usually located at sites of pressure or

stress such as the dorsal aspect of the hands and forearms (Fig. 14.23). Articular involvement in nodular rheumatoid arthritis distinguishes it from rheumatoid nodulosis, which consequently has a better prognosis.

Juvenile Rheumatoid Arthritis

Juvenile rheumatoid arthritis is a group of at least three chronic inflammatory synovial diseases that affect children; girls are more frequently affected than boys. The three defined subtypes are Still disease, polyarticular arthritis, and pauciarticular arthritis. Each of these subgroups has distinct clinical and laboratory findings and different natural histories. There is no pathognomonic laboratory test for any of them, and the diagnosis is based on the clinical spectrum exhibited by a given patient.

Still Disease

Still disease is well-known for sudden onset of spiking fever, lymphadenopathy, and an evanescent salmon-colored skin rash. Patients may exhibit hepatosplenomegaly, fatigue, anorexia, and weight loss. The majority of patients have chronic and recurrent arthralgias. A significant number of patients, depending on the series, may also subsequently have chronic polyarthritis. A poorly un-

Figure 14.22 Rheumatoid nodulosis. A 52-year-old man with a 15-year history of polyarthritis presented with large, fluctuant nodules on the dorsal aspect of the hands and elbows. A high titer of rheumatoid factor (1: 1280) was identified in his serum. **(A)** Dorsovolar view of both hands shows several soft-tissue nodules adjacent to joints. Note the lack of joint abnormalities. Anteroposterior **(B)** and lateral **(C)** radiographs of the left elbow demonstrate similar soft-tissue masses at the dorsal aspect of the proximal forearm. The elbow joint is intact. (From Greenspan A, et al., 1983, with permission.) *(continued)*

soft tissue nodules

Figure 14.22 **Rheumatoid nodulosis.** *Continued.*

erosion

pit erosions

rheumatoid nodules

Figure 14.23 **Rheumatoid nodules. (A)** A 39-year-old man with rheumatoid arthritis originally misdiagnosed as gout. Lateral radiograph of the right elbow demonstrates erosions of the olecranon process, olecranon bursitis on the left, and rheumatoid nodules on the dorsal aspect of the forearm. Note the characteristic pit-like cortical erosions at the site of the rheumatoid nodules. This presentation of rheumatoid arthritis should not be mistaken for rheumatoid nodulosis. **(B)** A 68-year-old woman with rheumatoid arthritis had a large rheumatoid nodule at the lateral side of the elbow joint. Note erosions at the radiocapitellar joint (*arrow*).

Figure 14.23 Rheumatoid nodules. *Continued.*

derstood Still-like disease with fever and arthralgias may develop in some adult patients.

Polyarticular Juvenile Rheumatoid Arthritis

Polyarticular juvenile rheumatoid arthritis consists of inflammation at four or more joints with associated findings of anorexia, weight loss, fatigue, and adenopathy. Growth retardation is common. This disorder also results in the following abnormalities: undergrowth of the mandible, early closure of the growth plates resulting in shortening of metacarpals and metatarsals, and overgrowths of the epiphyses at the knees, hips, and shoulders. A worse prognosis occurs in patients with positive rheumatoid factors.

Juvenile Rheumatoid Arthritis With Pauciarticular Onset

The third subtype of juvenile rheumatoid arthritis has pauciarticular onset, with four or fewer joints involved. Approximately 40% of patients with juvenile rheumatoid arthritis exhibit involvement of fewer than four joints in the first 6 months of the disease. Some of these patients may even present with negative rheumatoid factor whereas others may have positive antigen HLA-B27. Pediatric rheumatologists have attempted to define other subgroups within this pauciarticular subgroup, but, with the exception of HLA-B27-positive children with sacroiliitis, such definitions are broad and clinically dependent on unique systemic features such as iridocyclitis. However, involvement of the sacroiliac joints is not a feature of juvenile rheumatoid arthritis as was thought in the past; rather, it represents juvenile onset of ankylosing spondylitis. Similarly, some investigators believe that patients with pauciarticular arthritis, particularly those with positive histocompatibility antigen HLA-B27, may in fact have atypical ankylosing spondylitis syndrome or spondyloarthropathy; both these conditions are different from rheumatoid arthritis.

Other Types of Juvenile Rheumatoid Arthritis

It is worthwhile to note that two new diagnostic terms currently in use in childhood arthritides—*juvenile chronic arthritis* and *juvenile arthritis*—are not equivalent to each other or to classic juvenile rheumatoid arthritis. These conditions lack any characteristic radiographic features. Much research is needed to gain a better understanding of juvenile rheumatoid arthritis before we will clearly be able to define the number of different diseases involved.

Radiographic Features

Juvenile rheumatoid arthritis exhibits many of the features of adult rheumatoid arthritis. However, some additional features that are almost pathognomonic for this condition have been identified.

Periosteal Reaction. This feature is usually seen along the shafts of the proximal phalanges and metacarpals (Fig. 14.24).

Joint Ankylosis. Ankylosis may occur not only in the wrist but also in the interphalangeal articulations (Fig. 14.25). Fusion in the apophyseal joints of the cervical spine is also a characteristic finding (Fig. 14.26).

Growth Abnormalities. Because the onset of juvenile rheumatoid arthritis frequently occurs before completion of skeletal maturation, alterations in growth of the bones is a common finding. The involvement of epiphyseal sites often leads to fusion of the growth plate, with resultant retardation of bone growth (Fig. 14.27); it may also precipitate acceleration of growth caused by stimulation of the growth plates by hyperemia. Enlargement of the epiphysis of the distal femur leads to characteristic overgrowth of the condyles in the knee (Fig. 14.28).

Figure 14.24 Juvenile rheumatoid arthritis. Dorsovolar view of the wrist and hand of a 26-year-old woman with a 14-year history of juvenile rheumatoid arthritis shows severe destructive changes in the wrist and in the metacarpophalangeal and proximal interphalangeal articulations. Note the ankylosis of the third and fourth metacarpophalangeal joints and periostitis involving the proximal phalanges and metacarpals.

Figure 14.25 Juvenile rheumatoid arthritis. Dorsovolar projection of the left hand of a 25-year-old woman with a 10-year history of juvenile rheumatoid arthritis shows advanced destructive changes in multiple joints of the hand and wrist. Joint ankylosis is evident in several articulations.

Figure 14.26 Juvenile rheumatoid arthritis. Lateral radiograph of the cervical spine in a 25-year-old woman with a 15-year history of polyarthritis shows fusion of the apophyseal joints, a common finding in juvenile rheumatoid arthritis.

Figure 14.27 Juvenile rheumatoid arthritis. (A), (B) Dorsovolar view of the hands of a 24-year-old woman with advanced juvenile rheumatoid arthritis, which was diagnosed when she was 7 years old, shows retarded growth of the bones caused by early fusion of the growth plates. Multiple deformities of the digits include hitchhiker's thumb and a boutonnière configuration of the fingers.

Figure 14.28 Juvenile rheumatoid arthritis. Anteroposterior radiograph of both knees of a 20-year-old woman with juvenile rheumatoid arthritis shows overgrowth of the medial condyles, one of the characteristic features of this disorder.

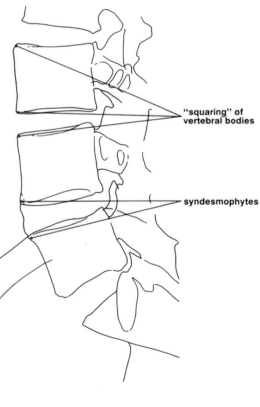

Figure 14.29 Ankylosing spondylitis. Lateral radiograph of the lumbar spine in a 28-year-old man demonstrates squaring of the vertebral bodies secondary to small osseous erosions at the corners. This finding is an early radiographic feature of ankylosing spondylitis. Note also the formation of syndesmophytes at the L4-5 disk space.

Seronegative Spondyloarthropathies

Ankylosing Spondylitis

Clinical Features

Ankylosing spondylitis, known in the European literature as *Bechterev disease* or *Marie-Strümpell disease,* is a chronic, progressive, inflammatory arthritis principally affecting the synovial joints of the spine and adjacent soft tissues as well as the sacroiliac joints; however, the peripheral joints such as the hips, shoulders, and knees may also be involved. It is seen seven-times more frequently in men than in women, and predominantly at a young age. Patients with ankylosing spondylitis frequently exhibit extraarticular features of disease including iritis, pulmonary fibrosis, cardiac conduction defects, aortic incompetence, spinal cord compression, and amyloidosis. Patients may also have low-grade fever, anorexia, fatigue, and weight loss.

Rheumatoid factor is negative in patients with ankylosing spondylitis, which is the prototype of the seronegative spondyloarthropathies. A high percentage of patients (up to 95%), however, possess histocompatibility antigen HLA-B27. Pathologically, ankylosing spondylitis is a diffuse proliferative synovitis of the diarthrodial joints exhibiting features similar to those seen in rheumatoid arthritis.

Radiographic Features

Squaring of the anterior border of the lower thoracic and lumbar vertebrae is one of the earliest radiographic features of ankylosing spondylitis, best demonstrated on the lateral radiograph of the spine (Fig. 14.29). As the condition progresses, syndesmophytes form, bridging the vertebral bodies (Fig. 14.30). The delicate appearance of these excrescences and their vertical rather than horizontal orientation distinguish them from the osteophytes of degenerative spine disease. Paravertebral ossifications are common in ankylosing spondylitis. When the apophyseal joints and vertebral bodies fuse late in the course of the disease, a radiographic hallmark of this condition, the "bamboo" spine, can be observed (Fig. 14.31); the sacroiliac joints are also invariably affected in this process (see Fig. 14.31B).

In the peripheral joints, inflammatory changes may be indistinguishable from those seen in rheumatoid arthritis (see Fig. 14.31B). In the foot, erosions characteristically occur at certain tendinous insertions, particularly in the os calcis (see Fig. 12.30). Involvement of the ischial tuberosities and iliac crests exhibits a lace-like formation of new bone called "whiskering."

Reiter Syndrome

Clinical Features

Reiter syndrome is a clinical infectious disease that affects five-times more males than females and is characterized by arthritis, conjunctivitis, and urethritis. It was first reported in 1916 by the German physician Hans Reiter, and in the same year it was described by the French physicians Fiessinger and LeRoy. Reiter syndrome is also well-known for the presence of mucocutaneous rash, keratoderma blenorrhagica. Like ankylosing spondylitis, eye involvement is com-

Figure 14.30 Ankylosing spondylitis. Lateral radiograph of the cervical spine in a 31-year-old man demonstrates delicate syndesmophytes bridging the vertebral bodies, a common feature of ankylosing spondylitis. Note the fusion of several apophyseal joints.

Figure 14.31 Ankylosing spondylitis.(A) Lateral radiograph of the cervical spine in a 53-year-old man with advanced ankylosing spondylitis shows anterior syndesmophytes bridging the vertebral bodies and posterior fusion of the apophyseal joints, together with paravertebral ossifications, producing a "bamboo-spine" appearance. The same phenomenon is seen on the anteroposterior **(B)** and lateral **(C)** radiographs of the lumbosacral spine. Note on the anteroposterior view the fusion of the sacroiliac joints and the involvement of both hip joints, which show axial migration of the femoral heads similar to that seen in rheumatoid arthritis. **(D)** Sagittal proton-density MRI shows anterior syndesmophytes, calcification of the posterior longitudinal ligament, and preservation of the intervertebral disks.

Figure 14.32 Reiter syndrome. (A) Anteroposterior radiograph of right hip joint of a 39-year-old man with Reiter syndrome shows characteristic changes of inflammatory arthritis. **(B)** Lateral radiograph of the foot of a 28-year-old man with Reiter syndrome demonstrates the "fluffy" periostitis of the os calcis and inflammatory changes of the metatarsophalangeal joints typical of this condition.

mon and can include conjunctivitis, iritis, uveitis, and episcleritis. Approximately 60% to 80% of patients are positive for HLA-B27. This frequency varies according to the ethnic origin of the patient. Unlike ankylosing spondylitis, Reiter syndrome may exhibit unilateral sacroiliac diseases.

Two types of this syndrome have been identified. First, the sporadic or endemic type, which is common in the United States, is associated with nongonococcal urethritis, prostatitis, or hemorrhagic cystitis. It occurs almost exclusively in males. In Europe, a second type has been identified, which is an epidemic form associated with bacillary (*Shigella*) dysentery. It may be seen in women as well. There has been considerable research on the putative role of *Yersinia enterocolitica* in inducing disease, particularly in Scandinavia, where such infections are more prevalent than in North America.

Radiographic Features

Radiographically, Reiter syndrome is marked by peripheral and usually asymmetric arthritis, with a predilection for the joints of the lower limb (Fig. 14.32). The foot is the most common site of involvement, particularly the metatarsophalangeal joints and the heels (Fig. 14.32B; see also Figs. 12.30 and 12.31). Periosteal new bone formation is not uncommon. Involvement of the sacroiliac joints, which is frequently encountered, may be either asymmetric (unilateral or bilateral) or symmetric (bilateral) (Fig. 14.33). In the thoracic and lumbar spine, coarse syndesmophytes or paraspinal ossifications may be present, characteristically bridging adjacent vertebrae (Fig. 14.34).

Psoriatic Arthritis

Clinical Features

Psoriasis is a dermatologic disorder that affects approximately 1% to 2% of the population. The macular and papular skin lesions of psoriasis display characteristic silver scales and are commonly located over extensor surfaces of the extremities. Nail abnormalities,

Figure 14.33 Reiter syndrome. Anteroposterior radiograph of the pelvis of the patient shown in Figure 14.32B demonstrates symmetric bilateral involvement of the sacroiliac joints.

Figure 14.34 Reiter syndrome. Anteroposterior radiograph of the lumbar spine of a 23-year-old man with Reiter syndrome demonstrates a single, coarse syndesmophyte bridging the L-2 and L-3 vertebrae.

Figure 14.35 Psoriatic arthritis. A 57-year-old woman with long-standing psoriasis developed resorption of the tufts of the distal phalanges (acroosteolysis) of both hands, typical of this condition.

including discoloration, fragmentation, pitting, and onycholysis, may provide an early diagnostic clue. Approximately 10% to 15% of patients with psoriasis develop inflammatory arthritis. Articular disease is more common in patients with moderate or severe skin abnormalities and, according to Wright, severe and mutilating arthropathy is often associated with extensive exfoliative skin abnormalities.

The cause of psoriatic arthritis is unknown, and its relationship to rheumatoid arthritis and spondyloarthropathies is still unsettled. The arthritis predominantly affects the distal interphalangeal joints of the

Figure 14.36 Psoriatic arthritis. Dorsovolar radiograph of both hands of a 55-year-old woman who presented with skin changes typical of psoriasis shows destructive changes in the proximal and distal interphalangeal joints. Note the spontaneous fusion of the distal interphalangeal joint of the small finger of the right hand and the distal interphalangeal joint of the ring finger of the left hand.

Table 14.3 **Most Common Causes of Acroosteolysis**

Trauma	Congenital (Hajdu-Cheney
Diabetic gangrene	syndrome)
Psoriasis	Leprosy
Scleroderma	Gout
Dermatomyositis	Pyknodysostosis
Rheumatoid arthritis	Sarcoidosis
Raynaud disease	Sjögren syndrome
Hyperparathyroidism	Polyvinyl chloride
(primary, secondary)	Pachydermoperiostosis
Frostbite	Thromboangiitis obliterans
Burn (thermal, electrical)	Syringomyelia

Modified from Reeder MM, Felson B, 1975, with permission.

hands and feet, although other sites of involvement—the proximal interphalangeal joints as well as the hips, knees, ankles, shoulders, and spine—may also be encountered.

Five specific subgroups of arthritic syndromes have been described in psoriatic arthritis.

Subgroup 1, or classic psoriatic arthritis, includes nail pathology with frequent erosion of the terminal tufts termed acroosteolysis (Fig. 14.35) and involvement of the distal and occasionally proximal interphalangeal joints of the hand (Fig. 14.36). It is important, however, to remember that other conditions may also exhibit acroosteolysis (Table 14.3).

Subgroup 2, well-known for the "opera glass" deformity of the hand, is termed *arthritis mutilans* because of the extensive destruction of the phalanges and metacarpal joints, including the "pencil-in-cup" deformity (Fig. 14.37). Other joints such as hip or elbow (Fig. 14.38) are also frequently affected. Patients with arthritis mutilans often will have sacroiliitis.

Figure 14.38 Psoriatic arthritis. A 49-year-old man presented with psoriatic arthritis mutilans. Anteroposterior (**A**) and lateral (**B**) radiographs of the right elbow show extensive articular erosions. Elevated anterior fat pad indicates a joint effusion.

Subgroup 3 is characterized by symmetric polyarthritis (Fig. 14.39) and may result in ankylosis of the proximal and distal interphalangeal joints. In this form, psoriatic arthritis is frequently indistinguishable from rheumatoid arthritis (Fig. 14.40).

Subgroup 4 is characterized by oligoarticular arthritis, and in contrast to subgroup 3 the joint involvement is asymmetric, generally including the proximal and distal interphalangeal and metacarpophalangeal articulations (Fig. 14.41). Patients with this oligoarticular arthritis form the most frequent subgroup of psoriatic arthritis and are known for the appearance of sausage-like swelling of digits (Fig. 14.42).

Subgroup 5 is a spondyloarthropathy that has features similar to those of ankylosing spondylitis.

Radiographic Features

In general, there are few characteristic radiographic features of psoriatic arthritis that help to make a correct diagnosis. In the phalanges of the hand or foot, a periosteal reaction in the form of a "fluffy" new bone apposition may often be noted (see Fig. 14.41). If this new bone is periarticular in location and associated with erosions of the inter-

Figure 14.37 Psoriatic arthritis. Dorsovolar radiograph of the hand of a 57-year-old woman shows the typical presentation of psoriatic polyarthritis. The "pencil-in-cup" deformity in the interphalangeal joint of the thumb is characteristic of this form of psoriasis.

Figure 14.39 Psoriatic arthritis. A 75-year-old woman presented with symmetric psoriatic polyarthritis affecting all joints of the hands and wrists. Unlike in adult-onset-type of rheumatoid arthritis the distal interphalangeal joints are also involved.

phalangeal joints, it exhibits a "mouse-ear" appearance (Fig. 14.43). In the advanced arthritis mutilans stage of psoriatic arthritis, severe deformities such as the "pencil-in-cup" configuration (see Fig. 14.37) and interphalangeal ankylosis may be observed (see Fig. 14.40). In the heel, late-stage changes may be seen in the formation of broad-based

osteophytes and in the presence of erosions and a fluffy periostitis (see Figs. 12.30 and 12.31C).

Psoriatic arthritis of the spine is associated with a particularly high incidence of sacroiliitis, which may be bilateral and symmetric, bilateral and asymmetric, or unilateral. As in Reiter syndrome, coarse

Figure 14.40 Psoriatic arthritis. Dorsovolar view of the left hand of a 67-year-old man with the polyarthritic form of psoriatic arthritis demonstrates erosions and fusion of multiple joints. The swan-neck deformity of the small finger is similar to that seen in patients with rheumatoid arthritis.

Figure 14.41 Psoriatic arthritis. A 39-year-old man with psoriasis presented with a painful and swollen middle finger of his right hand. The magnification radiograph shows subtle periarticular erosions, fluffy periosteal reaction, and soft tissue swelling, features characteristic of oligoarticular psoriatic arthritis.

Figure 14.42 Psoriatic arthritis. Dorsovolar radiograph of the hands of a 33-year-old man with psoriasis and oligoarticular involvement shows destructive changes in the distal interphalangeal joints of the right middle finger and the left index and small fingers. The right middle and left index fingers presented as "sausage digits."

Figure 14.43 Psoriatic arthritis. (A) Magnification study of the hand of a 48-year-old man who presented with documented psoriasis shows marginal erosions and new bone apposition in the proximal and distal interphalangeal joints, resembling mouse ears. Note the fluffy periostitis in the juxtaarticular areas of the phalanges and distal metacarpals. **(B)** In the feet, the same process has led to a "mouse-ear" appearance at the interphalangeal joints of the great toes.

Figure 14.44 Psoriatic arthritis. (A) Oblique radiograph of the lumbar spine in a 30-year-old man with psoriasis shows a characteristic single syndesmophyte bridging the bodies of L-3 and L-4. The right sacroiliac joint is also affected. **(B)** Anteroposterior radiograph of the lumbar spine in a 45-year-old man with psoriasis reveals paraspinal ossification at the level of L2-L3.

Figure 14.45 Psoriatic arthritis. A postmyelographic CT scan through the lumbar spine shows a paraspinal ossification in a 48-year-old man with psoriasis.

asymmetric syndesmophytes and paraspinal ossifications may form (Figs. 14.44 and 14.45) and, as Resnick pointed out, this may represent an early manifestation of the disease.

Enteropathic Arthropathies

This group comprises arthritides associated with inflammatory intestinal diseases such as ulcerative colitis, regional enteritis (Crohn disease), and intestinal lipodystrophy (Whipple disease), the last of which predominantly affects men in their fourth and fifth decades. The histocompatibility antigen HLA-B27 is present in most patients with enteropathic abnormalities. In all three conditions, the spine and the sacroiliac and peripheral joints may be affected. In the spine, squaring of the vertebral bodies and the formation of syndesmophytes are common features. Sacroiliitis, which is usually bilateral and sym-

metric, is radiographically indistinguishable from ankylosing spondylitis (Fig. 14.46). In addition, patients may also exhibit a peripheral arthritis, the activity of which generally approximates the activity of the bowel disease.

Finally, it should be noted that arthritis may follow intestinal bypass procedures. The synovitis is polyarticular and symmetric, but radiographically the lesions are nonerosive.

PRACTICAL POINTS TO REMEMBER

Erosive Osteoarthritis
[1] Erosive osteoarthritis, a condition seen predominantly in middle-aged women, combines the clinical manifestations of rheumatoid arthritis with the radiographic features of osteoarthritis.
[2] Erosive osteoarthritis can be recognized by:
  • involvement of the proximal and distal interphalangeal joints
  • a characteristic "gull-wing" configuration of articular erosions. Spontaneous fusion (ankylosis) in the interphalangeal joints may develop.

Rheumatoid Arthritis
[1] Rheumatoid arthritis has a predilection for:
  • the large joints (knees and hips)
  • the small joints in the hand (metacarpophalangeal and proximal interphalangeal)
  • the carpal articulations.
  The distal interphalangeal and sacroiliac joints are usually spared.
[2] The radiographic hallmarks of rheumatoid arthritis include:
  • diffuse, symmetric narrowing of the joint space
  • periarticular osteoporosis
  • fusiform soft-tissue swelling
  • marginal and central articular erosions
  • periarticular synovial cysts
  • subluxations and other joint deformities—swan-neck, boutonnière, hitchhiker's thumb.
[3] In the cervical spine, rheumatoid arthritis is characterized by:
  • erosion of the odontoid process associated with subluxation in the atlantoaxial joints and, frequently, cephalad translocation of C-2 (cranial settling)

Figure 14.46 Ulcerative colitis complicated by sacroiliitis. A 20-year-old woman with known ulcerative colitis developed severe low back pain localized to the sacroiliac joints. **(A)** Barium enema study shows extensive involvement of the transverse and descending colon, consistent with ulcerative colitis. **(B)** Posteroanterior radiograph of the pelvis shows symmetric, bilateral sacroiliitis similar to that seen in ankylosing spondylitis.

- involvement of the apophyseal joints
- erosions of vertebral bodies
- destruction of intervertebral disks
- erosions (whittling) of the spinous processess.

[4] In rheumatoid arthritis,
- axial or, less frequently, medial migration of the femoral head and acetabular protrusio are characteristic in the hip joint
- rotator cuff tear is a frequent complication in the shoulder joint
- the subtalar joint is most often affected in the foot, and a hallux valgus deformity is observed.

[5] Rheumatoid nodulosis, a condition occurring predominantly in men, is a variant of rheumatoid arthritis. It exhibits:
- a characteristic lack of joint abnormalities
- multiple subcutaneous nodules
- a high titer of rheumatoid factor.

[6] Juvenile rheumatoid arthritis displays several characteristic features that are not present in adult-onset disease:
- a periosteal reaction
- joint ankylosis, particularly affecting the apophyseal joints of the cervical spine
- growth abnormalities secondary to involvement of epiphyseal sites.

Other Inflammatory Arthritides

[1] Spondyloarthropathies comprise four distinctive entities: ankylosing spondylitis, psoriatic arthritis, Reiter syndrome, and arthritides associated with inflammatory bowel disease.

[2] Ankylosing spondylitis (Bechterev or Marie-Strümpell disease), a condition seen predominantly in young men, characteristically affects the spine and sacroiliac joints. Histocompatibility antigen HLA-B27 is invariably present in 95% of patients. The radiographic hallmarks of this condition include:
- squaring of the vertebral bodies
- the development of delicate syndesmophytes
- in a later stage of disease, complete fusion of the apophyseal joints and vertebrae, leading to "bamboo" spine.

[3] Reiter syndrome consists of inflammatory arthritis, urethritis, conjunctivitis, and mucocutaneous rash. Its radiographic features include:
- a peripheral, usually asymmetric arthritis that shows a predilection for the lower-limb joints, particularly in the foot
- coarse syndesmophytes and paraspinal ossifications bridging vertebral bodies
- sacroiliitis, which usually is asymmetric.

[4] Psoriatic arthritis has a predilection for the distal interphalangeal joints. Oligoarticular involvement may yield a phenomenon known as "sausage digit." Radiographically, psoriatic arthritis is marked by:
- fluffy periostitis
- "pencil-in-cup" deformity of the joints (arthritis mutilans)
- coarse syndesmophytes and paraspinal ossifications that are indistinguishable from those seen in Reiter syndrome
- involvement of the sacroiliac joints.

[5] Enteropathic arthropathies are associated with:
- ulcerative colitis
- regional enteritis (Crohn disease)
- intestinal lipodystrophy (Whipple disease)
- intestinal bypass procedures.

Characteristically, there is symmetric involvement of the sacroiliac joints.

SUGGESTED READINGS

Adam G, Dammer M, Bohndorf K, Christoph R, Fenke F, Günther RW. Rheumatoid arthritis of the knee: value of gadopentetate dimeglumine-enhanced MR imaging. *AJR Am J Roentgenol* 1991;156:125–129.

Ansell BM, Wigley RA. Arthritic manifestations in regional enteritis. *Ann Rheum Dis* 1964;23:64–72.

Arnett FC, Bias WB, Stevens MB. Juvenile-onset chronic arthritis. Clinical and roentgenographic features of a unique HLA-B27 subset. *Am J Med* 1980;69:369–376.

Arnett FC, Edworthy SM, Bloch DA, et al. The American Rheumatism Association 1987 revised criteria for the classification of rheumatoid arthritis. *Arthritis Rheum* 1988;31:315–324.

Azouz EM, Duffy CM. Juvenile spondyloarthropathies: clinical manifestations and medical imaging. *Skeletal Radiol* 1995;24:399–408.

Belhorn LR, Hess EV. Erosive osteoarthritis. *Semin Arthritis Rheum* 1993;22:298–306.

Beltran J, Caudill JL, Herman LA, et al. Rheumatoid arthritis: MR imaging manifestations. *Radiology* 1987;165:153–157.

Berens DL. Roentgen features of ankylosing spondylitis. *Clin Orthop* 1971;74:20–33.

Björkengren AG, Geborek P, Rydholm U, Holtas S, Petterson H. MR imaging of the knee in acute rheumatoid arthritis: synovial uptake of gadolinium-DOTA. *AJR Am J Roentgenol* 1990;155:329–332.

Björkengren AG, Pathria MN, Sartosis DJ, et al. Carpal alterations in adult-onset Still disease, juvenile chronic arthritis, and adult-onset rheumatoid arthritis: comparative study. *Radiology* 1987;165:545–548.

Bland JH, Brown EW. Seronegative and seropositive rheumatoid arthritis: clinical, radiological and biochemical differences. *Ann Intern Med* 1964;60:88–94.

Boden SD, Dodge LD, Bohlman HH, Rechtine GR. Rheumatoid arthritis of the cervical spine. *J Bone J Surg [Am]* 1993;75A:1282–1297.

Bollow M, Braun J, Biedermann T, et al. Use of contrast-enhanced MR imaging to detect sacroiliitis in children. *Skeletal Radiol* 1998;27:606–616.

Boutin RD, Resnick D. The SAPHO syndrome: an evolving concept for unifying several idiopathic disorders of bone and skin. *AJR Am J Roentgenol* 1998;170:585–591.

Breedveld FC, Algra PR, Vielvoye CJ, Cats A. Magnetic resonance imaging in the evaluation of patients with rheumatoid arthritis and subluxations of the cervical spine. *Arthritis Rheum* 1987;30:624–629.

Brower AC, Allman RM. Pencil pointing: a vascular pattern of deossification. *Radiographics* 1983;3:315–325.

Bundschuh C, Modic MT, Kearney F, Morris R, Deal C. Rheumatoid arthritis of the cervical spine: surface-coil MR imaging. *AJR Am J Roentgenol* 1988; 151: 181–187.

Burgos-Vargas R. Juvenile ankylosing spondylitis. *Rheum Dis Clin North Am* 1992;18:123–142.

Burgos-Vargas R, Vazquez-Mellado J. The early clinical recognition of juvenile-onset ankylosing spondylitis and its differentiation from juvenile rheumatoid arthritis. *Arthritis Rheum* 1995;38:835–844.

Calabro JJ, Gordon RD, Miller KI. Bechterew's syndrome in children: diagnostic criteria. *Scand J Rheumatol* 1980;32[Suppl]:45–48.

Cassidy JT, Levinson JE, Bass JC, et al. A study of classification criteria for a diagnosis of juvenile rheumatoid arthritis. *Arthritis Rheum* 1986;29:274–281.

Cassidy JT, Petty RE. Spondyloarthropathies. In: Cassidy JT, Petty RE, eds. *Text book of pediatric rheumatology*, 2nd ed. New York: Churchill Livingstone; 1990:221–259.

Chung C, Coley BD, Martin LC. Rice bodies in juvenile rheumatoid arthritis. *AJR Am J Roentgenol* 1998;170:698–700.

Clark RL, Muhletaler CA, Margulies SI. Colitic arthritis: clinical and radiographic manifestations. *Radiology* 1971;101:585–594.

Cobby M, Cushnaghan J, Creamer P, Dieppe P, Watt I. Erosive osteoarthritis: is it a separate disease entity? *Clin Radiol* 1990;42:258–263.

Dale K, Paus AC, Laires K. A radiographic classification in juvenile rheumatoid arthritis applied to the knee. *Eur Radiol* 1994;4:27–32.

Dihlmann W. Current radiodiagnostic concept of ankylosing spondylitis. *Skeletal Radiol* 1979;4:179–188.

Dixon AS. "Rheumatoid arthritis" with negative serological reaction. *Ann Rheum Dis* 1960;19:209–228.

Eastmond CJ, Woodrow JC. The HLA system and the arthropathies associated with psoriasis. *Ann Rheum Dis* 1977;36:112–121.

Ehrlich GE. Erosive osteoarthritis: presentation, clinical pearls, and therapy. *Curr Rheum Rep* 2001;3:484–488.

Ehrlich GE. Inflammatory osteoarthritis. II. The superimposition of rheumatoid arthritis. *J Chronic Dis* 1972;25:635–643.

El-Khoury GY, Larson RK, Kathol MH, Berbaum KS, Furst DE. Seronegative and seropositive rheumatoid arthritis: radiographic differences. *Radiology* 1988;168:517–520.

el-Noueam KI, Giuliano V, Schweitzer ME, O'Hara BJ. Rheumatoid nodules: MR/pathological correlation. *J Comput Assist Tomogr* 1997;21:796–799.

Fezoulidis I, Neuhold A, Wicke L, Seidl G, Eydokimidis B. Diagnostic imaging of the occipito-cervical junction in patients with rheumatoid arthritis. *Eur J Radiol* 1989;9:5–11.

Foley-Nolan D, Stack JP, Ryan M, et al. Magnetic resonance imaging in the assessment of rheumatoid arthritis: a comparison with plain film radiographs. *Br J Rheumatol* 1991;30:101–106.

Forrester DM. Imaging of the sacroiliac joints. *Radiol Clin North Am* 1990;28:1055–1072.

Galvez J, Sola J, Ortuno G, et al. Microscopic rice bodies in rheumatoid synovial fluid sediments. *J Rheum* 1992;19:1851–1858.

Ginsberg MH, Genant HK, Yü TF, McCarty D. Rheumatoid nodulosis: an unusual variant of rheumatoid disease. *Arthritis Rheum* 1975;18:49–58.

Giovagnoni A, Grassi W, Terilli F, et al. MRI of the hand in psoriatic and rheumatical arthritis. *Eur Radiol* 1995;5:590–595.

Gordon DA, Hastings DE. Rheumatoid arthritis: clinical features—early, progressive and late disease. In: Klippel JH, Dieppe PA, eds. *Rheumatology*. St. Louis: CV Mosby; 1994:3.4.1–3.4.14.

Gran JT, Husby G. The epidemiology of ankylosing spondylitis. *Semin Arthritis Rheum* 1993;22:319–334.

Graudal NA, Jurik AG, de Carvalho A, Graudal HK. Radiographic progression in rheumatoid arthritis: a long-term prospective study of 109 patients. *Arthritis Rheum* 1998;41:1470–1480.

Green L, Meyers OL, Gordon W, Briggs B. Arthritis in psoriasis. *Ann Rheum Dis* 1981;40:366–369.

Greenspan A. Erosive osteoarthritis. *Semin Musculoskel Radiol* 2003;7:155–159.

Greenspan A, Baker ND, Norman A. Rheumatoid arthritis simulating other lesions. *Bull Hosp Joint Dis Orthop Inst* 1983;43:70–77.

Gubler FM, Maas M, Dijkstra PF, de Jongh HR. Cystic rheumatoid arthritis: description of a nonerosive form. *Radiology* 1990;170:829–834.

Hazes JMW, Dijkmans BAC, Hoevers JM, et al. R4 prevalence related to the age at disease onset in female patients with rheumatoid arthritis. *Ann Rheum Dis* 1989;48:406–408.

Helliwell PS, Wright V. Clinical features of psoriatic arthritis. In: Klippel JH, Dieppe PA, eds. *Practical rheumatology*. London: Mosby; 1995:235–242.

Herve-Somma CMP, Sebag GH, Prieur AM, Bonnerot V, Lallemand DP. Juvenile rheumatoid arthritis of the knee: MR evaluation with Gd-DOTA. *Radiology* 1992;182:93–98.

Hoffman GS. Polyarthritis: the differential diagnosis of rheumatoid arthritis. *Semin Arthritis Rheum* 1978;8:115–141.

Kahn MF. Why the "SAPHO" syndrome? *J Rheumatol* 1995; 22: 2017–2019.

Kapasi OA, Ruby LK, Calney K. The psoriatic hand. *J Hand Surg [Am]* 1982;7A:492–497.

Karasick D, Schweitzer ME, O'Hara BJ. Distal fibular notch: a frequent manifestation of the rheumatoid ankle. *Skeletal Radiol* 1997;26:529–532.

Kaye BR, Kaye RL, Bobrove A. Rheumatoid nodules. *Am J Med* 1984;76:279–292.

Keat A. Reiter's syndrome and reactive arthritis in perspective. *N Engl J Med* 1983;309:1606–1615.

Kelly JJ 3rd, Weisiger BB. The arthritis of Whipple's disease. *Arthritis Rheum* 1963;25:615–632.

Kettering JM, Towers JD, Rubin DA. The seronegative spondyloarthropathies. *Semin Roentgenol* 1996;31:220–228.

Khan MA, van der Linden SM. A wider spectrum of spondyloarthropathies. *Semin Arthritis Rheum* 1990;20:107–113.

Klecker R, Weissman BN. Imaging features of psoriatic arthritis and Reiter's syndrome. *Semin Musculoskel Radiol* 2003;7:115–126.

Klenerman L. The foot and ankle in rheumatoid arthritis. *Br J Rheum* 1995;34:443–448.

König H, Sieper J, Wolf K-J. Rheumatoid arthritis: evaluation of hypervascular and fibrous pannus with dynamic MR imaging enhanced with Gd-DTPA. *Radiology* 1990;176:473–477.

Kumar R, Madewell JE. Rheumatoid and seronegative arthropathies of the foot. *Radiol Clin North Am* 1987;25:1263–1288.

Küster W, Lenz W. Morbus Crohn und Colitis ulcerosa. Häufigkeit, familiäres Vorkommen und Schwangerschaftsverlauf. *Ergeb Inn Med Kinderheilkd* 1984;53:103–132.

Laxer RM, Babyn P, Liu P, Silverman ED, Shore A. Magnetic resonance studies of the sacroiliac joints in children with HLA-B27 associated seronegative arthropathies. *J Rheumatol* 1992;19[Suppl 33]:123.

Leirisalo M, Skylv G, Kousa M, et al. Follow-up study on patients with Reiter's disease and reactive arthritis with special reference to HLA-B27. *Arthritis Rheum* 1982;25:249–259.

Lindsley CB, Schaller JG. Arthritis associated with inflammatory bowel disease in children. *J Pediatr* 1974;84:16–20.

Lund PJ, Heikal A, Maricic MJ, Krupinski EA, Williams CS. Ultrasonographic imaging of the hand and wrist in rheumatoid arthritis. *Skeletal Radiol* 1995;24:591–596.

Marsal L, Winblad S, Wollheim FA. *Yersinia enterocolitica* arthritis in Southern Sweden: a four-year follow-up study. *BMJ* 1981;283:101–103.

Martel W, Braunstein EM, Borlaza G, Good AE, Griffin PE. Radiologic features of Reiter disease. *Radiology* 1979;132:1–10.

Martel W, Holt JF, Cassidy JT. The roentgenologic manifestations of juvenile rheumatoid arthritis. *AJR Am J Roentgenol* 1962;88:400–423.

Martel W, Snarr JW, Horn JR. Metacarpophalangeal joints in interphalangeal osteoarthritis. *Radiology* 1973;108:1–7.

Martel W, Stuck KJ, Dworin AM, Hylland RG. Erosive osteoarthritis and psoriatic arthritis: a radiologic comparison in the hand, wrist, and foot. *AJR Am J Roentgenol* 1980;134:125–135.

Metzger AL, Morris RI, Bluestone R, Terasaki PI. HL-A W27 in psoriatic arthropathy. *Arthritis Rheum* 1975;18:111–115.

Michelson J, Easley M, Wigley FM, Hellmann D. Foot and ankle problems in rheumatoid arthritis. *Foot Ankle Int* 1994;15:608–613.

Nance EP, Kaye JJ. The rheumatod variants. *Semin Roentgenol* 1982;17:16–24.

Oloff-Solomon J, Oloff LM, Jacobs AM. Rheumatoid nodulosis in the foot: a variant of rheumatoid disease. *J Foot Surg* 1984;23:382–385.

Oudjhane K, Azouz EM, Hughes S, Paquin JD. Computed tomography of the sacroiliac joints in children. *Can Assoc Radiol J* 1993;44:313–314.

Paimela L. The radiographic criterion in the 1987 revised criteria for rheumatoid arthritis. *Arthritis Rheum* 1992;35:255–258.

Park WM, O'Neill M, McCall IW. The radiology of rheumatoid involvement of the cervical spine. *Skeletal Radiol* 1979;4:1–7.

Peterfy CG, Majumdar S, Lang P, van Dijke C, Sack K, Genant H. MR imaging of the arthritic knee: improved discrimination of cartilage, synovium, and effusion with pulsed saturation transfer and fat-suppressed T1-weighted sequences. *Radiology* 1994;191:413–419.

Peterson CC Jr, Silbiger ML. Reiter's syndrome and psoriatic arthritis. Their roentgen spectra and some interesting similarities. *AJR Am J Roentgenol* 1967;101:860–871.

Pettersson H, Larsson E-M, Holtas S, Cronquist S, Egund N, Zygmunt S, Brattstrom H. MR imaging of the cervical spine in rheumatoid arthritis. *AJNR* 1988;9:573–577.

Reith JD, Bauer TW, Schils JP. Osseous manifestations of SAPHO (synovitis, acne, pustulosis, hyperostosis, osteitis) syndrome. *Am J Surg Pathol* 1996;20:1368–1377.

Reiter H. Ueber eine bisher unerkannte Spirochaeteninfektion (Spirochaetosis arthritica). *Dtsch Med Wochenschr* 1916;42:1535–1536.

Resnick D. Common disorders of synovium-lined joints: pathogenesis, imaging abnormalities, and complications. *AJR Am J Roentgenol* 1988;151:1079–1093.

Resnick D. Rheumatoid arthritis of the wrist: why the ulnar styloid? *Radiology* 1974;112:29–35.

Resnick D, Niwayama G. On the nature and significance of bony proliferation in "rheumatoid variant" disorders. *AJR Am J Roentgenol* 1977;129:275–278.

Resnick D, Niwayama G. Rheumatoid arthritis and the seronegative spondyloarthropathies: radiographic and pathologic concepts. In: Resnick D, ed. *Diagnosis of bone and joint disorders*, 3rd ed. Philadelphia: WB Saunders; 1995:807–865.

Resnick D, Niwayama G, Goergen TG. Comparison of radiographic abnormalities of the sacroiliac joint in degenerative disease and ankylosing spondylitis. *AJR Am J Roentgenol* 1977;128:189–196.

Resnik CS, Resnick D. Radiology of disorders of the sacroiliac joints. *JAMA* 1985;253:2863–2866.

Reynolds H, Carter SW, Murtagh FR, Silbiger M, Rechtine GR. Cervical rheumatoid arthritis: value of flexion and extension views in imaging. *Radiology* 1987;164:215–218.

Rominger MB, Bernreuter WK, Kenney PJ, Morgan SL, Blackburn WD, Alarcon GS. MR imaging of the hands in early rheumatoid arthritis: preliminary results. *Radiographics* 1993;13:37–46.

Sanders KM, Resnik CS, Owen DS. Erosive arthritis in Cronkhite-Canada syndrome. *Radiology* 1985;156:309–310.

Sartoris DJ, Resnick D. The radiographic differential diagnosis of juvenile chronic arthritis. *Aust Paediatr J* 1987;23:273–275.

Sholkoff SD, Glickman MG, Steinbach HL. Roentgenology of Reiter's syndrome. *Radiology* 1970;97:497–503.

Smith D, Braunstein EM, Brandt KD, Katz BP. A radiographic comparison of erosive osteoarthritis and idiopathic nodal osteoarthritis. *J Rheumatol* 1992;19:896–904.

Solomon G, Winchester R. Immunogenetic aspects of inflammatory arthritis. In: Taveras JM, Ferrucci JT, eds. *Radiology—diagnosis, imaging, intervention*, vol. 5. Philadelphia: JB Lippincott; 1986:1–4.

Stiskal MA, Neuhold A, Szolar DH, et al. Rheumatoid arthritis of the craniocervical region by MR imaging: detection and characterization. *AJR Am J Roentgenol* 1995;165:585–592.

Sugimoto H, Takeda A, Hyodoh K. Early-stage rheumatoid arthritis: prospective study of the effectiveness of MR imaging for diagnosis. *Radiology* 2000;216:569–575.

Sugimoto H, Takeda A, Masuyama J-I, Furuse M. Early-stage rheumatoid arthritis: diagnostic accuracy of MR imaging. *Radiology* 1996;198:185–192.

Sundaram M, Patton JT. Paravertebral ossification in psoriasis and Reiter's disease. *Br J Radiol* 1975;48:628–633.

Swett HA, Jaffe RB, McIff EB. Popliteal cysts: presentation as thrombophlebitis. *Radiology* 1975;115:613–615.

Tehranzadeh J, Ashikyan O, Dascalos J. Magnetic resonance imaging in early detection of rheumatoid arthritis. *Semin Musculoskel Radiol* 2003;7:79–94.

Uhl M, Allmann KH, Ihling C, Hauer MP, Conca W, Langer M. Cartilage destruction in small joints by rheumatoid arthritis: assessment of fat-suppressed three-dimensional gradient-echo MR pulse sequences in vitro. *Skeletal Radiol* 1998;27:677–682.

Vinson EN, Major NM. MR imaging of ankylosing spondylitis. *Semin Musculoskel Radiol* 2003;7:103–113.

Wamser G, Bohndorf K, Vollert K, Bücklein W, Schalm J. Power Doppler sonography with and without echo-enhancing contrast agent and contrast-enhanced MRI for the evaluation of rheumatoid arthritis of the shoulder joint: differentiation between synovitis and joint effusion. *Skeletal Radiol* 2003;32:351–359.

Weissman BN. Imaging techniques in rheumatoid arthritis. *J Rheumatol (Suppl)* 1994;42:14–19.

Weissman BN. Spondyloarthropathies. *Radiol Clin North Am* 1987;25:1235–1262.

Wilkinson RH, Weissman BN. Arthritis in children. *Radiol Clin North Am* 1988;26:1247–1265.

Wisnieski JJ, Askari AD. Rheumatoid nodulosis. A relatively benign rheumatoid variant. *Arch Intern Med* 1981;141:615–619.

Wright V. Seronegative polyarthritis: a unified concept. *Arthritis Rheum* 1978;21:619–633.

Yamato M, Tamai K, Yamaguchi T, Ohno W. MRI of the knee in rheumatoid arthritis: Gd-DTPA perfusion dynamics. *J Comput Assist Tomogr* 1993;17:781–785.

MISCELLANEOUS ARTHRITIDES AND ARTHROPATHIES

Connective Tissue Arthropathies

An overview of the clinical and radiographic hallmarks of the forms of arthritis associated with connective tissue disorders is presented in Table 15.1.

Systemic Lupus Erythematosus

Systemic lupus erythematosus (SLE) is a chronic, inflammatory, connective tissue disorder of unknown cause characterized by significant immunologic abnormalities and involvement of multiple organs. Women, particularly adolescents and young adults, are affected four-times as frequently as men. The clinical manifestations of SLE vary according to the distribution and extent of systemic alterations. The most common symptoms are malaise, weakness, fever, anorexia, and weight loss. Consistent and characteristic features of this disease are serologic abnormalities, including a variety of serum autoantibodies to nuclear antigens, which have been historically associated with the presence of lupus erythematosus cells and neutrophilic leukocytes filled with cytoplasmic inclusion bodies.

Antinuclear antibodies are useful in the differential diagnosis of SLE, and changes in the titer of antibodies to DNA are useful in fol-

lowing disease activity. Antinuclear antibodies are a heterogeneous group of antibodies directed against a number of discrete nuclear macromolecular proteins. They represent what has classically been referred to as "autoantibodies," because they are directed against components normally present in all nucleated cells. They generally lack tissue or species specificity; therefore, they will cross-react with nuclei from different sources. The primary sources for study of these antibodies are patients with SLE and related systemic rheumatic diseases. Many studies have centered on defining the specificity of these antibodies and have contributed extensively to our understanding of their immunopathologic role in connective tissue disorders.

The musculoskeletal system is a frequent site of involvement in SLE, and joint abnormalities, exhibited by 90% of patients during the course of the disease, represent a significant part of the clinical and radiologic picture. Arthritic involvement is symmetric, and articular deformities without fixed contractures are a hallmark of this disorder. The hands are the predominant site of involvement. Typically, the lateral radiograph discloses malalignments, most commonly at the metacarpophalangeal and proximal interphalangeal joints of the fingers and the carpometacarpal, metacarpophalangeal and the interphalangeal joints of the thumb (Fig. 15.1). These abnormalities may not be apparent on a dorsovolar radiograph because the malalign-

Table 15.1 **Clinical and Radiographic Hallmarks of Connective Tissue Arthritides (Arthropathies)**

Type of Arthritis	Site	Crucial Abnormalities	Technique/Projection
Systemic lupus erythematosus (F> M; young adults; blacks > whites; skin changes: rash)	Hands Hips, ankles, shoulders	Flexible joint contractures Osteonecrosis	Lateral view Standard views of affected joints Scintigraphy Magnetic resonance imaging
Scleroderma (F> M; skin changes: edema, thickening)	Hands	Soft-tissue calcifications Acroosteolysis Tapering of distal phalanges Interphalangeal destructive changes	Dorsovolar and lateral views
	Gastrointestinal tract	Dilatation of esophagus Decreased peristalsis Dilatation of duodenum and small bowel	Esophagram Esophagram (cine or video study) Upper gastrointestinal and small bowel series
		Pseudodiverticulosis of colon	Barium enema
Polymyositis/Dermatomyositis	Upper and lower extremities (proximal parts)	Soft-tissue calcifications Periarticular osteoporosis	Xeroradiography; digital radiography
	Hands	Erosions and destructive changes in distal interphalangeal articulations	Dorsovolar and lateral views
Mixed connective tissue disease (overlap of clinical features of SLE, scleroderma, dermatomyositis, and rheumatoid arthritis)	Hands, wrists	Erosions and destructive changes in proximal interphalangeal, meta-carpophalangeal, radiocarpal and midcarpal articulations, associated with joint space narrowing Symmetric soft-tissue swelling Soft-tissue atrophy and calcifications	Dorsovolar and lateral views Magnetic resonance imaging
	Chest	Pleural and pericardial effusions	Posteroanterior and lateral views Ultrasound

Figure 15.1 Systemic lupus erythematosus. (A) Typical appearance of the thumb in a 43-year-old woman with systemic lupus erythematosus. Note subluxations in the first carpometacarpal and metacarpophalangeal joints without articular erosions. **(B)** In anther patient, a 32-year-old woman with SLE, the oblique radiograph of her left hand shows dislocation at the first carpometacarpal joint (*arrow*) and subluxations in the metacarpophalangeal joints of the index and middle fingers associated with swan-neck deformities (*open arrows*).

ments are flexible and are corrected by the pressure of the hand against the radiographic cassette (Fig. 15.2). These pathognomonic deformities usually occur secondary to a loss of support from the ligamentous and capsular structures about the joint, and at least in the early stage of disease are completely reducible. Only very seldom are

these abnormalities fixed and/or accompanied by articular erosions (Fig. 15.3).

Some patients present with sclerosis of the distal phalanges (acral sclerosis) (Fig. 15.4) or with resorption of the terminal tufts (acroosteolysis). Osteonecrosis, which is frequently seen, has been attributed

Figure 15.2 Systemic lupus erythematosus. (A) Lateral radiograph of both hands of a 42-year-old woman with documented systemic lupus erythematosus for the past 4 years demonstrates flexion deformities in the metacarpophalangeal joints. On the dorsovolar projection **(B)**, the flexion deformities have been corrected by the pressure of the hands against the radiographic cassette.

Figure 15.3 Systemic lupus erythematosus. A 62-year-old woman presented with a 15-year history of systemic lupus erythematosus. Dorsovolar view of both hands shows severe deformities, subluxations, and articular erosions. Note the advanced osteoporosis secondary to disuse of the extremities and treatment with corticosteroids.

to complications of treatment with corticosteroids (Fig. 15.5). However, current investigations suggest the vital role of the inflammatory process (vasculitis) in the development of this complication.

Scleroderma

Scleroderma (progressive systemic sclerosis) is a generalized disorder of unknown cause. It is seen predominantly in young women, usually becoming apparent in their third and fourth decades. Primarily a connective tissue disorder, it is characterized by thickening and fibrosis of the skin and subcutaneous tissues, with frequent involvement of the musculoskeletal system. Most patients have the so-called CREST syndrome, which refers to the coexistence of calcinosis, Raynaud phenomenon (episodes of intermittent pallor of the fingers and toes on exposure to cold, secondary to vasoconstriction of the small blood vessels), esophageal abnormalities (dilatation and hypoperistalsis), sclerodactyly, and telangiectasia; 30% to 40% of patients have a positive serologic test for rheumatoid factor and a positive antinuclear antibody (ANA) test.

Radiographically, scleroderma presents with characteristic abnormalities of the bone and soft tissues. The hands usually exhibit atrophy of the soft tissues at the tips of the fingers (Fig. 15.6), resorption of the distal phalanges, subcutaneous and periarticular calcifications (Figs. 15.7 and 15.8), and destructive changes of the small articulations, usually the interphalangeal joints (Fig. 15.9). Corroborative findings are seen in the gastrointestinal tract, where dilatation of the esophagus and small bowel, together with a pseudoobstruction pattern, are characteristic (Fig. 15.10). Pseudodiverticula in the colon are also commonly seen.

Polymyositis and Dermatomyositis

Polymyositis and dermatomyositis are disorders of striated muscle and skin and are characterized by diffuse, nonsuppurative inflammation, as well as degeneration. Early diagnosis and subsequent management of patients with any type of myopathy, including polymyositis and dermatomyositis, can be facilitated by the use of appropriate laboratory tests. The four tests most helpful in evaluating muscle disorders include: (A) serum enzymes; (B) urinary creatine and creatinine excretion; (C) electromyogram; and (D) muscle biopsy.

Figure 15.4 Systemic lupus erythematosus. Dorsovolar film of the hand of a 29-year-old woman with systemic lupus erythematosus demonstrates sclerosis of the distal phalanges (acral sclerosis). Similar sclerotic changes are also occasionally seen in rheumatoid arthritis and scleroderma.

Figure 15.5 Systemic lupus erythematosus complicated by osteonecrosis. Oblique radiograph (**A**) and lateral tomogram (**B**) of the ankle demonstrate osteonecrosis of the talus in a 26-year-old woman with lupus who was treated with massive doses of steroids.

Figure 15.6 Scleroderma. A 24-year-old woman with scleroderma presented with atrophy of the soft tissues at the distal phalanges of the index, middle, and ring fingers (*arrows*).

Figure 15.7 Scleroderma. A 32-year-old woman with progressive systemic sclerosis exhibits soft-tissue calcifications in the distal phalanges of the right hand, a typical feature of this disorder.

Figure 15.8 Scleroderma. A dorsovolar radiograph of the fingers of a 44-year-old woman reveals acroosteolysis (*arrow*), soft tissue calcifications, and destructive changes of the distal interphalangeal joint of the middle finger.

Different serum enzyme determinations have been advocated, but the most valuable tests include serum creatine phosphokinase (CPK), serum aldolase (ALD), serum lactate dehydrogenase (LDH), serum glutamic oxalacetic transaminase (SGOT), and serum glutamic pyruvic transaminase (SGPT). Further, the determination of serum enzyme levels and urinary creatine excretion are helpful for the clinical management of polymyositis and dermatomyositis, because the two tests provide a broader perspective than either test alone.

A positive biopsy may not only demonstrate that the disease process is myopathic, thus enabling the physician to rule out a neuro-genic lower motor neuron lesion, but may also identify those patients whose muscle disease is more severe pathologically than was suspected on clinical grounds. This is important with respect to prognosis. With the aid of histochemical and electron microscopic techniques, muscle biopsy will occasionally enable the pathologist to diagnose one of the rare forms of myopathy that can clinically mimic polymyositis. Such diseases include sarcoid myopathy, central core disease, and muscle diseases associated with abnormal mitochondria.

The pathologic changes found on muscle biopsy in polymyositis have been well described. The degree of pathologic change may vary widely; one patient may show only negligible pathologic changes in muscle fibers on biopsy results, whereas another patient presenting similar clinical features may show extensive necrosis and fiber replacement. This variability in histologic findings is probably responsible for the frequent normal muscle biopsy results from patients with otherwise classic polymyositis. The overall rate of positive findings from muscle biopsy in several studies of polymyositis was in the range of 55% to 80%.

Radiographic abnormalities in polymyositis and dermatomyositis are divided into two types: those involving soft tissues and those involving joints. The most characteristic soft-tissue abnormality in both conditions is soft-tissue calcifications. The favorite sites of intermuscular calcification are the large muscles in the proximal parts of upper and lower extremities. In addition, subcutaneous calcifications similar to those of scleroderma are seen.

Articular abnormalities are rare. The most frequently reported, however, is periarticular osteoporosis. Destructive joint changes have been reported only occasionally, and primarily in the distal interphalangeal articulations of the hands.

Mixed Connective Tissue Disease

Mixed connective tissue disease (MCTD) was first reported as a distinctive syndrome by Sharp and associates in 1972. This syndrome is characterized by clinical abnormalities that combine the features of SLE, scleroderma, dermatomyositis, and rheumatoid arthritis. The one feature that distinguishes MCTD as a separate entity is a positive serologic test for antibody to the ribonucleoprotein (RNP) component of extractable nuclear antigen (ENA). The typical clinical pattern consists of Raynaud phenomenon, polyarthralgia, swelling of the

Figure 15.9 Scleroderma. Dorsovolar radiograph of the hands of a 50-year-old man with documented systemic sclerosis shows destructive changes in the distal interphalangeal joints, as well as soft-tissue calcifications and resorption of the tip of the distal phalanx of the left middle finger.

Figure 15.10 Scleroderma. Upper gastrointestinal series and small bowel study in the patient shown in Figure 15.9 demonstrates dilatation of the second and third portions of the duodenum and jejunum, with a pseudoobstruction pattern.

dilated
duodenum

dilated
jejunum

hands, esophageal hypomotility, inflammatory myopathy, and pulmonary disease. Women constitute approximately 80% of affected patients. Patients with MCTD have prominent joint abnormalities, with typical involvement of the small articulations of the hand, wrist, and foot; large joints such as the knee, elbow, and shoulder may also be affected. The joint deformities mimic those seen in rheumatoid arthritis, but occasionally joint subluxation may be nonerosive, as in SLE. Soft-tissue abnormalities are identical to those encountered in scleroderma (Figs. 15.11 and 15.12).

Vasculitis

There is a diverse clinical spectrum of the vasculitides that includes systemic necrotizing vasculitis, hypersensitivity vasculitis, Wegener granulomatosis, lymphomatoid granulomatosis, giant cell arteritis, and a variety of miscellaneous syndromes (e.g., Kawasaki disease, Behçet disease, and others). A discussion of these diverse but often overlapping diseases is far beyond the scope of this volume, but the reader is referred to several key references at the end of this chapter. The demonstration of vasculitis by angiograms can often be documented by the presence of aneurysmal dilatation in affected vessels. Generally, an angiogram is performed when the diagnosis cannot be established by tissue biopsy.

Metabolic and Endocrine Arthritides

An overview of the clinical and radiographic hallmarks of the arthritides associated with metabolic and endocrine abnormalities is shown in Table 15.2.

Gout

Gout is a metabolic disorder characterized by recurrent episodes of arthritis associated with the presence of monosodium urate monohydrate crystals in the synovial fluid leukocytes and, in many cases, gross deposits of sodium urate (tophi) in periarticular soft tissues. Serum uric acid concentrations are elevated.

The great toe is the most common site of involvement in gouty arthritis; the condition known as *podagra*, which involves the first metatarsophalangeal joint, occurs in approximately 75% of patients. Other frequently affected sites include the ankle, knee, elbow, and wrist. Most patients are men, but gouty arthritis is seen in postmenopausal women as well.

Hyperuricemia

An increased miscible pool of uric acid with resulting hyperuricemia can occur in two principal ways. First, urate is produced in such large quantities that, even though excretion routes are of normal capacity, they are inadequate to handle the excessive load. Second, the capacity for uric acid excretion is critically reduced, so that even a normal quantity of uric acid cannot be eliminated.

In 25% to 30% of gouty patients, a primary defect in the rate of purine synthesis causes excessive uric acid formation, as reflected in excessive urinary uric acid excretion (more than 600 mg/day) measured while the patient is maintained on a standard purine-free diet. Increased production can also be seen in gout secondary to myeloproliferative disorders associated with increased destruction of cells and result in increased breakdown of nucleic acids. Decreased excretion occurs in primary gout in patients with a dysfunction in the renal tubular capacity to secrete urate and in patients with chronic renal

Figure 15.11 Mixed connective tissue disease. A 44-year-old woman presented with clinical and imaging features of rheumatoid arthritis. In addition, she had clinically documented dermatomyositis. A dorsovolar radiograph of her left hand shows extensive articular erosions at radiocarpal, metacarpophalangeal, and proximal interphalangeal joints, typical for rheumatoid arthritis. The muscle biopsy result was consistent with polymyositis.

disease. In most patients, however, there is evidence of both uric acid overproduction and diminished renal excretion of uric acid.

The chance of development of gouty arthritis in hyperuricemic individuals should increase in proportion to the duration and, even more, to the degree of hyperuricemia. Monosodium urate, however, has a marked tendency to form relatively stable supersaturated solutions; therefore, the proportion of hyperuricemic patients in whom gouty arthritis actually develops is relatively low. The clinical development of gouty arthritis in the hyperuricemic subject is also substantially influenced by other factors, such as binding of urate to plasma proteins or the presence of promoters or inhibitors of crystallization.

Examination of Synovial Fluid

A wet preparation of fresh synovial fluid is best for examination of crystals. Although crystals may often be seen by ordinary light microscopy, reliable identification requires polarization equipment. To differentiate between urate and pyrophosphate crystals—characteristics of gout and pseudogout, respectively—a compensated, polarized light microscope is advisable. Because both types of crystals are birefringent, they refract the polarized light that passes through them. The birefringence phenomenon is caused by the refractive index for light, which vibrates either parallel or perpendicular to the axis of the crystal being viewed. Color is the key to negative or positive birefringence. Urates are strongly birefringent; therefore, they are brightly colored in polarized light, with a red compensator. They are usually seen as needles. During an acute gouty attack, many intraleukocytic crystals are present. Monosodium urate crystals are negatively birefringent, i.e., they appear yellow when the longitudinal axis of the crystal is parallel to the axis of slow vibrations of the red compensator on the polarizing system, and they appear blue when perpendicular.

Monosodium urate crystals, the pathogens of gouty arthritis, range in length from 2 to 10 μ and are found within synovial leukocytes or extracellularly in virtually every case of acute gout, although the likelihood of finding such crystals varies inversely with the amount of time elapsed from onset of symptoms to the time of examination. Crystals from tophi may be larger.

Figure 15.12 Mixed connective tissue disease. A 26-year-old woman presented with swelling of both hands, polyarthralgia, and Raynaud phenomenon. She tested positively for the rheumatoid factors and antinuclear antibodies, and her clinical findings were characteristic for systemic lupus erythematosus (SLE) and scleroderma. Oblique radiograph (**A**) of the right hand and coned-down view (**B**) of the thumb and index finger of the left hand show flexion deformities and subluxations in the multiple joints. Deformities of both thumbs are characteristic for SLE, whereas soft-tissue calcifications (*arrows*) are typical for scleroderma. The clinical diagnosis was mixed connective tissue disease.

Table 15.2 Clinical and Radiographic Hallmarks of Metabolic, Endocrine, and Miscellaneous Arthritides

Type of Arthritis	Site	Crucial Abnormalities	Technique/Projection
Gout (M>F)	Great toe	Articular erosion with preservation of part of joint	Standard views of affected joints
	Large joints (knee, elbow)	Overhanging edge of erosion	
	Hand	Lack of osteoporosis	
		Periarticular swelling	
		Tophi	
CPPD Crystal deposition disease (M=F)	Variable joints	Chondrocalcinosis (calcification of articular cartilage and menisci)	Standard views of affected joints
		Calcifications of tendons, ligaments, and capsule	
	Femoropatellar joint	Joint space narrowing	Lateral (knee) and axial (patella) views
		Subchondral sclerosis	
		Osteophytes	
	Wrists, elbows, shoulders, ankles	Degenerative changes with chondrocalcinosis	Standard views of affected joints
CHA crystal deposition disease (F>M)	Variable joints, but predilection for shoulder joint (supraspinatus tendon)	Pericapsular calcifications	Standard views of affected joints
		Calcifications of tendons	
Hemochromatosis (M>F)	Hands	Involvement of second and third metacarpophalangeal joints with beak-like osteophytes	Dorsovolar view
	Large joints	Chondrocalcinosis	Standard views of affected joints
Alkaptonuria (ochronosis) (M=F)	Intervertebral disks, sacroiliac joints, symphysis pubis, large joints (knees, hips)	Calcification and ossification of intervertebral disks, narrowing of disks, osteoporosis, joint space narrowing, periarticular sclerosis	Anteroposterior and lateral views of spine; standard views of affected joints
Hyperparathyroidism (F>M)	Hands	Destructive changes in interphalangeal joints	Dorsovolar view
		Subperiosteal resorption	Dorsovolar and oblique views
	Multiple bones	Bone cysts (brown tumors)	Standard views specific for locations
	Skull	Salt-and-pepper appearance	Lateral view
	Spine	Rugger-jersey appearance	Lateral view
Acromegaly (M>F)	Hands	Widened joint spaces	Dorsovolar view
		Large sesamoid	
		Degenerative changes (beak-like osteophytes)	
	Skull	Large sinuses	Lateral view
	Facial bones	Large mandible (prognathism)	Lateral view
	Heel	Thick heel pad (>25 mm)	Lateral view
	Spine	Thoracic kyphosis	Lateral view (thoracic spine)
Amyloidosis (M>F)	Large joints (hips, knees, shoulders, elbows)	Articular and periarticular erosions, osteoporosis (periarticular), joint subluxations, pathologic fractures	Standard views of affected joints Radionuclide bone scan (scintigraphy)
Multicentric Reticulohistiocytosis (F>M)	Hands (distal and proximal interphalangeal joints)	Soft-tissue swelling, articular erosions, lack of osteoporosis	Dorsovolar view Norgaard ("Allstate") view
	Feet		Dorsoplantar view Oblique view
Hemophilia (M>F)	Large joints (hips, knees, shoulders)	Joint effusion, osteoporosis, symmetrical and concentric joint space narrowing, articular erosions, widening of intercondylar notch, squaring of patella; very similar to changes of juvenile rheumatoid arthritis	Standard views of affected joints Magnetic resonance imaging
	Elbows, ankles		

Radiographic Features

Gouty arthritis has several characteristic radiographic features. Erosions, which are usually sharply marginated, are initially periarticular in location and are later seen to extend into the joint (Fig. 15.13); an "overhanging edge" of erosion is a frequent identifying feature (Fig. 15.14). Occasionally, intraosseous defects are present secondary to formation of intraosseous tophi (Fig. 15.15). Usually, there is a striking lack of osteoporosis, which helps differentiate this condition from rheumatoid arthritis. The reason for the absence of osteoporosis is that the duration of an acute gouty attack is too short to allow the development of the disuse osteoporosis so often seen in patients with rheumatoid arthritis. If erosion involves the articular end of the bone and extends into the joint, part of the joint is usually preserved (Fig. 15.16). Unlike rheumatoid arthritis, periarticular and articular erosions are asymmetric in distribution (Fig. 15.17). In chronic tophaceous gout, sodium urate deposits in and around the joint are seen, creating a dense mass in the soft tissues called a tophus, which frequently exhibits calcifications (Fig. 15.18). Characteristically, tophi are randomly distributed and are usually asymmetric; if they occur in the hands or feet, they are more often seen on the dorsal aspect (Fig. 15.19).

CPPD Crystal Deposition Disease

Clinical Features

Resulting from the intraarticular presence of calcium pyrophosphate dihydrate (CPPD) crystals, CPPD crystal deposition disease affects men and women equally; most commonly, patients are middle-aged

Figure 15.13 Gouty arthritis. (A) Dorsovolar radiograph of the left hand of a 43-year-old man with tophaceous gout shows multiple sharply marginated periarticular erosions and soft tissue masses at the proximal interphalangeal joints of the index and middle fingers, representing tophi. **(B)** Dorsovolar radiograph of the fingers of a 70-year-old man with gouty arthritis shows multiple articular and periarticular erosions associated with large tophi (*arrows*).

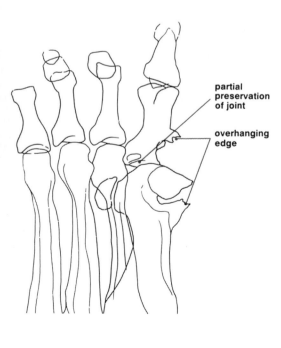

Figure 15.14 Gouty arthritis. Oblique radiograph of the right foot of a 58-year-old man with a 3-month history of gout shows the typical involvement of the first metatarsophalangeal joint. Note the characteristic "overhanging edge" of the erosive changes and preservation of the lateral portion of the joint.

Figure 15.15 **Gouty arthritis.** Dorsovolar radiograph of both hands of a 60-year-old man with gout shows articular and periarticular erosions. In addition, note the presence of intraosseous defects in the phalanges consistent with intraosseous tophi.

Figure 15.16 **Gouty arthritis.** Dorsoplantar radiograph of the left foot of a 62-year-old man with a long history of tophaceous gout shows multiple erosions involving the big and small toes and the base of the fourth and fifth metatarsals. The first metatarsophalangeal joint is partially preserved, a characteristic feature of gouty arthritis. A large soft-tissue swelling of the great toe represents a tophus.

Figure 15.17 Gouty arthritis. Dorsovolar radiograph of the hands of a 64-year-old woman with gout shows the typical asymmetric distribution of periarticular and articular erosions.

Figure 15.18 Gouty tophus. Lateral radiograph of the elbow of a 73-year-old man with a 30-year history of gout shows a tophus with dense calcifications adjacent to the olecranon process, which exhibits a small erosion.

Figure 15.19 Gouty tophus. Dorsoplantar **(A)** and lateral **(B)** radiographs of the great toe show articular and periarticular erosions (*arrows*) associated with a large tophus on the dorsal aspect of the first metatarsophalangeal joint (*arrow heads*).

and older. The condition may be asymptomatic, in which case the only radiologic finding may be *chondrocalcinosis* (see later). When symptomatic, it is called *pseudogout*. There is, however, a great deal of confusion about these terms, and they are often misused.

In an effort to explain the relationship between chondrocalcinosis, calcium pyrophosphate arthropathy, and the pseudogout syndrome, Resnick has proposed an integration of these terms under the rubric CPPD crystal deposition disease. *Chondrocalcinosis*, a condition in which calcification of the hyaline (articular) cartilage or fibrocartilage (menisci) occurs, may be seen in other conditions as well, such as gout, hyperparathyroidism, hemochromatosis, hepatolenticular degeneration (Wilson disease), and degenerative joint disease (Table 15.3). *Calcium pyrophosphate arthropathy* refers to CPPD crystal deposition disease affecting the joints and producing structural damage to the articular cartilage. It displays distinctive radiographic abnormalities such as narrowing of the joint space, subchondral sclerosis, and osteophytosis. The *pseudogout syndrome* represents a condition in which symptoms such as acute pain are similar to those seen in gouty arthri-

tis; however, it does not respond to the usual treatment (colchicine) for the latter disease.

Calcium pyrophosphate crystals, the pathogens in pseudogout, range up to 10 μ in length. As in gout, many intracellular crystals are seen during an acute episode. The colors are usually but not always much less intense than urates, i.e., they are weakly birefringent. Pyrophosphate crystals are generally chunkier and often show a line down the middle. The most common form of calcium pyrophosphate crystal is a rhomboid. Pyrophosphate crystals are positively birefringent in that they are blue when the longitudinal axis of the crystal is parallel to the slow vibrations axis of the red compensator and yellow when it is perpendicular.

Radiographic Features

Radiographically, the arthritic changes encountered in this condition are similar to those seen in osteoarthritis, but the wrist (Fig. 15.20), elbow (Fig. 15.21), shoulder, ankle, and femoropatellar joint compartment are characteristically involved. As mentioned, CPPD crystal deposition disease is characterized by calcification of the articular cartilage and fibrocartilage; the tendons, ligaments, and joint capsule may exhibit calcifications as well (Figs. 15.22 and 15.23).

Rarely, CPPD deposits can assume the form of bulky tumor-like masses located in the joint and paraarticular soft tissues. In these instances, it may mimic a malignant tumor; hence, this form of CPPD deposition was termed by Sissons and associates, "tumoral calcium pyrophosphate deposition disease." The mineral deposits are associated with a tissue reaction characterized by the presence of histiocytes and multinucleated giant cells, sometimes with bone and cartilage formation. The differential diagnosis should include tumoral calcinosis, a disorder characterized by the presence of single or multiple lobulated cystic masses in the soft tissues, usually near the major joints, containing chalky material consisting of calcium phosphate, calcium carbonate, or hydroxyapatite. The calcified deposits fail to show a crystalline appearance when examined by polarization microscopy. In this

Table 15.3 **Most Common Causes of Chondrocalcinosis**

Senescent (aging process)	Hemochromatosis
Idiopathic	Hyperparathyroidism
Osteoarthritis	Hypophosphatasia
Posttraumatic	Ochronosis
Calcium pyrophosphate arthropathy	Oxalosis
(CPPD crystal deposition disease)	Wilson disease
Gout	Acromegaly

Modified from Reeder MM, Felson B, 1975, with permission.

Figure 15.20 CPPD crystal deposition disease. A 63-year-old man with calcium pyrophosphate dihydrate (CPPD) crystal deposition disease presented with an acute onset of pain in the wrist. A dorsovolar radiograph shows chondrocalcinosis of the triangular fibrocartilage, cystic changes in the scaphoid and lunate, and narrowing of the radiocarpal joint.

Figure 15.21 CPPD crystal deposition disease. An anteroposterior **(A)** and radial **(B)** head–capitellum view of the right elbow of a 52-year-old woman with pseudogout syndrome demonstrate chondrocalcinosis (*open arrows*) but no other alterations of the joint space.

Figure 15.22 CPPD crystal deposition disease. A 70-year-old woman presented with acute onset of pain in her right knee and was treated with colchicine for acute gouty arthritis without relief of her pain. Synovial fluid yielded crystals of calcium pyrophosphate dihydrate (CPDD). Anteroposterior **(A)** and lateral **(B)** radiographs of the knee demonstrate calcification of the hyaline and fibrocartilage. Capsular calcifications are also apparent, as well as narrowing of the femoropatellar joint compartment, a characteristic feature of CPPD crystal deposition disease.

Figure 15.23 CPPD crystal deposition disease. A 51-year-old man presented with pain in the left knee. A frontal radiograph shows calcifications of the menisci, articular cartilage, and medial collateral ligament. Joint aspiration was diagnostic for CPPD crystal deposition disease.

condition, the masses are painless and usually occur in children and adolescents, a majority of whom are black.

CHA Crystal Deposition Disease

Resulting from abnormal deposition of calcium hydroxyapatite (CHA) crystals in and around the joints, CHA crystal deposition disease is more common in women and may at times simulate gout or pseudogout syndrome. Acute symptoms include pain, tenderness on palpation, and local swelling and edema. The syndrome may be associated with other disorders, such as scleroderma, dermatomyositis, mixed connective tissue disease, and chronic renal disease, particularly one treated by hemodialysis. Recent investigations suggested a genetic predisposition for this condition. Amor and associates raised the possibility of an inherited defect that might be responsible for the development of CHA crystal deposition disease by demonstrating an increased prevalence of the histocompatibility antigen of HLA-A2 and HLA-BW35 in patients affected by this disorder.

CHA crystals are most frequently deposited in periarticular locations, usually in and around tendons, joint capsule, or bursae. This is the feature that distinguishes the syndrome from CPPD crystal deposition disease, which affects primarily hyaline cartilage and fibrocartilage.

Radiographic features depend on the site of involvement, but usually cloud-like or dense homogeneous calcific deposits are seen around the joint and tendons. The most common location is around the shoulder joint at the site of the supraspinatus tendon (Fig. 15.24).

Hemochromatosis

Hemochromatosis is a rare disorder characterized by iron deposition in various organs, particularly the liver, skin, and pancreas. It may be primary (endogenous or idiopathic), caused by an error in metabolizing iron, or secondary, caused by iron overload. Idiopathic hemochromatosis may be familial and has been linked with histocompatibility antigens HLA-A3, HLA-B7, and HLA-B14. The secondary form of hemochromatosis is related to iron overload (such as transfusions or dietary intake) and may be associated with alcohol abuse. Hemochromatosis affects men 10-times more frequently than women. It is generally diagnosed between the ages of 40 and 60 on the basis of markedly elevated serum iron levels. For confirmation, biopsy of the liver or synovium may be performed. Fifty percent of patients with hemochromatosis will have a slowly progressing arthritis, starting in the small joints of the hands, but eventually the large joints (Fig. 15.25) and intervertebral disks in the cervical and lumbar region may become affected. Some investigators believe that the arthropathy seen in this condition differs from typical degenerative joint disease and warrants classification in the group of metabolic arthritides.

In the hand, the second and third metacarpophalangeal joints are characteristically affected (Fig. 15.26; see also Fig. 13.21), although other small joints such as the interphalangeal and carpal articulations may also be involved. Degenerative changes may also be seen in the shoulders, knees, hips, and ankles. Loss of the articular space, eburnation, subchondral cyst formation, and osteophytosis are the most prominent radiographic features of hemochromatosis. The changes may occasionally mimic those seen in CPPD crystal deposition disease and rheumatoid arthritis.

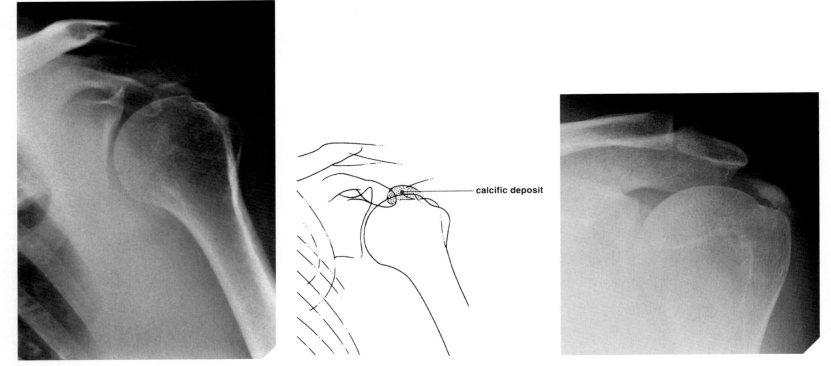

Figure 15.24 **CHA crystal deposition disease. (A)** Anteroposterior radiograph of the left shoulder of a 50-year-old woman who had been experiencing pain in this region for several months demonstrates an amorphous, homogenous calcific deposit in the soft tissues at the site of supraspinatus tendon. This finding is typical of calcium hydroxyapatite crystal deposition disease. **(B)** In another patient, a 38-year-old woman who presented with left shoulder pain, a similar calcific deposit is seen at the site of insertion of the supraspinatus tendon.

Figure 15.25 **Hemochromatosis.** A 67-year-old woman with hemochromatosis arthropathy. **(A)** Anteroposterior radiograph of the pelvis shows advanced arthritis of both hip joints. Severe concentric narrowing of joint space, subchondral sclerosis, and periarticular cysts are typical of hemochromatosis. Anteroposterior **(B)** and lateral **(C)** radiographs of the right knee demonstrate predilection for medial and femoropatellar compartments. Joint space narrowing and marked subarticular sclerosis with small osteophyte formation are characteristic. (From Baker ND, 1986, with permission.)

Figure 15.26 Hemochromatosis. (A) A dorsovolar radiograph of both hands of a 45-year-old man shows typical abnormalities of hemochromatosis predominantly affecting wrists and metacarpophalangeal joints. **(B)** A coned-down magnified radiograph of the second and third metacarpophalangeal joints of the right hand demonstrates characteristic involvement of the metacarpal heads.

Alkaptonuria (Ochronosis)

Alkaptonuria is a rare autosomal-recessive inherited disease characterized by the presence of homogentisic acid in the urine that turns black when oxidized. This metabolic abnormality results from the absence of the enzyme homogentisic acid oxidase, which plays a part in the normal degradation process of the aromatic amino acids tyrosine and phenylalanine. As a consequence, there is significant accumulation of homogentisic acid in various organs, with predilection for connective tissues. The deposition of an abnormal brown–black pigment,

a polymer of homogentisic acid, within the intervertebral disks and in the articular cartilage is termed ochronosis. This deposition leads to spondylosis and peripheral arthropathy. As a rule, ochronotic arthropathy is a manifestation of long-standing alkaptonuria. The condition affects men and women equally. The clinical signs consist of mild pain and a decreased range of motion in various joints. The radiographic presentation includes dystrophic calcifications, most commonly in the intervertebral disks and the articular cartilage, tendons, and ligaments (Fig. 15.27). Osteoporosis is usually present. Disk spaces are narrowed, with occasional vacuum phenomena. The ex-

Figure 15.27 Ochronosis. Anteroposterior radiograph of the lumbar spine **(A)** and lateral **(B)** radiograph of the thoracic spine of a 64-year-old woman with a clinical diagnosis of alkaptonuria demonstrate narrowing of several intervertebral disk spaces associated with marginal anterior osteophytes and moderate osteoporosis. Characteristic calcifications of multiple intervertebral disks are a hallmark of ochronosis (Courtesy of Dr. J. Tehranzadeh, Orange, CA).

Figure 15.28 Hyperparathyroidism arthropathy. Subchondral resorption resulted in widening of the sacroiliac joints in this patient with hyperparathyroidism arthropathy.

traspinal abnormalities are limited to involvement of the sacroiliac joints, the symphysis pubis, and the large peripheral joints, which are likewise narrowed and show periarticular sclerosis with occasional small osteophytes. Tendinous calcifications and ossifications may occur, at times leading to tendon rupture. The radiographic appearance may mimic that of degenerative joint disease or CPPD.

Hyperparathyroidism

Hyperparathyroidism is the result of overactivity of the parathyroid glands, which produce parathormone. Increased production of this hormone is secondary to either hyperplasia of glands or adenoma; only in very rare instances does hyperparathyroidism occur secondary to parathyroid carcinoma. Excessive secretion of parathormone, which acts on the kidneys and bones, leads to disturbances in calcium and phosphorus metabolism, resulting in hypercalcemia, hyperphosphaturia, and hypophosphatemia. Renal excretion of calcium and phosphate is increased, and serum levels of calcium are elevated while those of phosphorous are reduced; serum levels of alkaline phosphatase are also elevated. Most characteristic features of subperiosteal and subchondral bone resorption appear at the margins of certain joints, thus accounting for articular manifestation or "arthropathy" of hyperparathyroidism. This is frequently noted at the acromioclavicular joint, at the sternoclavicular and sacroiliac articulations (Fig. 15.28), at the symphysis pubis, and sometimes at the metacarpophalangeal and interphalangeal joints. The erosions can mimic rheumatoid arthritis, although they are usually asymptomatic, involve more commonly distal interphalangeal joints (Fig. 15.29), and almost invariably are associated with subperiosteal bone resorption, typical for hyperparathyroidism.

The other feature of hyperparathyroidism arthropathy is chondrocalcinosis, which involves calcium deposition in the articular cartilage and fibrocartilage. This finding may mimic degenerative joint disease and CPPD crystal deposition arthropathy. It may be distinguished from the calcification of degenerative joint disease by the absence of arthritic changes in the joint and from CPPD crystal deposition by the presence of osteopenia and other typical features of hyperparathyroidism. A more detailed description of hyperparathyroidism is provided in Part VI: Metabolic and Endocrine Disorders.

Acromegaly

Degenerative joint changes in acromegaly are the result of hypertrophy of articular cartilage, which is not adequately nourished by synovial fluid because of its abnormal thickness.

After initial overgrowth of cartilage, as reflected by widening of the radiographic joint spaces in the hand, particularly at the metacar-

Figure 15.29 Hyperparathyroidism arthropathy. Typical hyperparathyroidism arthropathy at the distal interphalangeal joints of the index and middle fingers. Note also beginning of the resorption of the distal tufts (acroosteolysis).

pophalangeal joints (Fig. 15.30), a later manifestation of this disorder is thinning of the joint cartilages with osteophyte formation caused by secondary osteoarthritis. Arthritis-like symptoms including pain and stiffness are common, and limitation of joint motion becomes apparent. Besides articulations of the hands, large joints such as the hip, knee, and

Figure 15.30 Acromegalic arthropathy. Characteristic abnormalities in acromegalic hand include prominence of the soft tissue, enlargement of the tufts and bases of the distal phalanges, widening of the metacarpophalangeal joints, and beak-like osteophytes at the radial aspect of the metacarpal heads. Note also markedly enlarged sesamoid bone at the first metacarpophalangeal joint.

Figure 15.31 **Amyloidosis. (A)** Anteroposterior radiograph of the right shoulder of an 80-year-old man with amyloidosis demonstrates a moderate degree of juxtaarticular osteoporosis, soft-tissue swelling, and a large osteolytic lesion in the humeral head. The glenohumeral joint space is relatively well-preserved. **(B)** Radionuclide bone scan shows an increased uptake of technetium-labeled MDP in the shoulder (Courtesy of Dr. A. Norman, New York, NY).

even shoulder or elbow may be affected. In particular, beak-like osteophytes on the inferior aspect of the humeral head, the lateral aspect of the acetabulum, the superior margin of the symphysis pubis, and radial aspects of the heads of metacarpals are characteristic (see Fig. 13.20).

Miscellaneous Conditions

Amyloidosis

Amyloidosis is a systematic disorder characterized by the infiltration of various organs by a homogeneous eosinophilic material consisting of protein fibers in a ground substance of mucopolysaccharides. Amyloid arthropathy is a sign of acquired idiopathic systemic amyloidosis and is a condition that results in noninflammatory arthropathy. Clinically, it bears a striking resemblance to rheumatoid arthritis, because the joints are stiff and painful and the arthropathy is bilateral and symmetric. There is a predilection for large joints such as the hips, knees, shoulders, and elbows. Subcutaneous nodules are noted over the extensor surfaces of the forearm and dorsum of the hand, often mimicking the rheumatoid nodules. Another characteristic feature is the massive involvement of the soft tissues, giving the patient an almost pathognomonic appearance known as "shoulder-pad sign" or "football player shoulders." Carpal tunnel syndrome is frequently an associated abnormality.

The bone abnormalities and arthropathy associated with deposition of B_2-microglobulin (B_2-MG) amyloid are well-recognized complications of long-term hemodialysis and chronic renal failure. B_2-MG, a low-molecular-weight serum protein, is not filtered by standard dialysis membranes. It therefore accumulates in the bones, joints, and soft tissues. Clinically, characteristic pain and decreased joint mobility occur in the shoulders, hips, and knees.

Regardless of cause, imaging studies show massive accumulation of amyloid around the joints, and there is invasion of the periarticular tissue, capsule, and joint. Also, deposits can be seen in the synovium. The articular ends of the bone can be destroyed, and both subluxations and pathologic fractures are frequently encountered. In addition, focal osteolytic lesions, particularly in the bones of the upper extremities and in the proximal ends of the femora, can be seen (Fig. 15.31).

Multicentric Reticulohistiocytosis

Multicentric reticulohistiocytosis is a rare systemic disorder of unknown cause seen in adulthood and is characterized by the proliferation of the histiocytes in the skin, the mucosa, the subcutaneous tissue, and the synovium. The disease has been also called lipoid dermatoarthritis, reticulohistiocytoma, lipid rheumatism, giant cell reticulo-

histiocytosis, giant cell histiocytoma, and giant cell histiocytosis. Women are more frequently affected than men. In approximately 60% to 70% of patients, polyarthralgia is the first manifestation of the disease. Clinical findings, like those of rheumatoid arthritis, consist of soft-tissue swelling, stiffness, and tenderness. Unlike rheumatoid arthritis, however, the distal interphalangeal joints are most frequently affected. Occasionally, the articular lesions may be marked by severe destruction similar to arthritis mutilans of rheumatoid arthritis or psoriatic arthritis. The characteristic absence of significant periarticular osteoporosis distinguishes this disorder from the inflammatory arthritides, and there is also no periosteal new bone formation, which distinguishes it from psoriatic arthritis or juvenile rheumatoid arthritis. Lack of osteophytes and interphalangeal ankylosis, and the presence of soft tissue nodules and atlantoaxial abnormalities including subluxation and erosion of the odontoid process distinguish this arthropathy from erosive osteoarthritis. At times, the pattern of bone erosions with sclerotic margins and overhanging edges may mimic those of gout (Fig. 15.32). Unlike gout, however, there is symmetrical

Figure 15.32 **Multicentric reticulohistiocytosis.** A 46-year-old woman with multicentric reticulohistiocytosis. Note sharply marginated erosions at the distal interphalangeal joints (*arrows*) resembling gout.

distribution of the lesions in the hands and feet and lack of calcification within soft tissue nodules.

Hemophilia

Hemophilia A is an inherited bleeding disorder characterized by an anomaly of blood coagulation caused by functional deficiency of antihemophilic factor (AHF) VIII. It is inherited as an X-linked recessive trait and essentially occurs only in males, although female carriers transmit the abnormal gene. In hemophilia B, also known as "Christmas disease," there is a deficiency of plasma thromboplastin component, factor IX. This disorder may also affect females.

The articular changes in hemophilia most often occur in the first and second decade of life and are secondary to chronic repetitive bleeding into the joints and bones. Repeated episodes of intraarticular bleeding and inflammatory tissue response cause proliferation of synovium and erosion of cartilage and subchondral bone.

Usually there is no problem in clinical recognition of this disorder; however, the changes of hemophilic arthropathy may radiographically mimic those of rheumatoid arthritis, particularly juvenile rheumatoid arthritis (Fig 15.33). Cartilage destruction, joint space narrowing, and erosions of the articular surfaces are identical to those seen in rheumatoid arthritis (Fig. 15.34, see also Fig. 12.17). The knee, ankle, and elbow are the most frequently involved articulations, and this involvement is usually bilateral. In the knee, the radiographic features include periarticular osteoporosis, joint effusion (hemarthrosis), overgrowth of femoral condyles with widening of the intercondylar notch, and squaring of the patella. Frequently, multiple subchondral cysts and articular erosions are evident. In the late stages of disease, the uniform narrowing of the joint space and secondary osteoarthritic changes may be observed. The differential diagnosis from juvenile rheumatoid arthritis is based on evidence that there is no bony ankylosis, no evidence of growth inhibition, and frequent presence of pseudotumors.

Figure 15.33 Hemophilic arthropathy. A 42-year-old man with hemophilia had several intraarticular bleeding episodes in his life. Anteroposterior **(A)** and lateral **(B)** radiographs of his left knee demonstrate advanced hemophilic arthropathy. Note involvement of all three joint compartments. Similar destructive changes in the left elbow are demonstrated on anteroposterior **(C)** and lateral **(D)** projections of this joint.

Figure 15.34 Hemophilic arthropathy. Anteroposterior (**A**) radiograph of the right shoulder and lateral (**B**) radiograph of the left ankle of a 49-year-old man with hemophilia A show destructive arthropathy of the glenohumeral, ankle, and subtalar joints.

Jaccoud Arthritis

Jaccoud arthritis is related to repeated attacks of rheumatic fever and migratory arthralgias. Usually there is complete recovery, but residual stiffness in metacarpophalangeal joints may develop with subsequent attacks. The lesion appears to be periarticular rather than articular, and the changes are caused by mild flexion at the metacarpophalangeal joints with ulnar deviation, most notably in the fourth and fifth fingers, although any finger may be affected. The articular changes are not erosive and patients can physically correct the deformity, particularly in the early course of the disease. The syndrome is rare and not well recognized in the United States.

Arthritis Associated with Acquired Immunodeficiency Syndrome

Recently, an increased prevalence of rheumatologic disorders has been described in patients with human immunodeficiency virus (HIV) infection. Berman and colleagues stated that 71% of patients infected with HIV virus had rheumatic symptoms, including arthralgias, Reiter syndrome, psoriatic arthritis, myositis, vasculitis, and undifferentiated spondyloarthropathy. Solomon and colleagues found that patients with HIV infection demonstrated a 144-fold increase in the prevalence of Reiter syndrome and a 10-fold to 40-fold increase in the prevalence of psoriasis compared with the general population. It is interesting to note that arthritis was seen during various stages of HIV infection and often preceded clinical manifestations of the acquired immunodeficiency syndrome (AIDS). The arthritis was more severe and was unresponsive to conventional treatment with nonsteroidal antiinflammatory medications. A few hypotheses have been suggested to explain the coexistence of inflammatory arthritis and HIV infection. One is that Reiter syndrome entails an interaction between a genetic predisposition (for example, HLA-B27 locus) and environmental factors, most often venereal infections. The immune sys-

tem also plays a role in the pathogenesis of Reiter syndrome. Likewise, the pathogenesis of psoriatic arthritis may entail genetic predisposition (for example, HLA-B27 or HLA-B38 loci). Because HIV infection is commonly followed by the development of immunodeficiency, it is possible that the altered immune mechanism noted in patients with AIDS triggered the onset of Reiter syndrome or psoriatic arthritis in genetically predisposed patients. The second hypothesis is that HIV-related immunodeficiency causes susceptibility to infection with a variety of bacterial and viral organisms, which in turn trigger the onset of arthritis in a genetically predisposed patient. A third hypothesis is that there may be yet-undiscovered causative factors that predispose an individual to arthritis when exposed to HIV. Finally, the arthritis may reflect the direct action of HIV infection on synovium. As Rosenberg and colleagues have pointed out, radiographic documentation of seronegative arthritis should raise the possibility of HIV-associated arthritis as part of the differential diagnosis, particularly in patients with known risk factors for HIV infection.

Infectious Arthritis

Most infectious arthritides demonstrate a positive radionuclide bone scan, particularly when using indium-labeled white cells as a tracer (see Chapter 2), and they also show a very similar radiographic picture, including joint effusion and destruction of cartilage and subchondral bone with consequent joint space narrowing. However, certain clinical and radiographic features are characteristic of individual infectious processes as demonstrated at various target sites. In general, however, infectious arthritis is characterized by the complete destruction of both articular ends of the bones forming the joint; all communicating joint compartments are invariably involved, with diffuse osteoporosis, joint effusion, and periarticular soft-tissue swelling. A detailed description of pyogenic arthritis, tuberculous arthritis, fungal arthritis, and other infectious arthritides caused by viruses and spirochetes is provided in Part V: Infections.

PRACTICAL POINTS TO REMEMBER

Connective Tissue Arthropathies

[1] Systemic lupus erythematosus (SLE) is characterized by flexible joint contractures and malalignments of the metacarpophalangeal and proximal interphalangeal joints. These abnormalities are better demonstrated on the lateral radiographs, because they can easily be reduced during positioning of the hand for the dorsovolar view.

[2] Osteonecrosis is a frequent complication of SLE.

[3] Radiographically, the musculoskeletal abnormalities associated with scleroderma are recognized by:
- atrophy of the soft tissues, particularly the tips of fingers
- resorption of the distal phalanges (acroosteolysis)
- subcutaneous and periarticular calcifications
- destructive changes in the interphalangeal joints.

[4] In scleroderma, corroborative findings are seen in the gastrointestinal tract, where characteristically there is:
- dilatation and hypomotility of the esophagus
- dilatation of the duodenum and small bowel, with a pseudoobstruction pattern
- pseudodiverticula of the colon.

[5] Mixed connective tissue disease is characterized by the clinical and radiologic features that combine the findings of systemic lupus erythematosus, scleroderma, dermatomyositis, and rheumatoid arthritis.

Metabolic and Endocrine Arthritides

[1] Gout is a metabolic disorder characterized by recurrent episodes of arthritis associated with the presence of monosodium urate monohydrate crystals in the synovial fluid.

[2] Hyperuricemia may result from either increased uric acid production or decreased renal excretion.

[3] Gouty arthritis can be recognized radiographically by:
- sharply marginated periarticular and articular erosions, with an "overhanging edge" phenomenon
- partial preservation of the joint space
- asymmetric joint involvement
- asymmetric distribution of tophi
- the absence of osteoporosis.

[4] CPPD crystal deposition disease consists of three distinct entities:
- chondrocalcinosis
- calcium pyrophosphate arthropathy
- the pseudogout syndrome.

[5] The presence of intraarticular crystals and calcifications of hyaline and fibrocartilage, occasionally associated with painful attacks similar to gout, are characteristic features of CPPD crystal deposition disease.

[6] Chondrocalcinosis may also be seen in other conditions, such as gout, hyperparathyroidism, hemochromatosis, Wilson disease, and degenerative joint disease.

[7] Calcium hydroxyapatite (CHA) crystal deposition disease results from abnormal deposition of mineral crystals in and around the joints. The most common location is around the shoulder joint, at the site of supraspinatus tendon.

[8] Hemochromatosis is a disorder resulting from an error of metabolism of iron or caused by iron overload. The arthropathy starts in the small joints of the hand with characteristic involvement of the heads of second and third metacarpals.

[9] Alkaptonuria (ochronosis) is characterized by narrowing of the intervertebral disk spaces, disk calcification and ossification, involvement of sacroiliac joints and symphysis pubis, and joint space narrowing with periarticular osteosclerosis. The radiographic appearance may occasionally mimic degenerative joint disease or CPPD crystal deposition disease.

[10] Hyperparathyroidism arthropathy results from subperiosteal and subchondral resorption at the site of small joints of the hand. This accounts for articular manifestation of this disorder.

[11] Acromegaly arthropathy is the result of overgrowth of the articular cartilage and secondary degenerative changes (secondary osteoarthritis). The characteristic findings include:
- beak-like osteophytes of the radial aspects of the metacarpal heads
- beak-like osteophytes of the inferior aspects of the humeral heads
- widening of the radiographic joint spaces.

Miscellaneous Arthropathies

[1] Amyloid arthropathy is a noninflammatory symmetric polyarthritis. It may complicate long-term hemodialysis and chronic renal failure. The articular ends of the bone can be destroyed and subluxations and pathologic fractures occur. Focal osteolytic lesions, particularly of the bones of the upper extremities and in the proximal ends of the femora, can be seen.

[2] Multicentric reticulohistiocytosis is characterized by proliferation of histiocytes in the skin, mucosa, subcutaneous tissue, and synovium. This may lead to severe articular destruction, but there is neither periarticular osteoporosis nor periosteal bone formation. The radiographic appearance may simulate gouty arthritis.

[3] The articular changes in hemophilia are due to repetitive bleeding into the joints and bone. The radiographic presentation is similar to that of juvenile rheumatoid arthritis. In the bones, pseudotumors are frequently encountered.

[4] Jaccoud arthritis is a poorly defined entity resulting in periarticular stiffness in patients with repeated attacks of rheumatic fever. The articular changes are not erosive.

[5] There is an increased prevalence of rheumatologic disorders in patients with acquired immune deficiency syndrome (AIDS), particularly Reiter syndrome, psoriatic arthritis, and vasculitis.

[6] Infectious arthritis is characterized by the complete destruction of both articular ends of the bones forming the joint. All communicating joint compartments are invariably involved, with diffuse osteoporosis, joint effusion, and periarticular soft-tissue swelling.

SUGGESTED READINGS

Adams PC, Searle J. Neonatal hemochromatosis: a case and review of the literature. *Am J Gastroenterol* 1988;83:422–425.

Adamson TC 3rd, Resnik CS, Guerra J Jr, Vint VC, Weisman MH, Resnick D. Hand and wrist arthropathies of hemochromatosis and calcium pyrophosphate deposition disease: distinct radiographic features. *Radiology* 1983;147:377–381.

Amor B, Cherot A. Delbarre F, Nunez Roldan A, Hors J. Hydroxyapatite rheumatism and HLA markers. *J Rheumatol* 1977;Suppl 3:101–104.

Anderson HC. Mechanisms of pathologic calcification. *Rheum Dis Clin North Am* 1988;14:303–319.

Arnett FC, Reveille JD, Duvic M. Psoriasis and psoriatic arthritis associated with human immunodeficiency virus infection. *Rheum Dis Clin North Am* 1991;17:59–78.

Baker ND. Hemochromatosis. In: Taveras JM, Ferrucci JT, eds. *Radiology—diagnosis, imaging, intervention.* Philadelphia: JB Lippincott; 1986:1–6.

Baker ND, Jahss MH, Leventhal GH. Unusual involvement of the feet in hemochromatosis. *Foot Ankle* 1984;4:212–215.

Barrow MV, Holubar K. Multicentric reticulohistiocytosis. A review of 33 patients. *Medicine* 1969;48:287–305.

Barthelemy CR, Nakayama DA, Carrera GF, Lightfoot RW Jr, Wortmann RL. Gouty arthritis: a prospective radiographic evaluation of sixty patients. *Skeletal Radiol* 1984;11:1–8.

Beltran J, Marty-Delfaut E, Bencardino J, et al. Chondrocalcinosis of the hyaline cartilage of the knee: MRI manifestations. *Skeletal Radiol* 1998;27:369–374.

Berman A, Espinoza LR, Diaz JD, et al. Rheumatic manifestations of human immunodeficiency virus infections. *Am J Med* 1988;85:59–64.

Bonavita JA, Dalinka MK, Schumacher HR Jr. Hydroxyapatite deposition disease. *Radiology* 1980;134:621–625.

Boskey AL, Vigorita VJ, Sencer O, Stuchin SA, Lane JM. Chemical, microscopic, and ultrastructural characterization of the mineral deposits in tumoral calcinosis. *Clin Orthop* 1983;178:258–269.

Brower AC, Resnick D, Karlin C, Piper S. Unusual articular changes of the hand in scleroderma. *Skeletal Radiol* 1979;4:119–123.

Burke BJ, Escobedo EM, Wilson AJ, Hunter JC. Chondrocalcinosis mimicking a meniscal tear on MR imaging. *AJR Am J Roentgenol* 1998;170:69–70.

Bywaters EGL, Dixon ASJ, Scott JT. Joint lesions of hyperparathyroidism. *Ann Rheum Dis* 1963;22:171–187.

Calabrese LH. The rheumatic manifestations of infection with human immunodeficiency virus. *Semin Arthritis Rheum* 1989;18:225–239.

Campbell SM. Gout: how presentation, diagnosis, and treatment differ in the elderly. *Geriatrics* 1988;43:71–77.

Chen C, Chandnani VP, Kang HS, Resnick D, Sartoris DJ, Haller J. Scapholunate advanced collapse: a common wrist abnormality in calcium pyrophosphate dihydrate crystal deposition disease. *Radiology* 1990;177:459–461.

Chen CK, Chung CB, Yeh L, Pan HB, Yang CF, Lai PH, Liang HL, Resnick D. Carpal tunnel syndrome caused by tophaceous gout: CT and MR imaging features in 20 patients. *AJR Am J Roentgenol* 2000;175:655–659.

Chen CKH, Yeh LR, Pan H-B, et al. Intra-articular gouty tophi of the knee: CT and MR imaging in 12 patients. *Skeletal Radiol* 1999;28:75–80.

Chung CB, Mohana-Borges A, Pathria M. Tophaceous gout in an amputation stump in a patient with chronic myelogenous leukemia. *Skeletal Radiol* 2003;32:429–431.

Currey HL, Key JJ, Mason RM, Swettenham KV. Significance of radiological calcification of joint cartilage. *Ann Rheum Dis* 1966;25:295–306.

Dalinka MK, Reginato AJ, Golden DA. Calcium deposition diseases. *Semin Roentgenol* 1982;17:39–48.

Dawn B, Williams JK, Walker SE. Prepatellar bursitis: a unique presentation of tophaceous gout in a normouricemic patient. *J Rheumatol* 1997;24:976–978.

Ellman MH, Levin B. Chondrocalcinosis in elderly persons. *Arthritis Rheum* 1975;18:43–47.

Escobedo EM, Hunter JC, Zink-Brody GC, Andress DL. Magnetic resonance imaging of dialysis-related amyloidosis of the shoulder and hip. *Skeletal Radiol* 1996;25:41–48.

Fam AG, Topp JR, Stein HB, Little AH. Clinical and roentgenographic aspects of pseudogout: a study of 50 cases and a review. *Can Med Assoc J* 1981;124:545–551.

Flemming DJ, Murphey MD, Shekitka KM, Temple HT, Jelinek JJ, Kransdorf MJ. Osseous involvement in calcific tendinitis: a retrospective review of 50 cases. *AJR Am J Roentgenol* 2003;181:965–972.

Gaary E, Gorlin JB, Jaramillo D. Pseudotumor and arthropathy in the knees of a hemophiliac. *Skeletal Radiol* 1996;25:85–87.

Genant HK. Roentgenographic aspects of calcium pyrophosphate dihydrate crystal deposition disease (pseudogout). *Arthritis Rheum* 1976;1[Suppl 3]:307–328.

Goldman AB, Pavlov H, Bullough P. Case report 137. Primary amyloidosis involving the skeletal system. *Skeletal Radiol* 1981;6:69–74.

Grossman RE, Hensley GT. Bone lesions in primary amyloidosis. *AJR Am J Roentgenol* 1967;101:872–875.

Hayes CW, Conway WF. Calcium hydroxyapatite deposition disease. *Radiographics* 1990;10:1031–1048.

Hirsch JH, Killien FC, Troupin RH. The arthropathy of hemochromatosis. *Radiology* 1976;118:591–596.

Huaux JP, Vandenbroucke JM, Noel H. Amyloidosis 1970–1985 with special reference to amyloid arthropathy. A discussion about 106 cases. *Acta Clin Belg* 1987;42:365–380.

Jensen PS. Chondrocalcinosis and other calcifications. *Radiol Clin North Am* 1988;26:1315–1325.

Jensen PS, Putman CE. Current concepts with respect to chondrocalcinosis and the pseudogout syndrome. *AJR Am J Roentenol* 1975;123:531–539.

Justesen P, Andersen PE Jr. Radiologic manifestations in alkaptonuria. *Skeletal Radiol* 1984;11:204–208.

Kerr R. Imaging of musculoskeletal complications of hemophilia. *Semin Musculoskel Radiol* 2003;7:127–136.

Laborde JM, Green DL, Ascari AD, Muir A. Arthritis in hemochromatosis. *J Bone Joint Surg [Am]* 1977;59A:1103–1107.

Lawson JP, Steere AC. Lyme arthritis: radiologic findings. *Radiology* 1985; 154: 37–43.

Lee DJ, Sartoris DJ. Musculoskeletal manifestations of human immunodeficiency virus infection: review of imaging characteristics. *Radiol Clin North Am* 1994;32:399–411.

Ling D, Murphy WA, Kyriakos M. Tophaceous pseudogout. *AJR Am J Roentgenol* 1982;138:162–165.

Madhok R, Bennett D, Sturrock RD, Forbes CD. Mechanisms of joint damage in an experimental model of hemophilic arthritis. *Arthritis Rheum* 1988;31:1148–1155.

Major NM, Tehranzadeh J. Musculoskeletal manifestations of AIDS. *Radiol Clin North Am* 1997;35:1167–1189.

Martel W. The overhanging margin of bone: a roentgenologic manifestation of gout. *Radiology* 1968;91:755–756.

Martel W, McCarter DK, Solsky MA, et al. Further observation of the arthropathy of calcium pyrophosphate dihydrate crystal deposition disease. *Radiology* 1981;141:1–15.

McCarty DJ. Calcium pyrophosphate dihydrate crystal deposition disease: pseudogout—articular chondrocalcinosis. In: McCarty DJ, ed. *Arthritis and allied conditions: a textbook of rheumatology*, 11th ed. Philadelphia: Lea & Febiger; 1989:1714–1720.

McCarty DJ Jr, Haskin ME. The roentgenographic aspects of pseudogout (articular chondrocalcinosis). An analysis of 20 cases. *AJR Am J Roentgenol* 1963;90:1248–1257.

McDonald SP, Coates PTH, Disney APS. Amyloid, age and dialysis arthropathy. *Ann Rheum Dis* 1998;57:193–195.

Melton JW 3rd, Irby R. Multicentric reticulohistiocytosis. *Arthritis Rheum* 1972;15:221–226.

Nägele M, Brüning R, Kunze V, Eickhoff H, Koch W, Reiser M. Hemophilic arthropathy of the knee joint: static and dynamic Gd-DTPA-enhanced MRI. *Eur Radiol* 1995;5:547–552.

Rachbauer F, Kreczy A, Bodner G: Case report. Amyloidoma of the clavicle. *AJR Am J Roentgenol* 2003;181:771–773.

Recht MP, Resnick D. MR imaging of articular cartilage: current status and future directions. *AJR Am J Roentgenol* 1994;163:282–290.

Reeder MM, Felson B. *Gamuts in radiology*. Cincinnati, OH: Audiovisual Radiology of Cincinnati, Inc.; 1975:D142–143.

Resnik CS, Resnick D. Crystal deposition disease. *Semin Arthritis Rheum* 1983;12:390–403.

Resnick D. Bleeding disorders. In: Resnick D, ed. *Diagnosis of bone and joint disorders*, 4th ed. Philadelphia: WB Saunders; 2002;2346–2373.

Resnick D. Calcium hydroxyapatite crystal deposition disease. In: Resnick D, ed. *Diagnosis of bone and joint disorders*, 3rd ed. Philadelphia: WB Saunders; 1995:1615–1648.

Resnick D. Hemochromatosis and Wilson's disease. In: Resnick D, ed. *Diagnosis of bone and joint disorders*, 3rd ed. Philadelphia: WB Saunders; 1995:1649–1669.

Resnick D. Alkaptonuria. In: Resnick D, ed. *Diagnosis of bone and joint disorders*, 3rd ed. Philadelphia: WB Saunders; 1995:1670–1685.

Resnick D, Niwayama G. Gouty arthritis. In: Resnick D, ed. *Diagnosis of bone and joint disorders*, 3rd ed. Philadelphia: WB Saunders; 1995:1511–1555.

Resnick D, Niwayama G. Calcium pyrophosphate dihydrate (CPPD) crystal deposition disease. In: Resnick D, ed. *Diagnosis of bone and joint disorders*, 3rd ed. Philadelphia: WB Saunders; 1995:1556–1614.

Resnick D, Niwayama G, Goergen TC, et al. Clinical, radiographic and pathologic abnormalities in calcium pyrophosphate dihydrate crystal deposition disease (CPPD): pseudogout. *Radiology* 1977;122:1–15.

Resnick D, Utsinger PD. The wrist arthropathy of "pseudogout" occurring with and without chondrocalcinosis. *Radiology* 1974;113:633–641.

Rosenberg ZS, Norman A, Solomon G. Arthritis associated with HIV infection: radiographic manifestations. *Radiology* 1989;173:171–176.

Ross LV, Ross GJ, Mesgarzadeh M, Edmonds PR, Bonakdarpur A. Hemodialysis-related amyloidomas of bone. *Radiology* 1991;178:263–265.

Rubenstein J, Pritzker KPH. Crystal-associated arthropathies. *AJR Am J Roentgenol* 1989;152:685–695.

Schumacher HR. Articular cartilage in the degenerative arthropathy of hemochromatosis. *Arthritis Rheum* 1982;25:1460–1468.

Schumacher HR Jr. Crystals, inflammation, and osteoarthritis. *Am J Med* 1987;83:11–16.

Schumacher HR, Straka PC, Krikker MA, Dudley AT. The arthropathy of hemochromatosis. Recent studies. *Ann NY Acad Sci* 1988;526:224–233.

Sharp GC, Irvin WS, Tan EM, Gould RG, Holman HR. Mixed connective tissue disease—an apparently distinct rheumatic disease syndrome associated with a specific antibody to an extractable nuclear antigen (ENA). *Am J Med* 1972;52:148–159.

Sissons HA, Steiner GC, Bonar F, May F, Rosenberg ZS, Samuels H, Present D. Tumoral calcium pyrophosphate deposition disease. *Skeletal Radiol* 1989;18:79–87.

Slavotinek JP, Coates PTH, McDonald SP, Disney APS, Sage MR. Shoulder appearances at MR imaging in long-term dialysis recipients. *Radiology* 2000;217:539–543.

Steinbach LS, Tehranzadeh J, Fleckenstein J, Vanarthos WJ, Pais MJ. Human immunodeficiency virus infection: musculoskeletal manifestations. *Radiology* 1993;186:833–838.

Steinbach LS, Resnick D. Calcium pyrophosphate dihydrate crystal deposition disease revisited. *Radiology* 1996;200:1–9.

Stoker DJ, Murray RO. Skeletal changes in hemophilia and other bleeding disorders. *Semin Roentgenol* 1974;9:185–193.

Talbott JH, Altman RD, Yu TF. Gouty arthritis masquerading as rheumatoid arthritis or vice versa. *Semin Arthritis Rheum* 1978;8:77–114.

Tehranzadeh J, Steinbach LS. *Musculoskeletal manifestations of AIDS*. St. Louis: Warren H. Green; 1994.

Udoff EJ, Genant HK, Kozin F, Ginsberg M. Mixed connective tissue disease: the spectrum of radiographic manifestations. *Radiology* 1977;124:613–618.

Wilkin E, Dieppe P, Maddison P, Evison G. Osteoarthritis and articular chondrocalcinosis in the elderly. *Ann Rheum Dis* 1983;42:280–284.

Wyatt SH, Fishman EK. CT/MRI of musculoskeletal complications of AIDS. *Skeletal Radiol* 1995;24:481–488.

Yamada T, Kurohori YN, Kashiwazaki S, Fujibayashi M, Ohkawa T. MRI of multicentric reticulohistiocytosis. *J Comput Assist Tomogr* 1996;20:838–840.

Yang BY, Sartoris DJ, Djukic S, Resnick D, Clopton P. Distribution of calcification in the triangular fibrocartilage region in 181 patients with calcium pyrophosphate dihydrate crystal deposition disease. *Radiology* 1995;196:547–550.

Yu JS, Chung CB, Recht M, Dailiana T, Jurdi R. MR imaging of tophaceous gout. *AJR Am J Roentgenol* 1997;168:523–527.

Yulish BS, Lieberman JM, Strandjord SE, Bryan PJ, Mulopulos GP, Modic MT. Hemophilic arthropathy: assessment with MR imaging. *Radiology* 1987;12:759–762.

Zitnan D, Si'taj S. Chondrocalcinosis articularis. Section L. Clinical and radiological study. *Ann Rheum Dis* 1963;22:142–152.

TUMORS AND TUMOR-LIKE LESIONS

CHAPTER 16

RADIOLOGIC EVALUATION OF TUMORS AND TUMOR-LIKE LESIONS

Classification of Tumors and Tumor-like Lesions

Tumors, including tumor-like lesions, can generally be divided into two groups: benign and malignant. The latter group can be further subclassified into primary malignant tumors, secondary malignant tumors (from the transformation of benign conditions) and metastatic tumors (Fig. 16.1). All of these lesions can be still further classified according to their tissue of origin (Table 16.1). Table 16.2 lists benign conditions that have the potential for malignant transformation.

To understand the terminology applied to tumors and tumor-like lesions of the bone, it is important to redefine certain terms pertinent to lesions and their location in the bone. The term *tumor* generally

means *mass;* in common radiologic and orthopedic parlance, however, it is the equivalent of the term *neoplasm.* By definition, a neoplasm demonstrates autonomous growth; if in addition it produces local or remote metastases, it is defined as a *malignant neoplasm* or *malignant tumor.* Beyond this (and not dealt with in this chapter) are specific histopathologic criteria for defining a tumor as benign or malignant. It is nevertheless worth mentioning that certain giant cell tumors, despite a "benign" histopathology, may produce distant metastases and that certain cartilage tumors, despite adhering to a "benign" histopathologic pattern, can behave locally like malignant neoplasms, even though this is detectable only radiologically. Moreover, certain lesions discussed here and termed *tumor-like lesions* are not true neoplasms, but rather have a developmental or inflammatory origin. They are included in this chapter because they display a radiographic

529

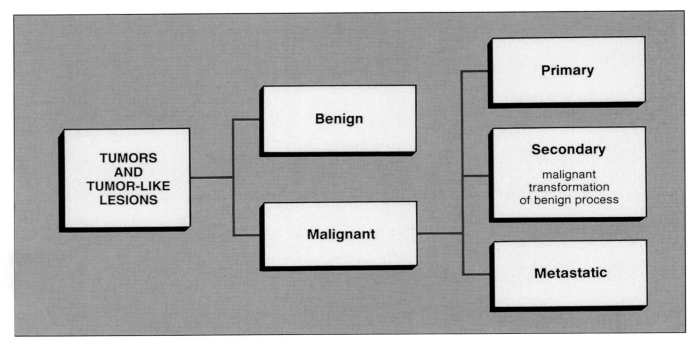

Figure 16.1 Classification of tumors and tumor-like lesions.

Table 16.1 **Classification of Tumors and Tumor-Like Lesions by Tissue of Origin**

Tissue of Origin	Benign Lesion	Malignant Lesion
Bone-forming (osteogenic)	Osteoma Osteoid osteoma Osteoblastoma	Osteosarcoma (and variants) Juxtacortical osteosarcoma (and variants)
Cartilage-forming (chondrogenic)	Enchondroma (chondroma) Periosteal (juxtacortical) chondroma Enchondromatosis (Ollier disease) Osteochondroma (osteocartilaginous exostosis, solitary or multiple) Chondroblastoma Chondromyxoid fibroma Fibrocartilaginous mesenchymoma	Chondrosarcoma (central) Conventional Mesenchymal Clear cell Dedifferentiated Chondrosarcoma (peripheral) Periosteal (juxtacortical)
Fibrous, osteofibrous, and fibrohistiocytic (fibrogenic)	Fibrous cortical defect (metaphyseal fibrous defect) Nonossifying fibroma Benign fibrous histiocytoma Fibrous dysplasia (mono- and polyostotic) Fibrocartilaginous dysplasia Focal fibrocartilaginous dysplasia of long bones Periosteal desmoid Desmoplastic fibroma Osteofibrous dysplasia (Kempson-Campanacci lesion) Ossifying fibroma (Sissons lesion)	Fibrosarcoma Malignant fibrous histiocytoma
Vascular	Hemangioma Glomus tumor Cystic angiomatosis	Angiosarcoma Hemangioendothelioma Hemangiopericytoma
Hematopoietic, reticuloendothelial, and lymphatic	Giant cell tumor (osteoclastoma) Langerhans cell histiocytosis Lymphangioma	Malignant giant cell tumor Histiocytic lymphoma Hodgkin lymphoma Leukemia Myeloma (plasmacytoma) Ewing sarcoma
Neural (neurogenic)	Neurofibroma Neurilemoma	Malignant schwannoma Neuroblastoma Primitive neuroectodermal tumor (PNET)
Notochordal		Chordoma
Fat (lipogenic)	Lipoma	Liposarcoma
Unknown	Simple bone cyst Aneurysmal bone cyst Intraosseous ganglion	Adamantinoma

Table 16.2 Benign Conditions With Potential for Malignant Transformation

Benign Lesion	Malignancy
Enchondroma (in the long or flat bones*; in the short, tubular bones almost always as a part of Ollier disease or Maffucci syndrome)	Chondrosarcoma
Osteochondroma	Peripheral chondrosarcoma
Synovial chondromatosis	Chondrosarcoma
Fibrous dysplasia (usually polyostotic, or treated with radiation)	Fibrosarcoma Malignant fibrous histiocytoma Osteosarcoma
Osteofibrous dysplasia† (Kempson-Campanacci lesion)	Adamantinoma
Neurofibroma (in plexiform neurofibromatosis)	Malignant schwannoma Liposarcoma Malignant mesenchymoma
Medullary bone infarct	Fibrosarcoma Malignant fibrous histiocytoma
Osteomyelitis with chronic draining sinus tract (usually more than 15–20 years duration)	Squamous cell carcinoma Fibrosarcoma
Paget disease	Osteosarcoma Chondrosarcoma Fibrosarcoma Malignant fibrous histiocytoma

*Some authorities believe that, at least in some "malignant transformations" of enchondroma to chondrosarcoma, there was in fact from the very beginning a malignant lesion masquerading as benign and not recognized as such.

†Some authorities believe that this is not a true malignant transformation, but rather independent development of malignancy in the benign condition.

Figure 16.3 Terminology used to describe the location of lesions in the bone.

pattern that is almost indistinguishable from that of true neoplasms. Their cause is, in some cases, still being debated.

Equally important is the redefinition of certain terms pertinent to the location of a lesion in the bone. In the growing skeleton, one can clearly distinguish the epiphysis, growth plate, metaphysis, and diaphysis (Fig. 16.2A), and when lesions are located at these sites they are named accordingly. The greatest confusion is in the use of the term *metaphysis*. The metaphysis is a histologically very thin zone of active bone growth, adjacent to the physis (growth plate). Consequently, for a lesion to be called metaphyseal in location, it must extend into and abut the growth plate. However, it is customary—however incorrect—to use the same term for locating a lesion after skeletal maturity has occurred. By the time of maturity, the growth plate is scarred, and neither the epiphysis nor metaphysis remains. More proper and less confusing would be a terminology (Fig. 16.2B) such as *articular end of the bone* and *shaft* for locating lesions in the bone whose growth plate has been obliterated and whose metaphysis has ceased to exist. Some other terms used to describe the location of bone lesions are illustrated in Fig. 16.3.

Radiologic Imaging Modalities

The radiologic modalities most often used in analyzing tumors and tumor-like lesions include:(a) conventional radiography; (b) tomography; (c) angiography (usually arteriography); (d) computed

Figure 16.2 Parts of the bone. (A) In the maturing skeleton, the epiphysis, growth plate, metaphysis, and diaphysis are clearly recognizable areas. **(B)** With skeletal maturity, distinct epiphyseal and metaphyseal zones have ceased to exist. The terminology for describing the location of lesions should alter accordingly. The inset illustrates an alternate terminology.

Figure 16.4 **Chondroblastoma.** Anteroposterior (**A**) and lateral (**B**) views of the right knee of a 13-year-old girl reveal a radiolucent lesion located eccentrically in the proximal epiphysis of the tibia, with sharply defined borders and a thin, sclerotic margin. Here, the standard projections led to the radiographic diagnosis of chondroblastoma.

tomography (CT); (e) magnetic resonance imaging (MRI); (f) scintigraphy (radionuclide bone scan); and (g) fluoroscopy- or CT-guided percutaneous soft tissue and bone biopsy.

In most instances, the standard radiographic views specific for the anatomic site under investigation, in conjunction with conventional tomography, suffice to make a correct diagnosis (Fig. 16.4), which can subsequently be confirmed by biopsy and histopathologic examination. Conventional radiography yields the most useful information about the location and morphology of a lesion, particularly concerning the type of bone destruction, calcifications, ossifications, and periosteal reaction. Conventional tomography can be a useful diagnostic tool, particularly on those occasions when questions arise regarding cortical destruction, periosteal reaction, or mineralization of the tumor matrix. It can also detect occult pathologic fracture. Chest radiography may also be required in cases of

suspected metastasis, the most frequent complication of malignant lesions. This should be done before any treatment of a malignant primary bone tumor, because most bone malignancies metastasize to the lung.

Although CT by itself is rarely helpful in making a specific diagnosis, it can provide a precise evaluation of the extent of a bone lesion and may demonstrate breakthrough of the cortex and involvement of surrounding soft tissues (Fig. 16.5). CT is moreover very helpful in delineating a bone tumor having a complex anatomic structure. The scapula (Fig. 16.6), pelvis (Fig. 16.7), and sacrum, for example, may be difficult to image fully with conventional radiographic techniques. CT examination is crucial in determining the extent and spread of a tumor in the bone if limb salvage is contemplated, so that a safe margin of resection can be planned (Fig. 16.8). It can effectively demonstrate the intraosseous extension of a tumor and its extraosseous in-

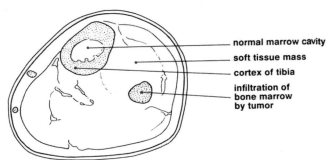

Figure 16.5 **Ewing sarcoma. (A)** Anteroposterior radiograph demonstrates a malignant lesion that proved to be Ewing sarcoma in the proximal diaphysis of the left fibula of a 12-year-old boy. **(B)** On CT examination, there is involvement of the bone marrow and extension of the tumor into the soft tissues.

Figure 16.6 **Chondrosarcoma.** Standard radiographs were ambiguous in this 70-year-old man with a palpable mass over the right scapula. However, two CT sections demonstrate a destructive lesion of the glenoid portion and body of the scapula **(A)**, with a large soft-tissue mass extending to the rib cage and containing calcifications **(B)**. The lesion proved to be a chondrosarcoma after biopsy.

rib

humerus

calcifications in soft tissue mass

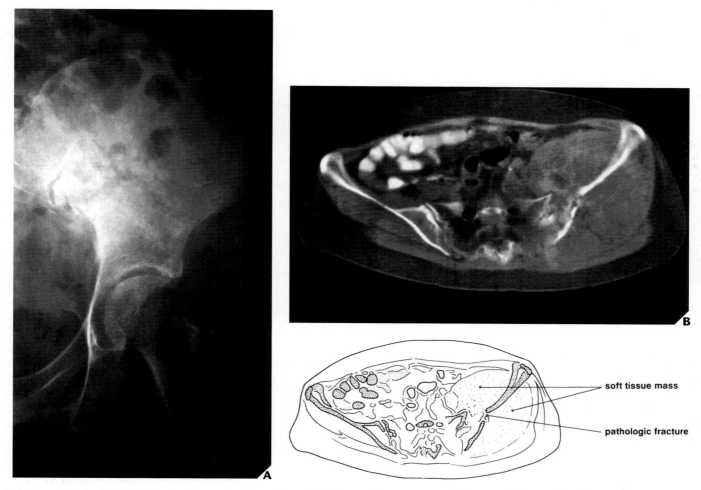

soft tissue mass

pathologic fracture

Figure 16.7 **Osteosarcoma. (A)** Standard anteroposterior radiograph of the pelvis was not sufficient to delineate the full extent of the destructive lesion of the iliac bone in this 66-year-old woman. **(B)** A CT scan, however, showed a pathologic fracture of the ilium and the full extent of soft-tissue involvement. The high Hounsfield values of the multiple soft-tissue densities suggested bone formation. Enhancement of the CT images with contrast agent showed an increased vascularity of the lesion. Collectively, the CT findings suggested a diagnosis of osteosarcoma that, although unusual for a person of this age, was confirmed by open biopsy.

Figure 16.8 Osteosarcoma—effectiveness of CT. (A) Anteroposterior radiograph of the left proximal femur of a 12-year-old boy demonstrates an osteolytic lesion in the intertrochanteric region, with a poorly defined margin and amorphous densities in the center associated with a periosteal reaction medially—features suggesting osteosarcoma, which was confirmed on biopsy. Because a limb-salvage procedure was contemplated, a CT scan was performed to determine the extent of marrow infiltration and the required level of bone resection. The most proximal section **(B)** shows obvious gross tumor involvement of the marrow cavity of the left femur. A more distal section **(C)** shows no gross marrow abnormality, but a positive Hounsfield value of 52 units indicates tumor involvement of the marrow, which was not shown on the standard radiographs. By comparison, the section of the right femur shows a normal Hounsfield value of −26 for bone marrow.

volvement of soft tissues such as muscles and neurovascular bundles. CT is also useful for monitoring the results of treatment, evaluating for recurrence of a resected tumor, and demonstrating the effect of nonsurgical treatment such as radiation therapy or chemotherapy (Fig. 16.9). It is also helpful in evaluating soft-tissue tumors (Fig. 16.10), which on standard radiographs are indistinguishable from one another (with the exception of lipomas, which usually demonstrate low-density features), blending imperceptibly into the surrounding normal tissue.

Contrast enhancement of CT images aids in the identification of major neurovascular structures and well-vascularized lesions. Evaluating the relationship between the tumor and the surrounding soft tissues and neurovascular structures is particularly important for planning limb-salvage surgery.

Arteriography is used mainly to map out bone lesions and to assess the extent of disease. It is also used to demonstrate the vascular supply of a tumor and to locate vessels suitable for preoperative intraarterial chemotherapy, as well as to demonstrate the area suitable for open biopsy, because the most vascular area of a tumor contains the most aggressive component. Occasionally, arteriography can be used to demonstrate abnormal tumor vessels, corroborating findings with plain-film radiography and tomography (Fig. 16.11). Arteriography is often useful in planning for limb-salvage procedures because it demonstrates the regional vascular anatomy and thus permits a plan to be drawn up for the resection procedure. It is also sometimes used to outline the major vessels before resection of a benign tumor (Fig. 16.12), and it can be combined with an interventional procedure, such as embolization of hypervascular tumors, before further

Figure 16.9 Osteosarcoma after chemotherapy. Before surgery, this 14-year-old girl with an osteosarcoma of the left femur underwent a full course of chemotherapy. **(A)** CT section before the therapy was begun shows involvement of the bone and marrow cavity. Note the soft-tissue extension of the tumor, with nonhomogeneous, amorphous tumor bone formation. After combined treatment with doxorubicin hydrochloride, vincristine, methotrexate, and cisplatin, a repeat CT scan **(B)** shows calcifications and ossifications in the periphery of the lesion, which represents reactive rather than tumor bone and demonstrates the success of chemotherapy. Radical excision of the femur and a subsequent histopathologic examination showed almost complete eradication of malignant cells, confirming the CT findings.

Figure 16.10 CT of malignant fibrous histiocytoma of the soft tissue. A 56-year-old woman presented with a soft-tissue mass on the posteromedial aspect of the right thigh. **(A)** Lateral radiograph of the femur demonstrates only a soft-tissue prominence posteriorly. **(B)** CT section shows an axial image of the mass, which is contained by a fibrotic capsule. The overlying skin is not infiltrated. Despite the benign appearance, the mass proved on biopsy to be a malignant fibrous histiocytoma.

Figure 16.11 Arteriography of dedifferentiated chondrosarcoma. (A) Anteroposterior radiograph of the pelvis in a 79-year-old woman with an 8-month history of pain in the right buttock and weight loss demonstrates a poorly defined destructive lesion of the right iliac bone, with multiple small calcifications and a soft-tissue mass extending into the pelvis. Note the effect of the mass on the urinary bladder filled with contrast. A chondrosarcoma was suspected, and a femoral arteriogram was performed as part of the diagnostic work-up. **(B)** Subtraction study of an arteriogram demonstrates hypervascularity of the tumor. Note the abnormal tumor vessels, encasement and stretching of some vessels, and "pulling" of contrast medium into small "lakes"—all characteristic signs of a malignant lesion. Biopsy revealed a highly malignant, dedifferentiated chondrosarcoma. In this case, the vascular study corroborated the radiographic findings of a malignant bone tumor.

Figure 16.12 Arteriography of osteochondroma. A 12-year-old boy with osteochondroma of the distal femur underwent arteriography to demonstrate the relationship of the distal superficial femoral artery to the lesion. This subtraction study shows no major vessels near the planned site of resection at the base of the lesion, important information for surgical planning.

Figure 16.13 **Vertebral arteriography and embolization of hemangioma.** A 73-year-old woman presented with a collapsed T-11 vertebra, which showed a corduroy-like pattern suggestive of hemangioma. Vertebral angiography was performed. **(A)** Arteriogram of the 11th right intercostal artery outlines a vascular paraspinal mass associated with hemangioma and indicating extension of the lesion into the soft tissues. **(B)** After embolization, the lesion shows a marked decrease in vascularity. Subsequently, the patient underwent decompression laminectomy and anterior fusion at T10-T11 using a fibular strut graft.

treatment (Fig. 16.13). In selected cases, arteriography may help make a differential diagnosis, such as of osteoid osteoma versus a bone abscess.

Myelography may be helpful in dealing with tumors that invade the vertebral column and thecal sac (Fig. 16.14), although recently this procedure has been almost completely replaced by MRI.

MRI is indispensable in evaluating bone and soft-tissue tumors. Particularly with soft-tissue masses, MRI offers distinct advantages over

CT. There is improved visualization of tissue planes surrounding the lesion, for example, and neurovascular involvement can be evaluated without the use of intravenous contrast.

In the evaluation of intraosseous and extraosseous extensions of a tumor, MRI is crucial because it can determine with high accuracy the presence or absence of soft-tissue invasion by a tumor (Fig. 16.15). MRI has often proved to be superior to CT in delineating the extraosseous and intramedullary extent of the tumor and its relationship

Figure 16.14 **Myelography of aneurysmal bone cyst.** Initial radiographic examination of the lumbar spine of this 14-year-old girl with an 18-month history of pain in the lower back and sciatica of the left leg did not disclose any abnormalities; myelography was performed because of suspected herniation of a lumbar disk, but it was inconclusive. A repeat study was requested when the symptoms became more severe after 3 months. **(A)** Posteroanterior radiograph of the lumbosacral spine shows destruction of the left pedicle and the left part of the L-5 body (note the residual contrast in the subarachnoid space). A repeat myelogram using a water-soluble contrast (metrizamide) shows, on the posteroanterior view **(B)**, extradural compression of the thecal sac on the left side with displacement of the nerve roots. Biopsy confirmed the radiographic diagnosis of an aneurysmal bone cyst.

Figure 16.15 MRI of chondrosarcoma. (A) Conventional radiograph in anteroposterior projection of a 67-year-old woman with chondrosarcoma of the left femur demonstrates a tumor in the distal shaft destroying the medullary portion of the bone and breaking through the cortex. The soft-tissue extension cannot be determined. **(B)** Axial T2-weighted MR image (SE; TR 2500/TE 70 msec) demonstrates a tumor infiltrating bone marrow, destroying the posterolateral cortex, and breaking into the soft tissues with formation of a large mass (*arrows*). Compare with a normal contralateral extremity.

to surrounding structures (Fig. 16.16). By showing sharper demarcation between normal and abnormal tissue than CT, MRI—particularly in evaluation of the extremities—reliably identifies the spatial boundaries of tumor masses (Fig. 16.17), the encasement and displacement of major neurovascular bundles, and the extent of joint involvement. Spin-echo T1-weighted images enhance tumor contrast with bone, bone marrow, and fatty tissue, whereas spin-echo T2-weighted images enhance tumor contrast with muscle and accentuate peritumoral edema. Axial and coronal images have been used in determining the extent of soft-tissue invasion in relation to important vascular structures. However, in comparison with CT, MR images do not clearly demonstrate calcification in the tumor matrix; in fact, large amounts of calcification or ossification may be almost undetectable. Moreover, MRI has been shown to be less satisfactory than CT in the demonstra-

Figure 16.16 MRI of parosteal osteosarcoma. (A) From this lateral film of the distal femur of a 22-year-old woman with parosteal osteosarcoma, it is difficult to evaluate if the tumor is on the surface of the bone or already infiltrated through the cortex. **(B)** Sagittal T1-weighted MRI (SE; TR 500/TE 20 msec) demonstrates invasion of the cancellous portion of the bone, as represented by an area of low signal intensity (*arrows*).

normal cortex

tumor

Invasion of cancellous bone

Figure 16.17 MRI of malignant fibrous histiocytoma. Coronal T1-weighted MRI (SE; TR 500/TE 20 msec) demonstrates involvement of the medullary cavity of the right femur in this 16-year-old girl with malignant fibrous histiocytoma. Note the excellent demonstration of the interface between normal bone displaying high-signal intensity and a tumor displaying intermediate signal intensity.

tion of cortical destruction. It is important to realize that both MRI and CT have advantages and disadvantages, and circumstances exist in which either can be the preferential or complementary study. But it is even more important that the surgeon tell the radiologist who is performing and interpreting the study what information is needed.

Several investigators have stressed the superior contrast enhancement of MR images using intravenous injection of gadopentetate dimeglumine [gadolinium diethylenetriamine-penta-acetic acid, (Gd-DTPA)]. Enhancement was found to give better delineation of the tumor's richly vascularized parts and of the compressed tissue immediately surrounding the tumor. It was also found to assist in differentiation of intraarticular tumor extension from joint effusion, and, as Erlemann pointed out, improved the differentiation of necrotic tissue from viable areas in various malignant tumors.

According to the recent investigations, MRI may have an additional application in evaluating both the tumor's response to radiation and chemotherapy and any local recurrence. On gadolinium-enhanced T1-weighted images, signal intensity remains low in avascular, necrotic areas of tumor while it increases in viable tissue. Although static MRI was of little value for assessment of response to the treatment, dynamic MRI using Gd-DTPA as a contrast enhancement, according to Erlemann, had the highest degree of accuracy (85.7%) and was superior to scintigraphy, particularly in patients who were receiving intraarterial chemotherapy. In general, drug-sensitive tumors display slower uptake of Gd-DTPA after preoperative chemotherapy than do nonresponsive lesions. As Vaupel contended, the rapid uptake of Gd-DTPA by malignant tissues may be due to increased vascularity and more rapid perfusion of the contrast material through an expanded interstitial space. The latest observation by Dewhirst and Kautcher suggests that MR spectroscopy may also be useful in the evaluation of patients undergoing chemotherapy.

It must be stressed, however, that most of the time MRI is not suitable for establishing the precise nature of a bone tumor. In par-

ticular, too much faith has been placed in MRI as a method of distinguishing benign lesions from malignant ones. An overlap between the classic characteristics of benign and malignant tumors is often observed. Moreover, some malignant bone tumors can appear misleadingly benign on MR images and, conversely, some benign lesions may exhibit a misleadingly malignant appearance. Attempts to formulate precise criteria for correlating MRI findings with histologic diagnosis have been largely unsuccessful. Tissue characterization on the basis of MRI signal intensities is still unreliable. Because of the wide spectrum of bone tumor composition and their differing histologic patterns, as well as in tumors of similar histologic diagnosis, signal intensities of histologically different tumors may overlap or there may be variability of signal intensity in histologically similar tumors.

Trials using combined hydrogen-1 MRI and P-31 MR spectroscopy also failed to distinguish most benign lesions from malignant tumors. Despite the use of various criteria, the application of MRI to tissue diagnosis has rarely brought satisfactory results. This is because, in general, the small number of protons in calcified structures renders MRI less effective in diagnosing bone lesions, and hence valuable evidence concerning the production of the tumor matrix can be missed. Moreover, as several investigations have shown, MRI is an imaging modality of low specificity. T1 and T2 measurements are generally of limited value for histologic characterization of musculoskeletal tumors. Quantitative determination of relaxation times has not proved to be clinically valuable in identifying various tumor types, although, as noted by Sundaram, it has proved to be an important technique in the staging of osteosarcoma and chondrosarcoma. T2-weighted images in particular are a crucial factor in delineating extraosseous tumor extension and peritumoral edema, as well as in assessing the involvement of major neurovascular bundles. Necrotic areas change from a low-intensity signal in the T1-weighted image to a very bright, intense signal in the T2-weighted image and can be differentiated from viable, solid tumor tissue. Although MRI cannot predict the histology of bone tumors, as Sundaram pointed out, it is a useful tool for distinguishing round cell tumors and metastases from stress fractures or medullary infarcts in symptomatic patients with normal radiographs, and, according to Baker, it can occasionally differentiate benign from pathologic fracture.

The radionuclide bone scan is an indicator of mineral turnover, and because there is usually enhanced deposition of bone-seeking radiopharmaceuticals in areas of bone undergoing change and repair, a bone scan is useful in localizing tumors and tumor-like lesions in the skeleton, particularly in such conditions as fibrous dysplasia, eosinophilic granuloma, or metastatic cancer, in which more than one lesion is encountered (Fig. 16.18). It also plays an important role in localizing small lesions such as osteoid osteomas, which may not always be seen on conventional radiographs (see Fig. 17.12B). Although in most instances a radionuclide bone scan cannot distinguish benign lesions from malignant tumors, because increased blood flow with increased isotope deposition and increased osteoblastic activity takes place in benign and malignant conditions, it is still occasionally capable of making such differentiation in benign lesions that do not absorb the radioactive isotope (Fig. 16.19). The radionuclide bone scan is sometimes also useful for differentiating multiple myeloma, which usually shows no significant uptake of the tracer, from metastatic cancer, which usually does.

Aside from routine radionuclide scans performed using technetium-99m-labeled phosphate compounds, occasionally gallium-67 is used for detection and staging of bone and soft tissue neoplasms. Gallium is handled by the body much like iron in that the protein transferrin carries it in the plasma, and it also competes for extravascular iron-binding proteins such as lactoferrin. The administered dose for adults ranges from 3 mCi (111 MBq) to 10 mCi (370 MBq) per study. The exact mechanism of tumor uptake of gallium remains unsettled, and its uptake varies with tumor type. In particular, Hodgkin lymphomas and histiocytic lymphomas are prone to significant gallium uptake.

Figure 16.18 Scintigraphy of the metastases. A radionuclide bone scan was performed on a 68-year-old woman with metastatic breast carcinoma to determine the distribution of metastases. After an intravenous injection of 15 mCi (555 MBq) of technetium-99m diphosphonate, an increased uptake of the radiopharmaceutical is seen in the skull and cervical spine **(A)** and lumbar spine and pelvis **(B)**, localizing the site of the multiple metastases.

Percutaneous bone and soft-tissue biopsy performed in the radiology department has in recent years gained its place in the diagnostic work-up for various neoplastic diseases, including bone tumors. In patients with primary bone neoplasms, it is a helpful diagnostic and evaluative tool, allowing rapid histologic diagnosis, which is now considered essential, particularly in the planning of a limb-salvage procedure. It also helps assess the effect of chemotherapy and radiation therapy and helps locate the site of the primary tumor in cases of metastatic disease (Fig. 16.20). In addition, percutaneous bone and soft-tissue biopsy performed in the radiology suite is simpler and costs less than a biopsy performed in the operating room.

Finally, it is important to compare recent radiographic studies with earlier films. This point cannot be emphasized enough. The comparison can reveal not only the nature of a bone lesion (Fig. 16.21) but also its aggressiveness, a critical factor in a diagnostic work-up.

Figure 16.19 Scintigraphy of enostosis. A 32-year-old woman presented with pain localized in the wrist area. **(A)** Dorsovolar radiograph of the wrist demonstrates a sclerotic round lesion in the scaphoid, and a diagnosis of osteoid osteoma was considered. **(B)** Radionuclide bone scan reveals normal isotope uptake, ruling out osteoid osteoma, which is invariably associated with an increased uptake of radiopharmaceutical. The lesion instead proved to be a bone island (enostosis), an asymptomatic developmental error of endochondral ossification without any consequence to the patient. The pain was unrelated to the island, coming instead from tenosynovitis; it disappeared after the patient was treated for the latter condition.

Figure 16.20 Percutaneous bone biopsy. (A) Anteroposterior radiograph of the lumbar spine in a 67-year-old woman with lower back pain for 4 months demonstrates destruction of the left pedicle of the L-4 vertebra. **(B)** CT section shows, in addition, involvement of the vertebral body by the tumor. **(C)** Percutaneous biopsy of the lesion, performed in the radiology suite for the purpose of rapid histopathologic diagnosis, revealed a metastatic adenocarcinoma from the colon.

Figure 16.21 Simple bone cyst—comparison radiography. (A) Anteroposterior radiograph of the humerus in a 26-year-old woman with vague pain in the left upper humerus for 2 months shows an ill-defined lesion in the medullary region, with a periosteal reaction medially and laterally. There appear to be scattered calcifications in the proximal portion of the lesion. The possibility of a cartilage tumor such as chondrosarcoma was considered, but a film made 17 years earlier **(B)** shows an unquestionably benign lesion (a simple bone cyst) that had been treated by curettage and the application of bone chips. In view of this, the later findings were interpreted as representing a healed bone cyst. The patient's pain was found to be related to muscular strain.

Tumors and Tumor-Like Lesions of the Bone

Diagnosis

Patient age and determination of whether a lesion is solitary or multiple are the starting approaches in the diagnosis of bone tumors (Fig. 16.22).

Clinical Information

The age of the patient is probably the single most important item of clinical data in radiographically establishing the diagnosis of a tumor (Fig. 16.23). Certain tumors have a predilection for specific age groups. Aneurysmal bone cysts, for example, rarely occur beyond age 20, and giant cell tumors as a rule are found only after the growth plate is closed. Other lesions may have different radiographic presentations or occur in different locations in patients of different ages. Simple bone cysts, which before skeletal maturity present almost exclusively in the long bones such as the proximal humerus and proximal femur, may appear in other locations (pelvis, scapula, os calcis) and have unconventional radiographic presentations with progressing age (Fig. 16.24).

Also important for clinically differentiating lesions of similar radiographic presentation—such as Langerhans cell histiocytosis (formerly called eosinophilic granuloma), osteomyelitis, and Ewing sarcoma—is the duration of the patient's symptoms. In Langerhans cell histiocytosis, for example, the amount of bone destruction seen radiographically after 1 week of symptoms is usually the same as that seen after 4 to 6 weeks of symptoms in osteomyelitis and 3 to 4 months in Ewing sarcoma.

Occasionally, race may also be an important differential diagnostic factor, because certain lesions, such as tumoral calcinosis or bone infarctions, are seen more commonly in blacks than in whites, whereas others, such as Ewing sarcoma, are almost never seen in blacks.

The growth rate of the tumor may be an additional factor in differentiating malignant tumors (usually rapid-growing) from benign tumors (usually slow-growing).

Laboratory data, such as an increased erythrocyte sedimentation rate or an elevated alkaline or acid phosphatase level in the serum, occasionally can be a corroborative factor in diagnosis.

Imaging Modalities

With so many imaging techniques available to diagnose and characterize the bone tumor further, radiologists and clinicians are frequently at a loss as to how to proceed in a given case, what modality to use for this particular problem, in what order of preference to use the modalities, and when to stop. It is important to keep in mind that the choice of techniques for imaging the bone or soft-tissue tumor should be dictated not only by the clinical presentation and the technique's expected effectiveness but also by equipment availability, expertise, cost, and restrictions applicable to individual patients (for example, allergy to ionic or nonionic iodinated contrast agents may preclude the use of arthrography; presence of a pacemaker may preclude the use of MRI; or physiologic states such as pregnancy warrant the use of ultrasound over the use of ionized radiation). Some of these problems were discussed in general in chapters 1 and 2.

Here, I give a general guideline related to the most effective modality for diagnosing and evaluating bone and soft-tissue tumors. In the evaluation of bone tumors, conventional radiography and tomography are still the standard diagnostic procedures. No matter what ancillary technique is used, the conventional radiograph should always be available for comparison. Most of the time, the choice of imaging technique is dictated by the type of suspected tumor. For instance, if osteoid osteoma is suspected based on the clinical history (see Fig. 1.5), conventional radiography followed by scintigraphy should be performed first, and after the lesion is localized to the particular bone, CT should be used for more specific localization and for obtaining quantitative information (measurements). However, if a soft-tissue tumor is suspected, MRI is the only technique able to localize and characterize the lesion accurately. Likewise, if radiographs are suggestive of a malignant bone tumor, MRI or CT should be used next to evaluate both the intraosseous extent of the tumor and the extraosseous involvement of the soft tissues.

The use of CT versus MRI is based on the radiographs: If there is no definite evidence of soft-tissue extension, then CT is superior to MRI for detecting subtle cortical erosions and periosteal reaction, while providing at the same time an accurate means of determining the intraosseous extension of the tumor; if, however, the radiographs suggest cortical destruction and soft-tissue mass, then MRI would be the preferred modality because it provides an excellent soft-tissue contrast and can determine the extraosseous extension of the tumor much better than CT.

In evaluating the results of malignant tumors treated by radiotherapy and chemotherapy, dynamic MRI using Gd-DTPA as a contrast enhancement is much superior to scintigraphy, CT, or even plain MRI.

Figure 16.25 depicts an algorithm for evaluating a bone lesion discovered on the standard plain radiographs. Note that the proper order of the various imaging modalities depends on two main factors: whether the radiographic findings are or are not diagnostic for any particular tumor and the lesion's uptake of a tracer on the radionuclide bone scan. Scintigraphy plays a crucial role here, dictating further steps in using the different techniques.

Radiographic Features of Bone Lesions

The radiographic features that help the radiologist diagnose a tumor or tumor-like bone lesion include: (a) the site of the lesion (location

Figure 16.22 Diagnosis of bone lesion. Analytic approach to evaluation of the bone neoplasm must include patient age, multiplicity of a lesion, location in the skeleton and in the particular bone, and radiographic morphology.

Figure 16.23 Peak age incidence of benign and malignant tumors and tumor-like lesions. (Sources: Dahlin DC, 1986, Dorfman HD, Czerniak B, 1998; Fechner RE, Mills SE, 1993; Huvos AG, 1979; Jaffe HL, 1968; Mirra JM, 1989; Moser RP, 1990; Schajowicz F, 1994; Unni KK, 1988; Wilner D, 1982.)

Figure 16.24 Simple bone cyst. (A) Anteroposterior radiograph of the right shoulder of a 69-year-old man with shoulder pain for 8 months demonstrates a well-defined radiolucent lesion with a sclerotic border in the glenoid portion of the scapula. Because the patient had a history of gout, the lesion was thought to represent an intraosseous tophus. In the differential diagnosis, an intraosseous ganglion and even a cartilage tumor were also considered. An excision biopsy, however, revealed a simple bone cyst, which is very unusual in the glenoid part of the scapula. **(B)** Lateral radiograph of the left hindfoot of a 50-year-old woman shows a radiolucent lesion in the calcaneus proven on the excision biopsy to be a simple bone cyst.

in the skeleton and in the individual bone); (b) the borders of the lesion (the so-called zone of transition); (c) the type of matrix of the lesion (composition of the tumor tissue); (d) the type of bone destruction; (e) the type of periosteal response to the lesion (periosteal reaction); (f) the nature and extent of soft-tissue involvement; and (g) the single or multiple nature of the lesion (Fig. 16.26).

Site of the Lesion. The site of a bone lesion is an important feature, because some tumors have a predilection for specific bones or specific sites in the bone (Table 16.3 and Fig. 16.27). The sites of some lesions are so characteristic that a diagnosis can be suggested on this basis alone, as in the case of parosteal osteosarcoma (Fig. 16.28) or chondroblastoma (see Fig. 16.4). Moreover, certain entities can be readily excluded from the differential diagnosis on the basis of the lesion's location. Thus, for example, the diagnosis of a giant cell tumor should not be made for a lesion that does not reach the articular end of the bone, because very few of these tumors develop in sites remote from the joint.

Borders of the Lesion. Evaluation of the borders or margins of a lesion is crucial in determining whether it is slow-growing or fast-growing (aggressive) (Fig. 16.29). Three types of lesion margins have been described: (a) a margin with sharp demarcation by sclerosis between the peripheral aspect of the tumor and the adjacent host bone (IA margin); (b) a margin with sharp demarcation without sclerosis around the periphery of the lesion (IB margin); and (c) a margin with an ill-defined region (either the entire circumference or only a portion of it) at the interface between lesion and host bone (IC margin). Slow-growing lesions, which are usually benign, have sharply outlined sclerotic borders (a narrow zone of transition) (Fig. 16.30A), whereas malignant or aggressive lesions typically have indistinct borders (a wide zone of transition) with either minimal or no reactive

sclerosis (Fig. 16.30B). Some lesions ordinarily lack a sclerotic border (Table 16.4), and some lesions commonly display a sclerotic border (Table 16.5). It must be emphasized that treatment can alter the appearance of malignant bone tumors; after radiation or chemotherapy, they may exhibit significant sclerosis as well as a narrow zone of transition (Fig. 16.31).

Type of Matrix. All bone tumors are composed of characteristic tissue components, the so-called tumor matrix. Only two of these—osteoblastic and cartilaginous tissue—can usually be clearly demonstrated radiographically. If one can identify bone or cartilage within a tumor, one can assume that it is osteoblastic or cartilaginous (Fig. 16.32). The identification of tumor bone within or adjacent to the area of destruction should alert the radiologist to the possibility of osteosarcoma. However, the deposition of new bone may also be the result of a reparative process secondary to bone destruction—so-called reactive sclerosis—rather than production of osteoid or bone by malignant cells. This new tumor bone is often radiographically indistinguishable from reactive bone; however, fluffy, cotton-like, or cloud-like densities within the medullary cavity and in the adjacent soft tissue should suggest the presence of tumorous bone and hence the diagnosis of osteosarcoma (Fig. 16.33).

Cartilage is identified by the presence of typically popcorn-like, punctate, annular, or comma-shaped calcifications (Fig. 16.34). Because cartilage usually grows in lobules, a tumor of cartilaginous origin can often be suggested by lobulated growth. A completely radiolucent lesion may be either fibrous or cartilaginous in origin, although hollow structures produced by tumor-like lesions, such as simple bone cysts or intraosseous ganglia, can also present as radiolucent areas (Table 16.6). The list of tumors and pseudotumors that may present as radiodense lesions is provided in Table 16.7.

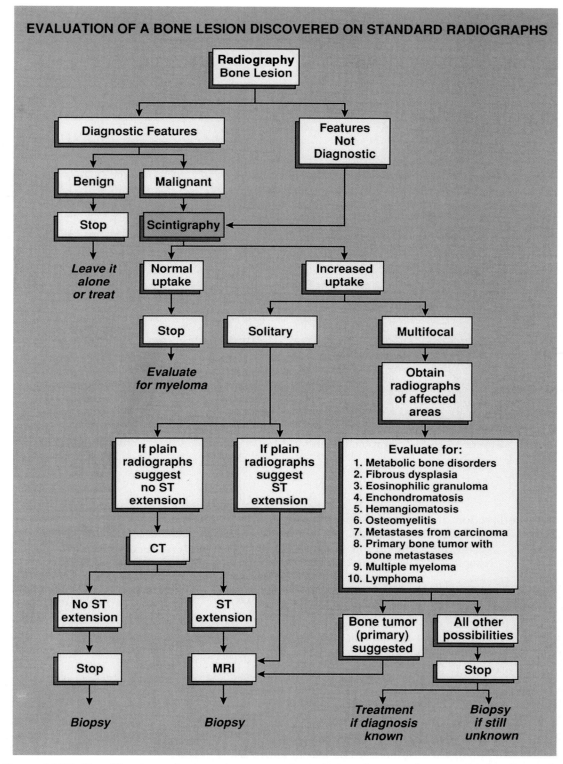

Figure 16.25 Algorithm to evaluate and manage a bone lesion discovered on standard radiographs.

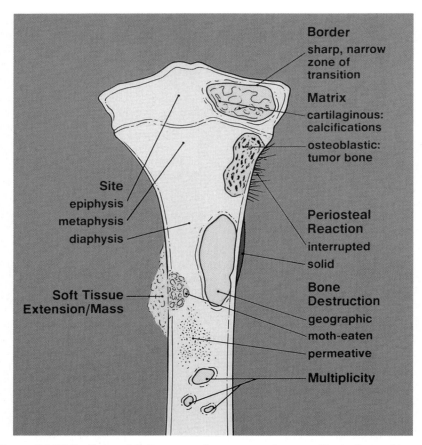

Figure 16.26 Radiographic features of tumors and tumor-like lesions of bone.

Table 16.3 **Predilection of Tumors for Specific Sites in the Skeleton**

	Skeletal Predilection of Benign Osseous Neoplasms and Tumor-Like Lesions	**Skeletal Predilection of Malignant Osseous Neoplasms**
Axial skeleton	*Skull and facial bones:* Osteoma, osteoblastoma, Langerhans cell histiocytosis, fibrous dysplasia, solitary hemangioma, osteoporosis circumscripta (lytic phase of Paget disease)	*Skull and facial bones:* Mesenchymal chondrosarcoma, multiple myeloma, metastatic neuroblastoma, metastatic carcinoma
	Jaw: Giant cell reparative granuloma, myxoma, ossifying fibroma, desmoplastic fibroma	*Mandible:* Osteosarcoma
	Spine: Aneurysmal bone cyst, osteoblastoma, Langerhans cell histiocytosis, hemangioma	*Spine:* Chordoma, myeloma, metastases
Appendicular skeleton	*Long tubular bones:* Osteoid osteoma, simple bone cyst, aneurysmal bone cyst, osteochondroma, enchondroma, periosteal chondroma, chondroblastoma, chondromyxoid fibroma, nonossifying fibroma, giant cell tumor, osteofibrous dysplasia, desmoplastic fibroma, intraosseous ganglion	*Long tubular bones:* Osteosarcoma (all variants), adamantinoma, malignant fibrous histiocytoma, primary lymphoma, chondrosarcoma, angiosarcoma, fibrosarcoma
	Hands and feet: Giant cell reparative granuloma, florid reactive periostitis, enchondroma, glomus tumor, epidermoid cyst, subungual exostosis, bizarre parosteal osteochondromatous lesion	*Hands and feet:* None
Specific predilections	Simple bone cyst—proximal humerus, proximal femur	Adamantinoma—tibia, fibula
	Osteofibrous dysplasia—tibia, fibula (anterior cortex)	Parosteal osteosarcoma—distal femur (posterior cortex)
	Osteoid osteoma—femur, tibia	Periosteal osteosarcoma—tibia
	Chondromyxoid fibroma—tibia, metaphyses	Clear cell chondrosarcoma—proximal femur and humerus
	Chondroblastoma—epiphyses	Chordoma—sacrum, clivus, C-2
	Giant cell tumor—articular ends of femur, tibia, radius	Multiple myeloma—pelvis, spine, skull

Modified from Fechner RE, Mills SE, 1993, with permission.

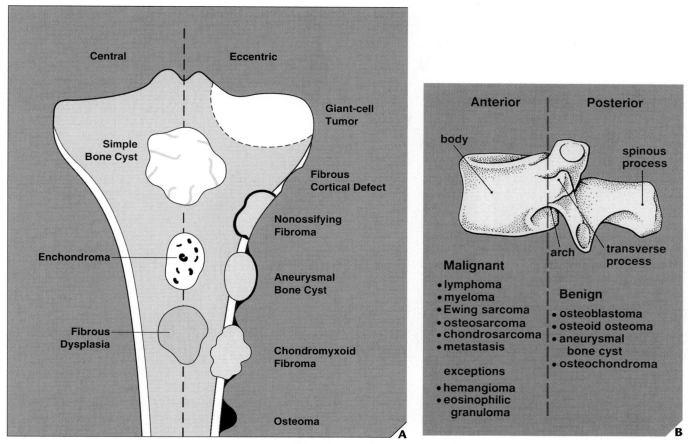

Figure 16.27 **Site of the lesion. (A)** Eccentric versus central location of the similar-appearing lesions is helpful in differential diagnosis. **(B)** Distribution of various tumors and tumor-like lesions in a vertebra. Malignant lesions are seen predominantly in its anterior part (body), while benign lesions predominate in its posterior elements (neural arch).

Figure 16.28 **Parosteal osteosarcoma.** Parosteal osteosarcoma has a predilection for the posterior aspect of the distal femur.

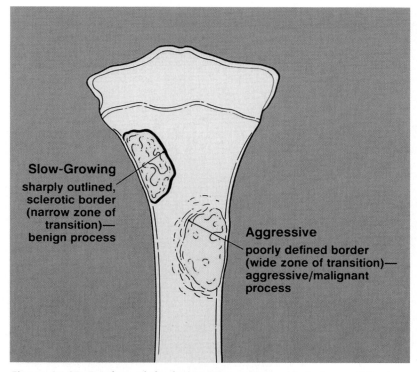

Figure 16.29 **Borders of the lesion.** The radiographic features of the borders of a lesion characterize it as either slow-growing (and most likely benign) or aggressive (and most likely malignant).

Figure 16.30 Borders of the lesion—benign vs. malignant. (A) A sclerotic border or narrow zone of transition from normal to abnormal bone typifies a benign lesion, as in this example of nonossifying fibroma. **(B)** A wide zone of transition typifies an aggressive/malignant lesion, in this case a solitary plasmacytoma involving the pubic bone and the supraacetabular portion of the right ilium.

Table 16.4 Bone Lesions Usually Lacking a Sclerotic Border

Benign	Malignant
Enchondroma in short tubular bone	Myeloma (plasmacytoma)
Giant cell tumor	Fibrosarcoma
Brown tumor of hyper-parathyroidism	Malignant fibrous histiocytoma
Osteolytic phase of Paget disease	Telangiectatic osteosarcoma
Acute osteomyelitis	Lymphoma
	Leiomyosarcoma of bone
	Angiosarcoma
	Metastatic tumor from primary in lung, gastrointestinal tract, kidney, breast, or thyroid

Table 16.5 Bone Lesions Commonly Displaying a Sclerotic Border

Benign	Malignant
Aneurysmal bone cyst	Chordoma
Benign fibrous histiocytoma	Clear-cell chondrosarcoma
Bone abscess	Low-grade central osteosarcoma
Chondroblastoma	Some malignant tumors after treatment with radiation or chemotherapy
Chondromyxoid fibroma	
Epidermoid inclusion cyst	
Fibrous cortical defect	
Fibrous dysplasia	
Intraosseous ganglion	
Medullary bone infarct	
Nonossifying fibroma	
Osteoblastoma	
Osteofibrous dysplasia	
Periosteal chondroma	
Simple bone cyst	

Figure 16.31 Osteosarcoma after chemotherapy. After 3 months of combined therapy with methotrexate, doxorubicin, hydrochloride, and vincristine, the anteroposterior radiograph of the knee of this 16-year-old boy with a conventional osteosarcoma of the right tibia reveals reactive sclerosis at the borders of the tumor and a narrow zone of transition, features more often seen in benign lesions. The patient underwent a limb-salvage procedure.

Figure 16.32 Tumor matrix. Radiographic features of the matrix of tumors and tumor-like lesions that characterize a lesion as cartilage-forming or bone-forming.

Figure 16.33 Osteoblastic matrix. The matrix of a typical osteoblastic lesion, in this case an osteosarcoma, is characterized by the presence of fluffy, cotton-like densities within the medullary cavity of the distal femur.

Figure 16.34 Chondroid matrix. The matrix of the typical cartilaginous tumor is characterized by punctate, annular, and popcorn-like calcifications within the radiolucent lesion. **(A)** Enchondroma. **(B)** Chondrosarcoma.

Table 16.6 **Tumors and Pseudotumors that May Present as Radiolucent Lesions**

Solid	Cystic
Osteoblastic (osteoid osteoma, osteoblastoma, telangiectatic osteosarcoma)	Simple bone cyst Aneurysmal bone cyst
Cartilaginous (enchondroma, chondroblastoma, chondromyxoid fibroma, chondrosarcoma)	Various bone cysts (synovial, degenerative) Intraosseous lipoma
Fibrous and histiocytic (nonossifying fibroma, fibrous dysplasia, osteofibrous dysplasia, desmoplastic fibroma, fibrosarcoma, malignant fibrous histiocytoma)	Brown tumor of hyperparathyroidism Vascular lesions Hydatid cyst
Lymphoma	Hemophilic pseudotumor
Myeloma (plasmacytoma)	Intraosseous ganglion
Ewing sarcoma	Bone abscess
Metastatic (from lung, breast, gastrointestinal tract, kidney, thyroid)	
Giant cell tumor	
Reparative giant cell granuloma	
Langerhans cell histiocytosis	
Paget disease (osteolytic phase—osteoporosis circumscripta)	

Table 16.7 **Tumors and Pseudotumors That May Present as Radiodense Lesions**

Benign	Malignant
Bone island	Adamantinoma
Caffey disease	Ewing sarcoma (after chemotherapy)
Calcifying enchondroma	Lymphoma
Condensing osteitis	Osteoblastic metastasis
Diskogenic vertebral sclerosis	Osteosarcoma
Healed fibrous cortical defect	Parosteal osteosarcoma
Healed nonossifying fibroma	
Healing or healed fracture	
Liposclerosing myxofibrous tumor	
Mastocytosis	
Medullary bone infarct	
Melorheostosis	
Osteoblastoma	
Osteofibrous dysplasia	
Osteoid osteoma	
Osteoma	
Osteonecrosis	
Osteopoikilosis	
Sclerosing hemangioma	

Type of Bone Destruction. The type of bone destruction caused by a tumor is primarily related to the tumor growth rate. While not pathognomonic for any specific neoplasm, the type of destruction, which can be described as geographic, moth-eaten, or permeative (Fig. 16.35),may suggest not only a benign or malignant neoplastic process (Fig. 16.36A,B) but also, at times, the histologic type of a tumor, as in the permeative type of bone destruction characteristically produced by the so-called round cell tumors—Ewing sarcoma (Fig. 16.36C) and lymphoma.

Periosteal Response. The periosteal reaction to a neoplastic process in the bone is usually categorized as uninterrupted or interrupted (Fig. 16.37 and Table 16.8). The first type of reaction is marked by solid layers of periosteal density, indicating a long-standing benign process, such as that seen in osteoid osteoma (Fig. 16.38) or osteoblastoma (see Fig. 17.32). Uninterrupted reaction is also seen in nonneoplastic processes such as Langerhans cell histiocytosis, osteomyelitis, bone abscess (Fig. 16.39), or pachydermoperiostosis, in fractures in the healing stage, or in hypertrophic pulmonary osteoarthropathy (Fig. 16.40). The interrupted type of periosteal reaction suggests malignancy or a highly aggressive nonmalignant process. It may present as a sunburst pattern, a lamellated (onion-skin) pattern, a velvet pattern, or a Codman triangle, and it is commonly seen in malignant primary tumors such as osteosarcoma or Ewing sarcoma (Fig. 16.41).

Soft-Tissue Extension. With few exceptions—such as giant cell tumors, aneurysmal bone cysts, osteoblastomas, or desmoplastic fi-

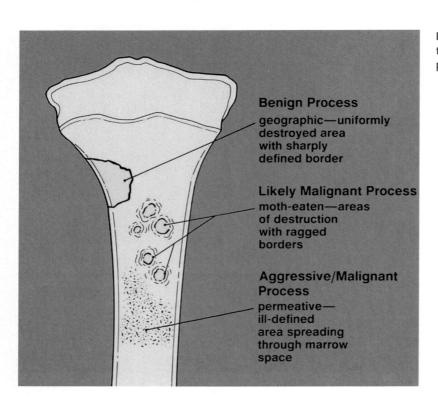

Benign Process
geographic—uniformly destroyed area with sharply defined border

Likely Malignant Process
moth-eaten—areas of destruction with ragged borders

Aggressive/Malignant Process
permeative—ill-defined area spreading through marrow space

Figure 16.35 Type of bone destruction. The radiographic features of the type of bone destruction may suggest a benign or malignant neoplastic process.

Figure 16.36 Types of bone destruction. (A) The geographic type of bone destruction, characterized by a uniformly affected area within sharply defined borders, typifies slow-growing benign lesions, in this case a chondromyxoid fibroma. **(B)** Moth-eaten bone destruction is characteristic of rapidly growing infiltrating lesions, in this case myeloma. **(C)** The permeative type of bone destruction is characteristic of round cell tumors, in this case Ewing sarcoma. Note the almost imperceptible destruction of the metaphysis of the femur by a tumor that has infiltrated the medullary cavity and cortex and extended into the surrounding soft tissues, forming a large mass. (Figure part A from Lewis MM, et al., 1987, with permission.)

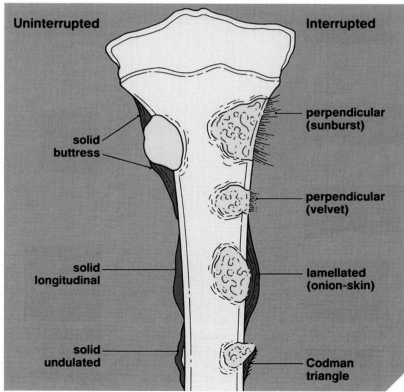

Figure 16.37 Types of periosteal reaction. Radiographic characteristics of uninterrupted and interrupted types of periosteal reaction. Uninterrupted periosteal reaction indicates a benign process, while interrupted reaction indicates a malignant or aggressive nonmalignant process.

Table 16.8 **Examples of Non-Neoplastic and Neoplastic Processes Categorized by Type of Periosteal Reaction**

UNINTERRUPTED PERIOSTEAL REACTION	
Benign Tumors and Tumor-Like Lesions	**Nonneoplastic Conditions**
Osteoid osteoma	Osteomyelitis
Osteoblastoma	Langerhans cell histiocytosis
Aneurysmal bone cyst	Healing fracture
Chondromyxoid fibroma	Juxtacortical myositis ossificans
Periosteal chondroma	Hypertrophic pulmonary osteoarthropathy
Chondroblastoma	Hemophilia (subperiosteal bleeding)
	Varicose veins and peripheral vascular insufficiency
Malignant Tumors	Caffey disease
Chondrosarcoma (rare)	Thyroid acropachy
	Treated scurvy
	Pachydermoperiostosis
	Gaucher disease

INTERRUPTED PERIOSTEAL REACTION	
Malignant Tumors	**Nonneoplastic Conditions**
Osteosarcoma	Osteomyelitis (occasionally)
Ewing sarcoma	Langerhans cell histiocytosis (occasionally)
Chondrosarcoma	
Lymphoma (rare)	Subperiosteal hemorrhage (occasionally)
Fibrosarcoma (rare)	
Malignant fibrous histiocytoma (MFH) (rare)	
Metastatic carcinoma	

bromas—benign tumors and tumor-like bone lesions usually do not exhibit soft-tissue extension; thus, almost invariably, a soft-tissue mass indicates an aggressive lesion and one that is in many instances malignant (Fig. 16.42). It should be kept in mind, however, that non-neoplastic conditions such as osteomyelitis also exhibit a soft-tissue

Figure 16.39 Solid periosteal reaction—bone abscess. A bone abscess located at the base of the fourth metatarsal bone elicits a solid type of periosteal reaction.

component, but the involvement of the soft tissues is usually poorly defined, with obliteration of fatty tissue layers. In malignant processes, however, the tumor mass is sharply defined, extending through the destroyed cortex with preservation of the tissue planes (Fig. 16.43).

In the case of a bone lesion associated with a soft-tissue mass, it is always helpful to determine which condition arose first. Is the soft tis-

Figure 16.38 Solid periosteal reaction—osteoid osteoma. An uninterrupted solid periosteal reaction is characteristic of benign lesions, in this case a cortical osteoid osteoma.

Figure 16.40 Solid periosteal reaction—hypertrophic pulmonary osteoarthropathy. An uninterrupted periosteal reaction typifies changes of hypertrophic pulmonary osteoarthropathy as seen here in the distal forearm and hand in a patient with carcinoma of the lung.

Figure 16.41 Interrupted type of periosteal reaction. (A) Highly aggressive and malignant lesions may present radiographically with a sunburst pattern of periosteal reaction, as seen in this case of osteosarcoma. **(B)** Another pattern of interrupted periosteal reaction is the lamellated or onion-skin type, as seen here in Ewing sarcoma involving the proximal femur. **(C)** Radiograph of the slab sections (coronal at left and transverse at right) of the resected specimen from Ewing sarcoma demonstrate lamellated type in more detail. **(D)** Codman triangle also reflects an aggressive, usually malignant type of periosteal reaction, as seen here in a patient with Ewing sarcoma and **(E)** in a patient with osteosarcoma.

Figure 16.42 Soft-tissue mass. Radiographic features of soft-tissue extension characterizing malignant/aggressive bone lesions and benign neoplastic processes.

sue lesion, in other words, an extension of a primary bone tumor or is it itself a primary lesion that has invaded the bone? Although not always applicable, certain radiographic criteria may help in deciding this issue (Fig. 16.44). In most instances, for example, a large soft-tissue mass and a smaller bone lesion indicate secondary skeletal involvement. Ewing sarcoma breaks this rule, however. Its destructive primary bone lesion may be small and often accompanied by a large soft-tissue mass. A destructive lesion of bone lacking a periosteal reaction and adjacent to a soft-tissue mass may indicate secondary invasion by a primary soft-tissue tumor, which usually destroys the neighboring periosteum. This contrasts with primary bone lesions, which usually prompt a periosteal reaction when they break through the cortex and extend into adjacent soft tissues. Because these observations are not

universally applicable, however, they should be taken only as indicators and not as pathognomonic features.

Multiplicity of Lesions. A multiplicity of malignant lesions usually indicates metastatic disease, multiple myeloma, or lymphoma (Fig. 16.45). Very rarely do primary malignant lesions, such as an osteosarcoma or Ewing sarcoma, present as multifocal disease. Benign lesions, however, tend to involve multiple sites, as in polyostotic fibrous dysplasia (Fig. 16.46), multiple osteochondromas, enchondromatosis, Langerhans cell histiocytosis, hemangiomatosis, and fibromatosis.

Benign Versus Malignant. Although it is sometimes very difficult to distinguish benign from malignant bone lesions on the basis of radiography alone, certain characteristic features favor one designation over the other (Fig. 16.47). Benign tumors usually present with well-defined, sclerotic borders, a geographic type of bone destruction, an uninterrupted, solid periosteal reaction, and no soft-tissue mass (see Figs. 16.24, 16.30A, 16.36A, and 16.38). Malignant lesions, however, tend to demonstrate poorly defined borders with a wide zone of transition, a moth-eaten or permeative pattern of bone destruction, an interrupted periosteal reaction of the sunburst or onion-skin type, and an adjacent soft-tissue mass (see Figs. 16.30B, 16.36B,C, 16.41, and 16.43A). It should be kept in mind, however, that some benign lesions may also exhibit aggressive features (Table 16.9).

Management

When all the clinical and radiographic information concerning a patient with a bone lesion has been analyzed, the most important diagnostic decision is whether the lesion is definitely benign and not to undergo biopsy, but rather merely monitored or completely ignored—a "don't touch" lesion (Fig. 16.48 and Table 16.10)—or whether it has an aggressive or ambiguous appearance and should be further investigated via percutaneous or open biopsy (Fig. 16.49). The results of the histopathologic examination of a specimen determine whether the further management in a given case should be surgical, chemotherapeutic, radiotherapeutic, or a combination of these.

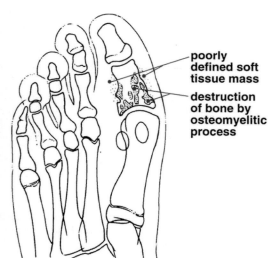

Figure 16.43 Soft-tissue mass. (A) A malignant tumor of the clavicle, in this case Ewing sarcoma, exhibits a distinct, sharply outlined soft-tissue mass. **(B)** In osteomyelitis, however, the tissue planes are obliterated and the soft-tissue mass has an indistinct border.

Figure 16.44 Primary soft-tissue tumor vs. primary bone tumor. Certain radiographic features of bone and soft-tissue lesions may help differentiate a primary soft-tissue tumor invading the bone from a primary bone tumor invading soft tissues.

Figure 16.45 Multiplicity of lesion. (A) Multiple myeloma is characterized by numerous osteolytic lesions. **(B)** Metastatic disease may also present with multiple foci, as seen in this 66-year-old man with carcinoma of the prostate. Note several osteoblastic lesions scattered throughout the pelvis and both femora.

Figure 16.46 Multiplicity of lesion—fibrous dysplasia. Anteroposterior view of the hip in a 10-year-old boy with polyostotic fibrous dysplasia shows numerous sites of involvement in the left femur and ilium. Scintigraphy (not shown here) demonstrated involvement of additional sites.

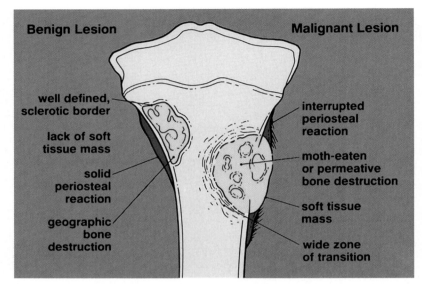

Figure 16.47 Benign vs. malignant lesion. Radiographic features that may help differentiate benign from malignant lesions.

Table 16.9 **Benign Lesions With Aggressive Features**

Lesion	Radiographic Presentation
Osteoblastoma (aggressive)	Bone destruction and soft tissue extension similar to osteosarcoma
Desmoplastic fibroma	Expansive destructive lesion, frequently trabeculated
Periosteal desmoid	Irregular cortical outline, mimics osteosarcoma or Ewing sarcoma
Giant cell tumor	Occasionally aggressive features such as osteolytic bone destruction, cortical penetration, and soft tissue extension
Aneurysmal bone cyst	Soft tissue extension, occasionally mimicking malignant tumor (i.e., telangiectatic osteosarcoma)
Osteomyelitis	Bone destruction, aggressive periosteal reaction
	Occasionally, features resembling osteosarcoma, Ewing sarcoma, or lymphoma
Langerhans cell histiocytosis	Bone destruction, aggressive periosteal reaction
	Occasionally, features resembling Ewing sarcoma
Pseudotumor of hemophilia	Bone destruction, periosteal reaction occasionally mimics malignant tumor
Myositis ossificans	Features of parosteal or periosteal osteosarcoma, soft tissue osteosarcoma, or liposarcoma
Brown tumor of hyperparathyroidism	Lytic bone lesion, resembling malignant tumor

Figure 16.48 "Don't touch" lesions. **(A)** A typical benign "don't touch" lesion, in this case a nonossifying fibroma in healing phase, should not be mistaken for a malignant tumor of bone. **(B)** Another "don't touch" lesion, a periosteal (cortical) desmoid (*arrows*) in a typical location at the distal femoral metaphysis, medially. **(C)** A fibrous cortical defect (*arrow*) is an innocent fibrous lesion that never requires biopsy. **(D)** A bone island (*arrows*) should be recognized by a characteristic brush border and is not to be mistaken for a sclerotic neoplasm.

Table 16.10 "Don't Touch" Lesions That Should Not Undergo Biopsy

Tumors and Tumor-Like Lesions	Nonneoplastic Processses
Fibrous cortical defect	Stress fracture
Nonossifying fibroma (healing phase)	Avulsion fracture (healing stage)
Periosteal (cortical) desmoid	Bone infarct
Small, solitary focus of fibrous dysplasia	Bone island (enostosis)
Pseudotumor of hemophilia	Myositis ossificans
Intraosseous ganglion	Degenerative and posttraumatic cysts
Enchondroma in a short, tubular bone	Brown tumor of hyperparathyroidism
Intraosseous hemangioma	Diskogenic vertebral sclerosis

Figure 16.49 Chronic osteomyelitis. A typical "ambiguous" lesion exhibiting aggressive characteristics requires biopsy. The radiographic differential diagnosis in this case included osteosarcoma, Ewing sarcoma, lymphoma, and bone infection. Biopsy revealed chronic osteomyelitis.

nidus of osteoid osteoma

Figure 16.50 Osteoid osteoma. (A) During surgery for resection of a nidus of osteoid osteoma in the proximal diaphysis of the tibia of a 10-year-old boy, needles are taped into the skin to localize the nidus. **(B)** Radiograph of the resected specimen demonstrates complete excision of the lesion.

Figure 16.51 Chondromyxoid fibroma. A 9-year-old boy was treated for a chondromyxoid fibroma, a benign cartilaginous lesion in the proximal left tibia. **(A)** Preoperative film shows a lesion exhibiting a thin sclerotic border with endosteal scalloping, a geographic-type bone destruction, and a solid buttress of periosteal new bone formation at its distal part. **(B)** Postoperative film shows the lesion's cavity packed with bone chips after curettage. **(C)** Two years later, the tumor recurred.

Monitoring the Results of Treatment

Five modalities—conventional radiography, CT, MRI, scintigraphy, and arteriography—are commonly used to monitor the results of treatment for bone tumors. Of these five, radiography is used mainly to document the results of surgical resection of benign lesions such as osteochondroma or osteoid osteoma (Fig. 16.50), or to follow-up after curettage of benign tumors or tumor-like lesions and application of bone graft (Fig. 16.51). In the case of malignant tumors, radiographic films permit one to demonstrate the position of endoprostheses (Fig. 16.52) or bone grafts (Fig. 16.53) in limb-salvage procedures. The effectiveness of chemotherapy is best mon-

itored by a combination of radiography, arteriography (Fig. 16.54), CT (see Fig. 16.9), and MRI. Recurrence or metastatic spread of a tumor can be effectively shown at an early stage on scintigraphy, CT, or MRI.

Complications

Although the most frequent direct complication of malignant bone tumors is metastasis, particularly to the lung, the most serious complication of some benign lesions is their potential for malignant transformation (Fig. 16.55; see also Table 16.2). Moreover, some benign lesions, such as those seen in multiple cartilaginous exostoses (Fig.

Figure 16.52 Osteosarcoma—endoprosthesis. After a course of chemotherapy, an 8-year-old girl with an osteosarcoma of the right femur **(A)** underwent radical resection of the distal three fourths of the femur, with insertion of an expandable (LEAP) prosthesis **(B)**, which can be lengthened as the child grows. (Courtesy of Dr. M.M. Lewis, New York, NY).

Figure 16.53 Ewing sarcoma—resection and bone grafting. After a course of radiotherapy and chemotherapy, a 9-year-old girl with a Ewing sarcoma in the diaphysis of the left humerus **(A)** underwent radical resection of the middle segment of the humerus. **(B)** Reconstruction was accomplished with the application of a fibular autograft.

Figure 16.54 Osteosarcoma after chemotherapy. (A) Anteroposterior radiograph of the proximal left tibia of a 15-year-old boy demonstrates an osteosarcoma in the metaphysis associated with a large soft-tissue mass. **(B)** An arteriogram done prior to treatment shows the soft-tissue mass to be hypervascular. After combination chemotherapy with methotrexate, vincristine, doxorubicin hydrochloride, and cisplatin, a repeated plain film **(C)** and arteriogram **(D)** show marked reduction of the tumor mass. Subsequently, a wide resection of the proximal tibia was performed, and a metallic spacer similar to the one shown in Fig. 16.52B was implanted.

Figure 16.55 Malignant transformation to chondrosarcoma. An enchondroma at the base of the ring finger of this 32-year-old man with multiple enchondromatosis underwent sarcomatous transformation to a chondrosarcoma.

Figure 16.56 Multiple cartilaginous exostoses—growth disturbance. Anteroposterior radiograph of the wrist of a 14-year-old boy with multiple cartilaginous exostoses (osteochondromas) shows marked growth disturbance of the distal ends of the radius and ulna.

Figure 16.57 Nonossifying fibroma complicated by a pathologic fracture. A 9-year-old boy with a giant nonossifying fibroma of the distal diaphysis of the right femur developed a pathologic fracture, a common complication of this lesion.

16.56) or enchondromatosis, may result in severe growth disturbance. The most common complication of tumors and tumor-like lesions in general, however, is pathologic fracture. Although not a diagnostic feature, this may complicate both benign and malignant lesions. Among lesions with a high potential for fracture are simple bone cysts, large nonossifying fibromas (Fig. 16.57), fibrous dysplasia, and enchondromas. Occasionally, pathologic fracture is the first sign of a neoplastic process. Other complications, such as pressure erosion of adjacent bone (Fig. 16.58) or compression of adjacent blood vessels or nerves (see Fig. 18.30B), may occur with growth of a lesion beyond the cortex.

Figure 16.58 Osteochondroma eroding the adjacent bone. Extension of a lesion arising from the posterolateral aspect of the distal tibia in a 24-year-old man with an osteochondroma erodes the adjacent fibula.

Table 16.11 **Most Common Benign and Malignant Soft Tissue Tumors**

Benign	**Malignant**
Ganglion	Rhabdomyosarcoma
Lipoma	Leiomyosarcoma
Myoma, leiomyoma	Malignant fibrous histiocytoma
Fibroma	Fibrosarcoma
Myxoma	Malignant schwannoma
Hemangioma, hemangiomatosis	Spindle-cell sarcoma
	Liposarcoma
Lymphangioma	Synovial sarcoma
Chondroma	Extraskeletal osteosarcoma
Neurofibroma	Extraskeletal chondrosarcoma
Desmoid	
Giant cell tumor of tendon sheath	
Morton's neuroma	

Soft-Tissue Tumors

Unlike tumors and tumor-like lesions of bone, most soft-tissue tumors (Table 16.11) lack specific radiographic characteristics that might be helpful in their diagnosis. Some findings, however, may point to a particular kind of lesion. For instance, calcified phleboliths in a soft-tissue mass suggest a hemangioma or hemangiomatosis (Fig. 16.59); radiolucency within a mass suggests a lipoma (Fig. 16.60); mottled lucencies within a dense mass, in association with bone formation, suggest liposarcoma (Fig. 16.61); popcorn-like calcifications suggest soft tissue chondroma or chondrosarcoma; similar calcifications in the vicinity of a joint, particularly when associated with bone destruction, suggest synovial sarcoma; and ill-defined, nonhomogeneous, smudgy bone in a soft-tissue mass may indicate a soft-tissue osteosarcoma (Fig. 16.62). Several investigators implied the efficacy of MRI in the characterization and evaluation of soft-tissue masses; its superiority over CT stems from lack of ionizing radiation, its capability of multidirectional and multiplanar imaging, and its excellent contrast resolution and accurate anatomic definition of soft-tissue tumors. On T1-weighted pulsing sequences, the majority of soft-tissue masses display low-to-intermediate signal in-

Figure 16.60 Soft-tissue lipoma. Oblique radiograph of the hand of a 27-year-old woman with a soft-tissue mass in the dorsal aspect shows a radiolucent lesion in the soft tissues adjacent to the radial aspect of the second metacarpal bone. Within the radiolucent area there is evidence of bone formation. The lesion proved to be a lipoma.

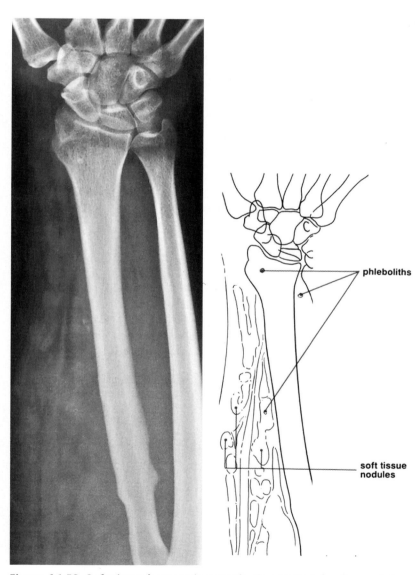

Figure 16.59 Soft-tissue hemangiomatosis. Conventional radiograph in a 39-year-old woman with a nodular swelling of the left forearm demonstrates multiple small calcified phleboliths, suggesting the diagnosis of hemangiomatosis.

tensity, whereas on T2-weighted images they display high-signal intensity. There are, however, masses that show high-signal intensity on T1-weighting because of blood or fat content, such as lipomas, hemangiomas, and chronic hematomas. One of the fatty tumors that does not show a high signal on T1 weighting is myxoid liposarcoma. At present, however, as Sundaram contended based on MRI results, neither visual characteristics nor signal intensity values permit one to distinguish or predict the histology of soft-tissue masses. Nevertheless, certain criteria are very helpful to predict the benign or malignant nature of the tumor; sharp margination and homogeneity of the mass favor benignity, whereas prominent peritumoral edema and necrosis suggest malignancy.

The main role of the radiologist is not to make a specific diagnosis, but rather to demonstrate the extent of the lesion and decide whether the lesion is a tumor or pseudotumor (Table 16.12), and in case of malignancy, whether it is a primary soft-tissue tumor invading the bone or an extracortical extension of a primary bone tumor (Fig. 16.44). Most often, this is achieved by using arteriography (Fig. 16.63), CT scan (Fig. 16.64), and MRI (Fig. 16.65). After this, the radiologist's role may become more active, involving fluoroscopy-guided or CT-guided percutaneous biopsy of the lesion. In this respect, arteriography helps select the proper area for biopsy, with the specimen usually taken from the most vascular part of the lesion (Fig. 16.66).

Figure 16.61 Soft-tissue liposarcoma. (A) Lateral radiograph in a 54-year-old man with a slowly enlarging mass on the posterior aspect of the thigh demonstrates a poorly defined soft-tissue mass with radiolucent areas and bone formation at the site of the posterior cortex of the femur. **(B)** CT section at the level of the radiolucency confirms the presence of fatty tissue. **(C)** A section through the bone formation discloses a denser mass infiltrating surrounding muscular structures. A liposarcoma was suggested as a possible diagnosis and was later confirmed on excision biopsy.

Figure 16.62 Soft-tissue osteosarcoma. A 51-year-old woman presented with a large suprapatellar soft-tissue mass. Lateral radiograph of the knee demonstrates a mass with ill-defined nonhomogeneous bone formation in the central part of the lesion. Biopsy revealed a soft-tissue osteosarcoma. (From Greenspan A, et al., 1987, with permission.)

Table 16.12 Most Common Benign Soft Tissue Masses That May Mimic Neoplasms

Abscess	
Amyloidoma	Nodular fasciitis
Calcific myonecrosis	Pigmented villonodular synovitis
Cyst	Pseudoaneurysm
Florid reactive periostitis	Reactive adenopathy
Foreign body granuloma	Rheumatoid nodule
Gouty tophus	Seroma
Hematoma	Synovial cyst
Myositis ossificans	Tumoral calcinosis

Figure 16.63 Soft-tissue malignant fibrous histiocytoma. Femoral arteriography was performed on a 56-year-old man with a tumor on the medial aspect of the right thigh, which proved to be a malignant fibrous histiocytoma of the soft-tissues. **(A)** The arterial phase demonstrates the displacement of the superficial femoral artery by the tumor, the extent of the tumor and area of neovascularity, and the accumulation of contrast medium within the tumor. **(B)** The venous phase shows the accumulation of contrast in abnormal vessels and a tumor "stain," as well as the topography of venous structures.

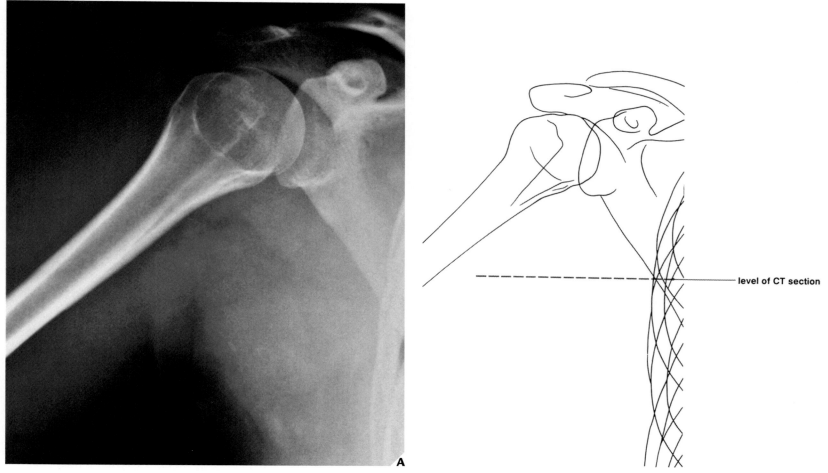

level of CT section

Figure 16.64 Soft-tissue fibrosarcoma. (A) Anteroposterior radiograph of the shoulder of a 40-year-old woman with a history of an enlarging mass in the right axilla shows an ill-defined mass adjacent to the lateral border of the scapula. **(B)** CT section with contrast enhancement shows the extent of the mass and the lack of bone involvement. The tumor proved to be a fibrosarcoma.

Figure 16.64 Soft-tissue fibrosarcoma. *Continued*

Figure 16.65 Intramuscular hemangioma. A 34-year-old woman presented with pain in the distal left forearm. The radiograph **(A)** demonstrates periosteal reaction at the ulnar border of the distal radius, associated with a phlebolith (*arrow*). **(B)** Coronal T2-weighted MRI (SE; TR 2000/TE 80 msec) shows a large mass situated in the pronator quadratus muscle of the distal forearm, displaying inhomogeneous signal ranging from intermediate to high intensity. The lesion proved to be an intramuscular hemangioma. (From Greenspan A, et al., 1992, with permission.)

Figure 16.66 Parosteal liposarcoma. Vascular study of the patient shown in Fig 16.61 shows that the lesion consists of two parts: the proximal part is more radiolucent and hypovascular, while the distal is denser and more hypervascular. The biopsy specimen on which the diagnosis of liposarcoma was made was obtained from the more vascular segment of the tumor. After radical resection and examination of the entire specimen, the more radiolucent hypovascular area revealed almost no malignant component. Had the biopsy been obtained only from that part of the tumor, the result probably would not have been consistent with the final diagnosis.

PRACTICAL POINTS TO REMEMBER

[1] The most helpful clinical data concerning patients presenting with suspected bone or soft tissue lesions are:
- the age of the patient
- the duration of the symptoms
- the growth rate of the tumor.

[2] In the evaluation of tumors or tumor-like bone lesions, several key radiographic features should be sought, including:
- the site of the lesion (the particular bone and site in the bone affected)
- the nature of the border of the lesion (narrow or wide zone of transition)
- the type of matrix (calcified, ossified, or hollow)
- the type of bone destruction (geographic, moth-eaten, or permeative)
- the periosteal reaction (solid or interrupted—sunburst, velvet, lamellated, Codman triangle)
- the presence or absence of soft-tissue extension.

[3] A lytic (radiolucent) lesion located in the epiphysis and showing a narrow zone of transition is most likely a chondroblastoma.

[4] A lytic lesion lacking a sclerotic border and extending into the articular end of a bone after closure of the growth plate is most likely a giant cell tumor. The absence of extension into the articular end of the bone virtually excludes giant cell tumor.

[5] A centrally located lesion having a sclerotic border and abutting the growth plate in the proximal humerus or proximal femur is most likely a simple bone cyst.

[6] A radiolucent lesion located in the lateral aspect of the calcaneus is most likely a simple bone cyst.

[7] An eccentrically located lesion ballooning out from the cortex and seen in a patient below 20 years of age is most likely an aneurysmal bone cyst or a chondromyxoid fibroma. If the patient is 30 or older, these possibilities are remote.

[8] A radiolucent lesion in a short tubular bone is most likely an enchondroma.

[9] A lesion with a sclerotic margin located in the anterior aspect of the tibia in a child is most likely an osteofibrous dysplasia (Kempson-Campanacci lesion). A similar lesion or multiple osteolytic lesions in the tibia in adults most likely represent adamantinoma.

[10] A lesion in the medial aspect of distal femur lying close to the linea aspera and showing cortical irregularity is most likely a periosteal desmoid.

[11] An intramedullary lesion in the posterior aspect of the distal femur having a scalloped, sclerotic margin is most likely a nonossifying fibroma.

[12] A sclerotic, lobulated lesion on the surface of the posterior aspect of distal femur should be considered to represent a parosteal osteosarcoma.

[13] An ill-defined lesion displaying calcifications and located on the anterior aspect of the tibia should raise the possibility of periosteal osteosarcoma.

[14] A lesion in a vertebral body is most often a metastasis, a myeloma, lymphoma, hemangioma, or Langerhans cell histiocytosis.

[15] A lesion in the posterior vertebral arch is most likely an aneurysmal bone cyst, osteoblastoma, or osteoid osteoma.

[16] A lesion most likely represents a benign tumor when it exhibits:
- geographic bone destruction
- a sclerotic margin
- solid, uninterrupted periosteal reaction, or no periosteal response
- no soft-tissue mass.

[17] A lesion most likely represents a malignant tumor when it shows
- poorly defined margins (a wide zone of transition)
- a moth-eaten or permeative type of bone destruction
- an interrupted periosteal reaction
- a soft tissue mass.

[18] A lesion most likely represents a cartilage tumor (e.g., enchondroma or chondrosarcoma) when it exhibits:
- lobulation (endosteal scalloping)
- punctate, annular, or comma-like calcifications in the matrix.

[19] An eccentric lesion displaying a solid buttress of periosteal reaction is most likely an aneurysmal bone cyst, chondromyxoid fibroma, or juxtacortical chondroma.

[20] A lesion exhibiting a moth-eaten or permeative type of bone destruction and associated with a large soft-tissue mass without ossifications or calcifications is most likely a Ewing sarcoma. If the patient is younger than age 5 years or is black, Ewing sarcoma is unlikely.

[21] When a soft-tissue mass and a destructive bone lesion coexist, certain radiographic features of the lesion may help differentiate a primary soft-tissue tumor invading bone from a primary bone tumor invading soft tissue:
- the epicenter of the lesion: if outside the bone, then it is probable that it is primary soft tissue; if within it, then it is probable that it is primary bone

- the bevel of cortical destruction: if toward the bone, then it is probable that it is primary soft tissue; if toward the soft tissue, then it is probable that it is primary bone
- the absence of periosteal reaction: probable primary soft tissue
- a large soft-tissue mass and a small bone lesion: probable primary soft tissue (with the exception of Ewing sarcoma).

[22] Benign lesions such as fibrous dysplasia, nonossifying fibroma, Langerhans cell histiocytosis, hemangioma, cartilaginous exostoses, and enchondroma tend to be multiple. Multiple malignant lesions, on the other hand, should raise the possibility of metastatic disease, multiple myeloma, and lymphoma.

[23] In the evaluation of soft-tissue lesions, some radiographic findings can help suggest a diagnosis.
Among these are:
- phleboliths (hemangioma)
- radiolucent areas within the mass (lipoma)
- dense areas dispersed with radiolucencies and ossifications (liposarcoma)
- ill-defined ossifications within the dense mass (osteosarcoma)
- mass near the joint with calcifications (synovial sarcoma)
- popcorn-like calcifications within the mass (chondroma or chondrosarcoma).

[24] MRI features suggesting a benign soft-tissue mass include sharp margination and homogeneity of the lesion, whereas prominent peritumoral edema and necrosis suggest malignant nature.

SUGGESTED READINGS

Aisen AM, Martel W, Braunstein EM, McMillin KI. MRI and CT evaluation of primary bone and soft tissue tumors. *AJR Am J Roentgenol* 1986;146:749–756.

Adler RS, Bell DS, Bamber JC, Moskovic E, Thomas JM. Evaluation of soft-tissue masses using segmented color Doppler velocity images: preliminary observations. *AJR Am J Roentgenol* 1999;172:781–788.

Arata MA, Peterson HA, Dahlin DC. Pathological fractures through nonossifying fibromas: review of the Mayo Clinic experience. *J Bone Joint Surg [Am]* 1981;63A:890–988.

Ayala AG, Zornosa J. Primary bone tumors: percutaneous needle biopsy. Radiology 1983;149:675–679.

Barnes G, Gwinn J. Distal irregularities of the femur simulating malignancy. *AJR Am J Roentgenol* 1974;122:180–185.

Berquist TH. Magnetic resonance imaging of primary skeletal neoplasms. *Radiol Clin North Am* 1993;31:411–424.

Berquist TH. Magnetic resonance imaging of musculoskeletal neoplasms. *Clin Orthop* 1989;244:101–118.

Bloem JL. *Radiological staging of primary malignant musculoskeletal tumors. A correlative study of CT, MRI, ^{99m}Tc scintigraphy and angiography.* The Hague: A. Jongbloed;1988.

Bloem JL, Bluemm RG, Taminiau AHM, van Oosterom AT, Stolk J, Doornbos J. Magnetic resonance imaging of primary malignant bone tumors. *Radiographics* 1987;7:425–445.

Bloem JL, Reiser MF, Vanel D. Magnetic resonance contrast agents in evaluation of the musculoskeletal system. *Magn Res Q* 1990;6:136–163.

Bloem JL, Taminiau AHM, Eulderink F, Hermans J, Pauwels EK. Radiologic staging of primary bone sarcoma: MR imaging, scintigraphy, angiography, and CT correlated with pathologic examination. *Radiology* 1988;169:805–810.

Bloem JL, Van der Woude HJ, Giernaerdt M, Hogentorn PC, Taminiau AHM, Hermans J. Does magnetic resonance imaging make a difference for patients with musculoskeletal sarcoma? *Br J Radiol* 1997;70:327–337.

Bodner G, Schocke MFH, Rachbauer F, et al. Differentiation of malignant and benign musculoskeletal tumors: combined color and power Doppler US and spectral wave analysis. *Radiology* 2002;223:410–416.

Bohndorf K, Reiser M, Lochner B. Magnetic resonance imaging of primary tumors and tumor-like lesions of bone. *Skeletal Radiol* 1986;15:511–517.

Boyko OB, Cory DA, Cohen MD, Provisor A, Mirkin D, DeRosa GP. MR imaging of osteogenic and Ewing's sarcoma. *AJR Am J Roentgenol* 1987;148:317–322.

Brown KT, Kattapuram SV, Rosenthal DI. Computed tomography analysis of bone tumors: patterns of cortical destruction and soft tissue extension. *Skeletal Radiol* 1986;15:448–451.

Chew FS, Hudson TM. Radionuclide bone scanning of osteosarcoma: falsely extended uptake patterns. *AJR Am J Roentgenol* 1982;139:49–54.

Coffre C, Vanel D, Contesso G, Kalifa C, Dubousset J, Genin J, Masselot J. Problems and pitfalls in the use of computed tomography for the local evaluation of long bone osteosarcoma. Report on 30 cases. *Skeletal Radiol* 1985;13:147–153.

Cohen EK, Kressel HY, Frank TS, et al. Hyaline cartilage-origin bone and soft-tissue neoplasms: MR appearance and histologic correlation. *Radiology* 1988;167:477–481.

Cohen MD, Weetman RM, Provisor AJ, et al. Efficacy of magnetic resonance imaging in 139 children with tumors. *Arch Surg* 1986;121:522–529.

Conrad EU 3rd, Enneking WF. Common soft tissue tumors. *Clin Symp* 1990;42:2–32.

Crim JR, Seeger LL, Yao L, Chandnani V, Eckardt JJ. Diagnosis of soft-tissue masses with MR imaging: can benign masses be differentiated from malignant ones? *Radiology* 1992;185:581–586.

Dahlin DC, Unni KK. *Bone tumors: general aspects and data on 8542 cases,* 4th ed. Springfield, IL: Charles C. Thomas; 1986.

Davies MA, Wellings RM. Imaging of bone tumors. *Curr Opin Radiol* 1992;4:32–38.

Dewhirst MW, Sostman HD, Leopold KA, et al. Soft-tissue sarcomas: MR imaging and MR spectroscopy for prognosis and therapy monitoring. Work in progress. *Radiology* 1990;174:847–853.

Dorfman HD, Czerniak B. *Bone tumors.* St. Louis: Mosby;1998:1–33.

Dwyer AJ, Frank JA, Sank VJ, Reinig JW, Hickey AM, Doppman JL. Short-TI inversion-recovery pulse sequence: analysis and initial experience in cancer imaging. *Radiology* 1988; 169: 827–836.

Edeiken J, Hodes PJ, Caplan LH. New bone production and periosteal reaction. *AJR Am J Roentgenol* 1966;97:708–718.

Ehman RL, Berquist TH, McLeod RA. MR imaging of the musculoskeletal system: a 5-year appraisal. *Radiology* 1988;166:313–320.

Elias DA, White LM, Simpson DJ, Kandel RA, Tomlinson G, Bell RS, Wunder JS. Osseous invasion by soft-tissue sarcoma: assessment with MR imaging. *Radiology* 2003; 229:145–152.

Enneking WF. Staging of musculoskeletal neoplasms. *Skeletal Radiol* 1985;13:183–194.

Enneking WF, Spanier SS, Goodman MA. A system for the surgical staging of musculoskeletal sarcoma. *Clin Orthop* 1980;153:106–120.

Enzinger FM, Weiss SW. *Soft tissue tumors,* 3rd ed. St. Louis: Mosby;1995: 3–56.

Erlemann R, Reiser MF, Peters PE, et al. Musculoskeletal neoplasms: static and dynamic Gd-DPTA-enhanced MR imaging. *Radiology* 1989;171:767–773.

Erlemann R, Sciuk J, Bosse A, et al. Response of osteosarcoma and Ewing sarcoma to preoperative chemotherapy: assessment with dynamic and static MR imaging and skeletal scintigraphy. *Radiology* 1990;175:791–796.

Erlemann R, Vassallo P, Bongartz G, et al. Musculoskeletal neoplasms: fast low-angle shot MR imaging with and without Gd-DTPA. *Radiology* 1990;176:489–495.

Ewing J. A review and classification of bone sarcomas. *Arch Surg* 1922;4:485–533.

Fechner RE, Mills SE. *Tumors of the bones and joints.* Washington, DC: Armed Forces Institute of Pathology;1993:1–16.

Frank JA, Ling A, Patronas NJ, et al. Detection of malignant bone tumors: MR imaging vs. scintigraphy. *AJR Am J Roentgenol* 1990;155:1043–1048.

Frouge C, Vanel D, Coffre C, Couanet D, Contesso G, Sarrazin D. The role of magnetic resonance imaging in the evaluation of Ewing sarcoma. *Skeletal Radiol* 1988;17: 387–392.

Galasko CS. The pathological basis for skeletal scintigraphy. *J Bone Joint Surg [Br]* 1975; 57B:353–359.

Gaskin CM, Helms CA. Lipomas, lipoma variants, and well-differentiated liposarcomas (atypical lipomas): results of MRI evaluations of 126 consecutive fatty masses. *AJR Am J Roentgenol* 2004;182:733–739.

Gatenby RA, Mulhern CB, Moldofsky PJ. Computed tomography guided thin needle biopsy of small lytic bone lesions. *Skeletal Radiol* 1984;11:289–291.

Gillespy T III, Manfrini M, Ruggieri P, Spanier SS, Pettersson H, Springfield DS. Staging of intraosseous extent of osteosarcoma: correlation of pre-operative CT and MR imaging with pathologic macroslides. *Radiology* 1988;167:765–767.

Gold RH, Bassett LW. Radionuclide evaluation of skeletal metastases: practical considerations. *Skeletal Radiol* 1986;15:1–9.

Golfieri R, Baddeley H, Pringle JS, et al. Primary bone tumors. MR morphologic appearance correlated with pathologic examinations. *Acta Radiol* 1991;32: 290–298.

Golfieri R, Baddeley H, Pringle JS, Leung AWL, Greco A, Souhami R. MR imaging in primary bone tumors: therapeutic implications. *Eur J Radiol* 1991;12:201–207.

Golfieri R, Baddeley H, Pringle JS, Souhami R. The role of the STIR sequence in magnetic resonance imaging examination of bone tumors. *Br J Radiol* 1990;63: 251–256.

Graif M, Pennock JM, Pringle J, et al. Magnetic resonance imaging: comparison of four pulse sequences in assessing primary bone tumors. *Skeletal Radiol* 1989;18: 439–444.

Greenfield GB, Warren DL, Clark RA. MR imaging of periosteal and cortical changes of bone. *Radiographics* 1991;11:611–623.

Greenspan A. Bone island (enostosis): current concept—a review. *Skeletal Radiol* 1995; 24:111–115.

Greenspan A. Pragmatic approach to bone tumors. *Semin Orthop* 1991;6:125–133.

Greenspan A, Klein MJ. Radiology and pathology of bone tumors. In: Lewis MM, ed. *Musculoskeletal oncology. A multidisciplinary approach.* Philadelphia: WB Saunders;1992:13–16.

Greenspan A, McGahan JP, Vogelsang P, Szabo RM. Imaging strategies in the elevation of soft-tissue hemangiomas of the extremities: correlation of the findings of plain radiography, angiography, CT, MRI, and ultrasonography in 12 histologically proven cases. *Skeletal Radiol* 1992;21:11–18.

Greenspan A, Stadalnik RC. Bone island: scintigraphic findings and their clinical application. *Can Assoc Radiol J* 1995;46:368–379.

Greenspan A, Stadalnik RC. Central versus eccentric lesions of long tubular bones. *Semin Nucl Med* 1996;26:201–206.

Greenspan A, Steiner G, Norman A, Lewis MM, Matlen J. Osteosarcoma of the soft tissues of the distal end of the thigh. *Skeletal Radiol* 1987;16:489–492.

Hanna SL, Fletcher BD, Parham DM, Bugg MR. Muscle edema in musculoskeletal tumors: MR imaging characteristics and clinical significance. *J Magn Reson Imaging* 1991;1:441–449.

Hanna SL, Langston JW, Gronemeyer SA, Fletcher BD. Subtraction technique for contrast-enhanced MR images of musculoskeletal tumors. *Magn Reson Imaging* 1990;8: 213–215.

Hayes CW, Conway WF, Sundaram M. Misleading aggressive MR imaging appearance of some benign musculoskeletal lesions. *Radiographics* 1992;12:1119–1134.

Helms C, Munk P. Pseudopermeative skeletal lesions. *Br J Radiol* 1990;63:461–467.

Helms CA. Skeletal "don't touch" lesions. In: Brant WE, Helms CA, eds. *Fundamentals of diagnostic radiology*. Baltimore: Williams & Wilkins;1994:963–975.

Hermann G, Abdelwahab IF, Miller TT, Klein MJ, Lewis MM. Tumor and tumor-like conditions of the soft tissue: magnetic resonance imaging features differentiating benign from malignant masses. *Br J Radiol* 1992;65:14–20.

Hudson TM. *Radiologic-pathologic correlation of musculoskeletal lesions*. Baltimore: Williams & Wilkins; 1987.

Huvos AG. *Bone tumors. Diagnosis, treatment and prognosis*. Philadelphia: WB Saunders; 1979.

Jaffe HL. *Tumors and tumorous conditions of the bones and joints*. Philadelphia: Lea & Febiger; 1968.

Jelinek JS, Murphey MD, Welker JA, Henshaw RM, Kransdorf MJ, Shmookler BM, Malawer MM. Diagnosis of primary bone tumors with image-guided percutaneous biopsy: experience with 110 tumors. *Radiology* 2002;223:731–737.

Johnson LC. A general theory of bone tumors. *Bull NY Acad Med* 1953;29:164–171.

Kloiber R: Scintigraphy of bone tumors. In: *Current concepts of diagnosis and treatment of bone and soft tissue tumors*. Berlin: Springer-Verlag; 1984:55–60.

Koutcher JA, Ballon D, Graham M, et al. ^{31}P NMR spectra of extremity sarcomas: diversity of metabolic profiles and changes in response to chemotherapy. *Magn Reson Med* 1990;16:19–34.

Kransdorf MJ. Malignant soft-tissue tumors in a large referral population: distribution of diagnoses by age, sex, and location. *AJR Am J Roentgenol* 1995;164:129–134.

Kransdorf MJ, Bancroft LW, Peterson JJ, Murphey MD, Foster WC, Temple HT. Imaging of fatty tumors: distinction of lipoma and well-differentiated liposarcoma. *Radiology* 2002;224:99–104.

Kransdorf M, Jelinek J, Moser RP Jr, et al. Soft-tissue masses. Diagnosis using MR imaging. *AJR Am J Roentgenol* 1989;153:541–547.

Kransdorf MJ, Murphey MD. *Imaging of soft tissue tumors*. Philadelphia: WB Saunders, 1997.

Kransdorf MJ, Murphey MD. Radiologic evaluation of soft-tissue masses: a current perspective. *AJR Am J Roentgenol* 2000;175:575–587.

Kransdorf MJ, Murphey MD, Sweet DE. Liposclerosing myxofibrous tumor: a radiologic-pathologic-distinct fibro-osseous lesion of bone with a marked predilection for the intertrochanteric region of the femur. *Radiology* 1999; 212:693–698.

Kransdorf MJ. Magnetic resonance imaging of musculoskeletal tumors. *Orthopedics* 1994;17:1003–1016.

Kricun ME. Radiographic evaluation of solitary bone lesions. *Orthop Clin North Am* 1983; 14:39–64.

Lang P, Honda G, Roberts T, et al. Musculoskeletal neoplasm: perineoplastic edema versus tumor on dynamic postcontrast MR images with spatial mapping of instantaneous enhancement rates. *Radiology* 1995;197:831–839.

Larsson SE, Lorentzon R. The incidence of malignant primary bone tumors in relation to age, sex and site. A study of osteogenic sarcoma, chondrosarcoma, and Ewing's sarcoma diagnosed in Sweden from 1958–1968. *J Bone Joint Surg [Br]* 1974;56B: 534–540.

Lee JK, Yao L, Wirth CR. MR imaging of solitary osteochondromas: report of eight cases. *AJR Am J Roentgenol* 1987;149–557.

Lewis MM. The use of an expandable and adjustable prosthesis in the treatment of childhood malignant bone tumors of the extremity. *Cancer* 1986;57:499–502.

Lewis MM, Sissons HA, Norman A, Greenspan A. Benign and malignant cartilage tumors. In: Griffin PP, ed. *Instructional course lectures*. Chicago: American Academy of Orthopaedic Surgeons; 1987:87–114.

Lichtenstein L. *Bone tumors*, 5th ed. St. Louis: Mosby; 1977.

Lodwick GS. Solitary malignant tumors of bone: the application of predictor variables in diagnosis. *Semin Roentgenol* 1966;1:293–313.

Lodwick GS. A systematic approach to the roentgen diagnosis of bone tumors. In: *M.D. Anderson Hospital and Tumor Institute—Clinical Conference on Cancer: Tumors of Bone and Soft Tissue*. Chicago: Year Book; 1965:49–68.

Lodwick GS, Wilson AJ, Farrell C, Virtama P, Dittrich F. Determining growth rates of focal lesions of bone from radiographs. *Radiology* 1980;134:577–583.

Lodwick GS, Wilson AJ, Farrell C, Virtama P, Smeltzer FM, Dittrich F. Estimating rate of growth in bone lesions. Observer performance and error. *Radiology* 1980;134: 585–590.

Ma LD, Frassica FJ, McCarthy EF, Bluenke DA, Zerhouni EA. Benign and malignant musculoskeletal masses: MR imaging differentiation with rim-to-center differential enhancement ratios. *Radiology* 1997;202:739–744.

Ma LD, Frassica FJ, Scott WW Jr, Fishman EK, Zerhouni EA. Differentiation of benign and malignant musculoskeletal tumors: potential pitfalls with MR imaging. *Radiographics* 1995;15:349–366.

Madewell JE, Ragsdale BD, Sweet DE. Radiologic and pathologic analysis of solitary bone lesions. Part I: Internal margins. *Radiol Clin North Am* 1981;19:715–748.

Magid D. Two-dimensional and three-dimensional computed tomographic imaging in musculoskeletal tumors. *Radiol Clin North Am* 1993;31:425–447.

Manaster BJ, Ensign MF. The role of imaging in musculoskeletal tumors. *Semin US CT MR* 1989;10:498–517.

Mankin HJ, Lange TA, Spanier SS. The hazards of biopsy in patients with malignant primary bone and soft-tissue tumors. *J Bone Joint Surg* 1982;64:1121–1127.

Martel W, Abell MR. Radiologic evaluation of soft tissue tumors: retrospective study. *Cancer* 1973;32:352–366.

McCook BM, Sandler MP, Powers TA, Weaver GR, Nance EP Jr. Correlative bone imaging. In: *Nuclear medicine annual*. New York: Raven Press; 1989:143–177.

McNeil BJ. Value of bone scanning in neoplastic disease. *Semin Nucl Med* 1984;14: 277–286.

Mink J. Percutaneous bone biopsy in the patient with known or suspected osseous metastases. *Radiology* 1986;161:191–194.

Mirowitz SA. Fast scanning and fat-suppression MR imaging of musculoskeletal disorders. *AJR Am J Roentgenol* 1993;161:1147–1157.

Mirowitz SA, Apicella P, Reinus WR, Hammerman AM. MR imaging of bone marrow lesions: relative conspicuousness on T1-weighted, fat-suppressed T2-weighted, and STIR images. *AJR Am J Roentgenol* 1994;162:215–221.

Mirra JM, Picci P, Gold RH. *Bone tumors: clinical, radiologic and pathologic correlations*. Philadelphia: Lea & Febiger; 1989.

Moore SG, Bisset GS, Siegel MJ, Donaldson JS. Pediatric musculoskeletal MR imaging. *Radiology* 1991;179:345–360.

Moser RP. Cartilaginous tumors of the skeleton. In: *AFIP atlas of radiologic-pathologic correlations*. Fascicle II. St. Louis: Mosby-Year Book; 1990.

Moser RP, Madewell JE. An approach to primary bone tumors. *Radiol Clin North Am* 1987;25:1049–1093.

Moulton JS, Blebea JS, Dunco DM, Braley SE, Bisset GS, Emery KH. MR imaging of soft tissue masses: diagnostic efficacy and value of distinguishing between benign and malignant lesions. *AJR AM J Roentgenol* 1995;164:1191–1199.

Mulder JD, Kroon HM, Schütte HE, Taconis WK. *Radiologic atlas of bone tumors*. Amsterdam: Elsevier; 1993:9–46.

Munk PL, Helms CA, Holt RG. Immature bone infarcts: findings on plain radiographs and MR scans. *AJR Am J Roentgenol* 1989;152:547–549.

Munk PL, Lee MJ, Janzen DL, et al. Lipoma and liposarcoma: evaluation using CT and MR imaging. *AJR Am J Roentgenol* 1997;169:589–594.

Murphy WA Jr. Imaging bone tumors in the 1990s. *Cancer* 1991;67:1169–1176.

Murray RO, Jacobson HG. *The radiology of bone diseases*, 2nd ed. New York: Churchill Livingstone; 1977.

Negendank WG, Crowley MG, Ryan JR, Keller NA, Evelhoch JL. Bone and soft-tissue lesions: diagnosis with combined H-1 MR imaging and P-31 MR spectroscopy. *Radiology* 1989;173:181–188.

Nelson MC, Stull MA, Teitelbaum GP, et al. Magnetic resonance imaging of peripheral soft tissue hemangiomas. *Skeletal Radiol* 1990;19:477–482.

Nelson SW. Some fundamentals in the radiologic differential diagnosis of solitary bone lesions. *Semin Roentgenol* 1966;1:244–267.

Norman A. The radiologic approach to bone tumors. In: *Bones and joints*. Baltimore: Williams & Wilkins; 1976:196–205.

Norman A. Tumor and tumor-like lesions of the bones of the foot. *Semin Roentgenol* 1970;5:407–418.

Norman A, Dorfman HD. Juxtacortical circumscribed myositis ossificans: evolution and radiographic features. *Radiology* 1970;96:301–306.

Norman A, Schiffman M. Simple bone cyst: factors of age dependency. *Radiology* 1977; 124:779–782.

Nuovo MA, Norman A, Chumas J, Ackerman LV. Myositis ossificans with atypical clinical, radiographic, or pathologic findings: a review of 23 cases. *Skeletal Radiol* 1992; 27:87–101.

Oliveira AM, Nascimento AG. Grading in soft tissue tumors: principles and problems. *Skeletal Radiol* 2001;30:543–559.

Olson P, Everson LI, Griffith HJ. Staging of musculoskeletal tumors. *Radiol Clin North Am* 1994;32:151–162.

Onitsuka H. Roentgenologic aspects of bone islands. *Radiology* 1977;124:607–612.

Panicek DM, Gatsonis C, Rosenthal DI, et al. CT and MR imaging in the local staging of primary malignant musculoskeletal neoplasms: report of the Radiology Diagnostic Oncology Group. *Radiology* 1997;202:237–246.

Petasnick JP, Turner DA, Charters JR, Gitelis S, Zacharias CE. Soft-tissue masses of the locomotor system: comparison of MR imaging with CT. *Radiology* 1986;160: 125–133.

Peterson JJ, Kransdorf MJ, Bancroft LW, O'Connor MI. Malignant fatty tumors: classification, clinical course, imaging appearance and treatment. *Skeletal Radiol* 2003;32: 493–503.

Pettersson H, Eliasson J, Egund N, et al. Gadolinium-DTPA enhancement of soft tissue tumors in magnetic resonance imaging—preliminary clinical experience in five patients. *Skeletal Radiol* 1988;14:319–323.

Pettersson H, Gillespie T III, Hamlin DJ, et al. Primary musculoskeletal tumors: examination with MR imaging compared with conventional modalities. *Radiology* 1987; 164:237–241.

Pettersson H, Slone RM, Spanier S, Gillespie T III, Fitzsimmons JR, Scott KN. Musculoskeletal tumors: T1 and T2 relaxation times. *Radiology* 1988;167:783–785.

Pettersson H, Spanier S, Fitzsimmons JR, Slone R, Scott KN. MR imaging relaxation measurements in musculoskeletal tumors and surrounding tissue. *Radiology* 1985; 157(P):109.

Pettersson H, Springfield DS, Enneking WF. *Radiologic management of musculoskeletal tumors*. New York: Springer-Verlag; 1987:9–13.

Pui MH, Chang SK. Comparison of inversion recovery fast spin-echo (FSE) with T2-weighted fat-saturated FSE and T1-weighted MR imaging in bone marrow lesion detection. *Skeletal Radiol* 1996;25:149–152.

Ragsdale BD, Madewell JE, Sweet DE. Radiologic and pathologic analysis of solitary bone lesions. Part II: Periosteal reactions. *Radiol Clin North Am* 1981;19:749–783.

Reinus WR, Wilson AJ. Quantitative analysis of solitary lesions of bone. *Invest Radiol* 1995;30:427–432.

Reiser M, Rupp N, Biehl T. MR in diagnosis of bone tumors. *Eur J Radiol* 1985;5:1–7.

Reuther G, Mutschler W. Detection of local recurrent disease in musculoskeletal tumors: magnetic resonance imaging versus computed tomography. *Skeletal Radiol* 1990;19:85.

Richardson ML, Kilcoyne RF, Gillespie T III, Genant HK. Magnetic resonance imaging of musculoskeletal neoplasms. *Radiol Clin North Am* 1987;24:259–267.

Rosenthal DI. Computed tomography of orthopedic neoplasms. *Orthop Clin North Am* 1985;16:461–470.

Rossleigh MA, Smith J, Yeh SD. Scintigraphic features of primary sacral tumors. *J Nucl Med* 1986;27:627–630.

Rotte KH, Schmidt-Peter P, Kriedemann E. CT-evaluation of osseous tumors. *Eur J Radiol* 1986;6:5–8.

Schajowicz F. *Tumors and tumorlike lesions of bone. Pathology, radiology, and treatment*, 2nd ed. Berlin: Springer-Verlag; 1994:1–21.

Seeger LL, Widoff BE, Bassett LW, Rosen G, Eckardt JJ. Preoperative evaluation of osteosarcoma: value of gadopentetate dimeglumine-enhanced MR imaging. *AJR Am J Roentgenol* 1991;157:347–351.

Selby S. Metaphyseal cortical defects in the tubular bones of growing children. *J Bone Joint Surg* 1961;43:395–400.

Sepponen RE, Sipponen JT, Tanttu JI. A method for chemical shift imaging: demonstration of bone marrow involvement with proton chemical shift imaging. *J Comput Assist Tomogr* 1984;8:585–587.

Shuman WP, Patten RM, Baron RL, Liddell RM, Conrad EU, Richardson ML. Comparison of STIR and spin-echo MR imaging at 1.5T in 45 suspected extremity tumors: lesion conspicuity and extent. *Radiology* 1991;179:247–252.

Sostman HD, Charles HC, Rockwell S, et al. Soft-tissue sarcomas: detection of metabolic heterogeneity with P-31 MR spectroscopy. *Radiology* 1990;176:837–843.

Spjut HJ, Dorfman HD, Fechner RE, Ackerman LV. Tumors of bone and cartilage. In: *Atlas of tumor pathology*, Fasicle 5. Washington, DC: Armed Forces Institute of Pathology; 1971.

Steinbach LS. MRI of musculoskeletal tumors. *Contemp Diagn Radiol* 1989;12:1–6.

Sundaram M, McDonald DJ. Magnetic resonance imaging in the evaluation of the solitary tumor of bone. *Radiology* 1990;2:697–702.

Sundaram M, McDonald DJ. The solitary tumor or tumor-like lesion of bone. *Top Magn Reson Imaging* 1989;1:17–29.

Sundaram M, McGuire MH. Computed tomography or magnetic resonance imaging for evaluating the solitary tumor or tumor-like lesion of bone. *Skeletal Radiol* 1988;17:393–401.

Sundaram M, McGuire MH, Herbold DR, Beshany SE, Fletcher JW. High signal intensity soft tissue masses on T_1-weighted pulsing sequences. *Skeletal Radiol* 1987;16:30–36.

Sundaram M, McGuire MH, Herbold DR, Wolverson MK, Heiberg E. Magnetic resonance imaging in planning limb-salvage surgery for primary malignant tumors of bone. *J Bone Joint Surg [Am]* 1986;68A:809–819.

Sundaram M, McLeod R. MR imaging of tumor and tumorlike lesions of bone and soft tissue. *AJR Am J Roentgenol* 1990;155:817–824.

Sweet DE, Madewell JE, Ragsdale BD. Radiologic and pathologic analysis of solitary bone lesions. Part III: Matrix patterns. *Radiol Clin North Am* 1981;19:785–814.

Szumowski J, Eisen JK, Vinitski S, Haake PW, Plewes DB. Hybrid methods of chemical shift-imaging. *Magn Reson Med* 1989;9:379–388.

Szumowski J, Plewes D. Fat suppression in the time domain in fast MR imaging. *J Magn Reson Med* 1988;8:345–354.

Tehranzadeh J, Mnaymneh W, Ghavam C, Morillo G, Murphy BJ. Comparison of CT and MR imaging in musculoskeletal neoplasms. *J Comput Assist Tomogr* 1989;13:466–472.

Unni KK, ed. *Bone tumors*. New York: Churchill Livingstone; 1988.

Vanel D, Verstraete KL, Shapeero LG. Primary tumors of the musculoskeletal system. *Radiol Clin North Am* 1997;35:213–237.

Vaupel P, Kallinowski F, Okunieff P. Blood flow, oxygen and nutrient supply, and metabolic microenvironment of human tumors: a review. *Cancer Res* 1989;49: 6449–6465.

Verstraete KL, De Deene Y, Roels H, Dierick A, Uyttendaele D, Kunnen M. Benign and malignant musculoskeletal lesions: dynamic contrast-enhanced MR imaging—parametric "first-pass" images depict tissue vascularization and perfusion. *Radiology* 1994;192:835–843.

Volberg FM Jr., Whalen JP, Krook L, Winchester P. Lamellated periosteal reactions: a radiologic and histologic investigation. *AJR Am J Roentgenol* 1977;128:85–87.

Watt I. Radiology in the diagnosis and management of bone tumours. Review article. *J Bone Joint Surg [Br]* 1985;67B:520–529.

Wetzel LH, Levine E. Soft tissue tumors of the foot: value of MR imaging for specific diagnosis. *AJR Am J Roentgenol* 1990;155:1025–1030.

Wetzel LH, Levine E, Murphey MD. A comparison of MR imaging and CT in the evaluation of musculoskeletal masses. *Radiographics* 1987;7:851–874.

Wilner D. *Radiology of bone tumors and allied disorders*, Philadelphia: Lea & Febiger; 1982.

Zimmer WD, Berquist TH, McLeod RA, et al. Bone tumors: magnetic resonance imaging versus computed tomography. *Radiology* 1985;155:709–718.

Zlatkin MB, Lenkinski RE, Shinkwin M, et al. Combined MR imaging and spectroscopy of bone and soft tissue tumors. *J Comput Assist Tomogr* 1990;14:1–10.

CHAPTER 17

BENIGN TUMORS AND TUMOR-LIKE LESIONS I

Bone-Forming Lesions

Benign Osteoblastic Lesions

Bone-forming neoplasms are characterized by the formation of osteoid or mature bone directly by the tumor cells. Only one malignant tumor, osteosarcoma, is capable of doing this. The other bone-forming tumors are benign: osteoma, osteoid osteoma, and osteoblastoma.

Osteoma

An osteoma is a slow-growing osteoblastic lesion commonly seen in the outer table of the calvarium and in the frontal and ethmoid sinuses. It is also occasionally encountered in long and short tubular bones, and at these sites is known as a parosteal osteoma. The lesion grows on the bone surface and has the radiographic appearance of a dense, ivory-like sclerotic mass attached to the cortex with sharply demarcated borders (Fig. 17.1). Osteomas have been reported in patients from ages 10 to 79 years, with most in the fourth and fifth decades. Men and women are equally affected (Fig. 17.2). Histologically, osteoma is composed primarily of bone, with a mature lamellar architecture consisting of concentric rings as in compact bone or, more commonly, parallel plates as in cancellous bone. An osteoma is an asymptomatic lesion that does not recur if excised surgically. Its importance lies in its similar radiographic presentation to the more aggressive parosteal osteosarcoma (see Fig. 16.28) and its common association with cutaneous and subcutaneous masses and intestinal polyps in the condition known as Gardner syndrome (Fig. 17.3). Intestinal adenomatous polyps, particularly in the colon, may undergo a malignant transformation to carcinoma. The syndrome is a familial, autosomal-dominant disorder, frequently seen in Mormons in Utah.

Figure 17.1 Parosteal osteoma. Dorsovolar radiograph of the hand demonstrates a parosteal osteoma of the proximal phalanx of the middle finger. A typical ivory-like mass is seen attached to the cortex.

Figure 17.2 Osteoma: skeletal sites of predilection, peak age range, and male-to-female ratio.

Figure 17.3 Gardner syndrome. (A) Frontal view of the skull of a 36-year-old man shows the typical appearance of osteomas in the left frontal and ethmoid sinuses. The dense, sclerotic masses are sharply demarcated from the surrounding structures by air. **(B)** This patient also had a parosteal osteoma of the distal left humerus, multiple polyps in the colon, and subcutaneous masses, features of Gardner syndrome.

osteoma in frontal sinus

osteoma in ethmoid sinus

Differential Diagnosis

The differential diagnosis of solitary parosteal osteoma should include parosteal osteosarcoma, sessile osteochondroma, juxtacortical myositis ossificans, periosteal osteoblastoma, ossified parosteal lipoma, and focus of melorheostosis (Fig. 17.4 and Table 17.1). Among these, parosteal osteosarcoma is the most important entity that needs to be excluded, which may be a difficult task radiographically, because both lesions appear as ivory-like masses attached to the bone's surface. The keys to recognizing osteoma, however, are its usually exquisitely smooth borders and well-circumscribed, intensely homogeneous sclerotic appearance on conventional radiographs. Parosteal osteosarcoma, in contrast, usually appears less dense and homogeneous than osteoma and may show a zone of decreased density at the periphery.

Sessile osteochondroma can usually be identified by its characteristic radiographic features: the cortex of the lesion merges without interruption with the cortex of the host bone, and the cancellous portion is continuous with the host medullary cavity of the adjacent metaphysis or diaphysis (see Fig. 18.26B).

A well-matured focus of myositis ossificans may occasionally mimic parosteal osteoma. The radiographic hallmark of myositis ossificans is the so-called zonal phenomenon, characterized by a radiolucent area in the center of the lesion that indicates immature bone formation and a dense zone of mature ossification at the periphery. Often a thin radiolucent cleft separates the ossific mass from the adjacent cortex. At times, however, a mature lesion may adhere to and fuse with the cortex, thus mimicking a parosteal osteoma. In these in-

stances, CT may demonstrate the classic zonal phenomenon of the lesion (see Figs. 4.56B and 4.57B).

Periosteal osteoblastoma and ossified parosteal lipoma rarely create a problem in terms of being mistaken for parosteal osteoma. Melorheostosis, a rare form of mixed sclerosing dysplasia, should be recognized on radiography by the characteristic appearance of segmental cortical thickening ("flowing hyperostosis"), often resembling wax dripping down one side of a candle. A typical focus of monostotic melorheostosis usually exhibits both parosteal and endosteal involvement, and the lesion commonly extends into the articular end of the bone, which are features that are almost never present in a parosteal osteoma (see Fig. 33.47).

Osteoid Osteoma

The most important clinical symptom of osteoid osteoma is pain that is more severe at night but is dramatically relieved by salicylates (aspirin) within approximately 20 to 25 minutes. This typical history holds in more than 75% of cases and serves as an important clue to the diagnosis. Osteoid osteoma occurs in the young, usually between the ages of 10 and 35, and its sites of predilection are the long bones, particularly the femur and tibia (Fig. 17.5).

Osteoid osteoma is a benign osteoblastic lesion characterized by a nidus of osteoid tissue, which may be purely radiolucent or have a sclerotic center. The nidus has limited growth potential and usually measures less than 1 cm in diameter. It is often surrounded by a zone of reactive bone formation (Fig. 17.6). Very rarely, an osteoid osteoma may have more than one nidus, in which case it is called a multicen-

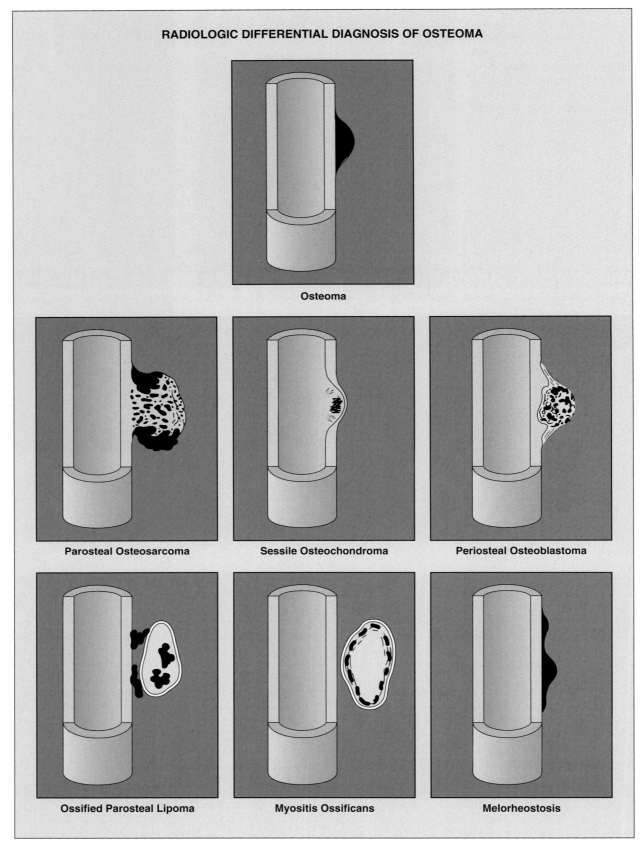

RADIOLOGIC DIFFERENTIAL DIAGNOSIS OF OSTEOMA

Osteoma

Parosteal Osteosarcoma

Sessile Osteochondroma

Periosteal Osteoblastoma

Ossified Parosteal Lipoma

Myositis Ossificans

Melorheostosis

Figure 17.4 Differential diagnosis of parosteal osteoma. Differential diagnosis of parosteal osteoma includes similarly appearing cortical and juxtacortical lesions.

Table 17.1 **Differential Diagnosis of Parosteal Osteoma**

Condition (Lesion)	Radiologic Features
Parosteal osteoma	Ivory-like, homogeneously dense sclerotic mass, with sharply demarcated borders, intimately attached to cortex; no cleft between lesion and adjacent cortex
Parosteal osteosarcoma	Ivory-like, frequently lobulated sclerotic mass, homogeneous or heterogeneous in density with more radiolucent areas at periphery; incomplete cleft between lesion and adjacent cortex occasionally present
Sessile osteochondroma	Cortex of host bone merges without interruption with cortex of lesion and respective cancellous portions of adjacent bone and osteochondroma communicate
Juxtacortical myositis ossificans	Zonal phenomenon: radiolucent area in center of lesion and dense zone of mature ossification at periphery; frequently thin radiolucent cleft separates ossific mass from adjacent cortex
Periosteal osteoblastoma	Round or ovoid heterogeneous in density mass attached to cortex
Ossified parosteal (periosteal) lipoma	Lobulated mass containing irregular ossifications and radiolucent area of fat; hyperostosis of adjacent cortex occasionally present
Melorheostosis (monostotic)	Cortical thickening resembling wax dripping down one side of a candle

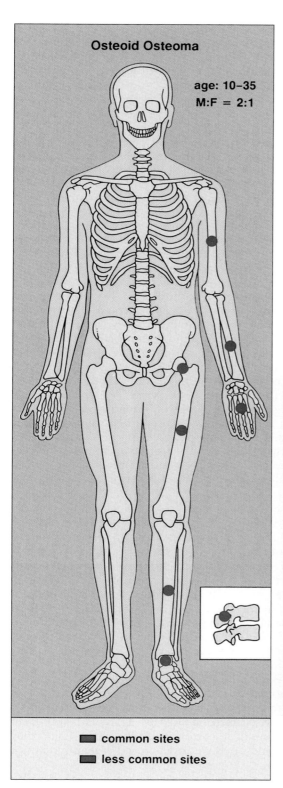

Osteoid Osteoma

age: 10–35
M:F = 2:1

■ common sites
■ less common sites

Figure 17.5 Skeletal sites of predilection, peak age range, and male-to-female ratio in osteoid osteoma.

Figure 17.6 Osteoid osteoma. (A) Anteroposterior radiograph of the right hip of a 12-year-old boy with a history of right groin pain that was more severe at night and was relieved promptly by aspirin shows the typical appearance and location of osteoid osteoma. The radiolucent nidus in the medial aspect of the femoral neck measures 1 cm in diameter and is surrounded by a zone of reactive sclerosis. Note the periarticular osteoporosis that usually accompanies this lesion. **(B)** Purely radiolucent nidus surrounded by a zone of reactive sclerosis is seen in the medial femoral cortex of an 18-year-old woman.

Figure 17.7 Multifocal osteoid osteoma. A 17-year-old boy presented with pain in the left lower leg for 3 months. It was promptly relieved by aspirin. Lateral radiograph of the lower leg shows two well-defined radiolucencies within a sclerotic area in the anterior aspect of the distal tibia. A resected specimen showed three nidi of osteoid osteoma, the two most distal of which were fairly close to one another, creating a single radiolucency on the radiograph. (From Greenspan A, et al., 1974, with permission.)

tric or multifocal osteoid osteoma (Fig. 17.7). Depending on its location in the particular part of the bone, the lesion can be classified as cortical, medullary (cancellous), or subperiosteal. Osteoid osteomas can be further subclassified as extracapsular or intracapsular (intraarticular) (Fig. 17.8).

Standard radiographs may demonstrate the lesion, but usually conventional tomography (Fig. 17.9) or computed tomography (CT) (Fig. 17.10) are required to demonstrate the nidus and localize it precisely. CT has the added advantage of allowing exact measurement of the size of the nidus (Fig. 17.11). Frequently, when the lesion cannot be demonstrated radiographically, a radionuclide bone scan is helpful, because osteoid osteoma invariably shows a marked increase in isotope uptake (Fig. 17.12). This modality can be particularly helpful in cases for which the symptoms are atypical and the initial radiographs appear normal. The use of a three-phase radionuclide bone scan has also been suggested. This technique can be especially valuable when intramedullary or intraarticular lesions are not clearly visualized by conventional radiography. Radionuclide tracer activity can be observed on both immediate and delayed images (Fig. 17.13). If the nidus is demonstrated radiographically, the diagnosis can usually be made with great assurance; only atypical presentations create diagnostic difficulty (Fig. 17.14).

The suitability of magnetic resonance imaging (MRI) for detection of osteoid osteoma remains unclear, and published reports have shown mixed results. Goldman and associates reported on four cases of intracapsular osteoid osteoma of the femoral neck, in which the le-

sions were evaluated with bone scintigraphy, CT, and MRI. Although in all cases abnormal findings were apparent in the MR images, the nidi could not be identified prospectively. On the basis of MRI findings of secondary bone marrow edema or synovitis, several incorrect diagnoses were made, which included Ewing sarcoma, osteonecrosis, stress fracture, and juvenile arthritis. In these cases, it is noteworthy that the correct diagnoses were made only after review of the radiographs and thin-section CT studies. Another report by Woods and associates involved three patients with a highly unusual association of osteoid osteoma with a reactive soft-tissue mass. In these cases, MRI studies might have led to confusion of osteoid osteoma with osteomyelitis or a malignant tumor. Moreover, in each case the nidus displayed different signal characteristics. In one case, the intensity of signal was generally low on all pulse sequences, but mild enhancement was seen after administration of gadolinium. In another case, the signal was of intermediate intensity, and administration of gadolinium revealed inhomogeneous enhancement of the nidus. For the third case in which radiographs showed the nidus to be intracortical, MRI could not identify the nidus distinctly.

However, some reports do suggest the effectiveness of MRI for demonstrating the nidus of osteoid osteoma (Figs. 17.15 and 17.16) Bell and colleagues clearly demonstrated an intracortical nidus on MRI that had not been seen on scintigraphy, angiography, or CT scans. In particular, imaging of osteoid osteoma with dynamic gadolinium-enhanced MR technique demonstrated greater conspicuity in detecting the lesion than with nonenhanced MR imaging.

Recently, Ebrahim and associates reported sonographic findings in patients with intraarticular osteoid osteoma. Ultrasound images revealed focal cortical irregularity and adjacent focal hypoechoic synovitis at the site of intraarticular lesions. The nidus was hypoechoic with posterior acoustic enhancement, and color Doppler imaging identified a vessel entering a focus of osteoid osteoma. It is noteworthy, however, that the authors concluded that the accuracy of sonography in diagnosis of intraarticular osteoid osteoma cannot be certain because other intraarticular pathologic conditions, e.g., inflammatory synovitis, may have a similar appearance. Therefore, one should seek corroborative features of this lesion using other imaging techniques, such as CT or MRI.

Histologically, the nidus is composed of osteoid or even mineralized immature bone. It is a small, well-circumscribed, and self-limited lesion. Its microtrabeculae and irregular islets of osteoid matrix and bone are surrounded by a richly vascular fibrous stroma in which osteoblastic and osteoclastic activity are often prominent. The perilesional sclerosis is composed of dense bone displaying a variety of maturation patterns.

Differential Diagnosis

It must be emphasized that even when dealing with an apparent cortical osteoid osteoma of classic radiographic appearance, the differential diagnosis should include a stress fracture, a cortical abscess, and an osteosarcoma (Fig. 17.17). In a stress fracture, the radiolucency is usually more linear than in an osteoid osteoma, and it runs perpendicular or at an angle to the cortex rather than parallel to it (Fig. 17.18). A cortical bone abscess may have a similar radiographic appearance to that of osteoid osteoma, but it can usually be differentiated by a linear, serpentine tract that extends away from the abscess cavity (Fig. 17.19). An intracortical osteosarcoma is a rare bone-forming malignancy that arises solely within the cortex of bone and grossly involves neither the medullary cavity nor the soft tissues. On radiography, it appears as a radiolucent focus within the cortex (femur or tibia), surrounded by zone of sclerosis, and varying in size from 1.0 cm to 4.2 cm in reported cases. The cortex at the site of the lesion may bulge slightly or may be thickened. Periosteal reaction may or may not be present.

In intramedullary lesions, the differential diagnosis must consider a bone abscess (Brodie abscess), and in a lesion with calcified nidus, a bone island (enostosis). The larger lesions must be also differentiated from osteoblastoma (see Fig. 17.17B). A bone abscess may have a similar

Figure 17.8 Types of osteoid osteoma. The radiographic presentation of osteoid osteoma differs according to its location in the bone. **(A)** In the cortical type, there is intense reactive sclerosis surrounding the nidus, as seen here in the medial cortex of the femur. **(B)** The medullary variant, as seen here in the distal fibula, exhibits a dense, sclerotic nidus surrounded by a halo of radiolucent osteoid tissue. Note the almost total lack of reactive sclerosis. **(C)** In subperiosteal osteoid osteoma, seen here on the surface of the talar bone, periosteal response is minimal and reactive sclerosis completely absent. **(D)** In the intracapsular osteoid osteoma, the radiolucent nidus seen here in the medial aspect of the proximal portion of the femoral neck shows only minimal reactive sclerosis.

Figure 17.9 Osteoid osteoma. A 15-year-old boy presented with a history of nocturnal pain in the shoulder relieved promptly by aspirin. **(A)** On the anteroposterior radiograph of the right shoulder, the lesion is not apparent. **(B)** Conventional tomogram clearly demonstrates the radiolucent nidus of osteoid osteoma and its surrounding zone of reactive sclerosis.

radiographic appearance, but one can usually detect a linear, serpentine tract extending from the abscess cavity toward the nearest growth plate (Fig. 17.20). A bone island is characterized on radiography by the lesion's brush borders, which blend with surrounding trabeculae in a pattern likened to "thorny radiation" or pseudopodia (Fig. 17.21). In addition, bone islands usually show no increased activity on radionuclide bone scan. To distinguish osteoid osteoma from osteoblastoma can be very difficult, if not impossible. In general, osteoblastoma is larger than osteoid osteoma (usually >2 cm in diameter) and exhibits less reactive sclerosis, but the periosteal reaction may be more prominent.

For detailed features of the differential diagnosis of osteoid osteoma, see Table 17.2.

Figure 17.10 CT of osteoid osteoma. (A) Anteroposterior radiograph of the hip of a 24-year-old man with pain in the right upper thigh shows a lesion in the lesser trochanter, but a diagnosis of osteoid osteoma cannot unequivocally be made. **(B)** CT section, however, clearly demonstrates the nidus.

Figure 17.11 CT of osteoid osteoma. (A) Anteroposterior radiograph of the left elbow of a 31-year-old man with the typical clinical symptoms of osteoid osteoma demonstrates periarticular osteoporosis. There is the suggestion of a lesion in the capitellum. **(B)** Conventional tomogram shows a radiolucent area surrounded by a zone of sclerotic reaction. **(C)** CT section unequivocally demonstrates a subarticular nidus, which measures 6.5 mm.

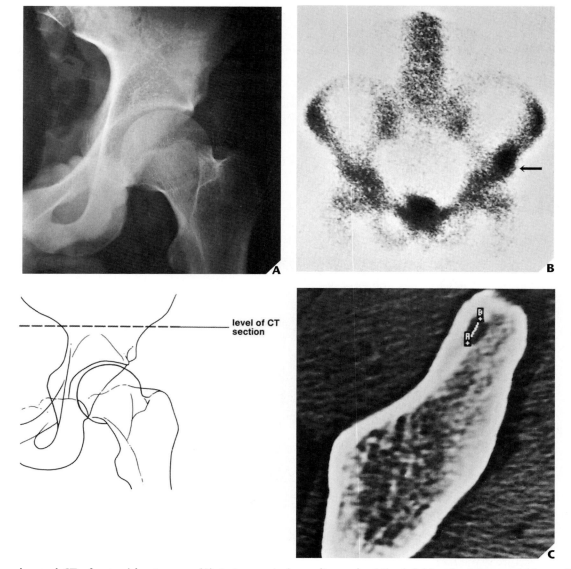

level of CT
section

Figure 17.12 Scintigraphy and CT of osteoid osteoma. (A) Anteroposterior radiograph of the left hip of a 16-year-old boy with a typical history of osteoid osteoma is equivocal, although there is the suggestion of radiolucency in the supraacetabular portion of the ilium. **(B)** Radionuclide bone scan shows an increased uptake of isotope in the supraacetabular portion of the left ilium (*arrow*). **(C)** Subsequent CT scan not only demonstrates the lesion but also allows its measurement (6.8 mm).

Figure 17.13 Scintigraphy of osteoid osteoma. **(A)** In the first phase of a three-phase radionuclide bone scan, 1 minute after intravenous injection of 15 mCi (555 MBq) technetium-99m-labeled MDP, there is increased activity in the iliac and femoral vessels. Discrete activity in the area of the medial femoral neck *(open arrows)* is related to the nidus of osteoid osteoma. **(B)** In the third phase, 2 hours after injection, there is accumulation of a bone-seeking tracer in the femoral neck lesion. (From Greenspan A, 1993, with permission.)

Figure 17.14 Osteoid osteoma. An anteroposterior radiograph of the right hip shows a radiolucent lesion in the femoral neck with a faintly outlined central density. There is no evidence of surrounding sclerosis. On the excisional biopsy, the lesion proved to be an osteoid osteoma.

Figure 17.15 MRI of osteoid osteoma. (A) Conventional radiograph shows a sclerotic area localized to the medial aspect of proximal femoral shaft. The nidus is not apparent. **(B)** Axial T1-weighted MRI clearly demonstrates the high-intensity nidus *(arrow)* within a low-intensity sclerotic cortex. (Courtesy of Lynne S. Steinbach, M.D., San Francisco, California. From Greenspan A, 1993, with permission.)

Figure 17.16 MRI of osteoid osteoma. (A) Coronal T1-weighted (SE; TR 600/TE 20 msec) MRI shows an osteoid osteoma (*curved arrow*) in the lateral aspect of the neck of the left femur. **(B)** Coronal T1-weighted (SE; TR 600/TE 20 msec) MRI shows an osteoid osteoma in the medial cortex of the left tibia (*arrow*). The *curved arrow* points to the perilesional sclerosis.

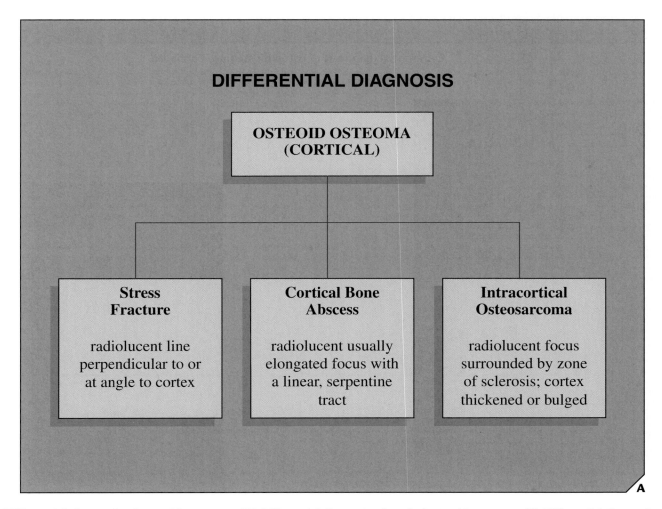

Figure 17.17 Differential diagnosis of osteoid osteoma. (A) Differential diagnosis of cortical osteoid osteoma. **(B)** Differential diagnosis of medullary osteoid osteoma. *(continued)*

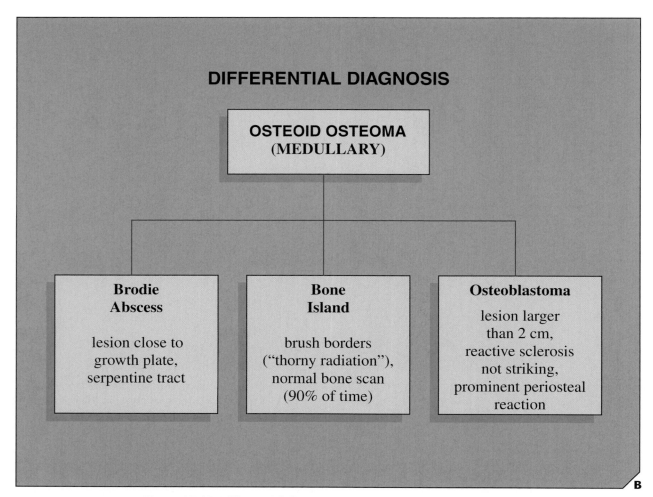

DIFFERENTIAL DIAGNOSIS

OSTEOID OSTEOMA
(MEDULLARY)

Brodie Abscess

lesion close to growth plate, serpentine tract

Bone Island

brush borders ("thorny radiation"), normal bone scan (90% of time)

Osteoblastoma

lesion larger than 2 cm, reactive sclerosis not striking, prominent periosteal reaction

B

Figure 17.17 **Differential diagnosis of osteoid osteoma.** *Continued.*

Figure 17.18 Stress fracture. Lateral magnification view demonstrates a stress fracture of the tibia. Note the perpendicular direction of the radiolucency to the long axis of the tibial cortex. In osteoid osteoma, the radiolucent nidus is oriented parallel to the cortex.

Figure 17.19 Cortical abscess. Lateral tomogram of the tibia shows a radiolucent, serpentine tract of a cortical bone abscess (*arrow*) that was originally misdiagnosed as osteoid osteoma.

Figure 17.20 Brodie abscess. In a bone abscess, seen here in the distal femoral diaphysis, a serpentine tract extends from an abscess cavity toward the growth plate. This feature distinguishes the lesion from osteoid osteoma.

Figure 17.21 Enostosis. A bone island in the medial aspect of the proximal tibia exhibits the brush borders characteristic of this lesion.

Table 17.2 **Differential Diagnosis of Osteoid Osteoma**

Condition (Lesion)	Radiologic Features
Cortical osteoid osteoma	Radiolucent nidus, round or elliptical, surrounded by radiodense reactive sclerosis; solid or laminated (but not interrupted) periosteal reaction; scintigraphy invariably shows increased uptake of radiotracer; "double-density" sign
Medullary osteoid osteoma	Radiolucent (or with central calcification) nidus, without or with only minimal perinidal sclerosis; usually no or only minimal periosteal reaction; scintigraphy—as above
Subperiosteal osteoid osteoma	Radiolucent or sclerotic nidus with or without reactive sclerosis; occasionally shaggy, crescent-like focus of periosteal reaction; scintigraphy—increased uptake of radiotracer
Intracapsular (periarticular) osteoid osteoma	Periarticular osteoporosis; premature onset of osteoarthritis; nidus may or may not be visualized; scintigraphy—as above
Osteoblastoma	Radiolucent lesion >2 cm, frequently with central opacities; perilesional sclerosis less intense than in osteoid osteoma; abundant periosteal reaction; scintigraphy—as above
Stress fracture (cortical)	Linear radiolucency runs perpendicular or at an angle to the cortex; scintigraphy—increased uptake of radiotracer
Bone abscess (Brodie)	Irregular in outline radiolucency, usually with a sclerotic rim, commonly associated with serpentine or linear tract; predilection for metaphysis and the ends of tubular bones; scintigraphy—increased uptake of radiotracer; MRI—on T1-weighted image a well-defined low-to-intermediate-signal lesion outlined by a low-intensity rim; on T2-weighted image a very bright homogeneous signal, outlined by a low-signal rim
Bone island (enostosis)	Homogeneously dense, sclerotic focus in cancellous bone with distinctive radiating streaks (thorny radiation) that blend with the trabeculae of the host bone; scintigraphy—usually no increased uptake; MRI—low-intensity signal on T1- and T2-weighted images
Intracortical osteosarcoma	Intracortical radiolucent focus surrounded by zone of sclerosis; occasionally central "fluffy" densities; cortex thickened or bulged; scintigraphy—increased uptake of radiotracer

Complications

Osteoid osteoma may be accompanied by a few complications. Accelerated bone growth may occur if the nidus is located near the growth plate, particularly in young children (Fig. 17.22). A vertebral lesion, particularly in the neural arch, may lead to painful scoliosis, with concavity of the curvature directed toward the side of the lesion (Fig. 17.23). An intracapsular lesion may result in arthritis of precocious onset (Fig. 17.24). As observed by Norman and associates, this latter complication may serve as an important diagnostic clue to an osteoid osteoma when a typical history of the condition is elicited from the patient but the nidus is not recognizable radiographically (Fig. 17.25).

Treatment

The treatment of osteoid osteoma consists of complete *en bloc* resection of the nidus. The resected specimen and the involved bone should be radiographed promptly (Fig. 17.26) so as to exclude the possibility of incomplete resection, which can lead to recurrence (Fig. 17.27).

A variety of techniques other than *en bloc* excision have been tried, among them intralesional curettage, excision with trephines after surgical exposure, fluoroscopically-guided or CT-guided percutaneous extraction, and percutaneous radiofrequency ablation. The latter technique, suggested by Rosenthal and colleagues, is a promising alternative to surgery in selected patients. It is performed through a small radiofrequency electrode that is introduced into the lesion through the biopsy track with CT guidance to produce thermal necrosis of an approximately 1 cm sphere of tissue.

Osteoblastoma

Osteoblastoma, which accounts for approximately 1% of all primary bone tumors and 3% of all benign bone tumors, is a lesion histologi-

nidus of osteoid osteoma

Figure 17.22 Complication of osteoid osteoma. A 2-year-old boy has been diagnosed with an osteoid osteoma of the distal femoral diaphysis. The proximity of the nidus to the growth plate caused accelerated growth of the bone, with marked widening of the distal end of the femur.

Figure 17.23 Complication of osteoid osteoma. Anteroposterior radiograph of the spine shows an osteoid osteoma in the left pedicle of L-1 in a 12-year-old boy. Note the shallow-curve scoliosis, with concavity directed toward the lesion.

Figure 17.24 Complication of osteoid osteoma. **(A)** Anteroposterior radiograph of the right hip demonstrates an intracapsular osteoid osteoma located in the medial aspect of the neck of the right femur in a 28-year-old man. **(B)** Tomographic cut shows the early changes of osteoarthritis. Note a collar osteophyte and slight narrowing of the weight-bearing segment of the hip joint. A radionuclide bone scan showed increased uptake not only at the site of the lesion but also at the site of the reactive bone formation resulting from the osteoarthritis.

Figure 17.25 Complication of osteoid osteoma. A 14-year-old boy presented with pain in the left hip for 8 months; it was more severe at night and was relieved by aspirin within 15 to 20 minutes. Several previous radiographic examinations, including conventional and computed tomographic scans, had failed to demonstrate the nidus. A frog-lateral view shows evidence of periarticular osteoporosis and early degenerative changes, both presumptive features of osteoid osteoma.

nidus of osteoid osteoma

Figure 17.26 Surgical treatment of osteoid osteoma. (A) Preoperative lateral radiograph of the ankle of a 13-year-old boy demonstrates the nidus of osteoid osteoma in the talar bone. Intraoperative films demonstrate the area of resection **(B)** and the resected specimen **(C)**, confirming that the lesion was totally excised.

Figure 17.27 Recurrence of osteoid osteoma. (A) Anteroposterior radiograph of the left hip in a 17-year-old boy with pain in the left groin relieved promptly by salicylates demonstrates a nidus of osteoid osteoma in the medial cortex of the femoral neck. **(B)** The lesion was incompletely resected; note its remnants (*arrow*). Two years later, the symptoms recurred. **(C)** Follow-up radiograph of the left hip shows a radiolucent area in the medial femoral cortex (*arrows*), and a CT section **(D)** demonstrates the nidus.

cally similar to osteoid osteoma but characterized by a larger size (more than 1.5 cm in diameter and usually more than 2 cm). The age range of its occurrence is also similar to that of osteoid osteoma: 75% of osteoblastomas are found in patients in their first, second, or third decade. Although the long bones are frequently involved, the lesion has a predilection for the vertebral column (Fig. 17.28). Its clinical presentation, however, is different from that of osteoid osteoma. Some patients are asymptomatic, but pain is not as readily relieved by salicylates. Their natural histories also differ. Whereas osteoid osteoma tends toward regression, osteoblastoma tends toward progression and even malignant transformation, although the possibility of the latter event remains controversial. Multifocal osteoblastomas have also been reported. Moreover, toxic osteoblastoma, a rare variant of this tumor, has recently been recognized. It is associated with systemic manifestations, including diffuse periostitis of multiple bones, fever, and weight loss.

Radiography and conventional tomography are usually sufficient to demonstrate the lesion and suggest the diagnosis (Figs. 17.29 and 17.30). On those rare occasions when the tumor penetrates the cortex and extends into the soft tissues, MRI may demonstrate these features (Fig. 17.31).

Osteoblastoma has four distinctive radiographic presentations:

1. A giant osteoid osteoma. The lesion is usually more than 2 cm in diameter and exhibits less reactive sclerosis and a possibly more prominent periosteal response than does osteoid osteoma (Fig. 17.32).
2. A blow-out expansion similar to an aneurysmal bone cyst with small radiopacities in the center. This pattern is particularly common in lesions involving the spine (Fig. 17.33).
3. An aggressive lesion simulating a malignant tumor (Fig. 17.34).
4. Periosteal lesion that lacks perifocal bone sclerosis but exhibits a thin shell of newly formed periosteal bone (Fig. 17.35).

Figure 17.28 **Skeletal sites of predilection, peak age range, and male-to-female ratio in osteoblastoma.**

similarity to osteoid osteoma, osteoblastoma represents a variant of clinical expression of the same pathologic process.

The differential radiologic diagnosis of osteoblastoma should include an osteoid osteoma, a bone abscess, an aneurysmal bone cyst, an enchondroma, and an osteosarcoma (Table 17.3). A bone abscess is usually marked by a serpentine tract (see Fig. 17.20) or it is seen to cross the growth plate (Fig. 17.36), phenomena almost never seen in osteoblastoma. An aneurysmal bone cyst occasionally can assume a similar appearance to osteoblastoma but lacks central radiopacities. An enchondroma will usually display a calcified matrix assuming the form of dots, rings, and arcs. In addition, unless there has been a pathologic fracture, an enchondroma (see Fig. 18.6), unlike osteoblastoma (Fig. 17.37), does not elicit a periosteal reaction.

Aggressive osteoblastoma should be differentiated from osteosarcoma, for which tomography may be helpful. CT may also help in the differential diagnosis of lesions located in complex anatomic regions

Figure 17.29 **Osteoblastoma. (A)** Anteroposterior radiograph of the right shoulder of a 28-year-old woman shows a faint radiolucent focus in the scapula surrounded by a sclerotic area, accompanied by shaggy periosteal reaction at the axillary border. **(B)** A conventional tomogram clearly demonstrates a radiolucent nidus with a sclerotic border, resembling an osteoid osteoma. However, the size of this lesion (3 cm × 3 cm) marks it as an osteoblastoma, a diagnosis proved by excisional biopsy.

Differential Diagnosis

Histologic differentiation between osteoid osteoma and osteoblastoma can be very difficult, and in a considerable number of patients it can be impossible. Both are osteoid-producing lesions, but in the typical osteoblastoma the bone trabeculae are broader and longer and seem less densely packed and less coherent than those in osteoid osteoma. Some authorities believe that because of its striking histologic

Figure 17.30 Osteoblastoma. Anteroposterior **(A)** and oblique **(B)** radiographs of the lumbosacral spine of an 18-year-old man show an expansive lesion in the left pedicle and lamina of L5 (*arrows*). Excisional biopsy revealed an osteoblastoma.

Figure 17.31 Scintigraphy and MRI of osteoblastoma. A 15-year-old girl presented with pain in her left shoulder. **(A)** Radiograph demonstrates a sharply demarcated sclerotic lesion in the proximal metaphysis of the left humerus abutting the growth plate. **(B)** Radionuclide bone scan obtained after injection of 15 mCi (555 MBq) of technetium-99m-labeled MDP shows an increased uptake of tracer localized to the site of the lesion. *(continued)*

Figure 17.31 Scintigraphy and MRI of osteoblastoma. *Continued.* **(C)** Axial spin-echo T1-weighted MR image (TR 700/TE 20 msec) demonstrates that the lesion is located posteriorly. The cortex is destroyed and the tumor extends into the soft tissues. **(D)** Axial spin-echo T2-weighted MR image (TR 2200/TE 60 msec) shows that the lesion remains of low signal intensity, indicating bony matrix. The rim of high-signal intensity adjacent to the posterolateral margin of the tumor reflects peritumoral edema. Biopsy confirmed the diagnosis of osteoblastoma.

Figure 17.32 Osteoblastoma. Osteoblastoma in the proximal humerus of this 8-year-old boy is similar to the lesion of osteoid osteoma. This lesion, however, is larger (2.5 cm in its largest dimension), and there is a more pronounced periosteal response in the medial and lateral humeral cortices. Conversely, the extent of reactive bone surrounding the radiolucent nidus is less than that usually seen in osteoid osteoma. This type of osteoblastoma is frequently called a giant osteoid osteoma.

Figure 17.33 Conventional tomography of osteoblastoma. Tomographic section of the cervical spine shows an expanding, blow-out lesion of osteoblastoma, with several small central opacities, in the lamina of C-6 (*arrows*).

Figure 17.34 Aggressive osteoblastoma. Posteroanterior (**A**) and lateral (**B**) radiographs of the hand demonstrate an aggressive osteoblastoma. Note the destruction of the entire fourth metacarpal with massive bone formation, particularly in the distal portion. Although very similar in appearance to osteosarcoma, the lesion still appears to be contained by a shell of periosteal new bone formation.

Figure 17.35 Periosteal osteoblastoma. (**A**) Periosteal osteoblastoma of the mandible and (**B**) periosteal osteoblastoma of the femur are covered by a thin shell of a new periosteal bone. (Courtesy of Prof. Dr. Wolfgang Remagen, Cologne, Germany.)

Table 17.3 **Differential Diagnosis of Osteoblastoma**

Condition (Lesion)	Radiologic Features
Cortical and medullary osteoid-osteoma-like osteoblastoma (giant osteoid osteoma)	Radiolucent lesion, spherical or oval, with well-defined margins; frequent perilesional sclerosis; abundant periosteal reaction; size of the nidus >2 cm
Aneurysmal bone cyst-like expansive osteoblastoma	Blow-out lesion, similar to aneurysmal bone cyst, but with central opacities
Aggressive osteoblastoma (simulating malignant neoplasm)	Ill-defined borders, destruction of the cortex; aggressive-looking periosteal reaction; occasionally soft-tissue extension
Periosteal osteoblastoma	Round or ovoid heterogeneous in density mass attached to cortex, covered by shell of periosteal new bone
Osteoid osteoma	Radiolucent nidus ≤1.5 cm, occasionally with a sclerotic center
Aneurysmal bone cyst	Blow-out, expansive lesion; in long bone buttress of periosteal reaction; thin shell of reactive bone frequently covers the lesion, but may be absent in rapidly growing lesions; soft-tissue extension may be present
Enchondroma	Radiolucent lesion with or without sclerotic border, frequently displaying central calcifications in form of dots, rings, and arcs
Osteosarcoma	Permeative or moth-eaten bone destruction; wide zone of transition; tumor-bone in form of cloud-like opacities; aggressive periosteal reaction; soft-tissue mass

Figure 17.36 Brodie abscess. (A) Anteroposterior radiograph of the right knee of a 10-year-old boy demonstrates an oval radiolucent lesion abutting and crossing the growth plate of the proximal tibia. Confirmation of extension of the lesion into the epiphysis is shown on an anteroposterior tomographic section **(B)**. The lesion proved to be a bone abscess.

Figure 17.37 Osteoblastoma. Dorsovolar **(A)** and lateral **(B)** radiographs of the small finger show enchondroma-like osteoblastoma. Note the periosteal reaction *(arrow)* and lack of chondroid matrix that is typical of enchondroma. Small radiopacities in the center of the lesion represent bone formation, a characteristic feature of osteoblastoma.

Figure 17.38 Aggressive osteoblastoma. (A) Anteroposterior radiograph of the lumbar spine shows a destructive lytic lesion affecting the right half of the vertebral body of L-3 in a 65-year-old man who presented with insidious onset of pain in the lower back radiating to the right lower extremity. **(B)** CT section demonstrates focal areas of bone formation within the lesion and invasion of the cortex. Subsequent biopsy revealed an aggressive osteoblastoma. (Courtesy of Ibrahim F. Abdelwahab, M.D., New York, NY.)

such as the vertebrae (Fig. 17.38). If there is tumor extension into the thecal sac, MRI may be needed.

Treatment

The treatment for osteoblastoma is similar to that for osteoid osteoma; en bloc resection should be performed. Larger lesions may require additional bone grafting and internal fixation.

PRACTICAL POINTS TO REMEMBER

[1] Parosteal osteoma, an asymptomatic bone-forming lesion, may be a part of the Gardner syndrome marked by sebaceous cysts, skin fibromas, desmoid tumors, and intestinal polyposis.

[2] In differential diagnosis of parosteal osteoma, the most important entity that needs to be excluded is parosteal osteosarcoma.

[3] The most characteristic clinical symptom of osteoid osteoma is pain that is most severe at night and is promptly relieved by salicylates (aspirin).

[4] In the radiographic evaluation of osteoid osteoma:
- the lesion (nidus) consists of a small radiolucent area, sometimes with a sclerotic center; the dense zone surrounding the nidus represents reactive sclerosis, not a tumor
- the radiographic characteristics depend on the location of the lesion: intracortical, intramedullary, subperiosteal, or periarticular (intracapsular)
- the differential diagnoses of osteoid osteoma should include osteoblastoma, stress fracture, bone abscess (Brodie abscess), bone island, and an intracortical osteosarcoma.

[5] The complications of osteoid osteoma include:
- recurrence of the lesion (if not completely resected)
- accelerated growth (if the lesion is close to the growth plate)
- scoliosis
- arthritis of precocious onset (if nidus is intracapsular).

[6] A well-prepared surgical approach to the treatment of osteoid osteoma requires:
- imaging localization of the lesion (by scintigraphy, radiography, conventional tomography, CT)
- verification of total excision of the lesion in vivo (by examination of the host bone) and in vitro (by examination of the resected specimen).

[7] A variety of techniques other than *en bloc* excision of osteoid osteoma are available, including intralesional curettage, excision with trephines after surgical exposure, percutaneous excision (usually CT-guided), and radiofrequency thermal ablation.

[8] CT-guided radiofrequency thermal ablation of osteoid osteoma is a promising technique and alternative to surgery in selected patients. It is performed through a small radiofrequency electrode that is introduced into the lesion percutaneously to produce thermal necrosis of an approximately 1 cm sphere of tissue.

[9] Osteoblastoma, histologically almost identical with osteoid osteoma, is nevertheless a distinct clinical entity. Its radiographic appearance is characterized by:
- features similar to a giant osteoid osteoma
- a "blow-out" type of expansive lesion with small radiopacities in the center, resembling aneurysmal bone cyst
- a lesion exhibiting aggressive features resembling a malignant tumor (osteosarcoma).

[10] The differential diagnosis of osteoblastoma includes osteoid osteoma, bone abscess, aneurysmal bone cyst, enchondroma, and osteosarcoma.

[11] Unusual presentation of osteoblastoma includes lesion associated with diffuse periostitis and systemic manifestations (so-called toxic osteoblastoma), and lesion in muticentric location (so-called multifocal osteoblastoma).

SUGGESTED READINGS

Adil A, Hoeffel C, Fikry T. Osteoid osteoma after a fracture of the distal radius. *AJR Am J Roentgenol* 1996;167:145–146.

Adler C-P. Multifocal osteoblastoma of the hand. *Skeletal Radiol* 2000;29:601–604.

Alani WO, Bartal E. Osteoid osteoma of the femoral neck stimulating an inflammatory synovitis. *Clin Orthop* 1987;223:308–312.

Anderson RB, McAlister JA Jr, Wrenn RN. Case report 585. Intracortical osteosarcoma of tibia. *Skeletal Radiol* 1989;18:627–630.

Assoun J, Railhac JJ, Bonnevialle P, et al. Osteoid osteoma: percutaneous resection with CT guidance. *Radiology* 1993;188:541–547.

Assoun J, Richardi G, Railhac JJ, et al. Osteoid osteoma: MR imaging versus CT. *Radiology* 1994;191:217–223.

Atar D, Lehman WB, Grant AD. Tips of the trade: computerized tomography—guided excision of osteoid osteoma. *Orthop Rev* 1992;21:1457–1458.

Azouz EM, Kozlowski K, Marton D, Sprague P, Zerhouni A, Assalah F. Osteoid osteoma and osteoblastoma of the spine in children. Report of 22 cases with brief literature review. *Pediatr Radiol* 1986;16:25–31.

Baron D, Soulier C, Kermabon C, Leroy JP, Le Goff P. Ostéomes ostéoides post-traumatique: á propos de deux cas et revue de la litérature. *Rev Rhum Mal Osteoartic* 1992;59:271–275.

Bauer TW, Zehr RJ, Belhobek GH, Marks KE. Juxta-articular osteoid osteoma. *Am J Surg Pathol* 1991;15:381–387.

Baum PA, Nelson MC, Lack EE, Bogumill GP. Case report 560. Parosteal osteoma of tibia. *Skeletal Radiol* 1989;18:406–409.

Bell RS, O'Conner GD, Waddell JP. Importance of magnetic resonance imaging in osteoid osteoma: a case report. *Can J Surg* 1989;32:276–278.

Bertoni F, Unni KK, Beabout JW, Sim FH. Parosteal osteoma of bones other than of the skull and face. *Cancer* 1995;75:2466–2473.

Bertoni F, Unni KK, McLeod RA, Dahlin DC. Osteosarcoma resembling osteoblastoma. *Cancer* 1985;55:416–426.

Bettelli G, Tigani D, Picci P. Recurring osteoblastoma initially presenting as a typical osteoid osteoma. Report of two cases. *Skeletal Radiol* 1991;20:1–4.

Biebuyck JC, Katz LD, McCauley T. Soft tissue edema in osteoid osteoma. *Skeletal Radiol* 1993;22:37–41.

Bullough PG. *Atlas orthopedic pathology with clinical and radiologic correlations*, 2nd ed. New York: Gower Medical Publishing; 1992.

Byers PD. Solitary benign osteoblastic lesions of bone. Osteoid osteoma and benign osteoblastoma. *Cancer* 1968;22:43–57.

Campanacci M. *Bone and soft tissue tumors*. New York: Springer-Verlag; 1990:355–373.

Campanacci M, Ruggieri P, Gasbarrini A, Ferraro A, Campanacci L. Osteoid osteoma: direct visual identification and intralesional excision of the nidus with minimal removal of bone. *J Bone Joint Surg [Br]* 1999;81B:814–820.

Campbell CJ, Papademetriou T, Bonfiglio M. Melorheostosis. A report of the clinical, roentgenographic, and pathological findings in fourteen cases. *J Bone Joint Surg [Am]* 1968;50A:1281–1304.

Carter TR. Osteoid osteoma of the hip: an alternate method of excision. *Orthop Rev* 1990;19:903–905.

Cassar-Pullicino VN, McCall IW, Wan S. Intra-articular osteoid osteoma. *Clin Radiol* 1992;45:153–160.

Cervilla V, Haghighi P, Resnick D, Sartoris DJ. Case report 596. Parosteal osteoma of the acetabulum. *Skeletal Radiol* 1990;19:135–137.

Chew FS. Benign bone-forming tumors. *Contemp Diagn Radiol* 2001;24:1–5.

Chamberlain BC, Mosher JF, Levinsohn EM, Greenberg JA. Subperiosteal osteoid osteoma of the hamate: a case report. *J Hand Surg [Am]* 1992;17A:462–465.

Chang CH, Piatt ED, Thomas KE, Watne AL. Bone abnormalities in Gardner's syndrome. *AJR Am J Roentgenol* 1968;103:645–652.

Cohen MD, Harrington TM, Ginsburg WW. Osteoid osteoma: 95 cases and a review of the literature. *Semin Arthritis Rheum* 1983;12:265–281.

Corbett JM, Wilde AH, McCormack LJ, Evarts CM. Intra-articular osteoid osteoma: a diagnostic problem. *Clin Orthop* 1974;98:225–230.

Crim JR, Mirra JM, Eckardt JJ, Seeger LL. Widespread inflammatory response to osteoblastoma: the flare phenomenon. *Radiology* 1990;177:835–836.

Dahlin DC. Osteoma. In: *Bone tumors. General aspects on 8,542 cases*, 4th ed. Springfield, IL: Charles C. Thomas; 1986:84–87, 308–321.

Dahlin DC, Johnson EW Jr. Giant osteoid osteoma. *J Bone Joint Surg [Am]* 1954;36A:559–572.

Dahlin DC, Unni KK. *Bone tumors: general aspects and data on 8,542 cases*, 4th ed. Springfield, IL: Charles C. Thomas; 1987:88–101.

Dale S, Breidahl WH, Baker D, Robbins PD, Sundaram M. Severe toxic osteoblastoma of the humerus associated with diffuse periostitis of multiple bones. *Skeletal Radiol* 2001;30:464–468.

Della Rocca C, Huvos AG. Osteoblastoma: varied histological presentations with a benign clinical course. 55 cases. *Am J Surg Pathol* 1996;20:841–850.

Denis F, Armstrong GW. Scoliogenic osteoblastoma of the posterior end of the rib: a case report. *Spine* 1984;9:74–76.

DeSouza Diaz L, Frost HM. Osteoid osteoma—osteoblastoma. *Cancer* 1974;33:1075–1081.

Dockerty MB, Ghormley RK, Jackson AE. Osteoid osteoma: clinicopathologic study of 20 cases. *Ann Surg* 1951;133:77–89.

Dolan K, Seibert J, Seibert R. Gardner's syndrome. *AJR Am J Roentgenol* 1973;119:359–364.

Dorfman HD, Weiss SW. Borderline osteoblastic tumors: problems in the differential diagnosis of aggressive osteoblastoma and low-grade osteosarcoma. *Semin Diagn Pathol* 1984;1:215–234.

Doyle T, King K. Percutaneous removal of osteoid osteomas using CT control. *Clin Radiol* 1989;40:515–517.

Ebrahim FS, Jacobson JA, Lin J, Housner JA, Hayes CW, Resnick D. Intraarticular osteoid osteoma: sonographic findings in three patients with radiographic, CT, and MR imaging correlation. *AJR Am J Roentgenol* 2001;177:1391–1395.

Edeiken J, DePalma AF, Hodes PJ. Osteoid osteoma (roentgenographic emphasis). *Clin Orthop* 1966;49:201–206.

Ehara S, Rosenthal DI, Aoki J, et al. Peritumoral edema in osteoid osteoma on magnetic resonance imaging. *Skeletal Radiol* 1999;28:265–270.

Fabris D, Trainiti G, Di Comun M, Agostini S. Scoliosis due to rib osteoblastoma: report of two cases. *J Pediatr Orthop* 1983;3:370–375.

Fanning JW, Lucas GL. Osteoblastoma of the scaphoid: a case report. *J Hand Surg [Am]* 1993;18A:663–665.

Farmlett EJ, Magid D, Fishman EK. Osteoblastoma of the tibia: CT demonstration. *J Comput Assist Tomogr* 1986;10:1068–1070.

Fechner RE, Mills SE. *Tumors of the bones and joints.* Washington, DC: Armed Forces Institute of Pathology, 1993:25–38.

Fleming RJ, Alpert M, Garcia A. Parosteal lipoma. *AJR Am J Roentgenol* 1962;87:1075–1084.

Freiberger RH, Loitman BS, Helpern M, Thompson TC. Osteoid osteoma: a report of 80 cases. *AJR Am J Roentgenol* 1959;82:194–205.

Gamba JL, Martinez S, Apple J, Harrelson JM, Nunley JA. Computed tomography of axial skeletal osteoid osteomas. *AJR Am J Roentgenol* 1984;142:769–772.

Gardner EJ, Plenk HP. Hereditary pattern for multiple osteomas in a family group. *Am J Hum Genet* 1952;4:31–36.

Gardner EJ, Richards RC. Multiple cutaneous and subcutaneous lesions occurring simultaneously with hereditary polyposis and osteomatosis. *Am J Hum Genet* 1953;5:139–147.

Gentry JF, Schechter JJ, Mirra JM. Case report 574. Periosteal osteoblastoma of rib. *Skeletal Radiol* 1989;18:551–555.

Geschickter CF, Copeland MM. Parosteal osteoma of bone: a new entity. *Ann Surg* 1951;133:790–807.

Gil S, Marco SF, Arenas J, et al. Doppler duplex color localization of osteoid osteoma. *Skeletal Radiol* 1999;28:107–110.

Gitelis S, Schajowicz F: Osteoid osteoma and osteoblastoma. *Orthop Clin North Am* 1989;20:313–325.

Glass RB, Poznanski AK, Fisher MR, Shkolnik A, Dias L. MR imaging of osteoid osteoma. *J Comput Assist Tomogr* 1986;10:1065–1067.

Goldberg VM, Jacobs B. Osteoid osteoma of the hip in children. *Clin Orthop* 1975;106:41–47.

Goldman AB, Schneider R, Pavlov H. Osteoid osteomas of the femoral neck: report of four cases evaluated with isotopic bone scanning, CT, and MR imaging. *Radiology* 1993;186:227–232.

Graham HK, Laverick MD, Cosgrove AP, Crone MD. Minimally invasive surgery for osteoid osteoma of the proximal femur. *J Bone Joint Surg [Br]* 1993;75B:115–118.

Greenspan A. Benign bone-forming lesions: osteoma, osteoid osteoma, and osteoblastoma. *Skeletal Radiol* 1993;22:485–500.

Greenspan A. Bone island (enostosis): current concept. *Skeletal Radiol* 1995;24:111–115.

Greenspan A. Sclerosing bone dysplasias—a target-site approach. *Skeletal Radiol* 1991;20:561–583.

Greenspan A, Elguezabal A, Bryk D. Multifocal osteoid osteoma. A case report and review of the lieterature. *AJR Am J Roentgenol* 1974;121:103–106.

Greenspan A, Remagen W. *Differential diagnosis of tumors and tumor-like lesions of bones and joints.* Philadelphia, PA: Lippincott-Raven; 1997;33–50.

Greenspan A, Stadalnik RC: Bone island: scintigraphic findings and their clinical application. *Can Assoc Radiol J* 1995;46:368–379.

Greenspan A, Steiner G, Knutzon R. Bone island (enostosis): clinical significance and radiologic and pathologic correlations. *Skeletal Radiol* 1991;20:85–90.

Griffith JF, Kumta SM, Chow LTC, Leung PC, Metreweli C. Intracortical osteosarcoma. *Skeletal Radiol* 1998;27:228–232.

Haibach H, Farrell C, Gaines RW. Osteoid osteoma of the spine: surgically correctable cause of painful scoliosis. *Can Med Assoc J* 1986;135:895–899.

Healey HJ. Ghelman B: Osteoid osteoma and osteoblastoma. *Clin Orthop* 1986;204:76–85.

Helms CA. Osteoid osteoma: the double density sign. *Clin Orthop* 1987;222:167–173.

Helms CA, Hattner RS, Vogler JB III: Osteoid osteoma: radionuclide diagnosis. *Radiology* 1984;151:779–784.

Herrlin K, Ekelund L, Lövdahl R, Persson B. Computed tomography in suspected osteoid osteomas of tubular bones. *Skeletal Radiol* 1982;9:92–97.

Houghton MJ, Heiner JP, DeSmet AA. Osteoma of the innominate bone with intraosseous and parosteal involvement. *Skeletal Radiol* 1995;24:445–457.

Huvos AG. *Bone tumors. Diagnosis, treatment, and prognosis,* 2nd ed. Philadelphia: WB Saunders; 1991.

Huvos AG. Osteoid osteoma. In: *Bone tumors.* Philadelphia: WB Saunders; 1979:18–32.

Iceton J, Rang M. An osteoid osteoma in an open distal femoral epiphysis. *Clin Orthop* 1986;206:162–165.

Jackson RP, Reckling FW, Mants FA. Osteoid osteoma and osteoblastoma. Similar histologic lesions with different natural histories. *Clin Orthop* 1977;128:303–313.

Jacobs P. Parosteal lipoma with hyperostosis. *Clin Radiol* 1972;23:196–198.

Jacobson HG. Dense bone—too much bone: radiological considerations and differential diagnosis. Part I. *Skeletal Radiol* 1985;13:1–20.

Jacobson HG. Dense bone—too much bone: radiological considerations and differential diagnosis. Part II. *Skeletal Radiol* 1985;13:97–113.

Jaffe HL. Benign osteoblastoma. *Bull Hosp Joint Dis* 1956;17:141–151.

Jaffe HL. Osteoid osteoma: a benign osteoblastic tumor composed of osteoid and atypical bone. *Arch Surg* 1935;31:709–728.

Jaffe HL. Osteoid osteoma of bone. *Radiology* 1945;45:319–334.

Jaffe HL, Mayer L. An osteoblastic osteoid tissue-forming tumor of a metacarpal bone. *Arch Surg* 1932;24:550–564.

Kayser F, Resnick D, Haghighi P, et al. Evidence of the subperiosteal origin of osteoid osteomas in tubular bones: analysis by CT and MR imaging. *AJR Am J Roentgenol* 1998;170:609–614.

Keim HA, Reina EG. Osteoid osteoma as a cause of scoliosis. *J Bone Joint Surg [Am]* 1975;57-A:159–163.

Kenan S, Floman Y, Robin GC, Laufer A. Aggressive osteoblastoma. A case report and review of the literature. *Clin Orthop* 1985;195:294–298.

Kendrick JL, Evarts CM. Osteoid osteoma: a critical analysis of 40 tumors. *Clin Orthop* 1967;54:51–59.

Kirchner B, Hillmann A, Lottes G, et al. Intraoperative, probe guided curettage of osteoid osteoma. *Eur J Nucl Med* 1993;20:609–613.

Klein MH, Shankman S. Osteoid osteoma: radiologic and pathologic correlation. *Skeletal Radiol* 1992;21:23–31.

Kneisl JS, Simon MA. Medical management compared with operative treatment for osteoid osteoma. *J Bone Joint Surg [Am]* 1992;74A:179–185.

Kransdorf MJ, Stull MA, Gilkey FW, Moser RP Jr. Osteoid osteoma. *Radiographics* 1991;11:671–696.

Kribbs S, Munk PL, Vellet AD, Levin MF. Diagnosis of osteoid osteoma using STIR magnetic resonance imaging. *Australas Radiol* 1993;37:292–296.

Kricun ME. *Imaging of bone tumors.* Philadelphia: WB Saunders; 1993:121–125, 114–116.

Kroon HM, Schurmans J. Osteoblastoma: clinical and radiologic findings in 98 new cases. *Radiology* 1990;175:783–790.

Kyriakos M. Intracortical osteosarcoma. *Cancer* 1980;46:2525–2533.

Lawrie TR, Aterman K, Sinclair AM. Painless osteoid osteoma: a report of two cases. *J Bone Joint Surg [Am]* 1970;52A:1357–1363.

Lee DH, Malawer MM. Staging and treatment of primary and persistent (recurrent) osteoid osteoma: evaluation of intraoperative nuclear scanning, tetracycline fluorescence, and tomography. *Clin Orthop* 1992;281:229–238.

Lichtenstein L. Benign osteoblastoma. A category of osteoid- and bone-forming tumors other than classical osteoid osteoma, which may be mistaken for giant-cell tumor or osteogenic sarcoma. *Cancer* 1956;9:1044–1052.

Lichtenstein L. *Bone tumors,* 5th ed. St. Louis: Mosby; 1977:11.

Lichtenstein L, Sawyer WR. Benign osteoblastoma: further observations and report of twenty additional cases. *J Bone Joint Surg [Am]* 1964;46A:755–765.

Lisbona R, Rosenthall L. Role of radionuclide imaging in osteoid osteoma. *AJR Am J Roentgenol* 1979;132:77–80.

Liu PT, Chivers FS, Roberts CC, Schultz CJ, Beauchamp CP. Imaging of osteoid osteoma with dynamic gadolinium-enhanced MR imaging. *Radiology* 2003;227:691–700.

Lucas DR, Unni KK, McLeod RA, O'Connor MI, Sim FH. Osteoblastoma: clinicopathologic study of 306 cases. *Hum Pathol* 1994;25:117–134.

Marcove RC, Alpert M. A pathologic study of benign osteoblastoma. *Clin Orthop* 1963;30:175–180.

Marinelli A, Giacomini S, Bianchi G, Pellacani A, Bertoni F, Mercuri M. Osteoid osteoma simulating an osteocartilaginous exostosis. *Skeletal Radiol* 2004;33:181–185.

Marsh BW, Bonfiglio M, Brady LP, Enneking WF. Benign osteoblastoma: range of manifestations. *J Bone Joint Surg [Am]* 1975;57A:1–9.

Mazoyer JF, Kohler R, Bossard D. Osteoid osteoma: CT-guided percutaneous treatment. *Radiology* 1991;181:269–271.

McDermott MB, Kyriakos M, McEnery K. Painless osteoid osteoma of the rib in an adult. *Cancer* 1996;77:1442–1449.

McGrath BE, Bush CH, Nelson TE, Scarborough MT. Evaluation of suspected osteoid osteoma. *Clin Orthop* 1996;327:247–252.

McLeod RA, Dahlin DC, Beabout JW. The spectrum of osteoblastoma. *AJR Am J Roentgenol* 1976;126:321–325.

Meltzer CC, Scott WW Jr, McCarthy EF. Case report 698. Osteoma of the clavicle. *Skeletal Radiol* 1991;20:555–557.

Mirra JM, Dodd L, Johnston W, Frost DB. Case report 700. Primary intracortical osteosarcoma of femur, sclerosing variant, grade 1 to 2 anaplasia. *Skeletal Radiol* 1991;20:613–616.

Mirra JM, Gold RH, Pignatti G, Remotti F. Case report 497. Compact osteoma of iliac bone. *Skeletal Radiol* 1988;17:437–442.

Mirra JM, Picci P, Gold RH. *Bone tumors: clinical, pathologic, and radiologic correlations.* Philadelphia: Lea & Febiger; 1989:226–248.

Mitchell ML, Ackerman LV. Metastatic and pseudomalignant osteoblastoma: a report of two unusual cases. *Skeletal Radiol* 1986;15:213–218.

Murphey MD, Andrews CL, Flemming DJ, Temple HT, Smith WS, Smirniotopoulos JG. Primary tumors of the spine: radiologic-pathologic correlation. *Radiographics* 1996;16:1131–1158.

Murphey MD, Johnson DL, Bhatia PS, Neff JR, Rosenthal HG, Walker CW. Parosteal lipoma: MR imaging characteristics. *AJR Am J Roentgenol* 1994;162:105–110.

Nakatani T, Yamamoto T, Akisue T, et al. Periosteal osteoblastoma of the distal femur. *Skeletal Radiol* 2004;33:107–111.

Nogues P, Marti-Bonmati L, Aparisi F, Saborido MC, Garci J, Dosda R. MR imaging assessment of juxtacortical edema in osteoid osteoma in 28 patients. *Eur Radiol* 1998;8:236–238.

Norman A. Persistence or recurrence of pain: a sign of surgical failure in osteoid osteoma. *Clin Orthop* 1978;130:263–266.

Norman A, Abdelwahab IF, Buyon J, Matzkin E. Osteoid osteoma of the hip stimulating an early onset of osteoarthritis. *Radiology* 1986;158:417–420.

O'Connell JX, Rosenthal DI, Mankin HJ, Rosenberg AE. Solitary osteoma of a long bone. *J Bone Joint Surg [Am]* 1993;75A:1830–1834.

Pettine KA, Klassen RA. Osteoid osteoma and osteoblastoma of the spine. *J Bone Joint Surg [Am]* 1986;68A:354–361.

Peyser AB, Makley JT, Callewart CC, Brackett B, Carter JR, Abdul-Karim FW. Osteoma of the long bones and the spine: a study of eleven patients and a review of the literature. *J Bone Joint Surg [Am]* 1996;78A:1172–1180.

Picci P, Campanacci M, Mirra JM. Osteoid osteoma. Differential clinicopathologic diagnosis. In: Mirra JM, ed. *Bone tumors. clinical, radiologic, and pathologic correlations.* Philadelphia: Lea & Febiger; 1989:411–414.

Picci P, Gherlinzoni F, Guerra A. Intracortical osteosarcoma: rare entity or early manifestation of classical osteosarcoma? *Skeletal Radiol* 1983;9:255–258.

Pinto CH, Taminiau AHM, Vanderschueren GM, Hogendoorn PCW, Bloem JL, Obermann WR. Technical considerations in CT-guided radiofrequency thermal ablation of osteoid osteoma: tricks of the trade. *AJR Am J Roentgenol* 2002;179:1633–1642.

Ramos A, Castello J, Sartoris DJ, Greenway GD, Resnick D, Haghighi P. Osseous lipoma: CT appearance. *Radiology* 1985;157:615–619.

Resnick D, Kyriakos M, Greenway G. Tumors and tumor-like lesions of bone: imaging and pathology of specific lesions. In: Resnick D, ed. *Diagnosis of bone and joint disorders,* 3rd ed. Philadelphia: WB Saunders; 1995:3629–3647.

Roger B, Bellin M-F, Wioland M, Grenier P. Osteoid osteoma: CT-guided percutaneous excision confirmed with immediate follow-up scintigraphy in 16 outpatients. *Radiology* 1996;201:239–242.

Rosenthal DI. Percutaneous radiofrequency treatment of osteoid osteomas. *Semin Musculoskelet Radiol* 1997;1:265–272.

Rosenthal DI, Alexander A, Rosenberg AE, Springfield D. Ablation of osteoid osteomas with a percutaneously placed electrode: a new procedure. *Radiology* 1992;183:29–33.

Rosenthal DI, Hornicek FJ, Wolfe MW, Jennings LC, Gebhardt MC, Mankin HJ. Percutaneous radiofrequency coagulation of osteoid osteoma compared with operative treatment. *J Bone Joint Surg [Am]* 1998;80A:815–821.

Rosenthal DI, Springfield DS, Gebhardt MC, Rosenberg AE, Mankin HJ. Osteoid osteoma: percutaneous radiofrequency ablation. *Radiology* 1995;197:451–454.

Sabanas AO, Bickel WH, Moe JH. Natural history of osteoid osteoma of the spine: review of the literature and report of three cases. *Am J Surg* 1956;91:880–889.

Sadry F, Hessler C, Garcia J. The potential aggressiveness of sinus osteomas. A report of two cases. *Skeletal Radiol* 1988;17:427–430.

Schai P, Friederich NB, Krüger A, Jundt G, Herbe E, Buess P. Discrete synchronous multifocal osteoid osteoma of the humerus. *Skeletal Radiol* 1996;25:667–670.

Schajowicz F. *Tumors and tumorlike lesions of bone: pathology, radiology and treatment,* 2nd ed. Berlin: Springer-Verlag; 1994:30–32, 48–56, 406–411.

Schajowicz F, Lemos C. Malignant osteoblastoma. *J Bone Joint Surg [Br]* 1976;58B:202–211.

Schajowicz F, Lemos C. Osteoid osteoma and osteoblastoma. Closely related entities of osteoblastic derivation. *Acta Orthop Scand* 1970;41:272–291.

Schlesinger AE, Hernandez RJ. Intracapsular osteoid osteoma of the proximal femur: findings on plain film and CT. *AJR Am J Roentgenol* 1990;154:1241–1244.

Schweitzer ME, Greenway G, Resnick D, Haghighi P, Snoots WE. Osteoma of soft parts. *Skeletal Radiol* 1992;21:177–180.

Shaikh MI, Saifuddin A, Pringle J, Natali C, Sherazi Z. Spinal osteoblastoma: CT and MR imaging with pathological correlation. *Skeletal Radiol* 1999;28:33–40.

Sherazi Z, Saifuddin A, Shaikh MI, Natali C, Pringle JAS. Unusual imaging findings in association with spinal osteoblastoma. *Clin Radiol* 1996;51:644–648.

Sim FH, Dahlin DC, Beabout JW. Osteoid-osteoma: diagnostic problems. *J Bone Joint Surg [Am]* 1975;57A:154–159.

Simm RJ. The natural history of osteoid osteoma. *Aust NZ J Surg* 1975;45:412–415.

Smith FW, Gilday DL. Scintigraphic appearances of osteoid osteoma. *Radiology* 1980;137:191–195.

Spencer MG, Mitchell DB. Growth of a frontal sinus osteoma. *J Laryngol Otol* 1987;101:726–728.

Spjut HJ, Dorfman HD, Fechner RE, Ackerman LV. Tumors of bone and cartilage. In: Firminger HI, ed. *Atlas of tumor pathology,* 2nd series, fascicle 5. Washington, DC: Armed Forces Institute of Pathology; 1971:117–119.

Steinberg GG, Coumas JM, Breen T. Preoperative localization of osteoid osteoma: a new technique that uses CT. *AJR Am J Roentgenol* 1990;155:883–885.

Steinberg I. Huge osteoma of the eleventh left rib. *JAMA* 1959;170:1921–1923.

Steiner GC. Ultrastructure of osteoblastoma. *Cancer* 1977;39:2127–2136.

Steiner GC. Ultrastructure of osteoid osteoma. *Hum Pathol* 1976;7:309–325.

Stern PJ, Lim EVA, Krieg JK. Giant metacarpal osteoma. A case report. *J Bone Joint Surg [Am]* 1985;67A:487–489.

Strach EH. Osteoid osteoma. *BMJ* 1953;1:1031.

Sundaram M, Falbo S, McDonald D, Janney C. Surface osteomas of the appendicular skeleton. *AJR Am J Roentgenol* 1996;167:1529–1533.

Swee RG, McLeod RA, Beabout JW. Osteoid osteoma. Detection, diagnosis, and localization. *Radiology* 1979;130:117–123.

Tamarito LV, Pardo J. Parosteal osteoma: a clinipathological approach. *Pathol Ann* 1977;1:373–387.

Thompson GH, Wong KM, Konsens RM, Vibhakars S. Magnetic resonance imaging of an osteoid osteoma of the proximal femur: a potentially confusing appearance. *J Pediatr Orthop* 1990;10:800–804.

Towbin R, Kaye R, Meza MP, Pollock AN, Yaw K, Moreland M. Osteoid osteoma: percutaneous excision using a CT-guided coaxial technique. *AJR Am J Roentgenol* 1995;164:945–949.

Unni KK, *Dahlin's bone tumors: general aspects and data on 11,087 cases.* 5th ed. Philadelphia: Lippincott-Raven Publishers; 1996.

Unni KK, Dahlin DC, Beabout JW, Ivins JC. Parosteal osteogenic sarcoma. *Cancer* 1976;37:2644–2675.

Vanderschueren GM, Taminiau AHM, Obermann WR, Bloem JL. Osteoid osteoma: clinical results with thermocoagulation. *Radiology* 2002;224:82–86.

Verstraete KL, Van der Woude HJ, Hogendoorn PC, De-Deene Y, Kunnen M, Bloem JL. Dynamic contrast-enhanced MR imaging of musculoskeletal tumors: basic principles and clinical applications. *J Magn Reson Imaging* 1996;6:311–321.

Voto SJ, Cook AJ, Weiner DS, Ewing JW, Arrington LE. Treatment of osteoid osteoma by computed tomography guided excision in the pediatric patient. *J Pediatr Orthop* 1990;10:510–513.

Ward WG, Eckardt JJ, Shayestehfar S, Mirra J, Grogan T, Oppenheim W. Osteoid osteoma diagnosis and management with low morbidity. *Clin Orthop* 1993;291:229–235.

Wilner D. *Radiology of bone tumors and allied disorders.* Philadelphia: WB Saunders; 1982:629–638.

Winter PF, Johnson PM, Hilal SK, Feldman F. Scintigraphic detection of osteoid osteoma. *Radiology* 1977;122:177–178.

Woods ER, Martel W, Mandell SH, Crabbe JP. Reactive soft-tissue mass associated with osteoid osteoma: correlation of MR imaging features with pathologic findings. *Radiology* 1993;186:221–225.

Worland AL, Ryder CT, Johnson AD. Recurrent osteoid osteoma. *J Bone Joint Surg [Am]* 1975;57A:277–278.

Yamamura S, Sato K, Sugiura H, Asano M, Takahasi M, Iwata H. Magnetic resonance imaging of inflammatory reaction in osteoid osteoma. *Arch Orthop Trauma Surg* 1994; 114:8–13.

Yeager BA, Schiebler ML, Wertheim SB, et al. Case report: MR imaging of osteoid osteoma of the talus. *J Comput Assist Tomogr* 1987;11:916–917.

Youssef BA, Haddad MC, Zahrani A, et al. Osteoid osteoma and osteoblastoma: MRI appearances and the significance of ring enhancement. *Eur Radiol* 1996;6: 291–296.

BENIGN TUMORS AND TUMOR-LIKE LESIONS II

Lesions of Cartilaginous Origin

Benign Chondroblastic Lesions

Diagnosis of a bone lesion as originating from cartilage is usually a simple task for the radiologist. The lesion's radiolucent matrix, scalloped margins, and annular, comma-shaped, or punctate calcifications usually suffice to establish its chondrogenic nature. However, whether a cartilage tumor is benign or malignant is sometimes extremely difficult for the radiologist to determine.

Enchondroma (Chondroma)

Enchondroma is the second most common benign tumor of bone, constituting approximately 10% of all benign bone tumors and representing the most common tumor of the short tubular bones of the hand. This benign lesion is characterized by the formation of mature hyaline cartilage. When it is located centrally in the bone, it is termed an *enchondroma* (Fig. 18.1); if it is extracortical (periosteal) in location, it is called a *chondroma* (periosteal or juxtacortical) (see Figs. 18.10

and 18.11). Although occurring throughout life, enchondromas are usually seen in patients in their second through fourth decades. There is no sex predilection. The short tubular bones of the hand (phalanges and metacarpals) are the most frequent sites of occurrence (Fig. 18.2), although the lesions may also be encountered in the long tubular bones (Fig. 18.3). According to recent investigations, enchondromas result from the continued growth of residual benign cartilaginous rests that are displaced from the growth plate. They are often asymptomatic; a pathologic fracture through the tumor (Figs. 18.4 and 18.5) often calls attention to the lesion.

Enchondroma protuberans is a rare variant. It is a lesion that arises in the intramedullary cavity of a long bone and forms a prominent exophytic mass on the cortical surface. This lesion must be distinguished from an osteochondroma or central chondrosarcoma that penetrates the cortex and forms a juxtacortical mass.

In most instances, radiography and conventional tomography suffice to demonstrate the lesion. In the short bones, the lesion is often entirely radiolucent (Fig. 18.6), whereas in the long bones it may

Figure 18.1 Enchondroma. A radiolucent lesion in the medullary portion of the proximal femur of a 22-year-old man is seen eroding the inner aspect of the lateral cortex. Note scalloped borders and matrix calcification. It proved on biopsy to be an enchondroma.

Figure 18.2 Enchondroma. (A) A radiolucent lesion in the proximal phalanx of the middle finger of a 40-year-old woman, and **(B)** a similar lesion with central calcification in the proximal phalanx of the ring finger of a 42-year-old man are typical examples of enchondroma in the short tubular bones.

Figure 18.3 Skeletal sites of predilection, peak age range, and male-to-female ratio in enchondroma.

Figure 18.4 Enchondroma. Radiograph of a 31-year-old man who had injured his left thumb reveals a pathologic fracture through an otherwise asymptomatic lesion.

Figure 18.6 Enchondroma. A typical, purely radiolucent lesion at the base of the proximal phalanx of the ring finger of a 37-year-old woman represents an enchondroma. Note the marked attenuation of the ulnar side of the cortex.

Figure 18.5 Enchondroma. Pathologic fracture through a large enchondroma is present in the proximal phalanx of the middle finger.

display visible calcifications. If the calcifications are extensive, enchondromas are called "calcifying" (Fig. 18.7). The lesions can also be recognized by shallow scalloping of the inner (endosteal) cortical margins, because the cartilage in general grows in a lobular pattern (see Fig. 18.1).

Computed tomography (CT) and magnetic resonance imaging (MRI) may further delineate the tumor and more precisely localize it in the bone. On spin-echo T1-weighted MR images, enchondromas demonstrate intermediate to low signal intensity, whereas on T2-weighted images they exhibit high signal intensity. The calcifications within the tumor will image as low-signal-intensity structures (Figs. 18.8 and 18.9). It must be stressed, however, that most of the time neither CT nor MRI is suitable for establishing the precise nature of a cartilaginous lesion, nor can CT or MRI distinguish benign from malignant lesions. Despite the use of various criteria, the application of MRI to the tissue diagnosis of cartilaginous lesions has not brought satisfactory results, although preliminary results of recent trials with fast contrast-enhanced MR imaging showed that this technique might assist in differentiation between benign and malignant cartilaginous tumors.

Skeletal scintigraphy usually reveals mild to moderate increased uptake of the tracer in uncomplicated enchondromas, whereas the presence of a pathologic fracture or malignant transformation is revealed by marked scintigraphic activity.

Intracortical chondroma is a very rare variant of conventional enchondroma. The lesion is located in cortical bone and is surrounded by sclerosis of the medullary bone and periosteal reaction. Some of these lesions may actually represent periosteal chondroma with an atypical radiographic appearance, as reported by Abdelwahab and associates. Intracortical chondroma can occasionally simulate an osteoid osteoma.

Periosteal chondroma is a slow-growing, benign cartilaginous lesion that arises on the surface of a bone in or beneath the periosteum. It oc-

Figure 18.7 Calcifying enchondroma. In this heavily calcified enchondroma of the proximal humerus of a 58-year-old woman, note the lobular appearance of the lesion and the scalloping of the endocortex.

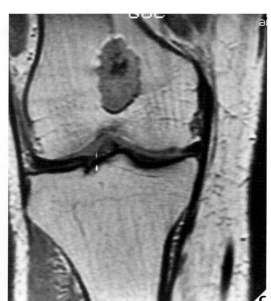

Figure 18.8 MRI of enchondroma. A 61-year-old man sustained a trauma to the left knee. Anteroposterior (**A**) and lateral (**B**) radiographs demonstrate only a few calcifications in the distal femur. The extent of the lesion cannot be determined. Coronal (**C**) and sagittal (**D**) T1-weighted MR images show a well-circumscribed, lobulated lesion displaying intermediate signal intensity. The darker area in the center represents calcifications. Coronal T2-weighted image (**E**) shows the lesion displaying a mixed-intensity signal: the brighter areas represent cartilaginous tumor and the darker areas show calcifications. The biopsy of the lesion revealed enchondroma.

Figure 18.9 MRI of enchondroma. (A) Lateral radiograph of the knee shows chondroid calcifications in the distal femur. Coronal **(B)** and sagittal **(C)** spin-echo T1-weighted MR images show the lesion being predominantly of low signal intensity. Coronal **(D)** inversion recovery T2-weighted with fat saturation and sagittal **(E)** fast-spin echo T2-weighted images demonstrate the full extent of enchondroma. Calcifications exhibit low signal intensity.

curs in children as well as adults, with no sex predilection. There is usually a history of pain and tenderness, often accompanied by swelling at the site of the lesion, which is most commonly located in the proximal humerus. As the tumor enlarges, it is seen radiographically eroding the cortex in a saucer-like fashion, producing a solid buttress of periosteal new bone (Fig. 18.10). The lesion has a sharp sclerotic inner

margin demarcating it from the buttress of periosteal new bone. Scattered calcifications are often seen within the lesion (Fig. 18.11).

CT may show to better advantage the scalloped cortex and matrix calcification (Fig. 18.12). It also may demonstrate the separation of a lesion from the medullary cavity, an important feature in differentiation from osteochondroma. MRI findings correspond to radiographic findings, depicting the cartilaginous soft-tissue component. If periosteal chondroma affects the medullary canal, MRI may be useful in depicting the extent of involvement (Fig. 18.13). Fat suppression or enhanced gradient-echo sequences may improve tumor-marrow contrast. The potential pitfall of MRI is marrow edema mimicking tumor invasion or vice versa. Unlike enchondroma and osteochondroma, periosteal chondroma may continue to grow after skeletal maturation. Some lesions may attain a large size (up to 6 cm) and may resemble osteochondromas (Figs. 18.14 and 18.15). Some lesions may mimic an aneurysmal bone cyst. Very rarely the lesion may encase itself intracortically, thus mimicking other intracortical lesions (such as intracortical angioma, intracortical fibrous dysplasia, or intracortical bone abscess).

Histologically, enchondroma consists of lobules of hyaline cartilage of varying cellularity and is recognized by the features of its intracellular matrix, which has a uniformly translucent appearance and contains relatively little collagen. The tissue is sparsely cellular, and the cells contain small and darkly staining nuclei. The tumor cells are located in rounded spaces known as lacunae. On histologic examination of periosteal chondroma, the findings are identical to those of en-

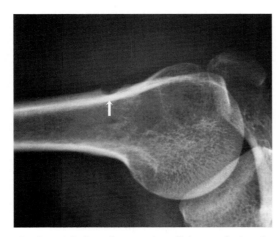

Figure 18.10 Periosteal chondroma. A radiolucent lesion (*arrow*) eroding the external surface of the cortex of the proximal humerus of a 24-year-old man proved on excision biopsy to be a periosteal chondroma.

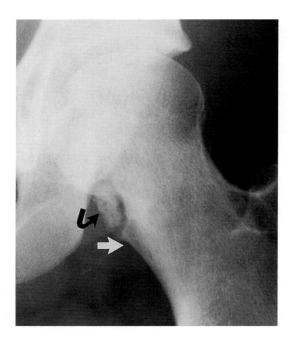

Figure 18.11 Periosteal chondroma. A periosteal chondroma at the medial aspect of the neck of the left femur eroded the cortex in a saucer-like fashion. The characteristic buttress of a periosteal reaction is seen at the inferior border of the lesion *(arrow)*. Note also cluster of calcification in the soft tissue *(curved arrow)*.

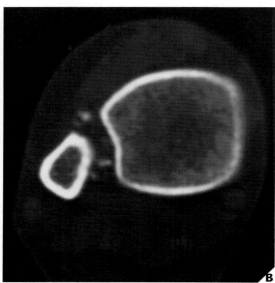

Figure 18.12 CT of periosteal chondroma. **(A)** An oblique radiograph of the right ankle shows a lesion containing calcifications eroding the medial cortex of the distal fibula. CT using a bone window **(B)** and a soft-tissue window **(C)** better demonstrates the extent of the lesion and the distribution of the calcifications. The excisional biopsy revealed a periosteal chondroma.

Figure 18.13 MRI of periosteal chondroma. (A) A large periosteal chondroma eroded the cortex of the proximal fibula and extended into the medullary cavity. Coronal **(B)** proton-density (SE; TR 2000/TE 19 msec) and sagittal **(C)** T2-weighted (SE; TR 2000/TE 70 msec) MRI show the lesion's extension into the bone marrow.

Figure 18.14 Periosteal chondroma. A large periosteal chondroma *(arrow)* mimics an osteochondroma. Note, however, the periosteal reaction and separation of the tumor from the medullary cavity by a cortex, features that helped in the differentiation from osteochondroma. (Courtesy of Dr. K.K. Unni, Rochester, Minnesota.)

Figure 18.15 Periosteal chondroma. (A) Lateral radiograph of the distal femur shows a lesion arising from the posterior cortex that resembles an osteo-chondroma. **(B)** Conventional tomography shows calcifications at the base of the lesion and continuity of the posterior cortex of the femur. **(C)** CT section demonstrates lack of communication between the medullary portion of the femur and the lesion, thus excluding the diagnosis of osteochondroma (**A** and **C** from Greenspan et al., 1993, with permission.)

chondroma, although the lesion sometimes exhibits higher cellularity, occasionally with atypical cells.

Differential Diagnosis

The main differential diagnosis of enchondroma, particularly in lesions of the long bones, is a medullary bone infarct (Fig. 18.16). At times, the two lesions may be difficult to distinguish from one another, particularly if the enchondroma is small, because both lesions present with similar calcifications. The radiographic features helpful in the differential diagnosis are the lobulation of the inner cortical margins in enchondroma, the annular, punctate, and comma-shaped calcifications in the matrix, and the lack of sclerotic rim that is usually seen in bone infarcts (Fig. 18.17).

The most difficult task for the radiologist is to distinguish a large solitary enchondroma from a slowly growing low-grade chondrosarcoma. One of the most significant findings pointing to a chondrosarcoma in the early stage of development is localized thickening of the cortex (Fig. 18.18). The size of the lesion should also be taken into consideration. Lesions longer than 4 cm are suggestive of malignancy. In more advanced tumors, destruction of the cortex and the presence of a soft-tissue mass are the hallmarks of malignancy.

Complications

The single most important complication of enchondroma, aside from pathologic fracture (see Fig. 18.4), is its malignant transformation to chondrosarcoma. With solitary enchondromas, this occurs almost exclusively in a long or flat bone and almost never in a short tubular bone. The radiographic signs of the transformation are thickening of the cortex, destruction of the cortex, and a soft-tissue mass. The development of pain in the absence of fracture at the site of the lesion is an important clinical sign.

Treatment

Curettage of the lesion with the application of bone graft is the most common course of treatment.

Enchondromatosis (Ollier Disease)

Enchondromatosis is a condition marked by multiple enchondromas, generally in the region of the metaphysis and diaphysis (Fig. 18.19). If the skeleton is extensively affected, with predominantly unilateral distribution, the term Ollier disease is applied. The clinical manifestations of multiple enchondromas, such as knobby swellings of the digits or gross disparity in the length of the forearms or legs, are frequently recognized in childhood and adolescence; the disease has a strong preference for one side of the body. The disorder has no hereditary or familial tendency. Some investigators claim that it is not a neoplastic lesion but rather a developmental bone dysplasia.

The pathogenesis of Ollier disease is unknown. There are two hypotheses for the mechanism of enchondroma formation—one attributes formation to ectopic nests of chondroblasts and the other to the failure of chondrocytes and the growth plate to mature.

Conventional radiography is usually sufficient to demonstrate the typical features of enchondromatosis. Characteristically, interference of the lesion with the growth plate causes foreshortening of the limbs. Deformity of the bones is marked by radiolucent masses of cartilage, often in the hand and foot, containing foci of calcification (Fig. 18.20). Enchondromas in this location may be intracortical and periosteal. They sometimes protrude from the shaft of the short or long tubular bone, thus resembling osteochondromas (Fig. 18.21). Linear columns of cartilage in the form of radiolucent streaks extend from the growth plate to the diaphysis, and a fan-like pattern is common in the iliac bones (Fig. 18.22).

Figure 18.16 Bone infarct. In a medullary bone infarct, seen here in the proximal humerus of a 36-year-old man with sickle-cell disease, there is no endosteal scalloping of the cortex, and the calcified area is surrounded by a thin, dense sclerotic rim, the hallmark of a bone infarct.

Figure 18.18 Low-grade chondrosarcoma. A 48-year-old woman presented with pain in the upper leg. A radiograph shows a radiolucent lesion in the proximal tibia with a wide zone of transition and central calcifications. Note the thickening of the cortex, an important feature that distinguishes chondrosarcoma from similarly appearing enchondroma. On the excisional biopsy the lesion proved to be a low-grade chondrosarcoma.

Figure 18.17 Bone infarct. (A) Conventional radiograph of the proximal tibia shows the typical coarse calcifications of medullary bone infarct. Note the sharply defined peripheral margin separating necrotic from viable bone, and the lack of characteristics for chondroid tumor annular and comma-shaped calcifications. **(B)** In another patient with a bone infarct in the distal femur, a CT section reveals central coarse calcifications and no endosteal scalloping of the cortex.

Enchondromatosis (Ollier Disease)

age: 10–30
M:F = 1:1

common sites

less common sites

Figure 18.19 Skeletal sites of predilection, peak age range, and male-to-female ratio in enchondromatosis (Ollier disease).

Figure 18.20 Ollier disease. Large, lobulated cartilaginous masses markedly deform the bones of the hand in this 20-year-old man with Ollier disease.

Figure 18.21 Enchondromatosis. In this 12-year-old boy with enchondromatosis, the intracortical lesion in the metaphysis of the fourth metacarpal protrudes from the bone, thus resembling an osteochondroma.

Figure 18.22 Ollier disease. The classic features of Ollier disease in a 17-year-old boy are exhibited in extensive involvement of multiple bones. **(A)** Anteroposterior radiograph of the pelvis demonstrates crescent-shaped and ring-like calcifications in tongues of cartilage extending from the iliac crests and proximal femora. **(B)** A radiograph of both legs shows growth stunting and deformities of the tibia and fibula. **(C)** In another patient, a 6-year-old boy with Ollier disease, note extensive involvement of the tibia and distal femur. **(A** from Norman A, Greenspan A, 1982, with permission.)

Figure 18.23 Chondrosarcoma in Ollier disease. In this case of sarcomatous transformation of enchondroma in the hand in a patient with Ollier disease, note the large, lobulated masses of cartilage in all fingers. The lesion of the middle phalanx of the ring finger shows destruction of the cortex and extension into the soft tissues.

Histologically, the lesions of enchondromatosis are essentially indistinguishable from those of solitary enchondromas, although on occasion they tend to be more cellular.

Complications

The most frequent and severe complication of Ollier disease is malignant transformation to chondrosarcoma. In contrast to solitary enchondromas, even lesions in the short tubular bones may undergo sarcomatous change (Fig. 18.23). This is particularly true in patients with Maffucci syndrome, a congenital, nonhereditary disorder manifested by enchondromatosis and soft-tissue hemangiomatosis (Fig. 18.24).

Figure 18.24 Maffucci syndrome. Radiograph of the hand of a patient with Maffucci syndrome reveals typical changes of enchondromatosis, accompanied by calcified phleboliths in soft-tissue hemangiomas. (From Bullough PG, 1992, with permission.)

The hemangiomas are mostly located in the subcutaneous soft tissues. The skeletal lesions in this syndrome show a predilection for involvement of the tubular bones and have the same distribution as those in Ollier disease, with a similarly strong predilection for one side of the body. Maffucci syndrome is recognized radiographically by multiple calcified phleboliths.

Osteochondroma

Also known as osteocartilaginous exostosis, this lesion is characterized by a cartilage-capped bony projection on the external surface of a

Figure 18.25 Skeletal sites of predilection, peak age range, and male-to-female ratio in osteochondroma (osteocartilaginous exostosis).

Figure 18.26 Osteochondroma. (A) The typical pedunculated type of osteochondroma is seen arising near the proximal growth plate of the right humerus in a 13-year-old boy. **(B)** In the typical sessile or broad-based variant, seen here arising from the medial cortex of the proximal diaphysis of the right humerus in a 14-year-old boy, the cortex of the host bone merges without interruption with the cortex of the lesion. The cartilaginous cap is not visible on the plain films, but dense calcifications in the stalk can be seen.

bone. It is the most common benign bone lesion, constituting approximately 20% to 50% of all benign bone tumors, and is usually diagnosed in patients before their third decade. Osteochondroma, which has its own growth plate, usually stops growing at skeletal maturity. The most common sites of involvement are the metaphyses of the long bones, particularly in the region around the knee and the proximal humerus (Fig. 18.25). Variants of osteochondroma include subungual exostosis, turret exostosis, traction exostosis, bizarre parosteal osteochondromatous proliferation, florid reactive periostitis, and dysplasia epiphysealis hemimelica (also called intraarticular osteochondroma).

The radiographic presentation of osteochondroma is characteristic according to whether the lesion is pedunculated, with a slender pedicle usually directed away from the neighboring growth plate (Fig. 18.26A), or sessile, with a broad base attached to the cortex (Fig. 18.26B). The most important characteristic feature of either type of lesion is uninterrupted merging of the cortex of the host bone with the cortex of the osteochondroma; additionally, the medullary portion of the lesion and the medullary cavity of the adjacent bone communicate. CT scanning can establish unequivocally the lack of cortical interruption and the continuity of cancellous portions of the lesion and the host bone (Fig. 18.27). These are important features that distinguish this le-

Figure 18.27 CT of osteochondroma. (A) Lateral radiograph of the knee shows a calcified lesion at the posterior aspect of the proximal tibia. The exact nature of this lesion cannot be ascertained. **(B)** CT clearly establishes the continuity of the cortex, which extends without interruption from the osteochondroma into the tibia. Note also that the medullary portion of the lesion and the tibia communicate.

LESIONS OF SIMILAR APPEARANCE TO OSTEOCHONDROMA

Osteochondroma

uninterrupted merging of cortex of host bone with cortex of lesion

Myositis Ossificans

lesion with dense periphery and lucent center, cleft separating lesion from cortex

Juxtacortical Osteosarcoma

lesion with lucent periphery and dense center, no cleft

Soft Tissue Osteosarcoma

lesion with smudgy densities in center, more lucent at periphery

Juxtacortical Osteoma

homogeneously dense (ivory) lesion, no cleft

Periosteal Chondroma

solid buttress of periosteal reaction, calcifications in center of lesion

Figure 18.28 Differential diagnosis of osteochondroma. Radiographic features characterizing lesions similar in appearance to osteochondroma.

sion from the occasionally similar looking bone masses of osteoma, periosteal chondroma, juxtacortical osteosarcoma, soft-tissue osteosarcoma, and juxtacortical myositis ossificans (Fig. 18.28). The other characteristic feature of osteochondroma involves calcifications in the chondro-osseous portion of the stalk of the lesion (see Fig. 18.26) and cartilaginous cap. The thickness of the cartilaginous cap ranges from 1 to 3 mm and rarely exceeds 1 cm. On MRI, the cartilaginous cap shows high signal intensity on T2-weighted and gradient-echo sequences. A

narrow band of low signal intensity surrounding the cap represents the overlying perichondrium (Fig. 18.29).

Histologically, the osteochondroma cap is composed of hyaline cartilage arranged similarly to that of a growth plate. A zone of calcification in the chondro-osseous portion of the stalk corresponds to the zone of provisional calcification in the physis. Beneath this zone, there is vascular invasion and replacement of the calcified cartilage by new bone formation, which undergoes maturation and merges with the cancellous bone of the host bone's medullary cavity.

Complications

Osteochondroma may be complicated by a number of secondary abnormalities, including pressure on nerves or blood vessels (Fig. 18.30), pressure on the adjacent bone, with occasional fracture (Fig. 18.31), fracture through the lesion itself, and inflammatory changes of the bursa exostotica ("exostosis bursata") covering the cartilaginous cap (Fig. 18.32).

The least common complication of osteochondroma, seen in solitary lesions in less than 1% of cases, is malignant transformation to chondrosarcoma. Nevertheless, it is important to recognize this complication at an early stage. The chief clinical features suggesting malignant transformation are pain (in the absence of a fracture, bursitis, or pressure on nearby nerves) and a growth spurt or continued growth of the lesion beyond the age of skeletal maturity. Certain radiologic features have also been identified that may help in the determination of malignancy (Table 18.1).

The most reliable imaging modalities for evaluating the possible malignant transformation of an osteochondroma are conventional radiography, conventional tomography, CT, and MRI; the results of a radionuclide bone scan, which may show increased uptake of radiopharmaceutical at the site of the lesion, may not be reliable. The radiography usually demonstrates whether the calcifications in an osteochondroma are contained within the stalk of the lesion—a clear indication of benignity (see Fig. 18.26)—but conventional tomography can occasionally also be helpful in this respect (Fig. 18.33). Similarly, CT can demonstrate both dispersed calcifications in the cartilaginous cap and increased thickness of the cap, cardinal signs of malignant transformation of the lesion, as Norman and Sissons have pointed out (Fig. 18.34).

The unreliability of radionuclide imaging is related to the fact that even benign exostoses exhibit increased uptake of radiopharmaceutical caused by endochondral ossification. Exostotic chondrosarcoma is also marked by isotope uptake, which is related to active ossification, osteoblastic activity, and hyperemia within the cartilage and bony stalk of the tumor. Thus, although the uptake is more intense in exostotic chondrosarcomas than in benign exostoses, various investigations show that this is not always a reliable feature distinguishing these lesions.

Treatment

Solitary lesions of osteochondroma usually can simply be monitored if they do not cause clinical problems. Surgical resection is indicated if the lesion becomes painful, if there is suspected encroachment on adjacent nerves or blood vessels, if pathologic fracture occurs, or if there is concern about the diagnosis.

Multiple Osteocartilaginous Exostoses

This condition, also known as multiple hereditary osteochondromata, familial osteochondromatosis, or diaphyseal aclasis, is classified by some authorities in the category of bone dysplasias. It is a hereditary, autosomal-dominant disorder with incomplete penetrance in females. Approximately two thirds of affected individuals have a positive family history. The specific genetic defect has been recently identified, with three distinct loci on chromosomes 8, 11, and 19. There is a decided 2:1 male predilection. The knees, ankles, and shoulders are the sites most frequently affected by the development of multiple osteochondromas (Fig. 18.35). The radiographic features are similar to those of single osteochondromas (see Fig. 18.26), but the lesions are more frequently of the sessile type (Figs. 18.36, 18.37, and 18.38). The

Figure 18.29 MRI of osteochondroma. (A) Radiograph of the right proximal humerus shows a sessile osteochondroma at the medial aspect of metadiaphysis. **(B)** T1-weighted coronal MRI reveals that the lesion exhibits low signal intensity because of extensive mineralization. **(C)** T2-weighted image shows the thin cartilaginous cap as a band of high signal intensity *(arrows)*, covered by a linear area of low signal representing perichondrium *(open arrow)*.

Figure 18.30 Complication of osteochondroma. A 14-year-old boy with a known osteochondroma of the right humerus complained of pain and numbness of the hand and fingers. **(A)** Radiograph of the right shoulder demonstrates a sessile-type osteochondroma arising from the medial aspect of the proximal diaphysis of the humerus. **(B)** Arteriography reveals compression and displacement of the brachial artery.

Figure 18.31 Complication of osteochondroma. A 9-year-old boy had a sessile osteochondroma of the distal tibia. The lesion produced pressure erosion, and later bowing and attenuation of the fibula, with subsequent fracture of the bone. (From Norman A, Greenspan A, 1982, with permission.)

Figure 18.32 Bursa exostotica. (A) A 25-year-old man with a known solitary osteochondroma of the distal right femur reported gradually increasing pain. The capillary phase of an arteriogram reveals a huge bursa exostotica. Inflammation of the bursa, with the accumulation of a large amount of fluid (bursitis), was the cause of the patient's symptoms. **(B)** Another patient, a 12-year-old girl, presented with pain in the popliteal fossa. Coronal T1-weighted MR image (SE; TR 650/TE 25 msec) demonstrates a large osteochondroma arising from the posterolateral aspect of distal femur. **(C)** Axial T2-weighted image (SE; TR 2200/TE 70 msec) demonstrates a bursa exostotica distended with fluid.

Table 18.1 Clinical and Radiologic Features Suggesting Malignant Transformation of Osteochondroma

Clinical Features	Radiologic Findings	Imaging Modality
Pain (in the absence of fracture, bursitis, or pressure on nearby nerves)	Enlargement of the lesion	Conventional radiography (comparison with earlier radiographs)
Growth spurt (after skeletal maturity)	Development of a bulky cartilaginous cap usually 2–3 cm thick	CT, MRI
	Dispersed calcifications in the cartilaginous cap	Conventional tomography
	Development of a soft-tissue mass with or without calcifications	Radiography, CT, MRI
	Increased uptake of isotope after closure of growth plate (not always reliable)	Scintigraphy

Figure 18.33 Complication of osteochondroma. (A) Lateral radiograph of the left ankle of a 26-year-old woman with a painful osteochondroma shows a sessile lesion arising from the posterior aspect of the distal tibia. In the interpretation of this radiograph, uncertainties were raised that some of the calcifications might not be contained within the stalk, and tomographic examination was suggested. **(B)** Tomographic section demonstrates lack of separation of calcifications from the main mass, suggesting a benign lesion. The osteochondroma was resected, and a histopathologic examination confirmed the lack of malignant transformation. The symptoms were apparently caused by pressure on a nerve.

Figure 18.34 Transformation of osteochondroma to chondrosarcoma. A 28-year-old man had pain in the popliteal region and also noticed an increase in a mass he had been aware of for 15 years—important clinical information that warranted further investigation to rule out the malignant transformation of an osteochondroma. **(A)** Lateral radiograph of the knee demonstrates a sessile-type osteochondroma arising from the posterior cortex of the distal femur. Note that calcifications are present not only in the stalk of the lesion but also are dispersed in the cartilaginous cap. **(B)** An arteriogram demonstrates displacement of the small vessels, which are draped over the invisible cartilaginous cap. **(C)** CT section confirms the increased thickness of the cartilaginous cap (2.5 cm) and dispersed calcifications within the cap. These radiologic features are consistent with a diagnosis of malignant transformation to chondrosarcoma, which was confirmed by histopathologic examination. *(continued)*

Figure 18.34 **Transformation of osteochondroma to chondrosarcoma.** *Continued.*

Figure 18.35 **Skeletal sites of predilection, peak age range, and male-to-female ratio in multiple osteocartilaginous exostoses (multiple osteochondromata, diaphyseal aclasis).**

Figure 18.36 Hereditary multiple exostoses. (A) Anteroposterior radiograph of the shoulder of a 22-year-old man with familial multiple osteochondromatosis demonstrates multiple sessile lesions involving the proximal humerus, scapula, and ribs. **(B)** Involvement of the distal femur and proximal tibia is characteristic of this disorder.

Figure 18.37 Hereditary multiple exostoses. An anteroposterior radiograph of both knees of a 17-year-old boy shows numerous sessile and pedunculated osteochondromas.

Figure 18.38 MRI of hereditary multiple exostoses. (A) Anteroposterior radiograph of the hips shows multiple sessile osteochondromas mainly affecting proximal femora. Some lesions are also present at the pubic bones. Coronal **(B)** and axial **(C)** T1-weighted (SE; TR 600/TE 20 msec) MR images demonstrate continuity of the lesions with the medullary portion of the femora. Note also dysplastic changes expressed by abnormal tubulation of the bones. *(continued)*

Figure 18.38 **MRI of hereditary multiple exostoses** *Continued.*

Figure 18.39 **Hereditary multiple exostoses— growth disturbance.** Posteroanterior radiograph of the forearm of an 8-year-old boy with multiple osteochondromas shows a growth disturbance in the distal radius and ulna, which is frequently seen as a complication in this disorder.

Figure 18.40 Malignant transformation. (A) Oblique radiograph of the right hand of a 22-year-old man shows multiple osteochondromas. A large soft-tissue mass situated between the index finger and thumb and containing chondroid calcifications indicates malignant transformation to chondrosarcoma. **(B)** Sagittal T1-weighted (SE; TR 600/TE 16 msec) MRI reveals volar extension of a large soft-tissue tumor. **(C)** Coronal inversion recovery (FMPIR/90; TR 4000/TE 64 msec/Ef) MR image shows malignant lobules of the cartilage invading the bones and soft tissues of the hand.

histopathologic features of multiple osteochondromas are the same as those of solitary lesions.

Complications

There is a greater incidence of growth disturbance in multiple osteo-cartilaginous exostoses than in solitary osteochondroma. Growth abnormalities are primarily seen in the forearms (Fig. 18.39) and legs. Malignant transformation to chondrosarcoma is also more common, seen in 5% to 15% of cases, with lesions at the shoulder girdle and around the pelvis at greater risk of undergoing transformation. The clinical and radiographic signs of this complication are identical to those in malignant transformation of a solitary osteochondroma (Fig. 18.40, see also Fig. 18.34 and Table 18.1).

Treatment

Multiple osteochondromas are treated individually. Like solitary lesions, they are likely to recur in younger children, and surgery may be deferred to a later date.

Chondroblastoma

Also known as a Codman tumor, chondroblastoma, representing fewer than 1% of all primary bone tumors, is a benign lesion occurring before skeletal maturity, characteristically presenting in the epiphyses of long bones such as the humerus, tibia, and femur (Fig. 18.41). Although secondary involvement of the metaphysis after skeletal maturity is recognized, a predominantly metaphyseal or diaphyseal location is exceedingly rare. Equally unusual is involvement of the vertebra or intracortical location in the long bones. Occasionally the patella, which is considered equivalent to an epiphysis, is affected. Ten percent of chondroblastomas involve the small bones of the hands and feet, with the talus and calcaneus representing the most common sites. Although the lesion is usually seen in growing bones, some cases have been reported after obliteration of the growth plate. Chondroblastoma is usually located eccentrically, shows a sclerotic border, and often demonstrates scattered calcifications of the matrix (25% of cases) (Fig. 18.42). Brower and col-

leagues noticed a distinctively thick, solid periosteal reaction distal to the lesion in 57% of chondroblastomas in long bones (Fig. 18.43). This most likely represents an inflammatory reaction to the tumor. In most cases, radiography and conventional tomography suffice to demonstrate the lesion (Fig. 18.44), but CT scan can help demonstrate the calcifications if they are not visible on the standard radiographs (Fig. 18.45). MRI usually reveals a larger area of involvement than can be seen on radiography, including regional bone marrow and soft-tissue edema (Fig. 18.46).

Histologically, chondroblastoma is composed of nodules of fairly mature cartilage matrix surrounded by a highly cellular tissue containing uniformly large round cells with ovoid nuclei and clear cytoplasm. Multinucleated osteoclast-like giant cells are a frequent finding. The matrix shows characteristic fine calcifications surrounding apposing chondroblasts, having a spatial arrangement resembling the hexagonal configuration of chicken wire.

Treatment and Complications

Chondroblastomas are usually treated by curettage and bone grafting. Only few reported cases have been treated with percutaneous radiofrequency ablation.

In rare cases, pulmonary metastases develop in the absence of any histologic evidence of malignancy in either the primary bone tumor or the pulmonary lesions.

Chondromyxoid Fibroma

Chondromyxoid fibroma is a rare tumor of cartilaginous derivation, characterized by the production of chondroid, fibrous, and myxoid tissues in variable proportions, and accounts for 0.5% of all primary bone tumors and 2% of all benign bone tumors. It occurs predominantly in adolescents and young adults (males more than females), most commonly in the patient's second or third decade. It has a predilection for the bones of the lower extremities, with preferred sites in the proximal tibia (32%) and distal femur (17%) (Fig. 18.47). Exceedingly rare, the lesion may be located in the vertebra. Few cases of chondromyxoid fibroma have been reported in juxtacortical

Figure 18.41 **Skeletal sites of predilection, peak age incidence, and male-to-female ratio in chondroblastoma.**

Figure 18.42 **Chondroblastoma.** A lesion located in the proximal tibia *(arrows)* of a 17-year-old boy exhibits faint sclerotic border and central calcifications.

Figure 18.43 **Chondroblastoma.** A lesion in the proximal humerus *(arrows)* elicited periosteal reaction along the lateral cortex *(open arrow).*

Figure 18.44 Chondroblastoma. Lateral (A) radiograph and anteroposterior (B) tomogram of the knee show the typical appearance of a chondroblastoma in the proximal epiphysis of the tibia. Note the radiolucent, eccentrically located lesion with a thin, sclerotic margin. There are small, scattered calcifications in the center of the lesion, which are better seen on the tomogram.

Figure 18.45 CT of chondroblastoma. (A) Anteroposterior radiograph of the right shoulder of a 16-year-old boy shows a lesion in the proximal humeral epiphysis, but calcifications are not well demonstrated. Note the well-organized layer of periosteal reaction at the lateral cortex. **(B)** CT section shows the calcifications clearly. The tumor was removed by curettage, and a histopathologic examination confirmed the radiographic diagnosis of chondroblastoma.

Figure 18.46 MRI of chondroblastoma. (A) Axial T2-weighted (SE; TR 2000/TE 80 msec) MRI of the shoulder in an 18-year-old man with chondroblastoma of the left humeral head shows sharply marginated lesion with sclerotic border and central calcifications. Note the small amount of joint effusion and peritumoral edema. In another patient, sagittal proton-density (SE; TR 2000/TE 28 msec) **(B)** and axial T2-weighted (SE; TR 2000/TE 80 msec) **(C)** MR images of the knee show extension of chondroblastoma located in the posterior aspect of proximal tibia into the soft tissues.

Figure 18.47 Skeletal sites of predilection, peak age range, and male-to-female ratio in chondromyxoid fibroma.

Figure 18.48 Chondromyxoid fibroma. Anteroposterior **(A)** and lateral **(B)** radiograph of the left leg of an 8-year-old girl with a chondromyxoid fibroma demonstrate a radiolucent lesion extending from the metaphysis into the diaphysis of the tibia, with a geographic type of bone destruction and a sclerotic scalloped border.

Figure 18.49 Chondromyxoid fibroma. Anteroposterior **(A)** and lateral **(B)** radiographs of the left knee of a 12-year-old girl show a radiolucent, slightly lobulated lesion with a thin sclerotic margin in the proximal tibial diaphysis. Note the lack of visible calcifications. Excisional biopsy revealed chondromyxoid fibroma.

location. Its clinical symptoms include local swelling and pain, which are occasionally caused by pressure on adjacent neurovascular structures by a peripherally located mass.

Its characteristic radiographic picture is that of an eccentrically located radiolucent lesion in the bone, with a sclerotic scalloped margin often eroding or ballooning out the cortex (Figs. 18.48 and 18.49). The lesion may range from 1 to 10 cm in size, with an average of 3 to 4 cm. Calcifications are not apparent radiographically, but focal microscopic calcifications have been reported in as many as 27% of cases. Frequently, a buttress of periosteal new bone can be ob-

served. MRI reveals characteristics of most cartilaginous tumors: intermediate to low signal intensity on T1-weighted and high signal on T2-weighted sequences (Fig. 18.50).

Pathologically, the most important feature of the lesion is its lobular or pseudolobular arrangement into zones of varying cellularity. The center of the lobule is hypocellular. Within the matrix, loosely arranged spindle-shaped and stellate cells with elongated processes are present. The periphery of the lobule is densely cellular, containing a mixture of mononuclear spindle-shaped and polyhedral stromal cells with a variable number of multinucleated giant cells.

Figure 18.50 MRI of chondromyxoid fibroma. (A) Sagittal T1-weighted (SE; TR 600/TE 19 msec) MRI in a 10-year-old girl shows a well-demarcated lesion in the plantar aspect of the calcaneus, displaying low signal intensity. **(B)** An axial T1-weighted (SE; TR 600/TE 17 msec) image shows significant amount of peritumoral edema. **(C)** Sagittal T2-weighted (SE; TR 2000/TE 80 msec) MRI shows the lesion displaying high signal intensity. A sclerotic border is imaged as a rim of low signal intensity. Excisional biopsy revealed chondromyxoid fibroma.

Figure 18.51 Chondromyxoid fibroma resembling an aneurysmal bone cyst. (A) Anteroposterior radiograph of the knee of an 18-year-old woman shows a chondromyxoid fibroma in the lateral aspect of the proximal tibia. The lesion balloons out from the cortex and is supported by a solid periosteal buttress resembling that seen in an aneurysmal bone cyst. The periosteal buttress is better appreciated on a tomographic cut **(B)**.

Differential Diagnosis

Commonly, one can observe a characteristic buttress of periosteal new bone formation (Fig. 18.51), in which case a chondromyxoid fibroma may be radiographically indistinguishable from an aneurysmal bone cyst. In unusual locations such as in short tubular or flat bones, it may mimic a giant cell tumor or desmoplastic fibroma.

Treatment

The treatment of this lesion usually consists of curettage and a bone graft. Recurrences are frequent, with the reported rate between 20% and 80% (see Fig. 16.51).

PRACTICAL POINTS TO REMEMBER

[1] Enchondroma is characterized by the formation of mature hyaline cartilage and is seen:
  • most commonly in the short tubular bones of the hand, where the lesion is usually radiolucent
  • in the long bones, where scattered calcifications may be seen, resembling a medullary bone infarct.
[2] The characteristic radiographic features of enchondroma include:
  • popcorn-like, annular, or punctate calcifications
  • a lobulated growth pattern with frequent shallow scalloping of the endosteal cortex.
[3] Important clinical and radiographic features of the malignant transformation of an enchondroma include:
  • the development of pain, in the absence of a fracture, in a previously asymptomatic lesion
  • thickening or destruction of the cortex
  • development of a soft-tissue mass.
[4] Enchondromatosis is a condition marked by multiple enchondromas, commonly in metaphysis and diaphysis. If skeleton is extensively affected and the lesions are distributed unilaterally, the term Ollier disease is applied.
[5] Ollier disease and Maffucci syndrome (an association of Ollier disease with soft-tissue hemangiomatosis) both carry an increased risk for malignant transformation to chondrosarcoma.
[6] In the radiographic evaluation of osteochondroma, the most common benign bone lesion, note that:

  • it can be seen as predunculated or sessile (broad-based) variants
  • its two important radiographic features are uninterrupted merging of the lesion's cortex with the host bone cortex and continuity of the cancellous portion of the lesion with the medullary cavity of the host bone.
[7] The most important differential diagnoses in suspected osteochondroma include:
  • juxtacortical osteoma
  • juxtacortical osteosarcoma
  • soft-tissue osteosarcoma
  • juxtacortical myositis ossificans.
[8] Osteochondroma may be complicated by:
  • pressure on adjacent nerves or blood vessels
  • pressure on the adjacent bone, frequently leading to fracture
  • bursitis exostotica
  • malignant transformation to chondrosarcoma.
[9] In the malignant transformation of osteochondroma, radiologic signs include:
  • enlargement of the lesion
  • marked thickening of the cartilaginous cap of the lesion
  • dispersion of calcifications into the cartilaginous cap
  • development of a soft-tissue mass
  • increased isotope uptake by the lesion after skeletal maturity.
[10] Variants of osteochondroma include subungual exostosis, turret exostosis, traction exostosis, bizarre parosteal osteochondromatous proliferation, florid reactive periostitis, and dysplasia epiphysealis hemimelica (Trevor-Fairbank disease).
[11] Multiple osteocartilaginous exostoses, a familial hereditary condition, carries the increased risk of malignant transformation of an osteochondroma to a chondrosarcoma, particularly in the shoulder girdle and pelvis.
[12] Chondroblastoma is characterized radiographically by:
  • its eccentric epiphyseal location
  • sclerotic margin
  • scattered calcifications
  • periosteal reaction (>50% cases).
[13] Chondromyxoid fibroma is characterized radiographically by:
  • its location close to the growth plate
  • its scalloped, sclerotic border
  • a buttress of periosteal new bone
  • lack of visible calcifications.
    It may mimic an aneurysmal bone cyst.

SUGGESTED READINGS

Abdelwahab IF, Hermann G, Lewis MM, Klein MJ. Case report 588. Intracortical chondroma of the left femur. *Skeletal Radiol* 1990;19:59–61.

Adams MJ, Spencer GM, Totterman S. Case report 776. Chondromyxoid fibroma of femur. *Skeletal Radiol* 1993;22:358–361.

Aoki JA, Sone S, Fujioka F, et al. MR of enchondroma and chondrosarcoma: rings and arcs of Gd-DTPA enhancement. *J Comput Assist Tomogr* 1991;15:1011–1016.

Azouz EM, Greenspan A, Marton D. CT evaluation of primary epiphyseal bone abscesses. *Skeletal Radiol* 1993;22:17–23.

Bandiera S, Bacchini P, Bertoni F. Bizarre parosteal osteochondromatous proliferation of bone. *Skeletal Radiol* 1998;27:154–156.

Bansal M, Goldman AB, DiCarlo EF, McCormack R. Soft tissue chondromas: diagnosis and differential diagnosis. *Skeletal Radiol* 1993;22:309–315.

Beggs IG, Stoker DJ. Chondromyxoid fibroma of bone. *Clin Radiol* 1982;33:671–679.

Berquist TH. Magnetic resonance imaging of primary skeletal neoplasms. *Radiol Clin North Am* 1993;31:411–424.

Björnsson J, Unni KK, Dahlin DC, Beabout JW, Sim FH. Clear-cell chondrosarcoma of bone: observation in 47 cases. *Am J Surg Pathol* 1984;8:223–230.

Bloem JL, Mulder JD. Chondroblastoma: a clinical and radiological study of 104 cases. *Skeletal Radiol* 1985;14:1–9.

Borges AM, Huvos AG, Smith J. Bursa formation and synovial chondrometaplasia associated with osteochondromas. *Am J Clin Pathol* 1981;75:648–653.

Boriani S, Bacchini P, Bertoni F, Campanacci M. Periosteal chondroma. A review of twenty cases. *J Bone Joint Surg [Am]* 1983;65A:205–212.

Braunstein E, Martel W, Weatherbee L. Periosteal bone apposition in chondroblastoma. *Skeletal Radiol* 1979;4:34–36.

Brien EW, Mirra JM, Luck JV Jr. Benign and malignant cartilage tumors of bone and joint: their anatomic and theoretical basis with an emphasis on radiology, pathology, and clinical biology. II. Juxtacortical cartilage tumors. *Skeletal Radiol* 1999;28:1–20.

Brower AC, Moser RP, Gilkey FW, Kransdorf MJ. Chondroblastoma. In: Moser RP, ed. *Cartilaginous tumors of the skeleton. AFIP atlas of radiologic-pathologic correlation,* Fascicle II. Philadelphia: Hanley & Belfus; 1990:74–113.

Brower AC, Moser RP, Kransdorf MJ. The frequency and diagnostic significance of periostitis in chondroblastoma. *AJR Am J Roentgenol* 1990;154:309–314.

Bruder E, Zanetti M, Boos N, von Hochstetter AR. Chondromyxoid fibroma of two thoracic vertebrae. *Skeletal Radiol* 1999;28:286–289.

Bullough PG. *Atlas of orthopedic pathology,* 2nd ed. New York: Gower; 1992:14.9.

Cannon CP, Nelson SD, Seeger L, Eckardt JJ. Clear cell chondrosarcoma mimicking chondroblastoma in a skeletally immature patient. *Skeletal Radiol* 2002;31:369–372.

Chung EB, Enzinger FM. Chondromas of soft parts. *Cancer* 1978;41:1414–1424.

Codman EA. Epiphyseal chondromatous giant cell tumors of the upper end of the humerus. *Surg Gynecol Obstet* 1931;52:543–548.

Cohen EK, Kressel HY, Frank TS, et al. Hyaline cartilage-origin bone and soft-tissue neoplasms: MR appearance and histologic correlation. *Radiology* 1988;167:477–481.

Collins PS, Han W, Williams LR, Rich N, Lee JF, Villavicencio JL. Maffucci's syndrome (hemangiomatosis osteolytica): a report of four cases. *J Vasc Surg* 1992;16:364–371.

Conway WF, Hayes CW. Miscellaneous lesions of bone. *Radiol Clin North Am* 1993;31:339–358.

Crim JR, Seeger LL, Yao L, Chandnani V, Eckardt JJ. Diagnosis of soft-tissue masses with MR imaging: can benign masses be differentiated from malignant ones? *Radiology* 1992;185:581–586.

Dahlin DC. Chondromyxoid fibroma of bone, with emphasis on its morphological relationship to benign chondroblastoma. *Cancer* 1956;9:195–203.

Dahlin DC, Ivins JC. Benign chondroblastoma: a study of 125 cases. *Cancer* 1972;30:401–413.

Dahlin DC, Salvador AH. Cartilaginous tumors of the soft tissues of the hands and feet. *Mayo Clin Proc* 1974;49:721–726.

Dahlin DC, Unni KK. *Bone tumors: general aspects and data on 8,542 cases,* 4th ed. Springfield, IL: Charles C. Thomas; 1986:18, 33–51, 227–259.

Davids JR, Glancy GL, Eilert RE. Fracture through the stalk of pedunculated osteochondromas. A report of three cases. *Clin Orthop* 1991;271:258–264.

De Beuckeleer LHL, De Schepper AMA, Ramon F. Magnetic resonance imaging of cartilaginous tumors: is it useful or necessary? *Skeletal Radiol* 1996;25:137–141.

De Beuckeleer LHL, De Schepper AMA, Ramon F. Magnetic resonance imaging of cartilaginous tumors: retrospective study of 79 patients. *Eur J Radiol* 1995;21:34–40.

deSantos LA, Spjut HJ. Periosteal chondroma: a radiographic spectrum. *Skeletal Radiol* 1981;6:15–20.

El-Khoury GY, Bassett GS. Symptomatic bursa formation with osteochondromas. *AJR Am J Roentgenol* 1979;133:895–898.

Enzinger FM, Weiss SW. Cartilaginous tumors and tumor-like lesions of soft tissue. In: *Soft tissue tumors,* 2nd ed. St. Louis: Mosby; 1988:861.

Epstein DA, Levin EJ. Bone scintigraphy in hereditary multiple exostoses. *AJR Am J Roentgenol* 1978;130:331–333.

Erickson JK, Rosenthal DI, Zaleske DJ, Gebhardt MC, Cates JM. Primary treatment of chondroblastoma with percutaneous radiofrequency heat ablation: report of three cases. *Radiology* 2001;221:463–468.

Fairbank TJ. Dysplasia epiphysealis hemimelica (tarso-epiphyseal aclasis). *J Bone Joint Surg [Br]* 1956;38B:237–257.

Fechner RE, Mills SE. *Tumors of the bones and joint.* Armed Forces Institute of Pathology, Washington DC; 1993.

Feldman F. Cartilaginous lesions of bones and soft tissues. *CRC Crit Rev Clin Radiol Nucl Med* 1974;4:477–554.

Feldman F. Cartilaginous tumors and cartilage-forming tumor-like conditions of the bones and soft tissues. In: Ranniger K, ed. *Bone tumors.* Berlin: Springer-Verlag; 1977:83–242.

Feldman F, Hecht HL, Johnston AD. Chondromyxoid fibroma of bone. *Radiology* 1970;94:249–260.

Flach HZ, Ginai AZ, Oosterhuis JW. Best cases from the AFIP. Maffucci syndrome: radiologic and pathologic findings. *Radiographics* 2001;21:1311–1316.

Flemming DJ, Murphey MD. Enchondroma and chondrosarcoma. *Semin Musculoskelet Radiol* 2000;4:59–71.

Fobben ES, Dalinka MK, Schiebler ML, et al. The MRI appearance at 1.5 Tesla of cartilaginous tumors involving the epiphysis. *Skeletal Radiol* 1987;16:647–651.

Freiberg TA, Hembree JL, Laine W. Periosteal chondroma: a review of the literature and case report. *J Foot Surg* 1986;25:54–57.

Fujiwara S, Nakamura I, Goto T, Motoi T, Yokokura S, Nakamura K. Intracortical chondromyxoid fibroma of humerus. *Skeletal Radiol* 2003;32:156–160.

Gardner DJ, Azouz EM. Solitary lucent epiphyseal lesions in children. *Skeletal Radiol* 1988;17:497–504.

Garrison RC, Unni KK, McLeod RA, Pritchard DJ, Dahlin DC. Chondrosarcoma arising in osteochondroma. *Cancer* 1982;49:1890–1897.

Geirnaerdt MJA, Bloem JL, Eulderink F, Hogendoorn PCW, Taminiau AH. Cartilaginous tumors: correlation of gadolinium-enhanced MR imaging and histopathologic findings. *Radiology* 1993;186:813–817.

Geirnaerdt MJA, Hogendoorn PCW, Bloem JJ, Taminiau AHM, van der Woude H-J. Cartilaginous tumors: fast contrast-enhanced MR imaging. *Radiology* 2000;214:539–546.

Giudici MA, Moser RP Jr, Kransdorf MJ. Cartilaginous bone tumors. *Radiol Clin North Am* 1993;31:237–259.

Gohel VK, Dalinka MK, Edeiken J. Ischemic necrosis of the femoral head simulating chondroblastoma. *Radiology* 1973;107:545–546.

González-Lois C, Garcia-de-la-Torre JP, SantosBriz-Terrón A, Vila J, Manrique-Chico J, Martinez-Tello FJ. Intracapsular and para-articular chondroma adjacent to large joints: report of three cases and review of the literature. *Skeletal Radiol* 2001;30:672–676.

Goodman SB, Bell RS, Fornasier VS, De Demeter D, Bateman JE. Ollier's disease with multiple sarcomatous transformation. *Hum Pathol* 1984;15:91–93.

Green P, Wittaker RP. Benign chondroblastoma. Case report with pulmonary metastasis. *J Bone Joint Surg [Am]* 1975;57A:418–420.

Greenfield GB, Arrington JA. *Imaging of bone tumors. A multimodality approach.* Philadelphia: JB Lippincott; 1995.

Greenspan A. Tumors of cartilage origin. *Orthop Clin North Am* 1989;20:347–366.

Greenspan A, Klein MJ. Radiology and pathology of bone tumors. In: Lewis MM, ed. *Musculoskeletal oncology. A multidisciplinary approach.* Philadelphia: WB Saunders; 1992:13–72.

Greenspan A, Unni KK, Matthews J II. Periosteal chondroma masquerading as osteochondroma. *Can Assoc Radiol J* 1993;44:205–210.

Griffiths HJ, Thompson RC Jr, Galloway HR, Everson LI, Suh J-S. Bursitis in association with solitary osteochondromas presenting as mass lesions. *Skeletal Radiol* 1991;20:513–516.

Hau MA, Fox EJ, Rosenberg AE, Mankin HJ. Chondromyxoid fibroma of the metacarpal. *Skeletal Radiol* 2001;30:719–721.

Hayes CW, Conway WF, Sundaram M. Misleading aggressive MR imaging: appearance of some benign musculoskeletal tumors. *Radiographics* 1992;12:1119–1134.

Helliwell TR, O'Connor MA, Ritchie DA, Feldberg L, Stilwell JH, Jane MJ. Bizarre parosteal osteochondromatous proliferation with cortical invasion. *Skeletal Radiol* 2001;30:282–285.

Helms C. Pseudocyst of the humerus. *AJR Am J Roentgenol* 1979;131:287–292.

Hensinger RN, Cowell HR, Ramsey PL, Leopold RG. Familial dysplasia epiphysealis hemimelica associated with chondromas and osteochondromas. Report of a kindred with variable presentations. *J Bone Joint Surg [Am]* 1974;56A:1513–1516.

Hofman S, Heeg M, Klein J-P, Krikke AP. Simultaneous occurrence of a supra- and infratentorial glioma in a patient with Ollier's disease: more evidence for non-mesodermal tumor predisposition in multiple enchondromatosis. *Skeletal Radiol* 1998;27:688–691.

Hudson TM, Chew FS, Manaster BJ. Scintigraphy of benign exostoses and exostotic chondrosarcoma. *AJR Am J Roentgenol* 1983;140:581–586.

Hudson TM, Hawkins IF Jr. Radiological evaluation of chondroblastoma. *Radiology* 1981;139:1–10.

Hudson TM, Spriengfield DS, Spanier SS, Enneking WF, Hamlin DJ. Benign exostoses and exostotic chondrosarcomas: evaluation of cartilage thickness by CT. *Radiology* 1984;152:595–599.

Huvos AG. Chondroblastoma and clear cell chondrosarcoma: In: Huvos AG, ed. *Bone tumors. Diagnosis, treatment and prognosis,* 2nd ed. Philadelphia: WB Saunders; 1991:295–318.

Huvos AG, Higinbotham NL, Marcove RC, O'Leary P. Aggressive chondroblastoma: review of the literature on aggressive behavior and metastases with a report of one new case. *Clin Orthop* 1977;126:266–272.

Ilaslan H, Sundaram M, Unni KK. Vertebral chondroblastoma. *Skeletal Radiol* 2003;32:66–71.

Ishida T, Goto T, Motoi N, Mukai K. Intracortical chondroblastoma mimicking intra-articular osteoid osteoma. *Skeletal Radiol* 2002;31:603–607.

Jaffe HL. Juxtacortical chondroma. *Bull Hosp Joint Dis* 1956;17:20–29.

Jaffe HL, Lichtenstein L. Benign chondroblastoma of bone: reinterpretation of so-called calcifying or chondromatous giant cell tumor. *Am J Pathol* 1942;18:969–991.

Jaffe HL, Lichtenstein L. Chondromyxoid fibroma of bone: a distinctive benign tumor likely to be mistaken especially for chondrosarcoma. *Arch Pathol* 1948;45:541–551.

Janzen L, Logan PM, O'Connell JX, Connel DG, Munk PL. Intramedullary chondroid tumors of bone: correlation of abnormal peritumoral marrow and soft-tissue MRI signal with tumor type. *Skeletal Radiol* 1997;26:100–106.

Kahn S, Taljanovic MS, Speer DP, Graham AR, Dennis PD. Kissing periosteal chondroma and osteochondroma. *Skeletal Radiol* 2002;31:235–239.

Kaim AH, Hügli R, Bonél HM, Jundt G. Chondroblastoma and clear cell chondrosarcoma: radiological and MRI characteristics with histopathological correlation. *Skeletal Radiol* 2002;31:88–95.

Karasick D, Schweitzer ME, Eschelman DJ. Symptomatic osteochondromas: imaging features. *AJR Am J Roentgenol* 1997;68:1507–1512.

Keating RB, Wright PW, Staple TW. Enchondroma protuberans of the rib. *Skeletal Radiol* 1985;13:55–58.

Kenan S, Abdelwahab I, Klein MJ, Lewis MM. Case report 837. Juxtacortical chondromyxoid fibroma of the proximal tibia. *Skeletal Radiol* 1994;23:237–239.

Kenney PJ, Gilula LA, Murphy WA. The use of computed tomography to distinguish osteochondroma and chondrosarcoma. *Radiology* 1981;139:129–137.

Kettelkamp DB, Campbell CJ, Bonfiglio M. Dysplasia epiphysealis hemimelica. A report of fifteen cases and a review of the literature. *J Bone Joint Surg [Am]* 1966;48A:746–766.

Kobayashi Y, Murakami R, Toba M, et al. Chondroblastoma of the temporal bone. *Skeletal Radiol* 2001;30:714–718.

Kransdorf MJ, Jelinek JS, Moser RP Jr, et al. Soft-tissue masses: diagnosis using MR imaging. *AJR Am J Roentgenol* 1989;153:541–547.

Kricun ME. *Imaging of bone tumors.* Philadelphia: WB Saunders; 1993.

Kricun ME, Kricun R, Haskin ME. Chondroblastoma of the calcaneus: radiographic features with emphasis on location. *AJR Am J Roentgenol* 1977;128:613–616.

Kroon HM, Bloem JL, Holscher HC, van der Woude HJ, Reijnierse M, Taminiau AHM. MR imaging of edema accompanying benign and malignant bone tumors. *Skeletal Radiol* 1994;23:261–269.

Kurt AM, Unni KK, Sim FH, McLeod RA. Chondroblastoma of bone. *Hum Pathol* 1989;20:965–976.

Lang IM, Azouz EM. MRI appearances of dysplasia epiphysealis hemimelica of the knee. *Skeletal Radiol* 1997;26:226–229.

Lange RH, Lange TA, Rao BK. Correlative radiographic, scintigraphic, and histological evaluation of exostoses. *J Bone Joint Surg [Am]* 1984;66A:1454–1459.

Lee JK, Yao L, Wirth CR. MR imaging of solitary osteochondromas: report of eight cases. *AJR Am J Roentgenol* 1987;149:557–560.

Leffler SG, Chew FS. CT-guided percutaneous biopsy of sclerotic bone lesions: diagnostic yield and accuracy. *AJR Am J Roentgenol* 1999;172:1389–1392.

Leung LYJ, Shu SJ, Chan MK, Chan CHS. Chondroblastoma of the lumbar vertebra. *Skeletal Radiol* 2001;30:710–713.

Lewis MM, Kenan S, Yabut SM, Norman A, Steiner G. Periosteal chondroma. A report of ten cases and review of the literature. *Clin Orthop* 1990;256:185–192.

Li C, Arger PH, Dalinka MK. Soft tissue osteochondroma. A report of three cases. *Skeletal Radiol* 1989;18:435–437.

Lichtenstein L, Hall JE. Periosteal chondroma: a distinctive benign cartilage tumor. *J Bone Joint Surg [Am]* 1952;34A:691–697.

Liu J, Hudkins PG, Swee RG, Unni KK. Bone sarcomas associated with Ollier's disease. *Cancer* 1987;59:1376–1385.

Ly JQ, Beall DP. A rare case of infantile Ollier's disease demonstrating bilaterally symmetric extremity involvement. *Skeletal Radiol* 2003;32:227–230.

Ly JQ, LaGatta LM, Beall DP. Calcaneal chondroblastoma with secondary aneurysmal bone cyst. *AJR Am J Roentgenol* 2004;182:130.

Macdonald D, Fornasier V, Holtby R. Chondromyxoid fibroma of the acromium with soft tissue extension. *Skeletal Radiol* 2000;29:168–170.

Maffucci A. Di un caso di encondroma el antioma multiplo. Contribuzone alla genesi embrionale dei tumori. *Movimento Med Chir Napoli* 1881;3:399–412.

Malghem J, Vande Berg B, Noël H, Maldague B. Benign osteochondromas and exostotic chondrosarcomas: evaluation of cartilage cap thickness by ultrasound. *Skeletal Radiol* 1992;21:33–37.

Marin C, Gallego C, Manjón P, Martinez-Tello FJ. Juxtacortical chondromyxoid fibroma: imaging findings in three cases and a review of the literature. *Skeletal Radiol* 1997;26:642–649.

McLeod RA, Beabout JW. The roentgenographic features of chondroblastoma. *AJR Am J Roentgenol* 1973;118:464–471.

Mellon CD, Carter JE, Owen DB. Ollier's disease and Maffucci's syndrome: distinct entities or a continuum? *J Neurol* 1988;235:376–378.

Meneses MF, Unni KK, Swee RG. Bizarre parosteal osteochondromatous proliferation of bone (Nora's lesion). *Am J Surg Pathol* 1993;17:691–697.

Milgram JW, Dunn EJ. Para-articular chondromas and osteochondromas. A report of three cases. *Clin Orthop* 1980;148:147–151.

Mills TD, Hiorns MP, Hall CM. Symmetrical enchondromatosis without vertebral involvement and with cone-shaped phalangeal epiphyses. *Skeletal Radiol* 2001;30:346–349.

Mirra JM, Gold R, Downs J, Eckardt JJ. A new histologic approach to the differentiation of enchondroma and chondrosarcoma of the bones: a clinicopathologic analysis of 51 cases. *Clin Orthop* 1987;2:89–107.

Mirra JM, Picci P, Gold RH. *Bone tumors: Clinical, radiologic and pathologic correlations.* Philadelphia: Lea & Febiger; 1989.

Mirra JM, Ulich TR, Eckardt JJ, Bhuta S. "Aggressive" chondroblastoma. Light and ultramicroscopic findings after *en bloc* resection. *Clin Orthop* 1983;178:276–284.

Mitchell ML, Ackerman LV. Case report 405. Ollier disease (enchondromatosis). *Skeletal Radiol* 1987;16:61–66.

Mitchell ML, Sartoris DJ, Resnick D. Case report 713. Chondromyxoid fibroma of the third metatarsal. *Skeletal Radiol* 1992;21:252–255.

Monda L, Wick MR. S-100 protein immunostaining in the differential diagnosis of chondroblastoma. *Hum Pathol* 1985;16:287–293.

Moser RP, Brockmole DM, Vinh TN, Kransdorf MJ, Aoki J. Chondroblastoma of the patella. *Skeletal Radiol* 1988;17:413–419.

Moser RP, Gilkey FW, Madewell JE. Enchondroma. In: Moser RP, ed. *Cartilaginous tumors of the skeleton. AFIP atlas of radiologic-pathologic correlation,* Fascicle II. Philadelphia: Hanley & Belfus; 1990:8–34.

Mulder JD, Schütte HE, Kroon HM, Taconis WK. *Radiologic atlas of bone tumors.* Amsterdam: Elsevier; 1993.

Murphey MD, Choi JJ, Kransdorf MJ, Flemming DJ, Gannon FH. Imaging of osteochondroma: variants and complications with radiologic-pathologic correlation. *Radiographics* 2000;20:1407–1434.

Murphey MD, Flemming DJ, Boyea SR, Bojescul JA, Sweet DE, Temple HT. From the archives of the AFIP. Enchondroma versus chondrosarcoma in the appendicular skeleton: differentiation features. *Radiographics* 1998;18:1213–1237.

Murphy NB, Price CHG. The radiological aspects of chondromyxoid fibroma of bone. *Clin Radiol* 1971;22:261–269.

Nguyen T, Burk D. Periosteal (juxtacortical) chondroma. *AJR Am J Roentgenol* 1995;165:203–205.

Nojima T, Unni KK, McLeod RA, Pritchard DJ. Periosteal chondroma and periosteal chondrosarcoma. *Am J Surg Pathol* 1985;9:666–677.

Nora FE, Dahlin DC, Beabout JW. Bizarre parosteal osteochondromatous proliferation of the hands and feet. *Am J Surg Pathol* 1983;7:245–250.

Norman A, Sissons HA. Radiographic hallmarks of peripheral chondrosarcoma. *Radiology* 1984;151:589–596.

O'Connor PJ, Gibbon WW, Hardy G, Butt WP. Chondromyxoid fibroma of the foot. *Skeletal Radiol* 1996;25:143–148.

Ollier L. De la dyschondroplasie. *Bull Soc Lyon Med* 1899;93:23–24.

Peh WCG, Shek TWH, Ip WY. Metadiaphyseal chondroblastoma of the thumb. *Skeletal Radiol* 2000;29:176–180.

Peterson HA. Multiple hereditary osteochondromata. *Clin Orthop* 1989;239:222–230.

Pösl M, Werner M, Amling M, Ritzel H, Delling G. Malignant transformation of chondroblastoma. *Histopathology* 1996;29:477–480.

Quint LE, Gross BH, Glazer GM, Braunstein EM, White SJ. CT evaluation of chondroblastoma. *J Comput Assist Tomogr* 1984;8:907–910.

Ragsdale BD, Sweet DE, Vinh TN. Radiology as gross pathology in evaluating chondroid tumors. *Hum Pathol* 1989;20:930–951.

Rahimi A, Beabout JW, Ivins JC, Dahlin DC. Chondromyxoid fibroma: clinicopathologic study of 75 cases. *Cancer* 1972;30:726–736.

Ramnath RR, Rosenthal DI, Cates J, Gebhardt M, Quinn RH. Intracortical chondroma simulating osteoid osteoma treated by radiofrequency. *Skeletal Radiol* 2002;31:597–602.

Raymond AK, Raymond PG, Edeiken J. Case report 531. Epiphyseal osteoblastoma distal end of femur. *Skeletal Radiol* 1989;18:143–146.

Resnik CS, Levine AM, Aisner SC, Young JW, Dorfman HD. Case report 522. Concurrent adjacent osteochondroma and enchondroma. *Skeletal Radiol* 1989;18:66–69.

Resnick D, Cone RO III. The nature of humeral pseudocysts. *Radiology* 1984;150:27–28.

Ribalta T, Ro JY, Carrasco CH, Heffelman C, Ayala AG. Case report 638. Chondromyxoid fibroma of a sesamoid bone. *Skeletal Radiol* 1990;19:549–551.

Robinson P, White LM, Sundaram M, et al. Periosteal chondroid tumors: radiologic evaluation with pathologic correlation. *AJR Am J Roentgenol* 2001;177:1183–1188.

Rudman DP, Damron TA, Vermont A, Mathur S. Intracortical chondroma. *Skeletal Radiol* 1998;27:581–583.

Schajowicz F. Chondromyxoid fibroma: report of three cases with predominant cortical involvement. *Radiology* 1987;164:783–786.

Schajowicz F. Cartilage-forming tumors. In: Schajowicz F, ed., *Tumors and tumorlike conditions of bone.* New York: Springer-Verlag; 1994:141–256.

Schajowicz F, Ackerman LV, Sissons HA. Histological typing of bone tumours. *International histological classification of tumors, no. 6.* Geneva: World Health Organization, 1972.

Schajowicz F, Gallardo H. Chondromyxoid fibroma (fibromyxoid chondroma) of bone. *J Bone Joint Surg [Br]* 1971;53B:198–216.

Schajowicz F, Gallardo H. Epiphyseal chondroblastoma of bone: a clinicopathological study of sixty-nine cases. *J Bone Joint Surg [Br]* 1970;52B:205–226.

Schajowicz F, McGuire M. Diagnostic difficulties in skeletal pathology. *Clin Orthop* 1989;240:281–308.

Schajowicz F, Sissons HA, Sobin LH. The World Health Organization's histologic classification of bone tumors. A commentary on the second edition. *Cancer* 1995;75:1208–1214.

Shapiro F. Ollier's disease. An assessment of angular deformity, shortening, and pathological fracture in twenty-one patients. *J Bone Joint Surg [Am]* 1982;64A:95–103.

Spjut HJ, Dorfman HD, Fechner RE, Ackerman LV. Tumors of bone and cartilage. In: *Atlas of Tumor pathology*, Second Series, Fascicle 5. Washington, DC: Armed Forces Institute of Pathology; 1971.

Springfield DS, Capanna R, Gherlinzoni F, Picci P, Campanacci M. Chondroblastoma: a review of seventy cases. *J Bone Joint Surg [Am]* 1985;67A:748–755.

Steiner GC. Benign cartilage tumors. In: Taveras JM, Ferrucci JT, eds. *Radiology: Diagnosis-imaging–intervention,* no 5. Philadelphia: JB Lippincott; 1986.

Sun TC, Swee RG, Shives TC, Unni KK. Chondrosarcoma in Maffucci's syndrome. *J Bone Joint Surg [Am]* 1985;67A:1214–1219.

Sundaram M, McLeod RA. MR imaging of tumor and tumor-like lesions of bone and soft tissue. *AJR Am J Roentgenol* 1990;155:817–824.

Unger EC, Kessler HB, Kowalyshyn MJ, Lackman RD, Morea GT. MR imaging of Maffucci syndrome. *AJR Am J Roentgenol* 1988;150:351–353.

Unni KK. Chondroma. In: Unni KK, ed. *Dahlin's bone tumors. General aspect and data on 11,087 cases, 5th* ed. Philadelphia: Lippincott–Raven Publishers; 1996:25–45.

Uri DS, Dalinka MK, Kneeland JB. Muscle impingement: MR imaging of a painful complication of osteochondromas. *Skeletal Radiol* 1996;25:689–692.

Ushigome S, Takakuwa T, Shinagawa T, Kishida H, Yamazaki M. Chondromyxoid fibroma of bone. An electron microscopic observation. *Acta Pathol Jpn* 1982;32:113–122.

Varma DGK, Kumar R, Carrasco CH, Guo S-Q, Richli WR. MR imaging of periosteal chondroma. *J Comput Assist Tomogr* 1991;15:1008–1010.

Weatherall PT, Maale GE, Mendelsohn DB, Sherry CS, Erdman WE, Pascoe HR. Chondroblastoma: classic and confusing appearance at MR imaging. *Radiology* 1994;190:467–474.

White PG, Saunders L, Orr W, Friedman L. Chondromyxoid fibroma. *Skeletal Radiol* 1996;25:79–81.

Wilson AJ, Kyriakos M, Ackerman LV. Chondromyxoid fibroma: radiographic appearance in 38 cases and in a review of the literature. *Radiology* 1991;179:513–518. [Erratum, *Radiology* 1991;180:586.]

Yamaguchi T, Dorfman HD. Radiologic and histologic patterns of calcification in chondromyxoid fibroma. *Skeletal Radiol* 1998;27:559–564.

Yamamura S, Sato K, Sugiura H, Iwata H. Inflammatory reaction in chondroblastoma. *Skeletal Radiol* 1996;25:371–376.

Zillmer DA, Dorfman HD. Chondromyxoid fibroma of bone: thirty-six cases with clinicopathologic correlation. *Hum Pathol* 1989;20:952–964.

Zlatkin MB, Lander PH, Begin LR, Hadjipavlou A. Soft-tissue chondromas. *AJR Am J Roentgenol* 1985;144:1263–1267.

BENIGN TUMORS AND TUMOR-LIKE LESIONS III

Fibrous, Fibroosseus, and Fibrohistiocytic Lesions

Fibrous Cortical Defect and Nonossifying Fibroma

Fibrous cortical defects and nonossifying (nonosteogenic) fibromas are the most common fibrous lesions of bone and are predominantly seen in children and adolescents. More common in boys than in girls, they have a predilection for the long bones, particularly the femur and tibia (Fig. 19.1). Some authors prefer the term fibroxanthoma for both lesions, whereas Schajowicz prefers the term histiocytic xanthogranuloma. These lesions are not true neoplasms and are considered by many investigators developmental defects.

Fibrous cortical defect (metaphyseal fibrous defect) is a small asymptomatic lesion found in 30% of normal individuals in the first and second decades of life. The radiolucent lesion is elliptical and confined to the cortex of a long bone near the growth plate; it is demarcated by a thin margin of sclerosis (Figs.19.2 and 19.3). Most of these lesions disappear spontaneously, but a few may continue to enlarge. When they encroach on the medullary region of a bone, they are designated nonossifying fibroma (Fig. 19.4).With continued growth, these lesions, which are typically located eccentrically in the bone, display a characteristic scalloped sclerotic border (Fig. 19.5).

Occasionally, nonossifying fibroma may involve several bones, in which case the condition is called disseminated nonossifying fibromatosis. Some of the patients with this presentation may exhibit on the skin café-au-lait spots with smooth ("coast of California") borders, similar to those seen in neurofibromatosis (see Chapter 33). This association is known as Jaffe-Campanacci syndrome.

Skeletal scintigraphy shows a minimal to mild increase in activity. During the healing phase, mild hyperemia may be seen on the blood

Figure 19.1 demonstrates the skeletal sites of predilection, peak age range, and male-to-female ratio.

Fibrous Cortical Defect and Nonossifying Fibroma

age: 2–20
M > F

■ common sites
■ less common sites

Figure 19.1 Skeletal sites of predilection, peak age range, and male-to-female ratio in fibrous cortical defect and nonossifying fibroma.

pool image, and the positive delayed scan reflects the osteoblastic activity. Computed tomography (CT) may demonstrate to better advantage the cortical thinning and medullary involvement and may delineate early pathologic fracture more precisely. Hounsfield attenuation values for nonossifying fibroma are higher than for normal bone marrow. Magnetic resonance imaging (MRI), usually performed for another reason, shows intermediate to low signal intensity on T1-weighted and T2-weighted sequences. After gadolinium-diethylenetriamine-pentaacetic acid (DTPA) injection, both fibrous cortical defects and nonossifying fibromas invariably exhibit a hyperintense border and signal en-

Figure 19.2 Fibrous cortical defect. Fibrous cortical defect, seen here in lateral cortex of the distal tibia in a 13-year-old boy, typically presents as a radiolucent lesion demarcated by a thin zone of sclerosis.

hancement. Mineralization of the lesion during healing appears predominantly as low signal intensity on MR images.

Histologically identical, regardless of size, fibrous cortical defect and nonossifying fibroma are composed of spindle and histiocytic cells that have a clear, foamy cytoplasm. In addition, osteoclast-like multinucleated giant cells are present, and varying numbers of inflammatory cells (lymphocytes) and plasma cells are scattered in the background. The cells are often arranged in a storiform pattern, typifying fibrohistiocytic lesions. Some lesions contain an excessive amount of fat within the foam cells, and the term *xanthoma* or *fibroxanthoma* may be applied to such lesions.

Complications and Treatment

Most lesions undergo spontaneous involution (healing) by sclerosis or remodeling (Fig. 19.6). Some larger lesions may be complicated by pathologic fracture (Fig. 19.7). Therefore, if a lesion is large, extending across 50% or more of the medullary cavity, then curettage and bone grafting is the treatment of choice.

Figure 19.3 Fibrous cortical defect. A 21-year-old woman with a fibrous cortical defect affecting medial cortex of the distal femur.

Figure 19.4 Nonossifying fibroma. When a fibrous cortical defect encroaches on the medullary cavity, it is called a nonossifying fibroma. Note the similarity of the lesion to that in the previous figure. The only difference is that the fibroma is larger and extends beyond the cortex.

Figure 19.5 Nonossifying fibroma. Nonossifying fibroma, seen here in the distal tibia in an asymptomatic 15-year-old boy, typically appears eccentrically located in the bone and has a scalloped sclerotic border.

Figure 19.6 Healing of nonossifying fibroma. (A) Spontaneous involution of nonossifying fibroma in the distal tibia is characterized by progressive sclerosis of peripheral parts of the lesion. **(B)** A nonossifying fibroma that healed completely may persist as a sclerotic patch. Nonossifying fibromas in this sclerosing phase should not be mistaken for osteoblastic tumors or for sclerosing dysplasia.

Figure 19.7 Complication of nonossifying fibroma. Pathologic fracture is a common complication of a large nonossifying fibroma, as seen here in the distal tibia of a 10-year-old boy. Lesions extending halfway or farther into the medullary region of a bone should be treated by curettage and bone grafting.

Benign Fibrous Histiocytoma

The term benign fibrous histiocytoma, although it may be controversial, is useful to subclassify lesions with histologic features similar to those of nonossifying fibroma but having an atypical clinical presentation and an atypical radiographic pattern. This lesion frequently has radiographic features very similar to those of nonossifying fibroma; it is radiolucent, with sharply defined and frequently sclerotic borders, without any mineralization of the matrix (Figs. 19.8 and 19.9). Its differentiation from nonossifying fibroma is made on purely clinical grounds, because the histologic features of both lesions are almost identical. Patients presenting with benign fibrous histiocytoma are older (usually older than 25 years) than those with nonossifying fibroma; unlike the latter lesion, benign fibrous histiocytomas may produce symptoms such as pain or discomfort in the involved bone. These lesions also seem to run a more aggressive clinical course and may recur after treatment, which consists of curettage and bone grafting.

Periosteal Desmoid

The periosteal desmoid is a tumor-like fibrous proliferation of the periosteum. It occurs in patients between the ages of 12 and 20 years and has a striking predilection for the posteromedial cortex of the medial femoral condyle. Many patients have a history of injury, although trauma is not necessarily a predisposing factor. The lesion simulates a fibrous cortical defect, except in the specificity of its location. Occasionally, it may simulate an aggressive and even malignant tumor. Radiographically, the hallmarks of a periosteal desmoid are its radiolucent saucer-shaped appearance, with sclerosis at the base eroding the cortex or producing cortical irregularity (Fig. 19.10). On MRI, the lesion appears hypointense on T1-weighted and hyperintense on T2-

weighted images, with a dark rim on both sequences at or near the sites of the bony attachment of the medial head of the gastrocnemius muscle. Periosteal desmoid belongs to the "don't touch" lesions (see Table 16.10), so it should not undergo biopsy. Most lesions disappear spontaneously by the time the patient reaches age 20.

The histologic appearance of the lesion demonstrates fibroblastic spindle cells that produce large amounts of collagen. Large areas of hyalinization and fibrocartilage and small fragments of bone may be scattered within the fibrous tissue.

Differential Diagnosis

Some authorities believe that periosteal desmoid should be differentiated from distal femoral cortical irregularity. This latter abnormality, which presents as cortical roughening just distal to the extension of the linea aspera, is a common finding in boys in the 10- to 15-year age group. Its cause is not settled. Although it was thought to represent an avulsion injury caused by traction of the adductor magnus aponeurosis, Brower and colleagues have shown that this lesion may exist in the area without any muscular or ligamentous attachment. Others consider periosteal desmoid and distal femoral cortical irregularity to be the same entity. Dahlin suggests that the periosteal desmoid is a hypocellular variant of nonossifying fibroma, and Schajowicz classifies it as a periosteal variant of desmoplastic fibroma. Other authors apply a broader definition to periosteal desmoid, considering it essentially a hypocellular variant of fibrous cortical defect. In any event, it is a self-limited benign lesion that requires no treatment.

Fibrous Dysplasia

Fibrous dysplasia is a fibroosseous lesion that some authorities classify among the group of developmental dysplasias. It may affect one bone (monostotic form) or several bones (polyostotic form). It is characterized by the replacement of normal lamellar cancellous bone by an abnormal fibrous tissue that contains small, abnormally arranged trabeculae of immature woven bone formed by metaplasia of the fibrous stroma.

Figure 19.8 Benign fibrous histiocytoma. A 37-year-old man presented with occasional pain in the right knee. Oblique radiograph of the knee demonstrates a lobulated radiolucent lesion with a well-defined sclerotic border, located eccentrically in the proximal tibia. Biopsy revealed benign fibrous histiocytoma.

Figure 19.9 Benign fibrous histiocytoma. (A) Anteroposterior radiograph of the left proximal humerus in a 26-year-old woman with chronic arm pain shows eccentric, well-defined, partially sclerotic lesion (*arrows*). (B) A radionuclide bone scan demonstrates a focal homogenous increased uptake of radiotracer. Excisional biopsy was consistent with healing benign fibrous histiocytoma.

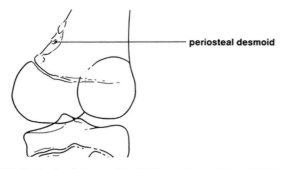

periosteal desmoid

Figure 19.10 Periosteal desmoid. Oblique view of the left knee of a 12-year-old boy shows the classic appearance of periosteal desmoid. Note the saucer-like radiolucency eroding the medial border of the distal femoral metaphysis at the linea aspera and producing cortical irregularity. This lesion should not be mistaken for a malignant bone tumor.

Monostotic Fibrous Dysplasia

Monostotic fibrous dysplasia most commonly affects the femur—particularly the femoral neck—as well as the tibia and ribs (Fig. 19.11). The lesion arises centrally in the bone, usually sparing the epiphysis in children, and it is very rarely seen in the articular end of the bone in adults (Fig. 19.12). As the lesion enlarges, it expands the medullary cavity. The radiographic appearance of monostotic fibrous dysplasia varies, depending on the proportion of osseous-to-fibrous content. Lesions with greater osseous content are more dense and sclerotic, whereas those with greater fibrous content are more radiolucent, with a characteristic ground-glass appearance (Figs. 19.13 and 19.14, see also Fig. 19.11B).

Scintigraphy is helpful in determining the activity (Fig. 19.15) and the potential multicentricity of the lesion. Machida and associates reported that although a high incidence of increased uptake of radiopharmaceutical was seen in 59 patients with fibrous dysplasia, 10% of the lesions with a ground-glass appearance failed to show similarly increased uptake.

The CT findings parallel those of conventional radiography. CT sections show areas of high attenuation in more sclerotic lesions and a low-attenuation matrix with an amorphous ground-glass texture in lesions with greater fibrous content (Fig. 19.16). As pointed out by Daffner and colleagues, CT is particularly useful to define the extent of craniofacial disease, including impingement on orbital structures. The lesion of fibrous dysplasia shows a variety of appearances on MRI caused by the histologic composition of these lesions. Some lesions show a decreased signal on T1 and T2 sequences, and some show low signal on T1-weighted but either mixed or high signal on T2-weighted images. The sclerotic rim (rind sign) is invariably imaged as a band of low signal intensity on T1 and T2 sequences.

Pathologic fracture of the structurally weakened bone is the most frequent complication of monostotic fibrous dysplasia.

Figure 19.11 Monostotic fibrous dysplasia. (A) Typically, the focus of fibrous dysplasia is located in the femoral neck, as seen here in a 13-year-old girl. Note a characteristic sclerotic "rind" encapsulating the lesion. **(B)** The rib is a frequent site of fibrous dysplasia. Note the expansive lesion exhibiting a ground-glass appearance.

Figure 19.12 Monostotic fibrous dysplasia. Oblique **(A)** and lateral **(B)** radiographs of the left leg of a 32-year-old woman demonstrate a large, trabeculated radiolucent lesion in the distal tibia. Because of its aggressive features, it was thought to be a desmoplastic fibroma; however, biopsy proved it to be a fibrous dysplasia, a rare lesion at this site in adults.

Figure 19.13 Monostotic fibrous dysplasia. (A) Anteroposterior radiograph of the distal leg of a 17-year-old girl shows a monostotic focus of fibrous dysplasia in the diaphysis of the tibia. Observe the slight expansion and thinning of the cortex and the partial loss of trabecular pattern in the cancellous bone, which gives the lesion a ground-glass or smoky appearance. **(B)** The focus of fibrous dysplasia in the femoral neck in this 25-year-old man exhibits a more sclerotic appearance than that seen in **A**.

Figure 19.14 Monostotic fibrous dysplasia. Anteroposterior radiographs of the left humerus in neutral **(A)** and external rotation **(B)** projections of a 13-year-old boy show a radiolucent focus of fibrous dysplasia in the diaphysis of the bone.

Figure 19.15 Scintigraphy of fibrous dysplasia. A 24-year-old woman presented with mild discomfort in the right leg. **(A)** Anteroposterior radiograph shows a radiolucent lesion in the midshaft of the tibia, with "smoky" appearance associated with thinning of the cortex and slight expansion, characteristic of fibrous dysplasia. **(B)** Radionuclide bone scan shows markedly increased uptake of the radiopharmaceutical tracer indicating an active lesion.

Figure 19.16 CT of fibrous dysplasia. A 24-year-old woman presented with pain in the left arm. **(A)** Anteroposterior radiograph of the proximal left humerus shows expansive, mostly radiolucent lesion (*arrows*) with focal sclerotic areas at the junction of the head and neck (*open arrow*). The cortex is thinned out. Another sclerotic focus is seen in the scapula (*curved arrow*). **(B)** CT section through the shaft of the humerus shows a low-attenuation lesion with minimal scalloping of the endocortex. **(C)** CT section through the shoulder joint reveals the high-attenuation areas of sclerosis in the humeral head and scapula (arrows).

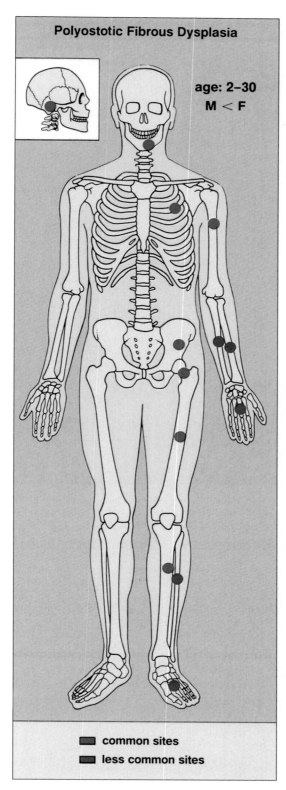

Figure 19.17 Skeletal sites of predilection, peak age range, and male-to-female ratio in polyostotic fibrous dysplasia, which is usually seen in only one side of the skeleton.

Polyostotic Fibrous Dysplasia

Although radiographically similar to the monostotic form, polyostotic fibrous dysplasia is a more aggressive disorder. It also has a different distribution in the skeleton and a striking predilection for one side of the body (Fig. 19.17), a tendency that has been noted in more than 90% of cases. The pelvis is frequently affected, followed by the long bones, skull, and ribs; the proximal end of the femur is a common site of involvement (Fig. 19.18). The lesions generally progress in number and size until the end of skeletal maturation, at which time they become quiescent. In only 5% of cases do they continue to enlarge.

Radiographically, the changes typical of fibrous dysplasia may occur in a limited segment or a major portion of the long bones affected by the polyostotic form of the disease, but as in the monostotic form, the articular ends are usually spared. The cortex, which is generally left intact, is often thinned by the expansive component of the lesion, and the inner cortical margins may show scalloping. The lesion has a

Figure 19.18 Polyostotic fibrous dysplasia. Anteroposterior radiograph of the right hip of an 18-year-old woman with polyostotic fibrous dysplasia shows unilateral involvement of the ilium and femur. There is a pathologic fracture of the femoral neck with a varus deformity.

Histologically, fibrous dysplasia presents as an aggregate of moderately dense fibrous connective tissue containing bony trabeculae in haphazard distribution instead of the stress-oriented distribution expected in normal cancellous bone. The trabeculae are curved and branching, with sparse interconnections. Low-power photomicrographs have been likened to "alphabet soup" or Chinese ideographs. They are composed of woven, immature bone and exhibit no evidence of osteoblastic activity ("naked trabeculae"). Occasionally, an area of cartilage formation may be present within the lesion.

Figure 19.19 Polyostotic fibrous dysplasia. A 13-year-old girl injured her right hip. **(A)** A radiograph of the hip, obtained to exclude a fracture, demonstrates a silent focus of fibrous dysplasia in the femoral neck. To determine other sites of involvement, a radionuclide bone scan was obtained. In addition to the focus in the femoral neck **(B)**, increased uptake of isotope was demonstrated at various other sites, but predominantly the right leg **(C)**. Subsequent radiograph of the right lower leg in the anteroposterior projection **(D)** confirms the presence of multiple foci of polyostotic fibrous dysplasia.

well-defined border. Occasionally, as in the monostotic form, the replacement of medullary bone by fibrous tissue leads to a loss of the trabecular pattern, giving the lesions a ground-glass, "milky," or "smoky" appearance (see Fig. 19.13A). More osseous lesions appear dense. The quickest means of determining the distribution of the lesion in the skeleton is radionuclide bone scan, which often discloses unsuspected sites of skeletal involvement (Fig. 19.19).

CT can accurately delineate the extent of bone involvement. Tissue attenuation values, as measured by Hounsfield units, are usually within the 70- to 400-HU range, apparently reflecting the presence of calcium and microscopic ossification throughout the abnormal tissue. On MRI, fibrous dysplasia exhibits homogeneous, moderately low signal intensity on T1-weighted images, whereas on T2-weighting, the signal is bright or mixed. After gadolinium infusion, most lesions show central contrast enhancement and some peripheral rim enhancement. In general, signal intensity on T1- and T2-weighted images and the degree of contrast enhancement on T1-weighted sequences depend on the amount and degree of bone trabeculae, collagen, and cystic and hemorrhagic changes in fibrous dysplasia.

The histologic appearance of polyostotic fibrous dysplasia is identical to that of the monostotic form. The presence of small trabeculae of woven bone of various sizes and shapes, scattered within a fibrous tissue without evidence of osteoblastic activity, is diagnostic for this disorder.

Complications

The most frequent complication of polyostotic fibrous dysplasia is pathologic fracture. If fracture occurs at the femoral neck, it commonly leads to a deformity called "shepherd's crook" (Fig. 19.20). Occasionally, accelerated growth of a bone or hypertrophy of a digit may be encountered (Fig. 19.21). Massive cartilage hyperplasia (cartilaginous differentiation) may also be seen in this disorder, resulting in the accumulation of cartilaginous masses in the medullary portion of the affected bone (Figs. 19.22, 19.23 and 19.24). This condition is commonly referred to as *fibrochondrodysplasia or fibrocartilaginous dysplasia*. However, it should not be confused with so-called *focal fibrocartilaginous dysplasia of long bones*. The latter occurs mainly in children and young adults. Characteristically, it affects the proximal tibia, although other long bones, such as the ulna and femur, may sometimes be involved. The lesion shows a variety of histopathological features, ranging from purely dense fibrous tissue to benign fibrocartilaginous tissue. The sarcomatous transformation of either form of fibrous dysplasia is extremely rare, but it may occur spontaneously (Fig. 19.25) or, more commonly, after radiation therapy (Fig. 19.26).

Associated Disorders

Albright-McCune Syndrome

When polyostotic fibrous dysplasia is associated with endocrine disturbances (premature sexual development, hyperparathyroidism, and other endocrinopathies) and abnormal pigmentation marked by café au lait spots of the skin, the disorder is called Albright-McCune syndrome (Fig. 19.27). Overall, this condition almost exclusively affects girls who present with true sexual precocity secondary to acceleration of the normal process of gonadotropin release by the anterior lobe of the pituitary gland. The café au lait spots seen in Albright-McCune syndrome have characteristically irregular ragged borders (commonly called "coast of Maine" borders), as opposed to the smoothly marginated ("coast of California") borders of the spots seen in neurofibromatosis.

Mazabraud Syndrome

This syndrome, which is characterized by an association of polyostotic fibrous dysplasia with soft-tissue myxomas (solitary or multiple), was first described by German pathologist F. Henschen in 1926, and later was re-emphasized by French physician A. Mazabraud in 1967. The

Figure 19.20 Polyostotic fibrous dysplasia. A "shepherd's crook" deformity, seen here in the proximal femur in a 12-year-old boy with polyostotic fibrous dysplasia, is often the result of multiple pathologic fractures.

cause of Mazabraud syndrome remains unsettled. A variety of pathological mechanisms have been suggested to explain the link between fibrous dysplasia and soft tissue myxomas. Some investigators have emphasized a common histiogenic origin or a shared abnormality in tissue metabolism. Others have suggested a collaborative developmental error, perhaps related to a genetic predisposition. In this syndrome, it is important to recognize the soft-tissue masses as benign myxomas and not to confuse them with malignant soft-tissue tumors that may develop *de novo* (e.g., malignant fibrous histiocytoma, malignant mesenchymoma, or liposarcoma) or those that may be present in cases of malignant transformation of fibrous dysplasia. MR imaging is very helpful, because it reveals typical features of benign myxomas, i.e., very sharply defined borders, homogeneous signal intensity before administration of contrast, and a heterogeneous pattern of enhancement after injection of gadolinium. As pointed out by several investigators, the signal characteristics of myxoma on T1-weighted and T2-weighted sequences are quite similar to those of fluid: low-to-intermediate signal intensity on T1-weighted and high signal intensity on T2-weighted images.

Figure 19.21 Complication of fibrous dysplasia. Posteroanterior radiograph of the hand **(A)** and dorsoplantar film of the foot **(B)** of a 20-year-old man with polyostotic fibrous dysplasia demonstrate a frequent complication of this condition—accelerated growth of affected bones. In the hand, observe the enlargement of the third and fourth rays, including the metacarpals and phalanges, and in the foot note the hypertrophy of the first metatarsal.

Figure 19.22 Fibrocartilaginous dysplasia. An anteroposterior radiograph of the right proximal femur in a 20-year-old man with polyostotic fibrous dysplasia shows foci of cartilage formation (*arrow*), identifying this lesion as fibrocartilaginous dysplasia.

Figure 19.23 Fibrocartilaginous dysplasia. An anteroposterior radiograph of the proximal right femur of a 10-year-old boy with polyostotic fibrous dysplasia exhibits typical appearance of a massive formation of cartilage, known as fibrocartilaginous dysplasia.

Figure 19.24 Fibrocartilaginous dysplasia. **(A)** An anteroposterior radiograph of the left humerus in a 19-year-old man with polyostotic fibrous dysplasia shows an extensive involvement of almost the entire bone, with cartilage formation in the midportion of the diaphysis. **(B)** A magnification radiograph demonstrates morphologic details of fibrocartilaginous dysplasia.

Figure 19.25 Complication of fibrous dysplasia. A 34-year-old man was noted to have a deformity of the left leg at age 5 years. Radiographic examination at that time showed typical involvement of the tibia by fibrous dysplasia, which subsequently was confirmed by biopsy. No treatment was given, and he was asymptomatic for 28 years until acute pain in his left leg developed. Conventional radiograph shows evidence of fibrous dysplasia affecting the proximal shaft of the tibia. A large osteolytic destructive lesion in the distal third of the tibia is also seen encroaching on the dense segment of bone and affecting the medullary portion and the cortex. There is a periosteal reaction and a soft-tissue mass. Biopsy revealed transformation of fibrous dysplasia to undifferentiated spindle-cell sarcoma.

sclerotic changes of fibrous dysplasia

destructive lesion

Figure 19.26 Complication of fibrous dysplasia. Eleven years before this examination, a 35-year-old woman with polyostotic fibrous dysplasia underwent radiation treatment of the mandible. **(A)** Lateral radiograph of the skull demonstrates predominant involvement of the frontal bones with a characteristic expansion of the outer table. The base of the skull, a frequent site of polyostotic fibrous dysplasia, is typically thickened, and the frontal and ethmoid sinuses are obliterated. The maxilla and mandible are also affected. This advanced stage of involvement of the skull and facial bones by polyostotic fibrous dysplasia is frequently termed leontiasis ossea. **(B)** Oblique radiograph shows an expansive lytic lesion in the body of the left mandible, with partial destruction of the cortex. Biopsy revealed an osteosarcoma.

with few exceptions in the proximal third or mid segment of the bone and often localized to its anterior cortex. In more than 80% of patients, there is some degree of anterior bowing. Larger lesions may destroy the cortex and invade the medullary cavity.

On radiography, the Kempson-Campanacci lesion exhibits a lobulated sclerotic margin and a striking resemblance to nonossifying fibroma and fibrous dysplasia (Figs. 19.28 and 19.29). MRI features are also similar to those two lesions (Fig. 19.30). Furthermore, osteofibrous dysplasia and fibrous dysplasia, as the similarity in their names

Figure 19.27 Albright-McCune syndrome. Polyostotic fibrous dysplasia typically affects one side of the skeleton, as seen here in a 5-year-old girl with precocious puberty whose left upper and lower extremities were affected (Albright-McCune syndrome). Radiograph of the lower leg shows expansion of the tibia and fibula associated with thinning of the cortex. Note the ground-glass appearance of the medullary portion of these bones.

Osteofibrous Dysplasia

Osteofibrous dysplasia (Kempson-Campanacci lesion), called "ossifying fibroma" in the past, is a rare, benign, fibroosseous lesion that occurs predominantly in children, although it may not be discovered until adolescence. It has a decided preference for the tibia, being located

Figure 19.28 Osteofibrous dysplasia. This lesion in the anterior aspect of the right tibia of a 14-year-old girl was originally thought to be a nonossifying fibroma. Although it is similar to a nonossifying fibroma and fibrous dysplasia, its site is typical of osteofibrous dysplasia, which was confirmed by biopsy. Note the characteristic anterior bowing of the tibia.

Figure 19.29 Osteofibrous dysplasia. Anteroposterior **(A)** and lateral **(B)** radiographs of the right leg in a 2-year-old boy show osteofibrous dysplasia affecting the distal tibia.

Figure 19.30 MRI of osteofibrous dysplasia. (A) Sagittal T1-weighted image shows an oblong lesion involving the anterior cortex of tibia, exhibiting nonhomogeneous, mixed signal intensity (*arrows*). **(B)** Sagittal T1-weighted fat-suppressed sequence after injection of gadolinium shows significant enhancement of the lesion.

Table 19.1 Differential Features of Various Fibroosseous Lesions With Similar Radiographic Appearance

Sex	Age	Location	Radiographic Appearance	Histopathology
		Fibrous Dysplasia		
M/F	Any age (monostotic) First to third decades (polyostotic)	Femoral neck (frequent) Long bones Pelvis Ends of bones usually spared Polyostotic: unilateral in skeleton	Radiolucent, ground-glass, or smoky lesion Thinning of cortex with endosteal scalloping "Shepherd's crook" deformity Accelerated growth	Woven (nonlamellar) type of bone in loose to dense fibrous stroma; bony trabeculae lacking osteoblastic activity ("naked trabeculae")
		Nonossifying Fibroma		
M/F	First to third decades	Long bones (frequently posterior femur)	Radiolucent, eccentric lesion Scalloped, sclerotic border	Whorled pattern of fibrous tissue containing giant cells, hemosiderin, and lipid-filled histiocytes
		Osteofibrous Dysplasia (Kempson-Campanacci Lesion)		
M/F	First to second decades	Tibia (frequently anterior aspect) Fibula Intracortical (frequent)	Osteolytic, eccentric lesion Scalloped, sclerotic border Anterior bowing of long bone	Woven and mature (lamellar) type of bone surrounded by cellular fibrous spindle-cell growth in whorled or matted pattern; bony trabeculae rimmed by osteoblasts ("dressed trabeculae")
		Ossifying Fibroma of Jaw		
F	Third to fourth decades	Mandible (90%) Maxilla	Expansive radiolucent lesion Sclerotic, well defined borders	Uniformly cellular fibrous spindle-cell growth with varying amounts of lamellar bone formation and small, round cementum-like bodies
		Ossifying Fibroma (Sissons Lesion)		
M/F	Second decade	Tibia Humerus	Radiolucent lesion Sclerotic border Similar to osteofibrous dysplasia	Fibrous tissue containing rounded and spindle-shaped cells with scant intercellular collegen and small, partially calcified spherules resembling cementum-like bodies of ossifying fibroma of jaw

might suggest, display a remarkable histopathologic similarity. Like a lesion of fibrous dysplasia, osteofibrous dysplasia is composed of a fibrous background containing deformed trabeculae. These trabeculae, however, unlike those of fibrous dysplasia, display woven bone only in the center, being surrounded by an outer zone of lamellar bone with prominent appositional osteoblastic activity ("dressed trabeculae").

This lesion should not be confused with the lesion, also called ossifying fibroma, that is seen almost exclusively in the jaw (mandible) of women in their third and fourth decades, although it is still uncertain whether some of the latter lesions represent an atypical form of fibrous dysplasia. Sissons and colleagues reported two cases of fibroosseous lesions that differed histologically from osteofibrous dysplasia and fibrous dysplasia. They proposed the term *ossifying fibroma* for these, suggesting that the term *osteofibrous dysplasia* continue to be used for lesions of the tibia and fibula (Kempson-Campanacci lesions). To avoid confusion in terminology, the differential features of the various lesions are summarized in Table 19.1.

A relationship of osteofibrous dysplasia with fibrous dysplasia and adamantinoma has been suggested by some investigators. Although this remains a controversial matter, adamantinoma—a malignant tumor—may contain a fibroosseous component that on pathologic examination resembles both fibrous and osteofibrous dysplasia. Moreover, in recent years, patients have presented with lesions that contained foci of epithelial tissue corresponding to adamantinoma within areas of osteofibrous dysplasia. Czerniak and associates have termed such lesions "differentiated (regressing) adamantinomas." According to these investigators, features characteristic of differentiated adamantinomas include onset during the first two decades of life, an exclusively intracortical location, uniform predominance of oste-

ofibrous dysplasia, and scattered foci of epithelial elements that are identical to those observed in classic adamantinoma. This suggests that a single disease entity may exhibit a spectrum of manifestations with benign osteofibrous dysplasia at one end of the spectrum and malignant adamantinoma at the other end.

Complications and Treatment

Osteofibrous dysplasia is known to be an aggressive lesion that frequently recurs after local excision. According to some researchers, it may coexist with another very aggressive lesion, adamantinoma (see previous discussion).

Desmoplastic Fibroma

Desmoplastic fibroma (also called intraosseous desmoid tumor) is a rare, locally aggressive tumor that occurs in individuals younger than age 40 years, with 50% of all cases occurring in the patient's second decade. It was first described as a distinct entity in 1958 by H. Jaffe. Pain and local swelling are the most common symptoms, but some patients may be asymptomatic. The long bones (femur, tibia, fibula, humerus, and radius), the pelvis, and the mandible are frequent sites of involvement (Fig. 19.31). In the long bones, the lesion occurs in the diaphysis but often extends into the metaphysis. Although the epiphysis is spared, the lesion may extend into the articular end of the bone after closure of the growth plate.

Desmoplastic fibroma has no characteristic radiographic features. The lesion is generally expansive and radiolucent, with sharply

Figure 19.31 Skeletal sites of predilection, peak age range, and male-to-female ratio in desmoplastic fibroma.

defined borders (Fig. 19.32); the cortex of the bone may be thickened or thinned, with no significant periosteal response. Usually a geographic pattern of bone destruction is noted, with narrow zones of transition and nonsclerotic margins (76%). Internal pseudotrabeculation is present in 90% of cases (Fig. 19.33). Pathologic fractures through the tumor are rare (9%). Aggressive lesions of this type are marked by bone destruction and invasion of the soft tissues and may simulate malignant bone tumors (Fig. 19.34).

In addition to conventional radiography, radiologic evaluation of desmoplastic fibroma should include bone scintigraphy, CT, and MRI. Radionuclide bone scan shows an increase in the uptake of the radiopharmaceutical agent at the site of the lesion. CT is useful for evaluating cortical breakthrough and tumor extension into the soft tissues. MRI, also helpful in assessing intraosseous and extraosseous extension, can further characterize the tumor (Fig. 19.35; see also Fig. 19.33). The lesion appears well defined on MR images, exhibiting an intermediate signal intensity on T1-weighting and a heterogeneous pattern on T2-weighting, marked by an area of increased signal intensity mixed with foci of intermediate and low signal intensity. The hypointensity of the signal reflects the dense connective tissue matrix and relative acellularity of the tumor. After intravenous administration of gadolinium contrast, a majority of the lesions demonstrate heterogenous enhancement, with peripheral areas enhancing more intensely than the central portions of the tumor.

Histologically, the lesion is composed of spindle-shaped and occasionally stellate fibroblasts associated with a densely collagenized matrix. Cells are almost always in a smaller proportion to the matrix. The stroma usually contains large, thin-walled vessels similar to those seen in desmoid tumors of soft tissues. Desmoplastic fibroma may be difficult to distinguish from other fibrous tumors, particularly low-grade fibrosarcoma.

Wide excision is the treatment of choice, although the recurrence rate is high even after complete excision of the tumor. Despite this aggressiveness, metastases have never been reported.

Figure 19.32 Desmoplastic fibroma. A radiolucent, trabeculated, sharply marginated lesion occupies the proximal end of the right fibula in a 17-year-old girl. Note lack of periosteal reaction. Excisional biopsy revealed desmoplastic fibroma.

Figure 19.33 Desmoplastic fibroma. A 67-year-old man presented with a large pelvic mass. **(A)** Anteroposterior radiograph of the pelvis demonstrates an expansive trabeculated lytic lesion that involves ischium and pubis and extends into the supra-acetabular portion of the ilium. **(B)** Conventional tomography shows the lytic nature of the tumor and its expansive character. The involvement of ilium is better demonstrated. **(C)** CT section of the tumor through the hip joint shows a lobulated appearance and a thick, sclerotic margin. The lesion extends into the pelvic cavity, displacing the urinary bladder. **(D)** Axial spin-echo T2-weighted MR image (TR 2000/TE 80 msec) demonstrates nonhomogeneity of the signal from the tumor: The bulk of the lesion displays low to intermediate signal intensity with central areas of high signal intensity. An incisional biopsy revealed desmoplastic fibroma. (From Greenspan A, et al., 1992, with permission.)

Figure 19.34 Desmoplastic fibroma. Anteroposterior **(A)** and lateral **(B)** radiographs of the distal forearm in a 31-year-old woman show aggressive destructive lesions involving the radius and ulna, extending into the articular surfaces, complicated by pathologic fractures (*arrows*). Histologic study of an excisional biopsy revealed desmoplastic fibroma.

Figure 19.35 MRI of desmoplastic fibroma. (A) Coronal T1-weighted MRI shows desmoplastic fibroma in the left femoral shaft breaking through the cortex and extending into the soft tissues (*arrows*). **(B)** Axial proton-density MR image demonstrates replacement of the bone marrow by the tumor, soft-tissue involvement, and peritumoral edema. (Courtesy of Prof. Dr. Wolfgang Remagen, Cologne, Germany.)

PRACTICAL POINTS TO REMEMBER

[1] A fibrous cortical defect (metaphyseal fibrous defect) and nonossifying fibroma are closely related lesions of similar histopathologic structure. They differ radiologically only in their size.

[2] Most of these lesions disappear spontaneously. With continued growth they are eccentrically located and display a characteristic scalloped sclerotic border.

[3] Association of disseminated nonossifying fibromatosis with café au lait spots is known the Jaffe-Campanacci syndrome.

[4] Benign fibrous histiocytoma has radiographic features similar to those of nonossifying fibroma; however, it affects older patients, may be symptomatic, and runs a more aggressive clinical course (may recur after surgical treatment).

[5] Periosteal desmoid has a characteristic predilection for the posteromedial cortex of the medial femoral condyle. It should not be mistaken for a malignant bone tumor.

[6] Fibrous dysplasia may be monostotic or polyostotic, with the latter having a decided preference for one side of the skeleton. The polyostotic form, if accompanied by precocious puberty and café au lait spots (with irregular, ragged, or "coast of Maine" borders), is called Albright-McCune syndrome and is seen predominantly in girls.

[7] Association of polyostotic fibrous dysplasia with intramuscular myxomas is known as the Mazabraud syndrome.

[8] Massive formation of cartilage may be observed in fibrous dysplasia, a condition known as fibrocartilaginous dysplasia. This variant can radiographically resemble a cartilaginous neoplasm, such as chondrosarcoma.

[9] Fibrocartilaginous dysplasia (cartilaginous differentiation in fibrous dysplasia) should not be confused with focal fibrocartilaginous dysplasia of long bones, a condition seen predominantly in children and young adults that characteristically affects the proximal tibia.

[10] The best radiologic technique for evaluating the distribution of fibrous dysplasia is radionuclide bone scan.

[11] Osteofibrous dysplasia, a benign fibroosseous lesion seen in children and adolescents, has a decided predilection for the anterior aspect of the tibia. This lesion may be associated with adamantinoma.

[12] Desmoplastic fibroma, a locally aggressive tumor, is frequently marked by bone destruction and invasion of the soft tissues, thus mimicking a malignant neoplasm.

SUGGESTED READINGS

Abdelwahab IF, Kenan S, Herman G, Lewis MM, Klein MJ. Intramuscular myxoma: magnetic resonance features. *Br J Radiol* 1992;65:485–490.

Albright F, Butler AM, Hampton AO, Smith P. Syndrome characterized by osteitis fibrosa disseminata, areas of pigmentation and endocrine dysfunction with precocious puberty in females. *N Engl J Med* 1937;216:727–731.

Alguacil-Garcia A, Alonso A, Pettigrew NM. Osteofibrous dysplasia (ossifying fibroma) of the tibia and fibula and adamantinoma. *Am J Clin Pathol* 1984;82:470–474.

Arata MA, Peterson HA, Dahlin DC. Pathological fractures through non-ossifying fibromas. *J Bone Joint Surg [Am]* 1981;63A:980–988.

Bahk W-J, Kang Y-K, Lee A-H, Mirra JM. Desmoid tumor of bone with enchondromatous nodules, mistaken for chondrosarcoma. *Skeletal Radiol* 2003;32:223–226.

Bancroft LW, Kransdorf MJ, Menke DM, O'Connor MI, Foster WC. Intramuscular myxoma: characteristic MR imaging features. *AJR Am J Roentgenol* 2002;178:1255–1259.

Barnes GR Jr, Gwinn JL. Distal irregularities of the femur simulating malignancy. *AJR Am J Roentgenol* 1974;122:180–185.

Bertoni F, Calderoni P, Bacchini P, Campanacci M. Desmoplastic fibroma of bone: a report of six cases. *J Bone Joint Surg [Br]* 1984;66B:265–268.

Bertoni F, Calderoni P, Bacchini P, Sudanese A. Benign fibrous histiocytoma of bone. *J Bone Joint Surg [Am]* 1986;68A:1225–1230.

Bertoni F, Unni KK, McLeod RA, Sim FH. Xanthoma of bone. *Am J Pathol* 1988;90:377–384.

Blau RA, Zwick DL, Westphal RA. Multiple nonossifying fibromas. *J Bone Joint Surg [Am]* 1988;70A:299–304.

Brower AC, Culver JE Jr, Keats TE. Histological nature of the cortical irregularity of the medial posterior distal femoral metaphysis in children. *Radiology* 1971;99:389–392.

Bufkin WJ. The avulsive cortical irregularity. *AJR Am J Roentgenol* 1971;112:487–492.

Bullough PG, Vigorita VJ. *Atlas of orthopaedic pathology with clinical and radiologic correlations*, 2nd ed. New York, Gowen Medical Publishing; 1992.

Cabral CEL, Guedes P, Fonseca T, Rezende JF, Cruz Jr LC, Smith J. Polyostotic fibrous dysplasia associated with intramuscular myxomas: Mazabraud's syndrome. *Skeletal Radiol* 1998;27:278–282.

Caffey J. On fibrous defects in cortical walls of growing tubular bone: their radiologic appearance, structure prevalence, natural course and diagnostic significance. *Adv Pediatr* 1955;7:13–51.

Camilleri AE. Craniofacial fibrous dysplasia. *J Laryngol Otol* 1991;105:662–666.

Campanacci M. Osteofibrous dysplasia of the long bones. A new clinical entity. *Ital J Orthop Traumatol* 1976;2:221–237.

Campanacci M, Laus M. Osteofibrous dysplasia of the tibia and fibula. *J Bone Joint Surg [Am]* 1981;63A:367–375.

Campanacci M, Laus M, Boriani S. Multiple non-ossifying fibromata with extraskeletal anomalies: a new syndrome? *J Bone Joint Surg [Br]* 1983;65-B:627–632.

Campbell CJ, Hawk T. A variant of fibrous dysplasia (osteofibrous dysplasia). *J Bone Joint Surg [Am]* 1982;64A:231–236.

Choi IH, Kim CJ, Cho T-J, Chung CY, Song KS, Hwang JK, Sohn YJ. Focal fibrocartilaginous dysplasia of long bones: report of eight additional cases and literature review. *J Ped Orthop* 2000;20:421–427.

Clarke BE, Xipell JM, Thomas DP. Benign fibrous histiocytoma of bone. *Am J Surg Pathol* 1985;9:806–815.

Cohen DM, Dahlin DC, Pugh DG. Fibrous dysplasia associated with adamantinoma of the long bones. *Cancer* 1962;15:515–521.

Creagh MF, Nunan TO. Positive Gallium-67 citrate uptake in a patient with polyostotic fibrous dysplasia. *Clin Nucl Med* 1988;13:241–242.

Crim JR, Gold RH, Mirra JM, Eckardt JJ, Bassett LW. Desmoplastic fibroma of bone: radiographic analysis. *Radiology* 1989;172:827–832.

Cunningham BJ, Ackerman LV. Metaphyseal fibrous defects. *J Bone Joint Surg* 1956;38:797–808.

Czerniak B, Rojas-Corona RR, Dorfman HD. Morphologic diversity of long bone adamantinoma. The concept of differentiated (regressing) adamantinoma and its relationship to osteofibrous dysplasia. *Cancer* 1989;64:2319–2334.

Dahlin DC, Unni KK. *Bone tumors: general aspects and data on 8,542 cases*, 4th ed. Springfield, IL: Charles C Thomas, 1986:141–148.

DeSmet A, Travers H, Neff JR. Chondrosarcoma occurring in a patient with polyostotic fibrous dysplasia. *Skeletal Radiol* 1981;7:197–201.

Dominok GW, Eisengarten W. Benignes fibroeses Histiozytom des Knochens. *Zentralbl Pathol* 1980;124:77–83.

Dorfman HD, Ishida T, Tsuneyoshi M. Exophytic variant of fibrous dysplasia (fibrous dysplasia protuberans). *Hum Pathol* 1994;25:1234–1237.

Evans GA, Park WM. Familial multiple non-osteogenic fibromata. *J Bone Joint Surg [Br]* 1978;60B:416–419.

Friedland JA, Reinus WR, Fisher AJ, Wilson AJ. Quantitative analysis of the plain radiographic appearance of nonossifying fibroma. *Invest Radiol* 1995;30:474–479.

Gebhardt MC, Campbell CJ, Schiller AL, Mankin HJ. Desmoplastic fibroma of bone. A report of eight cases and review of the literature. *J Bone Joint Surg [Am]* 1985;67A:732–747.

Greenspan A, Unni KK. Case report 787. Desmoplastic fibroma. *Skeletal Radiol* 1993;22:296–299.

Gross ML, Soberman N, Dorfman HD, Seimon LP. Case report 556. Multiple nonossifying fibromas of long bones in a patient with neurofibromatosis. *Skeletal Radiol* 1989;18:389–391.

Hamada T, Ito H, Araki Y, Fujii K, Inoue M, Ishida O. Benign fibrous histiocytoma of the femur: review of three cases. *Skeletal Radiol* 1996;25:25–29.

Henschen F. Fall von Ostitis fibrosa mit multiplen Tumoren in der umgebenden Muskulatur. *Verh Dtsch Ges Pathol* 1926;21:93–97.

Hermann G, Klein M, Abdelwahab IF, Kenan S. Fibrocartilaginous dysplasia. *Skeletal Radiol* 1996;25:509–511.

Hoshi H, Futami S, Ohnishi T, Nagamachi S, Jinnouchi S, Murai N, Watanabe K. Gallium-67 uptake in fibrous dysplasia of the bone. *Ann Nucl Med* 1990;4:35–38.

Hudson TM, Stiles RG, Monson DK. Fibrous lesions of bone. *Radiol Clin North Am* 1993;31:279–297.

Huvos A. *Bone tumors: diagnosis, treatment and prognosis*, 2nd ed. Philadelphia: WB Saunders; 1991:677–693.

Huvos AG, Higinbotham NL, Miller TR. Bone sarcomas arising in fibrous dysplasia. *J Bone Joint Surg [Am]* 1972;54A:1047–1056.

Inamo Y, Hanawa Y, Kin H, Okuni M. Findings on magnetic resonance imaging of the spine and femur in a case of McCune-Albright syndrome. *Pediatr Radiol* 1993;23:15–18.

Inwards CY, Unni KK, Beabout JW, Sim FH. Desmoplastic fibroma of bone. *Cancer* 1991;68:1978–1983.

Ishida T, Dorfman HD. Massive chondroid differentiation in fibrous dysplasia of bone (fibrocartilaginous dysplasia). *Am J Surg Pathol* 1993;17:924–930.

Iwasko N, Steinbach LS, Disler D, et al. Imaging findings in Mazabraud's syndrome: seven new cases. *Skeletal Radiol* 2002;31:81–87.

Jaffe HL. Fibrous cortical defect and non-ossifying fibroma. In: *Tumors and tumorous conditions of the bones and joints*. Philadelphia: Lea & Febiger; 1958:76–91.

Jaffe HL, Lichtenstein L. Non-osteogenic fibroma of bone. *Am J Pathol* 1942;18:205–221.

Jee W-H, Choe B-Y, Kang H-S, Suh K-J, Suh J-S, Ryu K-N, Lee Y-S, Ok I-Y, Kim J-M, Choi K-H, Shinn K-S. Nonossifying fibroma: characteristics at MR imaging with pathologic correlation. *Radiology* 1998;209:197–202.

Jee W-H, Choi K-H, Choe B-Y, Park J-M, Shinn K-S. Fibrous dysplasia: MR imaging characteristics with radiopathologic correlations. *AJR Am J Roentgenol* 1996;167: 1523–1527.

Johnson CB, Gilbert EE, Gottlieb LI. Malignant transformation of polyostotic fibrous dysplasia. *South Med J* 1979;72:353–356.

Kahn LB. Adamantinoma, osteofibrous dysplasia and differentiated adamantinoma. *Skeletal Radiol* 2003;32:245–258.

Kaushik S, Smoker WRK, Frable WJ. Malignant transformation of fibrous dysplasia into chondroblastic osteosarcoma. *Skeletal Radiol* 2002;31:103–106.

Keeney GL, Unni KK, Beabout JW, Pritchard DJ. Adamantinoma of long bones. *Cancer* 1989;64:730–737.

Kempson RL. Ossifying fibroma of the long bones. A light and electron microscopic study. *Arch Pathol* 1966;82:218–233.

Kimmelstiel P, Rapp I. Cortical defect due to periosteal desmoids. *Bull Hosp Joint Dis* 1951;12:286–297.

Kransdorf MJ, Moser RP, Gilkey FW. Fibrous dysplasia. *Radiographics* 1990;10:519–537.

Kransdorf MJ, Murphey MD. Case 12: Mazabraud syndrome. *Radiology* 1999;212: 129–132.

Kransdorf MJ, Murphey MD, Sweet DE. Liposclerosing myxofibrous tumor: a radiologic-pathologic-distinct fibro-osseous lesion of bone with a marked predilection for the intertrochanteric region of the femur. *Radiology* 1999;212:693–698.

Kransdorf MJ, Utz JA, Gilkey FW, Berrey BH. MR appearance of fibroxanthoma. *J Comput Assist Tomogr* 1988;12:612–615.

Kumar R, Madewell JE, Lindell MM, Swischuk LE. Fibrous lesions of bones. *Radiographics* 1990;10:237–256.

Kumar R, Swischuk LE, Madewell JE. Benign cortical defect: site for an avulsion fracture. *Skeletal Radiol* 1986;15:553–555.

Kyriakos M, McDonald DJ, Sundaram M. Fibrous dysplasia with cartilaginous differentiation ("fibrocartilaginous dysplasia"): a review, with an illustrative case followed for 18 years. *Skeletal Radiol* 2004;33:51–62.

Levine SM, Lambiase RE, Petchprapa CN. Cortical lesions of the tibia: characteristic appearances at conventional radiography. *Radiographics* 2003;23:157–177.

Lichtenstein L, Jaffe HL. Fibrous dysplasia of bone. *Arch Pathol* 1942;33:777–816.

Lichtman EA, Klein MJ. Case report 302. Desmoplastic fibroma of the proximal end of the left femur. *Skeletal Radiol* 1985;13:160–163.

Machida K, Makita K, Nishikawa J, Ohtake T, Ilio M. Scintigraphic manifestation of fibrous dysplasia. *Clin Nucl Med* 1986;11:426–429.

Markel SF. Ossifying fibroma of long bone. *Am J Clin Pathol* 1978;69:91–97.

Matsuno T. Benign fibrous histiocytoma involving the ends of long bone. *Skeletal Radiol* 1990;19:561–566.

Mazabraud A, Semat P, Roze R. A propos de l'association de fibromyxomes des tissus mous à la dysplasie fibreuse des os. *Presse Med* 1967;75:2223–2228.

Mesiter P, Konrad E, Hohne N. Incidence and histological structure of the storiform pattern in benign and malignant fibrous histiocytomas. *Virchows Arch [A]* 1981;393: 93–101.

Mirra JM. Fibrohistiocytic tumors of intramedullary origin. In: Mirra JM, Picci P, Gold RH, eds. *Bone tumors: clinical, pathologic, and radiologic correlations.* Philadelphia: Lea & Febiger; 1989:691–799.

Mirra JM, Gold RH. Fibrous dysplasia. In: Mirra JM, Picci P, Gold RH, eds. *Bone tumors.* Philadelphia: Lea & Febiger; 1989:191–226.

Mirra JM, Gold RH, Rand F. Disseminated nonossifying fibromas in association with café-au-lait spots (Jaffe-Campanacci Syndrome). *Clin Orthop* 1982;168:192–205.

Moser RP Jr, Sweet DE, Haseman DB, Madewell JE. Multiple skeletal fibroxanthomas: Radiologic-pathologic correlation of 72 cases. *Skeletal Radiol* 1987;16:353–359.

Mulder JD, Schütte HE, Kroon HM, Taconis WK. *Radiologic atlas of bone tumors.* Amsterdam: Elsevier, 1993:607–625.

Murphey MD, McRae GA, Fanburg-Smith JC, Temple HT, Levine AM, Aboulafia AJ. Imaging of soft-tissue myxoma with emphasis on CT and MR and comparison of radiologic and pathologic findings. *Radiology* 2002;225:215–224.

Okada K, Yoshida S, Okane K, Sageshima M. Cystic fibrous dysplasia mimicking giant cell tumor: MRI appearance. *Skeletal Radiol* 2000;29:45–48.

Park Y, Unni KK, McLeod RA, Pritchard DJ. Osteofibrous dysplasia: clinicopathologic study of 80 cases. *Hum Pathol* 1993;24:1339–1347.

Pennes DR, Braunstein EM, Glazer GM. Computed tomography of cortical desmoid. *Skeletal Radiol* 1984;12:40–42.

Rabhan WN, Rosai J. Desmoplastic fibroma. Report of ten cases and review of the literature. *J Bone J Surg [Am]* 1968;50A:487–502.

Ragsdale BD. Polymorphic fibro-osseous lesions of bone: an almost site-specific diagnostic problem of the proximal femur. *Hum Pathol* 1993;24:505–512.

Resnick D, Greenway G. Distal femoral cortical defects, irregularities, and excavations: A critical review of the literature with the addition of histologic and paleopathologic data. *Radiology* 1982;143:345–354.

Riley GM, Greenspan A, Poirier VC. Fibrous dysplasia of a parietal bone. *J Comput Assist Tomogr* 1997;21:41–43.

Ritschl P, Hajek PC, Pechmann U. Fibrous metaphyseal defects. Magnetic resonance imaging appearances. *Skeletal Radiol* 1989;18:253–259.

Ritschl P, Karnel F, Hajek PC. Fibrous metaphyseal defects—determination of their origin and natural history using a radiomorphological study. *Skeletal Radiol* 1988; 17:8–15.

Robbin MR, Murphey MD, Temple HT, Kransdorf MJ, Choi JJ. Imaging of musculoskeletal fibromatosis. *Radiographics* 2001;21:585–600

Ruggieri P, Sim FH, Bond JA, Unni KK. Malignancies in fibrous dysplasia. *Cancer* 1994;73:1411–1424.

Schajowicz F. Histological typing of bone tumors. *World Health Organization International Histological Classification of Tumors.* Berlin: Springer-Verlag; 1993.

Schajowicz F. *Tumors and tumorlike lesions of bone. Pathology, radiology, and treatment,* 2nd ed. Berlin: Springer-Verlag; 1994.

Schajowicz F, Sissons HA, Sobin LH. The World Health Organization's histologic classification of bone tumors. A commentary on the second edition. *Cancer* 1995;75:1208–1214.

Schwartz AM, Ramos RM. Neurofibromatosis and multiple nonossifying fibroma. *AJR Am J Roentgenol* 1980;135:617–619.

Schwartz DT, Alpert M. The malignant transformation of fibrous dysplasia. *Am J Med Sci* 1964;247:1–20.

Selby S. Metaphyseal cortical defects in the tubular bones of growing children. *J Bone Joint Surg [Am]* 1961;43A:395–400.

Shelton III CH, Nimityongskul P, Richardson PH, Brogdon BG. Progressive painful bowing of the right leg. *Acad Radiol* 1995;2:351–353.

Sissons HA, Kancherla PL, Lehman WB. Ossifying fibroma of bone. Report of two cases. *Bull Hosp Joint Dis Orthop Inst* 1983;43:1–14.

Spjut HJ, Dorfman HD, Fechner RE, Ackerman LV. *Tumors of bone pathology. Atlas of tumor pathology,* 2nd series, Fascicle 5. Washington, DC: Armed Forces Institute of Pathology; 1971:249–292.

Springfield DS, Rosenberg AE, Mankin HJ, Mindell ER. Relationship between osteofibrous dysplasia and adamantinoma. *Clin Orthop* 1994;309:234–244.

Steiner GC. Fibrous cortical defect and non-ossifying fibroma of bone: a study of the ultrastructure. *Arch Pathol* 1974;97:205–210.

Sugiura I. Desmoplastic fibroma. Case report and review of the literature. *J Bone Joint Surg [Am]* 1976;58A:126–130.

Sundaram M, McDonald DJ, Merenda G. Intramuscular myxoma: A rare but important association with fibrous dysplasia of bone. *AJR Am J Roentgenol* 1989;153:107–108.

Sweet DE, Vinh TN, Devaney K. Cortical osteofibrous dysplasia of long bone and its relationship to adamantinoma. *Am J Surg Pathol* 1992;16:282–290.

Taconis WK, Schütte HE, van der Heul RO. Desmoplastic fibroma of bone: a report of 18 cases. *Skeletal Radiol* 1994;23:283–288.

Totty WG, Murphy WA, Lee JKT. Soft tissue tumors: MR imaging. *Radiology* 1986;160:135–141.

Ueda Y, Blasius S, Edel G, Wuisman P, Bocker W, Roessner A. Osteofibrous dysplasia of long bones—a reactive process to adamantinomatous tissue. *J Cancer Clin Oncol* 1992;118:152–156.

Unni KK. Fibrous and fibrohistiocytic lesions of bone. *Semin Orthop* 1991;6:177–186.

Unni KK, Dahlin DC, Beabout JW, Ivins JC. Adamantinoma of long bones. *Cancer* 1974;34:1796–1805.

Utz JA, Kransdorf MJ, Jelinek JS, Moser RP, Berrey BH. MR appearance of fibrous dysplasia. *J Comput Assist Tomogr* 1989;13:845–851.

Vanhoenacker FM, Hauben E, De Beuckeleer LH, Willemen D, Van Marck E, De Schepper AM. Desmoplastic fibroma of bone: MRI features. *Skeletal Radiol* 2000;29: 171–175.

Velchik MG, Heyman S, Makler PT Jr, Goldstein HA, Alavi A. Bone scintigraphy: differentiating benign cortical irregularity of the distal femur from malignancy. *J Nucl Med* 1984;25:72–74.

Wang J, Shih C, Chen W. Osteofibrous dysplasia (ossifying fibromas of long bones). *Clin Orthop* 1992;278:235–243.

Weiss SW, Dorfman HD. Adamantinoma of long bones. *Hum Pathol* 1977;8:141–153.

Wold LE. Fibrohistiocytic tumors of bone. In: Unni KK, ed. *Bone tumors.* New York: Churchill Livingstone; 1988:183–197.

Yabut SM, Kenan S, Sissons HA, Lewis MM. Malignant transformation of fibrous dysplasia. *Clin Orthop* 1988;228:281–289.

Yamazaki T, Maruoka S, Takahashi S, Saito H, Takase K, Nakamura M, Sakamoto K. MR findings of avulsive cortical irregularity of the distal femur. *Skeletal Radiol* 1995;24:43–46.

You JS, Lawrence S, Pathria M, Resnick D, Haghighi P. Desmoplastic fibroma of the calcaneus. *Skeletal Radiol* 1995;24:451–454.

Young JWR, Aisner SC, Levine AM, Resnik CS, Dorfman HD. Computed tomography of desmoid tumors of bone: desmoplastic fibroma. *Skeletal Radiol* 1988;17:333–337.

BENIGN TUMORS AND TUMOR-LIKE LESIONS IV

Miscellaneous Lesions

Simple Bone Cyst

The simple bone cyst, also called a unicameral bone cyst, is a tumor-like lesion of unknown cause. It has been attributed to a local disturbance of bone growth. More common in males than in females, it is ordinarily seen during the first two decades of life. The majority of simple bone cysts are located in the proximal diaphysis of the humerus and femur, especially in patients younger than age 17 years (Fig. 20.1) In older patients, the incidence of bone cysts in atypical sites such as the calcaneus (Fig. 20.2), talus, and ilium increases significantly. Radiographically, a simple bone cyst appears as a radiolucent, centrally located, well-circumscribed lesion with sclerotic margins (Figs. 20.3 and 20.4). There is no periosteal reaction, a feature distinguishing a simple bone cyst from an aneurysmal bone cyst, which invariably shows some degree of periosteal response; however, in the presence of pathologic fracture, there is periosteal reaction. Conventional radiography usually suffices to make a diagnosis. Mag-

netic resonance imaging (MRI) of a simple bone cyst shows the signal characteristics of fluid: a low-to-intermediate signal on T1-weighted images and a bright, homogeneous signal on T2 weighting (Fig. 20.5).

Histologically, a simple bone cyst is a diagnosis of exclusion. A surgical curettage yields almost no solid tissue, but the walls of the cavity may show remnants of fibrous tissue or a flattened single-cell lining. The fluid content of the cyst contains elevated levels of alkaline phosphatase.

Complications and Differential Diagnosis

The most common complication of a simple bone cyst is pathologic fracture, which occurs in approximately 66% of cases (Fig. 20.6). Occasionally, one can identify a piece of fractured cortex in the interior of the lesion—the "fallen fragment" sign—indicating that the lesion is either hollow or fluid-filled, as most simple bone cysts are. This sign permits the differentiation of a bone cyst, particularly in a slender

Figure 20.2 Simple bone cyst. Lateral radiograph of the hindfoot **(A)** and Harris-Beath view of the calcaneus **(B)** in a 32-year-old man show a simple bone cyst in the os calcis. Typically, bone cysts occurring at this site are located in the anterolateral aspect of the bone, as shown here.

Figure 20.1 Skeletal sites of predilection, peak age range, and male-to-female ratio in simple bone cyst. The left half of the skeleton shows unusual sites of occurrence seen in an older patient population.

Figure 20.3 Simple bone cyst. Anteroposterior view of the right shoulder demonstrates the typical appearance of a simple bone cyst in a 6-year-old boy. Its location in the metaphysis and the proximal diaphysis of the humerus is also characteristic. The radiolucent lesion is centrally located and shows pseudosepta. Note the slight thinning of the cortex and lack of periosteal reaction.

Figure 20.4 Simple bone cyst. Anteroposterior radiograph of the left hip of an 11-year-old girl shows characteristic features of this lesion. Note the central location, narrow zone of transition, geographic type of bone destruction, pseudotrabeculation, and lack of periosteal reaction.

Figure 20.5 MRI of simple bone cyst. (A) Lateral radiograph of the foot of an 18-year-old man shows a radiolucent lesion in the calcaneus with a slightly sclerotic border. **(B)** Sagittal T1-weighted (SE; TR 850/TE 15 msec) MR image demonstrates homogeneous intermediate signal intensity within the lesion, rimmed by low signal intensity sclerotic margin. *(continued)*

Figure 20.5 MRI of simple bone cyst. *Continued.* **(C)** Sagittal STIR MR image shows that the lesion now is of homogeneous high signal intensity. (From Greenfield GB and Arrington JA, 1995, with permission.)

bone, such as the fibula (Fig. 20.7), from other radiolucent, radiographically similar lesions containing solid fibrous or cartilaginous tissue, such as fibrous dysplasia, nonossifying fibroma, or enchondroma (Fig. 20.8). A bone abscess may occasionally mimic a simple bone cyst, particularly if located in the upper humerus or upper femur, the sites of predilection for simple bone cysts. In such cases, the presence of a periosteal reaction and extension beyond the growth plate are important differentiating features favoring a bone abscess (Fig. 20.9). On rare occasions, an intraosseous ganglion may be mistaken for a simple bone cyst (Fig. 20.10).

Treatment

The treatment of simple bone cysts is based on the premise that the induction of osteogenesis results in complete healing of the lesion. The simplest inducement for bone repair is fracture, but this alone is insufficient to obliterate the lesion completely, and simple bone cysts usually do not disappear after spontaneous fracture. The most common treatment is curettage followed by grafting with small pieces of cancellous bone. With this procedure, however, there is a higher rate of recurrence in patients younger than age 10 years. Moreover, this approach may lead to damage to the growth plate, because most solitary bone cysts occur about the physis. Recently, Scaglietti reported treating bone cysts with simple injection of methylprednisolone acetate. In younger patients so treated, complete bone repair occurred more rapidly than in older patients, who sometimes had to be administered several injections.

Aneurysmal Bone Cyst

The term aneurysmal bone cyst (ABC) was first used by Jaffe and Lichtenstein to describe two examples of blood-filled cysts in which tissue from the cyst wall contained conspicuous spaces, areas of

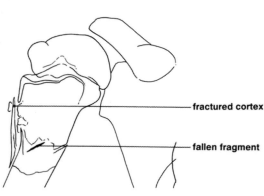

fractured cortex

fallen fragment

Figure 20.6 Simple bone cyst with pathologic fracture. One of the most common complications of simple bone cyst is pathologic fracture, as seen here in the proximal humeral metadiaphysis in a 6-year-old boy. The presence of the "fallen fragment" sign is characteristic of a simple bone cyst.

Figure 20.7 Fallen-fragment sign. Anteroposterior view demonstrates a radiolucent lesion in the distal diaphysis of the right fibula of a 5-year-old boy who sustained mild injury to the lower leg. Note the pathologic fracture through the lesion and the associated periosteal reaction. A radiodense cortical fragment in the center of the lesion represents the "fallen fragment" sign, identifying this lesion as a simple bone cyst.

Figure 20.8 Nonossifying fibroma. Anteroposterior radiograph of the right shoulder of a 10-year-old boy shows a radiolucent lesion in the metadiaphyseal region of the humerus, slightly eccentric in location, with a narrow zone of transition and a geographic type of bone destruction. The lateral cortex is significantly thinned and bulging. The lesion was believed to be a simple bone cyst; however, excisional biopsy revealed a nonossifying fibroma.

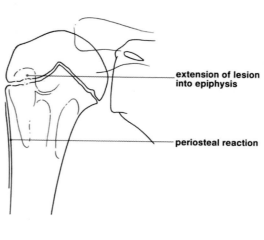

Figure 20.9 Bone abscess. A bone abscess may mimic a simple bone cyst, as seen here in the proximal humerus of a 12-year-old boy. The periosteal reaction in the absence of pathologic fracture and the extension of the lesion into the epiphysis favors the diagnosis of bone abscess.

Figure 20.10 Intraosseous ganglion. An 18-year-old woman presented with left shoulder pain. Anteroposterior radiograph shows a radiolucent, trabeculated lesion in the glenoid, with the appearance of a simple bone cyst. Excisional biopsy was consistent with an intraosseous ganglion (see also Fig. 16.24A).

hemosiderin deposition, giant cells, and occasional bone trabeculae. In a subsequent publication, Jaffe chose the designation aneurysmal bone cyst as a descriptive term for this lesion to emphasize the blown-out appearance. Although the cause of this lesion is unknown, alterations in local hemodynamics related to venous obstruction or arteriovenous fistula are believed to play an important role. Some investigators believe that the lesion is caused by a trauma. Dahlin and McLeod believe that it may be similar to and related to other reactive nonneoplastic processes, such as giant-cell reparative granuloma or traumatic reactions observed in periosteum and bone. ABC may arise *de novo* in bone, in which case no recognizable preexisting lesion can be demonstrated in the tissue, or it may be associated with various benign (e.g., giant-cell tumor, osteoblastoma, chondroblastoma, chondromyxoid fibroma, fibrous dysplasia) and malignant (e.g., osteosarcoma, fibrosarcoma, or chondrosarcoma) lesions. The concept of ABC as a secondary phenomenon occurring in a preexisting lesion has been validated by several researchers. Some investigators, however, regard ABC as a reparative process, probably the result of trauma or tumor-induced anomalous vascular process.

ABC constitutes approximately 6% of the primary lesions of bone and is seen predominantly in children; 90% of these lesions occur in patients younger than age 20 years. The metaphysis of long bones is a frequent site of predilection, although aneurysmal bone cysts may sometimes be seen in the diaphysis of a long bone, as well as in flat bones such as the scapula or pelvis and even in the vertebrae (Fig. 20.11). As already stated, these lesions can develop *de novo* or as a result of cystic changes in a preexisting lesion such as a chondroblastoma, osteoblastoma, giant cell tumor, or fibrous dysplasia (Fig. 20.12). The radiographic hallmark of an aneurysmal bone cyst is multicystic eccentric expansion (blow-out) of the bone, with a buttress or thin shell of periosteal response (Figs. 20.13 to 20.15). Although conventional radiographs usually suffice for evaluating the lesion, conventional tomography, computed tomography (CT), and radionuclide bone scan can be of further assistance. CT is particu-

larly helpful in determining the integrity of the cortex (Fig. 20.16). CT may also show internal ridges described on radiography as trabeculation or septation (Fig. 20.17). Fluid-fluid levels can also be demonstrated by this technique. These fluid levels are believed to

Figure 20.11 Skeletal sites of predilection, peak age range, and male-to-female ratio in aneurysmal bone cyst.

Figure 20.12 Secondary aneurysmal bone cyst. A 14-year-old boy had a painless swelling on the dorsum of the left hand. Dorsovolar film of the hand shows an expansive lesion in the distal segment of the third metacarpal. The lesion exhibits a well-organized periosteal reaction; the articular end of the bone is spared. Biopsy revealed an aneurysmal bone cyst engrafted on a monostotic focus of fibrous dysplasia.

Figure 20.13 Aneurysmal bone cyst. Anteroposterior **(A)** and lateral **(B)** radiographs of the lower leg in an 8-year-old girl with a history of lower leg pain demonstrate an expansive radiolucent lesion in the metaphysis of the distal tibia, extending into the diaphysis. Note its eccentric location in the bone and the buttress of periosteal response at the proximal aspect of the lesion. Biopsy revealed an aneurysmal bone cyst.

Figure 20.14 Aneurysmal bone cyst. Anteroposterior **(A)** and lateral **(B)** radiographs of the left proximal tibia of a 10-year-old girl show characteristic appearance of ABC, including eccentric location, expansive character, and a buttress of solid periosteal reaction proximally and distally (*arrows*).

Figure 20.15 Aneurysmal bone cyst. A large, radiolucent expansive lesion in the proximal fibula of an 11-year-old girl reveals a buttress of periosteal reaction (*arrows*).

Figure 20.16 Aneurysmal bone cyst. (A) Radiograph of the distal femur of an 8-year-old boy with a 6-month history of pain in the lower right thigh demonstrates a radiolucent expansive lesion located eccentrically in the femur and buttressed proximally and distally by a solid periosteal reaction, radiographic features consistent with an aneurysmal bone cyst. **(B)** CT section shows its intracortical location; the lesion balloons out from the lateral aspect of the femur but is contained within a thin uninterrupted shell of periosteal new bone. **(C)** Radionuclide bone scan obtained after injection of 10 mCi (375 MBq) of technetium-99m-labeled diphosphonate demonstrates increased uptake of radiopharmaceutical by the lesion.

represent the sedimentation of red blood cells and serum within the cystic cavities. To demonstrate this phenomenon, the patient must remain motionless for at least 10 minutes before scanning, and imaging must be performed in a plane perpendicular to the fluid levels.

MRI findings are rather characteristic and usually allow a specific diagnosis of ABC. These include a well-defined lesion, often with lobulated contours, cystic cavities with fluid–fluid levels, multiple internal septations, and an intact rim of low-intensity signal surrounding the lesion (Figs. 20.18 to 20.22). This rim has been described as an indicator of a benign process. The wide range of signal intensities within the cyst on T1- and T2-weighted sequences is probably caused by settling of degraded blood products and reflects intracystic hemorrhages of different ages.

Histologically, the ABC consists of multiple blood-filled sinusoid spaces alternating with more solid areas. The solid tissue is composed of fibrous elements containing numerous multinucleated giant cells and is richly vascular. The sinusoids have fibrous walls, often containing osteoid tissue or even mature bone. Focal or diffuse collections of hemosiderin or reactive foam cells may be seen in the fibrous septa.

Complications and Differential Diagnosis

The most common complication of an aneurysmal bone cyst is a pathologic fracture.

The conditions that should always be included in the differential diagnosis at any age are simple bone cyst (SBC), chondromyxoid fibroma, and giant cell tumor, which occurs after skeletal maturity when the lesion extends into the articular end of bone. The most critical points in differentiation of ABC from SBC are that the former is an eccentric, expansive lesion, invariably associated with some degree of periosteal reaction (usually a solid layer or solid buttress). The latter is a centrally located lesion, showing little if any expansion and exhibiting periosteal reaction only when a pathologic fracture has occurred. In thin bones, such as the ulna, fibula, metacarpals, or metatarsals, the characteristic eccentricity of ABC may be lost and, conversely, SBC may demonstrate expansive features (Fig. 20.23). Because the former contains solid tissue whereas SBC is a hollow structure filled with fluid, a fallen fragment sign (if present) is a good differential feature, pointing to the latter diagnosis. Chondromyxoid fibroma may be indistinguishable from ABC because both lesions are eccentric, expansive, and usually affect the metaphysis, exhibiting a

Figure 20.17 CT of aneurysmal bone cyst. Lateral **(A)** and oblique **(B)** radiographs of the right ankle of a 24-year-old woman show a radiolucent, trabeculated lesion in the talus. Coronal anterior **(C)** and coronal posterior **(D)** CT sections demonstrate the internal ridges of an aneurysmal bone cyst.

reactive sclerotic rim and the aforementioned solid periosteal reaction (usually in the form of a buttress). CT and MRI are sometimes effective in making this distinction if they identify fluid–fluid levels, a phenomenon that points to the diagnosis of ABC because chondromyxoid fibroma is a solid lesion. In the mature skeleton, giant cell tumor may closely mimic ABC, although it usually is not associated with a periosteal reaction and rarely exhibits a zone of reactive sclerosis. Giant cell reparative granuloma (so-called solid aneurysmal bone cyst) may be indistinguishable from the conventional ABC. This lesion, however, unlike true ABC, usually involves the short tubular bones of the hands and feet. The cortex is thin but is characteristically intact. Extension into the surrounding soft tissues is distinctly uncommon, and the periosteal reaction is usually absent (see later). In thinner bones, such as the fibula, metacarpals, or metatarsals, ABC caused by expansive growth may destroy the cortex, mimicking an aggressive tumor such as telangiectatic osteosarcoma. Conversely, it is important to remember that at times a telangiectatic osteosarcoma may masquerade as an ABC. Histopathologic differentiation is critical in these situations.

Treatment

The treatment for aneurysmal bone cyst consists of surgical removal of the entire lesion. At times, bone grafting to repair the resulting defect may be necessary (Fig. 20.24). Recently, percutaneous injections of Ethiblock®, an alcoholic (ethanol) solution of corn protein which has thrombogenic and fibrogenic properties, have been advocated. Recurrence of the lesion, however, is frequent.

Solid Variant of Aneurysmal Bone Cyst

In 1983, Sanerkin and colleagues described a variant of aneurysmal bone cyst in which the predominant histology was that of the solid components of a conventional aneurysmal bone cyst. The histopathologic appearance of this lesion was very similar to that of another condition, reported originally by Jaffe in 1953 and later by Lorenzo and Dorfman in 1980, that represented a nonneoplastic hemorrhagic process in bones, termed *giant cell reparative granuloma.*

Figure 20.18 MRI of aneurysmal bone cyst. (A) Anteroposterior radiograph of the left hip of a 4-year-old girl shows an expansive radiolucent lesion destroying the ischial bone (*arrows*). **(B)** CT section demonstrates that the lesion broke through the medial cortex (*open arrow*). **(C)** Axial T2-weighted MR image shows the lesion to be of high signal intensity. Multiple fluid-fluid levels characteristic of an aneurysmal bone cyst are well demonstrated.

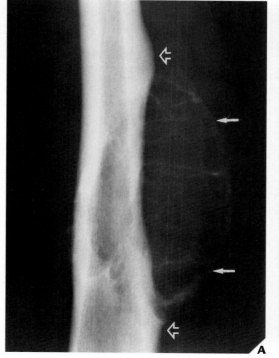

Figure 20.19 MRI of aneurysmal bone cyst. Anteroposterior **(A)** and lateral **(B)** radiographs of the midshaft of right femur of a 15-year-old girl show an expansive lesion arising eccentrically from the medial aspect of the bone. Note a thin shell of periosteal bone covering the lesion (*arrows*) and a buttress of periosteal reaction at its proximal and distal extent (*open arrows*), characteristic for aneurysmal bone cyst. (*continued*)

Figure 20.19 MRI of aneurysmal bone cyst. *Continued.* (C), (D) Coronal T1-weighted (SE; TR 600/TE 20 msec) MR images demonstrate nonhomogeneity of the lesion and internal septations. Axial T1-weighted **(E)** and T2-weighted **(F)** images show fluid-fluid levels (*arrowheads*).

Figure 20.20 MRI of aneurysmal bone cyst. (A) Radiograph of the right forearm of a 10-year-old boy shows a radiolucent lesion in the mid-diaphysis of the ulna exhibiting a narrow zone of transition and periosteal reaction. **(B)** Coronal T1-weighted MR image shows expansive lesion of low signal intensity (*arrow*). **(C)** Coronal proton-density MR image shows soft tissue extension (*arrow*). **(D)** Sagittal T2-weighted image demonstrates high signal of fluid and internal septa. **(E)** Axial T2-weighted image shows cortical breakthrough and soft-tissue extension of the lesion and peritumoral edema (*open arrows*). An excision biopsy revealed an aneurysmal bone cyst.

Figure 20.21 MRI of aneurysmal bone cyst. A 10-year-old boy presented with left foot pain for the previous 3 weeks. **(A)** Radiograph shows an expansive lesion of the second metatarsal abutting the growth plate, associated with well-organized periosteal reaction. **(B)** Axial T1-weighted (SE; TR 500/TE 17 msec) MR image shows the lesion to exhibit an intermediate to low signal intensity. **(C)** Coronal T2-weighted (FSE; TR 4500/TE 75 msec/Ef) image shows the lesion to become bright. Fluid–fluid level (*arrows*) is a typical finding in an aneurysmal bone cyst, a diagnosis confirmed by biopsy.

Figure 20.22 MRI of aneurysmal bone cyst. (A) Coronal T2-weighted (FSE; TR 2583/TE 110 msec/Ef) MR image of a distal femur in a 5-year-old girl shows a lesion extending into the growth plate that is nonhomogeneous in appearance. Axial **(B)** and sagittal **(C)** T2-weighted images demonstrate multiple fluid–fluid levels (*arrowheads*).

Figure 20.23 Simple bone cyst mimicking aneurysmal bone cyst. A radiolucent expansive lesion in the distal fibula of an 8-year-old girl exhibits periosteal reaction (*arrow*) secondary to a healing pathologic fracture (*open arrow*). Although diagnosis of an aneurysmal bone cyst was suggested, the excision biopsy was consistent with a simple bone cyst.

Figure 20.24 Aneurysmal bone cyst. (A) Anteroposterior radiograph of the shoulder of a 19-year-old woman shows a lesion in the right clavicle that was diagnosed on biopsy as an aneurysmal bone cyst. **(B)** The lesion was treated with curettage and the application of cancellous bone chips.

The terms *solid aneurysmal bone cyst* and *giant cell reparative granuloma* are now being used interchangeably. These lesions are considered reactive and nonneoplastic, although they can lead to a mistaken diagnosis of malignancy. Although these lesions are seen primarily in craniofacial and short tubular bones of the hands and feet, they may also occur in the long bones, such as femur, tibia, and ulna. Radiography reveals that most of these lesions are expansive and eccentric in location, with variably aggressive features. At times there is a thin shell of periosteal reaction indistinguishable from conventional aneurysmal bone cyst. MRI findings are variable, but most lesions show intermediate signal intensity on T1-weighted images, with heterogeneous but predominantly high signal intensity on T2 weighting. The areas of low signal on T2-weighted sequences represent mineralization within the lesion. Histopathologic examination of these lesions reveals fibrous stroma, an admixture of spindle cells, and many multinucleated giant cells. Occasional formation of osteoid and even mature bone trabeculae can be noted. Vascular spaces and hemorrhagic areas are also present. Some of these lesions have a histologic appearance similar to that of the so-called brown tumors of hyperparathyroidism. Treatment of these lesions usually consists of curettage. The recurrence rate, as recently reported from the Rizzoli Institute in Bologna, Italy, is close to 24%, whereas the Mayo Clinic reports approximately 39%.

Giant Cell Tumor

Also known as osteoclastoma, a giant cell tumor of bone is an aggressive lesion characterized by richly vascularized tissue containing proliferating mononuclear stromal cells and numerous uniformly distributed giant cells of osteoclast type. It represents approximately 5% to 8.6% of all primary bone tumors and approximately 23% of benign bone tumors; it is the sixth most common primary osseous neoplasm. Sixty percent of these lesions occur in long bones, and almost all are localized to the articular end of the bone. Preferred sites include the proximal tibia, distal femur, distal radius, and proximal humerus (Fig. 20.25). Giant cell tumors are seen almost exclusively after skeletal maturity, when the growth plate is obliterated.

Figure 20.25 Skeletal sites of predilection, peak age range, and male-to-female ratio in giant cell tumor.

Figure 20.26 Giant cell tumor. Anteroposterior **(A)** and lateral **(B)** radiographs of the knee of a 32-year-old man demonstrate a purely osteolytic lesion in the distal end of the femur. Note its eccentric location, the absence of reactive sclerosis, and the extension of the lesion into the articular end of the bone, all characteristic features of giant cell tumor.

Figure 20.27 Giant cell tumor. Anteroposterior radiograph of the right knee in a 28-year-old woman shows an expansive radiolucent lesion in the head of the fibula, shown by histology to be a giant cell tumor.

Most patients are between ages 20 and 40 years, and there is a female predominance of 2:1.

Multifocal giant cell tumors are rare, accounting for less than 1% of all cases of giant cell tumor of bone. They occur most commonly in patients with Paget disease. Multiple lesions can be discovered synchronously or metachronously. The preferential locations are skull and facial bones in Paget disease, and small bones of the hands and feet in other patients.

Clinical symptoms in patients with solitary lesions are nonspecific. They include pain (usually reduced by rest), local swelling, and limitation of range of motion in the adjacent joint. When a lesion is located in the spine, neurologic symptoms may be present.

The radiographic features of a giant cell tumor are characteristic. It is a purely osteolytic, radiolucent lesion with narrow zone of transition lacking sclerotic margins, revealing geographic bone destruction and usually no periosteal reaction (Figs. 20.26 to 20.28). Scintigraphy may show more intense uptake of the tracer around the periphery of the lesion than within the lesion itself, which Hudson calls a "donut configuration," and is presumably caused by hyperemic changes in the bone surrounding the tumor. A soft-tissue mass may also be present, and CT or MRI is usually required for sufficient evaluation (Figs. 20.29 to 20.31). Approximately 5% of giant cell tumors are malignant *de novo*. Having no characteristic radiographic features, however, malignant lesions cannot be diagnosed radiologically (Figs. 20.32 and 20.33). It is also well known that benign giant cell tumor may evolve into a malignant lesion. Several authors have reported cases of malignant transformation of giant cell tumor of bone. In most cases, this transformation occurs after radiation therapy. Only a few cases have been reported of spontaneous malignant transformation after initial surgical therapy. Histologically, the secondary malignancies include malignant fibrous histiocytoma, fibrosarcoma, osteosarcoma, and undifferentiated sarcoma.

Figure 20.28 Giant cell tumor. Anteroposterior radiograph of the right hip in a 31-year-old woman shows a radiolucent lesion in the supraacetabular portion of the ilium, with a narrow zone of transition and a geographic type of bone destruction.

Histologically, a giant cell tumor is composed of a related dual population of mononuclear stromal cells and multinucleated giant cells. The tumor background contains varying amounts of collagen. Morphologically, the giant cells bear some resemblance to osteoclasts, and they display increased acid phosphatase activity.

Historically, the radiologic appearance and staging of giant cell tumors have not accurately reflected the ultimate clinical outcome.

Several investigators, including Enneking, Campanacci, and Bertoni, have developed staging systems based on imaging and histologic appearance of this tumor. The stage 1 lesion has an indolent radiographic and histologic appearance. The stage 2 lesion demonstrates a more aggressive radiographic appearance, with extensive remodeling of bone but intact periosteum and a benign histologic pattern. Stage 3 giant cell tumor reveals aggressive growth and extension into adjacent soft tissues but remains histologically benign, although distant metastases may occur.

Differential Diagnosis

Various lesions may be mistaken for giant cell tumor and, conversely, giant cell tumor can mimic other lesions that affect the articular end of a bone. Primary ABC rarely affects the articular end of a bone and occurs in a younger age group. However, after obliteration of the growth plate at skeletal maturity, this lesion may extend into the subarticular region of a long bone, becoming indistinguishable from a giant cell tumor. Occasionally, if the fluid–fluid level is demonstrated either on CT or on MRI examination, this feature is more consistent with ABC. However, it should be noted that ABC might sometimes coexist with other lesions, among them the giant cell tumor. The so-called solid ABC, or a giant cell reparative granuloma at the articular end, may have the same radiologic characteristics as a conventional giant cell tumor. Benign fibrous histiocytoma, because of its frequent location at the end of a long bone, may appear identical to a giant cell tumor. Brown tumor of hyperparathyroidism is yet another lesion that can mimic GCT radiologically. However, the former lesion is usually accompanied by other skeletal manifestations of hyperparathyroidism, such as osteopenia, cortical or subperiosteal resorption, resorptive changes at the distal phalangeal tufts, or loss of the lamina dura of the teeth. Occasionally, an unusually large intraosseous ganglion may be mistaken for a giant cell tumor, although the former lesion invariably exhibits a sclerotic border. Some malignant lesions, such as chondrosarcoma, may extend into the articular end of bone and, particularly without radiographically identified calcifications, may closely mimic giant cell tumor. Myeloma and a lytic metastasis occupying subchondral segments of bone can usually be distinguished from giant cell tumor without much difficulty (the older age group in which the latter malignancies usually occur is a helpful hint), although at times the radiographic differences between the lesions may not be so obvious. Finally, on rare occasions, fibrosarcoma, malignant fibrous histiocytoma, or fibroblastic osteosarcoma (because of their purely lytic radiographic presentation) may exhibit some similarities to giant cell tumor.

Figure 20.29 CT of giant cell tumor. (A) Anteroposterior radiograph of the knee of a 33-year-old woman shows a giant cell tumor in the medial femoral condyle. There is no definite evidence of a soft-tissue mass. **(B)** CT, however, demonstrates destruction of the cortex and the presence of a soft-tissue mass.

Figure 20.30 MRI of giant cell tumor. A 45-year-old woman presented with pain in the left knee of 6 months' duration. Anteroposterior **(A)** and lateral **(B)** radiographs demonstrate a radiolucent lesion in the proximal tibia, extending into the articular end of the bone. Coronal **(C)** and sagittal **(D)** spin-echo T1-weighted MR images (TR 600/TE 20 msec) outline the lesion, which displays intermediate signal intensity, to the better advantage. Axial **(E)** proton-density image reveals that the lesion penetrates the cortex and extends laterally into the soft tissues. On this image, the lesion displays a nonhomogenous signal varying from intermediate to high intensity.

Figure 20.31 MRI of giant cell tumor. (A) Dorsovolar radiograph of the right wrist of a 36-year-old woman shows an osteolytic lesion in the distal radius. **(B)** Coronal T1-weighted (SE; TR 500/TE 20 msec) MR image shows the tumor to be of low signal intensity. **(C)** On coronal T2-weighted (SE; TR 2000/TE 80 msec) MRI, the lesion becomes bright, displaying low-signal septations.

Figure 20.32 Giant cell tumor. Dorsovolar radiograph of the left wrist of a 56-year-old woman shows a giant cell tumor of the distal radius that has destroyed the cortex and that extends into the soft tissues. Despite this aggressive radiographic presentation, on histopathologic examination the tumor had a typically benign appearance, without malignant features. After wide resection, a 5-year follow-up showed no evidence of recurrence or of distant metastases.

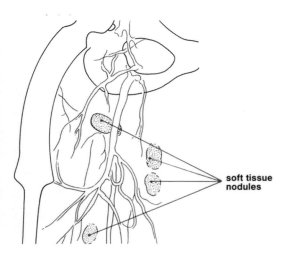

soft tissue nodules

Figure 20.33 Complication of giant cell tumor. A 28-year-old man had a 4-month history of right hip pain. **(A)** Anteroposterior radiograph of the hip shows a destructive radiolucent lesion involving the medial aspect of the femoral head and extending into the femoral neck. Biopsy revealed an aneurysmal bone cyst. Five months after curettage and packing of the cavity with cancellous bone chips, the lesion recurred. This time the histopathologic examination revealed a benign giant cell tumor with an engrafted aneurysmal bone cyst. The proximal femur was resected and an endoprosthesis was implanted. Eight months after this procedure, the patient was readmitted to the hospital with increased pain and a significant increase in the circumference of the thigh. **(B)** A femoral arteriogram demonstrates multiple soft-tissue nodules, which on biopsy proved to be metastases from the giant cell tumor. The patient also had pulmonary metastases.

Figure 20.34 Treatment of giant cell tumor. (A) Radiograph of the distal forearm of a 32-year-old woman shows a giant cell tumor in the distal radius. (B) After extensive curettage, postoperative film shows application of bone chips.

Treatment and Complications

The treatment of benign giant cell tumors consists of either surgical curettage and bone grafting (Fig. 20.34) or wide resection with secondary implantation of an allograft (Figs. 20.35 and 20.36) or an endoprosthesis (see Fig. 20.33). Good healing and lack of recurrence are recognized by incorporation of the bone graft into the normal bone (Fig. 20.37). Marcove recommends cryosurgery using liquid nitrogen, whereas other authorities recommend heat using methylmethacrylate to pack the tumor bed after intralesional excision. Recurrences are often encountered and are recognized radiographically by resorption of the bone graft and the appearance of radiolucent areas like those in the original tumor (Fig. 20.38). Especially after radiation therapy, recurrent lesions may exhibit malignant transformation to fibrosarcoma, malignant fibrous histiocytoma, or osteosarcoma. Occasionally, even histologically benign lesions produce distant (to the lung) metastases.

Fibrocartilaginous Mesenchymoma

Fibrocartilaginous mesenchymoma is an extremely rare tumor composed of two distinct tissues, one benign and cartilaginous, resembling an active growth plate, and the other resembling a low-grade fibrosarcoma. Mirra and associates classify this lesion as desmoid tumor with enchondroma-like nodules. The number of reported cases is probably less than 20, although several unpublished cases may exist. Fibrocartilaginous mesenchymoma has been reported in patients

Figure 20.35 Treatment of giant cell tumor. (A) Dorsovolar radiograph of the left wrist of a 38-year-old woman shows the classic appearance of a giant cell tumor of the distal radius. (B) Treatment consisted of resection of the distal radius and application of an allograft. In addition, a Suavé-Kapandji procedure was performed, creating a pseudoarthrosis of the distal ulna and fusion of the distal radioulnar joint.

Figure 20.36 Treatment of giant cell tumor. (A) Anteroposterior radiograph of the right shoulder of a 27-year-old woman shows a giant cell tumor affecting almost the entire proximal end of the humerus. (B) Wide resection was performed and the humerus was reconstructed by means of allograft.

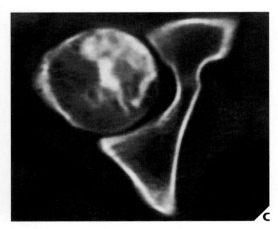

Figure 20.37 Treatment of giant cell tumor. (A) A 27-year-old woman had a giant cell tumor in the femoral head. (B) Two years after curettage and application of allograft there was no recurrence of the lesion. (C) CT demonstrates good incorporation of the graft into the normal bone (compare with Fig. 20.38).

Figure 20.38 Recurrence of giant cell tumor. A 30-year-old woman had a giant cell tumor of the proximal end of the right tibia **(A)** and was subsequently treated with curettage and application of cancellous bone chips. Twenty months after surgery, she began to experience progressive knee pain. **(B)** Follow-up radiograph shows that most of the bone chips have been resorbed; the osteolytic foci indicate recurrence of the tumor.

ranging from ages 9 to 23 years (mean age 13 years). Males were more frequently affected. The lesion is usually located in the epiphysis of a long bone, such as the fibula or humerus. The symptoms usually indicate a slow-growing tumor. They consist of slight discomfort and tenderness at the site of the lesion and occasionally a palpable mass.

On radiography, the lesion is radiolucent with scalloped borders, extending to or abutting the growth plate. After skeletal maturity, the lesion may extend into the articular end of bone (Fig. 20.39). Occasionally, the cortex is expanded and thinned. The cortex may be invaded, and in these cases the lesion extends into the soft tissues (Fig. 20.40). This can be effectively demonstrated with CT and MRI. Although a periosteal reaction is usually absent, when present it is sparse and of benign appearance. The tumor may contain visible calcifications typical of cartilaginous matrix.

By microscopy, the lesion is composed of a tissue made of intersecting bundles of spindle cells and collagen fibers. The tissue is fairly cellular, the nuclei are plump, and there is evidence of pleomorphism and hyperchromatism, with occasional mitotic figures. Superimposed on this background are well-defined islands of obviously benign cartilage. In its first description, the tumor was named fibrocartilaginous mesenchymoma with low-grade malignancy. However, because metastases have never been observed thus far, the group at the Mayo Clinic later deleted that addition, simply calling it fibrocartilaginous mesenchymoma.

Hemangioma

A hemangioma is a benign bone lesion composed of newly formed blood vessels. It comprises approximately 2% of all benign and 0.8%

of benign and malignant lesions of the skeletal system. Some investigators consider hemangiomas benign neoplasms; others put them into the category of congenital vascular malformations. They are classified, according to the type of vessels in the lesion, as capillary, cavernous, venous, or mixed.

Capillary hemangiomas are composed of small vessels that consist merely of a flat endothelium, surrounded only by a basal membrane. In bone, they most commonly occur in the vertebral body. *Cavernous hemangiomas* are composed of dilated, blood-filled spaces lined by the same flat endothelium with a basal membrane. Osseous cavernous hemangiomas most commonly involve the calvaria. *Venous hemangiomas* are composed of thick-walled vessels that possess a muscle layer. They frequently contain phleboliths. *Arteriovenous hemangiomas* are characterized by abnormal communications between arteries and veins. These are extremely rare in bone and almost exclusively involve the soft tissues. The biologic classification of vascular anomalies has recently gained renewed attention. Based on a system by Mulliken and Glowacki, who advocate regarding hemangiomas as hamartomas rather than true neoplasms, this classification takes into consideration cellular turnover and histology, as well as natural history and physical findings. It clearly separates hemangiomas of infancy, with their early proliferative and later involutional stages, from vascular malformations, which are characterized as arterial, venous, capillary, lymphatic, or combined. However, epithelioid hemangiomas have been observed that apparently are true tumors.

The incidence of hemangiomas seems to increase with age and is most frequent after middle age. Women are affected twice as often as men. The most common sites are the spine, particularly the thoracic segment, and the skull (Fig. 20.41). In the spine, the lesion typically involves a vertebral body, although it may extend into the pedicle or lam-

Figure 20.39 Fibrocartilaginous mesenchymoma. Anteroposterior **(A)** and lateral **(B)** radiographs of the right knee of a 23-year-old man show a radiolucent trabeculated lesion in the proximal tibia, bulging the anterolateral cortex and extending into the articular end of bone. Excision biopsy revealed fibrocartilaginous mesenchymoma.

Figure 20.40 MRI of fibrocartilaginous mesenchymoma. (A) Oblique radiograph of the left knee of a 14-year-old boy shows an osteolytic trabeculated lesion in the distal femur abutting the growth plate. The lateral cortex is destroyed. **(B)** CT section through the tumor shows destruction of the posterolateral cortex and a large soft-tissue mass containing calcifications. **(C)** Coronal T1-weighted MRI shows nonhomogeneous signal of the tumor that violated the growth plate and extended into the distal femoral epiphysis *(arrow). (continued)*

Figure 20.40 MRI of fibrocartilaginous mesenchymoma. *Continued.* **(D)** Axial T1-weighted MR image shows destruction of the cortex and a large soft-tissue mass of intermediate signal. Calcifications within the mass display low signal intensity. **(E)** On axial T2-weighted MR image, the tumor becomes of high signal intensity. Pseudoseptation of the mass and nonhomogeneous character is well demonstrated. (Courtesy Prof. Dr. Wolfgang Remagen, Cologne, Germany).

correlation between MRI signal intensity changes and patterns of uptake on bone imaging. Arteriography of the hemangioma is rarely indicated.

Histologically, most hemangiomas consist of simple endothelium-lined channels, morphologically identical with capillary endothelium. Some or all of the vascular channels may be enlarged and have a sinusoidal appearance, in which case the lesion is referred to as cavernous type. Occasionally, hemangiomas are composed of larger,

Figure 20.41 Skeletal sites of predilection, peak age range, and male-to-female ratio in hemangioma.

ina and, rarely, to the spinous process. Occasionally, multiple vertebrae may be affected. Most hemangiomas of the vertebral column are asymptomatic and discovered incidentally. Symptoms occur when the lesion in an affected vertebra compresses the nerve roots or spinal cord secondary to epidural extension. This neurologic complication is more commonly associated with lesions in the midthoracic spine (Fig. 20.42). Another mechanism considered responsible for compression of the cord, although seen less frequently, is fracture of the involved vertebral body with formation of an associated soft-tissue mass or hematoma.

Hemangioma is typified radiographically by the presence of multiloculated lytic foci or coarse vertical striations. In a vertebral body, this pattern is referred to as a "honeycomb" or "corduroy cloth" pattern, respectively (Fig. 20.43), and in the skull as a "spoke-wheel" configuration. When seen in the spine, this pattern is considered virtually pathognomonic for hemangioma. CT examination characteristically shows the pattern as multiple dots (often referred to as the "polka-dot" appearance), which represent a cross-section of reinforced trabeculae (Fig. 20.44). On MRI, T1- and T2-weighted images usually reveal areas of a high-intensity signal that correspond to the vascular components (Fig. 20.45). Areas of trabecular thickening exhibit a low signal intensity regardless of the pulse sequence used. Both CT and MR images obtained after intravenous administration of contrast material demonstrate lesion's enhancement. In the long and short tubular bones, hemangiomas are recognized by a typical lace-like pattern and honeycombing (Fig. 20.46).

On scintigraphy, the appearance of osseous hemangiomas ranges from photopenia to a moderate increase in the uptake of radiopharmaceutical tracer. A recent study of planar images and single-photon emission computed tomography (SPECT) of vertebral hemangiomas and their correlation with MRI showed that in most cases, hemangiomas exhibited normal uptake on planar images. SPECT images were also normal, particularly if the lesions were less than 3 cm in diameter. This study also showed a disparity between SPECT images and MRI: there was no

Figure 20.42 Vertebral hemangioma. A 39-year-old woman presented with back pain and decreased sensation and strength in the right upper extremity. Anteroposterior **(A)** and lateral **(B)** radiographs of the thoracic spine show a radiolucent lesion involving the body of T-6 and extending into the pedicle. **(C)** Lateral tomographic cut demonstrates ballooning of the posterior cortex of the vertebra and extension of the lesion into the posterior elements. **(D)** CT shows a soft-tissue mass encroaching on the spinal canal and displacing the spinal cord. Biopsy revealed a hemangioma. (From Greenspan A, et al., 1983, with permission.)

Figure 20.43 Vertebral hemangioma. (A) Lateral radiograph of the lumbar spine demonstrates a "honeycomb" pattern of hemangioma of L-2 vertebra. **(B)** Anteroposterior tomogram demonstrates vertical striations of hemangioma of L-1 vertebra (*arrows*), referred to as a "corduroy cloth" pattern.

Figure 20.44 CT of vertebral hemangioma. CT section of a T-10 vertebra demonstrates coarse dots that indicate reinforced vertical trabeculae of the cancellous bone, characteristic of hemangioma.

Figure 20.45 MRI of vertebral hemangioma. Sagittal T1-weighted (SE; TR 517/TE 12 msec) **(A)** and T2-weighted (SE; TR 2000/TE 80 msec) **(B)** MR images show high signal intensity of hemangioma of L-4 vertebra.

Figure 20.46 Hemangioma of a short tubular bone. Dorsovolar view of the hand of an 11-year-old girl with hemangioma involving the middle finger shows the lace-like pattern and honeycombing characteristic of this lesion. Overgrowth of the digit, as seen here, is a frequent complication of hemangioma.

Figure 20.47 Cystic angiomatosis. Several osteolytic lesions affect the shafts of the radius and ulna in this 25-year-old man with cystic angiomatosis.

Figure 20.48 Cystic angiomatosis. A radiograph of the pelvis of a 28-year-old man shows a honeycomb pattern in the right ilium and both pubic bones.

thick-walled arteries or veins and resemble arteriovenous malformations of the soft tissues.

Epithelioid hemangioma is a variant of conventional hemangioma. It has been previously described as *angiolymphoid hyperplasia with eosinophilia* and as *histiocytoid hemangioma* because of its morphologic features. Although it most commonly affects skin and subcutaneous tissue, epithelioid hemangioma may also involve bones, with a predilection for the vertebrae. The radiographic features of this lesion include expansive lytic areas with well-defined lobulated borders and marginal sclerosis. Rarely, the cortex is destroyed, causing formation of new periosteal bone. Histologically, as pointed out by Wenger and Wold, well-formed vessels with open lumina are observed, surrounded by multiple epithelioid endothelial cells with abundant eosinophilic cytoplasm. The vessels are usually of capillary size, and hemorrhage into the surrounding connective tissue may be present. The neighboring stroma may contain an inflammatory infiltrate. Occasionally, the histopathology of this lesion is similar to that of epithelioid hemangioendothelioma.

Diffuse involvement of bones by hemangiomatous lesions is defined as *hemangiomatosis* or *angiomatosis*. The radiographic presentation of angiomatosis is that of lytic lesions, often with a honeycomb or lattice work ("hole-within-hole") appearance. When bone is extensively involved, the term *cystic angiomatosis* is applied. Some other terms used for this condition include diffuse skeletal hemangiomatosis, cystic lymphangiectasia, and hamartous hemolymphangiomatosis. Schajowicz postulated that cystic hemangiomatosis should be distinguished from diffuse angiomatosis because of their different radiologic and macroscopic aspects. This is a rare bone disorder characterized by diffuse cystic lesions of bone, frequently (60% to 70% of cases) associated with visceral involvement. Patients with cystic angiomatosis usually present in the first three decades. There is 2:1 male-to-female predominance. The bones affected are most often those of the axial skeleton, as well as the femur, humerus, tibia, radius, and fibula. The bone-related symptoms

Figure 20.49 Cystic angiomatosis. Several confluent lesions with peripheral sclerosis and cortical thickening marked cystic angiomatosis in the right femur of a 20-year-old man.

are usually secondary to pathologic fractures through the cystic lesions. Most of the symptoms, however, are related to visceral involvement. On radiography, the osseous lesions are usually osteolytic (Fig. 20.47), occasionally with a honeycomb appearance (Fig. 20.48). They are well defined and surrounded by a rim of sclerosis, and they vary in size (Fig. 20.49). Although medullary involvement predominates, cortical invasion, osseous expansion, and periosteal reaction can occur. Rarely, sclerotic lesions may be present, and in these instances the condition may mimic osteoblastic metastases. On MRI, the lesions usually show intermediate signal intensity on T1-weighted images, and T2-weighted images with fat saturation show a mixture of high, intermediate, and low signal intensities. On histologic examination, cystic angiomatosis is characterized by cavernous angiomatous spaces, indistinguishable from benign hemangioma of bone.

A condition that must be distinguished from angiomatosis is *Gorham disease* of bone, also known as massive osteolysis, disappearing bone disease, and phantom bone disease. This entity is characterized by progressive, localized bone resorption, probably caused by multiple or diffuse cavernous hemangiomas or lymphangiomas of bone or by a combination of both. The radiographic presentation of Gorham disease consists of radiolucent areas in the cancellous bone or concentric destruction of the cortex, giving rise to a sucked-candy appearance. Eventually, the entire medullary cavity and the cortex are destroyed. On histologic examination, a marked increase is observed in intraosseous capillaries, which form an anastomosing network of endothelium-lined channels that are usually filled with erythrocytes or serum. Although some investigators claim that there is no evidence of

osteoclasts in areas of bone resorption, recent studies by Spieth and coworkers suggest that osteoclastic activity plays a role in the pathogenesis of Gorham disease.

Differential Diagnosis

The differential diagnosis of hemangioma, particularly in the spine, should include Paget disease, Langerhans cell histiocytosis, myeloma, and metastatic lesions. The characteristic "picture frame" appearance of a vertebra affected by Paget disease (see Fig. 29.5), as well as its larger than normal size, distinguishes it from hemangioma. Myeloma in a vertebra, unlike hemangioma, is purely radiolucent—as are most metastatic lesions—and shows no vertical striations.

Treatment

Asymptomatic hemangiomas do not require treatment. Symptomatic lesions are usually treated with radiation therapy to ablate the venous channels forming the lesions. Embolization, laminectomy, spinal fusion, or a combination of these is also used in treatment (see Fig. 16.13).

Intraosseous Lipoma

Lipomas can be categorized according to their location in the bone as intraosseous, cortical, or parosteal lesions. Intraosseous lipoma is considered to be an extremely rare tumor (with an incidence of less than 1 in 1,000 primary bone tumors). In recent years, an increasing number of reports of intraosseous lipoma have appeared, particularly located in the intertrochanteric and subtrochanteric regions of the femur and in the calcaneus. The tumor has no sex predilection and occurs in a wide range of ages, from 5 to 75 years. It is usually an asymptomatic lesion, found on radiographic examinations performed for other reasons. Some investigators report a higher incidence of symptomatic patients; however, even when a patient is symptomatic, the symptoms are not necessarily related to the lesion. In the large series of 61 intraosseous lipomas reported by Milgram, the most common sites were the intertrochanteric and subtrochanteric regions of the femur, followed by the calcaneus, ilium, proximal tibia, and sacrum.

Intraosseous lipoma has a rather characteristic radiographic appearance. It is invariably a nonaggressive radiolucent lesion with sharply defined borders, associated with thinning and bulging of the cortex, particularly in thin bones such as fibula or rib. The central calcifications and ossifications are frequently present (Fig. 20.50). CT

Figure 20.50 Intraosseous lipoma. Typical appearance of intraosseous lipoma in the calcaneus. Observe sharply marginated radiolucent lesion with central calcification.

may be helpful in the diagnosis of these lesions, because the Hounsfield units are consistent with fat. MRI shows the lesion to have a signal similar to subcutaneous fat on T1- and T2-weighted images (Fig. 20.51). A thin circumferential rim of low signal intensity on T1- and T2-weighted images, consistent with reactive sclerosis, is commonly present demarcating the margin of the fatty lesion. After administration of intravenous gadolinium, there is no enhancement

of the lesion. MRI is highly effective in demonstrating the exact intraosseous extension of the lesion.

Histologically, intraosseous lipomas are composed of lobules of mature adipose tissue and are characterized by the presence of mature lipocytes, which are slightly larger than nonneoplastic fat cells, in a background of fibroblasts with occasional foci of fat necrosis. A capsule may occasionally encompass all or part of the tumor mass, and in

Figure 20.51 Intraosseous lipoma. (A) Radiograph of the right ankle in a 42-year-old man shows a radiolucent lesion in the distal tibia sharply delineated by a thin sclerotic margin. **(B)** On the lateral radiograph, there is a suggestion of a faint calcific body in the center of the lesion (*arrow*). **(C)** Coronal T1-weighted (SE; TR 685/TE 20 msec) MRI demonstrates the lesion to be of a high signal intensity paralleling that of subcutaneous fat and thus consistent with intraosseous lipoma. A small focus of low signal is present within the lesion, corresponding to a calcific body seen on the conventional radiography. **(D)** Axial T2-weighted (SE; TR 2000/TE 70 msec) MR image shows that the lesion becomes of lower intensity, again paralleling the signal of subcutaneous fat. The central calcification exhibits low signal (*arrowhead*).

Figure 20.52 Intraosseous ganglion. A 28-year-old man sustained an injury to the right knee that tore the medial meniscus. Anteroposterior radiograph of the knee discloses an eccentric radiolucent lesion in the articular end of the proximal tibia. During surgery to remove the meniscus, the lesion was biopsied and histopathologic examination revealed it to be an intraosseous ganglion.

most cases reported, atrophic bone trabeculae are found throughout the lesion.

Nonneoplastic Lesions Simulating Tumors

Some nonneoplastic conditions that may mimic bone tumors include intraosseous ganglion, a "brown tumor" of hyperparathyroidism, Langerhans cell histiocytosis, Chester-Erdheim disease, encystified bone infarct, and myositis ossificans.

Intraosseous Ganglion

This lesion of unknown cause is frequently encountered in adults between ages 20 and 60 years. It has a predilection for the articular ends of the long bones, usually the non-weight-bearing segment. Radiographically, it exhibits the characteristic picture of a round or oval radiolucent area located eccentrically in the bone and rimmed by a sclerotic margin (Fig. 20.52). Its appearance is very similar to that of a degenerative cyst, but the adjacent joint does not show any degenerative changes; in most cases, the ganglion, in contrast to a degenerative cyst, does not communicate with the joint cavity. An intraosseous ganglion may also mimic chondroblastoma, osteoblastoma, enchondroma, pigmented villonodular synovitis, or bone abscess (Fig. 20.53).

Brown Tumor of Hyperparathyroidism

Hyperparathyroidism is a condition resulting from the excess secretion of parathormone by overactive parathyroid glands (see Chapter 28). Not infrequently, patients with this disorder present with solitary or multiple lytic lesions, most commonly in the long and short tubular bones; on radiographic examination, the lesions may resemble a tumor (Fig. 20.54). This lesion is called a brown tumor because, in addition to fibrous tissue, it contains decomposing blood, which gives specimens obtained for pathologic examination a brown coloration. The correct diagnosis can be made on radiography by observing associated abnormalities, including a decrease in bone density (osteopenia); subperiosteal bone resorption, which is best seen on the radial aspect of the proximal and middle phalanges of the second and third fingers; a granular "salt-and-pepper" appearance of the cranial vault; resorption of the acromial ends of the clavicles; and soft-tissue calcifications. Because of disturbed calcium and phosphorus metabolism, the serum calcium concentration is usually high (hypercalcemia) and the serum phosphorus concentration low (hypophosphatemia), which are laboratory findings that usually confirm the diagnosis.

Langerhans Cell Histiocytosis (Eosinophilic Granuloma)

A nonneoplastic condition, eosinophilic granuloma, currently termed Langerhans cell histiocytosis, belongs to the group of disorders known as reticuloendothelioses (or histiocytoses X, according to Lichtenstein's proposed name), which is a group that includes two other conditions, Hand-Schüller-Christian disease (xanthomatosis) and Letterer-Siwe disease (nonlipid reticulosis). The grouping has gained wide acceptance with the recognition that all three entities represent

Figure 20.53 Intraosseous ganglion. A 24-year-old man presented with an 8-week history of pain in the knee. Anteroposterior radiograph of the right knee **(A)** and CT section **(B)** demonstrate an oval radiolucent lesion eccentrically located in the proximal tibia with ramifications, rimmed by a zone of reactive sclerosis. The differential diagnosis included a bone abscess, osteoblastoma, chondroblastoma, and an intraosseous ganglion. Biopsy confirmed an intraosseous ganglion.

Figure 20.54 Brown tumors of hyperparathyroidism. Radiograph of the lower legs of a 28-year-old woman with hyperparathyroidism shows multiple brown tumors involving both tibiae. This condition can easily be misdiagnosed as multiple myeloma or metastatic disease.

different clinical manifestations of a single pathologic disorder, characterized by granulomatous proliferation of the reticulum cell.

Although its causes and pathogenesis remain unsettled, Langerhans cell histiocytosis is now considered a disorder of immune regulation rather than neoplastic process. The term Langerhans cell histiocytosis has been accepted because it has been verified that the primary proliferative element in this disease is the Langerhans cell, a mononuclear cell of the dendritic type that is found in the epidermis but is derived from precursors in the bone marrow. The disorder exhibits a broad spectrum of clinical and radiologic abnormalities. It is characterized by an abnormal proliferation of histiocytes in various parts of the reticuloendothelial system such as bone, lungs, central nervous system, skin, and lymph nodes.

Langerhans cell histiocytosis may manifest with solitary or with multiple lesions. It is usually seen in children, the common age of occurrence ranging from 1 to 15 years, with a peak incidence from 5 to 10 years. The most frequently affected sites are the skull, ribs, pelvis, spine, and long bones (Fig. 20.55). In the skull, the lytic lesions have a characteristic "punched-out" appearance, with sharply defined bor-

ders (Fig. 20.56). In the mandible or maxilla, the radiolucent lesions have the appearance of "floating teeth" (Fig. 20.57). In the spine, collapse of a vertebral body, the so-called vertebra plana, is a characteristic manifestation of the disease (Fig. 20.58). This finding was for a long time mistakenly interpreted as representing osteochondrosis of the vertebra and was called "Calve disease."

In the long bones, Langerhans cell histiocytosis presents as a destructive radiolucent lesion commonly associated with a lamellated periosteal reaction. It may mimic a malignant round cell tumor such as lymphoma or Ewing sarcoma (Fig. 20.59). In its later stages, the lesion becomes more sclerotic, with dispersed radiolucencies (Fig. 20.60). The distribution of the lesion and the detection of silent sites in the skeleton are best ascertained by a radionuclide bone scan; this may also be helpful in differentiating Langerhans cell histiocytosis from Ewing sarcoma, which rarely presents with multiple foci.

CT may be useful if conventional radiography inadequately defines the extent of the process, particularly in cases of spine and pelvic involvement. This modality effectively demonstrates periosteal reaction, beveled edges, and reactive sclerosis. There have been

Figure 20.55 Langerhans cell histiocytosis. Radiograph of the proximal femur of a 3-year-old boy with a limp and tenderness localized to the upper thigh shows an osteolytic lesion in the medullary portion of the bone, without sclerotic changes. There is fusiform thickening of the cortex and a solid periosteal reaction. The patient's age, the location of the lesion, and its radiographic appearance are typical of Langerhans cell histiocytosis.

Figure 20.56 Langerhans cell histiocytosis. Lateral radiograph of the skull of a 2.5-year-old boy with disseminated Langerhans cell histiocytosis shows an osteolytic lesion in the frontal bone with a sharply outlined margin, giving it a punched-out appearance. Uneven involvement of the inner and outer tables results in its beveled appearance.

Figure 20.57 Langerhans cell histiocytosis. A 3-year-old girl with extensive skeletal involvement of Langerhans cell histiocytosis had in addition a large destructive lesion in the mandible. Note the characteristic appearance of a floating tooth, which results from destruction of supportive alveolar bone.

Figure 20.58 Langerhans cell histiocytosis. (A) Vertebra plana in Langerhans cell histiocytosis represents collapse of a vertebral body secondary to the destruction of bone by a granulomatous lesion. Note the preservation of the adjacent intervertebral disk spaces. **(B)** In another patient, observe compression fractures of the vertebral bodies C-4 and C-6 (*arrows*).

Figure 20.59 Langerhans cell histiocytosis. Radiograph of the left lower leg of a 4-year-old boy demonstrates a lesion in the diaphysis of the tibia exhibiting a permeative type of bone destruction (*open arrows*) and a lamellated (onion skin) type of periosteal response (*arrows*) not infrequently seen in osteomyelitis or Ewing sarcoma. The duration of the patient's symptoms (fever and pain for 10 days), however, favored Langerhans cell histiocytosis.

Figure 20.60 Langerhans cell histiocytosis. The healing stage of Langerhans cell histiocytosis, seen here in the distal humerus of a 16-year-old girl, exhibits predominantly sclerotic changes with interspersed radiolucent foci, thickening of the cortex, and a well-organized periosteal reaction. In this stage, the lesion mimics chronic osteomyelitis.

Figure 20.61 MRI of Langerhans cell histiocytosis. (A) Anteroposterior radiograph of the right femur of a 13-year-old boy shows a radiolucent lesion in the proximal femoral diaphysis associated with a lamellated periosteal reaction. **(B)** Axial T1-weighted (SE; TR 600/TE 14 msec) MR image demonstrates the lesion to be of low signal intensity. The cortex is markedly thickened. **(C)** Coronal fat-suppressed T1-weighted (SE; TR 500/TE 15 msec) MR image obtained after intravenous injection of gadolinium shows marked enhancement of the lesion and the soft tissues adjacent to the thickened femoral cortex. **(D)** Axial T1-weighted (SE; TR 700/TE 18 msec) MR image obtained after intravenous injection of gadolinium shows enhancement of both granuloma and perilesional edema.

isolated reports of the usefulness of MRI in evaluating this condition. The MRI appearance varies and appears to correlate with the radiographic appearance. The MRI manifestations of Langerhans cell histiocytosis during the earlier stages are nonspecific and may simulate an aggressive lesion, such as osteomyelitis or Ewing sarcoma, and occasionally benign tumors, such as osteoid osteoma or chondroblastoma. After gadolinium-diethylene triamine pentaacetic acid (DTPA) injection, the lesions show marked enhancement on T1-weighted images (Fig. 20.61). Occasionally, MRI can demonstrate early bone marrow involvement in the absence of radiographic or scintigraphic abnormalities. In some studies, on T1-weighted sequences the lesions were isointense with adjacent structures. In the skull, lesions have been reported to show well-defined high-signal-intensity areas of marrow replacement on T2-weighted sequences. The most recent investigations have shown that the most common MRI appearance of Langerhans cell histiocyto sis is that of a focal lesion, surrounded by an extensive, ill-defined signal from bone marrow and by soft-tissue reaction with low signal intensity on T2-weighted images, considered to represent bone marrow and soft-tissue edema or the flare phenomenon.

Histologically, Langerhans cell histiocytosis is composed of a variable admixture of two types of cells: eosinophilic leukocytes possessing bilobate nuclei and coarse eosinophilic cytoplasmic granules and histiocytes, identical with the Langerhans histiocytes seen in the skin.

Infantile myofibromatosis is a condition that can be mistaken for Langerhans cell histiocytosis. It is a nodular myofibroblastic lesion of unknown cause that occurs in either a solitary (more commonly) or a multicentric form. In addition to bones, the dermis, subcutis, muscle, and viscera (heart, lungs, gastrointestinal tract) may be affected. Infantile myofibromatosis usually affects children younger than age 2 years. On radiography, radiolucent areas with or without sclerotic border are identified in the long bones, facial bones, and calvaria. MRI shows the lesions to be of low signal intensity on T1- and high signal intensity on T2-weighted sequences.

Chester-Erdheim Disease (Lipogranulomatosis)

Also known as Erdheim-Chester disease, this disseminated process of unknown cause affects the musculoskeletal system and various organs including heart, lungs, and skin. The clinical symptoms include bone pain, abdominal pain, shortness of breath, neurologic dysfunction, exophthalmos, fever, and generalized weakness. The imaging findings are characteristic. Radiographs show extensive medullary sclerosis and cortical thickening affecting predominantly the long bones, with sparing of the articular ends. The axial skeleton is usually not affected. MRI demonstrates decreased signal on T1-weighted images and increased signal on T2-weighting. The condition may mimic lymphoma and metastatic disease. Histologically, there is evidence of a dense infiltrate of lipid-laden foamy macrophages associated with cholesterol crystals, scattered giant cells, chronic inflammatory cells, and various amounts of fibrosis. Occasionally, Langerhans cells may

Figure 20.62 Encystified bone infarct. An expansive, radiolucent lesion in the proximal shaft of the left humerus was an incidental finding in a 31-year-old woman. The lesion exhibits the classic features of an encystified bone infarct: its location in the medullary portion of the bone with central coarse calcifications and a thin rim of reactive sclerosis. Note that although the cortex is thinned and expanded, there is no evidence of a periosteal reaction or soft tissue mass. (Courtesy of Dr. Alex Norman, New York, NY.)

be present, which raised the hypothesis of possible association of this disorder with Langerhans cell histiocytosis.

Medullary Bone Infarct

Radiographically, a medullary bone infarct presents with calcifications in the marrow cavity, usually surrounded by a well-defined hyalinized fibrotic or sclerotic border (see Figs. 18.16 and 18.17); occasionally, this presentation may be mistaken for a cartilage tumor such as an enchondroma. In the rare instances when a cyst develops in an infarcted segment of a long or flat bone, i.e., an encystified bone infarct, it is visualized radiographically as an expanding radiolucent lesion associated with thinning of the surrounding cortex. Usually, the cyst cavity is sharply outlined and the lesion is demarcated by a thin shell of reactive bone (Fig. 20.62). This encystification of a bone infarct can resemble an intraosseous lipoma or even a chondrosarcoma.

Myositis Ossificans

Myositis ossificans is a localized formation of heterotopic bone in the soft tissues that is initiated by trauma. Two types of these lesions have been identified. The first is a well-circumscribed lesion frequently seen adjacent to the cortex of a long tubular or flat bone, socalled juxtacortical myositis ossificans circumscripta; the other is a veil-like lesion that is less delineated. Radiographically, myositis ossificans circumscripta is characterized by a zonal phenomenon—dense, well-organized bone at the periphery of the lesion and less organized, immature bone at the center—and a radiolucent cleft that separates the lesion from the cortex of the adjacent bone (Fig. 20.63; see also Figs. 4.54 and 4.55). The appearance of this lesion may mimic a malignant bone tumor such as parosteal or periosteal osteosarcoma (see Figs. 21.21 and 21.22). Most errors in diagnosis occur when a biopsy of the lesion is performed too early in onset, when its histologic appearance may resemble sarcomatous tissue.

PRACTICAL POINTS TO REMEMBER

[1] Simple bone cysts have a predilection for:
- the proximal diaphysis of the humerus and femur in children and adolescents
- the pelvis and os calcis in adults.

[2] A simple bone cyst is characterized by:
- its central location in a long bone
- lack of periosteal reaction in the absence of fracture.

It may be complicated by pathologic fracture, in which case the "fallen fragment" sign is often present and may help in the differential diagnosis.

[3] An aneurysmal bone cyst, seen almost exclusively in children and adolescents younger than age 20, is characterized by:
- its eccentric location in a bone
- a buttress of periosteal reaction
- its usual containment by a thin shell of periosteum.

[4] An aneurysmal bone cyst *can* develop *de novo* or as a result of cystic changes in a preexisting benign (chondroblastoma, osteoblastoma, giant cell tumor, fibrous dysplasia) or malignant (osteosarcoma) tumors.

[5] MRI of an aneurysmal bone cyst usually shows rather characteristic fluid–fluid levels, which represent sedimentation of red blood cells and serum within cystic cavities.

[6] Solid variant of aneurysmal bone cyst is commonly termed giant cell reparative granuloma. This lesion is seen primarily in craniofacial bones and short tubular bones of the hands and feet.

[7] Giant cell tumor, seen characteristically at the articular ends of long bones, most often presents as a purely radiolucent lesion without any sclerotic reaction at the periphery. It is impossible to determine radiologically whether a giant cell tumor is benign or malignant.

Figure 20.63 Myositis ossificans. Characteristic appearance of posttraumatic myositis ossificans circumscripta, adjacent to the right ribs. Note that periphery of the lesion is denser than the center. The *arrowheads* point to the narrow radiolucent cleft that separates the lesion from the cortex of the ribs.

[8] Multifocal giant cell tumors are rare. Most commonly they occur in patients with Paget disease.

[9] Fibrocartilaginous mesenchymoma is a benign lesion composed of two distinct tissues, one cartilaginous, resembling an active growth plate, and one fibrous, resembling a low-grade fibrosarcoma.

[10] Hemangiomas are commonly seen in a vertebral body. Although most frequently asymptomatic, they may produce symptoms if they expand into the spinal canal.

[11] The characteristic MRI appearance of hemangioma includes high signal intensity on T1- and T2-weighted images.

[12] Epithelioid hemangioma represents a variant of conventional hemangioma with predilection to the vertebrae.

[13] Angiomatosis is defined as diffuse involvement of bones by hemangiomatous lesions. When bone is extensively involved, the term cystic angiomatosis is applied.

[14] Gorham disease of bone, also known as massive osteolysis or disappearing bone disease, is characterized by progressive, localized bone resorption, giving rise to a "sucked-candy" appearance.

[15] Intraosseous lipoma frequently presents with central calcification or ossification. The subtrochanteric region of the femur and the calcaneus are common sites for this lesion.

[16] Nonneoplastic conditions frequently mistaken for tumors include:
- an intraosseous ganglion
- the brown tumor of hyperparathyroidism
- Langerhans cell histiocytosis (eosinophilic granuloma)
- Chester-Erdheim disease
- an encystified medullary bone infarct
- posttraumatic myositis ossificans.

[17] Intraosseous ganglion resembles a degenerative cyst and has a predilection for the non-weight-bearing segments of the articular end of the long bones.

[18] Brown tumor of hyperparathyroidism appears on the radiographs as a lytic lesion, most commonly in the long and short tubular bones. The name derives from its pathologic appearance: the lesion contains decomposing blood, which gives specimens a brown coloration.

[19] Langerhans cell histiocytosis is seen predominantly in children and may be mistaken for Ewing sarcoma.

[20] Chester-Erdheim disease manifests on radiography by extensive medullary sclerosis and cortical thickening, mimicking lymphoma and osteoblastic metastases.

[21] Myositis ossificans is characterized by a zonal phenomenon (well-organized bone at the periphery of the lesion and immature bone at the center), and a radiolucent cleft that separates the lesion from the cortex of adjacent bone.

SUGGESTED READINGS

Abdelwahab IF. Sclerosing hemangiomatosis: a case report and review of the literature. *Br J Radiol* 1991;64:894–897.

Abdehvahab IF, Lewis MM, Klein MJ, Barbera C. Case report 515. Simple (solitary) bone cysts of the calcaneus. *Skeletal Radiol* 1989;17:607–610.

Adamsbaum C, Leclet H, Kalifa G. Intralesional Ethibloc injections in bone cysts. *Semin Musculoskelet Radiol* 1997;1:310–304.

Adamsbaum C, Mascard E, Guinebretière JM, Kalifa G, Dubousset J. Intralesional Ethibloc injections in primary aneurysmal bone cysts: an efficient and safe treatment. *Skeletal Radiol* 2003;10:559–566.

Aho HJ, Aho AJ, Einola S. Aneurysmal bone cyst, a study of ultrastructure and malignant transformation. *Virchows Arch (A)* 1982;395:169–179.

Aho HJ, Aho AJ, Pellineimi LJ, Ekfors TO, Foidart JM. Endothelium in aneurysmal bone cyst. *Histopathology* 1985;9:381–387.

Alles JU, Schulz A. Immunohistochemical markers (endothelial and histiocytic) and ultrastructure of primary aneurysmal bone cysts. *Hum Pathol* 1986;17:39–45.

Aoki J, Moriya K, Yamashita K, et al. Giant cell tumors of bone containing large amounts of hemosiderin: MR-pathologic correlation. *J Comput Assist Tomogr* 1991;15:1024–1027.

Aoki J, Moser RP Jr, Vinh TN. Giant cell tumor of the scapula. A review of 13 cases. *Skeletal Radiol* 1989;18:427–434.

Aoki J, Tanikawa H, Ishii K, et al. MR findings indicative of hemosiderin in giant-cell tumor of bone: frequency, cause, and diagnostic significance. *AJR Am J Roentgenol* 1996;166:145–148.

Apaydin A, OzkayTnak C, Yihnaz S, et al. Aneurysmal bone cyst of metacarpal. *Skeletal Radiol* 1996;25:76–78.

Asch MJ, Cohen AH, Moore TC. Hepatic and splenic lymphangiomatosis with skeletal involvement. Report of a case and review of the literature. *Surgery* 1974;76:334–339.

Assoun J, Richardi G, Railhac JJ, et al. CT and MRI of massive osteolysis of Gorham. *J Comput Assist Tomogr* 1994;18:981–984.

Athanasou NA, Bliss E, Gatter KC, Heryet A, Woods CG, McGee JO. An immunohistological study of giant-cell tumor of bone: evidence for an osteoclast origin of the giant cells. *J Pathol* 1985;147:153–158.

Averill R, Smith R, Campbell CJ. Giant cell tumors of the bones of the hand. *J Hand Surg* 1980;5:39–50.

Bacchini P, Bertoni F, Ruggieri P, Campanacci M. Multicentric giant cell tumor of skeleton. *Skeletal Radiol* 1995;24:371–374.

Backo M, Cindro L, Golouh R. Familial occurrence of infantile myofibromatosis. *Cancer* 1992;69:1294–1299.

Baker DM. Benign unicameral bone cyst. *Clin Orthop* 1970;71:140–151.

Baker ND, Greenspan A, Neuwirth M. Symptomatic vertebral hemangiomas: a report of four cases. *Skeletal Radiol* 1986;15:458–463.

Barcelo M, Pathria MN, Abdul-Karim FW. Intraosseous lipoma. A clinicopathological study of four cases. *Arch Pathol Lab Med* 1992;116:947–950.

Baudrez V, Galant C, Vande Berg BC. Benign vertebral hemangioma: MR-histological correlation. *Skeletal Radiol* 2001;30:442–446.

Beltran J, Simon DC, Levy M, Herman L, Weis L, Mueller CF. Aneurysmal bone cysts: MR imaging at 1.5 T. *Radiology* 1986;158:689–690.

Bergman AG, Rogero GW, Hellman B, Lones MA. Case report 841. Skeletal cystic angiomatosis. *Skeletal Radiol* 1994;23:303–305.

Bergstrand A, Hook 0, Lidvall H. Vertebral haemangiomas compressing the spinal cord. *Acta Neurol Scand* 1963;39:59–66.

Bertheussen KJ, Holck S, Schiodt T. Giant cell lesion of bone of the hand with particular emphasis on giant cell reparative granuloma. *J Hand Surg [Am]* 1983;8:46–49.

Bertoni F, Bacchini P, Capanna R, et al. Solid variant of aneurysmal bone cyst. *Cancer* 1993;71:729–734.

Bertoni F, Bacchini P, Staals EL. Malignancy in giant cell tumor. *Skeletal Radiol* 2003;32:143–146.

Bertoni F, Biscaglia R, Bacchini P. Giant cell reparative granuloma of the phalanx of the hand with aggressive radiographic features. *Skeletal Radiol* 1998;27:534–587.

Bertoni F, Present D, Enneking WF. Giant cell tumor of bone with pulmonary metastases. *J Bone Joint Surg [Am]* 1985;67A:890–900.

Bertoni F, Present D, Sudanese A, Baldini N, Bacchini P, Campanacci M. Giant cell tumor of bone with pulmonary metastases: six case reports and a review of the literature. *Clin Orthop* 1988;237:275–285.

Bhaduri A, Deshpande RB. Fibrocartilaginous mesenchymoma versus fibrocartilaginous dysplasia: are these a single entity? *Am J Surg Pathol* 1995;19:1447–1448.

Biesecker JL, Marcove RC, Huvos AG, Mike V. Aneurysmal bone cysts. A clinicopathologic study of 66 cases. *Cancer* 1970;26:615–625.

Blacksin MF, Ende N, Benevenia J. Magnetic resonance imaging of intraosseous lipomas: a radiologic-pathologic correlation. *Skeletal Radiol* 1995;24:37–41.

Blumberg ML. CT of iliac unicameral bone cysts. *AJR Am J Roentgenol* 1981;136:1231–1232.

Bohne WHO, Goldman AB, Bullough P. Case report 96. Chester-Erdheim disease (lipogranulomatosis). *Skeletal Radiol* 1979;4:164–167.

Bonakdarpour A, Levy WM, Aegerter E. Primary and secondary aneurysmal bone cysts: a radiological study of 75 cases. *Radiology* 1978;126:75–83.

Boseker EH, Bickel WH, Dahlin DC. A clinicopathologic study of simple unicameral bone cysts. *Surg Gynecol Obstet* 1968;127:550–560.

Boyle WJ. Cystic angiomatosis of bone. *J Bone Joint Surg [Br]* 1972;54B:626–636.

Brady TJ, Gebhardt MC, Pykett IL, et al. NMR imaging of forearms in healthy volunteers and patients with giant-cell tumor of bone. *Radiology* 1982;144:549–552.

Briccoli A, Malaguti C, Ianetti C, Rocca M, Bertoni F. Giant cell tumor of the rib. *Skeletal Radiol* 2003;32:107–110.

Bridge JA, Neff JR, Bhatia PS, Sanger WG, Murphey MD. Cytogenetic findings and biologic behavior of giant cell tumors of bone. *Cancer* 1990;65:2697–2703.

Broder HM. Possible precursor of unicameral bone cysts. *J Bone Joint Surg [Am]* 1968;50A:503–507.

Brower AC, Culver JE Jr, Keats TE. Diffuse cystic angiomatosis of bone: report of two cases. *Am J Roentgenol Ther Nucl Med* 1973;118:456–463.

Bruni L. The cockade image: a diagnostic sign of calcaneum intraosseous lipoma. *Rays* 1986;11:51–54.

Buetow PC, Kransdorf MJ, Moser RP jr, Jelinek JS, Berrey BH. Radiologic appearance of intramuscular hemangioma with emphasis on MR imaging. *AJR Am J Roentgenol* 1990;154:563–567.

Buirski G, Watt I. The radiological features of solid aneurysmal bone cysts. *Br J Radiol* 1984;57:1057–1065.

Bulichova LV, Unni KK, Bertoni F, Beabout JW. Fibrocartilaginous mesenchymoma of bone. *Am J Surg Pathol* 1993;17:830–836.

Bullough PG. *Atlas of orthopedic pathology with clinical and radiologic correlation*, 2nd ed. New York: Gower;1992:15.12–15.14.

Burmester GR, Winchester RJ, Dimitriu-Bona A, Klein MJ, Steiner G, Sissons HA. Delineation of four cell types comprising the giant cell tumor of bone. *J Clin Invest* 1983;71:1633–1648.

Burnstein MI, De Smet AA, Hafez GR, Heiner JP. Case report 611. Subperiosteal aneurysmal bone cyst of tibia. *Skeletal Radiol* 1990;4:294–297.

Campanacci M. *Bone and soft tissue tumors.* New York: Springer Verlag;1986:345–348.

Campanacci M, Baldini N, Boriani S, Sudanese A. Giant cell tumor of bone. *J Bone Joint Surg [Am]* 1987;69A:106–114.

Campanacci M, Capanna R, Picci P. Unicameral and aneurysmal bone cysts. *Clin Orthop* 1986;204:25–36.

Campanacci M, Giunti A, Olmi R. Giant-cell tumors of bone: a study of 209 cases with long-term follow-up in 130. *Ital J Orthop Traumatol* 1975;1:249–277.

Campbell RSD, Grainger AJ, Mangham DC, Beggs I, Teh J, Davies AM. Intraosseous lipoma: report of 35 new cases and a review of the literature. *Skeletal Radiol* 2003;32:209–222.

Capanna R, Van Horn J, Ruggieri P, Biagini R. Epiphyseal involvement in unicameral bone cysts. *Skeletal Radiol* 1986;15:428–432.

Carrasco CH, Murray JA. Giant cell tumors. *Orthop Clin North Am* 1989;20:395–405.

Caskey PM, Wolf MD, Fechner RE. Multicentric giant cell reparative granuloma of the small bones of the hand. A case report and review of the literature. *Clin Orthop* 1985;193:199–205.

Choma ND, Biscotti CV, Bauer TW, Betho AC, Licata, AA. Gorham's syndrome: a case report and review of the literature. *Am J Med* 1987;83:1151–1156.

Chow LT, Lee K. Intraosseous lipoma. A clinicopathological study of nine cases. *Am J Surg Pathol* 1992;16:401–410.

Chung EG, Enzinger FM. Infantile myofibromatosis. *Cancer* 1981;48:1807–1818.

Clough JR, Price CH. Aneurysmal bone cyst: pathogenesis and long term results of treatment. *Clin Orthop* 1973;97:52–63.

Cohen J. Etiology of simple bone cyst. *J Bone Joint Surg [Am]* 1970;52A:1493–1497.

Cohen J. Unicameral bone cysts: a current synthesis of reported cases. *Orthop Clin North Am* 1977;8:715–726.

Cohen JW, Weinreb JC, Redman HC. Arteriovenous malformations of the extremities: MR imaging. *Radiology* 1986;158:475–479.

Conway WF, Hayes CW. Miscellaneous lesions of bone. *Radiol Clin North Am* 1993;31:339–358.

Cooper PH. Is histiocytoid hemangioma a specific pathologic entity? *Am J Surg Pathol* 1988;12:815–817.

Dabska M, Buraczewski J. Aneurysmal bone cyst. Pathology, clinical course and radiologic appearances. *Cancer* 1969;23:371–389.

Dahlin DC. Giant cell tumor of bone: highlights of 407 cases. *AJR Am J Roentgenol* 1985;144:955–960.

Dahlin DC. Giant cell bearing lesions of bone of the hands. *Hand Clin* 1987;3:291–297.

Dahlin DC, Bertoni F, Beabout JW, Campanacci M. Fibrocartilaginous mesenchymoma with low grade malignancy. *Skeletal Radial* 1984;12:263–269.

Dahlin DC, Cupps RE, Johnson EW Jr. Giant cell tumor: a study of 195 cases. *Cancer* 1970;25:1061–1070.

Dahlin DC, McLeod RA. Aneurysmal bone cyst and other nonneoplastic conditions. *Skeletal Radiol* 1982;8:243–250.

Dahlin DC, Unni KK. *Bone tumors: general aspects and data on 8,542 cases,* 4th ed. Springfield, IL: Charles C Thomas;1986:181–185.

deSantos LA, Murray JA. Evaluation of giant cell tumor by computerized tomography. *Skeletal Radiol* 1978;2:205–212.

Donnelly LF, Adams DM, Bisset III GS. Vascular malformations and hemangiomas: a practical approach in a multidisciplinary clinic. *AJR Am J Roentgenol* 2000;174:597–608.

Dooms GC, Hricak H, Sollitto RA, Higgins CB. Lipomatous tumors and tumors with fatty component: MR imaging potential and comparison of MR and CT results. *Radiology* 1985;157:479–483.

Dumford K, Moore TE, Walker CW, Jaksha J. Multifocal, metachronous, giant cell tumor of the lower limb. *Skeletal Radiol* 2003;32:147–150.

Duncan CP, Morton KS, Arthur JS. Giant cell tumor of bone: its aggressiveness and potential for malignant change. *Can J Surg* 1983;26:475–476.

Eckhardt JJ, Grogan TJ. Giant cell tumor of bone. *Clin Orthop* 1986;204:45–58.

Egan AJM, Boardman LA, Tazelaar HD, et al. Erdheim-Chester disease. Clinical, radiologic, and histopathologic findings in five patients with lung disease. *Am J Surg Pathol* 1999;23:17–26.

Enzinger FM, Weiss SW. Benign tumors and tumorlike lesions of blood vessels. In: Enzinger FM, Weiss SW, eds. *Soft tissue tumors,* 3rd ed. St. Louis: CV Mosby;1995.

Fechner RE, Mills SE. *Tumors of the bones and joints.* Washington, DC: Armed Forces Institute of Pathology;1993:173–186, 203–209, 253–258.

Francis R, Lewis E. CT demonstration of giant cell tumor complicating Paget disease. *J Comput Assist Tomogr* 1983;7:917–918.

Freeby JA, Reinus WR, Wilson AJ. Quantitative analysis of the plain radiographic appearance of aneurysmal bone cyst. *Invest Radial* 1995;30:433–439.

Friedman DP. Symptomatic vertebral hemangiomas: MR findings. *AJR Am J Roentgenol* 1996;167:359–364.

Fush SE, Herndon JH. Aneurysmal bone cyst involving the hand: a review and report of two cases. *J Hand, Surg [Am]* 1979;4A:152–159.

Garg NK, Carty H, Walsh HPJ, Dorgan JC, Bruce CE. Percutaneous Ethibloc injection in aneurysmal bone cysts. *Skeletal Radiol* 2000;29:211–216.

Gerard PS, Wilck E. Spinal hemangioma. An unusual photopenic presentation on bone scan. *Spine* 1992;17:607–610.

Glass TA, Mills SE, Fechner RE, Dyer R, Martin W, Armstrong P. Giant-cell reparative granuloma of the hands and feet. *Radiology* 1983;149:65–68.

Godfry LW, Gresham GA. The natural history of aneurysmal bone cyst. *Proc R Soc Med* 1959;52:900–905.

Goldberg RP, Genant HK. Case report 67. Solitary bone cyst of the right ilium. *Skeletal Radiol* 1978;3:118–121.

Goldenberg RR, Campbell CJ, Bonfiglio M. Giant-cell tumor of bone. An analysis of two hundred and eighteen cases. *J Bone Joint Surg [Am]* 1970;52A:619–664.

Gorham UV, Stout AP. Massive osteolysis (acute spontaneous absorption of bone, phantom bone, disappearing bone): its relation to haemangiomatosis. *J Bone Joint Surg [Am]* 1955;37A:985–1004.

Gorham LW, WrightAW, Shultz HH, Mexon FC Jr. Disappearing bones: a rare form of massive osteolysis. *Am J Med* 1954;17:674–682.

Graham DY, Gonzales J, Kothari SM. Diffuse skeletal angiomatosis. *Skeletal Radiol* 1978;3:131–35.

Gramiak R, Ruiz G, Campeti FL. Cystic angiomatosis of bone. *Radiology* 1957;69:347–353.

Greenfield GB, Arrington JA. *Imaging of bone tumors.* Philadelphia: JB Lippincott; 1995:217–218.

Greenspan A, Klein MJ, Bennett AJ, Lewis MM, Neuwirth M, Camins MB. Case report 242. Hemangioma of the T6 vertebra with a compression fracture, extradural block and spinal cord compression. *Skeletal Radiol* 1978;10:183–188.

Grote HJ, Braun M, Kalinski T, et al. Spontaneous malignant transformation of conventional giant cell tumor. *Skeletal Radiol* 2004;33:169–175.

Gutierrez RM, Spjut HJ. Skeletal angiomatosis: report of three cases and review of the literature. *Clin Orthop* 1972;85:82–97.

Haims AH, Desai P, Present D, Beltran J. Epiphyseal extension of a unicameral bone cyst. *Skeletal Radiol* 1997;26:51–54.

Han BK, Ryu J-S, Moon DH, Shin MI, Kim YT, Lee HK. Bone SPECT imaging of vertebral hemangioma. Correlations with MR imaging and symptoms. *Clin Nucl Med* 1995;20:916–921.

Hasegawa M, Kida S, Yamashima T, Yamashima J, Takakuwa S. Multicentric infantile myofibromatosis in the cranium: case report. *Neurosurgery* 1995;36:1200–1203.

Hawnaur JM, Whitehouse RW, Jenkins JPR, Isherwood I. Musculoskeletal haemangiomas: comparison of MRI with CT. *Skeletal Radiol* 1990;19:251–258.

Herman SD, Mesgarzadeh M, Bonakdarpour A, Dalinka MK. The role of magnetic resonance imaging in giant cell tumor of bone. *Skeletal Radiol* 1987;16:635–643.

Hermann G, Abdelwahab IF, Klein MJ, Berson BD, Lewis MM. Case report 603. Giant cell reparative granuloma of the distal end of right femur. *Skeletal Radiol* 1990;19:367–369.

Heyman S, Treves S. Scintigraphy in pediatric bone tumors. In: Jaffe N, ed. *Bone tumors in children.* Littleton, MA: Wright;1979:79–96.

Hudson TM. Fluid levels in aneurysmal bone cysts: a CT feature. *AJR Am J Roentgenol* 1984;141:1001–1004.

Hudson TM. Scintigraphy of aneurysmal bone cysts. *AJR Am J Roentgenol* 1984;142:761–765.

Hudson TM. *Radiologic pathologic correlation of musculoskeletal lesions.* Baltimore: Williams & Wilkins;1987:209–237, 249–252, 261–265.

Hudson TM, Hamlin DJ, Fitzimmons JR. Magnetic resonance imaging of fluid levels in an aneurysmal bone cyst and in anticoagulated human blood. *Skeletal Radiol* 1985;13:267–270.

Hudson TM, Schiebler M, Springfield DS, et al. Radiology of giant cell tumors of bone: computed tomography, arthrotomography, and scintigraphy. *Skeletal Radiol* 1984;11:85–95.

Hutter RVP, Worcester, JN Jr, Francis KC, Foote FW Jr, Stewart FW. Benign and malignant giant cell tumors of bone. A clinicopathological analysis of the natural history of the disease. *Cancer* 1962;15:653–690.

Huvos AG. *Bone tumors: diagnosis, treatment, and prognosis,* 2nd ed. Philadelphia: WB Saunders;1991:713–743.

Ilaslan H, Sundaram M, Unni KK. Solid variant of aneurysmal bone cysts in long tubular bones: giant cell reparative granuloma. *AJR Am J Roentgenol* 2003;180:1681–1687.

Ishida T, Dorfman HD, Steiner GC, Norman A. Cystic angiomatosis of bone with sclerotic changes, mimicking osteoblastic metastases. *Skeletal Radiol* 1994;23:247–252.

Jacobs JE, Kimmelstiel P. Cystic angiomatosis of the skeletal system. *J Bone Joint Surg [Am]* 1953;35A:409–420.

Jaffe HL. Aneurysmal bone cyst. *Bull Hosp Joint Dis* 1950;11:3–13.

Jaffe HL. Giant-cell reparative granuloma, traumatic bone cyst, and fibrous (fibro-osseous) dysplasia of the jawbones. *Oral Surg* 1953;6:159–175.

Jaffe HL. *Tumors and tumorous conditions of the bones and joints.* Philadelphia: Lea & Febiger;1958.

Jaffe HL, Lichtenstein L. Solitary unicameral bone cyst with emphasis on the roentgen picture, the pathoogic appearance, and the pathogenesis. *Arch Surg* 1942;44:1004–1025.

Jaffe HL, Lichtenstein L, Perris RB. Giant cell tumor of bone. Its pathologic appearance, grading, supposed variants and treatment. *Arch Pathol* 1940;30:993–1031.

Joseph UA, Jhingran SG. Technetium-99m labeled red blood cells in the evaluation of hemangioma. *Clin Nucl Med* 1987;12:845–847.

Junghanns H. Lipomas (fatty marrow areas) in the vertebral column. In: *Handbuch de speziellen pathologischen Anatomic und Histologic,* Tome IX/4. Berlin: Springer-Verlag;1939:333–334.

Kaleem Z, Kyriakos M, Totty WG. Solitary skeletal hemangioma of the extremities. *Skeletal Radiol* 2000;29:502–513.

Kaplan PA, Murphy M, Greenway G, Resnick D, Sartoris DJ, Harms S. Fluid-fluid levels in giant cell tumors of bone: report of two cases. *Computed Tomogr* 1987;11: 151–155.

Karlin CA, Brower AC. Multiple primary hemangiomas of bone. *AJR Am J Roentgenol* 1977;129:162–164.

Keats TE. *Atlas of normal roentgen variants that may simulate disease,* 5th ed. St. Louis: Mosby Year Book;1992:637–648.

Keats TE, Harrison RB. The calcaneal nutrient foramen: a useful sign in the differentiation of true from simulated cysts. *Skeletal Radiol* 1979;3:239–240.

Kinley S, Wiseman F, Wertheimer ST. Giant cell tumor of the talus with secondary aneurysmal bone cyst. *J Foot Ankle Surg* 1993;32:38–46.

Kohler A, Zimmer EA. *Borderlands of normal and early pathologic findings in skeletal radiography,* 13th ed. Revised by Schmidt H, Freyschmidt J. Stuttgart: Thieme Verlag;1993:797–814.

Kransdorf MJ, Sweet DE. Aneurysmal bone cyst: concept, controversy, clinical presentation, and imaging. *AJR Am J Roentgenol* 1995;164:573–580.

Kransdorf MJ, Sweet DE, Buetow PC, Giudici MA, Moser RP Jr. Giant cell tumor in skeletally immature patients. *Radiology* 1992;184:233–237.

Kricun ME. *Imaging of bone tumors.* Philadelphia: WB Saunders, 1993:236-237.

Kricun ME. Tumors of the foot. In: Kricun ME, ed. *Imaging of bone tumors.* Philadelphia: WB Saunders;1993:221–225.

Kricum ME, Kricun R, Haskin ME. Chondroblastoma of the calcaneus: radiographic features with emphasis on location. *AJR Am J Roentgenol* 1977;128:613–616.

Kyriakos M, Hardy D. Malignant transformation of aneurysmal bone cyst, with an analysis of the literature. *Cancer* 1991;68:1770–1780.

Ladanyi M, Traganos F, Huvos AG. Benign metastasizing giant cell tumors of bone: a DNA flow cytometric study. *Cancer* 1989;64:1521–1526.

Lagier R. Calcaneus lipoma with bone infarct. *Fortschr Roentgenstr* 1985;142:472–474.

Laredo JD, Assouline E, Gelbert F, Wybier M, Merland JJ, Tubiana JM. Vertebral hamangiomas: fat content as a sign of aggressiveness. *Radiology* 1990;177:467–472.

Laredo JD, Reizine D, Bard M, Merland JJ. Vertebral hemangiomas: radiologic evaluation. *Radiology* 1986;161:183–189.

Lateur L, Simoens CJ, Gryspeerdt S, Samson I, Mertens V, van Damme B. Skeletal cystic angiomatosis. *Skeletal Radiol* 1996;25:92–95.

Lee JA, Bank WD, Gonzalez-Melendez M, Olan WJ, Tabbara SO. Giant cell tumor of the skull. *Radiographics* 1998;18:1295–1302.

Levey DS, MacCormack LM, Sartoris DJ, Haghighi P, Resnick D, Thorne R. Cystic angiomatosis: case report and review of the literature. *Skeletal Radiol* 1996;25:287–293.

Levey DS, Sartoris DJ, Resnick D. Advanced diagnostic imaging techniques for pedal osseous neoplasms. *Clin Podiatr Med Surg* 1993;10:655–682.

Levin DC, Gordon DH, McSweeney J. Arteriography of peripheral hemangiomas. *Radiology* 1976;121:625–630.

Levin MF, Vellet AD, Munk PL, McLean CA. Intraosseous lipoma of the distal femur: MRI appearance. *Skeletal Radiol* 1996;25:82–84.

Levine E, DeSmet AA, Neff JR. Role of radiologic imaging in management planning of giant cell tumor of bone. *Skeletal Radiol* 1984;12:79–89.

Levine E, DeSmet AA, Neff JR, Martin NL. Scintigraphic evaluation of giant cell tumor of bone. *AJR Am J Roentgenol* 1984;143:343–348.

Levy WM, Miller AS, Bonakdarpour A, Aegerter E. Aneurysmal bone cyst secondary to other osseous lesions. Report of 5 7 cases. *Am J Clin Pathol* 1975;63:1–8.

Lichtenstein L. Aneurysmal bone cyst. A pathological entity commonly mistaken for giant cell tumor and occasionally for hemangioma and osteogenic sarcoma. *Cancer* 1950;3:279–289.

Lichtenstein L. Aneurysmal bone cyst. Observations on fifty cases. *J Bone Joint Surg [Am]* 1957;39A:873–882.

Ling L, Klein MJ, Sissons HA, Steiner GC, Winchester RJ. Expression of Ia and monocyte-macrophage lineage antigens in giant cell tumor of bone and related lesions. *Arch Pathol Lab Med* 1988;112:65–69.

Lomasney LM, Basu A, Demos TC, Laskin W. Fibrous dysplasia complicated by aneurysmal bone cyst formation affecting multiple cervical vertebrae. *Skeletal Radiol* 2003;32:533–536.

Lomasney LM, Martinez S, Demos TC, Harrelson JM. Multifocal vascular lesions of bone: imaging characteristics. *Skeletal Radiol* 1996;25:255–261.

Lorenzo JC, Dorfman HD. Giant-cell reparative granuloma of short tubular bones of the hands and feet. *Am J Surg Pathol* 1980;4:551–563.

Makhija M, Bofill ER. Hemangioma: a rare cause of photopenic lesion on skeletal imaging. *Clin Nucl Med* 1988;13:661–662.

Maloney WJ, Vaughan LM, Jones HH, Ross J, Nagel DA. Benign metastasizing giant-cell tumor of bone. Report of three cases and review of the literature. *Clin Orthop* 1989;243:208–215.

Manaster BJ, Doyle AJ. Giant cell tumor of bone. *Radiol Clin North Am* 1993;31:299–323.

Martinat P, Cotten A, Singer B, Petyt L, Chastanet P. Solitary cystic lymphangioma. *Skeletal Radiol* 1995;24:556–558.

Martinez V, Sissons HA. Aneurysmal bone cyst. A review of 123 cases including primary lesions and those secondary to other bone pathology. *Cancer* 1988;61: 2291–2304.

Marui T, Yamamoto T, Yoshihara H, Kurosaka M, Mizuno K, Akamatsu T. De novo malignant transformation of giant cell tumor of bone. *Skeletal Radiol* 2001;30: 104–108.

Matsumoto K, Ishizawa M, Okabe H, Taniguchi I. Hemangioma of bone arising in the ulna: imaging findings with emphasis on MR. *Skeletal Radiol* 2000;29:231–234.

May DA, Good RB, Smith DK, Parsons T`W. MR imaging of musculoskeletal tumors and tumor mimickers with intravenous gadolinium: experience with 242 patients. *Skeletal Radiol* 1997;26:2–15.

McCarthy EF, Dorfman HD. Vascular and cartilaginous hamartoma of the ribs in infancy

with secondary aneurysmal bone cyst formation. *Am J Surg Pathol* 1980;4: 247–253.

McDonald DJ, Sim FH, McLeod RA, Dahlin DC. Giant cell tumor of bone. *J Bone Joint Surg [Am]* 1986;68A:235–242.

McGlynn FJ, Mickelson MR, El-Khoury GY. The fallen fragment sign in unicameral bone cyst. *Clin Orthop* 1981;156:157–159.

McGrath J. Giant-cell tumour of bone: an analysis of fifty-two cases. *J Bone Joint Surg [Br]* 1972;54B:216–229.

McInerney DP, Middlemis JH. Giant-cell tumors of bone. *Skeletal Radiol* 1978;2:195–204.

Meis JM, Dorfman HD, Nathanson SD, Haggar AM, Wu KK. Primary malig nant giant cell tumor of bone: dedifferentiated giant cell tumor. *Mod Pathol* 1989;2:541–546.

Meyer JS, Hoffer FA, Barnes PD, Mulliken JB. Biological classification of soft-tissue vascular anomalies: MR correlation. *AJR Am J Roentgenol* 1991;157:559–564.

Milgram JW. Intraosseous lipoma: radiologic and pathologic manifestations. *Radiology* 1988;167:155–160.

Milgram JW. Intraosseous lipomas. A clinicopathological study of 66 cases. *Clin Orthop* 1988;231:277–302.

Mintz MC, Dalinka MK, Schmidt R. Aneurysmal bone cyst arising in fibrous dysplasia during pregnancy. *Radiology* 1987;165:549–550.

Mirra JM, Arnold WD. Skeletal hemangiomatosis in association with hereditary hemorrhagic telangiectasia. *J Bone Joint Surg [Am]* 1973;55A:850–854.

Moore TE, King AR, Travis RC, Allen BC. Post-traumatic cysts and cyst-like lesions of bone. *Skeletal Radiol* 1989;18:93–97.

Moreno AJ, Reeves TA, Turnbull GL. Hemangioma of bone. *Clin Nucl Med* 1988;13:668–669.

Morton KS. The pathogenesis of unicameral bone cyst. *Can J Surg* 1964;7:140–150.

Moser RP Jr, Kransdorf MJ, Gilkey FW, Manaster BJ. Giant cell tumor of the upper extremity. *Radiographics* 1990;10:83–102.

Mueller MC, Robbins JL. Intramedullary lipoma of bone. Report of a case. *J Bone Joint Surg [Am]* 1960;42A:517–520.

Mulder JD, Kroon HM, SchCtte HE, Taconis WK. *Radiologic atlas of bone tumors.* Amsterdam: Elsevier; 1993:241–254, 507–516, 557–590.

Mulliken JB, Glowacki J. Hemangiomas and vascular malformations in infants and children: a classification based on endothelial characteristics. *Plast Reconstr Surg* 1982;69:412–420.

Mulliken JB, Zetter BR, Folkman J. In vitro characteristics of endothelium from hemangiomas and vascular malformations. *Surgery* 1982;92:348–353.

Munk PL, Helms CA, Holt RG, Johnston J, Steinbach L, Neumann C. MR imaging of aneurysmal bone cysts. *AJR Am J Roentgenol* 1989;153:99–101.

Murphey MD, Fairbairn KJ, Parman LM, Baxter KG, Parsa MB, Smith WS. Musculoskeletal angiomatous lesions: radiologic-pathologic correlation. *Radiographics* 1995;15:893–917.

Murphey MD, Nomikos GC, Flemming DJ, Gannon FH, Temple HT, Kransdorf MJ. From the archives of the AFIP. Imaging of giant cell tumor and giant cell reparative granuloma of bone: radiologic-pathologic correlation. *Radiographics* 2001;21: 1283–1309.

Nascimento AG, Huvos AG, Marcove RC. Primary malignant giant cell tumor of bone: a study of eight cases and review of the literature. *Cancer* 1979;44:1393–1402.

Neer CS II, Francis KC, Marcove RC, Tertz J, Carbonara PN. Treatment of unicameral bone cyst. A follow-up study of one hundred seventy-five cases. *J Bone Joint Surg [Am]* 1966;48A:731–745.

Netherlands Committee on Bone Tumors. *Radiological atlas of bone tumors,* vol 1. Baltimore: Williams & Wilkins;1966.

Nojima T, Takeda N, Matsuno T, Inoue K, Nagashima K. Case report 869. Benign metastasizing giant cell tumor of bone. *Skeletal Radiol* 1994;23:583–585.

Norman A, Schiffman M. Simple bone cyst: factors of age dependency. *Radiology* 1977;124:779–782.

Norman A, Steiner GC. Radiographic and morphological features of cyst formation in idiopathic bone infarction. *Radiology* 1983;146:335–338.

Nusbacher N, Sclafani SJ, Birla SR. Case report 155. Polyostotic Paget disease complicated by benign giant cell tumor of left clavicle. *Skeletal Radiol* 1981;6:233–235.

Oda Y, Tsuneyoshi M, Shinohara N. Solid variant of aneurysmal bone cyst (extragnatic giant cell reparative granuloma) in the axial skeleton and long bones: a study of its morphologic spectrum and distinction from allied giant cell lesions. *Cancer* 1992;70:2642–2649.

O'Reilly M, Chew FS. The scintigraphic features of giant-cell tumors in relation to other imaging modalities. *Clin Nucl Med* 1996;21:43–48.

Paley D, Evans DC. Angiomatous involvement of an extremity: a spectrum of syndromes. *Clin Orthop* 1986;206:215–218.

Park I-H, Jeon I-H. Multicentric giant cell tumor of bone: ten lesions at presentation. *Skeletal Radiol* 2003;32:526–529.

Pearce WH, Rutherford RB, Whitehill TA, Davis K. Nuclear magnetic resonance imaging: its diagnostic value in patients with congenital vascular malformations of the limbs. *J Vasc Surg* 1988;8:64–70.

Peimer CA, Schiller AL, Mankin HJ, Smith RJ. Multicentric giant cell tumor of bone. *J Bone Joint Surg [Am]* 1980;62A:652–656.

Picci P, Baldini N, Sudanese A, Boriani S, Campanacci M. Giant cell reparative granuloma and other giant cell lesions of the bones of the hand and feet. *Skeletal Radiol* 1986;15:415–421.

Picci P, Manfrini M, Zucchi V, et al. Giant cell tumor bone in skeletally immature patients. *J Bone Joint Surg [Am]* 1983:65A:486–490.

Posteraro RH. Radiographic evaluation of pedal osseous tumors. *Clin Podiatr Med Surg* 1993;10:633–653.

Potter HG, Schneider R, Ghelman B, Healey JH, Lane JM. Multiple giant cell tumors and Paget disease of bone: radiographic and clinical correlations. *Radiology* 1991;180:261–264.

Poussa M, Holmstrom T. Intraosseous lipoma of the calcaneus: report of a case and a short review of the literature. *Acta Orthop Scand* 1976;47:570–574.

Propeck T, Bullard MA, Lin J, Doi K, Martel W. Radiologic-pathologic correlation of intraosseous lipomas. *AJR Am J Roentgenol* 2000;175:673–678.

Ramos A, Castello J, Sartoris DJ, Greenway GD, Resnick D, Haghighi P. Osseous lipoma: CT appearance. *Radiology* 1985;157:615–619.

Ratcliffe PJ, Grimmer RJ. Aneurysmal bone cyst arising after tibial fracture. A case report. *J Bone Joint Surg [Am]* 1993;75A:1225–1227.

Ratner V, Dorfman HD. Giant-cell reparative granuloma of the hand and foot bones. *Clin Orthop* 1990;260:251–258.

Reid AB, Reid IL, Johnson G, Hamonic M, Major P. Familial diffuse cystic angiomatosis of bone. *Clin Orthop* 1989;238:211–218.

Remagen W. Pathologische Anatomic der Femurkopfnekrose. *Orthopäde* 1990;19: 174–181.

Remagen W, Lampérth BE, Jundt G, Schildt R. Das sogenannte osteolytische Dreieck de Calcaneus. Radiologische and pathoanatomische Befunde. *Osteologie* 1994;3: 275–283.

Resnick D, Greenway G, Genant H, Brower A, Haghighi P, Emmett M. Erdheim-Chester disease. *Radiology* 1982;142:289–295.

Resnick D, Kyriakos M, Greenway GD. Tumors and tumor-like lesions of bone: imaging and pathology of specific lesions. In: Resnick D, ed. *Bone and joint imaging.* Philadelphia: WB Saunders; 1989:1154–1156.

Resnick D, Kyriakos M, Greenway GD. Tumors and tumor-like lesions of bone: imaging and pathology of specific lesions. In: Resnick D, ed. *Diagnosis of bone and joint disorders,* 3rd ed. Philadelphia: WB Saunders; 1995:3628–3938.

Resnick D, Niwayama J. *Diagnosis of bone and joint disorders.* Philadelphia: WB Saunders;1988:3782–3786.

Resnik CS, Steffe JW, Wang SE. Case report 353. Giant cell tumor of distal end of the femur, containing a fluid level as demonstrated by computed tomography. *Skeletal Radiol* 1986;15:175–177.

Reynolds J. The fallen fragment sign in the diagnosis of unicameral bone cysts. *Radiology* 1969;92:949–953.

Rock MG, Pritchard DJ, Unni KK. Metastases from histologically benign giant-cell tumor of bone. *J Bone Joint Surg [Am]* 1984;66A:269–274.

Rock MG, Sim FH, Unni KK, et al. Secondary malignant giant-cell tumor of bone. Clinicopathological assessment of nineteen patients. *J Bone Joint Surg [Am]* 1986;68A: 1073–1079.

Rosai J. Carcinoma of pancreas simulating giant cell tumor of bone. Electronmicroscopic evidence of its acinar cell origin. *Cancer* 1968;22:333–344.

Ross JS, Masaryk TJ, Modic MT, Carter JR, Mapstone T, Dengel FH. Vertebral hemangioma: MR imaging. *Radiology* 1987;165:165–169.

Ruiter DJ, van Rijssel TG, van der Velde EA. Aneurysmal bone cysts. A clinicopathological study of 105 cases. *Cancer* 1977;39:2231–2239.

Sanerkin NG. Malignancy, aggressiveness and recurrence in giant cell tumor of bone. *Cancer* 1980;46:1641–1649.

Sanerkin NG, Mott MG, Roylance J. An unusual intraosseous lesion with fibromyxoid elements: solid variant of aneurysmal bone cyst. *Cancer* 1983;51:2278–2286.

Schajowicz F. *Tumors and tumorlike lesions of bone: pathology, radiology, and treatment,* 2nd ed. Berlin: Springer-Verlag, 1994:257–299.

Schajowicz F, Aiello CL, Francone MV, Giannini RE. Cystic angiomatosis (hamartous haemolymphlangiomatosis) of bone. *J Bone Joint Surg [Br]* 1978;60B:100–106.

Schajowicz F, Slullitel J. Giant cell tumor associated with Paget's disease of bone. *J Bone Joint Surg [Am]* 1966:48A:1340–1349.

Schoedel K, Shankman S, Desai P. Intracortical and subperiosteal aneurysmal bone cysts: a report of three cases. *Skeletal Radiol* 1996;25:455–459.

Scully SP, Temple HT, O'Keefe RJ, Gebhardt MC. Case report 830. Aneurysmal bone cyst. *Skeletal Radiol* 1994;23:157–160.

Shankman S, Greenspan A, Klein MJ, Lewis MM. Giant cell tumor of the ischium. A report of two cases and review of the literature. *Skeletal Radial* 1988;17:46–51.

Sharma P, Elangovan S, Ratnakar C. Case report: calcification within aneurysmal bone cyst. *Br J Radiol* 1994;67:306–308.

Sherman RS, Soong KY Aneurysmal bone cyst: its roentgen diagnosis. *Radiology* 1957;68:54–64.

Sherman RS, Wilner D. The roentgen diagnosis of hemangioma of bone. *AJR Am J Roentgenol* 1961;86:1146–1159.

Sim FH, Dahlin DC, Beabout JW. Multicentric giant cell tumors of bone. *J Bone Joint Surg [Am]* 1977;59A:1052–1060.

Simon MA, Kirchner PT. Scintigraphic evaluation of primary bone tumors. *J Bone, Joint Surg [Am]* 1980;62A:758–764.

Sirry A. The pseudo-cystic triangle in the normal os calcis. *Acta Radiol* 1951;36:516–520.

Smith RW, Smith CF. Solitary unicameral bone cyst of the calcaneus. A review of 20 cases. *J Bone Joint Surg [Am]* 1974;56A:49–56.

Soper JR, De Silva M. Infantile myofibromatosis: a radiological review. *Pediatr Radial* 1993;23:189–194.

Spieth ME, Greenspan A, Forrester DM, Ansari AN, Kimura RL, GleasonJordan I. Gorham's disease of the radius: radiographic, scintigraphic, and MRI findings with pathologic correlation. *Skeletal Radiol* 1997;26:659–663.

Spjut HJ, Dorfman HD, Fechner RE, Ackerman LV. *Tumors of bone and cartilage.* Washington, DC: Armed Forces Institute of Pathology, 1971.

Stacy GS, Peabody TD, Dixon LB. Pictorial essay. Mimics on radiography of giant cell tumor of bone. *AJR Am J Roentgenol* 2003;181:1583–1589.

Steiner GC, Ghosh L, Dorfman HD. Ultrastructure of giant cell tumor of bone. *Hum Pathol* 1972;3:569–586.

Steiner GM, Farman J, Lawson JP. Lymphangiomatosis of bone. *Radiology* 1969;93:1093–1098.

Struhl S, Edelson C, Pritzker H, Seimon LP, Dorfman HD. Solitary (unicameral) bone cyst. The fallen fragment sign revisited. *Skeletal Radial* 1989;18:261–265.

Suh JS, Hwang G, Hahn SB. Soft tissue hemangiomas: MR manifestations in 23 patients. *Skeletal Radial* 1994;23:621–625.

Taybi H, Lachman RS. *Radiology of syndromes, metabolic disorders, and skeletal dysplasias,* 4th ed. St. Louis: CV Mosby, 1996:580–581.

Tehranzadeh J, Murphy BJ, Mnaymneh W. Giant cell tumor of the proximal tibia: MR and CT appearance. *J Comput Assist Tomogr* 1989;13:282–286.

Thrall JH, Geslien GE, Corcoron RJ, Johnson MC. Abnormal radionuclide deposition patterns adjacent to focal skeletal lesions. *Radiology* 1975;115:659–663.

Tillman BP, Dahlin DC, Lipscomb PR, Stewart JR. Aneurysmal bone cyst: an analysis of ninety-five cases. *Mayo Clin Proc* 1968;43:478–495.

Torg JS, Steel HH. Sequential roentgenographic changes occurring in massive osteolysis. *J Bone Joint Surg [Am]* 1969;51A:1649–1655.

Tornberg DN, Dick HM, Johnston AD. Multicentric giant-cell tumors in the long bones. A case report. *J Bone Joint Surg [Am]* 1975;57A:420–422.

Tsai JC, Dalinka MK, Fallon MD, Zlatkin MB, Kresel HY. Fluid-fluid level: a nonspecific finding in tumors of bone and soft tissue. *Radiology* 1990;175:779–782.

Tubbs WS, Brown LR, Beabout JW, Rock MG, Unni KK. Benign giant-cell tumor of bone with pulmonary metastases: clinical findings and radiologic appearance of metastases in 13 cases. *AJR Am J Roentgenol* 1992;158:331–334.

Unni KK. *Dublin's bone tumors: general aspects and data on 11,087 cases,* 5th ed. New York: Lippincott-Raven Publishers;1996.

Van Linthoudt D, Lagier R. Calcaneal cysts: a radiological and anatomical-pathological study. *Acta Orthop Scand* 1978;49:310–316.

Van Nostrand D, Madewell JE, McNiesh LM, Kyle RW, Sweet D. Radionuclide bone scanning in giant cell tumor. *J Nucl Med* 1986;27:329–338.

Variend S, Bax MN, Van Gorp J. Are infantile myofibromatosis, congenital fibrosarcoma and congenital haemangiopericytoma histogenetically related? *Histopathology* 1995;26:57–62.

Vergel De Dios AM, Bond JR, Shives TC, McLeod RA, Unni KK. Aneurysmal bone cyst. A clinicopathologic study of 238 cases. *Cancer* 1992;69:2921–2931.

Vilanova JC, Barceló J, Smirniotopoulos JG, et al. Hemangioma from head to toe: MR imaging with pathologic correlation. *Radiographics* 2004;24:367–385.

Vinee P, Tanyu O, Havenstein KH, Sigmund G, Stover B, Adler CP. CT and MRI of Gorham syndrome. *J Comput Assist Tomogr* 1994;18:985–989.

Waldron RT, Zeller JA. Diffuse skeletal hemangiomatosis with visceral involvement. *J Can Assoc Radiol* 1969;20:119–123.

Weisel A, Hecht HL. Development of a unicameral bone cyst. *J Bone Joint Surg [Am]* 1980;62A:664–666.

Wenger DE, Wold LE. Benign vascular lesions of bone: radiologic and pathologic features. *Skeletal Radiol* 2000;29:63–74.

Williams AG Jr, Mettler FA Jr. Vertebral hemangioma. Radionuclide, radiographic, and CT correlation. *Clin Nucl Med* 1985;10:598.

Williams HT. Multicentric giant cell tumor of bone. *Clin Nucl Med* 1989;14:631–633.

Wilner D. *Radiology of bone tumors and allied disorders.* Philadelphia: WB Saunders; 1982:387.

Winterberger AR. Radiographic diagnosis of lymphangiomatosis of bone. *Radiology* 1972;102:321–324.

Wold LE, Dobyns JH, Swee RG, Dahlin DC. Giant cell reaction (giant cell reparative granuloma) of the small bones of the hands and feet. *Am J Surg Pathol* 1986;10:491–496.

Wold LE, Swee RG. Giant cell tumor of the small bones of the hands and feet. *Semin Diagn Pathol* 1984;1:173–184.

Wold LE, Swee RG, Sim FH. Vascular lesions of bone. *Pathol Annu* 1985;20/2:101–137.

Wray CC, MacDonald AW, Richardson RA. Benign giant-cell tumor with metastases to bone and lung. *J Bone Joint Surg [Br]* 1990;72B:486–489.

Yamamoto T, Marui T, Akisue T, Mizuno K. Solid aneurysmal bone cyst in the humerus. *Skeletal Radiol* 2000;29:470–473.

Yoo SY, Hong SH, Chung HW, Choi J-A, Kim CJ, Kang HS. MRI of Gorham's disease: findings in two cases. *Skeletal Radiol* 2002;31:301–306.

Zhu X, Steiner GC. Malignant giant cell tumor of bone: malignant transformation of a benign giant cell tumor treated by surgery. *Bull Hosp Joint Dis Orthop Inst* 1990;50: 169–176.

Zimmer WD, Berquist TH, McLeod RA, et al. Bone tumors: magnetic resonance imaging versus computed tomography. *Radiology* 1985;155:709–718.

Zimmer WD, Berquist TH, Sim FH, et al. Magnetic resonance imaging of aneurysmal bone cyst. *Mayo Clin Proc* 1984;59:633–636.

Zorn DT, Cordray DR, Randels PH. Intraosseous lipoma of bone involving the sacrum. *J Bone Joint Surg [Am]* 1971;53A:1201–1204.

MALIGNANT BONE TUMORS I

Osteosarcomas and Chondrosarcomas

Osteosarcomas

Osteosarcoma (osteogenic sarcoma) is one of the most common primary malignant bone tumors, comprising approximately 20% of all primary bone malignancies. There are several types of osteosarcoma (Fig. 21.1), each having distinctive clinical, radiographic, and histologic characteristics. The common feature of all types is that the osteoid and bone matrix are formed by malignant cells of connective tissue.

The majority of osteosarcomas are of unknown cause and can therefore be referred to as idiopathic, or *primary*. A smaller number of tumors can be related to known factors predisposing to malignancy, such as Paget disease, fibrous dysplasia, external ionizing irradiation, or ingestion of radioactive substances. These lesions are referred to as *secondary* osteosarcomas. All types of osteosarcomas may be further subdivided by anatomic site into lesions of the appendicular skeleton and axial skeleton. Furthermore, they may be classified on the basis of their location in the bone as central (medullary), intracortical, and juxtacor-

tical. A separate group consists of primary osteosarcoma originating in the soft tissues (so-called extraskeletal or soft-tissue osteosarcomas).

Histopathologically, osteosarcomas can be graded on the basis of their cellularity, nuclear pleomorphism, and degree of mitotic activity. According to Broder's system, the numerical grade (1 to 4) indicates the degree of malignancy (grade 1 indicating the least undifferentiated tumor and grade 4 the most undifferentiated tumor) (Table 21.1). For example, well-differentiated central osteosarcomas and parosteal osteosarcomas are regarded as grade 1 or, rarely, grade 2 tumors; periosteal osteosarcomas and gnathic osteosarcomas as grade 2 or, rarely, grade 3; and conventional osteosarcoma is grade 3 or 4. Telangiectatic osteosarcomas, osteosarcomas developing in pagetic bone, postirradiation osteosarcomas, and multifocal osteosarcomas are usually grade 4 tumors. This grading has clinical, therapeutic, and prognostic importance. Generally speaking, central osteosarcomas are much more frequent than juxtacortical tumors, and they tend to have a higher histologic grade. Although pulmonary metastasis is the most common and most significant complication in high-grade osteosarcoma, it is rare in two subtypes: osteosarcoma of the jaw and multicentric osteosarcoma.

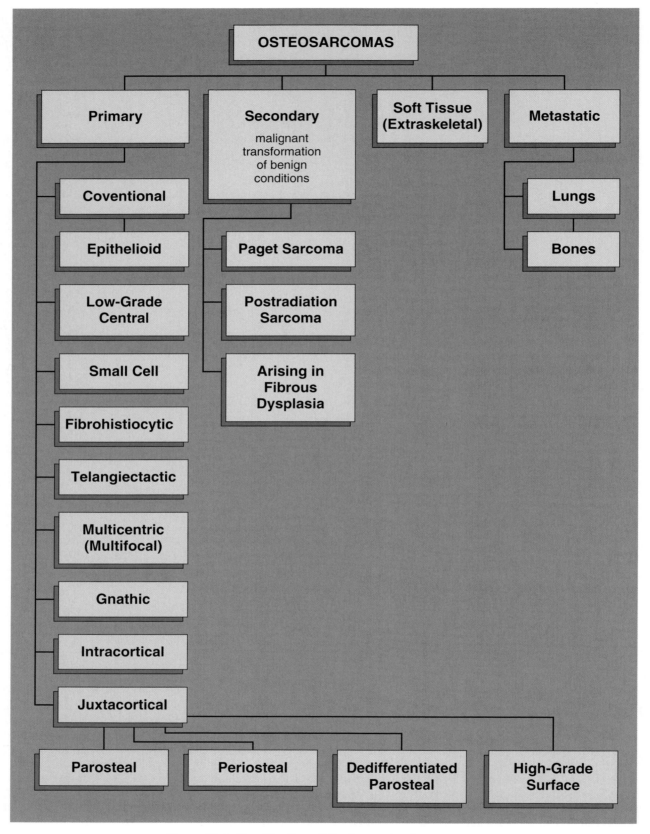

Figure 21.1 Classification of the types of osteosarcoma.

Table 21.1 **Histologic Grading of Osteosarcoma**

Grade	Histologic Features	Grade	Histologic Features
1	Cellularity: slightly increased Cytologic atypia: minimal to slight Mitotic activity: low Osteoid matrix: regular	3	Cellularity: increased Cytologic atypia: moderate to marked Mitotic activity: moderate to high Osteoid matrix: irregular
2	Cellularity: moderate Cytologic atypia: mild to moderate Mitotic activity: low to moderate Osteoid matrix: regular	4	Cellularity: markedly increased Cytologic atypia: markedly pleomorphic cells Mitotic activity: high Osteoid matrix: irregular, abundant

According to Unni KK, Dahlin DC, 1984

Primary Osteosarcomas

Conventional Osteosarcoma

Conventional osteosarcoma is the most frequent type, having its highest incidence in patients in their second decade and affecting males slightly more often than females. It has a predilection for the knee region (distal femur and proximal tibia), whereas the second most common site is the proximal humerus (Fig. 21.2). Patients usually present with bone pain, occasionally accompanied by a soft-tissue mass or swelling. At times, the first symptoms are related to pathologic fracture.

The distinctive radiologic features of conventional osteosarcoma, as demonstrated by radiography, are medullary and cortical bone destruction, an aggressive periosteal reaction, a soft-tissue mass, and tumor-bone either within the destructive lesion or at its periphery, as well as within the soft-tissue mass (Fig. 21.3). In some instances, the type of bone destruction may not be obvious on the conventional studies, but patchy densities representing tumor-bone and an aggressive periosteal reaction are clues to the diagnosis (Fig. 21.4).

The degree of radiopacity in the tumor reflects a combination of the amount of tumor bone production, calcified matrix, and osteoid. Tumors may present as purely sclerotic lesions or purely osteolytic lesions, but mostly a combination of both (Fig. 21.5). The borders are usually indistinct, with a wide zone of transition. The type of bone destruction is either moth-eaten or permeative, and only rarely geographic.

The most common types of periosteal response encountered with this tumor are the "sunburst" type and a Codman triangle; the lamellated (onionskin) type of reaction is less frequently seen (Fig. 21.6). In the past, computed tomography (CT) was an indispensable technique for evaluating these tumors (Fig. 21.7). This was particularly important if a limb-salvage procedure was contemplated, because extension of the tumor into the medullary cavity is crucial information for effective surgical planning (see Fig. 16.8). Recently, magnetic resonance imaging (MRI) has become an equally effective modality for evaluating these tumors, particularly for intraosseous tumor extension and soft-tissue involvement. On T1-weighted images, the solid non-mineralized parts of osteosarcoma generally present as areas of low to intermediate signal intensity. On T2-weighted images, the tumor demonstrates a high signal intensity (Fig. 21.8). Osteosclerotic tumors demonstrate low signal intensity on all imaging sequences (Fig. 21.9). MRI may also effectively demonstrate peritumoral edema. This feature displays an intermediate intensity signal on T1-weighted and a high intensity on T2-weighted images and is seen in the soft tissues surrounding the tumor. CT (see Fig. 16.9) and MRI are also essential in monitoring the results of treatment.

Based on the dominant histologic features, conventional osteosarcoma can be subdivided into three histologic subtypes: osteoblastic, chondroblastic, and fibroblastic. The last may occasionally mimic malignant fibrous histiocytoma. At times, the tumor cells may be so undifferentiated that on a purely cytologic basis, it is difficult to tell whether they are sarcomatous or epithelial. This variant of conventional osteosarcoma is sometimes referred to as epithelioid osteosarcoma. The diagnosis usually becomes evident from the patient's

Conventional Osteosarcoma

age: 10–20

M ≥ F

■ common sites
■ less common sites

Figure 21.2 **Skeletal sites of predilection, peak age range, and male-to-female ratio in conventional osteosarcoma.**

Figure 21.3 Osteosarcoma. Anteroposterior **(A)** and lateral **(B)** radiographs demonstrate the typical features of osteosarcoma in the femur of a 19-year-old woman. Medullary and cortical bone destruction can be seen in association with an aggressive periosteal response of the velvet and sunburst types, as well as with a soft-tissue mass containing tumor bone.

Figure 21.4 Osteosarcoma. Although there is no gross bone destruction evident in the distal femur of this 16-year-old girl, the patchy densities in the medullary portion of the femur and the sunburst appearance of the periosteal response are clues to the diagnosis of osteosarcoma. Note also the presence of a Codman triangle (*arrow*).

age, the production of obvious tumor matrix, and a radiographic appearance typical of osteosarcoma.

Complications and Treatment. The most frequent complications of conventional osteosarcoma are pathologic fracture and the development of pulmonary metastases.

If a limb-salvage procedure is feasible, a course of multidrug chemotherapy is used, followed by wide resection of the bone and insertion of an endoprosthesis (Fig. 21.10). Less frequently, amputation is performed, followed by chemotherapy. Currently, the 5-year survival rate after adequate therapy exceeds 50%.

Low-Grade Central Osteosarcoma

This rare form of osteosarcoma (1% of all osteosarcomas) has only recently been recognized. It usually occurs in patients older than those presenting with conventional osteosarcoma, although the sites of predilection are similar. Radiographically, it may be indistinguishable from conventional osteosarcoma, but it grows more slowly and has a better prognosis. At times its radiographic presentation clearly mimics fibrous dysplasia (Fig. 21.11) or other benign lesion (Fig. 21.12).

Telangiectatic Osteosarcoma

A very aggressive type of osteosarcoma, the telangiectatic variant, also called hemorrhagic osteosarcoma by Campanacci, is twice as common in males than in females and is seen predominantly in patients in their second and third decades of life. It is rare, comprising approximately 3% of all malignant bone tumors. It is characterized by a high degree of vascularity and large cystic spaces filled with blood, which account for its atypical radiographic presentation. It is an osteolytic destructive lesion with an almost complete absence of sclerotic changes; a soft-tissue mass may also be present (Figs. 21.13 to 21.16). Grossly, the tumor resembles a "bag" of blood and is characterized by blood-filled spaces, necrosis, and hemorrhage. Histologically, it is composed of loculated blood-filled spaces, partially lined by malignant cells producing sparse

Figure 21.5 Various presentations of a conventional osteosarcoma. Anteroposterior (**A**) and lateral (**B**) radiographs show sclerotic variant of osteosarcoma in the proximal tibia. (**C**) Anteroposterior radiograph shows a lytic variant of osteosarcoma in the distal humerus, which proved to be a fibroblastic osteosarcoma. (**D**) A radiograph of the distal femur shows a mixed variant of osteosarcoma: areas of bone formation are present within a destructive lytic lesion.

Figure 21.6 Periosteal reaction in osteosarcoma. Three types of periosteal reaction most commonly accompany osteosarcoma. The sunburst or perpendicular type of periosteal reaction (*arrows*) is seen here on the lateral radiograph of the forearm in an 18-year-old woman with osteosarcoma of the radius **(A)** and on the anteroposterior radiograph of the distal femur **(B)** in a 20-year-old man. **(C)** Codman triangle (*arrow*) may also be encountered, as seen here in a 15-year-old girl with osteosarcoma of the femur and in an 11-year-old boy **(D)** with osteosarcoma of the humerus (*arrows*). **(E)** The onion skin or lamellated type of periosteal response (*arrows*) is apparent in a 16-year-old girl with osteosarcoma of the femur. **(F)** Combination of lamellated (*arrows*) and sunburst (*open arrow*) periosteal reaction is present in a 16-year-old girl with osteosarcoma of the femur. (*continued*)

Figure 21.6 **Periosteal reaction in osteosarcoma.** *Continued.*

Figure 21.7 **CT of osteosarcoma. (A)** Standard anteroposterior radiograph reveals a destructive lesion with poorly defined borders extending from the metaphysis of the femur into the diaphysis. Note the aggressive periosteal reaction and the formation of tumor bone. These features are sufficient for making a diagnosis of osteosarcoma in this 14-year-old boy. **(B)** CT section demonstrates the extension of the soft-tissue mass. The tumor-bone in the medullary portion of the bone and in the soft-tissue mass is seen to better advantage.

Figure 21.8 MRI of osteosarcoma. (A) Conventional radiograph demonstrates involvement of the head of the fibula and extensive soft-tissue infiltration with significant tumor-bone formation in a 20-year-old man with osteosarcoma of the right proximal fibula. **(B)** Sagittal spin-echo T1-weighted MR image shows that the tumor displays a predominantly intermediate signal, blending with the muscular structures. **(C)** On axial T2-weighted image, the tumor shows high signal intensity in both its intramedullary component and its soft-tissue extension. The foci of tumor-bone formation are imaged as areas of low signal intensity.

osteoid tissue. It resembles an aneurysmal bone cyst, both radiologically and pathologically.

Small Cell Osteosarcoma

Described by Sim and associates, small cell osteosarcoma usually occurs as a radiolucent lesion with permeative borders and a large soft-tissue mass. Its radiographic appearance thus mimics that of a round cell bone sarcoma. These lesions usually exhibit small round cells in many histologic fields, much like Ewing sarcoma. The presence, however, of spindled tumor cells, as well as the focal production of osteoid or bone, helps to make a histologic diagnosis of osteosarcoma. The distal femur, proximal humerus, and proximal tibia are sites of predilection.

Figure 21.9 MRI of osteosarcoma. (A) Anteroposterior radiograph demonstrates a predominantly sclerotic tumor extending into the articular end of bone in this 17-year-old boy with osteosarcoma of the left proximal tibia. **(B)** The sclerotic parts of the lesion display low signal intensity on coronal spin-echo T2-weighted MR image. A nonmineralized part of the tumor, distally, shows high signal intensity. Likewise, the soft-tissue extension of the lesion displays high signal intensity.

Figure 21.10 Treatment of osteosarcoma. An 8-year-old boy underwent a limb-salvage procedure for osteosarcoma in the left tibia. After a full course of chemotherapy, consisting of a combination of methotrexate, doxorubicin hydrochloride, and cisplatin, a wide resection of the proximal tibia was performed and a LEAP metallic spacer inserted. This expandable prosthesis can be adjusted to maintain limb length with the normal contralateral limb as the child grows. (Courtesy of Dr. M. M. Lewis, Santa Barbara, California.)

Figure 21.11 Low-grade central osteosarcoma. Anteroposterior **(A)** and lateral **(B)** radiographs of the distal leg in an 18-year-old woman were originally interpreted as showing fibrous dysplasia of the distal tibia. Note a benign-appearing radiolucent lesion exhibiting a geographic type of bone destruction with a narrow zone of transition and no evidence of periosteal reaction. Sagittal **(C)** and axial **(D)** T1-weighted (SE; TR 600/TE 20 msec) MR images demonstrate intermediate to low signal intensity of the lesion and lack of a soft-tissue mass. Biopsy revealed a low-grade central osteosarcoma. (Courtesy of Dr. K. K. Unni, Rochester, Minnesota.) *(continued)*

Figure 21.11 **Low-grade central osteosarcoma.** *Continued.*

Figure 21.12 **Low-grade central osteosarcoma.** **(A)** A lytic lesion with geographic pattern of bone destruction and a narrow zone of transition is present in the intertrochanteric region of the left femur in a 24-year-old woman. **(B)** Lateral radiograph of the proximal tibia of a 30-year-old woman reveals a lytic lesion with well-defined borders and geographic type of bone destruction. (Reprinted with permission from Greenspan A, Remagen W, 1998.)

Figure 21.13 Telangiectatic osteosarcoma. A purely destructive lesion is present in the diaphysis of the femur of this 17-year-old girl. Note the velvet type of periosteal reaction (*arrows*). The sclerotic changes usually seen in osteosarcomas are absent, and there is no radiographic evidence of tumor-bone. Biopsy revealed a telangiectatic osteosarcoma, one of the most aggressive types of this tumor. (Courtesy of Dr. M. J. Klein, New York, NY.)

Fibrohistiocytic Osteosarcoma

Fibrohistiocytic osteosarcoma, which resembles malignant fibrous histiocytoma (MFH), has recently been described in the literature. It can sometimes be confused with true MFH of bone because both of these tumors tend to arise at a greater age than conventional osteosarcoma, usually after the third decade. Both tend to involve the articular ends of long bones, and less periosteal reaction is typically present than in conventional osteosarcoma. Although on radiography both of these lesions tend to be radiolucent and thus do resemble giant cell tumor and fibrosarcoma, the MFH-like osteosarcoma usually exhibits areas of bone formation resembling cotton balls or cumulus clouds, whereas MFH does not. When such areas are identified on radiologic studies, a diligent search should be made for tumor bone in the resected specimen. Histologically, MFH-like osteosarcoma is characterized by pleomorphic spindle cells and giant cells, many of which have bizarre nuclei. This lesion therefore resembles giant cell-rich osteosarcoma. An inflammatory background is not unusual, and the storiform or spiral nebular arrangement, characteristic of MFH, although sometimes a dominant feature, may be less prominent or may be replaced by areas of large pleomorphic cells arranged in diffuse sheets. As in all other subtypes of osteosarcoma, the distinction from other sarcomas depends on the demonstration of osteoid or bone formation by malignant cells in the very typical patterns seen in osteosarcomas.

Intracortical Osteosarcoma

Intracortical osteosarcoma is one of the rarest forms of osteosarcoma. Only 14 cases have thus far been reported, with an age range of 9 to 43 years (average 24 years) and a male predominance. The presenting symptom is pain, often associated with activity. In some patients, a history of previous trauma has been elicited. The tumor involves the cortex, without extension into the medullary portion of the bone or the soft tissues. The radiographic presentation is that of a radiolucent lesion with surrounding cortical sclerosis. The size of the lesion varies

Figure 21.14 MRI of telangiectatic osteosarcoma. (A) Lateral radiograph of the proximal tibia in a 21-year-old man shows a lesion with relatively narrow zone of transition and no visible periosteal reaction. Coronal **(B)** and sagittal **(C)** T1-weighted (SE; TR 400/TE 10 msec) MR images show the tumor to be predominantly of intermediate signal intensity with central areas of high signal. No definite soft-tissue mass is demonstrated. Coronal **(D)** and axial **(E)** inversion recovery (FM-PIR/90 msec; TR 4000/TE 54/TI 140 msec) images show the extension of the tumor into the soft tissues and presence of peritumoral edema.

Figure 21.14 **MRI of telangiectatic osteosarcoma.** *Continued.*

from 1.0 to 4.2 cm. In some instances, the lesion mimics osteoid osteoma or intracortical osteoblastoma.

Gnathic Osteosarcoma

Gnathic osteosarcoma is osteosarcoma arising in the maxilla or mandible. Unlike osteosarcoma arising elsewhere in the skeleton, this tumor occurs in older patients (fourth to sixth decades, with a mean age of 35 years). It is usually a well-differentiated tumor with a low mi-

totic rate, possessing a predominantly cartilaginous component in a high percentage of cases and with less malignant potential and a better prognosis than for other forms of osteosarcoma.

Multicentric (Multifocal) Osteosarcoma

The simultaneous development of foci of osteosarcoma in multiple bones is a rare occurrence (Figs. 21.17 and 21.18). Whether this entity is truly separate or represents multiple bone metastases from a pri-

Figure 21.15 **Telangiectatic osteosarcoma.** Anteroposterior **(A)** and lateral **(B)** radiographs of the right femur of a 41-year-old man show an ill-defined lesion that exhibits a permeative type of bone destruction *(arrows)*. Note the velvet type of aggressive periosteal reaction *(arrowheads)*. The biopsy revealed telangiectatic osteosarcoma.

Figure 21.16 **Telangiectatic osteosarcoma. (A)** A predominantly lytic tumor associated with periosteal reaction is seen in the distal femoral diaphysis of this 6-year-old girl. **(B)** Lateral radiograph demonstrates an oblique pathologic fracture *(arrows)*. (Courtesy of Dr. K. K. Unni, Rochester, Minnesota.)

Figure 21.17 Multicentric osteosarcoma. Multicentric osteosarcoma, a very rare bone tumor, is demonstrated here in the right hemipelvis **(A)**, right tibia **(B)**, and several bones of the right foot **(C)**.

Figure 21.18 MRI of multicentric osteosarcoma. Coronal T1-weighted image shows multiple low signal intensity lesions in both femora of a 12-year-old girl. (Reprinted with permission from Greenspan A, Remagen W, 1998).

mary conventional osteosarcoma remains a controversy. This type of osteosarcoma is currently recognized as having two variants: synchronous and metachronous. Multifocal osteosarcoma must be differentiated from osteosarcoma metastasized to other bones.

Juxtacortical Osteosarcomas

The term *juxtacortical* is a general designation for a group of osteosarcomas that arise on the bone surface (Fig. 21.19). Usually, these lesions are much rarer and occur a decade later than their intraosseous counterparts. The majority of juxtacortical osteosarcomas are low-grade tumors, although there are moderately and even highly malignant variants.

Parosteal Osteosarcoma. Parosteal tumors are seen largely in patients in their third and fourth decades, with a characteristic site of predilection in the posterior aspect of the distal femur (Fig. 21.20).

Conventional radiography is usually adequate for making a diagnosis of parosteal osteosarcoma. The lesion presents as a dense oval or spherical mass attached to the cortical surface of the bone and sharply demarcated from the surrounding soft tissues (Figs. 21.21 to 21.23).

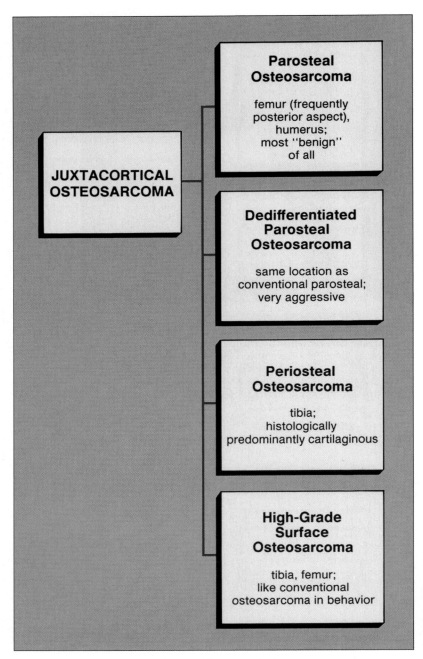

Figure 21.19 Variants of juxtacortical osteosarcoma.

Figure 21.20 Skeletal sites of predilection, peak age range, and male-to-female ratio in parosteal osteosarcoma.

CT (Fig. 21.23B) or MRI (see Fig. 16.16) are often necessary to determine whether the lesion has penetrated the cortex and invaded the medullary region of the bone.

Histologically, the lesion consists of fibrous stroma, probably derived from the outer fibrous periosteal layer. The bony component is often trabeculated but is at least partially immature, particularly at the periphery of the tumor. This is an important point in differentiating it from the sometimes similar-appearing myositis ossificans, which, however, matures in a centripetal fashion, with its most mature portion outermost.

Figure 21.21 Parosteal osteosarcoma. Typical presentation of parosteal osteosarcoma at the posterior aspect of the distal femur in a 23-year-old woman.

Figure 21.22 Parosteal osteosarcoma. Anteroposterior radiograph of the right hip shows a large ossific mass attached to the supra-acetabular portion of the ilium. (Reprinted with permission from Greenspan A, Remagen W, 1998.)

Figure 21.23 CT of parosteal osteosarcoma. (A) Lateral radiograph of the knee of a 37-year-old woman shows an ossific mass attached to the posterior cortex of the distal femur. Its location and appearance are typical of parosteal osteosarcoma. **(B)** Contrast-enhanced CT section demonstrates that the medullary portion of the bone has not been invaded.

Figure 21.24 Myositis ossificans. Juxtacortical myositis ossificans, seen here near the medial cortex of the femoral neck, typically presents as a more mature lesion at its periphery, with a center less dense than in parosteal osteosarcoma, and a clear zone representing complete separation of the lesion from the cortex.

Differential Diagnosis. Parosteal osteosarcoma must be differentiated from parosteal osteoma (see Fig. 17.4), myositis ossificans, soft-tissue osteosarcoma, parosteal liposarcoma with ossifications, and osteochondroma. Differentiation from myositis ossificans and osteochondroma is the most frequent source of confusion. Myositis ossificans is distinguished by a zonal phenomenon and by a cleft sep-

arating the ossific mass from the cortex (Fig. 21.24; see also Figs. 4.55, 4.56 and 18.28). In osteochondroma, however, the cortex of the lesion merges without interruption into the cortex of the host bone (see Figs. 18.26 and 18.28), a feature not seen in parosteal osteosarcoma. Because the lesion is relatively slow-growing and most often involves only the surface of the bone, the prognosis for patients with parosteal osteosarcoma is much better than for those with other types of osteosarcoma. Simple wide resection of the lesion often constitutes sufficient treatment.

Dedifferentiated Parosteal Osteosarcoma. A rare and unusual bone tumor, dedifferentiated parosteal osteosarcoma, was identified by a group from the Mayo Clinic. Most cases reportedly originate as conventional parosteal osteosarcomas that, after resection and multiple local recurrences, have undergone transformation to histologically high-grade sarcomas. Some cases, however, have presented as primary tumors arising on the cortical surface of a bone *de novo*. Radiographically and histologically, dedifferentiated parosteal osteosarcoma mimics the features of conventional parosteal osteosarcoma. There are, however, some traits of a high-grade sarcoma, such as radiographically identifiable cortical destruction (Fig. 21.25) and histologically identifiable pleomorphic tumor cells with hyperchromatic nuclei and a high mitotic rate. Hence, the prognosis is much worse than that of parosteal osteosarcoma.

Periosteal Osteosarcoma. Most often occurring in adolescence, periosteal osteosarcoma is a very rare tumor (accounting for 1% to 2% of all osteosarcomas) that grows on the bone surface, usually at the midshaft of a long bone such as the tibia. The characteristic feature of this tumor, which radiographically may resemble myositis ossificans, is a predominance of cartilaginous tissue (Fig. 21.26). This may lead to an erroneous diagnosis of periosteal chondrosarcoma. The radiologic characteristics of periosteal osteosarcoma were defined by deSantos and colleagues. These include an inhomogeneous tumor matrix with calcified spiculations interspersed with areas of radiolucency representing uncalcified matrix; occasional periosteal reaction in the form of a Codman triangle (Fig. 21.27); thickening of the periosteal surface

Figure 21.25 Dedifferentiated osteosarcoma. A 24-year-old woman presented with pain and palpable mass above the popliteal fossa of 2 months' duration. Three years before the current symptoms, a parosteal osteosarcoma had been resected from her distal femur. **(A)** Anteroposterior radiograph of the distal femur shows a destructive lesion *(arrows)* associated with an aggressive type of periosteal reaction *(curved arrows)* and a large soft-tissue mass *(open arrows)* with foci of bone formation. **(B)** Lateral radiograph shows in addition the remnants of the previously resected parosteal osteosarcoma *(arrow)*. *(continued)*

Figure 21.25 Dedifferentiated parosteal. *Continued.* **(C)** The proximal CT section shows a surface tumor exhibiting bone formation and a large soft-tissue mass with foci of tumor-bone. At this level the bone marrow is not invaded. **(D)** The more distal section reveals in addition the invasion of the medullary cavity, a feature not consistent with a conventional parosteal osteosarcoma. **(E)** Coronal T1-weighted (SE; TR 600/TE 25 msec) MR image demonstrates the extent of both intramedullary invasion and a soft-tissue mass. **(F)** Axial T2-weighted (SE; TR 2000/TE 90 msec) MR image shows nonhomogeneous signal of a large soft-tissue mass. At the level of this section the bone marrow is not infiltrated by a tumor.

Figure 21.26 Periosteal osteosarcoma. (A) Anteroposterior radiograph of the right knee of a 12-year-old girl with "discomfort" in the upper leg for 2 months demonstrates poorly defined calcifications and ossifications in a mass attached to the surface of the lateral tibial cortex. There appears to be no bone destruction. **(B)** CT section shows the extent of the soft-tissue mass. Note that the tumor, a periosteal osteosarcoma, is intimately attached to the cortex, a factor that virtually excludes myositis ossificans.

Figure 21.27 **Periosteal osteosarcoma.** (A) Anteroposterior radiograph of the right femur of a 16-year-old girl shows a surface lesion affecting the medial cortex, associated with a Codman triangle of periosteal reaction *(arrows)* and a large soft-tissue mass. (B) CT shows the soft-tissue component to better advantage. The medullary cavity is not invaded by the tumor; however, an increase in attenuation value, compared with the contralateral marrow cavity, indicates bone marrow edema.

of the cortex at the base of the lesion, with sparing of the endosteal surface; extension of the tumor into the soft tissues; and sparing of the medullary cavity (Fig. 21.28). By microscopy, these tumors have low-grade to medium-grade malignancy and are composed mainly of lobulated chondroid tissue with moderate cellularity. Periosteal osteosar-

coma is marked by a better prognosis than the conventional type but a worse one than the parosteal variant.

High-Grade Surface Osteosarcoma. High-grade surface osteosarcoma may exhibit radiographic features similar to those of parosteal or periosteal osteosarcoma (Fig. 21.29). Histologically, this

Figure 21.28 **Periosteal osteosarcoma.** Anteroposterior (A) and lateral (B) radiographs of the left leg in a 12-year-old boy show faint ossific densities on the anteromedial surface of the proximal tibia adjacent to the almost indistinct cortical destruction. An aggressive velvet type of periosteal reaction is evident *(arrows)*. (C) CT section through the tumor shows bone formation on the anterior surface of the tibia and lack of invasion of the medullary cavity. *(continued)*

Figure 21.28 Periosteal osteosarcoma *Continued.* **(D)** Axial spin-echo T1-weighted MRI shows that tumor displays slightly higher signal than the muscles. **(E)** On axial T2-weighted image (SE; TR 2000/TE 80 msec) the mass becomes bright, except for the central areas at which bone formation displays low signal intensity. The biopsy revealed a periosteal osteosarcoma.

lesion shows elements identical to those of conventional osteosarcoma. It also carries a high potential for metastasis.

Soft-Tissue (Extraskeletal) Osteosarcoma

Osteosarcoma of the soft tissues (extraskeletal, extraosseous) is an uncommon malignant tumor of mesenchymal origin. This tumor possesses the capacity to form neoplastic osteoid, bone, and cartilage. It usually targets middle-aged and elderly individuals, with a mean age at presentation of 54 years. Soft-tissue osteosarcoma is much less common than osteosarcoma of bone, accounting for only 4% of all osteosarcomas. It preferentially affects the lower extremities and buttocks. This lesion may also develop in a number of soft tissues, including breast, lung, thyroid, renal capsule, urinary bladder, and prostate, and even the pelvic retroperitoneum. A soft-tissue osteosarcoma may rarely arise after radiation therapy.

Patients most commonly present with a slowly enlarging mass that may or may not be accompanied by pain. Radiographic appearance is characterized by a soft-tissue mass with scattered amorphous calcifications and ossifications. The tumor exhibits a disorganized arrangement of osteogenic elements in its center (Fig. 21.30A,B). If the tumor develops close to bone, it may invade the cortex.

On CT, a heavily mineralized soft-tissue mass is usually seen, occasionally with necrotic areas. This technique is often better than radiography at revealing the pattern of central ossification, which is referred to as the "reverse zoning" phenomenon. CT also demonstrates a lack of attachment of the mass to the bone. On MRI, a mass with mixed low signal intensity on T1-weighted images and mixed but predominantly high signal intensity on T2-weighted and inversion recovery sequences is often seen. MRI may also reveal a pseudocapsule of tumor (Fig. 21.31A–D).

Figure 21.29 High-grade surface osteosarcoma. (A) Lateral radiograph of the distal leg demonstrates a tumor attached to the posterior cortex of tibia in a 24-year-old man. Poorly defined ossific foci are seen within a large soft-tissue mass. Note the similarity of the tumor to periosteal osteosarcoma (see Figs. 21.26 and 21.27). **(B)** CT section demonstrates the extent of the lesion. Characteristically, the marrow cavity is not affected.

Figure 21.30 Soft-tissue osteosarcoma. (A) Lateral radiograph of the knee of a 51-year-old woman shows a poorly defined soft-tissue mass above the patella, merging with the quadriceps muscle. The center of the lesion exhibits amorphous calcifications and ossifications. **(B)** Radiograph of the resected specimen of the tumor reveals foci of ossifications in the center of the mass, surrounded by a radiolucent zone at the periphery (so-called reverse zoning). (Reprinted with permission from Greenspan A, et al. *Skeletal Radiol* 1987; 16: 489–492.)

Figure 21.31 CT and MRI of soft-tissue osteosarcoma. A 68-year-old woman presented with a progressively enlarging soft-tissue mass in the popliteal region of the right knee. **(A)** Lateral radiograph shows a large soft-tissue mass, sharply outlined in its distal extent but poorly delineated at the proximal end. Calcifications and ossifications are present throughout the tumor. **(B)** Axial CT section reveals reverse zoning typical of soft-tissue osteosarcoma. **(C)** Axial T1-weighted MRI shows the mass to be slightly nonhomogeneous with low signal intensity. **(D)** Axial T2-weighted MRI reveals nonhomogeneity of the tumor, displaying variation of signals from high to intermediate intensity. Note lack of involvement of femoral bone marrow. (Reprinted with permission from Greenspan A, Remagen W, 1998.)

The histopathology of soft-tissue osteosarcoma is indistinguishable from that of a conventional osteosarcoma.

Differential Diagnosis. The differential diagnosis of extraskeletal osteosarcoma includes myositis ossificans, tumoral calcinosis, synovial sarcoma, extraskeletal chondrosarcoma, liposarcoma of soft tissues with ossification, and pseudomalignant osseous tumor of soft tissue.

Myositis ossificans is a benign, usually posttraumatic, lesion of the soft tissues that is observed predominantly in adolescents and young adults (see Figs. 4.55, 4.56, and 21.24). The zoning phenomenon reflects the maturation pattern of the lesion. The center of the lesion is undifferentiated and cellular, but increasingly mature ossification is observed toward the periphery constituting the histological hallmark of this condition. Radiography reveals that the zoning phenomenon of this lesion is characterized by a radiolucent center and a denser and more sclerotic periphery (see Fig. 4.55). The mass is often separated from the adjacent cortex by a radiolucent cleft. The evolution of myositis ossificans can be well correlated with the lapse of time since the trauma.

Synovial sarcoma has a predilection for adolescents and younger adults (13 to 55 years). This tumor is usually located near a joint, especially in the lower extremities and particularly in the area around the knee and foot. Radiography reveals a lobulated mass, and in 25% of cases, amorphous calcifications are present (see Fig. 23.15). Ossification is extremely rare in synovial sarcoma. In approximately 15% to 20% of patients, a periosteal reaction and/or erosion of adjacent bone structures can be observed. There may be osteoporosis of the affected limb secondary to disuse.

Chondrosarcoma of soft tissue is a rare malignant tumor and is much less common than extraskeletal osteosarcoma. It appears as a soft-tissue mass with ring-like or punctate calcifications. Soft-tissue chondrosarcoma can be distinguished from soft-tissue osteosarcoma on imaging studies by the lack of bone formation.

Liposarcoma of soft tissues tends to affect older adults and has a male prevalence. This tumor may closely mimic soft-tissue osteosarcoma, particularly when ossification is present. However, the ossification is usually more organized than that in osteosarcoma of soft tissues, and fatty tissue can usually be identified. This lesion commonly affects the thigh, leg, and gluteal region. Growth of the tumor may proceed very slowly, over many years, and erosion of adjacent bone is common.

Pseudomalignant osseous tumor of soft tissues was first described by Jaffe and later by Fine and Stout. These lesions are rare, are more common in females, and are located in the muscle and subcutaneous tissues. They are probably of infective origin, although this has not been unequivocally confirmed. Some lesions may represent unrecognized foci of myositis ossificans.

Secondary Osteosarcomas

In contrast to primary osteosarcomas, secondary lesions occur in an older population. Many of these tumors are responsible for the complications of Paget disease (osteitis deformans) and, characteristically, develop in pagetic bone (Fig. 21.32). The typical radiographic changes in malignant transformation of Paget disease include a de-

Figure 21.32 Secondary osteosarcoma. Radiograph in a 66-year-old man who had extensive skeletal involvement by Paget disease and who had pain in the right hip shows the typical features of osteitis deformans in the right ilium and ischium. There is also destruction of the cortex associated with a soft-tissue mass containing tumor-bone—characteristic features of malignant transformation to osteosarcoma.

cortical
destruction

soft tissue mass

structive lesion in the affected bone, the presence of tumor bone in the lesion, and an associated soft-tissue mass. Osteosarcoma in these patients must be differentiated from metastases to pagetic bone from primary carcinomas elsewhere in the body (most commonly the prostate, breast, and kidney). Secondary osteosarcoma may also develop spontaneously in fibrous dysplasia or after radiation therapy for benign bone lesions such as fibrous dysplasia and giant cell tumor, as well as after irradiation of malignant processes in the soft tissues such as breast carcinoma and lymphoma. (For further discussion of malignant transformation, see the sections in Chapter 22 on Paget disease and radiation-induced sarcoma under the heading Benign Conditions with Malignant Potential.)

Chondrosarcomas

Chondrosarcoma is a malignant bone tumor characterized by the formation of a cartilage matrix by tumor cells. As in osteosarcoma, there are several types of this tumor (Fig. 21.33), each with characteristic clinical, radiographic, and pathologic features.

Primary Chondrosarcomas

Conventional Chondrosarcoma

Also known as central or medullary chondrosarcoma, this tumor is seen twice as frequently in males than in females and more commonly in adults, usually in those past their third decade. The most frequent locations are the pelvis and long bones, particularly the femur and humerus (Fig. 21.34). Most conventional chondrosarcomas are slow-growing tumors, often discovered incidentally. Occasionally, local pain and tenderness may be present.

Radiographically, conventional chondrosarcoma appears as an expansive lesion in the medulla, with thickening of the cortex and characteristic endosteal scalloping; popcorn-like, annular or comma-shaped calcifications are seen in the medullary portion of the bone. A soft-tissue mass may sometimes be present (Figs. 21.35 and 21.36). In

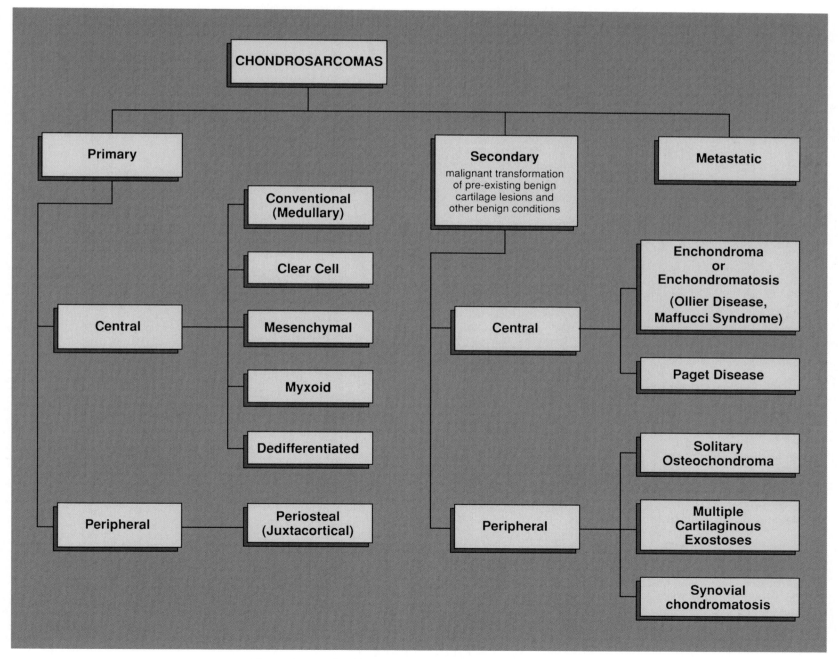

Figure 21.33 **Classification of the types of chondrosarcoma.**

Figure 21.34 Skeletal sites of predilection, peak age range, and male-to-female ratio in conventional chondrosarcoma.

chondroma and contains an appreciable number of plump cells, with large or double nuclei. Mitotic cells are infrequent. The histologic distinction among low-grade, intermediate, and high-grade lesions is based on the cellularity of the tumor tissue, the degree of pleomorphism of the cells and nuclei, and the number of mitoses present. Some investigators (e.g., Unni) disregard the last feature in grading these tumors (Table 21.2).

Differential Diagnosis. In exceptional cases, particularly in the early stage of development, chondrosarcoma can be indistinguishable from an enchondroma. For this reason, all centrally located cartilage tumors in long bones, particularly in adult patients, should be re-

Figure 21.35 Chondrosarcoma. Anteroposterior **(A)** and lateral **(B)** radiographs of the right elbow in a 55-year-old man show a tumor arising from the proximal ulna. Note a huge soft-tissue mass containing chondroid calcifications.

typical cases, conventional radiography is sufficient to make a diagnosis (Fig. 21.37). CT and MRI help delineate the extent of intraosseous and soft-tissue involvement (Figs. 21.38 to 21.40).

Histologically, chondrosarcoma is typified by the formation of cartilage by tumor cells. Present are lobules of hyaline cartilage with areas of matrix mineralization in distinctive ring-and-arc-like pattern. The tissue is more cellular and pleomorphic in appearance than en-

Figure 21.36 Chondrosarcoma. Anteroposterior radiograph of the pelvis in a 52-year-old man shows a large calcified mass arising from the left pubic bone and extending into the pelvic cavity.

garded as malignant until proven otherwise. At the articular ends of the bone, chondrosarcomas frequently lack characteristic calcifications and may mimic a giant cell tumor.

Complications and Treatment. Pathologic fractures through conventional chondrosarcomas are rare (Fig. 21.41). Moreover, conventional chondrosarcomas are slow-growing tumors, and only in rare cases do they metastasize to distant areas. Because they are not radiosensitive, surgical resection is the major means of therapy.

Clear Cell Chondrosarcoma

Clear cell chondrosarcoma is a rare (less than 4% of all chondrosarcomas in the Mayo Clinic series) variant of chondrosarcoma. First described by Unni and associates in 1976, it occurs twice as often in males than in females, usually in the third to fifth decades. It is predominantly a lytic lesion with a sclerotic border, which occasionally may contain calcifications. Many of these lesions resemble chondroblastomas or giant cell tumors, and many involve the proximal end of the humerus and femur (Fig. 21.42). Recently, Collins and colleagues reported MRI findings in 34 patients with pathologically documented cases of clear cell chondrosarcoma. The tumors revealed low signal intensity on T1-weighted sequences and moderately to significantly bright signal on T2 weighting. Heterogenic areas seen on T1- and T2-weighted images and on postgadolinium T1-weighted images correlated pathologically to areas of mineralization, intralesional hemorrhage, and cystic changes within the tumor.

Histologically, the clear cell variant exhibits larger and more rounded tumor cells than other chondrosarcomas with clear or vacuolated cytoplasm containing large amounts of glycogen. A chondroid matrix, trabeculae of reactive bone, and numerous osteoclast-like giant cells are distinctive features of this tumor.

Treatment. Clear cell chondrosarcoma is considered a low-grade malignancy, although distant metastases have been reported. It has been managed in a variety of ways, from simple observation or curettage to wide resection and even amputation. Although it is a less aggressive tumor than conventional chondrosarcoma, inadequate treatment may lead to recurrence. Therefore, en bloc resection with wide surgical margins of bone and soft tissue is the current treatment of choice.

Mesenchymal Chondrosarcoma

Mesenchymal chondrosarcoma is very uncommon (less than 1% of all malignant bone tumors) and tends to occur in the patient's second or third decade. It presents radiographically with the permeative type of bone destruction seen in round cell tumors, and calcifications in the cartilaginous portion of the tumor (Fig. 21.43). It may be indistinguishable from conventional chondrosarcoma and is a highly malignant lesion with a strong capacity to metastasize.

Histologically, the mesenchymal variant demonstrates a high degree of malignancy, typified by bimorphic pattern. The tumor is composed of, more or less, differentiated cartilage, together with highly vascular stroma of mesenchymal tissue containing spindle cells and round cells.

Dedifferentiated Chondrosarcoma

First described by Dahlin and Beabout in 1971, dedifferentiated chondrosarcoma is the most malignant of all chondrosarcomas and consequently carries a very poor prognosis; most patients die from the disease within 2 years of diagnosis. The patient typically has pain of long duration, followed by a more recent onset of rapid swelling and local tenderness. The prolonged pain probably reflects a slow-growing lesion, and the swelling and tenderness may be related to the develop-

Figure 21.37 Chondrosarcoma. Lateral radiograph in a 46-year-old man shows the characteristic features of a central chondrosarcoma of the right femur. Within the destructive lesion in the medullary portion of the bone are annular and comma-shaped calcifications. The thickened cortex, which is caused by periosteal new bone formation in response to destruction of the cortex by the chondroblastic tumor, shows the typical endosteal scalloping.

Figure 21.38 CT of chondrosarcoma. (A) Anteroposterior radiograph of the right shoulder of a 62-year-old man is not adequate for demonstrating the soft-tissue extension of the chondrosarcoma in the proximal humerus. **(B)** CT section through the lesion demonstrates cortical destruction and a large soft-tissue mass.

Figure 21.39 CT and MRI of chondrosarcoma. (A) A large calcified mass arises from the left anterior sixth rib. **(B)** Axial CT section reveals destruction of the rib and intrathoracic and extrathoracic extension of tumor. **(C)** Axial T2-weighted MRI demonstrates nonhomogeneity of the tumor. Areas of low-intensity signal represent calcified portions of the mass.

Figure 21.40 Scintigraphy and MRI of chondrosarcoma. Anteroposterior **(A)** and lateral **(B)** radiographs of the distal femur show typical appearance of central medullary chondrosarcoma. The cortex is destroyed, and there is a large soft-tissue mass projecting posteriorly. **(C)** Radionuclide bone scan obtained after intravenous injection of 15 mCi (555 MBq) of ^{99m}Tc-MDP (technetium-99m-labeled methylene diphosphonate) shows increased uptake of tracer localized to the site of the tumor. **(D)** Coronal T1-weighted (SE; TR 700/TE 20 msec) MR image shows the tumor to be of low signal intensity. The calcifications display signal void. **(E)** Axial T2-weighted (SE; TR 2000/TE 80 msec) image shows intramedullary tumor displaying a high signal intensity, whereas calcifications are of low signal. The soft-tissue mass shows heterogeneous signal.

Table 21.2 **Histologic Grading of Chondrosarcoma**

Grade	Histologic Features
0.5 (borderline)	Histologic features similar to enchondroma, but imaging features more aggressive
1 (low-grade)	Cellularity: slightly increased
	Cytologic atypia: slight increase in size and variation in shape of the nuclei; slightly increased hyperchromasia of the nuclei
	Binucleation: few binucleate cells are present
	Stromal myxoid change: may or may not be present
2 (intermediate)	Cellularity: moderately increased
	Cytologic atypia: moderate increase in size and variation in shape of the nuclei; moderately increased hyperchromasia of the nuclei
	Binucleation: large number of double-nucleated and tri-nucleated cells
	Stromal myxoid change: focally present
3 (high-grade)	Cellularity: markedly increased
	Cytologic atypia: marked enlargement and irregularity of the nuclei; markedly increased hyperchromasia of the nuclei
	Binucleation: large number of double- and multinucleated cells
	Stromal myxoid change: commonly present
	Other: small foci of spindling at the periphery of the lobules of chondrocytes; foci of necrosis present.

Modified from Dahlin and Unni, 1988.

Figure 21.41 Complication of chondrosarcoma. Pathologic fracture through a chondrosarcoma, as seen here in the right humerus in a 60-year-old man, is a rare complication of this lesion.

Figure 21.42 Clear cell chondrosarcoma. A 22-year-old man presented with left hip pain for 3 months. Anteroposterior radiograph demonstrates an osteolytic lesion located in the superolateral aspect of the femoral head and extending into the articular surface. The lesion, which is demarcated by a thin sclerotic border, closely resembles a chondroblastoma. On biopsy, however, it proved to be a clear cell chondrosarcoma.

Figure 21.43 Mesenchymal chondrosarcoma. Anteroposterior radiograph of the right lower leg of a 43-year-old woman with a 6-month history of intermittent pain in the right calf shows a destructive lesion at the midportion of the fibula associated with a large soft-tissue mass. The central portion of the lesion exhibits annular and comma-shaped calcifications typical of a cartilage tumor, but its periphery shows a permeative type of bone destruction characteristic of round cell tumors. Biopsy revealed mesenchymal chondrosarcoma.

void corresponding to matrix mineralization identified on the conventional radiography. The third MRI pattern consisted of relatively lower signal intensity of the tumor, accompanied by smaller areas revealing high signal and fluid–fluid levels on T2 weighting, presumably caused by tumor necrosis rather than chondroid tissue.

Histologically, dedifferentiated chondrosarcoma often shows a cartilaginous component of low-grade malignancy combined with highly cellular sarcomatous tissue.

Recently, the validity of the term "dedifferentiation" has been challenged. Studies using electron microscopy and immunohistochemistry indicate that sarcomatous dedifferentiation represents, in fact, the synchronous differentiation of separate clones of cells from a primitive spindle-cell sarcoma to various types of sarcoma.

Periosteal Chondrosarcoma

Generally, periosteal chondrosarcoma has the same radiographic and pathologic features as central chondrosarcoma. Because the lesion appears on the bone surface, it must be distinguished from periosteal osteosarcoma. The differentiation of this lesion may create problems for the radiologist and pathologist alike.

Secondary Chondrosarcomas

The most common types of secondary chondrosarcomas are tumors developing in preexisting enchondromas (see Fig. 18.23) or in multiple cartilaginous exostoses (see Figs. 18.34 and 18.40). These tumors develop in a slightly younger age group (age 20 to 40 years) than primary chondrosarcomas and have a more benign course. Because they are usually of low-grade malignancy, the prognosis is more favorable than in conventional chondrosarcoma. Total excision is the treatment

ment of a rapidly growing, more malignant component. The hallmark of this lesion is the appearance of an aggressive sarcoma engrafted on a benign chondral lesion or on a benign-appearing low-grade chondrosarcoma. Although it may radiographically resemble a conventional chondrosarcoma, its histologic composition differs. The dedifferentiated tissue may appear to be a fibrosarcoma, a MFH, or an osteosarcoma.

Radiographically, dedifferentiated chondrosarcomas exhibit calcific foci with aggressive bone destruction and are often accompanied by a large soft-tissue mass (Fig. 21.44). Recently reported by McSweeney and associates, MRI findings of dedifferentiated chondrosarcoma consisted of three distinct patterns. In one group of patients, clear demarcation was seen on T2-weighted images between the low-grade tumor that exhibited high signal intensity, and the high-grade tumor that showed relatively reduced signal, a so-called biphasic pattern. In another group of patients, the only MRI evidence of an underlying chondroid lesion was the presence of several areas of signal

Figure 21.44 Dedifferentiated chondrosarcoma. A 70-year-old woman had a destructive lesion in the medullary cavity of the proximal shaft of the left humerus with calcifications typical of a cartilage tumor; there was also a soft-tissue mass. However, although the lesion seen on this film exhibits features typical of medullary chondrosarcoma, biopsy revealed, in addition to typical chondrosarcomatous tissue, elements of a giant cell tumor and malignant fibrous histiocytoma, leading to a diagnosis of dedifferentiated chondrosarcoma—the most aggressive of all such tumors.

of choice. (For further discussion of malignant transformation, see the sections under the heading Benign Conditions with Malignant Potential in Chapter 22).

PRACTICAL POINTS TO REMEMBER

Osteosarcoma

[1] Osteosarcoma has the ability to produce osteoid tissue or bone. Its most characteristic radiographic features are:
- the presence of tumor bone in the lesion—the hallmark of this malignancy
- destruction of the medullary portion of the bone or cortex
- an aggressive periosteal reaction—sunburst, lamellated, or Codman triangle
- the presence of a soft-tissue mass.

[2] In the radiologic evaluation of the different types of osteosarcoma—conventional, telangiectatic, multifocal, and juxtacortical:
- Conventional radiography is usually sufficient to identify the radiographic characteristics of each type and make a definitive diagnosis
- CT and MRI are invaluable for defining the extent of the tumor in the bone and soft tissues, and for monitoring the results of presurgical chemotherapy and radiation therapy.

[3] Telangiectatic osteosarcoma, among the most aggressive of osteosarcomas, may present radiographically as a purely osteolytic lesion. It may resemble an aneurysmal bone cyst.

[4] Parosteal osteosarcoma, the least malignant type of osteosarcoma:
- has a predilection for the posterior aspect of the distal femur
- is usually seen attached to the cortex, without invasion of the medullary cavity.

[5] Periosteal osteosarcoma, like parosteal osteosarcoma, is a "surface" lesion. It is, however, more aggressive and contains an excessive amount of cartilaginous tissue. It may resemble periosteal chondrosarcoma and myositis ossificans.

[6] Extraskeletal (soft-tissue) osteosarcoma is a rare malignant tumor of mesenchymal origin, most often affecting middle-aged and elderly individuals. The preferential sites for this neoplasm are lower extremities and buttocks. It may resemble myositis ossificans, tumoral calcinosis, and synovial sarcoma.

[7] The most common form of secondary osteosarcoma is that complicating Paget disease. It is an extremely aggressive lesion; patients usually do not survive beyond 8 months after diagnosis.

Chondrosarcoma

[1] Chondrosarcoma is a malignant bone tumor capable of forming cartilage. Its most characteristic radiographic features are:
- an expansive, destructive lesion in the medullary portion of the bone
- the presence of annular and comma-shaped calcifications within the tumor matrix
- thickening of the cortex and endosteal scalloping
- the presence of a soft-tissue mass.

[2] Clear cell chondrosarcoma is characterized radiographically by lytic area occasionally containing calcifications and sclerotic border. It may resemble chondroblastoma.

[3] Mesenchymal chondrosarcoma demonstrates radiographically two different appearances: side-by-side present are areas of permeative type of bone destruction similar to round cell tumors, and areas resembling typical cartilaginous tumor with calcifications.

[4] Dedifferentiated chondrosarcoma, the most aggressive type of all cartilage tumors, carries a poor prognosis. In addition to chondrogenic tissue, it can contain elements of fibrosarcoma, MFH, or osteosarcoma.

[5] Periosteal chondrosarcoma may be indistinguishable from periosteal osteosarcoma.

[6] Secondary chondrosarcoma usually develops in a preexisting benign lesion such as an enchondromatosis or multiple cartilaginous exostoses. At risk are the patients with Ollier disease and Maffucci syndrome.

SUGGESTED READINGS

Abdulrahman RE, White CS, Templeton PA, Romney B, Moore EH, Aisner SC. Primary osteosarcoma of the ribs: CT findings. *Skeletal Radiol* 1995;24:127–129.

Abello R, Lomena F, Garcia A, et al. Unusual metastatic chondrosarcoma detected with bone scintigraphy. *Eur J Nucl Med* 1986;12:306–308.

Ackerman LV. Extra-osseous localized non-neoplastic bone and cartilage formation (so-called myositis ossificans). *J Bone Joint Surg [Am]* 1958;40A:279–298.

Ahuja SC, Villacin AB, Smith J, Bullough PG, Huvos AG, Marcove RC. Juxtacortical (parosteal) osteosarcoma: histological grading and prognosis. *J Bone Joint Surg [Am]* 1977;59A:632–647.

Aisen AM, Martel W, Braunstein EM, McMillin KI, Phillips WA, Kling TF. MRI and CT evaluation of primary bone and soft-tissue tumors. *Am J Roentgenol* 1986;146:749–756.

Aizawa T, Okada K, Abe E, Tsuchida S, Shimada Y, Itoi E. Multicentric osteosarcoma with long-term survival. *Skeletal Radiology* 2004;33:41–45.

Allan CJ, Soule EH. Osteogenic sarcoma of the somatic soft tissues. Clinicopathologic study of 26 cases and review of literature. *Cancer* 1971;27:11121–11133.

Alpert LI, Abaci IF, Werthamer S. Radiation-induced extraskeletal osteosarcoma. *Cancer* 1973;31:1359–1363.

Amendola MA, Glazer GM, Adha FP, Francis IR, Weatherbee L, Martel W. Myositis ossificans circumscripta: computed tomographic diagnosis. *Radiology* 1983;149:775–779.

Amir D, Amir G, Mogle P, Pogrund H. Extraskeletal soft tissue chondrosarcoma. Case report and review of the literature. *Clin Orthop* 1985;198:219–223.

Amstutz HC. Multiple osteogenic sarcomata—metastatic or multicentric? *Cancer* 1969;24:923–931.

Anderson RB, McAlister JA Jr, Wrenn RN. Case report 585. Intracortical osteosarcoma. *Skeletal Radiology* 1989;18:627–630.

Angervall L, Enerback L, Knutson H. Chondrosarcoma of soft tissue origin. *Cancer* 1973;32:507–513.

Angervall L, Stener B, Stener I, Ahren C. Pseudomalignant osseous tumor of soft tissue. A clinical, radiological and pathological study of five cases. *J Bone Joint Surg [Br]* 1969;51B:654–663.

Aoki J, Sone S, Fujioka F, et al. MR of enchondroma and chondrosarcoma: rings and arcs of Gd-DTPA enhancement. *J Comput Assist Tomogr* 1991;15:1011–1016.

Aprin H, Riseborough EJ, Hall JE. Chondrosarcoma in children and adolescents. *Clin Orthop* 1982;166:226–232.

Ayala AG, Ro JY, Raymond AK, et al. Small cell osteosarcoma. A clinicopathologic study of 27 cases. *Cancer* 1989;64:2162–2173.

Bagley L, Kneeland JB, Dalinka MK, Bullough P, Brooks J. Unusual behavior of clear cell chondrosarcoma. *Skeletal Radiol* 1993;22:279–282.

Ballance WA Jr, Mendelsohn G, Carter JR, Abdul-Karim FW, Jacobs G, Makley JT. Osteogenic sarcoma. Malignant fibrous histiocytoma subtype. *Cancer* 1988;62:763–771.

Bane BL, Evans HL, Ro JY, et al. Extra-skeletal osteosarcoma. A clinico-pathologic study of 26 cases. *Cancer* 1990;65:2762–2770.

Bathurst N, Sanerkin N, Watt I. Osteoclast-rich osteosarcoma. *Br J Radiol* 1986;59:667–673.

Berquist TH. Magnetic resonance imaging of primary skeletal neoplasms. *Radiol Clin North Am* 1993;31:411–424.

Bertoni F, Boriani S, Laus M, Campanacci M. Periosteal chondrosarcoma and periosteal osteosarcoma. Two distinct entities. *J Bone Joint Surg [Br]* 1982;64B:370–376.

Bertoni F, Picci P, Bacchini P, et al. Mesenchymal chondrosarcoma of bone and soft tissues. *Cancer* 1983;52:533–541.

Bertoni F, Present D, Bacchini P, et al. Dedifferentiated peripheral chondrosarcomas. A report of seven cases. *Cancer* 1989;63:2054–2059.

Bertoni F, Present D, Bacchini P, Pignatti G, Picci P, Campanacci M. The Instituto Rizzoli experience with small cell osteosarcoma. *Cancer* 1989;64:2591–2599.

Bertoni F, Present DA, Enneking WF. Staging of bone tumors. In: Unni KK, ed. *Bone tumors.* New York: Churchill Livingstone;1988:47–83.

Bertoni F, Unni KK, Beabout JW, Sim FH. Chondrosarcomas of the synovium. *Cancer* 1991;67:155–162.

Bertoni F, Unni KK, McLeod RA, Dahlin DC. Osteosarcoma resembling osteoblastoma. *Cancer* 1985;55:416–426.

Björnsson J, Unni KK, Dahlin DC, Beabout JW, Sim FH. Clear cell chondrosarcoma of bone: observation in 47 cases. *Am J Surg Pathol* 1984;8:223–230.

Blasius S, Link TM, Hillmann A, Rödl R, Edel G, Winkelmann W. Intracortical low grade osteosarcoma. A unique case and review of the literature on intracortical osteosarcoma. *Gen Diagn Pathol* 1996;141:273–278.

Bloem JL, Bluemm RG, Taminiau AH, van Oesterom AT, Stolk J, Doornbos J. Magnetic resonance imaging of primary malignant bone tumors. *Radiographics* 1987;7:425–445.

Bloem JL, Kroon HM. Osseous lesions. *Radiol Clin North Am* 1993;31:261–278.

Bohndorf K, Reiser M, Lochner B, Feaux de Lacroix W, Steinbrich W. Magnetic resonance imaging of primary tumors and tumor-like lesions of bone. *Skeletal Radiol* 1986;15:511–517.

Bonar SF, McCarthy S, Stalley P, et al. Epiphyseal osteoblastoma-like osteosarcoma. *Skeletal Radiology* 2004;33:46–50.

Boyko OB, Cory DA, Cohen MD, Provisor A, Mirkin D, DeRosa GP. MR imaging of osteogenic and Ewing's sarcoma. *AJR Am J Roentgenol* 1987;148:317–322.

Brien EW, Mirra JM, Herr R. Benign and malignant cartilage tumors of bone and joints: their anatomic and theoretical basis with an emphasis on radiology, pathology, and clinical biology. I. The intramedullary cartilage tumors. *Skeletal Radiol* 1997;26:325–353.

Brien EW, Mirra JM, Ippolito V, Vaughn L. Clear-cell chondrosarcoma with elevated alkaline phosphatase, mistaken for osteosarcoma on biopsy. *Skeletal Radiol* 1996;25:770–774.

Brien EW, Mirra JM, Luck JV Jr. Benign and malignant cartilage tumor of bone and joint: their anatomic and theoretical basis with an emphasis on radiology, pathology and clinical biology. II. Juxtacortical cartilage tumors. *Skeletal Radiol* 1999;28:1–20.

Broders AC. The microscopic grading of cancer. In: Pack CT, Ariel IM, eds. *Treatment of cancer and allied diseases*, vol 1, 2nd ed. New York: Paul B. Hoeber, 1958:55–59.

Burgener FA, Perry P. Solitary renal cell carcinoma metastasis in Paget's disease simulating sarcomatous degeneration. *AJR Am J Roentgenol* 1977;128:835–855.

Campanacci M, Cervellati G. Osteosarcoma: a review of 345 cases. *Ital J Orthop Traumatol* 1975;1:5–22.

Campanacci M, Picci P, Gherlinzoni F, Guerra A, Bertoni F, Nef JR. Parosteal osteosarcoma. *J Bone Joint Surg [Br]* 1984;66B:313–321.

Campanacci M, Pizzoferrato A. Osteosarcoma emorragico. *Chir Organi Mov* 1971;60:409–421.

Cannon CP, Nelson SD, Seeger LL, Eckardt JJ. Clear cell chondrosarcoma mimicking chondroblastoma in a skeletally immature patient. *Skeletal Radiol* 2002;31:369–372.

Capanna R, Bertoni F, Bettelli G, et al. Dedifferentiated chondrosarcoma. *J Bone Joint Surg [Am]* 1988;70A:60–69.

Cawte TG, Steiner GC, Beltran J, Dorfman HD. Chondrosarcoma of the short tubular bones of the hands and feet. *Skeletal Radiol* 1998;27:625–632.

Chan YF, Yeung SH, Chow TC, Ma L. Clear cell chondrosarcoma: case report and ultrastructural study. *Pathology* 1989;21:134–137.

Chung EB, Enzinger FM. Extraskeletal osteosarcoma. *Cancer* 1987;60:1132–1142.

Cohen EK, Kressel HY, Frank TS, et al. Hyaline cartilage-origin bone and soft-tissue neoplasms: MR appearance and histologic correlation. *Radiology* 1988;167:477–481.

Collins MS, Koyama T, Swee RG, Inwards CY. Clear cell chondrosarcoma: radiographic, computed tomographic, and magnetic resonance findings in 34 patients with pathologic correlation. *Skeletal Radiol* 2003;32:687–694.

Crim JR, Seeger LL. Diagnosis of low-grade chondrosarcoma. *Radiology* 1993;189:503–504.

Crim JR, Seeger LL, Yao L, Chandnani V, Eckardt JJ. Diagnosis of soft-tissue masses with MR imaging: can benign masses be differentiated from malignant ones? *Radiology* 1992;185:581–586.

Dahlin DC. Grading of bone tumors. In: Unni KK, ed. *Bone tumors*. New York: Churchill Livingstone, 1988:35–45.

Dahlin DC. Malignant osteoblastic tumors. In: Taveras JM, Ferucci JT, eds. *Radiology: diagnosis-imaging-intervention*, vol 5. Philadelphia: JB Lippincott; 1986:1–10.

Dahlin DC, Beabout JW. Dedifferentiation of low-grade chondrosarcomas. *Cancer* 1971;28:461–466.

Dahlin DC, Coventry MB. Osteogenic sarcoma: a study of six hundred cases. *J Bone Joint Surg [Am]* 1967;49A:101–110.

Dahlin DC, Unni KK. Osteosarcoma of bone and its important recognizable varieties. *Am J Surg Pathol* 1977;1:61–72.

Dahlin DC, Unni KK. *Bone tumors: general aspects and data on 8542 cases*, 4th ed. Springfield: Charles C. Thomas, 1986:227–259.

Dahlin DC, Unni KK, Matsuno T. Malignant (fibrous) histiocytoma of bone—fact or fancy? *Cancer* 1977;39:1508–1516.

Dardick I, Schatz JE, Colgan TJ. Osteogenic sarcoma with epithelial differentiation. *Ultrastruct Pathol* 1992;16:463–474.

De Beuckeleer LHL, De Schepper AMA, Ramon F. Magnetic resonance imaging of cartilaginous tumors: retrospective study of 79 patients. *Eur J Radiol* 1995;21:34–40.

deSantos LA, Edeiken B. Purely lytic osteosarcoma. *Skeletal Radiol* 1982;9:1–7.

deSantos LA, Edeiken BS. Subtle early osteosarcoma. *Skeletal Radiol* 1985;13:44–48.

deSantos LA, Murray JA, Finkelstein JB, Spjut HJ, Ayala AG. The radiographic spectrum of periosteal osteosarcoma. *Radiology* 1978;127:123–129.

DeSmet AA, Norris MA, Fisher DR. Magnetic resonance imaging of myositis ossificans: analysis of seven cases. *Skeletal Radiol* 1992;21:503–507.

Dickerson GR, Rossenberg AE. The ultrastructure of small cell osteosarcoma with a review of light microscopy and differential diagnosis. *Hum Pathol* 1991;221:267–275.

Doud TM, Moser RP Jr, Giudici MAI, Frauenhoffer EE, Maurer RJ. Case report 704. Extraskeletal osteosarcoma of the thigh. *Skeletal Radiol* 1991;20:628–632.

Edeiken J, Raymond AK, Ayala AG, Benjamin RS, Murray JA, Carrasco HC. Small-cell osteosarcoma. *Skeletal Radiol* 1987;16:621–628.

Edeiken-Monroe B, Edeiken J, Jacobson HG. Osteosarcoma. *Semin Roentgenol* 1989;24:153–173.

Ehman RL, Berquist TH, McLeod RA. MR imaging of the musculoskeletal system: a 5-year appraisal. *Radiology* 1988;166:313–320.

Ellis JH, Siegel CL, Martel W, Weatherbee L, Dorfman H. Radiologic features of well-differentiated osteosarcoma. *AJR Am J Roentgenol* 1988;151:739–742.

Enzinger F, Weiss S. *Soft tissue tumors*. St. Louis: CV Mosby; 1983.

Enzinger FM, Shiraki M. Extraskeletal myxoid chondrosarcoma—an analysis of 34 cases. *Hum Pathol* 1972;3:421–435.

Enzinger FM, Weiss SW. Cartilaginous tumors and tumorlike lesions of soft tissue. In: Enzinger FM, Weiss SW, eds. *Soft tissue tumors*. St. Louis: Mosby-Year Book; 1988:861–881.

Eustace S, Baker N, Lan H, Wadhwani A, Dorfman D. MR imaging of dedifferentiated chondrosarcoma. *Clin Imaging* 1997;21:170–174.

Evans HL, Ayala AG, Romsdahl MM. Prognostic factors in chondrosarcoma of bone. *Cancer* 1977;40:818–831.

Farr GH, Huvos AG, Marcove RC, Higinbotham NL, Foote FW Jr. Telangiectatic osteogenic sarcoma: a review of twenty-eight cases. *Cancer* 1974;34:1150–1158.

Fechner RE, Mills SE: *Tumors of the bones and joints*. Washington DC: Armed Forces Institute of Pathology; 1993.

Fechner RE, Mills SE. Osseous lesions. In: Rosai J, Sobin L, eds. *Atlas of tumor pathology: tumors of the bones and joints*. Washington DC: Armed Forces Institute of Pathology; 1993:25–77.

Feldman F. Cartilaginous tumors and cartilage-forming tumor-like conditions of the bones and soft tissues. In: Ranniger K, ed. *Bone tumors*. Berlin: Springer-Verlag; 1977:177–220.

Fine G, Stout AP. Osteogenic sarcoma of the extraskeletal soft tissues. *Cancer* 1956;9:1027–1043.

Fobben ES, Dalinka MK, Schiebler ML, et al. The MRI appearance at 1.5 Tesla of cartilaginous tumors involving the epiphysis. *Skeletal Radiol* 1987;16:647–651.

Frassica FJ, Unni KK, Beabout JW, Sim FH. Dedifferentiated chondrosarcoma. A report of the clinicopathological features and treatment of seventy-eight cases. *J Bone Joint Surg [Am]* 1986;68A:1197–1205.

Garrison RC, Unni KK, McLeod RA, Pritchard DJ, Dahlin DC. Chondrosarcoma arising in osteochondroma. *Cancer* 1981;49:1890–1897.

Geirnaerdt MJA, Bloem JL, Eulderink F, Hogendoorn PCW, Taminiau AHM. Cartilaginous tumors: correlation of gadolinium-enhanced MR imaging and histopathologic findings. *Radiology* 1993;186:813–817.

Geirnaerdt MJA, Bloem JL, van der Woude H-J, Taminiau AHM, Nooy MA, Hogendoorn PCW. Chondroblastic osteosarcoma: characterization by gadolinium-enhanced MR imaging correlated with histopathology. *Skeletal Radiol* 1998;27:145–153.

Geirnaerdt MJA, Hogendoorn PCW, Bloem JL, Taminiau AHM, van der Woude H-J. Cartilaginous tumors: fast contrast-enhanced MR imaging. *Radiology* 2000;214:539–546.

Gherlinzoni F, Antoci B, Canale V. Multicentric osteosarcomata (osteosarcomatosis). *Skeletal Radiol* 1983;10:281–285.

Gitelis S, Block JA, Inerot SE. Clonal analysis of human chondrosarcoma. The 35th Annual Meeting, Orthopedic Research Society. *Orthop Trans* 1989;13:443.

Glicksman AS, Toker C. Osteogenic sarcoma following radiotherapy for bursitis. *Mt Sinai J Med* 1976;43:163–167.

Goldman AB. Myositis ossificans circumscripta: a benign lesion with a malignant differential diagnosis. *AJR Am J Roentgenol* 1976;126:32–40.

Goldman RL, Lichtenstein L. Synovial chondrosarcoma. *Cancer* 1964;17:1233–1240.

Gomes H, Menanteau B, Gaillard D, Behar C. Telangiectatic osteosarcoma. *Pediatr Radiol* 1986;16:140–143.

Greenfield GB, Arrington JA. *Imaging of bone tumors. A multi-modality approach*. Philadelphia: JB Lippincott; 1955:48–91.

Greenspan A. Tumors of cartilage origin. *Orthop Clin North Am* 1989;20:347–366.

Greenspan A. Osteosarcoma. *Contemp Diagn Radiol* 1993;16:1–6.

Greenspan A, Klein MJ. Osteosarcoma: radiologic imaging, differential diagnosis, and pathological considerations. *Semin Orthop* 1991;6:156–166.

Greenspan A, Steiner G, Norman A, Lewis MM, Matlen JJ. Case report 436. Osteosarcoma of the soft tissues of the distal end of the thigh. *Skeletal Radiol* 1987;16:489–492.

Griffith JF, Kumta SM, Chow LTC, Leung PC, Metreweli C. Intracortical osteosarcoma. *Skeletal Radiol* 1998;27:228–232.

Hall RB, Robinson LH, Malawer MM, Dunham WK. Periosteal osteosarcoma. *Cancer* 1985;55:165–171.

Hamilton A, Davis RI, Hayes D, Mollan RA. Chondrosarcoma developing in synovial chondromatosis. *J Bone Joint Surg [Br]* 1987;69B:137–140.

Hasegawa T, Shimoda T, Yokoyama R, Beppu Y, Hirohashi S, Maeda S. Intracortical osteoblastic osteosarcoma with oncogenic rickets. *Skeletal Radiol* 1999;28:41–45.

Hatano H, Ogose A, Hotta T, Otsuka H, Takahashi HE. Periosteal chondrosarcoma invading the medullary cavity. *Skeletal Radiol* 1997;26:375–378.

Haygood TM, Teot L, Ward WG, Allen A, Monu JUV. Low-grade chondrosarcoma in a 12-year-old boy. *Skeletal Radiol* 1995;24:466–468.

Heinrich SD, Zembo MM, MacEwen GD. Pseudomalignant myositis ossificans. *Orthopedics* 1989;12:599–602.

Henderson ED, Dahlin DC. Chondrosarcoma of bone: a study of 280 cases. *J Bone Joint Surg [Am]* 1963;45A:1450–1458.

Hermann G, Abdelwahab IF, Kenan S, Lewis MM, Klein MJ. Case report 795. High-grade surface osteosarcoma of the radius. *Skeletal Radiol* 1993;22:383–385.

Hermann G, Klein MJ. Springfield D, Abdelwahab IF, Dan SJ. Intracortical osteosarcoma; two-year delay in diagnosis. *Skeletal Radiol* 2002;31:592–596.

Heul RO van der, Ronnen JR von. Juxtacortical osteosarcoma. Diagnosis, differential diagnosis, treatment, and an analysis of eighty cases. *J Bone Joint Surg [Am]* 1967;49A:415–439.

Hopper KD, Moser RP Jr, Haseman DB, Sweet DE, Madewell JE, Kransdorf MJ. Osteosarcomatosis. *Radiology* 1990;175:233–239.

Hudson TM. Medullary (central) chondrosarcoma. In: Hudson TM, ed. *Radiologic pathologic correlation of musculoskeletal lesions*. Baltimore, Williams & Wilkins; 1987: 153–175.

Hudson TM, Chew FS, Manaster BJ. Radionuclide scanning of medullary chondrosarcoma. *AJR Am J Roentgenol* 1982;139:1071–1076.

Hudson TM, Chew FS, Manaster BJ. Scintigraphy of benign exostoses and exostotic chondrosarcomas. *AJR Am J Roentgenol* 1983;140:581–586.

Hudson TM, Hamlin DJ, Enneking WF, Petterson H. Magnetic resonance imaging of bone and soft-tissue tumors: early experience in 31 patients compared with computed tomography. *Skeletal Radiol* 1985;13:134–146.

Hudson TM, Springfield DS, Benjamin M, Bertoni F, Present DA. Computed tomography of parosteal osteosarcoma. *AJR Am J Roentgenol* 1985;144:961–965.

Hudson TM, Springfield DS, Spanier SS, Enneking WF, Hamlin DJ. Benign exostoses and exostotic chondrosarcomas: evaluation of cartilage thickness by CT. *Radiology* 1984;152:595–599.

Huvos AG, Marcove RC. Chondrosarcoma in the young: a clinicopathologic analysis of 79 patients younger than 21 years of age. *Am J Surg Pathol* 1987;11:930–942.

Huvos AG, Rosen G, Bretsky SS, Butler A. Telangiectatic osteosarcoma: a clinicopathologic study of 124 patients. *Cancer* 1982;49:1679–1689.

Ilaslan H, Sundaram M, Unni KK, Shives TC. Primary vertebral osteosarcoma: imaging findings. *Radiology* 2004;230:697–702.

Ishida T, Dorfman HD, Habermann ET. Dedifferentiated chondrosarcoma of humerus with giant cell tumor-like features. *Skeletal Radiol* 1995;24:76–80.

Ishida T, Yamamoto M, Goto T, Kawano H, Yamamoto A, Machinami R. Clear cell chondrosarcoma of the pelvis in a skeletally immature patient. *Skeletal Radiol* 1999;28:290–293.

Jaffe HL. Intracortical osteogenic sarcoma. *Bull Hosp Joint Dis* 1960;21:180–197.

Jaffe HL. *Tumors and tumorous conditions of the bones and joints.* Philadelphia: Lea & Febiger;1968.

Janzen L, Logan PM, O'Connell JX, Connell DG, Munk PL. Intramedullary chondroid tumors of bone: correlation of abnormal peritumoral marrow and soft-tissue MRI signal with tumor type. *Skeletal Radiol* 1997;26:100–106.

Jee WH, Choe BY, Ok IY, et al. Recurrent parosteal osteosarcoma of the talus in a 2-year-old child. *Skeletal Radiol* 1998;27:157–160.

Jelinek JS, Murphey MD, Kransdorf MJ, Shmookler BM, Malawer MM, Hur RC. Parosteal osteosarcoma: value of MR imaging and CT in the prediction of histologic grade. *Radiology* 1996;201:837–842.

Johnson K, Davies AM, Mangham DC, Grimer RJ. Parosteal osteosarcoma of a metatarsal with intramedullary invasion. *Skeletal Radiol* 1999;28:111–115.

Johnson S, Tetu B, Ayala AG, Chawla SP. Chondrosarcoma with additional mesenchymal component (dedifferentiated chondrosarcoma). A clinical study of 26 cases. *Cancer* 1986;58:278–286.

Kaim AH, Hügli R, Bonél HM, Jundt G. Chondroblastoma and clear cell chondrosarcoma: radiological and MRI characteristics with histopathological correlation. *Skeletal Radiol* 2002;31:88–95.

Kaufman JH, Cedermark BJ, Parthasarathy KL, Didolkar MS, Bakshi SP. The value of ^{67}Ga scintigraphy in soft-tissue sarcoma and chondrosarcoma. *Radiology* 1977;123:131–134.

Kaufman RA, Towbin RB. Telangiectatic osteosarcoma simulating the appearance of an aneurysmal bone cyst. *Pediatr Radiol* 1981;11:102–104.

Kavanagh TG, Cannon SR, Pringle J, Stoker DJ, Kemp HB. Parosteal osteosarcoma: treatment by wide resection and prosthetic replacement. *J Bone Joint Surg [Br]* 1990;72B:959–965.

Kenan S, Abdelwahab IF, Klein MJ, Hermann G, Lewis MM. Lesions of juxtacortical origin surface lesions of bone. *Skeletal Radiol* 1993;22:337–357.

Kenan S, Abdelwahab IF, Klein MJ, Hermann G, Lewis MM. Case report 835. Parosteal osteosarcoma involving the left radius. *Skeletal Radiol* 1994;22:229–231.

Kersjes W, Grebe P, Runkel M, Störkel S, Schild H. Parosteal osteosarcoma of the talus. *Skeletal Radiol* 1995;24:217–219.

Kessler S, Mirra JM, Ishii T, Thompson JC, Brien EW. Primary malignant mesenchymoma of bone: case report, literature review, and distinction of this entity from mesenchymal and dedifferentiated chondrosarcoma. *Skeletal Radiol* 1995;24:291–295.

King JW, Spjut HJ, Fechner RE, Vanderpool DW. Synovial chondrosarcoma of the knee joint. *J Bone Joint Surg [Am]* 1967;49A:1389–1396.

Klein MJ. Chondrosarcoma. *Semin Orthop* 1991;6:167–176.

Klein MJ, Kenan S, Lewis MM. Osteosarcoma: clinical and pathological considerations. *Orthop Clin North Am* 1989;20:327–345.

Konishi E, Kusuzaki K, Murata H, Tsuchihashi Y, Beabout JW, Unni KK. Extraskeletal osteosarcoma arising in myositis ossificans. *Skeletal Radiol* 2001;30:39–43.

Kramer K, Hicks D, Palis J, et al. Epithelioid osteosarcoma of bone. Immunocytochemical evidence suggesting divergent epithelial and mesenchymal differentiation in a primary osseous neoplasm. *Cancer* 1993;71:2977–2982.

Kransdorf MJ, Jelinek JS, Moser RP Jr, et al. Soft-tissue masses: diagnosis using MR imaging. *AJR Am J Roentgenol* 1989;153:541–547.

Kransdorf MJ, Meis JM. Extraskeletal osseous and cartilaginous tumors of the extremities. *Radiographics* 1993;13:853–884.

Kransdorf MJ, Meis JM, Jelinek JS. Myositis ossificans: MR appearance with radiologic-pathologic correlation. *AJR Am J Roentgenol* 1991;157:1243–1248.

Kumar N, David R, Madewell JE, Lindell MM Jr. Radiographic spectrum of osteogenic sarcoma. *AJR Am J Roentgenol* 1987;148:767–772.

Kumar R, David R, Cierney G III. Clear cell chondrosarcoma. *Radiology* 1985;154:45–48.

Kumta SM, Griffith JF, Chow LTC, Leung PC. Primary juxtacortical chondrosarcoma dedifferentiating after 20 years. *Skeletal Radiol* 1998;27:569–573.

Kyriakos M. Intracortical osteosarcoma. *Cancer* 1980;46:2525–2533.

Kyriakos M, Gilula LA, Besich MJ, Schoeneker PL. Intracortical small cell osteosarcoma. *Clin Orthop* 1992;279:269–280.

Le Charpentier Y, Forest M, Postel M, Tomeno B, Abelanet R. Clear-cell chondrosarcoma: a report of five cases including ultrastructural study. *Cancer* 1979;44: 622–629.

Lee YY, Van Tassel P, Nauert C, Raymond AK, Edeiken J. Craniofacial osteosarcomas: plain film, CT and MR findings in 46 cases. *AJR Am J Roentgenol* 1988;150:1397–1402.

Levine E, De Smet AA, Huntrakoon M. Juxtacortical osteosarcoma: a radiologic and histologic spectrum. *Skeletal Radiol* 1985;14:38–46.

Lichtenstein L, Jaffe HL. Chondrosarcoma of the bone. *Am J Pathol* 1943;19:553–589.

Lin J, Yao L, Mirra JM, Balch WJ. Osteochondromalike parosteal osteosarcoma: a report of six cases of a new entity. *AJR Am J Roentgenol* 1998;170:1571–1577.

Lin W-Y, Wang S-J, Yeh S-H. Radionuclide imaging in extraskeletal myxoid chondrosarcoma. *Clin Nucl Med* 1995;20:524–527.

Lindell MM Jr, Shirkhoda A, Raymond AK, Murray JA, Harle TS. Parosteal osteosarcoma: radiologic-pathologic correlation with emphasis on CT. *AJR Am J Roentgenol* 1987;148:323–328.

Logan PM, Mitchell MJ, Munk PL. Imaging of variant osteosarcomas with an emphasis on CT and MR imaging. *AJR Am J Roentgenol* 1998;171:1531–1537.

Lopez BF, Rodriquez PJL, Gonzalez LJ, Sanchez HS, Sanchez DCM. Intracortical osteosarcoma. A case report. *Clin Orthop* 1991;278:218–222.

Lorigan JG, Lipshitz HI, Peuchot M. Radiation-induced sarcoma of bone: CT findings in 19 cases. *AJR Am J Roentgenol* 1989;153:791–794.

MacSweeney F, Darby A, Saifuddin A. Dedifferentiated chondrosarcoma of the appendicular skeleton: MRI-pathological correlation. *Skeletal Radiol* 2003;32:671–678.

Malcolm AJ. Osteosarcoma: classification, pathology, and differential diagnosis. *Semin Orthop* 1988;3:1–12.

Manivel JC, Dehner LP, Thompson R. Case report 460. Synovial chondrosarcoma of left knee. *Skeletal Radiol* 1988;17:66–71.

Mankin JH, Cantley KP, Lippiello L, Schiller AL, Campbell CJ. The biology of human chondrosarcoma. I. Description of the cases, grading, and biochemical analyses. *J Bone Joint Surg [Am]* 1980;62A:160–176.

Martinez-Tello FJ, Navas-Palacios JJ. The ultrastructure of conventional, parosteal, and periosteal osteosarcoma. *Cancer* 1982;50:949–961.

Matsuno T, Unni KK, McLeod RA, Dahlin DC. Telangiectatic osteogenic sarcoma. *Cancer* 1976;38:2538–2547.

McCarthy EF, Dorfman HD. Chondrosarcoma of bone with dedifferentiation: a study of eighteen cases. *Hum Pathol* 1982;13:36–40.

McFarland GB, McKinley LM, Reed RJ. Dedifferentiation of low-grade chondrosarcomas. *Clin Orthop* 1977;122:157–164.

McKenna RJ, Schwinn CP, Soong KY, Higinbotham NL. Osteogenic sarcoma arising in Paget's disease. *Cancer* 1964;17:42–66.

McLeod RA, Berquist TH. Bone tumor imaging: contribution of CT and MRI. In: Unni KK, ed. *Bone tumors.* New York: Churchill Livingstone; 1988:1–34.

McLeod RA, Dahlin DC, Beabout JW. The spectrum of osteoblastoma. *AJR Am J Roentgenol* 1976;126:321–325.

Meneses MF, Unni KK, Swee RG. Bizarre parosteal osteochondromatous proliferation of bone (Nora's lesion). *Am J Surg Pathol* 1993;17:691–697.

Mercuri M, Picci P, Campanacci M, Rulli E. Dedifferentiated chondrosarcoma. *Skeletal Radiol* 1995;24:409–416.

Mindell ER, Shah NK, Webster JH. Postradiation sarcoma of bone and soft tissues. *Orthop Clin North Am* 1977;8:821–834.

Mirra JM. Clinical guidelines for differentiating enchondroma from chondrosarcoma. *Complications Orthop* 1987;2:89–107.

Mirra JM, Gold R, Downs J, Eckardt JJ. A new histologic approach to the differentiation of enchondroma and chondrosarcoma of the bones. *Clin Orthop* 1985;201:214–237.

Mirra JM, Gold RH, Picci P. Osseous tumors of intramedullary origin. In: Mirra JM, ed. *Bone tumors.* Philadelphia: Lea & Febiger; 1989:143–438.

Mirra JM, Marcove RC. Fibrosarcomatous dedifferentiation of primary and secondary chondrosarcomas. *J Bone Joint Surg [Am]* 1974;56A:285–296.

Mirra JM, Picci P, Gold RH. *Bone tumors: clinical, radiologic and pathologic correlations.* Philadelphia: Lea & Febiger; 1989.

Mitchell A, Rudan JR, Fenton PV. Juxtacortical de-differentiated chondrosarcoma from a primary periosteal chondrosarcoma. *Mod Pathol* 1996;9:279–283.

Mitchell AD, Ayoub K, Mangham DC, Grimer RJ, Carter SR, Tillman RM. Experience in the treatment of dedifferentiated chondrosarcoma. *J Bone Joint Surg [Br]* 2000;82B:55–61.

Moore TE, King AR, Kathol MH, El-Khoury GY, Palmer R, Downey PR. Sarcoma in Paget disease of bone: clinical, radiologic, and pathologic features in 22 cases. *AJR Am J Roentgenol* 1991;156:1199–1203.

Moser RP. Cartilaginous tumors of the skeleton. *AFIP atlas of radiologic-pathologic correlation,* vol 2. Philadelphia: Hanley & Belfus; 1990:190–197.

Mulder JD, Schütte HE, Kroon HM, Taconis WK. *Radiologic atlas of bone tumors.* Amsterdam: Elsevier; 1993:51–76.

Mullins F, Berard CW, Eisenberg SH. Chondrosarcoma following synovial chondromatosis. A case study. *Cancer* 1965;18:1180–1188.

Murphey MD, Flemming DJ, Boyea SR, Bojescul JA, Sweet DE, Temple HT. Enchondroma versus chondrosarcoma in the appendicular skeleton: differentiating features. *Radiographics* 1998;18:1213–1237.

Murphey MD, Robbin MR, McRae GA, Flemming DJ, Temple HT, Kransdorf MJ. The many faces of osteosarcoma. *Radiographics* 1997;17:1205–1231.

Murphey MD, Walker EA, Wilson AJ, Kransdorf MJ, Temple HT, Gannon FH. From the archives of the AFIP. Imaging of primary chondrosarcoma: radiologic-pathologic correlation. *Radiographics* 2003;23:1245–1278.

Murphey MD, wan Joavisidha S, Temple HT, Gannon FH, Jelinek JS, Malawer MM. Telangiectatic osteosarcoma: radiologic-pathologic comparison. *Radiology* 2003;229:545–553.

Nakashima Y, Unni KK, Shives TC, Swee RG, Dahlin DC. Mesenchymal chondrosarcoma of bone and soft tissue. A review of 111 cases. *Cancer* 1986;57:2444–2453.

Noioma T, Unni KK, McLeod RA, Pritchard DJ. Periosteal chondroma and periosteal chondrosarcoma. *Am J Surg Pathol* 1985;9:666–677.

Nora FE, Dahlin DC, Beabout JW. Bizarre parosteal osteochondromatous proliferations of the hands and feet. *Am J Surg Pathol* 1983;7:245–250.

Norman A, Dorfman H. Juxtacortical circumscribed myositis ossificans: evolution and radiographic features. *Radiology* 1970;96:301–306.

Norman A, Sissons HA. Radiographic hallmarks of peripheral chondrosarcoma. *Radiology* 1984;151:589–596.

Norton KI, Hermann G, Abdelwahab IF, Klein MJ, Granowetter LF, Rabinowitz JG. Epiphyseal involvement in osteosarcoma. *Radiology* 1991;180:813–816.

Nuovo MA, Norman A, Chumas J, Ackerman LV. Myositis ossificans with atypical clinical, radiographic, or pathologic findings: a review of 23 cases. *Skeletal Radiol* 1992;21:87–101.

Okada K, Frassica FJ, Sim FH, Beabout JW, Bond JR, Unni KK. Parosteal osteosarcoma. A clinicopathological study. *J Bone Joint Surg [Am]* 1994;76A:366–378.

Okada K, Ito H, Miyakoshi N, Sageshima M, Nishida J, Itoi E. A low-grade extraskeletal osteosarcoma. *Skeletal Radiol* 2003;32:165–169.

Okada K, Kubota H, Ebina T, Kobayashi T, Abe E, Sato K. High-grade surface osteosarcoma of the humerus. *Skeletal Radiol* 1995;24:531–534.

Okamoto S, Hara K, Sumita S, Sato K, Hisaoka M, Aotei T, Hashimoto H. Extraskeletal myxoid chondrosarcoma arising in the finger. *Skeletal Radiol* 2002;31:296–300.

Onikul E, Fletcher BD, Parham DM, Chen G. Accuracy of MR imaging for estimating intraosseous extent of osteosarcoma. *AJR Am J Roentgenol* 1996;167:1211–1215.

Ontell F, Greenspan A. Chondrosarcoma complicating synovial chondromatosis: findings with magnetic resonance imaging. *Can Assoc Radiol J* 1994;45:318–323.

Park Y-K, Yang MH, Ryu KN, Chung DW. Dedifferentiated chondrosarcoma arising in an osteochondroma. *Skeletal Radiol* 1995;24:617–619.

Partovi S, Logan PM, Janzen DL, O'Connell JX, Connell DG. Low-grade parosteal osteosarcoma of the ulna with dedifferentiation into high-grade osteosarcoma. *Skeletal Radiol* 1996;25:497–500.

Pettersson H, Slone RM, Spanier S, Gillespy T III, Fitzsimmons JR, Scott KN. Musculoskeletal tumors: T1 and T2 relaxation times. *Radiology* 1988;167:783–785.

Picci P, Campanacci M, Bacci G, Capanna R, Ayala A. Medullary involvement in parosteal osteosarcoma: a case report. *J Bone Joint Surg [Am]* 1987;69A:131–136.

Picci P, Gherlinzoni F, Guerra A. Intracortical osteosarcoma: rare entity or early manifestation of classical osteosarcoma? *Skeletal Radiol* 1983;9:255–258.

Pignatti G, Bacci G, Picci P, et al. Telangiectatic osteosarcoma of the extremities. Results in 17 patients treated with neoadjuvant chemotherapy. *Clin Orthop* 1991;270:99–106.

Present DA, Bacchini P, Pignatti G, Picci P, Bertoni F, Campanacci M. Clear cell chondrosarcoma of bone. A report of eight cases. *Skeletal Radiol* 1991;20:187–191.

Present DA, Bonar SF, Greenspan A, Paonessa K. Clear-cell chondrosarcoma: an unusual case complicated by microinfiltrative pattern of bone marrow involvement and postsurgical myositis ossificans. *Clin Orthop* 1988;237:164–169.

Price CHG, Goldie W. Paget's sarcoma of bone: a study of eighty cases from the Bristol and Leeds bone tumor registries. *J Bone Joint Surg [Br]* 1969;51B:205–224.

Pritchard DJ, Lunke RJ, Taylor WF, Dahlin DC, Medley BE. Chondrosarcoma: clinicopathologic and statistical analysis. *Cancer* 1980;45:149–157.

Ragsdale BD, Sweet DE, Vinh TN. Radiology as gross pathology in evaluating chondroid lesions. *Hum Pathol* 1989;20:930–951.

Rao U, Cheng A, Didolkar MS. Extraosseous osteogenic sarcoma: clinicopathological study of eight cases and review of literature. *Cancer* 1978;41:1488–1496.

Raymond AK. Surface osteosarcoma. *Clin Orthop* 1991;270:140–148.

Reid RP. Bone neoplasms and tumor-like lesions on the bone surface. In: Helliwell TR, ed. *Pathology of bone and joint neoplasms*. Philadelphia: Saunders; 1999:215–235.

Reiter FB, Ackerman LV, Staple TW. Central chondrosarcoma of the appendicular skeleton. *Radiology* 1972;105:525–530.

Remagen W, Nidecker A, Dolanc B. Case report 368. Enchondroma of the tibia with extensive myxoid degeneration: recurrence with secondary highly differentiated chondrosarcoma. *Skeletal Radiol* 1986;15:330–333.

Resnick D, Kyriakos M, Greenway GD: Tumors and tumor-like lesions of bone: imaging and pathology of specific lesions. In: Resnick D, Niwayama G, eds. *Diagnosis of bone and joint disorders*, 3rd ed. Philadelphia: WB Saunders; 1988:3628–3917.

Richardson ML, Kilcoyne RF, Gillespy T III, Helms CA, Genant HK. Magnetic resonance imaging of musculoskeletal neoplasms. *Radiol Clin North Am* 1986;24:259–267.

Ritts GD, Pritchard DJ, Unni KK, Beabout JW, Eckardt JJ. Periosteal osteosarcoma. *Clin Orthop* 1987;219:299–307.

Robinson LH, Pitt MJ, Jaffe KA, Siegal GP. Small cell osteosarcoma of the soft tissue. *Skeletal Radiol* 1995;24:462–465.

Robinson P, White LM, Sundaram M, et al. Periosteal chondroid tumors: radiologic evaluation with pathologic correlation. *AJR Am J Roentgenol* 2001;177:1183–1188.

Roessner A, Hobik HP, Grundmann E. Malignant fibrous histiocytoma of bone and osteosarcoma: a comparative light and electron microscopic study. *Pathol Res Pract* 1979;164:385–401.

Rosenberg ZS, Leu S, Schmahmann S, Steiner GC, Beltran J, Present D. Osteosarcoma: subtle, rare, and misleading plain film features. *AJR Am J Roentgenol* 1995;165:1209–1214.

Rosenthal DJ, Schiller AL, Mankin HJ. Chondrosarcoma: correlation of radiological and histological grade. *Radiology* 1984;150:21–26.

Ruiter DJ, Cornelisse CJ, van Rijssel TG, van der Velde EA. Aneurysmal bone cyst and telangiectatic osteosarcoma. A histopathological and morphometric study. *Virchows Arch [A]* 1977;373:311–325.

Saifuddin A. The accuracy of imaging in the local staging of appendicular osteosarcoma. *Skeletal Radiol* 2002;31:191–201.

Salvador AH, Beabout JW, Dahlin DC. Mesenchymal chondrosarcoma—observations on 30 new cases. *Cancer* 1971;28:605–615.

Sanerkin NG. Definitions of osteosarcoma, chondrosarcoma and fibrosarcoma of bone. *Cancer* 1980;46:178–185.

Sanerkin NG. The diagnosis and grading of chondrosarcoma of bone. *Cancer* 1980;45:582–594.

Sanerkin NG, Gallagher P. A review of the behaviour of chondrosarcoma of bone. *J Bone Joint Surg [Br]* 1979;61B:395–400.

Sauer DD, Chase DR. Case report 461. Dedifferentiated parosteal osteosarcoma. *Skeletal Radiol* 1988;17:72–76.

Saunders C, Szabo RM, Mora S. Chondrosarcoma of the hand arising in a young patient with multiple hereditary exostoses. *J Hand Surg [Br]* 1997;22B:237–242.

Schajowicz F. Juxtacortical chondrosarcoma. *J Bone Joint Surg [Br]* 1978;59B:473–480.

Schajowicz F. *Tumors and tumorlike lesions of bone. Pathology, radiology, and treatment*, 2nd ed. Berlin: Springer-Verlag; 1994:103–106.

Schajowicz F, Araujo ES, Berenstein M. Sarcoma complicating Paget's disease of bone: a clinicopathological study of 62 cases. *J Bone Joint Surg [Br]* 1983;65B:299–307.

Schajowicz F, McGuire M. Diagnostic difficulties in skeletal pathology. *Clin Orthop* 1989;240:281–308.

Schajowicz F, McGuire MH, Araujo ES, Muscolo DL, Gitelis S. Osteosarcomas arising on the surfaces of long bones. *J Bone Joint Surg [Am]* 1988;70A:555–564.

Schajowicz F, Sissons HA, Sobin LH. The World Health Organization's histologic classification of bone tumors. A commentary on the second edition. *Cancer* 1995;75:1208–1214.

Scheele PM, von Kuster LC, Krivchenia G. Primary malignant mesenchymoma of bone. *Arch Pathol Lab Med* 1990;114:614–617.

Schiller AL. Diagnosis of borderline cartilage lesions of bone. *Semin Diagn Pathol* 1985;1:42–62.

Schreiman JS, Crass JR, Wick MR, Maile CW, Thompson RC Jr. Osteosarcoma: role of CT in limb-sparing treatment. *Radiology* 1986;161:485–488.

Sciot R, Samson I, Dal Cin P, et al. Giant cell rich parosteal osteosarcoma. *Histopathology* 1995;27:51–55.

Seeger LL, Eckardt JJ, Bassett LW. Cross-sectional imaging in the evaluation of osteogenic sarcoma: MRI and CT. *Semin Roentgenol* 1989;24:174–184.

Seeger LL, Farooki S, Yao L, Kabo JM, Eckardt JJ. Custom endoprotheses for limb salvage: a historical perspective and image evaluation. *AJR Am J Roentgenol* 1998;171:1525–1529.

Seeger LL, Yao L, Eckardt JJ. Surface lesions of bone. *Radiology* 1998;206:17–33.

Shapeero LG, Vanel D, Couanet D, Contesso G, Ackerman LV. Extraskeletal mesenchymal chondrosarcoma. *Radiology* 1993;186:819–826.

Sheth DS, Yasko AW, Raymond AK, et al. Conventional and dedifferentiated parosteal osteosarcoma: diagnosis, treatment and outcome. *Cancer* 1996;78:2136–2145.

Shuhaibar H, Friedman L. Dedifferentiated parosteal osteosarcoma with high-grade osteoclast-rich osteogenic sarcoma at presentation. *Skeletal Radiol* 1998;27:574–577.

Sim FH, Kurt A-M, McLeod RA, Unni KK. Case report 628. Low-grade central osteosarcoma. *Skeletal Radiol* 1990;19:457–460.

Sim FH, Unni KK, Beabout JW, Dahlin DC. Osteosarcoma with small cells simulating Ewing's tumor. *J Bone Joint Surg [Am]* 1979;61A:207–215.

Simon MA, Bos GD. Epiphyseal extension of metaphyseal osteosarcoma in skeletally immature individuals. *J Bone Joint Surg [Am]* 1980;62A:195–204.

Sirsat MV, Doctor VM. Benign chondroblastoma of bone. Report of a case of malignant transformation. *J Bone Joint Surg [Br]* 1970;52B:741–745.

Sissons HA, Greenspan A. Paget's disease. In: Taveras JM, Ferrucci JT, eds. *Radiology: diagnosis, imaging, intervention*, vol 5. Philadelphia: JB Lippincott; 1986:1–14.

Sissons HA, Matlen JA, Lewis MM. Dedifferentiated chondrosarcoma. Report of an unusual case. *J Bone Joint Surg [Am]* 1991;73A:294–300.

Smith J, Ahuja SC, Huvos AG, Bullough PG. Parosteal (juxtacortical) osteogenic sarcoma: a roentgenological study of 30 patients. *J Can Assoc Radiol* 1978;29:167–174.

Smith J, Botet JR, Yeh SDJ. Bone sarcomas in Paget's disease. A study of 85 patients. *Radiology* 1984;152:583–590.

Sordillo PP, Hajdu SI, Magill GB, Goldbey RB. Extraosseous osteogenic sarcoma. A review of 48 patients. *Cancer* 1983;51:727–734.

Spjut HJ, Dorfman HD, Fechner RE, Ackerman LV. Tumors of bone and cartilage. In: Firminger HI, ed. *Atlas of tumor pathology*, 2nd series, fascicle 5. Washington: Armed Forces Institute of Pathology; 1971.

Steiner GC, Mirra JM, Bullough PG. Mesenchymal chondrosarcoma. A study of the ultrastructure. *Cancer* 1973;32:926–939.

Stevens GM, Pugh DG, Dahlin DC. Roentgenographic recognition and differentiation of parosteal osteogenic sarcoma. *AJR Am J Roentgenol* 1957;78:1–12.

Stout AP, Verner EW. Chondrosarcoma of the extraskeletal soft tissues. *Cancer* 1953;6:581–590.

Sun TC, Swee RG, Shives TC, Unni KK: Chondrosarcoma in Maffucci's syndrome. *J Bone Joint Surg [Am]* 1985;67A:1214–1219.

Sundaram M, McGuire MH, Herbold DR. Magnetic resonance imaging of osteosarcoma. *Skeletal Radiol* 1987;16:23–29.

Sundaram M, McGuire MH, Herbold DR, Wolverson MK, Heiberg E. Magnetic resonance imaging in planning limb-salvage surgery for primary malignant tumors of bone. *J Bone Joint Surg [Am]* 1986;68A:809–819.

Sundaram M, Percelay S, McDonald DJ, Janney C. Case report 799. Extraskeletal chondrosarcoma. *Skeletal Radiol* 1993;22:449–451.

Taconis WK. Osteosarcoma and its variants. *J Med Imaging* 1988;2:276–285.

Tetu B, Ordonez NG, Ayala AG, Mackay B. Chondrosarcoma with additional mesenchymal component (dedifferentiated chondrosarcoma). *Cancer* 1986;58: 287–298.

Torres FX, Kyriakos M. Bone infarct-associated osteosarcoma. *Cancer* 1992;70: 2418–2430.

Troup JB, Dahlin DC, Coventry MB. The significance of giant cells in osteogenic sarcoma: do they indicate a relationship between osteogenic sarcoma and giant cell tumor of bone. *Mayo Clin Proc* 1960;35:179–186.

Tsuneyoshi M, Dorfman HD. Epiphyseal osteosarcoma: distinguishing features from clear cell chondrosarcoma, chondroblastoma and epiphyseal enchondroma. *Hum Pathol* 1987;18:644–651.

Unni KK: Osteosarcoma of bone. In: Unni KK, ed. *Bone tumors.* New York: Churchill Livingstone; 1988:107–133.

Unni KK. *Dahlin's bone tumors: general aspects and data on 11,087 cases,* 5th ed. Philadelphia: Lippincott-Raven; 1996:185–196.

Unni KK, Dahlin DC. Grading of bone tumors. *Semin Diagn Pathol* 1984;1:165–172.

Unni KK, Dahlin DC. Osteosarcoma: pathology and classification. *Semin Roentgenol* 1989;24:143–152.

Unni KK, Dahlin DC. Premalignant tumors and conditions of bone. *Am J Surg Pathol* 1979;3:47–60.

Unni KK, Dahlin DC, Beabout JW. Periosteal osteogenic sarcoma. *Cancer* 1976;37: 2476–2485.

Unni KK, Dahlin DC, Beabout JW, Ivins JC. Parosteal osteogenic sarcoma. *Cancer* 1976; 37:2644–2675.

Unni KK, Dahlin DC, Beabout JW, Sim FH. Chondrosarcoma: clear-cell variant: a report of 16 cases. *J Bone Joint Surg [Am]* 1976;58A:676–683.

Unni KK, Dahlin DC, McLeod RA. Intraosseous well-differentiated osteosarcoma. *Cancer* 1977; 40: 1337–1347.

Vanel D, De Paolis M, Monti C, Mercuri M, Picci P. Radiological features of 24 periosteal chondrosarcomas. *Skeletal Radiol* 2001;30:208–212.

Vanel D, Picci P, De Paolis M, Mercuri M. Radiological study of 12 high-grade surface osteosarcomas. *Skeletal Radiol* 2001;30:667–671.

van Trommel MF, Kroon HM, Bloem JL, Hogendoorn PCW, Taminiau AHM. MR imaging based strategies in limb salvage surgery for osteosarcoma of the distal femur. *Skeletal Radiol* 1997;26:636–641.

Varma DGK, Ayala AG, Carrasco CH, Guo S-Q, Kumar R, Edeiken J. Chondrosarcoma: MR imaging with pathologic correlation. *Radiographics* 1992;12:687–704.

Varma DGK, Ayala AG, Guo S-Q, Moulopoulos LA, Kim EE, Charnsangavej C. MRI of extraskeletal osteosarcoma. *J Comput Assist Tomogr* 1993;17:414–417.

Verela-Duran J, Enzinger FM. Calcifying synovial sarcoma. *Cancer* 1982;50:345–352.

Vigorita VJ, Jones JK, Ghelman B, Marcove RC. Intracortical osteosarcoma. *Am J Surg Pathol* 1984;8:65–71.

Waxman M, Vuletin JC, Saxe BI, Monteleone FA. Extraskeletal osteosarcoma. Light and electron microscopic study. *Mt Sinai J Med* 1981;48:322–329.

Weiss AC, Dorfman HD. Clear cell chondrosarcoma: a report of 10 cases and review of the literature. *Surg Pathol* 1988;1:123–129.

Wenger DE, Sundaram M, Unni KK, Janney CG, Merkel K. Acral synovial chondrosarcoma. *Skeletal Radiol* 2002;31:125–129.

Wenger DE, Sundaram M, Unni KK, Janney CG, Merkel K. Microscopic correlation of radiographically disparate appearing well differentiated osteosarcoma. *Skeletal Radiol* 2002;31:488–492.

West OC, Reinus WR, Wilson AJ. Quantitative analysis of the plain radiographic appearance of central chondrosarcoma of bone. *Invest Radiol* 1995;30:440–447.

Wines A, Bonar F, Lam P, McCarthy S, Stalley P. Telangiectatic dedifferentiation of a parosteal osteosarcoma. *Skeletal Radiol* 2000;29:597–600.

Wold LE: Fibrohistiocytic tumors of bone. In: Unni KK, ed. *Bone tumors.* New York: Churchill Livingstone; 1988:183–197.

Wold LE, Unni KK, Beabout JW, Pritchard DJ. High-grade surface osteosarcomas. *Am J Surg Pathol* 1984;8:181–186.

Wold LE, Unni KK, Beabout JW, Sim FH, Dahlin DC. Dedifferentiated parosteal osteosarcoma. *J Bone Joint Surg [Am]* 1984;66A:53–59.

Wong KT, Haygood T, Dalinka MK, Kneeland B. Chondroblastic, grade 3 periosteal osteosarcoma. *Skeletal Radiol* 1995;24:69–71.

Wu KK, Collon DJ, Guise ER. Extra-osseous chondrosarcoma. Report of five cases and review of the literature. *J Bone Joint Surg [Am]* 1980;62A:189–194.

Wurlitzer F, Ayala A, Romsdahl M. Extraosseous osteogenic sarcoma. *Arch Surg* 1972; 105:691–695.

Yaghmai I. Angiographic features of chondromas and chondrosarcomas. *Skeletal Radiol* 1978;3:91–98.

Yamaguchi H, Nojima T, Yagi T, Masuda T, Sasaki T. High-grade surface osteosarcoma of the left ilium. A case report and review of the literature. *Acta Pathol Jpn* 1988;38: 235–240.

Young CL, Sim FH, Unni KK, McLeod RA. Chondrosarcoma of bone in children. *Cancer* 1990;66:1641–1648.

Zimmer WD, Berquist TH, McLeod RA, et al. Bone tumors: magnetic resonance imaging versus computed tomography. *Radiology* 1985;155:709–718.

MALIGNANT BONE TUMORS II

Miscellaneous Tumors

Fibrosarcoma and Malignant Fibrous Histiocytoma

Fibrosarcoma and malignant fibrous histiocytoma (MFH) are malignant fibrogenic tumors that have very similar radiographic presentations and histologic patterns. Both typically occur in the third to sixth decades, and both have a predilection for the pelvis, femur, humerus, and tibia (Fig. 22.1).

Because there is no essential difference in the radiologic features, clinical behavior, and survival data for these tumors, it is justified to regard them as a single group. Both fibrosarcoma and MFH can be either primary tumors or secondary to a preexisting benign condition, such as Paget disease, fibrous dysplasia, bone infarct, or chronic draining sinuses of osteomyelitis. These lesions may also arise in bones that were previously irradiated. Such lesions are termed secondary fibrosarcomas (or secondary malignant fibrous histiocytomas). Rarely, fibrosarcoma can arise in a periosteal location (periosteal fibrosarcoma). Some investigators postulate, however, that in this location these lesions represent primary soft-tissue tumors abutting the bone and invading the underlying periosteum.

Histologically, fibrosarcoma and MFH are characterized by tumor cells that produce collagen fibers. In fibrosarcoma, however, there is a herringbone pattern of fibrous growth with mild cellular pleomorphism, whereas histiocytic features of a characteristic storiform or pinwheel arrangement of fibrogenic tissue typify MFH. In addition, numerous large bizarre polyhedral cells (histiocytic component) are present. Neither tumor is capable of producing osteoid matrix or bone, a factor distinguishing them from osteosarcoma.

Radiographically, fibrosarcoma and MFH are recognized by an osteolytic area of bone destruction and a wide zone of transition; the lesions are usually eccentrically located close to or in the articular end of the bone. They exhibit little or no reactive sclerosis and in most cases no periosteal reaction (Figs. 22.2 and 22.3); a soft-tissue mass, however, is frequently present.

On computed tomography (CT) examination, fibrosarcoma and MFH show a predominant density similar to that of normal muscle and exhibit the nonspecific tissue attenuation values of Hounsfield units encountered in most nonmineralized tissues. Hypodense areas reflect areas of necrosis within tumor. Magnetic resonance imaging (MRI) is useful to outline the intraosseous and extraosseous extension of these tumors, but there are no characteristic MRI findings for

Figure 22.1 **Skeletal sites of predilection, peak age range, and male-to-female ratio in fibrosarcoma and malignant fibrous histiocytoma.**

Figure 22.2 **Fibrosarcoma.** Oblique radiograph of the right knee of a 28-year-old woman shows a purely destructive osteolytic lesion in the inter-condylar fossa of the distal femur. Note the absence of reactive sclerosis and periosteal response. Biopsy proved it to be a fibrosarcoma.

sidered to represent a small group of undifferentiated pleomorphic sarcomas with no definable line of differentiation, and the term is used with reluctance.

Differential Diagnosis

Fibrosarcoma and MFH may resemble a giant cell tumor (Fig. 22.5) or telangiectatic osteosarcoma (see Fig. 21.13). They are also often mistaken for metastatic lesions (Fig. 22.3). Some authorities believe that an almost pathognomonic sign of fibrosarcoma are small sequestrum-

Figure 22.3 **Fibrosarcoma.** A 62-year-old man sustained a pathologic fracture through an osteolytic lesion in the proximal shaft of the left humerus. A metastatic lesion was suspected, but biopsy revealed a primary fibrosarcoma of the bone.

either one (Fig. 22.4). Some investigators found the signal characteristics comparable to those of other lytic bone tumors. Signal intensity is intermediate to low on T1-weighted images and high on T2 weighting, frequently nonhomogeneous, and varying with the degree of necrosis and hemorrhage within the tumor.

It should be stressed, however, that the entity of MFH has recently fallen out of favor and into disrepute. For example, in the new World Health Organization classification of soft tissue tumors, MFH is con-

Figure 22.4 Malignant fibrous histiocytoma. (A) Oblique radiograph of the right femur of a 16-year-old girl shows fusiform thickening of the cortex and permeative type of medullary bone destruction (*arrows*). **(B)** Radionuclide bone scan (^{99m}Tc-MDP) shows increased uptake of the tracer in the right femur. **(C)** Coronal T1-weighted (SE; TR 500/TE 20 msec) MR image demonstrates the extent of the tumor that involves about 75% of the length of the femur. **(D)** Coronal T2-weighted (SE; TR 2000/TE 80 msec) MR image shows that the tumor exhibits high signal intensity. The soft-tissue extension medially is also accurately depicted. Excision biopsy revealed malignant fibrous histiocytoma.

like fragments of cortical bone and spongy trabeculae, which may be demonstrated on conventional radiography or CT scan.

Immunohistochemical studies have been helpful in the diagnosis of MFH by demonstrating certain nonspecific markers of histiocytic enzymes such as lysozyme, α_1-antitrypsin, and α_1-antichymotrypsin in the tumor. Other antigens reported to variably stain MFH included vimentin, actin, desmin, and keratin.

Complications and Treatment

Because these tumors do not respond satisfactorily to radiation or chemotherapy, surgical resection is the treatment of choice. Pathologic fracture may occur and, as a palliative measure, internal splinting with a metallic implant may be justified. The tumor has been reported to recur after local excision and may spread to regional lymph

Figure 22.5 Malignant fibrous histiocytoma. Anteroposterior radiograph of the left knee **(A)** and a magnification study in the oblique projection **(B)** demonstrate an expansive, lytic lesion in the proximal end of the fibula in a 13-year-old girl. The cortex has been partially destroyed, and there is a buttress of periosteal new bone formation secondary to pathologic fracture. Biopsy revealed a malignant fibrous histiocytoma. The differential diagnosis of this malignancy at this site should include giant cell tumor and aneurysmal bone cyst.

nodes. As already stated previously, fibrosarcoma and MFH may complicate benign conditions such as fibrous dysplasia, Paget disease, bone infarction, or chronic draining sinuses of osteomyelitis. They may also arise in bones that were previously irradiated (see the discussion under the heading Benign Conditions with Malignant Potential). The 5-year survival rate after treatment varies according to different studies from 29% to 67%.

Figure 22.6 Skeletal sites of predilection, peak age range, and male-to-female ratio in Ewing sarcoma.

Ewing Sarcoma

Ewing sarcoma, a highly malignant neoplasm predominantly affecting children and adolescents, with decisive male predominance, is representative of the so-called round cell tumors. Its precise histogenesis is unknown, but it is generally thought that Ewing sarcoma originates from bone marrow cells. Some authorities, however, believe that Ewing sarcoma is a neurally derived small round cell malignancy very similar to the so-called primitive neuroectodermal tumor (PNET). Approximately 90% of Ewing sarcomas occur before age 25, and the disease is extremely rare in black persons. Ewing sarcoma has a predilection for the diaphysis of the long bones, as well as the ribs and flat bones such as the scapula and pelvis (Fig. 22.6). Clinically, it may present as a localized painful mass or with systemic symptoms such as fever, malaise, weight loss, and an increased erythrocyte sedimentation rate. These systemic symptoms may lead to an erroneous diagnosis of osteomyelitis.

The radiographic presentation of this malignancy is usually rather characteristic; the lesion is poorly defined, marked by a permeative or moth-eaten type of bone destruction, and associated with an aggressive periosteal response that has an onionskin (or "onion peel") or, less commonly, a "sunburst" appearance, and a large soft-tissue mass (Fig. 22.7). Occasionally, the bone lesion itself is almost imperceptible, with the soft-tissue mass being the only prominent radiographic finding (Fig. 22.8).

On radionuclide bone scan, Ewing sarcoma shows an intense increase of technetium-99m methylene diphosphonate (^{99m}Tc-MDP) uptake. Gallium-67-citrate (^{67}Ga-citrate) more readily identifies soft-tissue tumor extension. Although scintigraphic findings are nonspecific, this technique provides reliable information concerning the presence of skeletal metastases. CT reveals the pattern of bone destruction, and attenuation values (Hounsfield units) provide information about the medullary extension. In addition, CT may help to delineate extraosseous involvement (Fig. 22.7). MRI is essential for definite demonstration of the extent of intraosseous and extraosseous involvement by this tumor (Fig. 22.9). In particular, MRI may effectively reveal extension through the epiphyseal plate. T1-weighted images show intermediate to low signal intensity, which becomes bright on T2 weighting. Hypocellular regions and areas of necrosis are of lesser intensity. Imaging after injection of gadolinium-diethylene triamine pentaacetic acid (Gd-DTPA) reveals signal enhancement of the tumor on T1-weighted sequences. Enhancement occurs only in the cellular areas, allowing differentiation of the tumor from the peritumoral edema.

Histologically, Ewing sarcoma consists of a uniform array of small cells with round hyperchromatic nuclei, scant cytoplasm, and poorly defined cell borders. The mitotic rate is high, and necrosis is frequently extensive. Usually, the cytoplasm contains a moderate amount of glycogen, demonstrable with the periodic acid-Schiff (PAS) stain. This PAS-positive material is washed away after digestion with diastase, confirming that in fact it represents glycogen. The demonstration of glycogen, which at one time was considered an absolutely distinctive marker for Ewing sarcoma, has fallen into disfavor because in some Ewing sarcoma, glycogen is not found. Moreover, malignant lymphoma and primitive neural tumors may at times contain glycogen. Since the advent of immunohistochemistry, lymphomas are usually differentiated from Ewing sarcomas by demonstrating leukocyte-common antigen, a pathognomic marker for lymphomas, and primitive neural tumors differ from Ewing sarcomas by the fact that they contain neural protein antibodies.

Differential Diagnosis

Ewing sarcoma may often mimic metastatic neuroblastoma or osteomyelitis (Fig. 22.10). At times, Ewing sarcoma exhibits a feature once thought to be almost pathognomonic, the "saucerization" of the

Figure 22.7 Ewing sarcoma. (A) Lateral radiograph in a 12-year-old boy shows the typical appearance of Ewing sarcoma in the fibula. The poorly defined lesion exhibits permeative bone destruction associated with an aggressive periosteal reaction (*arrows*). **(B)** CT section through the lesion demonstrates a large soft-tissue mass, which is not clear on the conventional study. Note the complete obliteration of the marrow cavity by tumor.

Figure 22.8 Ewing sarcoma. (A) Bone destruction is almost imperceptible on this magnification study in a 10-year-old girl with Ewing sarcoma of the distal femoral diaphysis. **(B)** Lateral radiograph of distal femur, however, shows a large soft-tissue mass. **(C)** CT using a bone "window" demonstrates destruction of the medullary portion of the bone and invasion of the cortex.

Figure 22.9 MRI of Ewing sarcoma. Anteroposterior **(A)** and lateral **(B)** radiographs of the right distal femur of a 7-year-old girl show permeative type of bone destruction in the metaphysis and diaphysis associated with a large soft-tissue mass. Coronal **(C)** and sagittal **(D)** T1-weighted (SE; TR 750/TE 20 msec) MR images demonstrate the intraosseous and extraosseous extent of the tumor. **(E)** Axial T2-weighted (SE; TR 2000/TE 80 msec) MR image shows heterogeneous but mostly high signal intensity of the soft-tissue mass.

Figure 22.10 Ewing sarcoma. A 24-year-old man presented with pain and swelling of the left ankle for 8 weeks; he also had a fever. Anteroposterior radiograph of the ankle demonstrates a destructive lesion of the distal fibula exhibiting a permeative type of bone destruction and a lamellated periosteal reaction; a soft-tissue mass is also evident. The appearance is that of infection (osteomyelitis), but biopsy revealed Ewing sarcoma.

ious stages of maturation. Once called "reticulum cell sarcoma," "non-Hodgkin lymphoma," "lymphosarcoma," or "osteolymphoma," bone lymphoma is now known as *large cell* or *histiocytic* lymphoma. Primary bone lymphoma is a rare tumor that accounts for less than 5% of all primary bone tumors. It occurs in the second to seventh decades, with a peak age of occurrence from 45 to 75 years; it has a slightly greater prevalence in males. The lesion develops in the long bones, vertebrae, pelvis, and ribs (Fig. 22.14). Patients may present with local symptoms, such as pain and swelling, or with systemic symptoms, such as fever and weight loss.

Radiographically, histiocytic lymphoma produces a permeative or moth-eaten pattern of bone destruction or is a purely osteolytic lesion with or more commonly without a periosteal reaction (Fig. 22.15). The affected bone can also present with an "ivory" appearance, as is often the case in lesions of the vertebrae or flat bones. Because lymphoma usually does not evoke significant periosteal new bone formation, this is an important feature in differentiating it from Ewing sarcoma.

Histologically, lymphomas may be subdivided into non-Hodgkin lymphomas and Hodgkin lymphomas (Table 22.1). Although secondary involvement of bones is relatively common in Hodgkin lymphoma, primary Hodgkin bone lymphoma is extremely rare. Non-Hodgkin bone lymphomas are considered primary only if a complete systemic work-up reveals no evidence of extraosseous involvement. Histologically, the tumor consists of aggregates of malignant lymphoid cells replacing marrow spaces and osseous trabeculae. The cells contain irregular or even cleaved nuclei. As mentioned in the section on Ewing sarcoma, the most important single procedure used to dis-

cortex (Fig. 22.11), which may be related to destruction of the periosteal surface by the tumor combined with the effect of extrinsic pressure by the large soft-tissue mass. Although this sign has recently been reported in other tumors, and even in osteomyelitis, its presence in association with a permeative lesion and a soft-tissue mass favors the diagnosis of Ewing sarcoma. The radiographic distinction of Ewing sarcoma from metastatic neuroblastoma may occasionally be difficult; however, the latter usually occur in the first 3 years, whereas Ewing sarcoma is uncommon in the first 5 years.

Occasionally, Ewing sarcoma may resemble an osteosarcoma, particularly when the former is accompanied by abundant periosteal new bone formation. Moreover, dystrophic calcifications in the soft-tissue mass may mimic tumor-bone formation in osteosarcoma (Fig. 22.12). Lymphoma must also be included in the differential diagnosis, although this lesion usually occurs in an older age group. The important radiologic difference is usually the absence of a soft-tissue mass in lymphoma, whereas in Ewing sarcoma a soft-tissue mass is almost invariably present, often being disproportionally large compared with the amount of bone destruction (see Figs. 22.8 and 22.9). The distinction between Ewing sarcoma and PNET cannot be made on the basis of radiography. Differentiation between these two tumors must rely entirely on histologic examination.

Treatment

Ewing sarcoma is usually treated with a preoperative course of chemotherapy, either alone or combined with radiation therapy, to shrink the tumor, followed by wide resection (Fig. 22.13). Sometimes the affected limb can be reconstructed with an endoprosthesis or an allograft.

Malignant Lymphoma

The term *malignant lymphoma* refers to a group of neoplasms that are composed of lymphoid or histiocytic cells of different subtypes in var-

Figure 22.11 Ewing sarcoma. Anteroposterior radiograph of the right femur of a 12-year-old girl shows "saucerization" of the medial cortex of the diaphysis, often seen in Ewing sarcoma; there is also an associated soft-tissue mass.

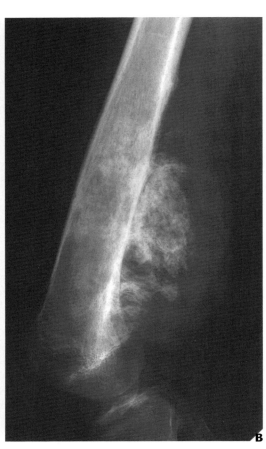

Figure 22.12 Ewing sarcoma. Anteroposterior **(A)** and lateral **(B)** radiographs of the left femur of a 17-year-old boy show a tumor displaying a significant degree of sclerosis that was originally interpreted as osteosarcoma. Biopsy revealed Ewing sarcoma.

Figure 22.13 Ewing sarcoma. (A) Radiograph of the shoulder of an 11-year-old boy shows the typical appearance of Ewing sarcoma involving the distal half of the left clavicle. The poorly defined destructive lesion is associated with an aggressive periosteal reaction and a large soft-tissue mass. **(B)** Tomographic cut gives a better picture of the periosteal response and soft-tissue mass. **(C)** After a 4-month course of chemotherapy, the lesion has become sclerotic, the periosteal reaction has disappeared, and the soft-tissue mass has shrunk substantially. **(D)** The clavicle was then removed en bloc.

Figure 22.14 **Skeletal sites of predilection, peak age range, and male-to-female ratio in primary bone lymphoma.**

Figure 22.15 Lymphoma. An 18-year-old woman presented with low-back pain for several months, which was attributed to herniation of an intervertebral disk. **(A)** Myelogram shows that the disk is normal, but the body of L-5 exhibits a mottled appearance and its posterior border is indistinct. **(B)** CT section demonstrates a large, osteolytic lesion extending from the anterior to the posterior margins of the vertebral body. Biopsy revealed a histiocytic lymphoma.

Table 22.1 **Revised European-American Lymphoma Classification**

B-Cell Lymphomas	T-Cell and Natural Killer Cell Neoplasms	Hodgkin Disease
Precursor B-cell neoplasm • Precursor B-lymphoblastic leukemia or lymphoma Mature B-cell neoplasm • B-cell chronic lymphocytic leukemia, prolymphocytic leukemia, small lymphocytic leukemia • Lymphoplasmacytoid lymphoma • Mantle cell lymphoma • Follicle center lymphoma • Marginal zone B-cell lymphoma • Hairy cell lymphoma • Diffuse large cell B-cell lymphoma • Burkitt lymphoma • High-grade B-cell lymphoma	Precursor T-cell neoplasm • Precursor T-lymphoblastic lymphoma or leukemia Peripheral T-cell and natural killer cell neoplasm • T-cell chronic lymphocytic leukemia • Large granular lymphocyte leukemia • Mycosis fungoides, Sezary syndrome • Peripheral T-cell lymphoma • Angioimmunoblastic T-cell lymphoma • Angiocentric lymphoma • Adult T-cell lymphoma • Anaplastic large cell lymphoma	Nodular lymphocyte predominance (paragranuloma) Nodular sclerosis Mixed cellularity Lymphocyte depletion Lymphocyte-rich classic Hodgkin disease

Modified from Krishnan A, et al., Radiographics 2003;23:1371–1387 with permission

tinguish lymphoma from the other round cell tumors is the stain for leukocyte-common antigen, because lymphoid cells are the only cells that stain positively.

Differential Diagnosis

Histiocytic lymphoma must be distinguished from secondary involvement of the skeleton by systemic lymphoma. It may resemble Ewing sarcoma, particularly in younger patients (Fig. 22.16), or Paget disease if the articular end of a bone is involved and there is a mixed sclerotic and osteolytic pattern (Fig. 22.17).

Treatment

The treatment for primary bone lymphoma is controversial, and there is no consensus with regard to radiotherapy, although this tumor is radiosensitive. Some cases require chemotherapy as the mainstay and additional adjuvant radiation therapy. The optimal treatment has not been determined and is still being debated.

Myeloma

Myeloma, also known as "multiple myeloma" or "plasma cell myeloma," is a tumor originating in the bone marrow and is the most common primary malignant bone tumor. It is usually seen between the fifth and seventh decades and is more frequent in men than women. The axial skeleton (skull, spine, ribs, and pelvis) are the most commonly affected sites, but no bone is exempt from involvement (Fig. 22.18). Rarely, the presentation can be that of a solitary lesion, in which case it is called a *solitary myeloma* or *plasmacytoma;* far more commonly, however, it presents with widespread involvement, in which case the name *multiple myeloma* is applied. Mild and transient pain exacerbated by heavy lifting or other activity is present in approximately 75% of cases and may be the initial symptom. Because of this, in its early course and before diagnosis, the disease may resemble sciatica or intercostal neuralgia. Rarely, a pathologic fracture through the lesion is the first sign of disease. The patient's urine in cases of myeloma contains Bence Jones protein; the serum albumin-to-globulin ratio is reversed and the total serum protein is elevated. Monoclonal γ-globulin is also present, with IgG and IgA peaks demonstrated on serum electrophoresis.

Histologically, the diagnosis is made by finding sheets of atypical plasmacytoid cells replacing the normal marrow spaces. The plasma cell is recognized by the presence of eccentrically situated nucleus within a large amount of cytoplasm that stains either light blue or pink. The neoplastic cells contain double or even multiple nuclei, usually hyperchromatic and enlarged, with prominent nucleoli.

Multiple myeloma may present in a variety of radiographic patterns (Fig. 22.19). Particularly in the spine, it may be seen only as diffuse osteoporosis with no clearly identifiable lesion; multiple compression fractures of the vertebral bodies may also be evident. More commonly, it exhibits multiple lytic lesions scattered throughout the skeleton. In the skull, characteristic "punched-out" areas of bone destruction, usually of uniform size, are noted (Fig. 22.20), whereas the ribs may contain lace-like areas of bone destruction and small osteolytic lesions, sometimes accompanied by adjacent soft-tissue masses. Areas of medullary bone destruction are noted in the flat and long bones, and if these appear about the cortex, they are accompanied by scalloping of the inner cortical margin (Fig. 22.21). Ordinarily, there is no evidence of sclerosis and no periosteal reaction. Fewer than 1% of myelomas may be of a sclerosing type called *sclerosing myelomatosis.*

Whereas in osteolytic myeloma only 3% of patients have polyneuropathy, the incidence of polyneuropathy in the osteosclerotic variant has been reported as 30% to 50%. Compared with classic myeloma, this variant usually occurs in younger individuals and shows fewer plasma cells in the bone marrow, lower levels of monoclonal protein, and a better prognosis.

An interesting variant of sclerosing myeloma is the so-called POEMS syndrome, first described in 1968 but gaining wide acceptance only more recently. It consists of polyneuropathy (P), organomegaly (O), particularly of the liver and the spleen, endocrine disturbances (E) such as amenorrhea and gynecomastia, monoclonal gammopathy (M), and skin changes (S) such as hyperpigmentation and hirsutism.

Differential Diagnosis

If the spine is involved, as is frequently the case, multiple myeloma must be differentiated from metastatic carcinoma. In this respect, the "vertebral pedicle" sign identified by Jacobson and colleagues may be helpful. They contend that in the early stages of myeloma, the pedicle (which does not contain as much red marrow as the vertebral body) is not involved, whereas even in an early stage of metastatic cancer the pedicle and vertebral body are both affected (Fig. 22.22). In the late stages of multiple myeloma, however, both the pedicle and vertebral body may be destroyed. Radionuclide bone scan can more reliably distinguish these two malignancies at this stage. It is invariably positive in cases of metastatic carcinoma, whereas in most cases of multiple myeloma there is no increased uptake of radiopharmaceutical. This phenomenon appears to reflect the purely lytic nature of most myelomatous lesions and the absence of significant reactive new bone formation in response to the tumor.

A solitary myeloma may create even greater diagnostic difficulty. As a purely osteolytic lesion, it may mimic such other purely destructive processes as the brown tumor of hyperparathyroidism, giant cell

Figure 22.16 Lymphoma. Conventional radiograph of the right femur of a 7-year-old girl with groin pain and a fever reveals a destructive lesion of the diaphysis extending to the growth plate; there is also a lamellated type of periosteal reaction. Because of the age of the patient, the primary differential diagnosis included Ewing sarcoma, osteomyelitis, and Langerhans cell histiocytosis, all three of which may have a similar radiographic presentation in a long bone. The main factor differentiating these lesions is the duration of the patient's symptoms. In this case, however, biopsy revealed a histiocytic lymphoma.

Figure 22.17 Lymphoma. Anteroposterior **(A)** and lateral **(B)** radiographs of the right knee of a 47-year-old woman who had knee pain and initially was diagnosed with Paget disease, show a destructive lesion of the proximal tibia extending into the articular end of the bone. The mixed sclerotic and osteolytic character of this lesion may resemble the coarse trabecular pattern of Paget disease; however, there is a lack of cortical thickening. There is a pathologic fracture, but only a minimal periosteal response is evident. Biopsy revealed a histiocytic lymphoma.

Figure 22.18 Skeletal sites of predilection, peak age range, and male-to-female ratio in myeloma.

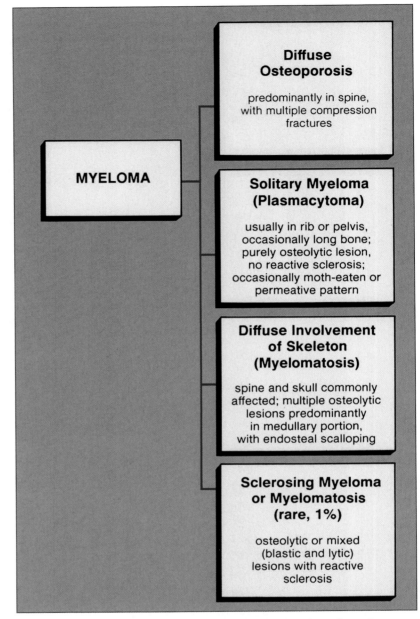

Figure 22.19 Variants in the radiographic presentation of myeloma.

Figure 22.20 Multiple myeloma. Involvement of the skull is prominent in this 60-year-old woman. Note the characteristic "punched-out," lytic lesions, most of which are uniform in size and lack sclerotic borders. Occasionally, this pattern may be seen in metastatic disease.

Figure 22.21 Multiple myeloma. Lateral radiograph of the distal femur **(A)** and anteroposterior film of the elbow **(B)** in a 65-year-old woman show endosteal scalloping of the cortex typical of diffuse myelomatosis.

Figure 22.22 Multiple myeloma. Anteroposterior **(A)** and lateral **(B)** radiographs of the spine in a 70-year-old man with multiple myeloma involving both the spine and appendicular skeleton show a compression fracture of the body of T-8; several other vertebrae show only osteoporosis. The pedicles are preserved in contrast to metastatic disease of the spine, which usually also affects the pedicles, as seen on this anteroposterior radiograph of the cervical spine **(C)** in a 65-year-old man with colon carcinoma and multiple lytic metastases. Note the involvement of the right pedicle of C-7 (*open arrows*).

Figure 22.23 Adamantinoma. Lateral radiograph of the left tibia in a 64-year-old woman shows a lesion in the midshaft, which proved on biopsy to be an adamantinoma. The destructive lesion is multifocal and slightly expansile, with mixed osteolytic and sclerotic areas creating a "soap-bubble" appearance resembling that of osteofibrous dysplasia (see Fig. 19.28).

tumor, fibrosarcoma, MFH, or a solitary metastatic focus of carcinoma from the kidney, thyroid, gastrointestinal tract, or lung.

Complications and Treatment

A common complication of bone myelomas is pathologic fracture, especially in lesions of the long bones, ribs, sternum, and vertebrae. The development of amyloidosis has also been reported in approximately 15% of patients.

Treatment consists of radiotherapy and systemic chemotherapy. The 5-year survival rate is approximately 10%.

Adamantinoma

Adamantinoma is a rare malignant tumor occurring equally in males and females between the second and fifth decades of life; 90% of cases involve the tibia. Radiographically, the disease is marked by well-defined and elongated osteolytic defects of varying size, separated by areas of sclerotic bone, which occasionally give the lesion a "soap bubble" appearance; ordinarily, there is no periosteal reaction (Fig. 22.23). At times, adamantinoma may affect an entire bone with multiple satellite lesions (Fig. 22.24); "saw-tooth" areas of cortical destruction in the tibia are quite distinctive of this tumor.

Figure 22.24 Adamantinoma. Lateral radiograph of the right tibia of a 28-year-old woman shows multiple, confluent lytic lesions involving almost the entire bone; only the articular ends are spared. The anterior cortex exhibits a predominantly saw-tooth type of destruction.

Histologically, the tumor is biphasic and consists of an epithelial component intimately admixed in varying proportions with a fibrous component. Although it has been speculated that adamantinoma represents a form of vascular neoplasm, ultrastructural and immunohistochemical evidence points toward an epithelial derivation.

A relationship of adamantinoma with osteofibrous dysplasia and fibrous dysplasia has been postulated, and its coexistence with either of these lesions has been suggested. However, this is still controversial, with some investigators maintaining that the lesions of adamantinoma may contain a fibro-osseous component that can resemble a Kempson-Campanacci lesion or fibrous dysplasia on histopathologic examination. (See also discussion in Chapter 19 in the section on Osteofibrous Dysplasia.)

Treatment

Because adamantinoma is insensitive to radiotherapy, the treatment of choice is en bloc surgical resection with application of bone graft. Recurrences have been reported.

Chordoma

A chordoma is a malignant bone tumor arising from developmental remnants of the notochord. Consequently, these tumors occur almost exclusively in the midline of the axial skeleton. Chordomas represent from 1% to 4% of all primary malignant bone tumors. They arise between the fourth and seventh decades and affect men slightly more often than women. The three most common sites for a chordoma are the sacrococcygeal area, the spheno-occipital area, and the C-2 vertebra (Fig. 22.25).

The radiographic appearance is that of a highly destructive lesion with irregular scalloped borders; it is sometimes accompanied by calcifications in the matrix, probably as a result of extensive tumor necrosis (Fig. 22.26A). Bone sclerosis has been reported in 64% of cases. Soft-tissue masses are commonly associated with the lesion (Fig. 22.26B). Conventional radiography and tomography usually suffices to delineate the tumor (Fig. 22.27), but CT or MRI is required to demonstrate soft-tissue extension and invasion of the spinal canal.

Histologically, the tumor consists of loose aggregates of mucoid material separating cord-like arrays and lobules of large polyhedral cells, along with vacuolated cytoplasm and vesicular nuclei referred to as physaliphorous cells.

Complications and Treatment

Invasion of the spinal canal by tumor may cause neurologic complications. Metastases are rare and usually late. The treatment for chordoma consists of complete resection, followed by radiation therapy. Cryosurgery with liquid nitrogen is occasionally used when complete tumor removal proves impossible.

Primary Leiomyosarcoma of Bone

Primary leiomyosarcomas of bone are very rare, with fewer than 100 cases reported in the world literature. More common are skeletal metastases from primary soft-tissue leiomyosarcoma. Therefore, an extraosseous primary tumor, mainly from the gastrointestinal tract or uterus, must be ruled out before a confident diagnosis of primary leiomyosarcoma of bone can be made. Leiomyosarcoma is a malignant, predominantly spindle-cell, neoplasm that exhibits smooth muscle differentiation. Although the patients reported range from 9 to 80 years of age, occurrence before age 20 is uncommon. Males are affected more often than females. The usual clinical presentation is pain of variable intensity and duration. A soft-tissue mass is occasionally observed. The most common sites are the distal femur, proximal tibia, proximal humerus, and iliac bone. Other bones occasionally may be affected, including the clavicle, ribs, and mandible.

Figure 22.25 Skeletal sites of predilection, peak age range, and male-to-female ratio in chordoma.

Although leiomyosarcoma exhibits no characteristic radiographic features, the tumor most often presents either as a lytic area of geographic bone destruction (Fig. 22.28) or with aggressive-looking, ill-defined borders and a permeative or moth-eaten pattern. Approximately 50% of reported lesions exhibit fine periosteal reaction. On MR imaging, the lesions are isointense to muscle on T1-weighted sequences, whereas on T2 weighting they exhibit a heterogeneous signal.

Microscopy reveals interlacing fascicles of spindle-shaped cells with eosinophilic cytoplasm, which resemble leiomyosarcoma of soft

Figure 22.26 Chordoma. (A) This destructive lesion in the sacrum of a 60-year-old woman proved to be a chordoma. Note its scalloped borders and the amorphous calcifications in the tumor matrix. **(B)** CT shows extensive bone destruction and a large soft tissue mass.

Figure 22.27 Chordoma. Open-mouth anteroposterior tomogram of the cervical spine of a 52-year-old man demonstrates an osteolytic lesion in the body of C-2, proven by biopsy to be a chordoma.

osteolytic lesion in body of C-2

destroyed pedicle

tissue. The degree of cellularity, nuclear pleomorphism, and necrosis varies from case to case. Rarely, a storiform-like pattern, reminiscent of malignant fibrous histiocytoma, is seen. Immunohistochemical staining is positive for vimentin and actin.

Because leiomyosarcoma of bone does not have a characteristic radiologic presentation, several possibilities should be considered in the differential diagnosis. The findings of aggressive bone destruction suggest that fibrosarcoma, malignant fibrous histiocytoma, and lymphoma should be considered. In younger patients, Ewing sarcoma is a possibility, as is a solitary metastasis in older patients.

Hemangioendothelioma and Angiosarcoma

These tumors represent the most common malignant vascular lesions. The present nomenclature used to describe malignant vascular tumors is not uniform and is therefore rather confusing. Different terms, including hemangiosarcoma (angiosarcoma), hemangioendothelioma, and hemangioendothelial sarcoma, have been used as synonyms. The tumors have also been classified into different grades, from grade I hemangioendothelioma (well-differentiated) to grade III hemangiosarcoma (poorly differentiated). Because of the prevailing confusion, the World Health Organization (WHO) classification system, although recently revised, continues to categorize these lesions as intermediate or indeterminate (including hemangioendothelioma and hemangiopericytoma) and clearly malignant (angiosarcoma). Unequivocal distinction among these tumors is sometimes difficult.

Hemangioendothelioma and a recently identified lesion called *epithelioid hemangioendothelioma* are considered to represent true neoplasms because of their independent growth potential, the histopathologic demonstration of nuclear atypia accompanied by occasional mitotic activity, and because they commonly recur after inadequate local excision. They can arise at any age within the range of 10 to 75 years, with a slight predilection for males. The lesion may be solitary or (usually epithelioid variant) multicentric. Patients with multifocal disease are usually 10 years younger than those with a solitary lesion. The most commonly affected sites are the calvaria, spine, and bones of the lower extremities. Clinical symptoms include dull local pain and tenderness. Some swelling and hemorrhagic joint effusion may sometimes be observed.

On radiography, hemangioendothelioma exhibits an osteolytic appearance, either well circumscribed or with a wide zone of transition. Variable degrees of peripheral sclerosis may sharply demarcate the lesion. Occasionally, a soap-bubble appearance with expansion of bone is observed, with extension into the soft tissues. MRI reveals a mixed signal on T1-weighted sequences, with moderately increased signal intensity on T2 weighting (Fig. 22.29). On radiologic studies, it is very difficult to differentiate hemangioendothelioma from other vascular lesions, either benign or malignant. A solitary osteolytic lesion may mimic a metastasis, fibrosarcoma, MFH, plasmacytoma, or lymphoma, and lesions that extend to the articular end of bone can be mistaken for giant cell tumor. Because the radiologic presentation of hemangioendothelioma is usually nonspecific, clinical information may be helpful in narrowing the differential diagnosis.

On histologic examination, hemangioendothelioma reveals markedly pleomorphic endothelial cells with abundant faintly eosinophilic or amphophilic cytoplasm and hyperchromatic nuclei with prominent nucleoli. The interanastomosing vascular channels, often arranged in an antler-like pattern, are delimited by a basal membrane. The stroma typically varies from fibrous to myxoid and small foci of hemorrhage or necrosis may be observed.

Angiosarcoma of bone represents the most malignant end of the spectrum of vascular tumors. This is an aggressive neoplasm, characterized by frequent local recurrence and distant metastases. The lesion occurs typically during the second to the seventh decade, with a peak in the fifth decade. Males are affected twice as frequently as females. Most common sites of occurrence are the long bones, particularly the tibia, femur, and humerus, and the most common symptoms are local pain and swelling. Metastases to the lungs and other internal organs occur in approximately 66% of cases.

On radiologic studies, it is impossible to distinguish angiosarcoma from other aggressive vascular lesions. Angiosarcoma has imaging features similar to those of hemangioendothelioma, although more commonly it exhibits a wide zone of transition between the tumor and uninvolved bone (Fig. 22.30). Cortical permeation and associated soft tissue masses are frequently observed.

Microscopically, angiosarcoma is composed of poorly formed blood vessels that exhibit complicated infoldings and irregular anastomoses. The endothelial cells that line these blood vessels display features of frank malignancy, with plump intraluminal cells showing nuclear hyperchromation and atypical mitoses. Solid areas of tumor may contain spindle and epithelioid cells.

Figure 22.28 Leiomyosarcoma of bone. (A) Anteroposterior radiograph of the right knee of a 12-year-old boy reveals an osteolytic lesion in the proximal tibial metaphysis destroying the medial cortex and extending into the soft tissues. **(B)** Axial CT section shows destruction of the medial aspect of the tibia and an associated soft tissue mass. (From Greenspan A, Remagen W, 1998, with permission).

Figure 22.29 Hemangioendothelioma of bone. (A) Anteroposterior radiograph of the right proximal tibia shows an osteolytic lesion destroying medial aspect of the bone. **(B)** Coronal T1-weighted MRI reveals a low-signal-intensity tumor replacing bone marrow. **(C)** Coronal T2-weighted MRI shows an increase in the signal intensity of the tumor, which exhibits nonhomogeneous appearance. (From Greenfield GB, Arrington JA, 1995, with permission).

Figure 22.30 Angiosarcoma of bone. An osteolytic lesion with a wide zone of transition is present in the proximal right humerus (*arrows*) in a 42-year-old man. Note a pathologic fracture through the tumor (*open arrows*). (From Greenspan A, Remagen W, 1998, with permission).

Benign Conditions With Malignant Potential

Several benign conditions have the potential for malignant transformation (see Table 16.2). Some benign tumors and tumor-like lesions that are in this category, such as enchondroma, osteochondroma, and fibrous dysplasia, are discussed in previous chapters (Chapters 18 and 19). Several of the conditions discussed have also been touched on in previous chapters (see the sections on Secondary Osteosarcomas and Secondary Chondrosarcomas).

Medullary Bone Infarct

The development of a sarcoma in association with a medullary bone infarct is a rare event. The clinical sign that should alert the radiologist to this possibility is the development of bone pain in a previously asymptomatic patient. The radiographic findings of bone destruction in the area of the medullary infarct in conjunction with a periosteal reaction and soft-tissue mass confirm the diagnosis of malignant transformation (Fig. 22.31).

Chronic Draining Sinus Tract of Osteomyelitis

Malignant transformation should be suspected when a long-standing sinus tract of osteomyelitis suddenly becomes painful and discharges purulent, foul material. In most patients with osteomyelitis, the history of the disease dates to childhood, and sinuses draining for more than 20 years are generally the precursors of malignant neoplasms. The development of squamous cell carcinoma is most commonly seen (Fig. 22.32), but fibrosarcoma and osteosarcoma may also be encountered. The incidence of neoplastic transformation, however, is low, ranging from 0.2% to 1.7%. The radiographic features of malignant transformation may occasionally be indistinguishable from those of

Figure 22.31 Malignant fibrous histiocytoma arising in a bone infarct. A 39-year-old woman with known multiple idiopathic medullary bone infarcts had pain above the left knee. **(A)** Anteroposterior radiograph of both knees shows the typical appearance of medullary bone infarcts in the lower femora. In the left femur there is evidence of a lamellated periosteal reaction along the lateral cortex. **(B)** Magnification study shows cortical destruction. On biopsy the suspicious lesion proved to be a malignant fibrous histiocytoma complicating the bone infarct.

Figure 22.32 Squamous cell carcinoma arising in a chronic draining sinus of osteomyelitis. A 59-year-old man was admitted for treatment of an ulcer of the right leg that was present for 5 years. At age 13 years, he had an open fracture of the tibia that became infected, and he developed chronic osteomyelitis. Anteroposterior **(A)** and lateral **(B)** radiographs of the right leg show a large saucerized defect of the anterior cortex of the middle third of the tibia, with dense compact bone lining its base. A large sharply circumscribed soft-tissue mass is also evident at this site. Above the defect, which is postsurgical, are medullary sclerosis and cortical thickening, both characteristic of chronic osteomyelitis. Open biopsy of the lesion revealed squamous cell carcinoma arising in a chronic draining sinus tract of osteomyelitis. (From Greenspan A, et al., 1981, with permission.)

chronic osteomyelitis, but an increase in the extent of bone destruction usually indicates the onset of sarcoma or carcinoma.

Plexiform Neurofibromatosis

A spectrum of neoplastic disorders is associated with neurofibromatosis as the most serious complication of this disease. Sarcoma of the peripheral nerves and somatic soft tissues is well recognized in neurofibromatosis, with its incidence varying from 3% to 16%. Most such sarcomas are neural in origin, including neurosarcoma, neurofibrosarcoma, and malignant schwannoma; nonneurogenic sarcomas such as rhabdomyosarcoma and liposarcoma are less common. The precise origin of the sarcomas arising in neurofibromatosis is uncertain; in some instances, the mass clearly originates in a nerve trunk, whereas in others there is no obvious relation to the nerve. The most frequent clinical features of malignant degeneration in a patient with neurofibromatosis are the development of pain, the rapid growth of a pre-existing neurofibroma, and a new soft-tissue mass. Radiographically, the diagnosis of sarcomatous transformation is almost certain if abnormal tumor vessels (Fig. 22.33) or a "tumor stain" are demonstrated on arteriography.

Paget Disease

The development of a sarcoma in pagetic bone is a serious complication of Paget disease. Although Paget sarcoma is rare (less than 1%), individuals with Paget disease are 20-times more likely to have a malignant bone tumor develop than are other persons of comparable age. Radiographically, sarcomatous transformation is indicated by the development of a lytic lesion, often with evidence of cortical breakthrough and a soft-tissue mass (Fig. 22.34); a periosteal reaction is uncommon. The bones commonly affected include the pelvis, femur, and humerus. Histologically, the most common type of tumor is osteosarcoma, followed by MFH, fibrosarcoma, and chondrosarcoma, in that order. The prognosis for patients with Paget sarcoma is poor; few survive beyond 6 to 8 months.

Radiation-Induced Sarcoma

Radiation-induced sarcomas may arise in areas of normal bone exposed to radiation fields or may be caused by benign conditions treated by irradiation, such as fibrous dysplasia or giant cell tumor. Generally, a sarcoma can develop only if at least 3,000 rads are

Figure 22.33 Liposarcoma arising in plexiform neurofibromatosis. An 18-year-old man with known neurofibromatosis since early childhood presented with an enlarging, painful pretibial mass of more than 10 months' duration. **(A)** Anteroposterior radiograph of the left knee shows instability with lateral subluxation. The medial cortex of the medial femoral condyle and the lateral cortex of the lateral femoral condyle are eroded at the site of a soft-tissue mass. **(B)** Anteroposterior radiograph of the pelvis shows asymmetry of the pelvis with a large deformed acetabulum, enlargement of the left obturator foramen, and superolateral subluxation of the left hip—all features typical of neurofibromatosis. **(C)** A femoral arteriogram shows the pretibial mass to be hypervascular, with numerous small tortuous tumor vessels. Biopsy of the mass disclosed pleomorphic liposarcoma arising in plexiform neurofibromatosis. (From Baker ND, Greenspan A, 1981, with permission.)

administered within a 4-week span, although cases have been reported after exposure to only 800 rads. The latency period for radiation-induced tumors varies from 4 to 40 years, with an average of 11 years. Their incidence is rather low, not exceeding 0.5%.

The criteria for diagnosis of postirradiation sarcoma are as follows:

1. The initial lesion and the postirradiation sarcoma must not be of the same histologic type.
2. The site of the new tumor must be within the field of irradiation.
3. At least 3 years must have elapsed since the previous radiation therapy.

Postirradiation osteosarcoma may also develop after the ingestion and intraosseous accumulation of radioisotopes, as has been described in painters of radium watch dials. Regardless of the source of radiation, the most common of such tumors is osteosarcoma, followed by fibrosarcoma and malignant fibrous histiocytoma (Fig. 22.35).

Skeletal Metastases

Skeletal metastases are the most frequent malignant bone tumors and consequently should always be considered in the differential diagno-

sis of malignant lesions, particularly in older patients. Most metastatic lesions involve the axial skeleton—the skull, spine, and pelvis—as well as the proximal segments of the long bones; only very rarely is a metastasis seen distal to the elbows or knees (Fig. 22.36). These lesions result from the hematogenous spread of a malignancy, the usual mechanism by which a primary neoplasm erodes regional blood vessels, seeding malignant cells to the capillary beds of the lung and liver. Tumor emboli become lodged in the axial skeleton through communication with the vertebral venous plexus.

The incidence of metastases to bone varies with the type of primary neoplasm and the duration of disease. Some malignant tumors have a far greater propensity for osseous metastatic involvement than do others. Because of their frequency, cancers of the breast, lung, and prostate are responsible for the majority of bone metastases, although primary tumors of the kidney, small and large intestines, stomach, and thyroid may also metastasize to bone. Carcinoma of the prostate has been reported to underlie nearly 60% of all bone metastases in men, whereas in women carcinoma of the breast is responsible for nearly 70% of all metastatic skeletal lesions.

Most skeletal metastases are asymptomatic. When metastases are symptomatic, pain is the major clinical symptom, with a pathologic fracture through a lesion only occasionally calling attention to the disease. Metastasis to bone can be solitary or multiple and can be fur-

Figure 22.34 Malignant fibrous histiocytoma arising in pagetic bone. A 66-year-old woman with known Paget disease had pain in the left hip joint radiating to the buttock. **(A)** Anteroposterior radiograph of the pelvis shows extensive involvement of the left hemipelvis by Paget disease. There is also an osteolytic area of bone destruction in the left ischium. CT sections, one through the femoral heads and acetabula **(B)** and a second through the ischium and pubic symphysis **(C)**, demonstrate cortical destruction and a large soft-tissue mass—both signs of malignant transformation to sarcoma. Note the displacement of the rectum and urinary bladder. Biopsy revealed a malignant fibrous histiocytoma arising in pagetic bone.

urinary bladder
soft tissue mass
destroyed acetabulum
rectum

Figure 22.35 Radiation-induced malignant fibrous histiocytoma. A 63-year-old woman had been treated 15 years earlier with radium for carcinoma of the cervix. **(A)** Anteroposterior radiograph of the pelvis shows a large, destructive lesion involving the right ilium and extending into the supra-acetabular region, with destruction of the right wing of the sacral bone. **(B)** CT section, in addition to the changes seen on radiography, demonstrates a soft-tissue mass. Biopsy revealed a malignant fibrous histiocytoma. The tumor developed in the ilium that had been exposed to radiation, extending into the soft tissue and invading the sacrum secondarily.

Figure 22.36 Skeletal sites of predilection and peak age range of metastatic lesions. The occurrence of such lesions distal to the elbow and knee is uncommon, and in those sites a primary malignancy of the breast or lung is usually the origin.

The detection of skeletal metastases is not always possible on conventional radiographs, because destruction of the bone may not be visible with this technique. Radionuclide bone scan is the best means of screening for early metastatic lesions whether they are lytic or blastic, although recently several investigators have pointed out the usefulness of MRI in detecting metastases, particularly in the spine. The accuracy of MRI in identifying intramedullary lesions and assessing spinal cord and soft-tissue involvement has been demonstrated. Most recent investigations by Daldrup-Link and associates, who compared the diagnostic accuracy of whole-body MR imaging, skeletal scintigraphy, and 18F-fluorodeoxyglucose (FDG) positron emission tomogra-

ther divided into purely lytic, purely blastic, and mixed lesions. The primary tumors that give rise to purely osteolytic metastases are usually those of the kidney, lung, breast, thyroid, and gastrointestinal tract, although purely lytic lesions may become sclerotic after radiation therapy, chemotherapy, or hormonal therapy. Primary tumors responsible for purely osteoblastic metastases are generally those of the prostate gland, although other primary neoplasms may also be responsible (Fig. 22.37).

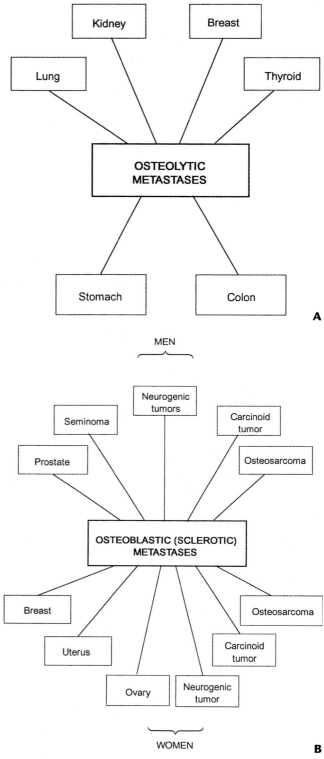

Figure 22.37 Skeletal metastases. Origin of osteolytic **(A)** and osteoblastic **(B)** metastases. (From Greenspan A, Remagen W, 1998, with permission.)

Figure 22.38 Skeletal metastases. (A) A 63-year-old man with bronchogenic carcinoma developed a single metastatic lesion in the proximal phalanx of the left thumb. **(B)** A 50-year-old woman with breast carcinoma had a solitary metastatic lesion in the distal phalanx of the right thumb.

phy (PET) for the detection of bone metastases in children and young adults, suggest the superiority of FDG PET scan. The latter technique had 90% sensitivity compared with 82% for whole-body MRI and 71% for skeletal scintigraphy.

In general terms, skeletal metastases may appear highly similar, irrespective of their primary source. However, there are instances in which the morphologic appearance, location, and distribution of metastatic lesions may suggest their site of origin. Thus, for instance, 50% of skeletal metastases distal to the elbows and knees—rare sites for metastases—are secondary to breast or bronchogenic carcinomas (Fig. 22.38). Lesions that have an expansive, "blown-out" appearance on radiographs and are highly vascular on arteriography are characteristic of metastatic renal carcinoma (Fig. 22.39). Moreover, Choi and associates recently reported a flow-void sign on MRI resulting from relatively rapid blood flow through dilated arteries that supply the hypervascular lesion and through dilated veins that drain the lesion, apparently characteristic for osseous metastases from renal cell carcinoma. Multiple round dense foci or diffuse bone density is often seen in metastatic carcinoma of the prostate (Fig. 22.40); in females, sclerotic metastases are usually from breast carcinoma.

Recently, characteristic cortical metastases have been described as originating from bronchogenic carcinoma; these metastases cause what Resnick has called "cookie bite" or "cookie cutter" lesions of the cortices of the long bones (Fig. 22.41). Because the bulk of metastases that reach the skeleton via hematogenous spread lodge in the bone marrow and in spongy bone, the initial radiographic appearance of metastatic lesions in the skeleton is that of destruction of cancellous bone; only with further growth do such lesions affect the cortex. The anastomosing vascular systems of the cortex, originating in the overlying periosteum, probably serve as the pathway by which malignant cells from the lung reach the compact bone to produce destruction of the cortex. Occasionally, other primary tumors (for example, breast and kidney) may also metastasize to the cortex.

Single metastatic lesions in a bone must be distinguished from primary malignant and benign bone tumors. A few characteristic features of metastatic lesions may be helpful in making the distinction: (a) metastatic lesions usually present without or with only a small adjacent soft-tissue mass and (b) they usually lack a periosteal reaction unless they have broken through the cortex. The latter feature, how-

ever, is not invariably reliable, because in some series more than 30% of metastatic lesions—particularly metastases from carcinoma of the prostate—have been accompanied by a periosteal response. Metastatic lesions to the spine usually destroy the pedicle, a useful feature for distinguishing them from myeloma or neurofibroma invading the vertebra (Fig. 22.42).

Histologically, metastatic tumors are easier to diagnose than many primary tumors because of their essential epithelial pattern. Although biopsies of suspected metastases are useful for diagnosis in patients with unknown primary tumors, these procedures are seldom helpful in specifying an exact site of an unknown primary tumor. Occasionally, if gland formation is present, a specific diagnosis of metastatic adenocarcinoma can be made, but rarely will a specific type of the tumor be detected. On occasion, a metastatic lesion may demonstrate a morphologic pattern that strongly suggests the site of a primary tumor, such as the clear cells of renal carcinoma or the pigment production of melanoma.

Complications

Although metastases are themselves complications of a primary malignant process, it must be emphasized that they can cause secondary complications such as pathologic fracture (Fig. 22.43) or, when occurring in the spine, compression of the thecal sac and spinal cord, thus producing neurologic symptoms (Fig. 22.44).

Figure 22.39 Angiography of metastatic lesion. A 52-year-old man with renal cell carcinoma (hypernephroma) presented with a solitary metastatic lesion in the acromial end of the left clavicle. **(A)** Radiograph shows an expansive "blown-out" lesion associated with a soft-tissue mass destroying the acromial end of the clavicle. **(B)** Subtraction study of a selective left subclavian arteriogram demonstrates hypervascularity of the tumor, a characteristic feature of metastatic hypernephroma.

Figure 22.40 Osteoblastic metastases. Anteroposterior radiograph of the left hemipelvis and femur of a 55-year-old man with carcinoma of the prostate shows extensive blastic skeletal metastases. Multiple sclerotic foci are scattered through the ilium, pubis, ischium, and proximal femur.

Figure 22.41 Cortical metastases. Anteroposterior (A) and lateral magnification (B) radiographs of the left femur in an 82-year-old man with progressive femoral pain demonstrate multiple sharply marginated osteolytic areas of bone destruction, predominantly affecting the cortical bone. There is no evidence of periosteal reaction. Note the characteristic "cookie bite" appearance of the lesion on the lateral radiograph. On the basis of this feature, attention was focused on the chest, where tomographic examination demonstrated bronchogenic carcinoma. (From Greenspan A, et al., 1984, with permission.)

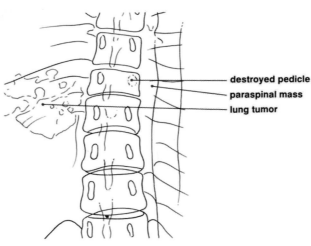

destroyed pedicle
paraspinal mass
lung tumor

Figure 22.42 Vertebral metastasis. Anteroposterior radiograph of the thoracolumbar spine in a 59-year-old woman with bronchogenic carcinoma shows a metastatic lesion in the body of T-7. Note the destroyed left pedicle and associated paraspinal mass, features helpful in distinguishing this lesion from myeloma or neurofibroma. The lung tumor is obvious.

Figure 22.43 Skeletal metastases complicated by pathologic fracture. Pathologic fracture may complicate metastatic disease of the skeleton, as seen here in the proximal shaft of the left femur in a 74-year-old man with multiple skeletal metastases from a prostate carcinoma.

Figure 22.44 Neurologic complication of skeletal metastasis. (A) Anteroposterior radiograph of the lumbar spine in a 47-year-old woman with breast carcinoma shows destruction of the body of L-3 with a pathologic fracture. Note the involvement of the left pedicle. **(B)** A myelogram demonstrates compression of the thecal sac. **(C)** On CT section, compression fracture of the vertebral body and involvement of the left pedicle are evident; the tumor extends into the soft tissue and compresses the ventral aspect of the thecal sac.

PRACTICAL POINTS TO REMEMBER

[1] Fibrosarcoma and malignant fibrous histiocytoma:
- characteristically present as purely osteolytic lesions, frequently in the long bones
- may resemble giant cell tumor, lymphoma, or telangiectatic osteosarcoma
- may develop in certain benign conditions, such as fibrous dysplasia and bone infarct.

[2] Ewing sarcoma, a round cell tumor, usually presents with characteristic radiographic features including:
- a permeative type of bone destruction
- cortical saucerization
- an aggressive periosteal reaction
- a soft-tissue mass.

The diaphysis of long bones, and the pelvis, ribs, and scapula are the most common sites of involvement.

[3] In the differential diagnosis of Ewing sarcoma, osteomyelitis and Langerhans cell histiocytosis should always be considered, as well as metastatic neuroblastoma, particularly in patients in their first decade. The most important distinguishing feature is the duration of symptoms. The amount of bone destruction seen radiographically in patients with Ewing sarcoma reporting symptoms for 4 to 6 months is usually the same as that:
- in patients with osteomyelitis reporting symptoms for 4 to 6 weeks
- in patients with Langerhans cell histiocytosis reporting symptoms for 1 to 2 weeks.

[4] Myeloma, the most common primary malignant bone tumor, has a predilection for the axial skeleton. Four distinctive forms of this lesion can be distinguished radiographically:
- a solitary lesion (plasmacytoma), usually affecting the pelvis or ribs
- diffuse myelomatosis
- diffuse osteoporosis, usually seen in the vertebral column
- sclerosing myeloma, the rarest manifestation of this tumor.

[5] Primary myeloma of the spine can usually be distinguished from radiographically similar metastatic disease by the preservation of the pedicles (vertebral-pedicle sign) in the early stages of the disease.

[6] In myeloma, radionuclide bone scan usually shows no increase in uptake of radiopharmaceutical.

[7] Adamantinoma, a malignant tumor with a strong predilection for the tibia, is characterized radiographically by:
- a "soap-bubble" appearance of the lesion combining lytic and sclerotic areas
- a "saw-tooth" appearance of cortical destruction.

[8] Chordoma, which arises from the remnants of the notochord, is located almost exclusively in the midline of the axial skeleton. It tends to arise in the spheno-occipital and sacrococcygeal areas and in the body of C-2.

[9] Primary leiomyosarcoma of bone, a rare bone malignancy, exhibits no characteristic radiographic features, although most often presents either as a lytic area of geographic bone destruction or with aggressive-looking, ill-defined borders and permeative or moth-eaten pattern.

[10] Hemangioendothelioma of bone may be solitary or multicentric. The radiographic features include an osteolytic appearance, either well-circumscribed or with a wide zone of transition, and occasionally a "soap-bubble" character with extension into the soft tissues.

[11] Angiosarcoma of bone represents the most malignant end of the spectrum of vascular tumors. The radiographic features include a wide zone of transition, cortical permeation, and soft tissue mass.

[12] Benign conditions with malignant potential include medullary bone infarct, the chronic draining sinus tract of osteomyelitis, plexiform neurofibromatosis, Paget disease, normal tissue undergoing radiation, enchondroma, osteochondroma, synovial chondromatosis, and fibrous dysplasia.

[13] Prostatic carcinoma is the primary tumor most often responsible for blastic metastases to bone. The primary tumors most often responsible for osteolytic skeletal metastases are carcinomas of the kidney, lung, breast, thyroid, and gastrointestinal tract.

[14] Bronchogenic carcinoma frequently produces cortical metastases ("cookie bite" lesions) and is responsible for metastases in sites distal to the elbow, including lesions of the phalanges.

[15] Carcinoma of the kidney usually produces lytic, "blown-out," hypervascular metastatic lesions.

[16] The best technique for mapping metastatic lesions in the skeleton is radionuclide bone scan.

SUGGESTED READINGS

Abdelwahab IF, Hermann G, Kenan S, Klein MJ, Lewis MM. Case report 794. Primary leiomyosarcoma of the right femur. *Skeletal Radiol* 1993;22:379–381.

Abdelwahab IF, Kenan S, Hermann G, Klein MJ, Lewis MM. Radiation-induced leiomyosarcoma. *Skeletal Radiol* 1995;24:81–83.

Abenoza P, Sibley RK. Chordoma: an immunohistochemical study. *Hum Pathol* 1987;17:744–747.

Abrahams TG, Bula W, Jones W. Epithelioid hemangioendothelioma of bone. *Skeletal Radiol* 1992;21:509–513.

Abrams HL. Skeletal metastases in carcinoma. *Radiology* 1950;55:534–538.

Abrams HL, Spiro R, Goldstein N. Metastases in carcinoma. Analysis of 1000 autopsied cases. *Cancer* 1950;3:74–85.

Adler C-P. Case report 587. Adamantinoma of the tibia mimicking osteofibrous dysplasia. *Skeletal Radiol* 1990;19:55–58.

Aggarwal S, Goulatia RK, Sood A, et al. POEMS syndrome: a rare variety of plasma cell dyscrasia. *AJR Am J Roentgenol* 1990;155:339–341.

Aisen AM, Martel W, Braunstein EM, McMillin KI, Phillips WA, Kling TF. MRI and CT evaluation of primary bone and soft-tissue tumors. *AJR Am J Roentgenol* 1986;146:749–756.

Alazraki N. Radionuclide techniques. In: Resnick D, ed. *Bone and joint imaging*. Philadelphia: WB Saunders; 1989:185–198.

Algra PR, Bloem JL. Magnetic resonance imaging of metastatic disease and multiple myeloma. In: Bloem JL, Sartoris DJ, eds. *MRI and CT of the musculoskeletal system*. Baltimore: Williams & Wilkins; 1992:218.

Algra PR, Bloem JL, Tissing H, Falke TH, Arndt JW, Verboom LJ. Detection of vertebral metastases: comparison between MR imaging and bone scintigraphy. *Radiographics* 1991;11:219–232.

Algra PR, Heimans JJ, Valk J, Nauta JJ, Lachniet M, Van Kooten B. Do metastases in vertebrae begin in the body or the pedicles? Imaging study in 45 patients. *AJR Am J Roentgenol* 1992;158:1275–1279.

Alquacil-Garcia A, Alonso A, Pettigrew NM. Osteofibrous dysplasia (ossifying fibroma) of the tibia and fibula and adamantinoma. *Am J Clin Pathol* 1984;82:470–474.

Ardran GM. Bone destruction not demonstrable by radiography. *Br J Radiol* 1951;24:107–109.

Asdourian PL, Weidenbaum M, Dewald RL, Hammerberg KW, Ramsey RG. The pattern of vertebral involvement in metastatic vertebral breast cancer. *Clin Orthop* 1991;250:164–170.

Avrahami E, Tadmor R, Dally O, Hadar H. Early MR demonstration of spinal metastases in patients with normal radiographs and CT and radionuclide bone scans. *J Comput Assist Tomogr* 1989;13:598–602.

Avrahami E, Tadmor R, Kaplinsky N. The role of T2-weighted gradient echo in MRI demonstration of spinal multiple myeloma. *Spine* 1993;18:1812–1815.

Azzarelli A, Quagliuolo V, Cerasoli S, et al. Chordoma: natural history and treatment results in 33 cases. *J Surg Oncol* 1988;37:185–191.

Bachman AS, Sproul EE. Correlation of radiographic and autopsy findings in suspected metastases in the spine. *Bull NY Acad Med* 1940;44:169–175.

Baker ND, Greenspan A. Case report 172: pleomorphic liposarcoma, grade IV, of the soft tissue, arising in generalized plexiform neurofibromatosis. *Skeletal Radiol* 1981;7:150–153.

Baker PL, Dockerty MD, Coventry MB. Adamantinoma (so-called) of the long bones. *J Bone Joint Surg [Am]* 1954;36A:704–720.

Baraga JJ, Amrani KK, Swee RG, Wold L, Unni KK. Radiographic features of Ewing's sarcoma of the bones of the hands and feet. *Skeletal Radiol* 2001;30:121–126.

Bardwick PA, Zvaifler NJ, Gill GN, Newman D, Greenway GD, Resnick D. Plasma-cell dyscrasia with polyneuropathy, organomegaly, endocrinopathy, M-protein and skin changes: the POEMS syndrome. Report on two cases and review of the literature. *Medicine* 1980;59:311–322.

Bataille R, Chevalier J, Rossi M, Sany J. Bone scintigraphy in plasma-cell myeloma. *Radiology* 1982;145:801–804.

Bataille R, Sany J. Solitary myeloma: clinical and prognostic features of a review of 114 cases. *Cancer* 1981;48:845–851.

Bator SM, Bauer TW, Marks KE, Norris DG. Periosteal Ewing's sarcoma. *Cancer* 1986;58:1781–1784.

Baur A, Stäbler A, Lamerz R, Bartl R, Reiser M. Light chain deposition disease in multiple myeloma: MR imaging features correlated with histopathologic findings. *Skeletal Radiol* 1998;27:173–176.

Beackley MC, Lau BP, King ER. Bone involvement in Hodgkin's disease. *AJR Am J Roentgenol* 1972;114:559–563.

Beaugié JM, Mann CV, Butler ECB. Sacrococcygeal chordoma. *Br J Surg* 1969;56:586–588.

Belza MG, Urich H. Chordoma and malignant fibrous histiocytoma. Evidence of transformation. *Cancer* 1986;589:1082–1087.

Berlin O, Angervall L, Kindblom LG, Berlin IC, Stener B. Primary leiomyosarcoma of bone. A clinical, radiographic, pathologic-anatomic, and prognostic study of 16 cases. *Skeletal Radiol* 1987;16:364–376.

Bernstein SC, Perez-Atayde AR, Weinstein HJ. Multiple myeloma in a child. *Cancer* 1985;56:2143–2147.

Berrettoni B, Carter JR. Mechanisms of cancer metastasis to bone. *J Bone Joint Surg [Am]* 1986;68A:308–312.

Bertoni F, Bacchini P, Ferruzzi A. Small round-cell malignancies of bone: Ewing's sarcoma, malignant lymphoma, and myeloma. *Semin Orthop* 1991;6:186–195.

Bertoni F, Capanna R, Calderoni P, Bacchini P, Campanacci M. Primary central (medullary) fibrosarcoma of bone. *Semin Diagn Pathol* 1984;1:185–198.

Bessler W, Antonucci F, Stamm B, Stuckmann G, Vollrath T. Case report 646. POEMS syndrome. *Skeletal Radiol* 1991;20:212–215.

Bloem JL, Taminiau AH, Eulderink F, Hermans J, Pauwels EK. Radiologic staging of primary bone sarcoma: MR imaging, scintigraphy, angiography, and CT correlated with pathologic examination. *Radiology* 1988;169:805–810.

Bloom RA, Libson E, Husband JE, Stoker DJ. The periosteal sunburst reaction to bone metastases. A literature review and report of 20 additional cases. *Skeletal Radiol* 1987;16:629–634.

Boland PJ, Huvos AG. Malignant fibrous histiocytoma of bone. *Clin Orthop* 1986;204:130–134.

Boston HC Jr, Dahlin DC, Ivins JC, Cupps RE. Malignant lymphoma (so-called reticulum cell sarcoma) of bone. *Cancer* 1974;34:1131–1137.

Boutin RD, Speath HJ, Mangalic A, Sell JJ. Epithelioid hemangioendothelioma of bone. *Skeletal Radiol* 1996;25:391–395.

Boyko OB, Cory DA, Cohen MD, Provisor A, Mirkin D, DeRosa GP. MR imaging of osteogenic and Ewing's sarcoma. *AJR Am J Roentgenol* 1987;148:317–322.

Bradwey TM, Murphy DA, Eyster RL, Cannon MW. Multiple myeloma in a 25-year-old woman. *Clin Orthop* 1993;294:290–293.

Bragg DG, Colby TV, Ward JH. New concepts in the non-Hodgkin lymphomas: radiologic implications. *Radiology* 1986;159:289–304.

Brandon C, Martel W, Weatherbee L, Capek P. Case report 572. Osteosclerotic myeloma (POEMS syndrome). *Skeletal Radiol* 1989;18:542–546.

Braunstein EM. Hodgkin's disease of bone: radiographic correlation with the histologic classification. *Radiology* 1980;137:643–646.

Braunstein EM, Kuhns LR. Computed tomographic demonstration of spinal metastases. *Spine* 1983;8:912–915.

Brown B, Laorr A, Greenspan A, Stadalnik R. Negative bone scintigraphy with diffuse osteoblastic breast carcinoma metastases. *Clin Nucl Med* 1994;19:194–196.

Brown TS, Paterson CR. Osteosclerosis in myeloma. *J Bone Joint Surg [Br]* 1973;55B:621–623.

Bullough PG. *Atlas of orthopedic pathology with clinical and radiologic correlations*, 2nd ed. New York: Gower; 1992:17.1–17.29.

Bush CH, Reith JD, Spanier SS. Mineralization in musculoskeletal leiomyosarcoma: radiologic-pathologic correlation. *AJR Am J Roentgenol* 2003;180:109–113.

Bushnell DL, Kahn D, Huston B, Bevering CG. Utility of SPECT imaging for determination of vertebral metastases in patients with known primary tumors. *Skeletal Radiol* 1995;24:13–16.

Byers PD. A study of histological features distinguishing chordoma from chondrosarcoma. *Br J Cancer* 1981;43:229–232.

Callstrom MR, Charboneau JW, Goetz MP, et al. Painful metastases involving bone: feasibility of percutaneous CT- and US-guided radio-frequency ablation. *Radiology* 2002;224:87–97.

Caluser CI, Scott AM, Schnieder J, Macapinlac HA, Yeh SD, Larson SM. Value of lesion location and intensity of uptake in SPECT bone scintigraphy of the spine in patients with malignant tumors. *Radiology* 1992;185(S):315.

Campanacci M. Osteofibrous dysplasia of long bones. A new clinical entity. *Ital J Orthop Traumatol* 1976;2:221–237.

Campanacci M. Plasmacytoma. In: *Bone and soft tissue tumors*. New York: Springer-Verlag; 1990:560.

Campanacci M, Laus M, Giunti A, Gitelis S, Bertoni F. Adamantinoma of the long bones. The experience at the Istituto Ortopedico Rizzoli. *Am J Surg Pathol* 1981;5:533–542.

Campbell SE, Filzen TW, Bezzant SM, Beall DP, Burton MP, Sanders TG, Parsons TW. Primary periosteal lymphoma: an unusual presentation of non-Hodgkin's lymphoma with radiographic, MR imaging, and pathologic correlation. *Skeletal Radiol* 2003;32:231–235.

Capanna R, Bertoni F, Bacchini P, Gacci G, Guerra A, Campanacci M. Malignant fibrous histiocytoma of bone: the experience at the Rizzoli Institute. Report of 90 cases. *Cancer* 1984;54:177–187.

Castellino RA. Hodgkin disease: practical concepts for the diagnostic radiologist. *Radiology* 1986;159:305–310.

Cavazzana AO, Miser JS, Jefferson J, Triche TJ. Experimental evidence for a neural origin of Ewing's sarcoma of bone. *Am J Pathol* 1987;127:507–518.

Chan K-W, Rosen G, Miller DR, Tan CTC. Hodgkin's disease in adolescents presenting as a primary bone lesion. A report of four cases and review of the literature. *Am J Pediatr Hematol Oncol* 1982;4:11–17.

Choi J-A, Lee KH, Jun WS, Yi MG, Lee S, Kang HS. Osseous metastasis from renal cell carcinoma: "flow-void" sign at MR imaging. *Radiology* 2003;228:629–634.

Chu TA. Chondroid chordoma of the sacrococcygeal region. *Arch Pathol Lab Med* 1987;111:861–864.

Citrin DL, Bessent RG, Greig WR. A comparison of the sensitivity and accuracy of the 99m Tc-phosphate bone scan and skeletal radiograph in the diagnosis of bone metastases. *Clin Radiol* 1977;28:107–117.

Clayton F, Butler JJ, Ayala AG, Ro JY, Zornoza J. Non-Hodgkin's lymphoma in bone: pathologic and radiologic features with clinical correlates. *Cancer* 1987;60:2494–2500.

Coerkamp EG, Kroon HM. Cortical bone metastases. *Radiology* 1988;169:525–528.

Cohen MD, Klatte EC, Smith JA, et al. Magnetic resonance imaging of lymphomas in children. *Pediatr Radiol* 1985;15:179–183.

Coindre JM, Rivel J, Trojan M, De Mascarel J, De Mascarel A. Immunohistological study in chordomas. *J Pathol* 1986;150:61–63.

Coldwell DM, Baron RL, Charnsangavej C. Angiosarcoma: diagnosis and clinical course. *Acta Radiol* 1989;30:627–631.

Coles WC, Schultz MD. Bone involvement in malignant lymphoma. *Radiology* 1948;50:458–462.

Coombs RJ, Coiner L. Sacral chordoma with unusual posterior radiographic presentation. *Skeletal Radiol* 1996;25:679–681.

Coombs RJ, Zeiss J, McKann K, Phillips E. Multifocal Ewing's tumor of the skeletal system. *Skeletal Radiol* 1986;15:254–257.

Crawford T. The staining reactions of chordoma. *J Clin Pathol* 1958;11:110–113.

Cumming J, Hacking N, Fairhurst J, Ackery D, Jenkins JD. Distribution of bony metastases in prostatic carcinoma. *Br J Urol* 1990;66:411–414.

Czerniak B, Rojas-Corona RR, Dorfman HD. Morphologic diversity of long bone adamantinoma. The concept of differentiated (regressing) adamantinoma and its relationship to osteofibrous dysplasia. *Cancer* 1989;64:2319–2334.

Dabska M. Parachordoma. A new clinicopathologic entity. *Cancer* 1977;40:1586–1592.

Dahlin DC. Grading of bone tumors. In: Unni KK, ed. *Bone tumors*. New York: Churchill Livinstone; 1988:35–45.

Dahlin DC, Ivins JC. Fibrosarcoma of bone: a study of 114 cases. *Cancer* 1969;23:35–41.

Dahlin DC, MacCarty CS. Chordoma. A study of fifty-nine cases. *Cancer* 1952;5:1170–1178.

Dahlin DC, Unni KK. *Bone tumors. General aspects and data on 8,542 cases,* 4th ed. Springfield, IL: Charles C. Thomas; 1986:193–336, 208–226, 379–393.

Dahlin DC, Unni KK, Matsuno T. Malignant (fibrous) histiocytoma of bone—fact or fancy? *Cancer* 1977;39:1508–1516.

Daldrup-Link HE, Franzius C, Link TM, et al. Whole-body MR imaging for detection of bone metastases in children and young adults: comparison with skeletal scintigraphy and FDG PET. *AJR Am J Roentgenol* 2001;177:229–236.

Dalinka MK, Turner ML, Thompson JJ, Lee RE. Lipid granulomatosis of the ribs: focal Erdheim-Chester disease. *Radiology* 1982;142:297–299.

Dardick I, Schatz JE, Colgan TJ. Osteogenic sarcoma with epithelial differentiation. *Ultrastruct Pathol* 1992;16:463–474.

Datz FL, Patch GG, Arias JM, Morton KA. *Nuclear medicine. A teaching file.* St. Louis: Mosby Year Book; 1992:28–29.

deBruine FT, Kroon HM. Spinal chordoma: radiologic features of 14 cases. *AJR Am J Roentgenol* 1988;150:861–863.

Dehner LP. Primitive neuroectodermal tumor and Ewing's sarcoma. *Am J Surg Pathol* 1993;17:1–13.

Delbeke D, Powers TA, Sandler MP. Negative scintigraphy with positive magnetic resonance imaging in bone metastases. *Skeletal Radiol* 1990;19:113–116.

Dellagi K, Lipinski M, Paulin D, Portier MM, Lenoir GM, Brouet JC. Characterization of intermediate filaments expressed by Ewing tumor cell lines. *Cancer* 1987;47:1170–1173.

Deutsch A, Resnick D. Eccentric cortical metastases to the skeleton from bronchogenic carcinoma. *Radiology* 1980;137:49–52.

Deutsch A, Resnick D, Niwayama G. Case report 145. Bilateral, almost symmetrical skeletal metastases (both femora) from bronchogenic carcinoma. *Skeletal Radiol* 1981;6:144–148.

Dimopoulos MA, Moulopoulos A, Delasalle K, Alexanian R. Solitary plasmacytoma of bone and asymptomatic multiple myeloma. *Hematol Oncol North Am* 1992;6:359–369.

Dorfman HD, Norman A, Wolff H. Fibrosarcoma complicating bone infarction in a caisson worker: case report. *J Bone Joint Surg [Am]* 1966;48A:528–532.

Durie BGM, Salmon SE. A clinical staging system for multiple myeloma. *Cancer* 1975;36:842–854.

Dwyer AJ, Frank SL, Sank VJ, Reinig JW, Hickey AM, Doppman SL. Short TI inversion recovery pulse sequence: analysis and initial experience in cancer imaging. *Radiology* 1988;168:827–836.

Eggli KD, Quiogue T, Moser RP. Ewing's sarcoma. *Radiol Clin North Am* 1993;31:325–337.

Enzinger FM, Weiss SW. Hemangioendothelioma: vascular tumors of intermediate malignancy. In: Enzinger FM, Weiss SW, eds. *Soft tissue tumors*, 3rd ed. St. Louis: CV Mosby; 1995.

Enzinger FM, Weiss SW. *Soft tissue tumors*. St. Louis: Mosby; 1988:951–958.

Estes DN, Magill HL, Thompson EL, Hayes FA. Primary Ewing sarcoma: follow-up with Ga-67 scintigraphy. *Radiology* 1990;177:449–453.

Eustace S, Tello R, DeCarvalho V, et al. A comparison of whole-body turboSTIR MR imaging and planar 99mTc-methylene diphosphonate scintigraphy in the examination of patients with suspected skeletal metastases. *AJR Am J Roentgenol* 1997;169:1655–1661.

Even-Sapir E, Martin RH, Barnes DC, Pringle CR, Iles SE, Mitchell MJ. Role of SPECT in differentiating malignant from benign lesions in the lower thoracic and lumbar vertebrae. *Radiology* 1993;187:193–198.

Evison G, Pizey N, Roylance J. Bone formation associated with osseous metastases from bladder carcinoma. *Clin Radiol* 1981;32:303–309.

Eyre-Brook AL, Price CHG. Fibrosarcoma of bone: review of 50 consecutive cases from the Bristol Bone Tumor Registry. *J Bone Joint Surg [Br]* 1969;51B:20–37.

Fechner RE, Mills SE. *Atlas of tumor pathology. Tumors of the bones and joints*, 3rd series, fascicle 8. Washington DC: Armed Forces Institute of Pathology; 1993:239–244.

Feldman F, Lattes R. Primary malignant fibrous histiocytoma (fibrous xanthoma) of bone. *Skeletal Radiol* 1977;1:145–160.

Feldman F, Norman D. Intra- and extraosseous malignant histiocytoma (malignant fibrous xanthoma). *Radiology* 1972;104:497–508.

Fig LM, Gross MD: Metastatic prostate carcinoma mimicking Paget's disease on bone imaging. *Clin Nucl Med* 1989;14:777–778.

Firooznia H, Printo RS, Lin JP, Baruch HH, Zausner J. Chordoma: radiologic evaluation of 20 cases. *AJR Am J Roentgenol* 1976;127:797–805.

Fischer B. Über ein primäres Adamantinom der Tibia. *Frankfurter Z Pathol* 1913;12:422–441.

Fishman EK, Kuhlman JE, Jones RJ. CT of lymphoma: spectrum of disease. *Radiographics* 1991;11:647–669.

Fletcher CD, Unni KK, Mertens F. *World Health Organization classification of tumors. Pathology and genetics of tumours of soft tissue and bone.* Lyon: IARC Press; 2002.

Flickinger FW, Salahattin SM. Bone marrow MRI: techniques and accuracy for detecting breast cancer metastases. *Magn Reson Imaging* 1994;12:829–835.

Foster D. Cortical skeletal metastasis in malignant melanoma. *Australas Radiol* 1982;20:545–560.

Frassica DA, Frassica FJ, Schray MF, Sim FH, Kyle RA. Solitary plasmacytoma of bone: Mayo Clinic experience. *Int J Radiat Oncol Biol Phys* 1989;16:43–48.

Friedman B, Hanoaka H. Round cell sarcoma of bone. *J Bone Joint Surg [Am]* 1971;53A:1118–1136.

Friedman I, Harrison DFN, Bird ES. The fine structure of chordoma with particular reference to the physaliphorous cell. *J Clin Pathol* 1962;15:116–125.

Frouge C, Vanel D, Coffre C, Couanet D, Contesso G, Sarrazin D. The role of magnetic resonance imaging in the evaluation of Ewing's sarcoma. A report of 27 cases. *Skeletal Radiol* 1988;17:387–392.

Fruehwald FX, Tschalakoff D, Schwaighofer B, et al. Magnetic resonance imaging of the lower vertebral column in patients with multiple myeloma. *Invest Radiol* 1988;23:193–199.

Galasko CSB. Mechanisms of lytic and blastic metastatic disease of bone. *Clin Orthop* 1982;69:20–27.

Galasko CSB. The anatomy and pathways of skeletal metastases. In: Weiss L, Gilbert H, eds. *Bone Metastasis.* Boston: GK Hall; 1981:49–63.

Galli SJ, Weintraub HP, Proppe KH. Malignant fibrous histiocytoma and pleomorphic sarcoma in association with medullary bone infarcts. *Cancer* 1978;41:607–619.

Garber CZ. Reactive bone formation in Ewing's sarcoma. *Cancer* 1951;4:839–845.

Ghandur-Mnaymneh L, Broder LE, Mnaymneh WA. Lobular carcinoma of the breast metastatic to bone with unusual clinical, radiologic, and pathologic features mimicking osteopoikilosis. *Cancer* 1984;53:1801–1803.

Gherlinzoni F, Antoci B, Canale V. Multicentric osteosarcomata (osteosarcomatosis). *Skeletal Radiol* 1983;10:281–285.

Gold RH, Mirra JM. Case report 101. Primary Hodgkin disease of humerus. *Skeletal Radiol* 1979;4:233–235.

Gold RI, Seeger LL, Bassett LW, Steckel RJ. An integrated approach to the evaluation of metastatic bone disease. *Radiol Clin North Am* 1990;28:471–483.

Gosfield E, Alavi A, Kneeland B. Comparison of radionuclide bone scans and magnetic resonance imaging in detecting spinal metastases. *J Nucl Med* 1993;34:2191–2198.

Granger W, Whitaker R. Hodgkin's disease in bone, with special reference to periosteal reaction. *Br J Radiol* 1967;40:939–948.

Greco A, Jelliffe AM, Maher EJ, Leung AWL. MR imaging of lymphomas: impact on therapy. *J Comput Assist Tomogr* 1988;12:785–791.

Greco A, Steiner GC, Fazzini E. Ewing's sarcoma with epithelial differentiation. Fine structural and immunocytochemical study. *Ultrastruct Pathol* 1988;12:317–325.

Greenfield GB, Arrington JA. *Imaging of bone tumors. A multimodality approach.* Philadelphia: JB Lippincott; 1995.

Greenspan A. Sclerosing bone dysplasias—a target-site approach. *Skeletal Radiol* 1991;20:561–584.

Greenspan A. *Orthopedic radiology. A practical approach*, 2nd ed. New York: Gower; 1992:15.15.

Greenspan A, Gerscovich EO, Szabo RM, Matthews II JG. Condensing osteitis of the clavicle: a rare but frequently misdiagnosed condition. *AJR Am J Roentgenol* 1991;156:1011–1015.

Greenspan A, Klein MJ. Radiology and pathology of bone tumors. In: Lewis MM, ed. *Musculoskeletal oncology. A multidisciplinary approach.* Philadelphia: WB Saunders; 1992:13–72.

Greenspan A, Klein MJ. Giant bone island. *Skeletal Radiol* 1996;25:67–69.

Greenspan A, Klein MJ, Lewis MM. Case report 272. Skeletal cortical metastases in the left femur arising from bronchogenic carcinoma. *Skeletal Radiol* 1984;11:297–301.

Greenspan A, Klein MJ, Lewis MM. Case report 284. Osteolytic cortical metastasis in the femur from bronchogenic carcinoma. *Skeletal Radiol* 1984;12:146–150.

Greenspan A, Norman A. Osteolytic cortical destruction: an unusual pattern of skeletal metastases. *Skeletal Radiol* 1988;17:402–406.

Greenspan A, Remagen W. *Differential diagnosis of tumors and tumor-like lesions of bones and joints.* Philadelphia: Lippincott-Raven; 1998:369–371.

Greenspan A, Stadalnik RC. Bone island: scintigraphic findings and their clinical application. *Can Assoc Radiol J* 1995;46:368–379.

Greenspan A, Steiner G, Knutzon R. Bone island (enostosis): clinical significance and radiologic and histologic correlations. *Skeletal Radiol* 1991;20:85–90.

Grover SB, Dhar A. Imaging spectrum in sclerotic myelomas: an experience in three cases. *Eur Radiol* 2000;10:1828–1831.

Guermazi A, Brice P, de Kerviler E, Fermé C, Hennequin C, Meignin V, Frija J. Extranodal Hodgkin disease: spectrum of disease. *Radiographics* 2001;21:161–179.

Hall FM, Gore SM. Osteosclerotic myeloma variant. *Skeletal Radiol* 1988;17:101–105.

Healey JH, Turnbull AD, Miedema B, Lane JM. Acrometastases. A study of twenty-nine patients with osseous involvement of the hands and feet. *J Bone Joint Surg [Am]* 1986;68A:743–746.

Hendrix RW, Rogers LF, Davis TM Jr. Cortical bone metastases. *Radiology* 1991;181:409–413.

Herman G, Klein MJ, Abdelwahab AF, Kenan S. MRI appearance of primary non-Hodgkin's lymphoma of bone. *Skeletal Radiol* 1997;26:629–632.

Hermann H, Abdelwahab IF, Berson BD, Greenberg ML, Palestro CJ. Case report 621. Multiple myeloma (IgD) in a 28 year old woman. *Skeletal Radiol* 1990;19:379–381.

Hicks DG, Gokan T, O'Keefe RJ, et al. Primary lymphoma of bone. Correlation of MRI features with cytokine production by tumor cells. *Cancer* 1995;75:973–980.

Higinbotham NL, Phillips RF, Farr HW, Hustu HO. Chordoma. Thirty-five-year study at Memorial Hospital. *Cancer* 1967;20:1841–1850.

Hillemanns M, McLeod RA, Unni KK. Malignant lymphoma. *Skeletal Radiol* 1996;25:73–75.

Hindman BW, Gill HK, Zuppan CW. Primitive neuroectodermal tumor in a child with tuberous sclerosis. *Skeletal Radiol* 1997;26:184–187.

Hoane BR, Shields AF, Porter BA, Schulman HM. Detection of lymphomatous bone marrow involvement with magnetic resonance imaging. *Blood* 1991;78:728–738.

Hove B, Gyldensted C. Spiculated vertebral metastases from prostatic carcinoma. *Neuroradiology* 1990;32:337–339.

Hruban RH, Traganos F, Reuter VE, Huvos AG. Chordomas with malignant spindle cell components. *Am J Pathol* 1990;137:435–447.

Hudson TM. *Radiologic-pathologic correlation of musculoskeletal lesions.* Baltimore: Williams & Wilkins, 1987:287–303, 359–397, 421–440.

Huvos AG. *Bone Tumors: Diagnosis, Treatment, and Prognosis*, 2nd ed. Philadelphia: WB Saunders; 1991:599–624, 695–711.

Huvos AG. Primary malignant fibrous histiocytoma of bone: clinicopathologic study of 18 patients. *NY State J Med* 1976;552–559.

Huvos AG, Heilweil M, Bretsky SS. The pathology of malignant fibrous histiocytoma of bone. A study of 130 patients. *Am J Surg Pathol* 1985;9:853–871.

Huvos AG, Higinbotham NL. Primary fibrosarcoma of bone: a clinico-pathologic study of 130 patients. *Cancer* 1975;35:837–847.

Huvos AG, Higinbotham NL, Miller TR. Bone sarcomas arising in fibrous dysplasia. *J Bone Joint Surg [Am]* 1972;64A:1047–1056.

Huvos AG, Marcove RC. Adamantinoma of long bones: a clinicopathological study of fourteen cases with vascular origin suggested. *J Bone Joint Surg [Am]* 1975;57A:148–154.

Huvos AG, Woodard HQ, Heilweil M. Postradiation malignant fibrous histiocytoma of bone. A clinicopathologic study of 20 patients. *Am J Surg Pathol* 1986;10:9–18.

Ignacio EA, Palmer KM, Mathur SC, Schwartz AM, Olan WJ. Residents' teaching files. Epithelioid hemangioendothelioma of the lower extremity. *Radiographics* 1999;19:531–537.

Igou D, Sundaram M, McDonald DJ, Janney C, Chalk DE. Appendicular metastatic prostate cancer simulating osteosarcoma, Paget's disease, and Paget's sarcoma. *Skeletal Radiol* 1995;24:447–449.

Isayama T, Iwasaki H, Kikuchi M, Yoh S, Takagishi N. Neuroectodermal tumor of bone. Evidence for neural differentiation in a cultured cell line. *Cancer* 1990;65:1771–1781.

Ishida T, Dorfman HD. Plasma cell myeloma in unusually young patients: a report of two cases and review of the literature. *Skeletal Radiol* 1995;24:47–51.

Ishida T, Dorfman HD, Steiner GC, Normatz A. Cystic angiomatosis of bone with sclerotic changes mimicking osteoblastic metastases. *Skeletal Radiol* 1994;23:247–252.

Ishida T, Iijima T, Kikuchi F, et al. A clinicopathological and immunohistochemical study of osteofibrous dysplasia, differentiated adamantinoma, and adamantinoma of long bones. *Skeletal Radiol* 1992;21:493–502.

Jacobson HG, Poppel MH, Shapiro JH, Grossberger S. The vertebral pedicle sign: a roentgen finding to differentiate metastatic carcinoma from multiple myeloma. *AJR Am J Roentgenol* 1958;80:817–821.

Jaffe H. Tumors metastatic to the skeleton. In: *Tumors and tumorous conditions of the bones and joints.* Philadelphia: Lea & Febiger; 1958:594–595.

Jaffe HL. *Metabolic, degenerative, and inflammatory diseases of bones and joints.* Philadelphia: Lea & Febiger; 1972:877.

Jaffe R, Santamaria M, Yunis EJ, et al. The neuroectodermal tumor of bone. *Am J Surg* 1984;8:885–898.

Johnston AD. Pathology of metastatic tumors in bone. *Clin Orthop* 1970;73:8–32.

Jundt G, Moll C, Nidecker A, Schilt R, Remagen W. Primary leiomyosarcoma of bone: report of eight cases. *Hum Pathol* 1994;25:1205–1212.

Jundt G, Remberger K, Roessner A, Schulz A, Bohndorf K. Adamantinoma of long bones. A histopathological and immunohistochemical study of 23 cases. *Pathol Res Pract* 1995;191:112–120.

Kahn LB, Webber B, Mills E, Anstey L, Heselson NG. Malignant fibrous histiocytoma (malignant fibrous xanthoma: xanthosarcoma) of bone. *Cancer* 1978;42:640–651.

Kaplan H. *Hodgkin disease,* 2nd ed. Cambridge, MA: Harvard University Press; 1980:85–92.

Kattapuram SV, Khurana JS, Scott JA, el-Khoury GY. Negative scintigraphy with positive magnetic resonance imaging in bone metastases. *Skeletal Radiol* 1990;19:113–116.

Keeney GL, Unni KK, Beabout JW, Pritchard DJ. Adamantinoma of long bones. A clinicopathologic study of 85 cases. *Cancer* 1989;64:730–737.

Kelly JJ Jr, Kyle RA, Miles JM, Dyck PJ. Osteosclerotic myeloma and peripheral neuropathy. *Neurology* 1983;33:202–210.

Kim EE, Deland FH, Maruyama Y. Decreased uptake in bone scans ("cold lesions") in metastatic carcinoma. *J Bone Joint Surg [Am]* 1978;60A:844–846.

Kim JH, Chu FC, Woodard HQ, Melamed MR, Huvos A, Cantin J. Radiation-induced soft-tissue and bone sarcoma. *Radiology* 1978;129:501–508.

Kissane JM, Askin PB, Foulkes M, Stratton LB, Shirley SF. Ewing's sarcoma of bone. Clinicopathological aspects of 303 cases from the intergroup Ewing's sarcoma study. *Hum Pathol* 1983;14:773–779.

Kleer CG, Unni KK, McLeod RA. Epithelioid hemangioendothelioma of bone. *Am J Surg Pathol* 1996;20:1301–1311.

Klein MJ, Rudin BJ, Greenspan A, Posner M, Lewis MM. Hodgkin disease presenting as a lesion in the wrist. *J Bone Joint Surg [Am]* 1987;69A:1246–1249.

Knapp RH, Wick MR, Scheithauer BW, Unni KK. Adamantinoma of bone. An electron microscopic and immunohistochemical study. *Virchows Arch (A)* 1982;398:75–86.

Kori SH. Computed tomographic evaluation of bone and soft tissue metastases. In: Weiss L, Gilbert H, eds. *Bone metastasis.* Boston: GK Hall; 1981:245–257.

Kramer K, Hicks D, Palis J, et al. Epithelioid osteosarcoma of bone. Immunocytochemical evidence suggesting divergent epithelial and mesenchymal differentiation in a primary osseous neoplasm. *Cancer* 1993;71:2977–2982.

Krishnan A, Shirkhoda A, Tehranzadeh J, Armin AR, Irwin R, Les K. Primary bone lymphoma: radiographic-MR imaging correlation. *Radiographics* 2003;23:1371–1387.

Kumar N, David R, Madewell JE, Lindell MM Jr. Radiographic spectrum of osteogenic sarcoma. *AJR Am J Roentgenol* 1987;148:767–772.

Kyle RA. Multiple myeloma: review of 869 cases. *Mayo Clinic Proc* 1975;50:29–40.

Kyle RA. Diagnostic criteria of multiple myeloma. *Hematol Oncol Clin North Am* 1992;6:347–358.

Kyle RA, Bayrd ED. Amyloidosis: review of 236 cases. *Medicine* 1975;54:271–299.

Lawson CW, Fisher C, Gatter KC. An immunohistochemical study of differentiation in malignant fibrous histiocytoma. *Histopathology* 1987;11:375–383.

Lazarus HM, Kellermeyer RW, Aikawa M, Herzig RH. Multiple myeloma in young men: clinical course and electron microscopic studies of bone marrow plasma cells. *Cancer* 1980;46:1397–1400.

Lecouvet FE, Vande Berg BC, Malghem J, Maldague BE. Magnetic resonance and computed tomography imaging in multiple myeloma. *Semin Musculoskelet Radiol* 2001;5:43–55.

Lehrer HZ, Maxfield WS, Nice CM. The periosteal sunburst pattern in metastatic bone tumors. *AJR Am J Roentgenol* 1970;108:154–161.

Libson E, Bloom RA, Husband JE, Stocker DJ. Metastatic tumours of the bones of the hand and foot. A comparative review and report of 43 additional cases. *Skeletal Radiol* 1987;16:387–392.

Lin WY, Kao CH, Hsu CY, Liao SQ, Wang SH, Yeh SH. The role of Tc-99m MDP and Ga-67 imaging in the clinical evaluation of malignant fibrous histiocytoma. *Clin Nucl Med* 1994;19:996–1000.

Linden A, Zankovich R, Theissen P, Diehl V, Schicha H. Malignant lymphoma: bone marrow imaging versus biopsy. *Radiology* 1989;173:335–339.

Link TM, Haeussler MD, Poppek S, Woertler K, Blasius S, Lindner N, Rummeny EJ. Malignant fibrous histiocytoma of bone: conventional X-ray and MR imaging features. *Skeletal Radiol* 1998;27:552–558.

Lipshitz HI, Malthouse SR, Cunningham D, MacVicar AD, Husband JE. Multiple myeloma: appearance at MR imaging. *Radiology* 1992;182:833–837.

Llombart-Bosch A, Contesso G, Henry-Amar M, et al. Histopathological predictive factors in Ewing's sarcoma of bone and clinicopathologic correlations. A retrospective study of 261 cases. *Virchows Arch (A)* 1986;409:627–640 (erratum published in *Virchows Arch (A)* 1986;410:263).

Llombart-Bosch A, Lacombe MJ, Peydro-Olaya A, Perez-Bacete M, Contesso G. Malignant peripheral neuroectodermal tumors of bone other than Askin's neoplasm: characterization of 14 new cases with immunohistochemistry and electron microscopy. *Virchows Arch (A)* 1988;412:421–430.

Llombart-Bosch A, Ortuno-Pacheco G. Ultrastructural findings supporting the angioblastic nature of the so-called adamantinoma of the tibia. *Histopathology* 1978;2:189–200.

Llombart-Bosch A, Terrier LMJ, Peydro-Olaya A, Contesso G. Peripheral neuroectodermal sarcoma of soft tissue (peripheral neuroepithelioma): a pathologic study of ten cases with differential diagnosis regarding other small, round cell sarcomas. *Hum Pathol* 1989;20:273–280.

Lukes RJ, Buttler JJ. Pathology and nomenclature of Hodgkin disease. *Cancer Res* 1966;26:1063–2083.

Mahnken AH, Wildberger JE, Gehbauer G, Schmitz-Rode T, Blaum M, Fabry V, Günther RW. Multidetector CT of the spine in multiple myeloma: comparison with MR imaging and radiography. *AJR Am J Roentgenol* 2002;178:1429–1436.

Markel SF. Ossifying fibroma of long bone. Its distinction from fibrous dysplasia and its association with adamantinoma of long bone. *Am J Clin Pathol* 1978;69:91–97.

Martin RF, Melnick PJ, Warner NE, Terry R, Bullock WK, Schwinn CP. Chordoid sarcoma. *Am J Clin Pathol* 1973;59:623–635.

McCarthy EF, Matsuno T, Dorfman HD. Malignant fibrous histiocytoma of bone: a study of 35 cases. *Hum Pathol* 1979;10:57–70.

McDougall IR, Kriss JP. Screening for bone metastases. Are only scans necessary? *JAMA* 1975;231:46–50.

Medeiros LJ, Jaffe ES. Pathology of non-Hodgkin's lymphomas and Hodgkin's disease. In: Wiernik PH, Canellos GP, Dutcher JP, Kyle RA, eds. *Neoplastic diseases of the blood,* 3rd ed. New York: Churchill Livingstone; 1996.

Mehta RC, Wilson MA, Perlman SB. False negative bone scan in extensive metastatic disease: CT and MR findings. *J Comput Assist Tomogr* 1989;13:717–719.

Meis JM, Butler JJ, Osborne BM, Ordonez NG. Solitary plasmacytomas of bone and extramedullary plasmacytomas. A clinicopathologic and immunohistochemical study. *Cancer* 1987;59:1475–1485.

Meis JM, Giraldo AA. Chordoma. An immuno-histochemical study of 20 cases. *Arch Pathol Lab Med* 1988;112:553–556.

Meis JM, Raymond AK, Evans HL, Charles RE, Giraldo AA. "Dedifferentiated" chordoma. A clinicopathologic and immunohistochemical study of three cases. *Am J Surg Pathol* 1987;11:516–525.

Melamed JW, Martinez S, Hoffman CJ. Imaging of primary multifocal osseous lymphoma. *Skeletal Radiol* 1997;26:35–41.

Meyer JE, Lepke RA, Lindfors KK, et al. Chordomas: their CT appearance in the cervical, thoracic and lumbar spine. *Radiology* 1984;153:693–696.

Meyer JE, Schulz MD. "Solitary" myeloma of bone: a review of 12 cases. *Cancer* 1974;34:438–440.

Miettinen M, Karaharju E, Järvinen H. Chordoma with a massive spindle-cell sarcomatous transformation. A light- and electron-microscopic and immunohistological study. *Am J Surg Pathol* 1987;11:563–570.

Mirra JM. Lymphoma and lymphoma-like disorders. In: Mirra JM, Picci P, Gold RH, eds. *Bone tumors: clinical, radiologic, and pathologic correlations.* Philadelphia: Lea & Febiger; 1989.

Mirra JM, Bullough PG, Marcove RC, Jacobs B, Huvos AG. Malignant fibrous histiocytoma and osteosarcoma in association with bone infarcts. *J Bone Joint Surg [Am]* 1974;56A:932–940.

Mirra JM, Gold RH, Marafiote R. Malignant (fibrous) histiocytoma arising in association with a bone infarct in sickle-cell disease: coincidence or cause-and-effect? *Cancer* 1977;39:186–194.

Mirra JM, Picci P, Gold RH. *Bone tumors: Clinical, radiologic, and pathologic correlations.* Philadelphia, Lea & Febiger, 1989.

Moll RH, Lee I, Gould VE, Berndt R, Roessner A, Franke WW. Immunocytochemical analysis of Ewing's tumors. Patterns of expression of intermediate filaments and desmosomal proteins indicate cell type heterogeneity and pluripotential differentiation. *Am J Pathol* 1987;127:288–304.

Moon NF, Mori H. Adamantinoma of the appendicular skeleton—updated. *Clin Orthop* 1986;204:215–237.

Moulopoulos LA, Varma DGK, Dimopoulos MA, et al. Multiple myeloma: spinal MR imaging in patients with untreated newly diagnosed disease. *Radiology* 1992;185:833–840.

Mulder JD, Kroon HM, Schütte HE, Taconis WK. *Radiologic atlas of bone tumors.* Amsterdam: Elsevier, 1993;267–274, 607–625.

Mulligan ME. Myeloma and lymphoma. *Semin Musculoskelet Radiol* 2000;4:127–135.

Mulligan ME, Kransdorf MJ. Sequestra in primary lymphoma of bone: prevalence and radiologic features. *AJR Am J Roentgenol* 1993;160:1245–1248.

Mulligan ME, McRae GA, Murphey MD. Imaging features of primary lymphoma of bone. *AJR Am J Roentgenol* 1999;173:1691–1697.

Mulvey RB. Peripheral bone metastases. *AJR Am J Roentgenol* 1964;91:155–160.

Mundy GR, Spiro TP. The mechanisms of bone metastasis and bone destruction by tumor cells. In: Weiss L, Gilbert HA, eds. *Bone metastasis.* Boston: GK Hall; 1981:64–82.

Murphey MD, Gross TM, Rosenthal HG. Musculoskeletal malignant fibrous histiocytoma: radiologic-pathologic correlation. *Radiographics* 1994;14:807–826.

Murray RO, Jacobson HG. *The radiology of bone diseases,* 2nd ed. New York: Churchill Livingstone; 1977:585.

Myers JL, Arocho J, Bernreuter W, Dunham W, Mazur MT. Leiomyosarcoma of bone. A clinicopathologic, immunohistochemical, and ultrastructural study of five cases. *Cancer* 1991;67:1051–1056.

Nair M. Bone scanning in Ewing's sarcoma. *J Nucl Med* 1985;26:349–352.

Napoli LD, Hansen HH, Muggia FM, et al. The incidence of osseous involvement in lung cancer, with special reference to the development of osteoblastic changes. *Radiology* 1973;108:17–21.

Nascimento AG, Unni KK, Cooper KL, Dahlin DC. A clinicopathologic study of 20 cases of large cell (atypical) Ewing's sarcoma of bone. *Am J Surg Pathol* 1980;4:29–36.

Negendank W, Weissman D, Bey TM, et al. Evidence for clonal disease by magnetic resonance imaging in patients with hypoplastic marrow disorders. *Blood* 1991;78:2872–2879.

Nesbit ME Jr, Gehan EA, Burgert EO Jr, et al. Multimodal therapy for the management of primary, nonmetastatic Ewing's sarcoma of bone: a long-term follow-up of the First Intergroup study. *J Clin Oncol* 1990;8:1664–1674.

Newcomer LN, Silverstein MB, Cadman EC, Farber LR, Bertino JR, Prosnitz LR. Bone involvement in Hodgkin's disease. *Cancer* 1982;49:338–342.

Norman A, Greenspan A, Steiner G. Case report 173. Metastases from a bronchial carcinoid tumor. *Skeletal Radiol* 1981;7:155–157.

Norman A, Ulin R. A comparative study of periosteal new-bone response in metastatic bone tumors (solitary) and primary bone sarcomas. *Radiology* 1969;92:705–708.

Nystrom JS, Weiner JM, Wolf RM, Bateman JR, Viola MV. Identifying the primary site in metastatic cancer of unknown origin. *JAMA* 1979;241:381–383.

Ohgi S, Ehara S, Satoh T, Kato S, Shimosegawa K, Ishida Y. Spontaneous regression of malignant lymphoma of the lumbar spine. *Skeletal Radiol* 2002;31:99–102.

Onitsuka H. Roentgenologic aspects of bone islands. *Radiology* 1977;123:607–612.

Ontell FK, Greenspan A. Blastic osseous metastases in ovarian carcinoma. *Can Assoc Radiol J* 1995;46:231–234.

Orzel JA, Sawaf NW, Richardson ML. Lymphoma of the skeleton: scintigraphic evaluation. *AJR Am J Roentgenol* 1988;150:1095–1099.

Ostrowski ML, Unni KK, Banks PM, et al. Malignant lymphoma of bone. *Cancer* 1986;58:2646–2655.

Panebianco AC, Kaupp HA. Bilateral thumb metastasis from breast carcinoma. *Arch Surg* 1968;96:216–218.

Papac RJ. Bone marrow metastases: a review. *Cancer* 1994;74:2403–2413.

Pardo-Mindán FJ, Guillen FJ, Villas C, Vasquez JJ. A comparative ultrastructural study of chondrosarcoma, chordoid sarcoma, and chordoma. *Cancer* 1981;47:2611–2619.

Peavy PW, Rogers JV Jr, Clements JL Jr, Burns JB. Unusual osteoblastic metastases from carcinoid tumors. *Radiology* 1973;107:327–330.

Perlman EJ, Dickman PS, Askin FB, Grier HE, Miser JS, Link MP. Ewing's sarcoma routine diagnostic utilization of MIC2 analysis: a Pediatric Oncology Group/Children's Cancer Group Intergroup Study. *Hum Pathol* 1994;25:304–307.

Pettersson H, Gillespy T, Hamlin DJ, et al. Primary musculoskeletal tumors: examination with MR imaging compared with conventional modalities. *Radiology* 1987;164:237–241.

Petterson H, Slone RM, Spanier S, Gillespy T III, Fitzsimmons JR, Scott KN. Musculoskeletal tumors: T1 and T2 relaxation times. *Radiology* 1988;167:783–785.

Pettit CK, Zukerberg LR, Gray MH, et al. Primary lymphoma of bone. A B-cell neoplasm with a high frequency of multilobated cells. *Am J Surg Pathol* 1990;14:329–334.

Powell JM. Metastatic carcinoid of bone. Report of two cases and review of the literature. *Clin Orthop* 1988;230:266–272.

Pritchard DJ, Sim FH, Ivins JC, Soule EH, Dahlin DC. Fibrosarcoma of bone and soft tissues of the trunk and extremities. *Orthop Clin North Am* 1977;8:869–881.

Rafii M, Firooznia H, Kramer E, Golimbu C, Sanger J. The role of computed tomography in evaluation of skeletal metastases. *J Comput Tomogr* 1988;12:19–24.

Rahmouni A, Divine M, Mathieu D, et al. Detection of multiple myeloma involving the spine: efficacy of fat-suppression and contrast-enhanced MR imaging. *AJR Am J Roentgenol* 1993;160:1049–1052.

Reinus WR, Gilula LA. Ewing's sarcoma. In: Taveras JM, Ferruci JT, eds. *Radiology: diagnosis, imaging, intervention,* vol 5. Philadelphia: JB Lippincott; 1987.

Reinus WR, Kyriakos M, Gilula LA, Brower AC, Merkel K. Plasma cell tumors with calcified amyloid deposition mistaken for chondrosarcoma. *Radiology* 1993;189:505–509.

Resnick D, Greenway GD, Bardwick PA, Zvaifler NJ, Gill GN, Newman DR. Plasma cell dyscrasia with polyneuropathy, organomegaly, endocrinopathy, M-protein, and skin changes: the POEMS syndrome. *Radiology* 1981;140:17–22.

Resnick D, Niwayama G. Skeletal metastases. In: Resnick D, ed. *Diagnosis of bone and joint disorders,* 3rd ed. Philadelphia: WB Saunders; 1995:3991–4065.

Ricci C, Cova M, Kang YS, et al. Normal age-related patterns of cellular and fatty bone marrow distribution in the axial skeleton: MR imaging study. *Radiology* 1990;177:83–88.

Rice RW, Cabot A, Johnston A. The application of electron microscopy to the diagnostic differentiation of Ewing's sarcoma and reticulum cell sarcoma of bone. *Clin Orthop* 1973;97:174–184.

Rich TA, Schiller A, Suit HD, Mankin HJ. Clinical and pathologic review of 48 cases of chordoma. *Cancer* 1985;56:182–187.

Rock MG, Beabout JW, Unni KK, Sim FH. Adamantinoma. *Orthopedics* 1983;6:472–477.

Ros PR, Viamonte M Jr, Rywlin AM. Malignant fibrous histiocytoma: mesenchymal tumor of ubiquitous origin. *AJR Am J Roentgenol* 1984;142:753–759.

Rosai J. Adamantinoma of the tibia: electron microscopic evidence of its epithelial origin. *Am J Clin Pathol* 1969;51:786–792.

Rosai J, Pinkus GS. Immunohistochemical demonstration of epithelial differentiation in adamantinoma of the tibia. *Am J Surg Pathol* 1982;6:427–434.

Rosenberg AE. Malignant fibrous histiocytoma: past, present, and future. *Skeletal Radiol* 2003;32:613–618.

Rosenthal DI, Scott JA, Mankin HJ, Wismer GL, Brady TJ. Sacrococcygeal chordoma: magnetic resonance imaging and computed tomography. *AJR Am J Roentgenol* 1985;145:143–147.

Rosenthal DI, Treat ME, Mankin HJ, Rosenberg AE, Jennings CL. Treatment of epithelioid hemangioendothelioma of bone using a novel combined approach. *Skeletal Radiol* 2001;30:219–222.

Rousselin B, Vanel D, Terrier-Lacombe MJ, Istria BJM, Spielman M, Masselot J. Clinical and radiologic analysis of 13 cases of primary neuro-ectodermal tumors of the bone. *Skeletal Radiol* 1989;18:115–120.

Ruzek KA, Wenger DE. The multiple faces of lymphoma of the musculoskeletal system. *Skeletal Radiol* 2004;33:1–8.

Saifuddin A, Whelan J, Pringle JAS, Cannon SR. Malignant round cell tumours of bone: atypical clinical and imaging features. *Skeletal Radiol* 2000;29:646–651.

Sartoris DJ, Pate D, Haghighi P, Greenway G, Resnick D. Plasma cell sclerosis of bone: a spectrum of disease. *Can Assoc Radiol J* 1986;37:25–34.

Schajowicz F. Ewing's sarcoma and reticulum cell sarcoma of bone: with special reference to the histochemical demonstration of glycogen as an aid to differential diagnosis. *J Bone Joint Surg [Am]* 1959;41A:349–356.

Schajowicz F. *Tumors and tumorlike lesions of bone, pathology, radiology, and treatment,* 2nd ed. Berlin: Springer-Verlag; 1994:301–367, 468–481, 552–566.

Schajowicz F, Santini-Araujo E. Adamantinoma of the tibia masked by fibrous dysplasia. Report of three cases. *Clin Orthop* 1989;238:294–301.

Schajowicz F, Velan O, Santini Araujo E, et al. Metastases of carcinoma in pagetic bone. *Clin Orthop* 1988;228:290–296.

Schweitzer ME, Levine C, Mitchell DG, Gannon FH, Gomella LG. Bull's-eyes and halos: useful MR discriminators of osseous metastases. *Radiology* 1993;188:249–252.

Seiss SW, Enzinger FM. Malignant fibrous histiocytoma: an analysis of 200 cases. *Cancer* 1978;41:2250–2260.

Shih WJ, Riley C, Magoun S, Ryo UY. Paget's disease mimicking skeletal metastases in a patient with coexisting prostatic carcinoma. *Eur J Nucl Med* 1988;15:422–423.

Shimpo S. Solitary myeloma causing polyneuritis and endocrine disorders. *Jpn J Clin Med* 1968;26:2444–2456.

Shirley SK, Gilula LA, Segal GP, Foulkes MA, Kissane JM, Askin FB. Roentgenographic-pathologic correlation of diffuse sclerosis in Ewing's sarcoma of bone. *Skeletal Radiol* 1984;12:69–78.

Sim FH, Frassica FJ. Metastatic bone disease. In: Unni KK, ed. *Bone tumors.* New York: Churchill Livingstone; 1988:226.

Simon MA, Bartucci EJ. The search for the primary tumor in patients with skeletal metastases of unknown origin. *Cancer* 1986;58:1088–1095.

Smith J. Radiation-induced sarcoma of bone: clinical and radiographic findings in 43 patients irradiated for soft tissue neoplasms. *Clin Radiol* 1982;33:205–221.

Smith J, Ludwig RL, Marcove RC. Sacrococcygeal chordoma. A clinicoradiological study of 60 patients. *Skeletal Radiol* 1987;16:37–44.

Smith J, Reuter V, Demas B. Case report 576. Anaplastic sacrococcygeal chordoma (dedifferentiated chordoma). *Skeletal Radiol* 1989;18:561–564.

Smoker WR, Godersky JC, Knutzon RK, Keyes WD, Norman D, Bergman W. The role of MR imaging in evaluating metastatic spinal disease. *AJR Am J Roentgenol* 1987;149:1241–1248.

Söderlund V. Radiological diagnosis of skeletal metastases. *Eur Radiol* 1996;6:587–595.

Soule EH, Enriquez P. Atypical fibrous histiocytoma, malignant fibrous histiocytoma, malignant histiocytoma, and epithelioid sarcoma. A comparative study of 65 tumors. *Cancer* 1972;30:128–143.

Spanier SS, Enneking WF, Enriquez P. Primary malignant fibrous histiocytoma of bone. *Cancer* 1975;36:2084–2098.

Spjut HJ, Dorfman HD, Fechner RE, Ackerman LV. *Atlas of tumor pathology. Tumors of bone and cartilage,* 2nd series, fascicle 5. Washington DC: Armed Forces Institute of Pathology, 1971:347–390.

Springfield DS, Rosenberg AE, Mankin HJ, Mindell ER. Relationship between osteofibrous dysplasia and adamantinoma. *Clin Orthop* 1994;309:234–244.

Stäbler A, Baur A, Bartl R, Munker R, Lamerz R, Reiser MF. Contrast enhancement and quantitative signal analysis in MR imaging of multiple myeloma: assessment of focal and diffuse growth patterns in marrow correlated with biopsies and survival rates. *AJR Am J Roentgenol* 1996;167:1029–1036.

Stein H, Kaiserling E, Lennert K. Evidence for B-cell origin of reticulum cell sarcoma. *Virchows Arch (A)* 1974;A364:51–67.

Steiner GC. Neuroectodermal tumor versus Ewing's sarcoma. Immuno histochemical and electron microscopic observations. *Curr Top Pathol* 1989;80:1–29.

Steiner GC, Matano S, Present D. Ewing's sarcoma of humerus with epithelial differentiation. *Skeletal Radiol* 1995;24:379–382.

Steiner RM, Mitchell DG, Rao VM, Schweitzer ME. Magnetic resonance imaging of diffuse bone marrow disease. *Radiol Clin North Am* 1993;31:383–409.

Stiglbauer R, Augustin I, Kramer J, Schurawitzki H, Imhof H, Rodaszkiewicz T. MRI in the diagnosis of primary lymphoma of bone: correlation with histopathology. *J Comput Assist Tomogr* 1992;16:248–253.

Strauchen JA, Dimitriu-Bona A. Malignant fibrous histiocytoma: expression of monocyte-macrophage differentiation antigens detected with monoclonal antibodies. *Am J Pathol* 1986;124:303–309.

Stout AP, Lattes R. Tumors of the soft tissues. In: *Atlas of tumor pathology,* 2nd fascicle, series 1. Washington DC: Armed Forces Institute of Pathology; 1967.

Sundaram M, Akduman I, White LM, McDonald DJ, Kandel R, Janney C. Primary leiomyosarcoma of bone. *AJR Am J Roentgenol* 1999;172:771–776.

Sundaram M, McLeod RA. MR imaging of tumor and tumorlike lesions of bone and soft tissue. *AJR Am J Roentgenol* 1990;155:817–824.

Sweet DE, Vinh TN, Devaney K. Cortical osteofibrous dysplasia of long bone and its relationship to adamantinoma. A clinicopathologic study of 30 cases. *Am J Surg Pathol* 1992;16:282–290.

Sze G, Uichanco LS III, Brant-Zawadzki MN, et al. Chordomas: MR imaging. *Radiology* 1988;166:187–191.

Taconis WK, Mulder JD. Fibrosarcoma and malignant fibrous histiocytoma of long bones: radiographic features and grading. *Skeletal Radiol* 1984;11:237–245.

Taconis WK, Van Rijssel TG. Fibrosarcoma of long bones: a study of the significance of areas of malignant fibrous histiocytoma. *J Bone Joint Surg [Br]* 1985;67B:111–116.

Taylor JR. Persistence of the notochondral canal in vertebrae. *J Anat* 1982;11:211–217.

Tehranzadeh J, Fanney D, Ghandur-Mnaymneh L, Ganz W, Mnaymneh W. Case report 517. Ulcerating adamantinoma of the tibia. *Skeletal Radiol* 1989;17:614–619.

Tertti R, Alanen A, Remes K. The value of magnetic resonance imaging in screening myeloma lesions of the lumbar spine. *Br J Haematol* 1995;91:658–660.

Thiery JP, Mazabraud A, Mignot J, Durigon M. Electron microscopic study of a sacral chordoma. Characterization of various evolutive stages of the tumoral cells. *Ann Anat Pathol* 1977;22:193–204.

Traill Z, Richards MA, Moore NR. Magnetic resonance imaging of metastatic bone disease. *Clin Orthop* 1995;312:76–88.

Thrall JH, Ellis BI. Skeletal metastases. *Radiol Clin North Am* 1987;25:1155–1170.

Trias A, Fery A. Cortical circulation of long bones. *J Bone Joint Surg [Am]* 1979;61A:1052–1059.

Triche T, Cavazzana A. Round cell tumors of bone. In: Unni KK, ed. *Bone tumors.* New York: Churchill Livingstone; 1988:199–223.

Triche TJ, Askin FB, Kissane JM. Neuroblastoma, Ewing's sarcoma and the differential diagnosis of small, round blue cell tumors. In: Finegold M, ed. *Pathology of neoplasia in children and adolescents*. Philadelphia: WB Saunders; 1986:145–156.

Trillet V, Revel D, Combaret V. Bone marrow metastases in small cell lung cancer: detection with magnetic resonance imaging and monoclonal antibodies. *Br J Cancer* 1989;60:83–88.

Turner ML, Mulhern CB, Dalinka MK. Lesions of the sacrum. Differential diagnosis and radiological evaluation. *JAMA* 1981;245:275–277.

Ueda Y, Roessner A, Bosse A, Edel G, Bocker W, Wuisman P. Juvenile intracortical adamantinoma of the tibia with predominant osteofibrous dysplasia-like features. *Pathol Res Pract* 1991;187:1039–1043.

Uhrenholt L, Stimpel H. Histochemistry of sacrococcygeal chordoma. *APMIS (A)* 1985;93:203–204.

Unni KK. Osteosarcoma of bone. In: Unni KK, ed. *Bone tumors*. New York: Churchill Livingstone; 1988:107–133.

Unni KK. Fibrous and fibrohistiocytic lesions of bone. *Semin Orthop* 1991;6:177–186.

Unni KK. *Dahlin's bone tumors: General aspects and data on 11,087 cases*, 5th ed. New York: Lippincott-Raven; 1996.

Unni KK, Dahlin DC, Beabout JW, Ivins JC. Adamantinoma of long bones. *Cancer* 1974;34:1796–1805.

Vanel D, Contesso G, Couanet D, Piekarski JD, Sarrazin D, Masselot J. Computed tomography in the evaluation of 41 cases of Ewing's sarcoma. *Skeletal Radiol* 1982;9:8–13.

Vanel D, Couanet D, Leclerc J, Patte C. Early detection of bone metastases of Ewing's sarcoma by magnetic resonance imaging. *Diagn Imaging Clin Med* 1986;55:381–383.

Vieco PT, Azouz EM, Hoeffel J-C. Metastases to bone in medulloblastoma. A report of five cases. *Skeletal Radiol* 1989;18:445–449.

Vilar JL, Lezena AH, Pedrosa CS. Spiculated periosteal reaction in metastatic lesions in bone. *Skeletal Radiol* 1979;3:230–233.

Vincent JM, Ng YY, Norton AJ, Armstrong PA. Case report. Primary lymphoma of bone: MRI appearances with pathological correlation. *Clin Radiol* 1992;45:407–409.

Voss SD, Murphey MD, Hall FM. Solitary osteosclerotic plasmacytoma: association with demyelinating polyneuropathy and amyloid deposition. *Skeletal Radiol* 2001; 30:527–529.

Weiss SW. Ultrastructure of the so-called "chordoid sarcoma." Evidence supporting cartilaginous differentiation. *Cancer* 1976;37:300–306.

Weiss SW, Bratthauer GL, Morris PA. Post-radiation malignant fibrous histiocytoma expressing cytokeratin: implications for the immunodiagnosis of sarcomas. *Am J Surg Pathol* 1988;12:554–558.

Weiss SW, Dorfman HD. Adamantinoma of long bone. An analysis of nine new cases with emphasis on metastasizing lesions and fibrous dysplasia-like changes. *Hum Pathol* 1977;8:141–153.

Weiss SW, Enzinger FM. Malignant fibrous histiocytoma: an analysis of 200 cases. *Cancer* 1978;41:2250–2266.

Wenger DE, Wold LE. Malignant vascular lesions of bone: radiologic and pathologic features. *Skeletal Radiol* 2000;29:619–631.

White LM, Schweitzer ME, Khalili K, Howarth DJC, Wunder JS, Bell RS. MR imaging of primary lymphoma of bone: variability of T2-weighted signal intensity. *AJR Am J Roentgenol* 1998;170:1243–1247.

Wilkins RM, Pritchard DJ, Burgert EO, Unni KK. Ewing's sarcoma of bone. Experience with 140 patients. *Cancer* 1986;58:2551–2555.

Wilner D. *Cancer metastasis to bone. In: Radiology of bone tumors and allied disorders*. Philadelphia: WB Saunders; 1982:3641–3908.

Wilner D. *Radiology of bone tumors and allied disorders*. Philadelphia: Lea & Febiger, 1982.

Wippold FJ III, Koeller KK, Smirniotopoulos JG. Clinical and imaging features of cervical chordoma. *AJR Am J Roentgenol* 1999;172:1423–1426.

Wood GS, Beckstead JH, Turner RR, Hendrickson MR, Kempson RL, Warnke RA. Malignant fibrous histiocytoma tumor cells resemble fibroblasts. *Am J Surg Pathol* 1986;10:323–335.

Woolfenden JM, Pitt MJ, Durie BGM, Moon TE. Comparison of bone scintigraphy and radiography in multiple myeloma. *Radiology* 1980;134:723–728.

Yamaguchi T, Tamai K, Yamato M, Honma K, Ueda Y, Saotome K. Inter trabecular pattern of tumors metastatic to bone. *Cancer* 1996;78:1388–1394.

Yochum TR, Rowe LJ. Tumor and tumor-like processes. In: Yochum TR, Rowe LJ, eds. *Essentials of skeletal radiology*, vol 2, Baltimore: Williams & Wilkins; 1987:699–919.

Yoneyama T, Winter WG, Milsow L. Tibial adamantinoma: its histogenesis from ultrastructural studies. *Cancer* 1977;40:1138–1142.

Yuh WT, Flickinger FW, Barloon TJ, Montgomery WJ. MR imaging of unusual chordomas. *J Comput Assist Tomogr* 1988;12:30–35.

Zehr RJ, Recht MP, Bauer TW. Adamantinoma. *Skeletal Radiol* 1995;24:553–555.

CHAPTER 23

TUMORS AND TUMOR-LIKE LESIONS OF THE JOINTS

Benign Lesions

Synovial (Osteo)Chondromatosis

Synovial (osteo)chondromatosis (also known as synovial chondromatosis or synovial chondrometaplasia) is an uncommon benign disorder marked by the metaplastic proliferation of multiple cartilaginous nodules in the synovial membrane of the joints, bursae, or tendon sheaths. It is almost invariably monoarticular; rarely, multiple joints may be affected. The disorder is twice as common in men as in women and is usually discovered in the third to fifth decade. The knee is a preferential site of involvement, with the hip, shoulder, and elbow accounting for most of the remaining cases (Fig. 23.1). Patients usually report pain and swelling. Joint effusion, tenderness, limited motion in the joint, and a soft-tissue mass are common clinical findings.

Three phases of articular disease have been identified: an initial phase, characterized by metaplastic formation of cartilaginous nodules in the synovium; a transitional phase, characterized by detach-

ment of those nodules and formation of free intraarticular bodies; and an inactive phase, in which synovial proliferation has resolved but loose bodies remain in the joint, usually with variable amounts of joint fluid.

The radiographic findings depend on the degree of calcification within the cartilaginous bodies, ranging from mere joint effusion to visualization of many radiopaque joint bodies, usually small and uniform in size (Fig. 23.2). The best proof that the bodies are indeed intraarticular is achieved by arthrography or computed tomography (CT) (Fig. 23.3). These modalities can visualize even noncalcified bodies. Magnetic resonance imaging (MRI) may also be helpful, although MRI appearance is variable and depends on the relative preponderance of synovial proliferation, loose bodies formation, and extent of calcification or ossification. Unmineralized hyperplastic synovial masses exhibit high signal intensity on T2-weighted images, whereas calcifications can be seen as signal void against the high-signal-intensity fluid (Figs. 23.4 and 23.5). In addition to revealing loose bodies in the joint, CT and MRI may demonstrate bony erosion.

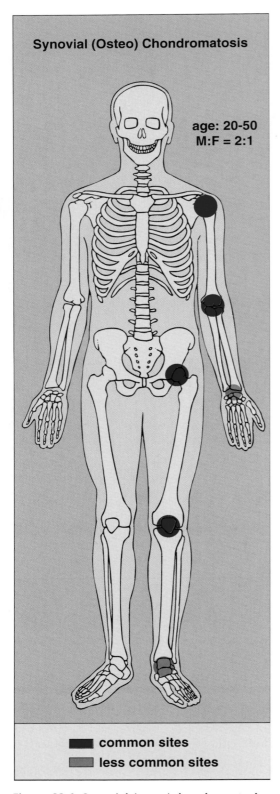

Figure 23.1 Synovial (osteo)chondromatosis: skeletal sites of predilection, peak age range, and male-to-female ratio.

Figure 23.2 Synovial chondromatosis. A 23-year-old man reported pain and occasional locking in the elbow joint; he had no history of trauma. Anteroposterior (**A**) and lateral (**B**) radiographs demonstrate multiple osteochondral bodies in the elbow joint, which are regularly shaped and uniform in size. This finding is characteristic of synovial chondromatosis.

Figure 23.3 CT of synovial chondromatosis. (A) Anteroposterior radiograph of the right hip of a 27-year-old woman shows multiple osteochondral bodies around the femoral head and neck. Note preservation of the joint space, a characteristic feature of synovial (osteo)chondromatosis. **(B), (C)** Two CT sections, one through the femoral head and another through the femoral neck, demonstrate unquestionably the intraarticular location of multiple osteochondral bodies.

Figure 23.4 MRI of synovial chondromatosis. (A) Oblique radiograph of the left ankle of a 14-year-old boy shows faint radiopaque foci projecting over the tibiotalar joint *(arrows)*. **(B)** CT section shows the location of calcified bodies in the anterior aspect of the joint. **(C)** Sagittal T1-weighted (SE; TR 640/TE 20 msec) MR image shows intermediate signal intensity of the fluid in the ankle joint and dispersed low-signal-intensity osteochondral bodies. **(D)** Coronal T2-weighted (SE; TR 2000/TE 80 msec) MR image of the ankle joint clearly defines low-signal-intensity osteochondral bodies within bright fluid. These findings are consistent with a diagnosis of synovial (osteo)chondromatosis.

Figure 23.5 MRI of synovial chondromatosis. (A) Lateral radiograph of the left knee of a 50-year-old man shows multiple osteochondral bodies in and around the joint. **(B)** Axial T2*-weighted (MPGR; TR 500/TE 20 msec, flip angle 30°) MR image demonstrates high-signal joint effusion and multiple bodies of intermediate signal intensity, primarily located in a large popliteal cyst. Coronal **(C)** fast spin-echo (TR 2400/TE 85 Ef msec) and sagittal **(D)** fast spin-echo (TR 3400/TE 85 Ef msec) MR images show to better advantage the distribution of numerous osteochondral bodies.

By microscopy, many cartilaginous nodules are observed as they form beneath the thin layer of cells that line the surface of the synovial membrane. These nodules are highly cellular, and the cells themselves may exhibit a moderate pleomorphism, with occasional plump and double nuclei. The cartilaginous nodules, which often are undergoing calcification and endochondral ossification, may detach and become loose bodies. The loose bodies continue to be viable and may increase in size as they receive nourishment from the synovial fluid.

Differential Diagnosis

Synovial (osteo)chondromatosis should be differentiated from the secondary osteochondromatosis caused by osteoarthritis, particularly in the knee and hip joints, and from synovial chondrosarcoma, either primary (arising *de novo* from the synovial membrane) or secondary (caused by malignant transformation). Distinguishing *primary* from *secondary osteochondromatosis* usually presents no problems. In the latter condition, there is invariably

radiographic evidence of osteoarthritis with all of its typical features, such as narrowing of the radiographic joint space, subchondral sclerosis, and, occasionally, periarticular cysts or cyst-like lesions (Fig. 23.6). The loose bodies are fewer, larger, and invariably of different sizes. Conversely, in primary synovial (osteo)chondromatosis the joint is not affected by any degenerative changes. In some cases, however, the bone may show erosions secondary to pressure of the calcified bodies on the outer aspects of the cortex. The intraarticular bodies are numerous, small, and usually of uniform size (see Fig. 23.2).

It is more difficult to distinguish synovial chondromatosis from *synovial chondrosarcoma*. The clinical and radiographic features have not been useful in this differentiation and are equally ineffective in distinguishing a secondary malignant lesion arising in synovial (osteo)chondromatosis. In addition, both entities tend to have a protracted clinical course, and local recurrence is common after synovectomy for synovial chondromatosis or local resection of synovial

Figure 23.6 Secondary osteochondromatosis. (A) Lateral radiograph of the knee in a 58-year-old man with advanced osteoarthritis of the femoropatellar joint compartment shows multiple osteochondral bodies in the suprapatellar bursa and within the popliteal cyst. **(B)** Radiograph of the left shoulder in a 68-year-old woman with osteoarthritis of the glenohumeral joint shows multiple intraarticular osteochondral bodies. **(C)** Sagittal T2-weighted fat-suppressed MRI of the knee in a 54-year-old woman reveals osteoarthritis and numerous osteochondral bodies (arrows).

chondrosarcoma. The presence of frank bone destruction rather than merely erosions, and the association of a soft-tissue mass, should always raise a concern for malignancy (see Fig. 23.17). Although extension beyond the joint capsule should heighten the suspicion of malignancy, some cases of synovial chondromatosis have been reported to have extraarticular extension.

The other conditions that can radiologically mimic synovial chondromatosis include pigmented villonodular synovitis, synovial hemangioma, and lipoma arborescens. In *pigmented villonodular synovitis* (discussed in detail later in this chapter), the filling defects in the joint are more confluent and less distinct. Magnetic resonance imaging (MRI) may show foci of decreased intensity of the synovium in all sequences because of the paramagnetic effects of deposition of hemosiderin (see Figs. 23.10 and 23.11). *Synovial hemangioma* usually presents as a single soft-tissue mass. On MRI, T1-weighted images show that the lesion is either isointense or slightly higher (brighter) in signal intensity than surrounding muscles, but much lower in intensity than subcutaneous fat.

On T2-weighted images, the mass is invariably much brighter than fat (see Fig. 23.13). Phleboliths and fibrofatty septa in the mass are common findings that show low-signal characteristics. *Lipoma arborescens* is a villous lipomatous proliferation of the synovial membrane. This rare condition usually affects the knee joint but has occasionally been reported in other joints, including the wrist and ankle. The disease has been variously reported to have a developmental, traumatic, inflammatory, or neoplastic origin, but its true cause is still unknown. The clinical findings include slowly increasing but painless synovial thickening as well as joint effusion with sporadic exacerbation. Radiographic studies reveal a joint effusion accompanied by various degrees of osteoarthritis. Histologic examination demonstrates complete replacement of the subsynovial tissue by mature fat cells and the formation of proliferative villous projections (see text below).

Treatment of synovial chondromatosis usually consists of removal of the intraarticular bodies and synovectomy, but local recurrence is not uncommon.

Pigmented Villonodular Synovitis

Pigmented villonodular synovitis (PVNS) is a locally destructive fibro-histiocytic proliferation, characterized by many villous and nodular synovial protrusions, which affects joints, bursae, and tendon sheaths. PVNS was first described by Jaffe, Lichtenstein, and Sutro in 1941, who used this name to identify the lesion because of its yellow–brown, villous, and nodular appearance. The yellow–brown pigmentation is caused by excessive deposits of lipid and hemosiderin. This condition can be diffuse or localized. When the entire synovium of the joint is affected, and when there is a major villous component, the condition is referred to as *diffuse pigmented villonodular synovitis*. When a discrete intraarticular mass is present, the condition is called *localized pigmented villonodular synovitis*. When the process affects the tendon sheaths, it is called *localized giant cell tumor of the tendon sheaths*. The diffuse form usually occurs in the knee, hip, elbow, or wrist and accounts for 23% of cases. The localized nodular form is often regarded as a separate entity. It consists of a single polypoid mass attached to the synovium. Nodular tenosynovitis is most often seen in the fingers and is the second most common soft-tissue tumor of the hand, exceeded only by the ganglion.

Both the diffuse and the localized form of villonodular synovitis usually occur as a single lesion, mainly in young and middle-aged individuals of either sex. One of the most characteristic findings in PVNS is the ability of the hyperplastic synovium to invade the subchondral bone, producing cysts and erosions. Although the cause is unknown and is often controversial, some investigators have suggested an autoimmune pathogenesis. Trauma is also a suspected cause, because similar effects have been produced experimentally in animals by repeated injections of blood into the knee joint. Some investigators have suggested a disturbance in lipid metabolism as a causative factor. It has also been postulated by Jaffe and colleagues that these lesions may represent an inflammatory response to an unknown agent. Ray, Stout, and Lattes postulated that they are true benign neoplasms. Although the latter theory was presumed to be supported by pathologic studies indicating that the histiocytes present in PVNS may function as facultative fibroblasts and that foam cells may derive from histiocytes, thus relating PVNS to a benign neoplasm of fibrohistiocytic origin, these findings do not constitute definite proof that PVNS is a true neoplasm. They are rather indicative of a special form of a chronic proliferative inflammation process, as has already been postulated by Jaffe and colleagues.

Clinically, PVNS is a slowly progressive process that manifests as mild pain and joint swelling with limitation of motion. Occasionally, increased skin temperature is noted over the affected joint. The knee joint is most commonly affected and 66% of patients present with a bloody joint effusion. In fact, the presence of a serosanguinous synovial fluid in the absence of a history of recent trauma should strongly suggest the diagnosis of PVNS. The synovial fluid contains elevated levels of cholesterol, and fluid reaccumulates rapidly after aspiration. Other joints may be affected, including the hip, ankle, wrist, elbow, and shoulder. There is a 2:1 predilection for females. Patients range from 4 to 60 years of age, with a peak incidence in the third and fourth decades (Fig. 23.7). The duration of symptoms can range from 6 months to as long as 25 years.

Radiography reveals a soft-tissue density in the affected joint, frequently interpreted as joint effusion. However, the density is greater than that of simple effusion, and it reflects not only a hemorrhagic fluid but also lobulated synovial masses (Fig. 23.8). A marginal, well-defined erosion of subchondral bone with a sclerotic margin may be present (incidence reported from 15% to 50%), usually on both sides of the affected articulation. Narrowing of the joint space has also been reported. In the hip, multiple cyst-like or erosive areas involving non-weight-bearing regions of the acetabulum, as well as the femoral head and neck, are characteristic. Calcifications are encountered only in exceptional cases.

Arthrography reveals multiple lobulated masses with villous projections, which appear as filling defects in the contrast-filled suprapatellar bursa (Fig. 23.9). CT effectively demonstrates the extent of the

Figure 23.7 Pigmented villonodular synovitis: sites of predilection, peak age range, and male-to-female ratio.

disease. The increase in iron content of the synovial fluid results in high Hounsfield values, a feature that can help in the differential diagnosis. MRI is extremely useful in making a diagnosis, because on T2-weighted images the intraarticular masses demonstrate a combination of high-signal-intensity areas, representing fluid and congested synovium, interspersed with areas of intermediate to low signal intensity, secondary to random distribution of hemosiderin in the synovium (Fig. 23.10). In general, MRI shows a low signal on T1- and T2-weighted images because of hemosiderin deposition and thick fibrous

Figure 23.8 Pigmented villonodular synovitis. Lateral radiograph of the knee of a 58-year-old man shows a large suprapatellar joint effusion and a dense, lumpy soft-tissue mass eroding the posterior aspect of the lateral femoral condyle. These features suggest pigmented villonodular synovitis. Note that posteriorly the density is greater than that of a suprapatellar fluid.

Figure 23.9 Arthrography of pigmented villonodular synovitis. (A) Lateral radiograph of another patient shows what appears to be a suprapatellar effusion (*arrows*). The density of the "fluid," however, is increased, and there is some lobulation evident. **(B)** Contrast arthrogram of the knee shows lobulated filling defects in the suprapatellar pouch, representing lumpy synovial masses. Joint puncture yielded thick bloody fluid, which explains the increased density of the soft-tissue mass seen on the plain film. Biopsy confirmed the diagnosis of pigmented villonodular synovitis.

Figure 23.10 MRI of pigmented villonodular synovitis. A 22-year-old woman had several episodes of knee pain and swelling. Bloody fluid was aspirated from the knee joint on two occasions. **(A)** Lateral radiograph of the right knee shows fullness in the suprapatellar bursa that was interpreted as "joint effusion." Note also the increased density in the region of the popliteal fossa and subtle erosion of the posterior aspect of the distal femur (*arrow*). **(B)** Sagittal MRI (SE; TR 800/TE 20 msec) shows a lobulated mass in the suprapatellar bursa, extending into the knee joint and invading the infrapatellar fat. Note also the lobulated mass in the posterior aspect of the joint capsule, extending toward the proximal tibia. These masses demonstrate an intermediate to low signal intensity. The erosion at the posterior aspect of the distal femur (supracondylar) is clearly demonstrated by an area of low signal intensity. **(C)** Coronal MRI (SE; TR 1800/TE 80 msec) demonstrates areas of high signal intensity that represent fluid and congested synovium, interspersed with areas of intermediate to low signal intensity, characteristic of hemosiderin deposits.

tissue (Fig. 23.11). In addition, within the mass, signals consistent with fat can be noted, which are caused by clumps of lipid-laden macrophages. Other MRI findings include hyperplastic synovium and occasionally bone erosions. Administration of gadolinium in the form of Gd-DTPA leads to a notable increase in overall heterogeneity, which tends toward an overall increase in signal intensity of the capsule and septae. This enhancement of the synovium allows it to be differentiated from the fluid invariably present, which does not enhance. Apart from its diagnostic effectiveness, MRI is also useful in defining the extent of the disease.

On histologic examination, PVNS reveals a tumor-like proliferation of the synovial tissue. A dense infiltration of mononuclear histio-

cytes is observed, accompanied by plasma cells, xanthoma cells, lymphocytes, and variable numbers of giant cells. Long-standing lesions show fibrosis and hyalinization.

Differential Diagnosis

The most common diagnostic possibilities include *hemophilic arthropathy, synovial chondromatosis,* and *synovial hemangioma.* MRI is very effective in distinguishing these entities because it can reveal hemosiderin deposition in PVNS. Although this feature may also be present in *hemophilic arthropathy,* detection of diffuse hemosiderin clumps, synovial irregularity and thickening, and distention of the synovial sac favor the diagnosis of PVNS. In addition, hemophilia,

Figure 23.11 MRI of pigmented villonodular synovitis. Coronal **(A)** and sagittal **(B)** T1-weighted (SE; TR 600/TE 12 msec) MR images of the knee of a 40-year-old man show lobulated low-signal-intensity masses mainly localized to the popliteal fossa. **(C)** Sagittal T2-weighted (SE; TR 2300/TE 80 msec) MR image shows high-intensity fluid in the suprapatellar bursa. The lobulated masses of pigmented villonodular synovitis remain of low signal intensity.

unlike PVNS, commonly affects multiple joints and is associated with growth disturbance at the articular ends of the affected bones. *Synovial chondromatosis* may manifest with pressure erosions of the bone similar to those of PVNS. However, it can be distinguished by the presence of multiple joint bodies, calcified or uncalcified. *Synovial hemangioma* is commonly associated with formation of phleboliths.

Treatment

Treatment usually consists of surgical or arthroscopic synovectomy. Occasionally, intraarticular radiation synovectomy is used when the abnormal synovial tissue is less than 5 mm thick. Local recurrence is not uncommon and is reported in approximately 50% of cases.

Synovial Hemangioma

Synovial hemangioma is a rare benign lesion that most commonly affects the knee joint, usually involving the anterior compartment. This lesion has also been found in the elbow, wrist, and ankle joints, as well as in tendon sheaths. Most cases affect children and adolescents. Almost all patients with synovial hemangioma are symptomatic, frequently presenting with a swollen knee or with mild pain or limitation of movement in the joint. Sometimes patients report a history of recurrent episodes of joint swelling and various degrees of pain of several years' duration. Synovial hemangioma is often associated with an adjacent cutaneous or deep soft-tissue hemangioma. For this reason, some investigators classify knee joint lesions as intraarticular, juxta-articular, or intermediate, depending on the extent of involvement. Synovial hemangioma is frequently misdiagnosed. According to one estimate, a correct preoperative diagnosis is made in only 22% of cases.

Until recently, synovial hemangiomas were evaluated by a combination of conventional radiography, arthrography, angiography, and contrast-enhanced CT. Although radiographs appear normal in at least half of the patients, they may reveal soft-tissue swelling, a mass around the joint, joint effusion, or erosions (Fig. 23.12). Phleboliths, periosteal thickening, advanced maturation of the epiphysis, and arthritic changes are also occasionally noted on conventional radiographs. Arthrography usually shows nonspecific filling defects with a villous configuration. Angiograms yield much more specific information than radiography. They can often reveal a vascular lesion and can demonstrate pathognomonic features of hemangioma. Contrast-enhanced CT of the joint typically reveals a heterogeneous-appearing soft-tissue mass that displays tissue attenuation approximating that of skeletal muscle and containing areas of decreased attenuation, some approaching that of fat. CT is effective for demonstrating phleboliths and revealing patchy enhancement around them, as well as enhancement of tubular areas and contrast pooling within the lesion. In some cases, CT reveals enlarged vessels feeding and draining the mass, as well as enlarged adjacent subcutaneous veins.

Recently, MRI has become the modality of choice for evaluation of hemangiomas because with this modality, a presumptive diagnosis can be made. The soft-tissue mass typically exhibits an intermediate signal intensity on T1-weighted sequences, appearing isointense with or slightly brighter than muscle but much less bright than fat. The mass is usually much brighter than subcutaneous fat on T2-weighted images and on fat suppression sequences (Fig. 23.13) and shows thin, often serpentine, low-intensity septa within it. In general, the signal intensity characteristics of hemangiomas appear to be related to a number of factors, including slow flow, thrombosis, vessel occlusion, and increased free water in stagnant blood that pools in larger vessels and dilated sinuses, as well as to the variable amounts of adipose tissue in the lesion. After intravenous injection of gadolinium, there is evidence of enhancement of the hemangioma. In patients with a cavernous hemangioma of the knee, fluid–fluid levels are also observed (Fig. 23.13B), a finding recently reported also in soft-tissue hemangiomas of this type.

Originating in the subsynovial layer mesenchyme of the synovial membrane, synovial hemangioma is a vascular lesion that contains variable amounts of adipose, fibrous, and muscle tissue, as well as thrombi in the vessels. When the lesion is completely intraarticular, it is usually well circumscribed and apparently encapsulated, attached to the synovial membrane by a pedicle of variable size, and adherent to the synovium on one or more surfaces by separable adhesions.

Figure 23.12 Synovial hemangioma. Anteroposterior (**A**) and lateral (**B**) radiographs of the right knee of a 7-year-old boy with synovial hemangioma show articular erosions at femoropatellar and femorotibial joint compartments. Soft-tissue masses are seen anteriorly and posteriorly. An incidental finding is a nonossifying fibroma in the posterior tibia (*arrowheads*).

Figure 23.13 MRI of synovial hemangioma. (A) Sagittal T1-weighted (SE; TR 400/TE 11 msec) MR image in a 9-year-old boy shows masses isointense with muscle involving the suprapatellar bursa and infrapatellar Hoffa fat. **(B)** With fat suppression technique the mass becomes very bright. The fluid–fluid level seen in the popliteal region is typical for the cavernous type of synovial hemangioma. **(C)** In another patient, a 16-year-old girl, axial T2*-weighted (MPGR; TR 500/TE 15 msec, flip angle 30°) MR image and **(D)** axial fast-spin echo (TR 5000/TE 85 Ef msec) image with fat suppression technique show the size and extent of the synovial hemangioma.

Grossly, the tumor is a lobulated soft, brown, doughy mass with overlying villous synovium that is often stained mahogany brown by hemosiderin. On microscopic examination, the lesion exhibits arborizing vascular channels of different sizes and a hyperplastic overlying synovium, which may show abundant iron deposition in chronic cases with repeated hemarthrosis.

Differential Diagnosis

The differential diagnosis of synovial hemangioma includes *PVNS* and *synovial chondromatosis*. All proliferative chronic inflammatory processes, such as rheumatoid arthritis, tuberculous arthritis, and hemophilic arthropathy, should also be considered in the differential, but these conditions, when involving the knee, can usually be distinguished clinically. Because it is extremely uncommon, lipoma arborescens is rarely included in the differential diagnosis. MRI is diagnostic for the latter condition, showing typical frond-like projections of the lesion and fat characteristics (bright on T1- and intermediate on T2-weighted images). In *PVNS*, radiography commonly reveals findings similar to those of synovial hemangioma, such as joint effusion and a mass in the suprapatellar bursa or popliteal fossa region. Radiographs may also demonstrate bone erosions on both sides of the joint. MRI, however, is usually diagnostic for PVNS, demonstrating that the synovium exhibits nodular thickening and masses of heterogeneous signal intensity. Most of the lesion will display a higher signal intensity than muscle on both T1- and T2-weighted sequences, with other portions exhibiting a low signal intensity on all sequences, reflecting the hemosiderin content of the

tumor. *Synovial chondromatosis* can be distinguished from synovial hemangioma if radiography shows calcified bodies. Intraarticular osteochondral fragments of uniform size are almost pathognomonic for this condition. CT may be helpful in demonstrating faint calcifications not otherwise seen.

Lipoma Arborescens

Lipoma arborescens, also known as villous lipomatous proliferation of the synovial membranes, is a rare intraarticular disorder characterized by non-neoplastic lipomatous proliferation of the synovium. The cause of this condition remains uncertain, although association with osteoarthritis, rheumatoid arthritis, psoriasis, and diabetes mellitus has been postulated. This lesion most commonly affects the knee joint, although involvement of other joints, such as shoulder, hip, wrist, elbow, and ankle, has been sporadically reported by various authors. It is more prevalent in males, usually in the fourth and fifth decades. These patients present with slowly increasing but painless joint effusion accompanied by synovial thickening.

Imaging studies, particularly MRI, are very characteristic and allow definite diagnosis of this condition. Joint effusion is invariably present, associated with frond-like masses arising from the synovium that have the signal intensity of fat on all imaging sequences (Fig. 23.14). Occasionally, a chemical shift artifact is present at the fat–fluid interface. Histopathologically, lipoma arborescens is characterized by hyperplasia of subsynovial fat, formation of mature fat cells, and the presence of proliferative villous projections.

Figure 23.14 MRI of lipoma arborescens. A 54-year-old woman reports fullness in the left knee for the past 5 months. Conventional radiography (not shown here) revealed knee joint effusion. **(A)** Sagittal proton-density MRI shows numerous structures within suprapatellar bursa exhibiting signal intensity consistent with fat (*arrows*). Coronal **(B)** and sagittal **(C)** T2-weighted fat-suppressed images demonstrate high-signal-intensity joint effusion. Hypertrophic synovial villa (*arrows*) again shows signal consistent with fat. Histopathologic examination of resected tissue was diagnostic for lipoma arborescens.

Figure 23.15 Synovial sarcoma. Lateral radiograph of the left ankle of a 71-year-old woman shows a large calcified mass located in the soft tissues anteriorly to the Achilles tendon, not affecting the adjacent bones. Excision biopsy revealed synovial sarcoma.

Differential diagnosis should include pigmented villonodular synovitis, synovial chondromatosis, synovial hemangioma, hemophilic arthropathy, and a variety of intraarticular inflammatory conditions.

Treatment usually consists of surgical or arthroscopic synovectomy.

Malignant Tumors

Synovial Sarcoma

Synovial sarcoma (synovioma) is an uncommon mesenchymal neoplasm, comprising approximately 8% to 10% of soft-tissue sarcomas. Despite its name (which was designated because of histologic resemblance of synovial sarcoma to normal synovial tissue), it does not arise from synovium, although it may originate from any other structure, including joint capsules, bursae, and tendon sheaths. The tumor usually occurs before age 50, most commonly between ages 16 and 36 years. There is no sex predilection. The extremities account for 83% of synovial sarcomas, and the most common sites are around the knee and foot. In exceptional instances, the tumor may be intraarticular. Synovial sarcoma is usually slow-growing, with an indolent course, although in late stages it may demonstrate aggressiveness. Metastases to the lung by the hematogenous route and to the soft tissue have been reported. Schajowicz cites a local recurrence rate of more than 50%. The clinical symptoms usually include soft-tissue swelling or a mass and progressive pain. On physical examination, a diffuse or discrete soft-tissue mass is present, usually tender on palpation.

The radiographic features of synovial sarcoma include a soft-tissue mass, usually in close proximity to a joint (Fig. 23.15) and occasionally associated with bone invasion. A periosteal reaction may also be observed. The soft-tissue calcifications, usually amorphous in type, are present in approximately 25% to 30% of cases.

CT effectively demonstrates the extent of the soft-tissue mass, calcifications, and bone invasion. MRI shows the tumor to be heterogeneous, septated mass of low to intermediate signal intensity with infiltrative margins on T1-weighted sequences, displaying a high signal on T2-weighting (Fig. 23.16).

On histopathologic examination, several subtypes of synovial sarcoma have been recognized. Among them are biphasic (fibrous and epithelial), monophasic, and poorly differentiated types. The classical biphasic type exhibits distinct spindle cell and epithelial components arranged in glandular or nest-like patterns. The monophasic synovial sarcoma is composed of interdigitating fascicles and "ball-like" structures formed by the spindle cells. Foci of calcification may also be observed, usually localized in areas of hyalinization within the spindle cell elements of the tumor.

Synovial Chondrosarcoma

Synovial chondrosarcoma is a rare tumor that originates from the synovial membrane. It may arise as a primary synovial tumor or it may develop as a malignant transformation of synovial (osteo)chondromatosis. The concept of malignant degeneration of synovial chondromatosis is still controversial and the entity is rare, with only 21 well-documented cases on record.

Most synovial chondrosarcomas are located in the knee joint. Rarely, other joints such as the hip, elbow, or ankle are affected. These

Figure 23.16 Scintigraphy and MRI of synovial sarcoma. (A) Anteroposterior radiograph of the left hip of a 37-year-old man shows an osteolytic lesion in the femoral neck bordered laterally by sclerotic margin. **(B)** Scintigraphic (blood pool) examination demonstrates increased vascularity to the left hip joint. **(C)** Delayed radionuclide bone scan with technetium-99m methylene diphosphonate (MDP) shows increased uptake of the radiopharmaceutical tracer in the femoral head and neck and around the hip joint. *(continued)*

Figure 23.16 Scintigraphy and MRI of synovial sarcoma. *Continued* **(D)** Coronal T1-weighted (SE; TR 850/TE 20 msec) MR image shows a low-signal-intensity lesion affecting the medial aspect of the femoral neck. **(E)** Coronal T2-weighted (SE; TR 2000/TE 80 msec) MR image demonstrates increased signal in the femoral neck and in the medial and lateral aspects of the hip joint. Excision biopsy revealed intraarticular synovial sarcoma.

malignancies show a slight predominance in men, and patients range in age from 25 to 70 years. The symptoms include pain and swelling, with duration in most patients exceeding 12 months. In patients with primary synovial (osteo)chondromatosis, malignant transformation to synovial chondrosarcoma should be clinically suspected if there is development of soft-tissue mass at the site of the affected joint.

Radiologically, the presence of chondroid calcifications within the joint, destruction of the adjacent bones, and a soft-tissue mass are highly suggestive of a synovial chondrosarcoma. In patients with documented primary synovial (osteo)chondromatosis, a soft-tissue mass and destructive changes in the joint should suggest the development of a secondary synovial chondrosarcoma (Fig. 23.17). Note, however, that frequently both uncomplicated synovial chondromatosis and synovial chondrosarcoma may exhibit similar features on radiography and MRI.

The histopathologic distinction between primary synovial chondromatosis and secondary malignancy in synovial chondromatosis has been a matter of dispute. Manivel and associates suggested that histologic features equivalent to those of grade 2 or 3 central chondrosarcoma must be present before chondrosarcoma arising in synovial chondromatosis can be diagnosed. Occasional foci of increased cellu-

larity showing hyperchromatic atypical cells, consistent with grade 1 chondrosarcoma, should not be sufficient evidence for a malignant change in synovial chondromatosis. However, evidence of aggressive growth (invasion) and a lesion's lack of attachment to the synovial lining, combined with hypercellularity and pleomorphisms of the cells, should support the diagnosis of malignancy. Bertoni and coworkers have attempted to develop criteria for making this crucial distinction. They identified several microscopic features indicative of malignancy. The distinguishing features of synovial chondrosarcoma include the following: tumor cells arranged in sheets, myxoid changes in the matrix, hypercellularity with crowding and spindling of nuclei at the periphery, necrosis, and permeation of bone trabeculae. Remarking on the danger of misinterpreting synovial chondromatosis as chondrosarcoma on both radiographic and histopathologic examination, Bertoni and colleagues singled out pulmonary metastases as the only distinguishing feature.

Differential Diagnosis

The main differential diagnosis is between synovial chondrosarcoma and synovial (osteo)chondromatosis. Frequently, the radiologic findings in both conditions are similar, although the development of de-

Figure 23.17 Malignant transformation of synovial osteochondromatosis to synovial chondrosarcoma. Anteroposterior **(A)** and lateral **(B)** radiographs of the right ankle of a 64-year-old man with a long history of synovial chondromatosis show a large soft-tissue mass on the dorsal aspect of the ankle joint, eroding the talus. Multiple calcifications, uniform in size and shape, are noted laterally. **(C)** After injection of 15 mCi (555 MBq) of technetium-99m-labeled methylene diphosphonate (MDP), there is increased uptake of radiopharmaceutical tracer in the right ankle. *(continued)*

Figure 23.17 Malignant transformation of synovial osteochondromatosis to synovial chondrosarcoma. *Continued* **(D)** Sagittal T1-weighted (SE; TR 400/TE 20 msec) MR image shows the mass displaying intermediate signal intensity, isointense with the muscles. **(E)** Parasagittal T1-weighted (SE; TR 400/TE 20 msec) MR image demonstrates the mass to be well encapsulated. **(F)** Coronal proton density (SE; TR 1800/TE 29 msec) MR image shows that the mass is continuous with the ankle joint. **(G)** Coronal T2-weighted (SE; TR 2000/TE 80 msec) MR image demonstrates the mass to be of high signal intensity. Punctate areas of low signal intensity within the mass represent calcifications.

structive changes around the affected joint favors synovial chondrosarcoma. However, these destructive changes should be differentiated from periarticular erosions occasionally present in synovial chondromatosis. PVNS can usually be excluded without much difficulty, because it does not exhibit calcifications and, in addition, shows rather characteristic MRI features (see previous text).

Malignant Pigmented Villonodular Synovitis

Recently, Kalil and Unni reported a case of malignancy in pigmented villonodular synovitis (PVNS) and cited eight other cases from the literature. Enzinger and Weiss defined malignant PVNS as a malignant lesion occurring with concomitant or previously documented benign PVNS at the same location. Bertoni and coworkers documented histologic evolution from benign to malignant PVNS in three cases. The malignancy in PVNS is an extremely rare occurrence, yet this is a controversial issue, mainly because other synovium-centered lesions, such as clear cell sarcoma or epithelioid sarcoma, may be mistaken for malignant PVNS.

PRACTICAL POINTS TO REMEMBER

[1] Characteristic radiographic findings of synovial (osteo)chondromatosis include joint effusion, numerous radiopaque osteochondral bodies (usually small and uniform in size), and bone erosions.

[2] Arthrography, CT, or MRI are effective imaging modalities to demonstrate noncalcified intraarticular bodies.

[3] Pigmented villonodular synovitis is invariably accompanied by serosanguinous synovial fluid. Radiography reveals a soft-tissue density in the affected joint caused by hemorrhagic fluid and lobulated synovial masses.

[4] MRI is very effective in diagnosis of PVNS because on T2 weighting, the intraarticular masses demonstrate a characteristic combination of high-signal-intensity areas representing fluid and congested synovium, interspersed with areas of intermediate to low signal intensity secondary to the presence of hemosiderin.

[5] Synovial hemangioma is best diagnosed by MRI. Characteristic imaging findings include a soft-tissue mass exhibiting an intermediate signal intensity on T1-weighted images (isointense with or slightly brighter than muscle but not as bright as fat), and high

signal on T2 weighting associated with serpentine low-intensity septa.

[6] Lipoma arborescens, a very rare intraarticular disorder, is characterized by non-neoplastic lipomatous proliferation of the synovium. MRI shows joint effusion and frond-like masses arising from the synovium that have the signal intensity of fat on all sequences.

[7] Synovial sarcoma is frequently located in close proximity to the joint. Calcifications and bone erosion are common findings.

[8] Synovial chondrosarcoma, a very rare tumor that originates from the synovial membrane, may be primary lesion or may develop in synovial chondromatosis.

SUGGESTED READINGS

Abdelwahab IF, Kenan S, Steiner GC, Abdul-Quader M. True bursal pigmented villonodular synovitis. *Skeletal Radiol* 2002;31:354–358.

Abrahams TG, Pavlov H, Bansal M, Bullough P. Concentric joint space narrowing of the hip associated with hemosiderotic synovitis (HS) including pigmented villonodular synovitis (PVNS). *Skeletal Radiol* 1988;17:37–45.

Ackerman LV. Extra-osseous localized non-neoplastic bone and cartilage formation (so-called myositis ossificans). Clinical and pathological confusion with malignant neoplasms. *J Bone Joint Surg [Am]* 1958;40A:279–298.

Aglietti P, Di Muria GV, Salvati EA, Stringa G. Pigmented vollonodular synovitis of the hip joint (review of the literature and report of personal case material). *Ital J Orthop Traumatol* 1983;9:487–496.

Armstrong SJ, Watt I. Lipoma arborescens of the knee. *Br J Radiol* 1989;62:178–180.

Atmore WG, Dahlin DC, Ghormley RK. Pigmented villonodular synovitis: a clinical and pathologic study. *Minn Med* 1956;39:196–202.

Azouz EM, Vicker DB, Brown KLB. Computed tomography of synovial sarcoma of the foot. *J Can Assoc Radiol* 1984;35:85–87.

Baker ND, Klein JD, Weidner N, Weissman BN, Brick GW. Pigmented villonodular synovitis containing coarse calcifications. *AJR Am J Roentgenol* 1989;153:1228–1230.

Balsara ZN, Staiken BF, Martinez AJ. MR image of localized giant cell tumor of the tendon sheath involving the knee. *J Comput Assist Tomogr* 1989;13:159–162.

Bertoni F, Unni KK, Beabout JW, Sim FH. Chondrosarcomas of the synovium. *Cancer* 1991;67:155–162.

Bertoni F, Unni KK, Beabout JW, Sim FH. Malignant giant cell tumor of the tendon sheaths and joints (malignant pigmented villonodular synovitis). *Am J Surg Path* 1997;21:153–163.

Besette PR, Cooley PA, Johnson RP, Czarnecki DJ. Gadolinium-enhanced MRI of pigmented villonodular synovitis of the knee. *J Comput Assist Tomogr* 1992;16:992–994.

Blacksin M, Adesokan A, Benevenia J. Case report 871. Synovial sarcoma, monophasic type. *Skeletal Radiol* 1994;23:589–591.

Blacksin MF, Ghelman B, Freiberger RH, Salvata E. Synovial chondromatosis of the hip: evaluation with air computed arthrotomography. *Clin Imaging* 1990;14:315–318.

Boyd AD Jr, Sledge CB. Evaluation of the hip with pigmented villonodular synovitis. A case report. *Clin Orthop* 1992;275:180–186.

Bravo SM, Winalski CS, Weissman BN. Pigmented villonodular synovitis. *Radiol Clin North Am* 1996;34:311–326.

Brodsky AE. Synovial hemangioma of the knee joint. *Bull Hosp Jt Dis Orthop Inst* 1956;17: 58–69.

Buetow PC, Kransdorf MJ, Moser RP Jr, Jelinek JS, Berrey BH. Radiologic appearance of intramuscular hemangioma with emphasis on MR imaging. *AJR Am J Roentgenol* 1990;154:563–567.

Bullough PG. *Atlas of orthopaedic pathology with clinical and radiologic correlations,* 2nd ed. New York: Gower; 1992:17.25–17.28.

Burnstein MI, Fisher DR, Yandow DR, Hafez GR, DeSmet AA. Case report 502. Intra-articular synovial chondromatosis of shoulder with extra-articular extension. *Skeletal Radiol* 1988;17:458–461.

Butt WP, Hardy G, Ostlere SJ. Pigmented villonodular synovitis of the knee: computed tomographic appearances. *Skeletal Radiol* 1990;19:191–196.

Cadman NL, Soule EH, Kelly PJ. Synovial sarcoma: an analysis of 134 tumors. *Cancer* 1965;18:613–627.

Campanacci M. *Bone and soft-tissue tumors.* New York: Springer-Verlag; 1990:998–1012.

Chen A, Shih S-L, Chen B-F, Sheu C-Y. Primary synovial osteochondromatosis of the first metatarsophalangeal joint. *Skeletal Radiol* 2002;31:122–124.

Chen DY, Lan JL, Chou SJ. Treatment of pigmented villonodular synovitis with yttrium-90: changes in immunologic features. Tc-99m uptake measurements, and MR imaging of one case. *Clin Rheumatol* 1992;11:280–285.

Conway WF, Hayes CW. Miscellaneous lesions of bone. *Radiol Clin North Am* 1993;31: 339–358.

Cotten A, Flipo R-M, Chastanet P, Desvigne-Noulet M-C, Duquesnoy B, Delcambre B. Pigmented villonodular synovitis of the hip: review of radiographic features in 58 patients. *Skeletal Radiol* 1995;24:1–6.

Cotten A, Flipo RM, Herbaux B, Gougeon F, Lecomte-Houcke M, Chastanet P. Synovial haemangioma of the knee: a frequently misdiagnosed lesion. *Skeletal Radiol* 1995;24:257–261.

Crosby EB, Inglis A, Bullough PG. Multiple joint involvement with pigmented villonodular synovitis. *Radiology* 1977;122:671–672.

Crotty JM, Monu JUV, Pope TL Jr. Synovial osteochondromatosis. *Radiol Clin North Am* 1996;34:327–342.

Dahlin DC, Unni KK. Chondrosarcoma. In: *Bone tumors. General aspects and data on 8,542 cases,* 4th ed. Springfield, IL: Charles C Thomas; 1986:227–259.

De Beuckeleer L, De Schepper A, De Belder F, et al. Magnetic resonance imaging of localized giant cell tumour of the tendon sheath (MRI of localized GCTTS). *Eur Radiol* 1997;7:198–201.

Descamps F, Yasik E, Hardy D, Lafontaine M, Delince P. Pigmented villonodular synovitis of the hip. A case report and review of the literature. *Clin Rheumatol* 1991;10: 184–190.

Devaney K, Vinh TN, Sweet DE. Synovial hemangioma: report of 20 cases with differential diagnostic considerations. *Hum Pathol* 1993;24:737–745.

Dinauer P, Bojeseul JA, Kaplan KJ, Litts C. Bilateral lipoma arborescens of the bicipitoradial bursa. *Skeletal Radiol* 2002;31:661–665.

Docken WP. Pigmented villonodular synovitis: a review with illustrative case reports. *Semin Arthritis Rheum* 1979;9:1–22.

Dorwart RH, Genant HK, Johnston WH, Morris JM. Pigmented villonodular synovitis of the shoulder: radiologic-pathologic assessment. *AJR Am J Roentgenol* 1984;143: 886–888.

Dorwart RH, Genant HK, Johnston WH, Morris JM. Pigmented villonodular synovitis of synovial joints: clinical, pathologic, and radiologic features. *AJR Am J Roentgenol* 1984;143:877–885.

Doyle AJ, Miller MV, French JG. Lipoma arborescens in the bicipital bursa of the elbow: MRI findings in two cases. *Skeletal Radiol* 2002;31:656–660.

Dunn EJ, McGavran MH, Nelson P, Greer RB III. Synovial chondrosarcoma. Report of a case. *J Bone Joint Surg [Am]* 1974;56A:811–813.

Enzinger FM, Weiss SW. Benign tumors and tumor-like lesions of synovial tissue. In: *Soft tissue tumors.* St. Louis: CV Mosby; 1988:638–658.

Enzinger FM, Weiss SW. *Soft tissue tumors,* 3rd ed. St. Louis: CV Mosby, 1995:749–751, 757–786.

Eustace SE, Harrison M, Srinivasen U, Stack J. Magnetic resonance imaging in pigmented villonodular synovitis. *Can Assoc Radiol J* 1994;45:283–286.

Evans HL. Synovial sarcoma: a study of 23 biphasic and 17 probably monophasic examples. *Pathol Annu* 1980;15:309–313.

Farris KB, Reed RJ. Monophasic, glandular, synovial sarcomas and carcinomas of the soft tissues. *Arch Pathol Lab Med* 1982;106:129–132.

Fechner RE, Mills SE. *Tumors of the bones and joints.* Washington, DC: Armed Forces Institute of Pathology; 1993.

Feldman F. Cartilaginous tumors and cartilage-forming tumor-like conditions of the bones and soft tissues. In: Ranniger K, ed. *Bone tumors.* Berlin: Springer-Verlag; 1977:83–242.

Flandry F, Hughston JC. Pigmented villonodular synovitis. *J Bone Joint Surg [Am]* 1987;69A:942–949.

Fletcher AG Jr, Horn RC Jr. Giant-cell tumor of tendon sheath origin: a consideration of bone involvement and report of 2 cases with extensive bone destruction. *Ann Surg* 1951;133:374–385.

Fraire AE, Fechner RE. Intra-articular localized nodular synovitis of the knee. *Arch Pathol* 1972;93:473–476.

Georgen TG, Resnick D, Niwayama G. Localized nodular synovitis of the knee: a report of two cases with abnormal arthrograms. *AJR Am J Roentgenol* 1976;126:647–650.

Ginaldi S. Computed tomography feature of synovial osteochondromatosis. *Skeletal Radiol* 1980;5:219–222.

Goldman AB, DiCarlo EF. Pigmented villonodular synovitis. Diagnosis and differential diagnosis. *Radiol Clin North Am* 1988;26:1327–1347.

Goldman RL, Lichtenstein L. Synovial chondrosarcoma. *Cancer* 1964;17:1233–1240.

Granowitz SP, D'Antonio J, Mankin HL. The pathogenesis and long-term end results of pigmented villonodular synovitis. *Clin Orthop* 1976;114:335–351.

Granowitz SP, Mankin HJ. Localized pigmented villonodular synovitis of the knee. Report of five cases. *J Bone Joint Surg [Am]* 1967;49A:122–128.

Greenfield GB, Arrington JA, Kudryk BT. MRI of soft tissue tumors. *Skeletal Radiol* 1993;22:77–84.

Greenfield MM, Wallace KM. Pigmented villonodular synovitis. *Radiology* 1950;54: 350–356.

Greenspan A, Azouz EM, Matthews J II, Décarie J-C. Synovial hemangioma: imaging features in eight histologically proved cases, review of the literature, and differential diagnosis. *Skeletal Radiol* 1995;24:583–590.

Grieten M, Buckwalter KA, Cardinal E, Rougraff B. Case report 873. Lipoma arborescens (villous lipomatous proliferation of the synovial membrane). *Skeletal Radiol* 1994;23:652–655.

Hallel T, Lew S, Bansal M. Villous lipomatous proliferation of the synovial membrane (lipoma arborescens). *J Bone Joint Surg [Am]* 1988;70A:264–270.

Hamilton A, Davis RI, Hayes D, Mollan RA. Chondrosarcoma developing in synovial chondromatosis. A case report. *J Bone Joint Surg [Br]* 1987;69B:137–140.

Hawnaur JM, Whitehouse RW, Jenkins JP, Isherwood I. Musculoskeletal haemangiomas: comparison of MRI with CT. *Skeletal Radiol* 1990;19:251–258.

Hermann G, Abdelwahab IF, Klein MJ, Kenan S, Lewis M. Synovial chondromatosis. *Skeletal Radiol* 1995;24:298–300.

Hermann G, Klein MJ, Abdelwahab IF, Kenan S. Synovial chondrosarcoma arising in synovial chondromatosis of the right hip. *Skeletal Radiol* 1997;26:366–369.

Hiraga H, Nojima T, Isu K, Yamashiro K, Yamawaki S, Nagashima K. Histological and molecular evidence of synovial sarcoma of bone. A case report. *J Bone Joint Surg [Am]* 1999;81A:558–563.

Horowitz AL, Resnick D, Watson RC. The roentgen features of synovial sarcomas. *Clin Radiol* 1973;24:481–484.

Huang G-S, Lee C-H, Chan WP, Chen C-Y, Yu JS, Resnick D. Localized nodular synovitis of the knee: MR imaging appearance and clinical correlates in 21 patients. *AJR Am J Roentgenol* 2003;181:539–543.

Hughes TH, Sartoris DJ, Schweitzer ME, Resnick DL. Pigmented villonodular synovitis: MRI characteristics. *Skeletal Radiol* 1995;24:7–12.

Ishida T, Iijima T, Moriyama S, Nakamura C, Kitagawa T, Machinami R. Intra-articular calcifying synovial sarcoma mimicking synovial chondromatosis. *Skeletal Radiol* 1996;25:766–769.

Jaffe HL, Lichtenstein L, Sutro CJ. Pigmented villonodular synovitis, bursitis and tenosynovitis. *Arch Pathol Lab Med* 1941;31:731–765.

Jelinek JS, Kransdorf MJ, Shmookler BM, Aboulafia AA, Malawer MM. Giant cell tumor of the tendon sheath: MR findings in nine cases. *AJR Am J Roentgenol* 1994;162: 919–922.

Jelinek JS, Kransdorf MJ, Utz JA, et al. Imaging of pigmented villonodular synovitis with emphasis on MR imaging. *AJR Am J Roentgenol* 1989;152:337–342.

Jergesen HE, Mankin HJ, Schiller AL. Diffuse pigmented villonodular synovitis of the knee mimicking primary bone neoplasms. A report of two cases. *J Bone Joint Surg [Am]* 1978;60A:825–829.

Jones BC, Sundaram M, Kransdorf MJ. Synovial sarcoma: MR imaging findings in 34 patients. *AJR Am J Roentgenol* 1993;161:827–830.

Jones FE, Soule EM, Coventry MB. Fibrous xanthoma of synovium (giant-cell tumor of tendon sheath, pigmented nodular synovitis). A study of 118 cases. *J Bone Joint Surg [Am]* 1969;51A:76–86.

Kaiser TE, Ivins JC, Unni KK. Malignant transformation of extra-articular synovial chondromatosis: report of a case. *Skeletal Radiol* 1980;5:223–226.

Kalil RK, Unni KK. Malignancy in pigmented villonodular synovitis. *Skeletal Radiol* 1998;27:392–395.

Karasick D, Karasick S. Giant cell tumor of tendon sheath: spectrum of radiologic findings. *Skeletal Radiol* 1992;21:219–224.

Keenan MG. Computed tomography in pigmented villonodular synovitis of the hip. *J Rheumatol* 1987;14:1181–1183.

Kerr R. Diffuse pigmented villonodular synovitis. *Orthopedics* 1989;12:1008–1012.

Khan S, Neumann CH, Steinback LS, Harrington KD. MRI of giant cell tumor of tendon sheath of the hand: a report of three cases. *Eur Radiol* 1995;5:467–470.

Kindblom L-G, Angervall L. Myxoid chondrosarcoma of the synovial tissue: a clinicopathologic, histochemical, and ultrastructural analysis. *Cancer* 1983;52:1886–1895.

Kindblom LG, Gunterberg B. Pigmented villonodular synovitis involving bone. Case report. *J Bone Joint Surg [Am]* 1978;60A:830–832.

King JW, Spjut HJ, Fechner RE, Vanderpool DW. Synovial chondrosarcoma of the knee joint. *J Bone Joint Surg [Am]* 1967;49A:1389–1396.

Kloen P, Keel SB, Chandler HP, Geiger RH, Zarins B, Rosenberg AE. Lipoma arborescens of the knee. *J Bone Joint Surg [Br]* 1998;80-B:298–301.

Klompmaker J, Veth RPH, Robinson PH, Molenaar WM, Nielsen HKL. Pigmented villonodular synovitis. *Arch Orthop Trauma Surg* 1990;109:205–210.

Kottal AR, Vogler JB, Matamoros A, Alexander AH, Cookson JL. Pigmented villonodular synovitis: a report of MR imaging in two cases. *Radiology* 1987;163:551–553.

Krall RA, Kostinovsky M, Patchefsky AS. Synovial sarcoma: a clinical, pathological, and ultrastructural study of 26 cases supporting the recognition of monophasic variant. *Am J Surg Pathol* 1981;5:137–151.

Kransdorf MJ, Jelinek JS, Moser RP, et al. Soft-tissue masses: diagnosis using MR imaging. *AJR Am J Roentgenol* 1989;153:541–547.

Laorr A, Helms CA. *MRI of musculoskeletal masses: a practical text and atlas.* New York: Igaku-Shoin; 1997.

Laorr A, Peterfy CG, Tirman PF, Rabassa AE. Lipoma arborescens of the shoulder: magnetic resonance imaging findings. *Can Assoc Radiol J* 1995;46:311–313.

Larson IJ, Landry RN. Hemangioma of the synovial membrane. *J Bone Joint Surg [Am]* 1969;51A:1210–1215.

Lee Fy-I, Keel SB, Gebhardt MC, Rosenthal DI. Intra-articular lipoma with osteochondroid metaplasia in the knee joint. *Skeletal Radiol* 2001;30:230–233.

Lenchik L, Poznanski AK, Donaldson JS, Sarwark JF. Case report 681. Synovial hemangioma of the knee. *Skeletal Radiol* 1991;20:387–389.

Lin J, Jacobson JA, Jamadar DA, Ellis JH. Pigmented villonodular synovitis and related lesions: the spectrum of imaging findings. *AJR Am J Roentgenol* 1999;172:191–197.

Llauger J, Monill JM, Palmer J, Clotet M. Synovial hemangioma of the knee: MRI findings in two cases. *Skeletal Radiol* 1995;24:579–581.

Llauger J, Palmer J, Rosón N, Bagué S, Camins A, Cremades R. Nonseptic monoarthritis: imaging features with clinical and histopathologic correlation. *Radiographics* 2000;20:S263–S278.

Llauger J, Palmer J, Rosón N, Cremades R, Bagué S. Pigmented villonodular synovitis and giant cell tumors of the tendon sheath: radiologic and pathologic features. *AJR Am J Roentgenol* 1999;172:1087–1091.

Madewell JE, Sweet DE. Tumors and tumor-like lesions in or about joints. In: Resnick D, ed. *Bone and joint imaging.* Philadelphia: WB Saunders; 1989:1182–1192.

Mahajan H, Lorigan JG, Shirkhoda A. Synovial sarcoma: MR imaging. *Magn Reson Imaging* 1989;7:211–216.

Majeste RM, Beckman EN. Synovial sarcoma with an overwhelming epithelial component. *Cancer* 1988;61:2527–2531.

Mandelbaum BR, Grant TT, Hartzman S, et al. The use of MRI to assist in the diagnosis of pigmented villonodular synovitis of the knee. *Clin Orthop* 1988;231:135–139.

Manivel JC, Dehner LP, Thompson R. Case report 460. Synovial chondrosarcoma of left knee. *Skeletal Radiol* 1988;17:66–71.

Maurice H, Crone M, Watt I. Synovial chondromatosis. *J Bone Joint Surg [Br]* 1988;70B:807–811.

McCarville MB, Spunt SL, Skapek SX, Pappo AS. Pictorial essay. Synovial sarcoma in pediatric patients. *AJR Am J Roentgenol* 2002;179:797–801.

McKinney CD, Mills SE, Fechner RE. Intraarticular synovial sarcoma. *Am J Surg Pathol* 1992;16:1017–1020.

McMaster PE. Pigmented villonodular synovitis with invasion of bone. Report of six cases. *J Bone Joint Surg [Am]* 1960;42A:1170–1183.

Meyer CA, Kransdorf MJ, Moser PP Jr, Jelinek JS. Case report 716. Soft-tissue metastasis in synovial sarcoma. *Skeletal Radiol* 1992;21:128–131.

Miettinen M, Virtanen I. Synovial sarcoma—a misnomer. *Am J Pathol* 1984;117:18–25.

Milchgrub S, Ghandur-Mnaymneh L, Dorfman HD, Albores-Saavedra J. Synovial sarcoma with extensive osteoid and bone formation. *Am J Surg Pathol* 1993;17:357–363.

Milgram JW. Synovial osteochondromatosis. A histopathological study of thirty cases. *J Bone Joint Surg [Am]* 1977;59A:792–801.

Milgram JW, Addison RG. Synovial osteochondromatosis of the knee. Chondromatous recurrence with possible chondrosarcomatous degeneration. *J Bone Joint Surg [Am]* 1976;58A:264–266.

Miller WE. Villonodular synovitis: pigmented and nonpigmented variations. *South Med J* 1982;75:1084–1086.

Morton MJ, Berquist TH, McLeod RA, Unni KK, Sim FH. MR imaging of synovial sarcoma. *AJR Am J Roentgenol* 1991;156:337–340.

Mulder JD, Kroon HM, Schütte HE, Taconis WK. *Radiologic atlas of bone tumors.* Amsterdam: Elsevier; 1993.

Mullins F, Berard CW, Eisenberg SH. Chondrosarcoma following synovial chondromatosis. A case study. *Cancer* 1965;18:1180–1188.

Murphy FP, Dahlin DC, Sullivan CR. Articular synovial chondromatosis. *J Bone Joint Surg [Am]* 1962;44A:77–86.

Myers BW, Masi AT. Pigmented villonodular synovitis and tenosynovitis, a clinical epidemiologic study of 166 cases and literature review. *Medicine* 1980;59:224–238.

Narváez JA, Narváez J, Ortega R, De Lama E, Roca Y, Vidal N. Pictorial essay. Hypointense synovial lesions on T2-weighted images: differential diagnosis with pathologic correlation. *AJR Am J Roentgenol* 2003;181:761–769.

Nisolle J-F, Blovard E, Baudrez V, Bautsen Y, De Cloedt P, Esselinckx W. Subacromial-subdeltoid lipoma arborescens associated with a rotator cuff tear. *Skeletal Radiol* 1999;28:283–285.

Norman A, Steiner GC. Bone erosion in synovial chondromatosis. *Radiology* 1986;161:749–752.

Ontell F, Greenspan A. Chondrosarcoma complicating synovial chondromatosis: findings with magnetic resonance imaging. *Can Assoc Radiol J* 1994;45:318–323.

Osburn AW, Bassett LW, Seeger LL, Mirra JM, Eckhardt JJ. Case report 609. Synovial (osteo)chondromatosis. *Skeletal Radiol* 1990;19:237–241.

Parsonage S, Mehr A, Davies MD. Lipoma arborescense: a definitive MR imaging diagnosis. *Osteol Közlem* 2001;9:80–82.

Patel MR, Zinberg EM. Pigmented villonodular synovitis of the wrist invading bone; report of a case. *J Hand Surg* 1984;9:854–858.

Peh WCG, Shek TWH, Davies AM, Wong JWK, Chien EP. Osteochondroma and secondary synovial osteochondromatosis. *Skeletal Radiol* 1999;28:169–174.

Perry BE, McQueen DA, Lin JJ. Synovial chondromatosis with malignant degeneration to chondrosarcoma. Report of a case. *J Bone Joint Surg [Am]* 1988;70A:1259–1261.

Poletti SC, Gates HS III, Martinez SM, Richardson WJ. The use of magnetic resonance imaging in the diagnosis of pigmented villonodular synovitis. *Orthopedics* 1990;13:185–190.

Rao AS, Vigorita VJ. Pigmented villonodular synovitis (giant-cell tumor of the tendon sheath and synovial membrane). A review of eighty-one cases. *J Bone Joint Surg [Am]* 1984;66A:76–94.

Resnick D, Oliphant M. Hemophilia-like arthropathy of the knee associated with cutaneous and synovial hemangiomas. *Radiology* 1975;114:323–326.

Rosenthal DI, Aronow S, Murray WT. Iron content of pigmented villonodular synovitis detected by computed tomography. *Radiology* 1979;133:409–411.

Ryu KN, Jaovisidha S, Schweitzer M, Motta AO, Resnick D. MR imaging of lipoma aborescens of the knee joint. *AJR Am J Roentgenol* 1996;167:1229–1232.

Sánchez Reyes JM, Alcaraz Mexia M, Quiñones Tapia D, Aramburu JA. Extensively calcified synovial sarcoma. *Skeletal Radiol* 1997;26:671–673.

Schajowicz F. Synovial chondromatosis. In: *Tumors and tumorlike lesions of bones and joints.* New York: Springer-Verlag; 1981:541–545.

Schumacher HR, Lotke P, Athreya B, Rothfuss S. Pigmented villonodular synovitis: light and electron microscopic studies. *Semin Arthritis Rheum* 1982;12:32–43.

Schwartz GB, Coleman DA. Pigmented villonodular synovitis of the wrist and adjacent bone. *Orthop Rev* 1986;15:526–530.

Sherry JB, Anderson W. The natural history of pigmented villonodular synovitis of tendon sheath. *J Bone Joint Surg [Am]* 1956;37A:1005–1011.

Silit E, Mutlu H, Pekkafali Z, Kizilkaya E, Basekim CC. Synovial hemangioma of the knee invading the femur. *Skeletal Radiol* 2002;31:612–614.

Soule EH. Synovial sarcoma. *Am J Surg Pathol* 1986;10:78–82.

Spritzer CE, Dalinka MK, Kressel HY. Magnetic resonance imaging of pigmented villonodular synovitis: a report of two cases. *Skeletal Radiol* 1987;16:316–319.

Steinbach LS, Neumann CH, Stoller DW, et al. MRI of the knee in diffuse pigmented villonodular synovitis. *Clin Imaging* 1989;13:305–316.

Stiehl JB, Hackbarth DA. Recurrent pigmented villonodular synovitis of the hip joint, case report and review of the literature. *J Arthroplasty* 1991;6:S85–S90.

Stout AP, Lattes R. Tumors of the soft tissue. In: *Atlas of tumor pathology,* 2nd series, fascicle 1. Washington, DC: Armed Forces Institute of Pathology; 1967.

Strickland B, Mackenzie DH. Bone involvement in synovial sarcoma. *J Faculty Radiol* 1959;10:64–72.

Sugimoto K, Iwai M, Kawate K, Yajima H, Takakura Y. Tenosynovial osteochondromatosis of the tarsal tunnel. *Skeletal Radiol* 2003;32:99–102.

Suh J, Griffith HJ, Galloway HR, Everson LI. MRI in the diagnosis of synovial disease. *Orthopedics* 1992;15:778–781.

Suh J-S, Swang G, Hahn S-B. Soft tissue hemangiomas: MR manifestations in 23 patients. *Skeletal Radiol* 1994;23:621–625.

Sundaram M, Chalk D, Merenda J, Verde JM, Salinas-Madrigal L. Case report 563. Pigmented villonodular synovitis (PVNS) of knee. *Skeletal Radiol* 1989;18:463–465.

Sundaram M, McGuire MH, Fletcher J, Wolverson MK, Heiberg E, Shields JB. Magnetic resonance imaging of lesions of synovial origin. *Skeletal Radiol* 1986;15: 110–116.

Sundaram M, McLeod RA. MR imaging of tumor and tumorlike lesions of bone and soft tissue. *AJR Am J Roentgenol* 1990;155:817–824.

Taconis WK, van der Heul RO, Taminiau AMM. Synovial chondrosarcoma: report of a case and review of the literature. *Skeletal Radiol* 1997;26:682–685.

Trias A, Quintana O. Synovial chondrometaplasia: review of world literature and study of 18 Canadian cases. *Can J Surg* 1976;19:151–158.

Tuckman G, Wirth CZ. Synovial osteochondromatosis of the shoulder: MR findings. *J Comput Assist Tomogr* 1989;13:360–361.

Ushijima M, Hashimoto H, Tsuneyoshi M, Enjoji M. Giant cell tumor of the tendon sheath (nodular tenosynovitis). A study of 207 cases to compare the large joint group with the common digit group. *Cancer* 1986;57:875–884.

van Rijswijk CSP, Hogendoorn PCW, Taminiau AHM, Bloem JL. Synovial sarcoma: dynamic contrast-enhanced MR imaging features. *Skeletal Radiol* 2001;30:25–30.

Varela-Duran J, Enzinger FM. Calcifying synovial sarcoma. *Cancer* 1982;50:345–352.

Villanova JC, Barceló J, Villalón M, Aldomà J, Delgado E, Zapater I. MR imaging of lipoma arborescens and the associated lesions. *Skeletal Radiol* 2003;32:504–509.

Wagner ML, Spjut HJ, Dutton RV, Glassman AL, Askew JB. Polyarticular pigmented villonodular synovitis. *AJR Am J Roentgenol* 1981;143:877–885.

Weisz GM, Gal A, Kitchener PN. Magnetic resonance imaging in the diagnosis of aggressive villonodular synovitis. *Clin Orthop* 1988;236:303–306.

Weitzman G. Lipoma arborescens of the knee. *J Bone Joint Surg [Am]* 1965;47A:1030–1033.

Wiss DA. Recurrent villonodular synovitis of the knee: successful treatment with yttrium-90. *Clin Orthop* 1982;169:128–129.

Witkin GB, Miettinen M, Rosai J. A biphasic tumor of the mediastinum with features of synovial sarcoma. *Am J Surg Pathol* 1989;13:490–499.

Wittkop B, Davies AM, Mangham DC. Primary synovial chondromatosis and synovial chondrosarcoma: a pictorial review. *Eur Radiol* 2002;12:2112–2119.

Wolfe RD, Giuliano VJ. Double-contrast arthrography in the diagnosis of pigmented villonodular synovitis of the knee. *AJR Am J Roentgenol* 1970;110:793–799.

Wright PH, Sim FH, Soule EH, Taylor WF. Synovial sarcoma. *J Bone Joint Surg [Am]* 1982;64A:112–122.

Young JM, Hudacek AG. Experimental production of pigmented villonodular synovitis in dogs. *Am J Pathol* 1981;19:379–392.

Yudd AP, Velchik MG. Pigmented villonodular synovitis of the hip. *Clin Nucl Med* 1985;10:441–442.

Zwass A, Abdelwahab IF, Klein MJ. Case report 463. Pigmented villonodular synovitis (PVNS) of the knee. *Skeletal Radiol* 1988;17:81–84.

Zwass A, Greenspan A, Green SM. Giant cell tumor of the tendon sheath with a pathologic phalangeal fracture: a rare association. *Bull Hosp Jt Dis Orthop Inst* 1985;45: 87–93.

INFECTIONS

RADIOLOGIC EVALUATION OF MUSCULOSKELETAL INFECTIONS

Musculoskeletal Infections

Infections of the musculoskeletal system can be subdivided into three categories: (a) those involving bones (osteomyelitis); (b) those involving joints (infectious arthritis); and (c) those involving soft tissues (cellulitis). Because of the complexity of the vertebrae and their soft-tissue structures, infectious processes of the spine are considered under a separate heading.

Osteomyelitis

Three basic mechanisms allow an infectious organism—whether bacterium, virus, mycoplasma, rickettsia, or fungus—to reach the bone: (a) *hematogenous spread* via the bloodstream from a remote site of infection, such as the skin, tonsils, gallbladder, or urinary tract; (b) spread from a *contiguous source* of infection, as from the soft tissues, teeth, or sinuses; and (c) *direct implantation*, such as through a puncture or missile wound or an operative procedure (Fig. 24.1).

Hematogenous spread is common in children, and the usual focus of infection develops in the metaphysis. The metaphyseal location of infection in children is related to an osseous–vascular anatomy that differs in the infant, child, and adult (Fig. 24.2). In the child (ages 1 to 16 years), there is separation of the blood supply to the metaphysis and epiphysis, each having its own source. Moreover, the arteries and capillaries of the metaphysis turn sharply without penetrating the open growth plate; in the region where capillaries become venules, the rate of blood flow is sluggish. Also contributing to the greater incidence of metaphyseal osteomyelitis in children is secondary thrombosis of end arteries with bacteria during transient bacteremia. In the infant (up to 1 year), however, osteomyelitis may sometimes have its focus in the epiphysis, because some metaphyseal vessels may penetrate the growth plate and reach the epiphysis (see Fig. 24.2). With obliteration of the growth plate in the adult, there is vascular continuity between the shaft and the articular ends of the bone; hence, the focus of osteomyelitis can develop in any part of a bone.

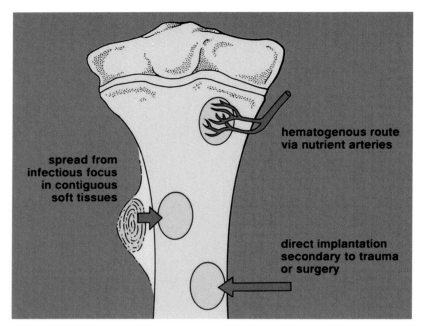

Figure 24.1 Entry routes of an infectious organism into a bone. Infectious agents may gain entry to a bone through hematogenous spread, a source of infection in the contiguous soft tissues, or through direct implantation secondary to trauma or surgery.

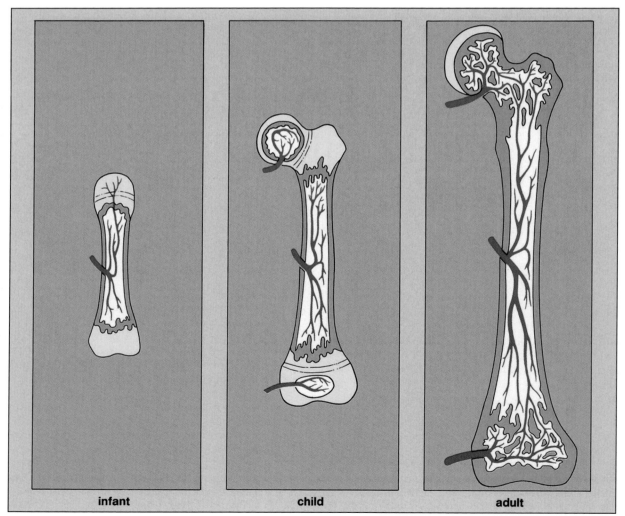

Figure 24.2 Vascular anatomy of long bone. The vascular anatomy of a long bone differs in an infant, a child, and an adult. These differences account for the various locations of infection in each age group. In an infant, nutrient, transphyseal, and foveal arteries are abundant. In a child, the physis becomes avascular when the foveal and transphyseal arteries recede. After the growth plate closes, the foveal arteries and periarticular arteries again become prominent.

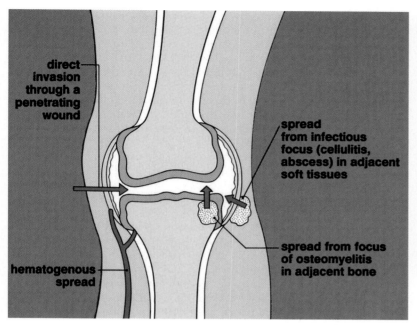

Figure 24.3 Entry routes of an infectious organism into a joint. The routes of infection in infectious arthritis are similar to those of osteomyelitis, which itself may be a source of spread.

Figure 24.4 Entry routes of an infectious organism into a vertebra. The potential routes of infection of a vertebra or an intervertebral disk are direct invasion, hematogenous spread, and extension from a focus of infection in the adjacent soft tissues.

Contiguous spread and direct implantation are more common in adults. The sites of bone infection via either of these routes are directly related to the focus of soft-tissue infection or the location of the wound.

Infectious Arthritis

An infectious agent may enter the joint by the same basic routes as in osteomyelitis: by direct invasion of the synovial membrane, either secondary to a penetrating wound or after a joint-replacement procedure; from an infection of the adjacent soft tissues; or indirectly via a blood-borne infection. Infectious arthritis may also occur secondary to a focus of osteomyelitis in the adjacent bone (Fig. 24.3).

Cellulitis

Soft-tissue infections most commonly result from a break in the skin leading to direct introduction of an infectious agent. Some patients, such as those with diabetes, are particularly prone to cellulitis caused by a combination of factors, including skin breakdown and local ischemia.

Infections of the Spine

Infections in the spine may be located in a vertebral body, an intervertebral disk, the paravertebral soft tissues, or the epidural compartment; very rarely, an infection may involve the contents of the spinal canal or the spinal cord. The mechanisms of infection are the same as those of osteomyelitis and infectious arthritis. An intervertebral disk infection, for example, may result from a puncture of the canal or of the disk itself during a procedure, as well as from a penetrating injury. It can also spread from a contiguous source of infection such as a paraspinal abscess. Most common, however, is hematogenous spread after surgical procedures such as laminectomy or spinal fusion, or during generalized bacteremia or sepsis (Fig. 24.4). Regardless of the primary location of the infectious process, *Staphylococcus aureus* is responsible for more than 90% of all infections of the spine.

Radiologic Evaluation of Infections

The radiologic modalities used to evaluate infections of the musculoskeletal system include the following:

1. Conventional radiography (including magnification studies)
2. Conventional tomography
3. Computed tomography (CT)
4. Arthrography
5. Myelography and diskography
6. Fistulography (sinogram)
7. Arteriography
8. Radionuclide imaging (scintigraphy, bone scan)
9. Ultrasound
10. Magnetic resonance imaging (MRI)
11. Percutaneous aspiration and biopsy (fluoroscopy-guided or CT-guided)

In most instances, radiography is sufficient to demonstrate the pertinent features of a bone or joint infection (Fig. 24.5; see also Figs. 4.49 and Fig. 4.50A). Magnification radiography is helpful in delineating subtle changes representing cortical destruction or periosteal new bone formation (Fig. 24.6) and is occasionally required for differentiating osteoporosis from the early stages of infection, which may appear radiographically similar. Conventional tomography using multi-directional motion (trispiral tomography) is particularly effective in demonstrating sequestra or subtle sinus tracts in the bone (Fig. 24.7; see also Fig. 4.50B). CT plays a determining role in demonstrating the extent of infection in bones and soft tissues and at times may be very helpful in making a specific diagnosis (Fig. 24.8).

Arthrography has rather limited application in the diagnosis of joint infections (see Fig. 25.16B). Scintigraphy, however, has a much more prominent role. In suspected osteomyelitis, radionuclide bone scan using technetium-99m-labeled phosphonate is routinely used, because there is an accumulation of tracer in the infected areas. A three- or four-phase technique is particularly useful for distinguishing infected joint tissues from infected periarticular soft tissues if radiography is not diagnostic. With cellulitis, diffuse increased uptake is present in the first two phases, but there is no significant increase in uptake in the bone in the third and fourth phases. Conversely, osteomyelitis causes focally increased uptake in all four phases (Fig. 24.9). In addition, the three-phase bone scan can accurately diagnose osteomyelitis within 3 days of the development of symptoms, much earlier than can be seen with conventional radiography. The three-phase bone scan can also be useful in diagnosing septic arthritis in situ or with extension into the adjacent bone.

Once the bone sustains an injury, such as surgery, fracture, or neuropathic osteoarthropathy, that causes increased bone turnover, routine scintigraphy with technetium-labeled phosphonate becomes less specific for infection. However, radionuclide studies using gal-

Figure 24.5 Chronic osteomyelitis. Anteroposterior radiograph of the right humerus demonstrates the classic features of chronic active osteomyelitis. There is destruction of the medullary portion of the bone, reactive sclerosis, and periosteal new bone formation. Note also a large sequestrum on the medial aspect of the humerus, the hallmark of an active infectious process.

leukocytes is used as a sensitive and specific test in the general diagnosis of infection of the musculoskeletal system, and in specific instances when infection complicates previous fracture or surgery. Like other imaging procedures in nuclear medicine, this test monitors the internal distribution of a tracer agent to provide diagnostic information. The inherent ability of white blood cells to localize at sites of inflammation makes their use in this test particularly effective in the diagnosis of infections. Merkel reported the sensitivity of indium scintigraphy in detecting infections to be 83%, with a specificity of 94% and an accuracy of 88%.

It must be stressed, however, that because the ^{111}In-labeled leukocytes also accumulate in active bone marrow, the sensitivity for detection of chronic osteomyelitis is reduced. To improve the diagnostic ability of this technique, a combined ^{99m}Tc-sulfur colloid bone marrow/^{111}In-labeled leukocyte study is advocated. A particularly difficult problem is the patient with diabetic foot neuropathy in whom superimposed infection is suspected. In this circumstance, radiography and even MRI are not very specific. Although soft-tissue infection can be detected by the latter technique, early changes of osteomyelitis may be missed. Often, no single imaging method can provide the correct diagnosis, and a combination of imaging techniques should be used. The traditional sequential use of ^{67}Ga citrate in conjunction with the ^{99m}Tc MDP bone scan as an aid to diagnose osteomyelitis in the diabetic foot has been supplanted in recent years by the use of ^{111}In-labeled leukocytes. The drawback of this technique is that there remain difficulties in differentiating infection in the bone (osteomyelitis) from that in the adjacent tissue (cellulitis). A more recent attempt

lium (a ferric analog) and indium are more specific in these instances. There is still no general agreement on the exact mechanism of gallium localization in infected tissues. After intravenous injections of gallium, more than 99% is bound to various plasma proteins, including transferrin, haptoglobin, lactoferrin, albumin, and ferritin. At least five mechanisms of gallium transfer from the plasma into inflammatory exudates and cells have been suggested. These include direct leukocyte uptake, direct bacteria uptake, the protein-bound tissue uptake, increased vascularity, and increased bone turnover. Because gallium binds to the iron-binding molecule transferrin, the mechanism of gallium uptake in infectious processes is best explained by hyperemia and elevated permeability that increase delivery of the protein-bound tracer transferrin into the area of inflammation. Cells associated with the inflammatory response, particularly polymorphonuclear white cells in which lactoferrin is carried within intracytoplasmic granules, deposit iron-binding proteins extracellularly at the site of inflammation, serving to combat the infection by sequestering needed iron from bacteria. Lactoferrin, which has a high binding affinity for iron, takes the gallium away from the transferrin.

Gallium can also be used to assess the patient's response to therapy. Particularly in osteomyelitis, gallium concentrations enhance the specificity of an abnormal bone scan, and decreased gallium uptake closely follows a good response to therapy.

The other tracer used in infections is indium. Because indium-labeled white blood cells are usually not incorporated into areas of increased bone turnover, scintigraphy with indium-111 oxine-labeled

Figure 24.6 Acute osteomyelitis. Magnification study of the right femur demonstrates subtle changes representative of cortical destruction and formation of periosteal new bone in an early stage of osteomyelitis. These findings were not well delineated on the conventional radiographs.

Figure 24.7 Tomography of active osteomyelitis. (A) Radiograph of the left femur shows thickening of the cortex, reactive sclerosis, and foci of destruction in the medullary cavity. Faint calcifications in the soft tissue suggest the presence of a fistula. **(B)** Conventional tomogram enhanced by magnification clearly demonstrates a sequestrum and a sinus tract in the cortex, the characteristic features of active osteomyelitis.

Figure 24.8 CT of bone abscess. A 7-year-old boy had intermittent pain in the left knee for 3 weeks; the pain was worse at night and was promptly relieved by salicylates. **(A)** Initial anteroposterior radiograph of the left knee demonstrates a radiolucent lesion with a well-defined, partly sclerotic border in the lateral portion of the distal femoral epiphysis. Osteoid osteoma and chondroblastoma were considered in the differential diagnosis. **(B)** CT examination, however, reveals cortical disruption at the posterolateral aspect of the lateral femoral condyle, a finding not seen on the standard radiographs. The serpentine configuration of the radiolucent tract and its extension into the cartilage prompted a diagnosis of epiphyseal bone abscess, which was confirmed on bone biopsy.

A

B

C

Figure 24.9 Application of radionuclide bone scan in infection. A 52-year-old woman with pain in her right ankle had cellulitis around the ankle joint. Although radiographs did not reveal changes in the joint suggestive of infectious arthritis, this possibility could not be ruled out clinically because early changes of infection may not be detected on standard radiographs. A three-phase radionuclide bone scan was performed. **(A)** In the first phase, 1 minute after intravenous injection of a 15 mCi (555 MBq) bolus of technetium-99m-labeled methylene diphosphonate, there is increased activity in the major vessels of the right leg. **(B)** In the second phase, 3 minutes after injection, a blood pool scan demonstrates increased uptake in the area of the infected soft tissues. **(C)** In the third phase, 2 hours after injection, almost complete washout of the radiopharmaceutical, with no evidence of localization in the bones on both sides of the joint, excludes the diagnosis of infectious arthritis. (Courtesy of Dr. R. Goldfarb, New York, NY.)

portant role in the guidance of percutaneous biopsy and aspiration of infectious lesions, as well as the therapeutic drainage of abscesses.

At the present time MRI established its place in the evaluation of bone and soft-tissue infections. As several studies have indicated, osteomyelitis, soft-tissue abscesses, joint and tendon sheath effusions, and various forms of cellulitis are well depicted by this modality. MRI is as sensitive as ^{99m}Tc-methylene diphosphonate (MDP) in demonstrating osteomyelitis and more sensitive and more specific than other scintigraphic techniques in demonstrating soft-tissue infections, primarily because of its superior spatial resolution. The proper evaluation of musculoskeletal infections with MRI requires both T1- and T2-weighted images in at least two imaging planes. In anatomically complex areas such as the pelvis, spine, foot, and hand, three planes may be necessary. Diagnostic criteria for MRI in diagnosing osteomyelitis are findings of decreased signal intensity in the bone marrow cavity on short spin-echo TR/TE sequences (T1 weighting) along with increased signal intensity in the bone marrow cavity on long TR/TE sequences (T2 weighting) (Fig. 24.11). Increased signal intensity of the soft tissues on long TR/TE sequences with poorly defined margins is considered indicative of edema and/or nonspecific inflammatory changes. Well-demarcated collections of decreased signal intensity on T1-weighted sequences and increased signal intensity surrounded by zones of decreased signal intensity on T2-weighted images are considered indicative of soft-tissue abscesses (Fig. 24.12). Decreased signal intensity on short TR/TE sequences and increased signal intensity on long TR/TE sequences in the area of the joint capsule or tendon sheath are consistent with synovial effusions and fluid in the tendon sheath.

Contrast enhancement using intravenous injection of gadolinium is routinely used for diagnosis of musculoskeletal infections. This technique allows differentiation of osteomyelitis from bone marrow edema

Figure 24.10 Fistulography in osteomyelitis. A 48-year-old man who had sustained a fracture of the femur was treated with open reduction and internal fixation using an intramedullary rod. Chronic osteomyelitis developed postoperatively. The rod was removed and the infection was treated with antibiotics. Subsequently, a draining sinus developed. **(A)** Radiograph of the left femur demonstrates changes typical of chronic osteomyelitis. There is focal destruction of the medullary portion of the bone, reactive sclerosis, and a periosteal reaction. **(B)** A sinogram performed to evaluate the extent of the draining fistula demonstrates a sinus tract with multiple ramifications.

to improve this situation is use of a combined ^{99m}Tc-bone scan/^{111}In-labeled leukocyte study to determine whether the leukocyte collection is in the bone or in the soft tissue. A new challenger to ^{111}In leukocyte scanning is the ^{99m}Tc-hexamethylpropylene amino oxine (HMPAO)-labeled leukocyte scan. At the time of this writing, other methods are being tested, namely, isotope-labeled (^{99m}Tc, ^{111}In, or ^{123}I) monoclonal antigranulocyte antibodies, isotope-labeled polyclonal IgG, isotope-labeled monocytes, isotope-labeled chemotactic polypeptide analogs, and isotope-labeled specific antibodies against bacteria.

Arteriography is important in the evaluation of the patient's vascular supply, particularly if a reconstructive procedure is planned. Myelography is still useful in evaluating infections within the spinal canal, as well as in vertebral osteomyelitis and disk infection (see Fig. 25.30). Fistulography (sinogram) is an important examination for outlining sinus tracts in the soft tissues and for evaluating their extension into the bone (Fig. 24.10).

Ultrasound can occasionally be used in diagnosing soft-tissue and joint infections, as well as osteomyelitis. This modality has the advantage of being easily accessible and available at relatively reasonable cost. In addition, this technique does not expose the patient to ionizing radiation. Real-time capability of ultrasound is unique in providing a means to evaluate structures under dynamic conditions. In diffuse soft-tissue infection, ultrasound may be helpful in distinguishing primary disease from that associated with underlying abscess such as in pyomyositis or osteomyelitis. Furthermore, ultrasound plays an im-

Figure 24.11 MRI of osteomyelitis. Sagittal T2-weighted MR image (SE; TR 2000/TE 80 msec) shows a well-defined area of increased signal intensity in the medullary space of the midshaft of the femur (*arrows*), indicating acute hematogenous osteomyelitis in this intravenous drug user. There are soft-tissue inflammatory changes with multiple small abscesses adjacent to the cortex (*arrowheads*). (From Beltran J, 1990, with permission.)

Figure 24.12 MRI of soft-tissue abscess. Axial T2-weighted MR image (SE; TR 2000/TE 80 msec) shows high signal intensity of soft-tissue fluid collection anterior to the tibia, with a focus of lower signal intensity in the center, representing the soft-tissue abscess (*arrows*). The abscess is surrounded by a thick low-signal-intensity capsule. Note the high-signal-intensity edema diffusely involving the subcutaneous fat and muscles (*open arrow*). (From Beltran J, 1990, with permission.)

Figure 24.13 Treatment of osteomyelitis. A 3-year-old girl had osteomyelitis of the left tibia after chronic tonsillitis. **(A)** Anteroposterior radiograph of the left leg shows extensive destruction of the tibia with sequestration of the diaphysis. Extensive and long-standing conservative treatment using broad-spectrum antibiotics failed to produce any improvement. **(B)** One year later, the dead sequestered segment of the tibial diaphysis was resected as a first stage in reconstruction of the limb. **(C)** Two months later, a fibular graft was attached to the proximal stump of the tibial diaphysis, and bone chips were applied proximally and distally to ensure bony union and stability.

or an abscess from cellulites or phlegmon in the soft tissues. The abscess demonstrates high-signal-intensity enhancement of its capsule, whereas the central portion remains of low signal intensity. Conversely, cellulites and phlegmon exhibit diffuse contrast enhancement.

Percutaneous aspiration and ultrasound-guided, CT-guided, or fluoroscopy-guided biopsy of a suspected focus of infection may be performed in the radiology suite. It can rapidly confirm a suspected diagnosis of infection and reveal the causative organism.

Monitoring the Treatment and Complications of Infections

Radiology plays an indispensable role in monitoring the treatment of infectious disorders of bone and associated soft tissues (Fig. 24.13).

Follow-up radiographs and radionuclide bone scans should be obtained at regular intervals to evaluate the disease state (acute, subacute, chronic, or inactive) (Fig. 24.14) and any complications that may arise (Fig. 24.15). The differentiation of active from inactive osteomyelitis may, however, be extremely difficult by radiologic techniques. The extensive osteosclerotic changes in inactive infection may obscure small foci of osteolytic change signifying reactivation. Tomography may at times be helpful in delineating fluffy periostitis, poorly marginated areas of osteolysis, or sequestra.

The main complication of osteomyelitis in infants and children is growth disturbance if the focus of infection is in the vicinity of the growth plate (Fig. 24.16). Pathologic fracture is another common complication of osteomyelitis (Fig. 24.17). In adults, the most serious, although rare, complication is the development of a malignant neoplasm in a chronically draining sinus tract (see Fig. 22.32).

Figure 24.14 Treatment of osteomyelitis. A 17-year-old girl had an acute pyogenic infection of the first metatarsal bone after a puncture injury of her right foot. **(A)** Anteroposterior radiograph demonstrates changes typical of active osteomyelitis: cortical and medullary bone destruction, a periosteal reaction, and diffuse soft-tissue swelling (*arrowheads*). Note also the significant periarticular osteoporosis. After extensive treatment with antibiotics, a radiograph of the foot **(B)** shows complete healing of the infection, which is in an inactive phase. There is residual endosteal sclerosis, but no destructive changes are evident and the soft-tissue planes are normal.

Figure 24.16 Complication of osteomyelitis. Anteroposterior radiograph of the right knee of an 8-year-old girl shows a growth disturbance as a sequela of metaphyseal osteomyelitis. Note the hypoplasia of the femur secondary to disuse of the limb and the deformity of the distal epiphysis. The cone-shaped growth plate shows almost complete fusion.

Figure 24.15 Treatment of joint infection after a total knee arthroplasty. A 62-year-old woman had an infection of the right knee joint after total knee arthroplasty. **(A)** Anteroposterior radiograph shows the joint replacement with a condylar-type cemented prosthesis. Active infection is still evident, as demonstrated by the soft-tissue swelling, joint effusion, and periosteal reaction. Small foci of bone destruction are seen in the proximal tibia. **(B)** An aspiration arthrogram (subtraction study) demonstrates abnormal extension of contrast medium into osteolytic areas of the tibia. The irregular outline on the lateral aspect of the joint is caused by synovitis. Bacteriologic examination of the aspirated material yielded *Staphylococcus aureus.* **(C)** After unsuccessful treatment of the infection with broad-spectrum antibiotics, the prosthesis had to be removed. Note the typical appearance of active osteomyelitis. **(D)** The treatment at this stage consisted of methylmethacrylate cement balls soaked with antibiotics and applied to the infected joint and medullary cavity of the femur and tibia.

Figure 24.17 Complication of osteomyelitis. Radiograph of the right leg of a 6-year-old boy with chronic active osteomyelitis shows a pathologic fracture, a complication of the infectious process.

PRACTICAL POINTS TO REMEMBER

[1] Three basic mechanisms allow an infectious organism to reach a bone or joint:
- hematogenous spread
- spread from a contiguous source
- direct implantation.

[2] The metaphysis is the most common site of an infectious focus in children, primarily because of the nature of the osseous–vascular anatomy at this stage of development, whereas the shaft of a long bone is a common site of infection in adult patients.

[3] Radionuclide bone scan using ^{99m}Tc-labeled phosphonates is a very useful radiologic modality for distinguishing a joint infection from cellulitis of the periarticular soft tissues.

[4] The scintigraphic radiopharmaceuticals most specific for detection of musculoskeletal infection are gallium-67 citrate and indium-111 oxine.

[5] MRI is more specific and more sensitive than scintigraphic techniques in demonstrating bone and soft-tissue infections, primarily because of its superior spatial resolution. Both T1- and T2-weighted sequences in at least two imaging planes should be obtained.

[6] Percutaneous aspiration biopsy of a suspected focus of infection is the most direct route for confirming a diagnosis and identifying the causative organism.

SUGGESTED READINGS

Abiri MM, Kirpekar M, Ablow RC. Osteomyelitis: detection with US. *Radiology* 1988;169:795–797.

Alazraki NP. Radionuclide imaging in the evaluation of infectious and inflammatory disease. *Radiol Clin North Am* 1993;31:783–794.

Al-Sheikh W, Sfakianakis GN, Mnaymneh W, et al. Subacute and chronic bone infections: diagnosis using In-111, Ga-67 and Tc-99m MDP bone scintigraphy, and radiography. *Radiology* 1985;155:501–506.

Bassett LW, Gold RH, Webber MM. Radionuclide bone imaging. *Radiol Clin North Am* 1981;19:675–702.

Becker W, Goldenberg DM, Wolf F. The use of monoclonal antibodies and antibody fragments in the imaging of infectious lesions. *Semin Nucl Med* 1994;24:142–153.

Beltran J. *MRI: musculoskeletal system.* Philadelphia: JB Lippincott; 1990.

Beltran J, McGhee RB, Shaffer PB, et al. Experimental infections of the musculoskeletal system: evaluation with MR imaging and Tc-99m MDP and Ga-67 scintigraphy. *Radiology* 1988;161:167–172.

Beltran J, Noto AM, McGhee RB, Freedy RM, McCalla MS. Infections of the musculoskeletal system: high field-strength MR imaging. *Radiology* 1987;164:449–454.

Butt WP. The radiology of infection. *Clin Orthop* 1973;96:20–30.

Capitanio MA, Kirkpatrick JA. Early roentgen observations in acute osteomyelitis. *AJR Am J Roentgenol* 1970;108:488–496.

Chandnani VP, Beltran J, Morris CS, et al. Acute experimental osteomyelitis and abscesses: detection with MR imaging versus CT. *Radiology* 1990;174:233–236.

Chhem R, Cardinal E, Cho KH. Skeletal and superficial soft tissues. In: McGahan JP, Goldberg BB, eds. *Diagnostic ultrasound. A logical approach.* Philadelphia: Lippincott-Raven; 1998:1115–1134.

Dagirmanjian A, Schills J, McHenry M, Modic MT. MR imaging of vertebral osteomyelitis revisited. *AJR Am J Roentgenol* 1996;167:1539–1543.

Dangman BC, Hoffer FA, Rand FF, O'Rourke EJ. Osteomyelitis in children: gadolinium-enhanced MR imaging. *Radiology* 1992;182:743–747.

Datz FL. Indium-111-labeled leukocytes for the detection of infection: current status. *Semin Nucl Med* 1994;24:92–109.

Datz FL. The current status of radionuclide infection imaging. In: Freeman LM, ed. *Nuclear medicine annual.* New York: Raven Press, 1993:47–76.

Datz FL, Morton KA. New radiopharmaceuticals for detecting infection. *Invest Radiol* 1993;28:356–365.

Erdman WA, Tamburro F, Jayson HT, Weatherall PT, Ferry KB, Peshock RM. Osteomyelitis: characteristics and pitfalls of diagnosis with MR imaging. *Radiology* 1991;180:533–539.

Fox IN, Zeiger L. Tc-99m-HMPAO leukocyte scintigraphy for the diagnosis of osteomyelitis in diabetic foot infections. *J Foot Ankle Surg* 1993;32:591–594.

Gold RH, Hawkins RA, Katz RD. Bacterial osteomyelitis: findings on plain radiography, CT, MR, and scintigraphy. *AJR Am J Roentgenol* 1991;157:365–370.

Guhlmann A, Brecht-Krauss D, Suger G, et al. Chronic osteomyelitis: detection with FDG PET and correlation with histopathologic findings. *Radiology* 1998;206:749–754.

Harcke HT, Grissom LE. Musculoskeletal ultrasound in pediatrics. *Semin Musculoskel Radiol* 1998;2:321–329.

Hoffer P. Gallium: mechanisms. *J Nucl Med* 1980;21:282–285.

Hopkins KL, Li KCP, Bergman G. Gadolinium-DTPA-enhanced magnetic resonance imaging of musculoskeletal infectious processes. *Skeletal Radiol* 1995;24:325–330.

Howie DW, Savage JP, Wilson TG, Paterson D. The technetium phosphate bone scan in the diagnosis of osteomyelitis in childhood. *J Bone Joint Surg [Am]* 1983;65A:431–437.

Israel O, Gips S, Jerushalmi J, Frenkel A, Front D. Osteomyelitis and soft-tissue infection: Differential diagnosis with 24 hour/4 hour ratios of Tc-99m MDP uptake. *Radiology* 1987;163:725–726.

Jacobson AF, Harley JD, Lipsky BA, Pecoraro RE. Diagnosis of osteomyelitis in the presence of soft-tissue infection and radiologic evidence of osseous abnormalities: value of leukocyte scintigraphy. *AJR Am J Roentgenol* 1991;157:807–812.

Jaramillo D, Treves ST, Kasser JR, Harper M, Sundel R, Laor T. Osteomyelitis and septic arthritis in children: appropriate use of imaging to guide treatment. *AJR Am J Roentgenol* 1995;165:399–403.

Kaim A, Maurer T, Ochsner P, Jundt G, Kirsch E, Mueller-Brandt J. Chronic complicated osteomyelitis of the appendicular skeleton: diagnosis with technetium-99m labelled monoclonal antigranulocyte antibody-immunoscintigraphy. *Eur J Nucl Med* 1997;24:732–738.

King AD, Peters AM, Stuttle AWJ, Lavender JP. Imaging of bone infection with labeled white cells: role of contemporaneous bone marrow imaging. *Eur J Nucl Med* 1990;17:148–151.

Krznaric E, DeRoo M, Verbruggen A, Stuyck J, Mortelmans L. Chronic osteomyelitis: diagnosis with technetium-99m-d, 1-hexamethylpropylene amine oxime labelled leucocytes. *Eur J Nucl Med* 1996;23:792–797.

Lantto T, Kaukonen J-P, Kokkola A, Laitinen R, Vorne M. Tc-99m HMPAO labeled leukocytes superior to bone scan in the detection of osteomyelitis in children. *Clin Nucl Med* 1992;17:7–17.

Lee SK, Suh KJ, Kim YW, et al. Septic arthritis versus transient synovitis at MR imaging: preliminary assessment with signal intensity alterations in bone marrow. *Radiology* 1999;211:459–465.

Lewin JS, Rosenfield NS, Hoffer PB, Downing D. Acute osteomyelitis in children: combined Tc-99m and Ga-67 imaging. *Radiology* 1986;158:795–804.

Loyer EM, DuBrow RA, David CL, Coan JD, Eftekhari F. Imaging of superficial soft-tissue infections: sonographic findings in cases of cellulitis and abscess. *AJR Am J Roentgenol* 1996;166:149–152.

Mason MD, Zlatkin MB, Esterhai JL, Dalinka MK, Velchik MG, Kressel HY. Chronic complicated osteomyelitis of the lower extremity: evaluation with MR imaging. *Radiology* 1989;173:355–359.

Merkel KD, Brown ML, Dewanjee MK, Fitzgerald RH Jr. Comparison of indium-labeled-leukocyte imaging with sequential technetium-gallium scanning in the diagnosis of low-grade musculoskeletal sepsis. A prospective study. *J Bone Joint Surg [Am]* 1985;57A:465–476.

Miller TT, Randolph DA Jr, Staron RB, Feldman F, Cushin S. Fat-suppressed MR of musculoskeletal infection: fast T2-weighted techniques versus gadolinium-enhanced T1-weighted images. *Skeletal Radiol* 1997;26:654–658.

Modic MT, Feiglin DH, Piraino DW, et al. Vertebral osteomyelitis: assessment using MR. *Radiology* 1985;157:157–166.

Modic MT, Pflanze W, Feiglin DHI, Belhobek G. Magnetic resonance imaging of musculoskeletal infections. *Radiol Clin North Am* 1986;24:247–258.

Morrison WB, Schweitzer ME, Bock GW, Mitchell DG. Diagnosis of osteomyelitis: utility of fat-suppressed contrast-enhanced MR images. *Radiology* 1993;189:251–257.

Morrison WB, Schweitzer ME, Wapner KL, Hecht PJ, Gannon FH, Behm WR. Osteomyelitis in feet of diabetics: clinical accuracy, surgical utility, and cost-effectiveness of MR imaging. *Radiology* 1995;196:557–564.

Numaguchi Y, Rigamonti D, Rothman MI, Sato S. Spinal epidural abscess: evaluation with gadolinium-enhanced MR imaging. *Radiographics* 1993;13:545–559.

Paajanen H, Brasch RC, Schmiedl U, Ogan M. Magnetic resonance imaging of local soft tissue inflammation using gadolinium-DTPA. *Acta Radiol* 1987;28:79–83.

Paajanen H, Grodd W, Revel D, Engelstad B, Brasch RC. Gadolinium-DTPA enhanced MR imaging of intramuscular abscesses. *Magn Reson Imaging* 1987;5:109–115.

Palestro CJ, Roumanas P, Swyer AJ, Kim CK, Goldsmith SJ. Diagnosis of musculoskeletal infection using combined In-111 labeled leukocyte and Tc-99m SC marrow imaging. *Clin Nucl Med* 1992;17:269–273.

Peters AM. The utility of [^{99m}Tc] HMPAO-leukocytes for imaging infection. *Semin Nucl Med* 1994;24:110–127.

Schauerwecker DS. The role of nuclear medicine in osteomyelitis. In: Collier BD Jr, Fogelman I, Rosenthall L, eds. *Skeletal nuclear medicine.* St. Louis: CV Mosby; 1996:183–202.

Schauwecker DS. Osteomyelitis: diagnosis with In-111-labeled leukocytes. *Radiology* 1989;171:141–146.

Schauwecker DS. The scintigraphic diagnosis of osteomyelitis. *AJR Am J Roentgenol* 1992;158:9–18.

Seabold JE, Flickinger FW, Kao SCS, et al. Indium-111 leukocyte/technetium-99m-MDP bone and magnetic resonance imaging: difficulty of diagnosing osteomyelitis in patients with neuropathic osteoarthropathy. *J Nucl Med* 1990;31:549–556.

Smith AS, Weinstein MA, Mizushima A, et al. MR imaging characteristics of tuberculosis spondylitis vs vertebral osteomyelitis. *AJR Am J Roentgenol* 1989;153:399–405.

Sorsdahl OA, Goodhart GL, Williams HT, Hanna LJ, Rodriquez J. Quantitative bone gallium scintigraphy in osteomyelitis. *Skeletal Radiol* 1993;22:239–242.

Stöver B, Sigmund G, Langer M, Brandis M. MRI in diagnostic evaluation of osteomyelitis in children. *Eur Radiol* 1994;4:347–352.

Tang JSH, Gold RH, Bassett LW, Seeger LL. Musculoskeletal infection of the extremities: evaluation with MR imaging. *Radiology* 1988;166:205–209.

Tigges S, Stiles RG, Roberson JR. Appearance of septic hip prostheses on plain radiographs. *AJR Am J Roentgenol* 1994;163:377–380.

Tsan M. Mechanism of gallium-67 accumulation in inflammatory lesions. *J Nucl Med* 1985;26:88–92.

Tumeh SS, Aliabadi P, Weissman BN, McNeil BJ. Chronic osteomyelitis: bone and gallium scan patterns associated with active disease. *Radiology* 1986;158:685–688.

Unger E, Moldofsky P, Gatenby R, Hartz W, Broder G. Diagnosis of osteomyelitis by MR imaging. *AJR Am J Roentgenol* 1988;150:605–610.

Van Holsbeeck M, Introcaso JH. *Musculoskeletal ultrasound.* St. Louis: Mosby-Year Book; 1991:207–229.

Wang A, Weinstein D, Greenfield L, et al. MRI and diabetic foot infections. *Magn Reson Imaging* 1990;8:805–809.

Wukich DK, Abreu SH, Callaghan JJ, et al. Diagnosis of infection by preoperative scintigraphy with indium-labeled white blood cells. *J Bone Joint Surg [Am]* 1987;69:1353–1360.

Yuh WT, Corson JD, Baraniewski HM, et al. Osteomyelitis of the foot in diabetic patients: evaluation with plain film, ^{99m}Tc-MDP bone scintigraphy, and MR imaging. *AJR Am J Roentgenol* 1989;152:795–800.

Zeiger LS, Fox IN. Use of indium-111 labeled white blood cells in the diagnosis of diabetic foot infections. *J Foot Ankle Surg* 1990;29:46–51.

OSTEOMYELITIS, INFECTIOUS ARTHRITIS, AND SOFT-TISSUE INFECTIONS

Osteomyelitis

Osteomyelitis can generally be divided into pyogenic and nonpyogenic types. The former may be further classified, on the basis of clinical findings, as subacute, acute, or chronic (active and inactive), depending on the intensity of the infectious process and its associated symptoms. From the viewpoint of anatomic pathology, osteomyelitis can be divided into diffuse and localized (focal) forms, with the latter referred to as bone abscesses.

Pyogenic Bone Infections

Acute and Chronic Osteomyelitis

The earliest radiographic signs of bone infection are soft-tissue edema and loss of fascial planes. These are usually encountered within 24 to 48 hours of the onset of infection. The earliest changes in the bone are evidence of a destructive lytic lesion, usually within 7 to 10 days after the onset of infection (Fig. 25.1), and a positive radionuclide bone scan. Within 2 to 6 weeks, there is progressive destruction of cortical and medullary bone, an increased endosteal sclerosis indicating reactive new bone formation, and a periosteal reaction (Fig. 25.2). In 6 to 8 weeks, sequestra indicating areas of necrotic bone usually become apparent; they are surrounded by a dense involucrum, representing a sheath of periosteal new bone (Fig. 25.3). The sequestra and involucra develop as the result of an accumulation of inflammatory exudate (pus), which penetrates the cortex and strips it of periosteum, thus stimulating the inner layer to form new bone. The newly formed bone is in turn infected, and the resultant barrier causes the cortex and spongiosa to be deprived of a blood supply and to become necrotic. At this stage, termed *chronic osteomyelitis,* a draining sinus tract often

Figure 25.1 Acute osteomyelitis. A 7-year-old boy had a fever and a painful knee for 1 week. Anteroposterior radiograph of the left knee demonstrates the earliest radiographic signs of bone infection: a poorly defined osteolytic area of destruction in the metaphyseal segment of the distal femur (*arrow*) and soft-tissue swelling (*open arrows*).

forms (Fig. 25.4; see also Figs. 24.7 and 24.10B). Small sequestra are gradually resorbed, or they may be extruded through the sinus tract.

Subacute Osteomyelitis

Brodie Abscess. This lesion, originally described by Brodie in 1832, represents a subacute localized form of osteomyelitis, commonly caused by Staphylococcus aureus. The highest incidence (approximately 40%) is in the second decade. More than 75% of cases occur in male patients. Its onset is often insidious, and systemic manifestations are generally mild or absent. The abscess, which is usually localized in the metaphysis of the tibia or femur, is typically elongated, with a well-demarcated margin and surrounded by reactive sclerosis. As a rule, sequestra are absent, but a radiolucent tract may be seen extending from the lesion into the growth plate (Fig. 25.5). A bone abscess may often cross the epiphyseal plate, but seldom does an abscess develop in and remain localized to the epiphysis (Fig. 25.6; Fig. 24.8).

Nonpyogenic Bone Infections.

The most common nonpyogenic bone infections are tuberculosis, syphilis, and fungal infections.

Tuberculous Infections

Tuberculous bone infection usually occurs secondarily as a result of hematogenous spread from a primary focus of infection such as the lung or genitourinary tract. Skeletal tuberculosis represents approximately 3% of all cases of tuberculosis and approximately 30% of all extrapulmonary tuberculous infections. In 10% to 15% of cases, bone involvement without articular disease is encountered. In children, tuberculous osteomyelitis has a predilection for the metaphyseal segment of the long bones; in adults, the joints are more often affected.

In the long and short bones, progressive destruction of the medullary region with abscess formation is apparent on radiography. Typically, there is evidence of osteoporosis but, at least in the early stage of the disease, little or no reactive sclerosis is usually present (Fig. 25.7). Occasionally, destruction in the mid diaphysis of a short tubular bone of the hand or foot (*tuberculous dactylitis*) may produce a fusiform enlargement of the entire diaphysis, a condition known as spina ventosa (Fig. 25.8). The appearance of multiple disseminated lytic lesions in short tubular bones is termed cystic tuberculosis, a form of skeletal tuberculosis seen particularly in children.

Fungal Infections

Fungal bone infections are infrequent, the most common being coccidioidomycosis, blastomycosis, actinomycosis, cryptococcosis, and nocardiosis. The infection is usually low-grade, with the formation of an abscess and a draining sinus. The lesion may resemble a tuberculous skeletal infection, because the abscess is usually found in cancellous bone with little or no reactive sclerosis or periosteal response (Fig. 25.9). The location of a lesion at a point of bony prominence—such as along the edges of the patella, the ends of the clavicles, or in the acromion, coracoid process, olecranon, or styloid process of the radius or ulna—may also suggest a fungal infection. Solitary marginal lesions of the ribs and lesions involving the vertebrae in an indiscriminate fashion, including the body, neural arch, and spinous and transverse processes, also favor fungal infectious process.

Among the fungal infections, coccidioidomycosis is of particular importance, not only because of an increase in the number of these infections in recent years but also because it may closely resemble skeletal tuberculosis. It is a systemic disease caused by the soil fungus *Coccidioides immitis*. This infection is endemic throughout the southwestern United States and the bordering regions of northern Mexico. Infection occurs through inhalation of dust containing the organism. The primary site of infection is the lung, and disease is commonly asymptomatic. Dissemination of coccidioidomycosis is rare, but the incidence is increased in patients with specific risk factors. Those at increased risk include Filipinos, blacks, Mexicans, males, pregnant women, children younger than 5 years, adults older than 50 years, and immunosuppressed patients. Patients with disseminated coccidioidomycosis usually present during the course of primary pulmonary infection. However, some patients with disseminated disease may have no clinical history or radiographic evidence of pulmonary disease. The skin and subcutaneous tissues are the most common sites of disseminated coccidioidal infection, followed by mediastinal involvement. The skeletal system is the third most common site of dissemination, and osseous manifestations occur in 10% to 50% of patients with disseminated disease.

Radiographic presentation of the lesion of coccidioidomycosis is variable, but it is usually characterized by well-marginated, punched-out osteolytic lesions, typically involving long and flat bones. The lesions are typically unilocular but occasionally may be multiloculated. The other pattern frequently observed is a permeative type of bone destruction, only occasionally accompanied by periosteal reaction. Soft-tissue swelling and osteoporosis are much more common with the permeative pattern than with the punched-out lesions. The third most common pattern is joint involvement (septic arthritis), usually monoarticular and almost invariably associated with osseous involvement. Changes typically seen in joints include periarticular osteoporosis, a permeative/destructive pattern involving both articular surfaces, soft-tissue swelling, and occasional periostitis. Joint involvement in coccidioidomycosis is indistinguishable from that seen with tuberculosis. Involvement of the spine most commonly manifests as vertebral osteomyelitis or rarely as disk space infection (spondylodiskitis). In the former variant, both punched-out and permeative lesions are observed in the vertebral bodies. Cases with almost complete vertebral destruction have also been reported. Coccidioidomycosis often involves the vertebral appendages, and paraspinal soft-tissue extension is common. Disk space narrowing and gibbous deformity, although previously re-

Figure 25.2 Acute osteomyelitis. Anteroposterior **(A)** and lateral **(B)** radiographs of the knee of an 8-year-old boy with acute osteomyelitis show widespread destruction of the cortical and medullary portions of the metaphysis and diaphysis of the distal femur, together with periosteal new bone formation. Note the pathologic fracture. On the lateral view, a large subperiosteal abscess is evident.

ported, are unusual findings in coccidioidomycosis, whereas both these findings are common in tuberculosis.

Scintigraphy is valuable in the evaluation of patients with disseminated coccidioidomycosis. Radionuclide scans using gallium-67 (^{67}Ga) citrate and technetium-99m (^{99m}Tc) methylene diphosphonate (MDP) have been used to localize disease and can identify disseminated lesions that are clinically unsuspected. No false-negative bone scans have been reported. Computed tomography (CT) and magnetic resonance imaging (MRI) are helpful in defining bony involvement and in determining the extent of soft-tissue disease (Fig. 25.10). The lesions exhibit low attenuation, often appearing bubbly

and expansive. On MRI, the lesions show decreased signal on T1-weighted images, with a corresponding increase on T2-weighted and gradient-echo sequences.

Syphilitic Infection

Syphilis is a chronic systemic infectious disease caused by a spirochete, *Treponema pallidum. Congenital syphilis,* which is transmitted from mother to fetus, may manifest as a chronic osteochondritis, periostitis, or osteitis. The lesions, which most frequently involve the tibia, are characteristically widespread and symmetric in appearance; destructive changes are usually seen in the metaphysis at the junction with the

Figure 25.3 Active osteomyelitis. Sequestra surrounded by involucrum, as seen here in the left leg of a 2-year-old child, is a feature of advanced osteomyelitis, usually apparent after 6 to 8 weeks of active infection. (Courtesy of Dr. R.H. Gold, Los Angeles, CA.)

Figure 25.4 Chronic osteomyelitis. A 28-year-old man with sickle-cell disease had osteomyelitis, a frequent complication of this condition. A sinogram enhanced by magnification shows a draining sinus typical of chronic osteomyelitis. Note the extent of the serpentine tract in the medullary portion of the bone.

Figure 25.5 Bone absess. Anteroposterior radiograph of the left knee of an 11-year-old boy with a subacute Brodie abscess in the proximal diaphysis and metaphysis of the tibia shows a radiolucent tract extending into the growth plate.

Figure 25.6 Bone abscess. Anteroposterior radiograph of the left knee of a 13-year-old boy demonstrates a well-defined osteolytic lesion surrounded by reactive sclerosis in the distal epiphysis of the femur. This is a rare site for a bone abscess.

Figure 25.7 Tuberculosis of bone. A 20-month-old girl had progressive swelling of the right foot. Anteroposterior radiograph of the foot shows a well-defined lytic defect in the medial aspect of the second metatarsal; there is no evidence of reactive sclerosis or periosteal new bone formation, but soft-tissue swelling is apparent. Aspiration of a mass yielded 1 mL of pus-like fluid, which on bacteriologic examination revealed acid-fast bacteria. The causative agent proved to be *Mycobacterium tuberculosis*.

Figure 25.8 Tuberculosis of bone. Oblique film of the right hand of a 7-year-old boy with skeletal tuberculosis shows expansive fusiform lesions of the first and fifth metacarpals associated with soft-tissue swelling; there is no evidence of a periosteal reaction. Such diaphyseal enlargement secondary to tuberculosis is known as spina ventosa.

Figure 25.9 Cryptococcosis of bone. Anteroposterior radiograph of the right shoulder of an 18-year-old man demonstrates a destructive osteolytic lesion in the medial aspect of the humeral head, with minimal sclerosis and no periosteal reaction—the typical appearance of a fungal infection. Aspiration biopsy showed the abscess to be caused by a cryptococcal infection.

other conditions. Particularly in its acute form, it may resemble Langerhans cell histiocytosis or Ewing sarcoma (Fig. 25.13). The soft-tissue changes in each of these conditions, however, are characteristic and different. In osteomyelitis, soft-tissue swelling is diffuse, with obliteration of the fascial planes, whereas Langerhans cell histiocytosis, as a rule, is not accompanied by significant soft-tissue swelling or a mass. The extension of a Ewing sarcoma into the soft tissues presents as a well-defined soft-tissue mass with preservation of the fascial planes. The duration of a patient's symptoms also plays an important diagnostic role. It takes a tumor such as a Ewing sarcoma from 4 to 6 months to destroy the bone to the same extent that osteomyelitis does in 4 to 6 weeks and that Langerhans cell histiocytosis does in only 7 to 10 days. Despite these differentiating features, however, the radiographic pattern of bone destruction, periosteal reaction, and location in the bone may be very similar in all three conditions (see Fig. 22.10).

A bone abscess, particularly in the cortex, may closely simulate a nidus of osteoid osteoma (see Fig. 17.20). In the medullary region, however, the presence of a serpentine tract favors the diagnosis of bone abscess over osteoid osteoma (Fig. 25.14).

Infectious Arthritides

Most infectious arthritides demonstrate a positive radionuclide bone scan and a very similar radiographic picture, including joint effusion and destruction of cartilage and subchondral bone with consequent joint space narrowing (see Figs. 12.21 and 12.24). However, certain clinical and radiographic features are characteristic of individual infectious processes as demonstrated at various target sites (Table 25.1).

Pyogenic Joint Infections

The clinical signs and symptoms of pyogenic (septic) arthritis depend on the site and extent of involvement as well as the specific infectious organism. Although most cases of septic arthritis are caused by *Staphylococcus aureus* and *Neisseria gonorrhoeae*, other pathogens—including *Pseudomonas aeruginosa*, *Enterobacter cloacae*, *Klebsiella pneumoniae*, *Candida albicans*, and *Serratia marcescens*—are being encountered with increasing frequency in joint infections in drug users caused by the contamination of injected drugs or needles.

Any small or large joint can be affected by septic arthritis, and hematogenous spread in drug addicts is characterized by unusual locations of the lesion, such as the spine (vertebrae and intervertebral

growth plate, producing what is called the Wimberger sign (Fig. 25.11). In the later stages of disease, involvement of the tibia results in a characteristic anterior bowing known as "saber-shin" deformity.

Acquired syphilis may manifest either as a chronic osteitis exhibiting irregular sclerosis of the medullary cavity or as syphilitic abscesses known as gumma (Fig. 25.12). The latter form of the disease may simulate pyogenic osteomyelitis, but the absence of sequestra typically found in bacterial osteomyelitis allows the distinction to be made.

Differential Diagnosis of Osteomyelitis

Usually, the radiographic appearance of osteomyelitis is so characteristic that the diagnosis is easily made with the clinical history, and ancillary radiologic examinations such as scintigraphy, CT, and MRI are rarely needed. Nevertheless, osteomyelitis may at times mimic

Figure 25.10 Coccidioidomycosis of bone. A 42-year-old man presented with a 4-week history of pain and decreased range of motion in the left shoulder. He had been previously hospitalized for pulmonary coccidioidomycosis. **(A)** Anteroposterior radiograph shows several osteolytic lesions affecting the superolateral aspect of the humeral head and glenoid (*arrows*). Small punched-out lesion is noted in the body of the scapula (*arrowhead*). The *curved arrow* points to periosteal reaction along the medial humeral shaft. **(B)** A CT section reveals erosions of the anterior and posterolateral aspects of the humeral head. Also apparent are destruction of the articular surfaces of the humeral head and glenoid and narrowing of the glenohumeral joint. *(continued)*

Figure 25.10 Coccidioidomycosis of bone. *Continued* Sagittal **(C)** and **(D)** axial fast-spin echo (TR 4000/TE 102 msec) MR images show multiple, well-defined soft-tissue abscesses displaying high signal intensity *(arrows)*. H, humeral head.

Figure 25.11 Congenital syphilis of bone. (A) Anteroposterior radiograph of the lower legs of a 7-week-old infant with congenital syphilis demonstrates characteristic periostitis affecting the femora and tibiae. In addition, destructive changes are evident in the medullary portion of the proximal tibiae. **(B)** Two months later, the infectious process has progressed, with destruction of the tibial metaphysis and marked periostitis. The characteristic erosion of the medial surface of the proximal tibial metaphysis is termed the Wimberger sign.

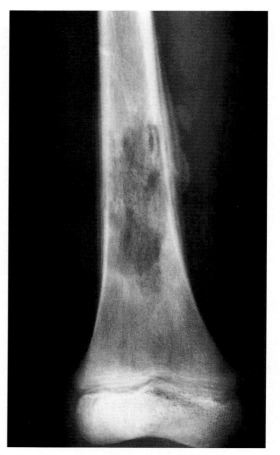

Figure 25.12 Acquired syphilis of bone. Oblique radiograph of the distal forearm of a 51-year-old man with acquired syphilis shows a lytic abscess (gumma) in the lateral aspect of the distal radius.

Figure 25.13 Osteomyelitis resembling Ewing sarcoma. A 7-year-old boy presented with pain in his right leg for 3 weeks. Anteroposterior radiograph demonstrates a lesion in the medullary portion of the distal femoral diaphysis with a moth-eaten type of bone destruction, associated with a lamellated periosteal reaction and a small soft-tissue prominence. These radiographic features suggest a diagnosis of Ewing sarcoma. The absence of a definite soft-tissue mass and the short symptomatic period, however, point to the correct diagnosis of osteomyelitis, which was confirmed by biopsy.

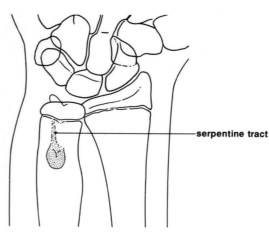

serpentine tract

Figure 25.14 Bone abscess resembling osteoid osteoma. A 17-year-old boy had a typical history of osteoid osteoma: nocturnal bone pain relieved promptly by salicylates. Anteroposterior radiograph of the distal forearm demonstrates a radiolucent lesion in the distal ulnar diaphysis. The presence of a serpentine tract extending from the radiolucent focus into the growth plate indicates a diagnosis of bone abscess.

Table 25.1 **Clinical and Radiographic Hallmarks of Infectious Arthritis at Various Target Sites**

Type	Site	Crucial Abnormalities	Techniques/Projections
Pyogenic Infections*			
	Peripheral joints	Periarticular osteoporosis	Radionuclide bone scan (early)
		Joint effusion	Standard views specific for site of involvement
		Destruction of subchondral bone (on both sides of joint)	Aspiration and arthrography
	Spine	Narrowing of disk space	Anteroposterior and lateral views
		Loss of definition of vertebral end plate	
		Paraspinal mass	CT, MRI
		Partial or complete obstruction of intrathecal contrast flow	Myelogram
		Destruction of disk	Diskogram and aspiration
Nonpyogenic Infections			
Tuberculosis	Large joints	Monoarticular involvement (similar to rheumatoid arthritis)	Radionuclide bone scan
		"Kissing" sequestra (knee)	Standard views
		Sclerotic changes in subchondral bone	Tomography, CT
	Spine	Gibbous formation	Anteroposterior and lateral views
		Lytic lesion in vertebral body	
		Destruction of disk	Diskogram and aspiration
		Paraspinal mass	CT, MRI
		Soft-tissue abscess ("cold" abscess)	
		Obstruction of intrathecal contrast flow	Myelogram
Lyme disease	Knee	Narrowing of femoropatellar compartment	Lateral view
		Edematous changes in infrapatellar fat pad	CT, MRI

* In IV drug users, unusual sites of infection are encountered, including the vertebra; the sacroiliac, sternoclavicular, and acromioclavicular joints; and the pubic symphysis. The radiologic techniques used to evaluate infections at these sites, as well as the crucial radiographic abnormalities, are the same as those for the more common sites.

disks), sacroiliac joints, sternoclavicular and acromioclavicular articulations, and pubic symphysis.

Standard radiography usually suffices to demonstrate septic arthritis. Certain characteristic radiographic features may be helpful in arriving at the correct diagnosis. Generally, a single joint is affected, most commonly a weight-bearing joint like the knee or hip. The early stage of joint infection may be seen simply as joint effusion, soft-tissue swelling, and periarticular osteoporosis (Fig. 25.15).

In the later phase of pyogenic arthritis, articular cartilage is destroyed; characteristically, both subarticular plates are involved and the joint space narrows (Fig. 25.16A). Arthrography, which is often performed after aspiration of the joint to obtain a fluid specimen for

Figure 25.15 Septic arthritis. Anteroposterior (**A**) and lateral (**B**) radiographs of the left knee of a 4-year-old child demonstrate a significant degree of periarticular osteoporosis and a large joint effusion. Note the small erosions of the distal epiphysis of the femur and the preservation of the joint space. Aspiration revealed hematogenous spread of a staphylococcal urinary tract infection.

Figure 25.16 Septic arthritis. A 64-year-old woman had had an upper respiratory infection 6 months before pain developed in her left hip. **(A)** Antero-posterior radiograph of the hip demonstrates complete destruction of the articular cartilage on both sides of the joint and erosion of the femoral head. Note the significant degree of osteoporosis. **(B)** Contrast arthrography was performed primarily to obtain joint fluid for bacteriologic examination, which yielded *Staphylococcus aureus.* The contrast agent outlines the destroyed joint, showing a synovial irregularity consistent with chronic synovitis.

bacteriologic examination, helps determine the extent of joint destruction and demonstrate the presence of synovitis (Fig. 25.16B). Radionuclide bone scan is often effective in distinguishing a joint infection from a periarticular soft-tissue infection (see Fig. 24.9). It is also useful in monitoring the progress of treatment, although several weeks may be required before the scan demonstrates a completely normal appearance.

Complications

Infectious arthritis of peripheral joints in children may lead to the destruction of the growth plate, with resulting growth arrest (see Fig. 24.16). The infection may also spread to an adjacent bone, causing osteomyelitis. Degenerative arthritis and intraarticular bony ankylosis may also occur.

Nonpyogenic Joint Infections

Tuberculous Arthritis

Tuberculous arthritis represents 1% of all forms of extrapulmonary tuberculosis, although the number of cases has recently been on the rise. The acid-fast tubercle bacilli *Mycobacterium tuberculosis* and *Mycobacterium bovi* are the causative organisms. The infection may be found in all groups, but more frequently in children and young adults. Predisposing factors such as trauma, alcoholism, drug abuse, intraarticular injection of steroids, or prolonged systemic illness are found in most patients with tuberculous arthritis. The joint infection usually is caused by either direct invasion from an adjacent focus of osteomyelitis or hematogenous dissemination of the tubercle bacillus. Large weight-bearing joints such as the hip or knee are most often affected, and monoarticular involvement is the rule.

Conventional radiography is usually sufficient to demonstrate the identifying features of tuberculous arthritis, although its early radiographic appearance is often indistinguishable from that of monoarticular rheumatoid arthritis. However, the involvement of only one joint, as demonstrated by scintigraphy, favors an infectious process (Fig. 25.17). A triad of radiographic abnormalities (Phemister triad),

comprised of periarticular osteoporosis, peripherally located osseous erosions, and gradual diminution of the joint space, should suggest the correct diagnosis; CT examination, however, can be helpful in delineating subtle features (Fig. 25.18). Occasionally, wedge-shaped necrotic foci, so-called kissing sequestra, may be present on both sides of the affected joint, especially in the knee. At a later stage of the disease, there may be complete destruction of the joint, and sclerotic changes in adjacent bones are more frequently encountered (Fig. 25.19).

Other Infectious Arthritides

Less frequently encountered than pyogenic or tuberculous arthritis are joint infections caused by fungi (actinomycosis, cryptococcosis, coccidioidomycosis, histoplasmosis, sporotrichosis, and candidiasis), viruses (smallpox), and spirochetes (syphilis, yaws).

Of interest is *Lyme arthritis,* an infectious articular condition caused by the spirochete *Borrelia burgdorferi,* which is transmitted by the tick *Ixodes dammini* or related ticks such as *Ixodes pacificus* and *Ixodes ricinus.* The illness usually begins in the summer with a characteristic skin lesion (erythema chronicum migrans) at the site of a tick bite, and flu-like symptoms; within weeks to months, a chronic arthritis develops that is characterized by erosions of cartilage and bone. The joint involvement has some similarities to juvenile rheumatoid arthritis and Reiter syndrome. A joint effusion may be present in the early stages of the disease, and characteristic edematous changes of the infrapatellar fat pad may be noted in the knee (Fig. 25.20). MR imaging may show ribbon-like folds of hypertrophied synovium and frond-like extensions of synovium and synovial fluid into infrapatellar fat pad (Fig. 25.21).

Infections of the Spine

Pyogenic Infections

Infectious organisms may reach the spine by several routes. Hematogenous spread occurs by way of arterial and venous routes (the Batson paravertebral venous system), and the organism lodges in

Figure 25.17 Tuberculous arthritis. A 29-year-old woman with chronic alcoholism presented with right hip pain. **(A)** Anteroposterior radiograph of the hip demonstrates diminution of the joint space, particularly in the weight-bearing region, as well as periarticular osteoporosis. **(B)** Radionuclide bone scan using technetium-99m-labeled diphosphonate demonstrates increased isotope uptake only in the right hip. The increased activity at both sacroiliac joints is a normal finding. The diagnosis of tuberculous arthritis was confirmed by joint aspiration.

Figure 25.18 Tuberculous arthritis. A 70-year-old man from India had pain in the left elbow for 4 months. According to his daughter, he had been treated for chronic lung disease. Anteroposterior **(A)** and lateral **(B)** radiographs of the elbow demonstrate a large joint effusion, as indicated by positive anterior and posterior fat pad signs on the lateral projection. Small periarticular erosions are not clear on these views. **(C)** CT section shows narrowing of the joint and peripheral erosions typical of tuberculous infection.

Figure 25.19 Tuberculous arthritis. Posteroanterior radiograph of the left wrist and hand of a 52-year-old woman with pulmonary tuberculosis shows advanced tuberculous arthritis involving the left carpus. There is complete destruction of the radiocarpal, midcarpal, and carpometacarpal articulations, as well as whittling and sclerotic changes in the distal radius and ulna. Note the osteoporosis distal to the affected joints and the soft-tissue swelling.

Figure 25.20 Lyme arthritis. Lateral radiograph of the right knee of a 13-year-old boy, who presented with intermittent soft-tissue swelling and knee effusion for several months, shows periarticular osteoporosis, joint effusion, soft-tissue swelling, and areas of mottled density at the site of infrapatellar fat pad. (Reprinted with permission from Lawson JP, Rahn, DW. Lyme disease and radiologic findings in Lyme arthritis. *AJR Am J Roentgenol* 1992; 158:1065–1069.)

Figure 25.21 MRI of Lyme arthritis. Sagittal T2-weighted MRI of the left knee of a 17-year-old boy, who presented with knee swelling for 7 months, reveals joint effusion that displaced medial meniscus anteriorly (*white arrow*). Note ribbon-like folds of hypertrophied synovium and frond-like extensions of synovium and synovial fluid into infrapatellar fat pad (*black arrows*). (Reprinted with permission from Lawson JP, Rahn DW. Lyme disease and radiologic findings in Lyme arthritis. *AJR Am J Roentgenol* 1992; 158:1065–1069.)

Figure 25.22 Sequential stages of involvement of a vertebral body and disk by an infectious process.

the vertebral body, commonly in the anterior subchondral region. This osteomyelitic focus can spread to the intervertebral disk through perforation of the vertebral end-plate, causing disk space infection (diskitis) (Fig. 25.22). Disk space infection can also be induced directly by the implantation of an organism through puncture of the spinal canal, either during spinal surgery or, rarely, by spread from a contiguous site of infection such as a paravertebral abscess (see Fig. 24.4). Disk infection may also occur in children via a hematogenous route, because there is still a blood supply to the disk.

Radiographically, disk infection is characterized by narrowing of the disk space, destruction of the adjacent vertebral end plates, and a paraspinal mass. Although most cases are obvious on standard anteroposterior and lateral radiographs of the spine (Fig. 25.23), conventional and computed tomography (Fig. 25.24) may yield additional information. Radionuclide bone scan can detect early infection before any changes noticed radiographically (Fig. 25.25). Occasionally, diskography is performed but, as in the use of arthrography in joint infections, the primary objective is obtaining a specimen for bacteriologic examination. A contrast study, however, may outline the extent of a disk infection (Fig. 25.26).

MRI has become the modality of choice in diagnosing and evaluating infections of the spine. Characteristic findings of disk space narrowing, disk destruction, paraspinal soft-tissue thickening, and edematous changes in the paraspinal musculature are well demonstrated by this technique (Fig. 25.27).

Nonpyogenic Infections

Tuberculosis of the Spine

Infection of the spine by the tubercle bacillus is known as *tuberculous spondylitis* or *Pott disease*. The vertebral body or intervertebral disk may be involved, with the lower thoracic and upper lumbar vertebrae being the preferred sites of infection. The disease constitutes 25% to 50% of all cases of skeletal tuberculosis.

The radiographic features of tuberculous infection of the spine are similar to those seen in pyogenic infections. There is disk space narrowing, and the vertebral end plates adjacent to the involved disk show evidence of destruction. A paraspinal mass is common (Fig. 25.28). Rarely, the infectious process may destroy a single vertebra or part of a vertebra (pedicle) without invasion of the disk.

Complications. Tuberculosis of the spine may cause collapse of a partially or completely destroyed vertebra, leading to kyphosis and a gibbous formation. Extension of infection to the adjacent ligaments and soft tissues is also rather frequent; the psoas muscles are often the site of secondary tuberculous infections, commonly called "cold" abscesses (Fig. 25.29). The most common complication of tuberculous spondylitis, however, is compression of the thecal sac and spinal cord with resulting paraplegia. Myelography and MRI are very helpful diagnostically if compression is suspected (Fig. 25.30).

Figure 25.23 Intervertebral disk infection. Lateral radiograph of the lumbar spine in a 32-year-old man demonstrates the typical radiographic changes of disk infection. There is narrowing of the disk space at L4-5, and the inferior end plate of L-4 and superior end plate of L-5 are indistinctly outlined. Note the normal end plates at the L3-4 disk space.

Figure 25.24 Intervertebral disk infection. A 40-year-old man presented with lower back pain for 8 weeks, which he attributed to lifting a heavy object. **(A)** Lateral radiograph of the lumbosacral spine shows narrowing of the L5-S1 disk space and suggests some fuzziness of the adjacent vertebral end plates. **(B)** CT section through the disk space clearly shows destructive changes of the disk and vertebral end plate characteristic of infection.

Figure 25.25 Intervertebral disk infection. Standard anteroposterior (**A**) and lateral (**B**) radiographs of the lumbar spine of a 40-year-old man who had back pain for 4 weeks show no definite abnormalities. (**C**) Radionuclide bone scan, however, reveals increased uptake of radiopharmaceutical at the L3-4 level. (**D**) On a subsequent diskogram, using the oblique approach, partial disk destruction is evident. (**E**) The extent of destruction is revealed by CT. Bacteriologic examination of aspirated fluid yielded *Escherichia coli.*

Figure 25.26 Disk space infection and vertebral osteomyelitis. A 22-year-old intravenous drug user with back pain for 2 months had an intervertebral disk infection. A diskogram was performed primarily to aspirate fluid for bacteriologic examination, which revealed *Pseudomonas aeruginosa.* Before the puncture, the patient received an intravenous injection of iodine contrast medium to visualize the kidneys, as a precautionary step before spine biopsy at that level. **(A)** Lateral radiograph of the lumbar spine shows narrowing of the disk space at L1-2 and destruction of the adjacent vertebral end plates. The spinal needle is located in the center of the disk. **(B)** Lateral radiograph obtained during the injection of metrizamide demonstrates extension of the contrast medium into the body of L-2, indicating the presence of vertebral osteomyelitis.

Figure 25.27 MRI of disk space infection and vertebral osteomyelitis. A 48-year-old man who is an intravenous drug user had disk infection at L1-2. **(A)** Lateral radiograph demonstrates classic changes of disk space infection: narrowing of the disk space and destruction of the vertebral end plates. **(B)** Sagittal spin-echo T1-weighted MR image (TR 600/TE 20 msec) demonstrates, in addition to the destruction of the disk, a large inflammatory mass extending anteriorly, destroying anterior longitudinal ligament and infiltrating paraspinal soft tissues. Posteriorly, it invades the content of spinal canal. **(C)** Sagittal T2*-weighted gradient (MPGR) MR image shows more clearly the fragmentation of the posterior aspect of adjacent vertebral bodies and compression of the thecal sac by a large abscess.

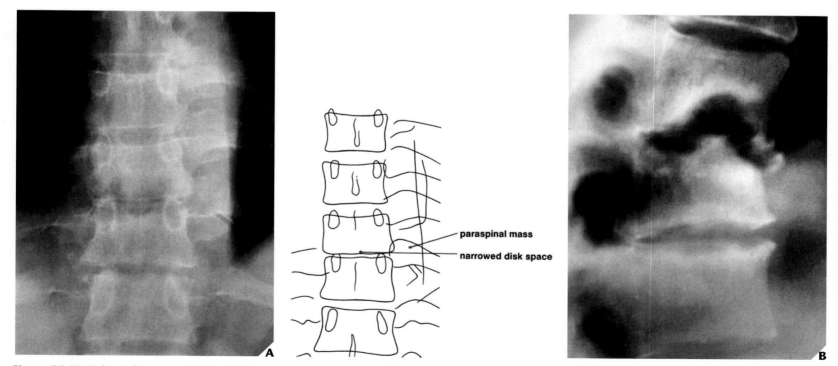

Figure 25.28 Tuberculous spondylitis. (A) Anteroposterior radiograph of the thoracic spine in a 50-year-old man shows narrowing of the T8-9 disk space, associated with a paraspinal mass on the left side. **(B)** Lateral tomogram shows destruction of the disk and extensive erosions of the inferior aspect of the body of T-8 and the superior end-plate of T-9.

Figure 25.29 **Tuberculous "cold" abscess.** Anteroposterior radiograph of the pelvis in a 35-year-old woman with spinal tuberculosis shows an oval radiodense mass with spotted calcifications overlapping the medial part of the ilium and right sacroiliac joint (right psoas muscle). This is the typical appearance of a "cold" abscess.

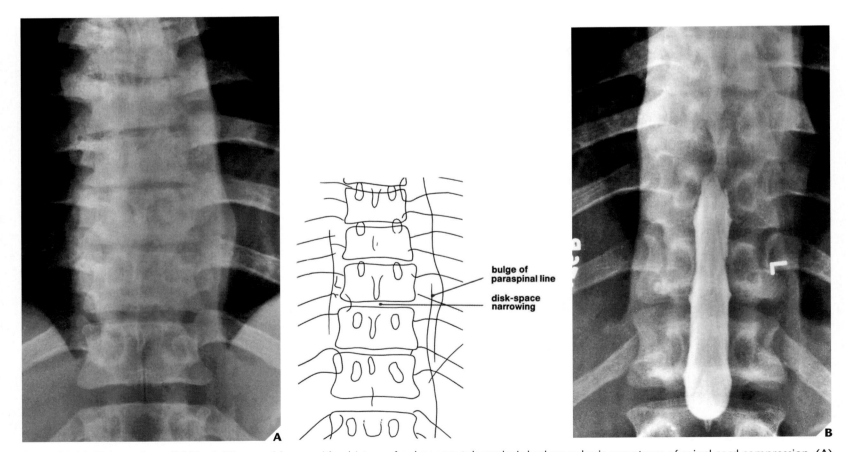

bulge of
paraspinal line

disk-space
narrowing

Figure 25.30 **Tuberculous diskitis.** A 39-year-old man with a history of pulmonary tuberculosis had neurologic symptoms of spinal cord compression. **(A)** Anteroposterior radiograph of the thoracic spine shows minimal disk space narrowing at T9-10 and a large left paraspinal mass. **(B)** A myelogram shows complete obstruction of the flow of contrast in the subarachnoid space at the level of the disk infection.

Figure 25.33 MRI of soft-tissue abscess. Sagittal spin-echo T2-weighted MR image (TR 2000/TE 80 msec) reveals a high-signal-intensity fluid collection adjacent to the medial malleolus in this diabetic patient with a foot infection. (From Beltran J, 1990, with permission.)

Soft-Tissue Infections

Soft-tissue infections (cellulitis) usually result from direct introduction of organisms through a skin puncture; they are also seen as a complication of systemic disorders such as diabetes. The most frequently encountered organisms are *Staphylococcus aureus*, *Clostridium novyi*, and *Clostridium perfringens*. These gas-forming organisms may cause an accumulation of gas in the soft tissues that can easily be recognized on plain films as radiolucent bubbles or streaks in the subcutaneous tissues or muscles. This finding usually indicates gangrene caused by anaerobic bacteria. Soft-tissue edema and obliteration of fat and fascial planes are also evident on the standard radiographic examination (Fig. 25.31). CT is effective in this respect, and in addition can differentiate pure cellulitis from that associated with bone infection (Fig. 25.32).

Currently, MRI is considered to be a gold standard to evaluate soft-tissue infection. In particular, soft-tissue abscesses, as well as involvement of tendon sheaths and muscles, are accurately depicted with this modality. Soft-tissue abscesses appear as rounded or elongated—but always well-demarcated—areas of decreased signal intensity on T1-weighted images, changing to increased signal intensity on T2-weighted images (Fig. 25.33). Occasionally, a peripheral band of decreased signal intensity is seen that represents the fibrous capsule surrounding the abscess (see Fig. 24.12). Infected fluid collection within the tendon sheath is always hyperintense on T2-weighting and hypointense on T1 weighting, but this cannot be differentiated from noninfected fluid.

Figure 25.31 Gangrene of soft tissues. Oblique radiograph of the foot of a 59-year-old man with long-standing diabetes mellitus shows marked soft-tissue swelling and edema, particularly in the region of the fourth and fifth digits. Radiolucent streaks of gas are typical of gangrenous infection.

Figure 25.32 Soft-tissue abscess. A 26-year-old man had an infection of the anterior aspect of the left lower leg. Axial **(A)** CT section and oblique **(B)** sagittal reformatted image show an abscess and its relation to the tibia. Note that the cortex is not affected.

PRACTICAL POINTS TO REMEMBER

Osteomyelitis

[1] The radiographic hallmarks of osteomyelitis include:
- cortical and medullary bone destruction
- reactive sclerosis and a periosteal reaction
- the presence of sequestra and involucra.

[2] The metaphysis is a characteristic site of osteomyelitis in children.

[3] Acute osteomyelitis of a long bone frequently mimics Ewing sarcoma and Langerhans cell histiocytosis. The clinical history, especially the duration of symptoms before the discovery of bone changes, usually serves as a clue to the correct diagnosis.

[4] A destructive metaphyseal lesion extending into the epiphysis usually indicates a bone abscess.

[5] A Brodie abscess may clinically and radiographically mimic an osteoid osteoma. In the differential diagnosis, the presence of a radiolucent tract extending from the lesion into the growth plate favors an infectious process.

In congenital syphilis:
- osteochondritis, periostitis, and osteitis are typical features
- destruction at the medial aspect of the metaphysis of a long bone (Wimberger sign) is characteristic.

Infectious Arthritis

[1] The characteristic radiographic features of septic arthritis of the peripheral joints include:
- periarticular osteoporosis, joint effusion, and soft-tissue swelling (early phase)
- destruction of cartilage and the subchondral plates on both sides of the joint (late phase).

[2] In tuberculosis of a peripheral joint, which usually manifests as a monoarticular disease (strongly resembling rheumatoid arthritis), the Phemister triad of radiographic abnormalities is characteristic and includes:
- periarticular osteoporosis
- peripheral osseous erosions
- gradual narrowing of the joint space.

[3] Lyme arthritis exhibits some similarities to juvenile rheumatoid arthritis and Reiter syndrome. Characteristic edematous changes of the infrapatellar fat pad and folds of hypertrophied synovium are demonstrated on MRI.

Infections of the Spine

[1] In the imaging evaluation of spine infections:
- radionuclide bone scan can detect disk infection prior to the appearance of any radiographic signs
- the diskogram is a valid examination performed primarily to obtain aspirate fluid for bacteriologic study
- MRI is the modality of choice to diagnose and evaluate spine infection.

[2] Pyogenic infection of the spine is recognized radiographically by:
- narrowing of the disk space
- destruction of both vertebral end plates adjacent to the involved disk
- a paraspinal mass.

[3] The radiographic hallmarks of tuberculous infection of an intervertebral disk are:
- narrowing of the disk space
- loss of the sharp outline of the adjacent vertebral end plates.

[4] Tuberculous infection of the spine may:
- destroy the disk and vertebra, leading to kyphosis and a gibbus formation
- extend into the soft tissues, forming a "cold" abscess.

Soft-Tissue Infections

[1] Cellulitis caused by gas-forming bacteria in soft tissues (gangrene) is recognized radiographically by:
- soft-tissue edema and swelling
- radiolucent bubbles or streaks representing accumulations of gas.

[2] Diabetic subjects are particularly prone to soft-tissue infections, the feet being common sites.

[3] Scintigraphy using indium-111-labelled white cells is useful in detecting and localizing the site of infection, whereas MRI is ideal in evaluating the extent of infection in the soft tissues.

[4] MRI using contrast enhancement with gadolinium allows differentiation of abscess from cellulitis or phlegmon.

SUGGESTED READINGS

Abdelwahab IF, Present DA, Zwass A, Klein MJ, Mazzara J. Tumorlike tuberculosis granulomas of bone. *AJR Am J Roentgenol* 1987;149:1207–1208.

Alexander GH, Mansuy MM. Disseminated bone tuberculosis (so-called multiple cystic tuberculosis). *Radiology* 1950;55:839–842.

Al-Shahed MS, Sharif HS, Haddad MC, Aabed MY, Sammak BM, Mutairi MA. Imaging features of musculoskeletal brucellosis. *Radiographics* 1994;14:333–348.

Armbuster TG, Goergen TG, Resnick D, Catanzaro A. Utility of bone scanning in disseminated coccidioidomycosis: a case report. *J Nucl Med* 1977;18:450–454.

Bayer AS, Guze LB. Fungal arthritis. II. Coccidioidal synovitis: clinical, diagnostic, therapeutic, and prognostic considerations. *Semin Arthritis Rheum* 1979;8:200–211.

Behrman RE, Masci JR, Nicholas P. Cryptococcal skeletal infections: case report and review. *Rev Infect Dis* 1990;12:181–190.

Beltran J. *MRI: musculoskeletal system* Philadelphia: JB Lippincott; 1990.

Benninghoven CD, Miller ER. Coccidioidal infection in bone. *Radiology* 1942;38:663–666.

Birsner JW, Smart S. Osseous coccidioidomycosis: a chronic form of dissemination. *AJR Am J Roentgenol* 1956;76:1052–1060.

Brodie BC. An account of some cases of chronic abscess of the tibia. *Trans Med Chir Soc* 1832;17:238–239.

Bruno MS, Silverberg TN, Goldstein DH. Embolic osteomyelitis of the spine as a complication of infection of the urinary tract. *Am J Med* 1960;29:865–878.

Carter RA. Infectious granulomas of bones and joints, with special reference to coccidioidal granuloma. *Radiology* 1934;23:1–16.

Chelboun J, Sydney N. Skeletal cryptococcosis. *J Bone Joint Surg [Am]* 1977;59A:509–514.

Cremin BJ, Fisher RM. The lesions of congenital syphilis. *Br J Radiol* 1970;43:333–341.

Crim JR, Seeger LL. Imaging evaluation of osteomyelitis. *Crit Rev Diagn Imaging* 1994;35:201–256.

Dalinka MK, Greendyke WH. The spinal manifestations of coccidioidomycosis. *J Can Assoc Radiol* 1971;22:93–99.

David R, Barron BJ, Madewell JE. Osteomyelitis, acute and chronic. *Radiol Clin North Am* 1987;25:1171–1201.

Drutz DJ, Catanzaro A. Coccidioidomycosis. Part I. *Am Rev Respir Dis* 1978;117:559–585.

Drutz DJ, Catanzaro A. Coccidioidomycosis. Part II. *Am Rev Respir Dis* 1978;117:727–771.

Erdman WA, Tamburo F, Jayson HT, Weatherall PT, Ferry KB, Peshock RM. Osteomyelitis: characteristics and pitfalls of diagnosis with MR imaging. *Radiology* 1991;180:533–539.

Ehrlich I, Kricum ME. Radiographic findings in early acquired syphilis: case report and critical review. *AJR Am J Roentgenol* 1976;127:789–792.

Fialk MA, Marcove RC, Armstrong D. Cryptococcal bone disease: a manifestation of disseminated cryptococcosis. *Clin Orthop* 1981;158:219–223.

Fletcher BD, Scoles PV, Nelson AD. Osteomyelitis in children: detection by magnetic resonance. *Radiology* 1984;150:57–60.

Gilmour WM. Acute haematogenous osteomyelitis. *J Bone Joint Surg [Br]* 1962;44B:841–853.

Gold RH, Hawkins RA, Katz RD. Bacterial osteomyelitis: findings on plain radiography, CT, MR, and scintigraphy. *AJR Am J Roentgenol* 1991;157:365–370.

Goodhart GL, Zakem JF, Collins WC, Meyer JD. Brucellosis of the spine. *Spine* 1985;12:414–416.

Graves VB, Schreiber MN. Tuberculosis psoas muscle abscess. *J Can Assoc Radiol* 1973;24:268–271.

Guyot DR, Manoli A II, Kling GA. Pyogenic sacroiliitis in IV drug users. *AJR Am J Roentgenol* 1987;149:1209–1211.

Haygood TM, Williamson SL. Radiographic findings of extremity tuberculosis in childhood: back to the future? *Radiographics* 1994;14:561–570.

Hoffman E, Crosier J, Cremin B. Imaging in children with spinal tuberculosis. *J Bone Joint Surg [Br]*, 1993:75-B:233–239.

Hopkins KL, Li KC, Bergman G. Gadolinium-DPTA-enhanced magnetic resonance imaging of musculoskeletal infectious processes. *Skeletal Radiol* 1995;24:325–330.

Jain R, Sawhney S, Berry M. Computed tomography of vertebral tuberculosis: patterns of bone destruction. *Clin Radiol* 1993;47:196–199.

Karchevsky M, Schweitzer ME, Morrison WB, Parellada JA. MRI findings of septic arthritis and associated osteomyelitis in adults. *AJR Am J Roentgenol* 2004;182:119–122.

Kido D, Bryan D, Halpern M. Hematogeneous osteomyelitis in drug addicts. *AJR Am J Roentgenol* 1973;118:356–363.

Lawson JP, Rahn DW. Lyme disease and radiologic findings in Lyme arthritis. *AJR Am J Roentgenol* 1992;158:1065–1069.

Lawson JP, Steere AC. Lyme arthritis: radiologic findings. *Radiology* 1985;154:37–43.

Lewis J, Rabinovich S. The wide spectrum of cryptococcal infections. *Am J Med* 1972;53:315–322.

Lund PJ, Chan KM, Unger EC, Galgiani TN, Pitt MJ. Magnetic resonance imaging in coccidioidal arthritis. *Skeletal Radiol* 1996;25:661–665.

May DA, Disler DG. Case 50: primary coccidioidal synovitis of the knee. *Radiology* 2002;224:665–668.

McGahan JP, Graves DS, Palmer PES. Coccidioidal spondylitis: usual and unusual roentgenographic manifestations. *Radiology* 1980;136:5–9.

McGahan JP, Graves DS, Palmer PES, Stadalnik RC, Dublin AB. Classic and contemporary imaging of coccidioidomycosis. *AJR Am J Roentgenol* 1981;136:393–404.

Modic MT, Feiglin DH, Piriano DW, et al. Vertebral osteomyelitis: assessment using MR. *Radiology* 1985;157:157–166.

Noh HM, Kuszyk BS, Fishman EK. Cryptococcoma of the sacrum. *Skeletal Radiol* 1999;28:49–51.

Paterson DC. Acute suppurative arthritis in infancy and childhood. *J Bone Joint Surg [Br]* 1970;52B:474–482.

Phemister DB, Hatcher CM. Correlation of pathological and roentgenological findings in the diagnosis of tuberculosis arthritis. *AJR Am J Roentgenol* 1933;29:736–752.

Resnik CS, Ammann AM, Walsh JW. Chronic septic arthritis of the adult hip: computed tomographic features. *Skeletal Radiol* 1987;16:513–516.

Resnik CS, Resnick D. Pyogenic osteomyelitis and septic arthritis. In: Taveras JM, Ferrucci JT, eds. *Radiology—diagnosis, imaging, intervention.* Philadelphia: JB Lippincott; 1986.

Resnick D, Niwayama G. Osteomyelitis, septic arthritis, and soft tissue infection: mechanisms and situations. In: Resnick D, ed. *Diagnosis of bone and joint disorders*, 3rd ed. Philadelphia: Saunders; 1995:2325–2418.

Resnick D, Niwayama G. Osteomyelitis, septic arthritis, and soft tissue infection: organisms. In: Resnick D, ed. *Diagnosis of bone and joint disorders*, 3rd ed. Philadelphia: Saunders, 1995:2448–2558.

Schauwecker D. Osteomyelitis: diagnosis with In-111-labeled leukocytes. *Radiology* 1989;171:141–146.

Stadalnik RC, Goldstein E, Hoeprich PD, dos Santos PA, Lee KK. Diagnostic value of gallium and bone scans in evaluation of extrapulmonary coccidioidal lesions. *Am Rev Respir Dis* 1980;121:673–676.

Theodorou DJ, Theodorou SJ, Kakitsubata Y, Sartoris DJ, Resnick D. Imaging characteristics and epidemiologic features of atypical mycobacterial infections involving the musculoskeletal system. *AJR Am J Roentgenol* 2001;176:341–349.

Trueta J. The three types of acute, haematogenous osteomyelitis. *J Bone Joint Surg [Br]* 1959;41B:671–680.

Waldvogel FA, Vasey MD. Osteomyelitis: the past decade. *N Engl J Med* 1980;303:360–370.

Wall SD, Fisher MR, Amparo EG, Hricak H. Higgins CB. Magnetic resonance imaging in the evaluation of abscesses. *AJR Am J Roentgenol* 1985;144:1217–1221.

Wolfgang GL. Tuberculosis joint infection. *Clin Orthop* 1978;136:225–263.

Young LW. Neonatal and infantile osteomyelitis and septic arthritis. In: Taveras JM, Ferrucci JT, eds. *Radiology—diagnosis, imaging, intervention*, vol. 5. Philadelphia: JB Lippincott; 1986:1–15.

Zeppa MA, Laorr A, Greenspan A, McGahan JP, Steinbach LS. Skeletal coccidioidomycosis: imaging findings in 19 patients. *Skeletal Radiol* 1996;25:337–343.

METABOLIC AND ENDOCRINE DISORDERS

CHAPTER 26

RADIOLOGIC EVALUATION OF METABOLIC AND ENDOCRINE DISORDERS

Composition and Production of Bone

Bone tissue consists of two types of material: (a) an extracellular material, which includes *organic matrix* or *osteoid tissue* (collagen fibrils within a mucopolysaccharide ground substance) and an *inorganic crystalline component* (calcium phosphate or hydroxyapatite); and (b) a cellular material, which includes *osteoblasts* (cells that induce bone formation), *osteoclasts* (cells that induce bone resorption), and *osteocytes* (inactive cells).

Bone is a living, dynamic tissue. Old bone is constantly being removed and replaced with new bone. Normally, this continuous process of bone resorption and formation is in balance (Fig. 26.1A), and the mineral content of the bones remains relatively constant. In some abnormal circumstances, however, when the metabolism of the bone is disturbed, this balance may be upset. If, for example, osteoblasts are

more active than usual, or if osteoclasts are less active, more bone is produced (a state known as "too much bone") (Fig. 26.1B). If, however, osteoclasts are normal or overactive and osteoblasts underactive, then less bone is produced ("too little bone") (Fig. 26.1C). A generalized reduction in bone mass may also be caused by decreased mineralization of osteoid, with equilibrium in the rate of bone resorption and production (Fig. 26.1D).

The growth and mineralization of bone are influenced by a variety of factors, the most important of which are the levels of growth hormone produced by the pituitary gland, of calcitonin produced by the thyroid gland, and of parathormone produced by the parathyroid glands, along with the dietary intake, intestinal absorption, and urinary excretion of vitamin D, calcium, and phosphorus.

It should be remembered, however, that normal bone density changes with age, increasing from infancy until age 35 to 40, and then

Figure 26.1 Bone production and bone resorption. (A) In normal bone, the relationship between bone resorption and bone production is in balance. **(B)** One abnormal state ("too much bone") is characterized by decreased bone resorption and normal bone production, or by normal bone resorption and increased bone production. **(C)** The other abnormal state ("too little bone") is characterized by increased bone resorption and normal bone production, by normal bone resorption and decreased bone production, or by increased bone resorption and decreased bone production. **(D)** Too little bone may also be caused by a decrease in bone mineralization, with bone resorption and production in balance.

progressively decreasing at the rate of 8% per decade in women and 3% in men.

Evaluation of Metabolic and Endocrine Disorders

Most metabolic and endocrine disorders are characterized radiographically by abnormalities in bone density that are generally related to increased bone production, increased bone resorption, or inadequate bone mineralization. The bones affected by these conditions appear abnormally radiolucent (osteopenia) or abnormally radiodense (osteosclerosis) (Table 26.1).

Radiologic Imaging Modalities

The radiologic modalities most often used to evaluate metabolic and endocrine bone disorders are:
1. Conventional radiography
2. Magnification radiography

Table 26.1 Metabolic and Endocrine Disorders Characterized by Abnormalities in Bone Density

Increased Radiodensity	Increased Radiolucency
Secondary hyperparathyroidism	Osteoporosis
Renal osteodystrophy	Osteomalacia
Hyperphosphatasia	Rickets
Idiopathic hypercalcemia	Scurvy
Paget disease	Primary hyperparathyroidism
Osteopetrosis*	Hypophosphatasia
Pycnodysostosis*	Hypophosphatemia
Melorheostosis*	Acromegaly
Hypothyroidism	Gaucher disease
Mastocytosis	Homocystinuria
Myelofibrosis	Osteogenesis imperfecta*
Gaucher disease (reparative stage)	Fibrogenesis imperfecta
Fluorine poisoning	Cushing syndrome
Intoxication with lead, bismuth, or phosphorus	Ochronosis (alkaptonuria)
Osteonecrosis	Wilson disease (hepatolenticular degeneration)
	Hypogonadism

* These conditions are discussed in Part VII: Congenital and Developmental Anomalies.

Cortical-Thickness Measurement

ab + cd = combined cortical thickness

$$\frac{ab + cd}{ad} = \text{index of bone mass}$$

$$ab + cd \cong \frac{ad}{2}$$

(the sum of the cortices approximates one-half the bone's diameter)

Figure 26.2 Measurement of cortical thickness. Determination of cortical thickness is based on the measurement of the cortices of the metacarpals (usually the second or third). It may be expressed either as the simple sum of the two cortices or as that sum divided by the total thickness of the bone, in which case it is considered an index of bony mass. Normally, the sum of the cortices should be approximately one-half the overall diameter of the metacarpal bone.

3. Computed tomography (CT)
4. Radionuclide imaging (scintigraphy, bone scan)
5. Magnetic resonance imaging (MRI).

Conventional and Magnification Radiography

Radiography is the simplest and most widely used method of evaluating bone density. This technique can easily detect even very small increases in bone density; however, it generally fails to detect decreases in overall skeletal mineralization unless the reduction reaches at least 30%. It must be pointed out that normal bone can easily acquire an abnormal radiographic appearance as a result of technical errors, such as improper settings for kilovoltage and milliamperage. Overexposure, for instance, creates the appearance of increased bone radiolucency, whereas underexposure creates an artificially increased bone radiodensity.

For these reasons, inspection of a standard radiograph should focus less on apparent increases or decreases in bone density than on the thickness of the bone cortex. Cortical thickness is directly correlated with skeletal mineralization; it can be objectively measured and compared either with a normal standard or with subsequent studies in the same patient. The cortical thickness measurement is obtained by adding the width of the two cortices in the midpoint of a given bone, a sum that should be approximately one-half the overall diameter of the bone; it may also be expressed as an index of bony mass, derived by dividing the combined cortical thickness by the total diameter of the bone (Fig. 26.2). The second or third metacarpal bone is frequently used to obtain these measurements (Fig. 26.3).

A related method for assessing bone density that also uses radiography is the photodensitometry technique. This technique is based

Figure 26.3 Cortical thickness of the hand. Dorsovolar radiographs of the hand show normal **(A)** and abnormal **(B)** thickness of the cortex of the second and third metacarpal bones.

Figure 26.4 **Osteopenia.** Increased radiolucency of bone on a standard radiograph is best termed osteopenia or bone rarefaction rather than osteoporosis, and it is a typical feature not only of osteoporosis but also of osteomalacia and hyperparathyroidism, which are clinically distinct conditions.

on the observation that the photographic density of a bone on a radiographic film is proportional to its mass. Through use of a photodensitometer, the photographic density of a given bone can be compared with that of known standard wedges, giving an accurate assessment of the degree of bone density.

The appearance of relative increased bone radiolucency on standard radiographs should not be called osteoporosis, because such a finding is not specific for osteoporosis, osteomalacia, or hyperparathyroidism. Most authorities agree that increased radiolucency is best termed *osteopenia* (poverty of bone). *Osteoporosis* refers specifically to a reduction in the amount of bone tissue (deficient bone matrix) and *osteomalacia* refers to a reduction in the amount of mineral in the matrix (deficient mineralization); both conditions are characterized by increased bone radiolucency (Fig. 26.4). As Resnick has pointed

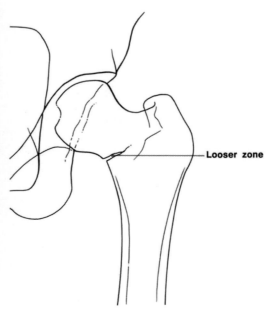

Figure 26.5 **Osteomalacia.** Looser zone or pseudofracture, seen here in the femoral neck, is represented by a radiolucent defect in the cortical bone that reflects accumulation of nonmineralized osteoid tissue and is a characteristic finding in osteomalacia.

out, any condition in which bone resorption exceeds bone formation results in osteopenia, regardless of the specific pathogenesis of the condition. In fact, diffuse osteopenia is found in osteoporosis, osteomalacia, hyperparathyroidism, neoplastic conditions such as multiple myeloma, and in a wide variety of other disorders.

Although osteopenia is a nonspecific finding, radiography can help detect other important radiographic features leading to a specific diagnosis. Among these are: Looser zones, representing pseudofractures that are characteristic of osteomalacia (Fig. 26.5); widening of the growth plate and flaring of the metaphysis, which are typical findings in rickets (Fig. 26.6); subperiosteal bone resorption, an identifying feature of hyperparathyroidism (Fig. 26.7); and focal areas of osteolytic destruction and endosteal scalloping, which are characteristic of multiple myeloma (Fig. 26.8).

Magnification radiography is useful in metabolic disorders for demonstrating the details of bone structure. The subperiosteal bone resorption characteristic of hyperparathyroidism, or cortical tunnel-

Figure 26.7 Hyperparathyroidism. Anteroposterior radiograph of the left knee of a 42-year-old woman with primary hyperparathyroidism caused by hyperplasia of the parathyroid glands demonstrates increased bone radiolucency and areas of subperiosteal bone resorption on the medial aspect of the proximal tibia, characteristic of the condition.

Figure 26.6 Rickets. Radiograph of the lower leg of a 2.5-year-old child with rickets shows the characteristic widening of the growth plate, specifically the zone of provisional calcification, and "cupping" of the metaphysis.

ing (Fig. 26.9), which may be seen in any process that causes increased bone resorption, can be well delineated on magnification studies. Cortical tunneling occurs very early in a pathologic process and may be found even in the absence of other radiographic abnormalities.

Computed Tomography

Although conventional tomography is occasionally useful for demonstrating lesions that are not well visualized on conventional radiographs, CT plays an important role in the evaluation of metabolic and endocrine disorders. The ability of CT to define a specific volume and

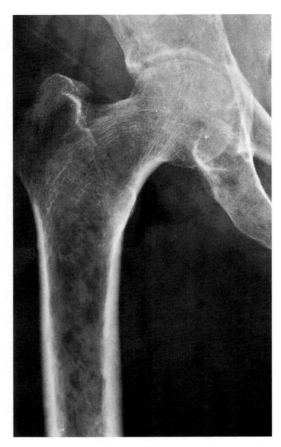

Figure 26.8 Multiple myeloma. Radiograph of the hip of a 58-year-old woman with multiple myeloma shows increased radiolucency of the bones. Focal radiolucencies and endosteal scalloping can also be seen in the femur.

to measure the density of that volume accurately makes it possible to perform quantitative analysis of bone mineral content (see later text). As Genant has pointed out, CT also has the unique ability to measure the cancellous bone of the axial skeleton, particularly that of the vertebrae, a site that is especially sensitive to metabolic stimuli.

Scintigraphy

Radionuclide imaging is a nonspecific modality, but it is a very sensitive detector of active bone turnover. For this reason, it is frequently effective in the evaluation of various metabolic diseases. It is particularly valuable in screening patients with Paget disease to determine the distribution of the lesion and activity of the disease (Fig. 26.10). The insufficiency-type stress fractures frequently seen in osteomalacia may be identified by this modality. In renal osteodystrophy, radionuclide bone scan may reveal the absence of renal images, confirming poor renal function. In hyperparathyroidism, it may detect silent sites of brown tumors. In the reflex sympathetic dystrophy syndrome, it may reveal abnormalities in the affected bone even before positive changes seen on standard radiography. Similarly, in regional migratory osteoporosis, focal abnormalities may be present on the radionuclide bone scan long before radiographic changes become prominent.

Magnetic Resonance Imaging

Magnetic resonance imaging (MRI) is occasionally helpful in evaluating metabolic and endocrine disorders. This technique may provide important information about bone marrow status in such disorders as transient regional osteoporosis, regional migratory osteoporosis, idiopathic juvenile osteoporosis, and reflex sympathetic dystrophy syndrome. It may effectively demonstrate bone marrow abnormalities in Gaucher disease, particularly medullary bone infarctions and osteonecrosis. In osteomalacia, MRI may outline so-called pseudofractures or Looser zones. In Paget disease, MRI is very effective in revealing early stages of emerging complications, particularly development of sarcoma in pagetic bone.

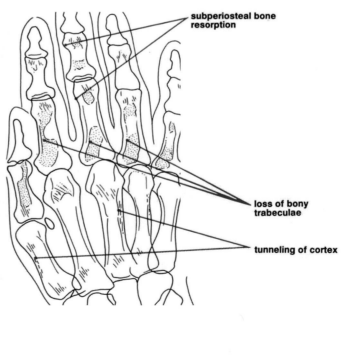

Figure 26.9 Hyperparathyroidism. (A) Dorsovolar radiograph of the hand of a 52-year-old man with hyperparathyroidism demonstrates the typical changes of this condition: increased bone radiolucency (osteopenia), subperiosteal resorption, loss of bony trabeculae, and tunneling of the cortices, which reflects a rapid bone turnover. *(continued)*

Figure 26.9 Hyperparathyroidism. *Continued* **(B)** Magnification study of the femur of the same patient shows the fine details of bone structure. The tunneling of the cortices is better appreciated.

Imaging Techniques for Measurement of Bone Mineral Density

During the past decade, the development of noninvasive technologies that allow accurate measurements of bone mass has revolutionized the study of osteoporosis and related disorders. Accurate detection and quantification of changes in bone mineralization became extremely valuable for the diagnosis and management of metabolic bone disorders. Several different techniques using different energy sources have been developed to measure bone mineral density, including radionuclide and X-ray methods, CT, and ultrasound.

Radionuclide and X-Ray Techniques

Several radionuclide and X-ray techniques are used to determine bone mineral density. These include single photon absorptiometry, dual photon absorptiometry, single X-ray absorptiometry, and dual-energy X-ray absorptiometry. These methods are used in clinical practice to assess patients with metabolic disease affecting the skeleton, to establish a diagnosis of osteoporosis or assess its severity, and to monitor response to therapy.

Single Photon Absorptiometry. Single photon absorptiometry (SPA) is used to determine bone mineral density at peripheral sites, such as a finger or the radius, and measures primarily cortical bone. A single energy source is used, either 125-iodine or 241-americium. The drawbacks of this technique include the need to replace decaying isotopes and inadequate spatial resolution. Moreover, the measurements are relatively insensitive to metabolic stimuli, and variations in thickness of soft tissue may lead to underestimation or overestimation of bone mineral density.

Dual Photon Absorptiometry. Dual photon absorptiometry (DPA) was introduced to overcome some of the limitations of SPA and to permit measurement of central bone sites such as the spine and the hip. The radionuclide source is 153-gadolinium, which produces photons at two energy levels (44 KeV and 100 KeV). The scans are obtained with a whole-body rectilinear scanner. The measurement re-

flects compact and trabecular bone in the scan path. The primary advantages of DPA are low radiation dose, diagnostic accuracy, and the availability of many accessible measurement sites. Its disadvantages include a relatively long scanning time.

Single X-Ray Absorptiometry. Single X-ray absorptiometry (SXA), unlike SPA and DPA, uses an X-ray system as a photon source. It is applicable mainly to peripheral bone sites such as the radius and calcaneus. SXA has the advantages of being portable and inexpensive. Its disadvantages include the need for a water bath to determine soft tissue equivalencies.

Dual-Energy X-Ray Absorptiometry. At present, the most effective technique for measuring bone mineral density is dual-energy

Figure 26.10 Paget disease. Radionuclide bone scan in this 72-year-old man with obvious clinical and radiographic evidence of Paget disease in the pelvis and proximal femora shows additional silent sites of involvement in patellae and humeri, as well as in several thoracic and lumbar vertebrae.

X-ray absorptiometry (DEXA), which uses photons produced from a low-dose energy source. The physical principles of DEXA are similar to those of DPA. However, the gadolinium source is replaced by an X-ray source with two energy levels that enable discrimination between bone and surrounding soft tissue. Therefore, an area-based two-dimensional image is generated, and measurements of bone mineral density can be calculated and compared with normal ranges matched for chronological age (Fig. 26.11). Because of the increased flux from an X-ray tube rather than from an isotope source, scanning time and the collimation of the X-ray beam can be decreased. DEXA can be used for spine, hip, and whole-body measurements, enabling patients to be classified as normal, osteopenic, or osteoporotic.

Computed Tomography Technique

Quantitative Computed Tomography. Quantitative computed tomography (QCT) is a method for measuring the lumbar spine mineral content in which the average density values of a region of interest are referenced to that of a calibration material scanned at the same time as the patient. Measurements are performed on a CT scanner and use a mineral standard for simultaneous calibration, a computed radiograph (scout view) for localization, and either single-energy or dual-energy techniques. In quantitative CT scanning, a cross-sectional image of the vertebral body is obtained, allowing differentiation of cortical and trabecular bone. The attenuation, referenced to a mineral equivalent phantom, is expressed as a trabecular bone density in mg/cm^3 of calcium hydroxyapatite. The standard examination procedure consists of taking CT scans through the midplane line of three or four adjacent vertebral bodies, usually from T-12 to L-3 or L-1 to L-4.

Axial images of the vertebral bodies are obtained by scanning the midplane of vertebral bodies while the patient is supine on a standard phantom. The average density from all vertebrae is calculated. The patient's values are compared with the values of bone density calibrated in the phantom (Fig. 26.12). For measuring the spine, QCT has advantages over other methods because of its great sensitivity and precise three-dimensional anatomic localization, its ability to distinguish cancellous bone from cortical bone, and its ability to exclude extraosseous minerals from the measurement. In particular, this method is useful for measurement of spinal bone mineral density in postmenopausal women, in patients with existing osteoporosis, and in patients being treated with corticosteroids.

Quantitative Ultrasound Technique

Ultrasound visualization is based on a mechanical wave vibrating at a frequency range from 20 kHz to 100 MHz. Passage of this wave through bone causes cortex and trabecular component to vibrate on a microscale. The physical and mechanical properties of the bone then progressively alter the shape, intensity, and speed of the propagating wave, which, as Haus et al. pointed out, allows characterization of bone tissue in terms of ultrasound velocity (speed of sound) and broadband ultrasound attenuation. These parameters allow determination of bone mineral density, predominantly at the calcaneus. Although this method is not as accurate as the methods listed in the previous text, the absence of ionizing radiation with ultrasound, the portability of the equipment, and its cost-effectiveness make ultrasound assessment of bone mineral density an attractive option for screening patients suspected of having osteoporosis.

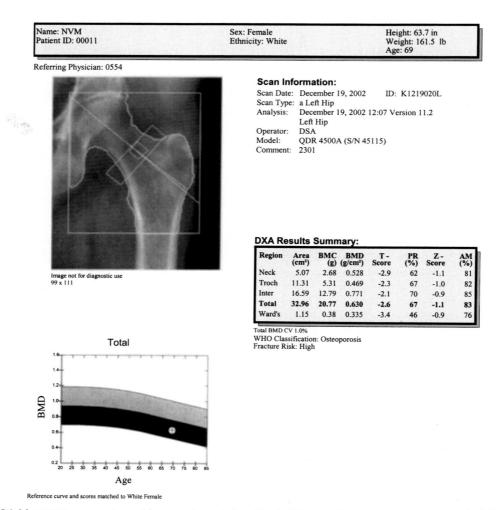

Name: NVM	Sex: Female	Height: 63.7 in
Patient ID: 00011	Ethnicity: White	Weight: 161.5 lb
		Age: 69

Referring Physician: 0554

Scan Information:

Scan Date: December 19, 2002   ID: K1219020L
Scan Type: a Left Hip
Analysis: December 19, 2002 12:07 Version 11.2
Left Hip
Operator: DSA
Model: QDR 4500A (S/N 45115)
Comment: 2301

Image not for diagnostic use
99 x 111

DXA Results Summary:

Region	Area (cm²)	BMC (g)	BMD (g/cm²)	T-Score	PR (%)	Z-Score	AM (%)
Neck	5.07	2.68	0.528	-2.9	62	-1.1	81
Troch	11.31	5.31	0.469	-2.3	67	-1.0	82
Inter	16.59	12.79	0.771	-2.1	70	-0.9	85
Total	**32.96**	**20.77**	**0.630**	**-2.6**	**67**	**-1.1**	**83**
Ward's	1.15	0.38	0.335	-3.4	46	-0.9	76

Total BMD CV 1.0%
WHO Classification: Osteoporosis
Fracture Risk: High

Total

BMD

Age

Reference curve and scores matched to White Female

Figure 26.11 DEXA measuring of bone mineral density. A 69-year-old woman was suspected of developing osteoporosis. DEXA scan of her left hip confirmed this diagnosis, indicating in addition high risk for a fracture.

Figure 26.12 Quantitative computed tomography. A 62-year-old woman was evaluated for degree of osteoporosis. Anteroposterior **(A)** and lateral **(B)** radiographs of the lumbar spine show diffuse osteopenia with multiple compression fractures. Quantitative computed tomography (QCT) measurements were obtained in the following fashion: The patient was supine on a standard bone mineral calibration phantom. Values were referenced to a translucent calibration phantom scanned with the patient, which contains tubes filled with standard solutions of potassium phosphate (representing minerals), ethanol (representing fat), and water (representing soft tissue). For each axial image, the regions of interest were positioned over the center portion of the phantom calibration compartments, as well as over the central portion of the vertebral body. Transverse (axial) CT scans were made through L-1, L-2, L-3, and L-4, with phantom included. Bone density values in mg/cm^3 were calculated for each vertebral body using the CT numbers (Hounsfield units) obtained from the calibrated density phantom **(C)**, **(D)**. Readings are averaged and compared with normal values for given age and sex. Average of readings for vertebral mineral content are also expressed in mg/cm^3. In this particular case, the average values of 77.4 mg of mineral/cm^3 are below the average values for the patient's age (97.5 mg/cm^3), as well as below the levels of fracture threshold (110 mg/cm^3).

PRACTICAL POINTS TO REMEMBER

[1] On a standard radiograph, increased bone radiolucency (osteopenia) or increased bone density (osteosclerosis) is related to the process of bone formation and resorption, which under normal circumstances is in equilibrium.

- If bone resorption exceeds bone production, either because of an increase in osteoclast activity or because of a decrease in osteoblast activity, or if there is insufficient mineral deposition in the matrix, then the result is increased radiolucency of the bone.
- If bone production surpasses bone resorption, either because of an increase in osteoblast activity or because of a decrease in

osteoclast activity, then the result is increased radiodensity of the bone.

[2] Instead of the specific term *osteoporosis*, the nonspecific descriptive term *osteopenia* is used to refer to any generalized or regional rarefaction of the skeleton, expressed radiographically as increased bone radiolucency, regardless of the specific pathogenesis. The main reason for this usage is that it is usually impossible to distinguish between the various causes of increased bone radiolucency. The term *osteosclerosis* refers to any increase in bone density, again regardless of the cause of the condition.

[3] Osteoporosis is a specific term defining a state in which bone tissue (bone matrix) is reduced but mineralization of the organic matrix is normal. Osteomalacia is a specific term defining a state in which there is insufficient mineralization of osteoid tissue.

[4] The important radiologic techniques used in evaluation of various metabolic and endocrine conditions include:
- conventional radiography
- magnification radiography
- computed tomography
- radionuclide imaging (scintigraphy, bone scan)
- magnetic resonance imaging.

[5] Scintigraphy is a nonspecific but highly sensitive modality to detect bone turnover in various metabolic and endocrine disorders.

[6] MRI provides important information of the status of the bone marrow in such disorders as transient regional osteoporosis, regional migratory osteoporosis, idiopathic juvenile osteoporosis, and reflex sympathetic dystrophy syndrome. This technique is also effective in evaluation of Gaucher disease and Paget disease.

[7] Several methods have been developed for accurate assessment of mineral content of the bone, including single photon absorptiometry (SPA), dual photon absorptiometry (DPA), dual-energy X-ray absorptiometry (DEXA), and quantitative computed tomography (QCT).

[8] At present, DEXA is considered the most effective technique providing measurement of bone mineral density that can be compared with normal ranges matched for chronological age.

[9] QCT is an accurate method for measuring mineral content of cancellous (trabecular) bone of the vertebrae. In this method, the average density of a measured region is referenced to that of a calibration phantom exposed simultaneously with a patient undergoing examination.

SUGGESTED READINGS

Adams JE. Single and dual energy X-ray absorptiometry. *Eur Radiol* 1997;7[Suppl 2]:S20–S31.

Baran DT, Faulkner KG, Genant HK, Miller PD, Pacifici R. Diagnosis and management of osteoporosis: guidelines for the utilization of bone densitometry. *Calcif Tissue Int* 1997;61:433–440.

Cann CE. Quantitative CT applications: comparison of newer CT scanners. *Radiology* 1987;162:257–261.

Cann CE. Quantitative CT for determination of bone mineral density: a review. *Radiology* 1988;166:509–522.

Cann CE, Genant HK. Precise measurement of vertebral mineral content using computed tomography. *J Comput Assist Tomogr* 1980;4:493–500.

Gamble CL. Osteoporosis: making the diagnosis in patients at risk for fracture. *Geriatrics* 1995;50:24–33.

Garn SM, Poznanski AX, Nagy JM. Bone measurement in the differential diagnosis of osteopenia and osteoporosis. *Radiology* 1971;100:509–518.

Genant HK. Current state of bone densitometry for osteoporosis. *Radiographics* 1998;18:913–918.

Genant HK, Block JE, Steiger P, Glüer CC, Ettinger B, Harris ST. Appropriate use of bone densitometry. *Radiology* 1989;170:817–822.

Genant HK, Glüer C-C, Steiger P, Faulkner KG. Quantitative computed tomography for the assessment of osteoporosis. In: Moss AA, Gamsu G, Genant HK, eds. *Computed tomography of the body with magnetic resonance imaging*, 2nd ed, Philadelphia: WB Saunders; 1992:523–549.

Gramp S, Jergas M, Glüer CC, Lang P, Brastow P, Genant HK. Radiologic diagnosis of osteoporosis: current methods and perspectives. *Radiol Clin North Am* 1993;31:1133–1145.

Gramp S, Steiner E, Imhof H. Radiological diagnosis of osteoporosis. *Eur Radiol* 1997;7[Suppl 2]:S11–S19.

Griffith HJ, Zimmerman R, Bailey G, Snider R. The use of photon absorptiometry in the diagnosis of renal osteodystrophy. *Radiology* 1973;109:277–281.

Guglielmi G, Schneider P, Lang TF, Giannatempo GM, Cammisa M, Genant HK. Quantitative computed tomography at the axial and peripheral skeleton. *Eur Radiol* 1997;7[Suppl 2]:S32–S42.

Hans D, Fuerst T, Duboeuf F. Quantitative ultrasound bone measurement. *Eur Radiol* 1997;7[Suppl 2]:S43–S50.

Hui SL, Slemenda CW, Johnston CC. Age and bone mass as predictors of fracture in a prospective study. *J Clin Invest* 1988;81:1804–1809.

Jergas M, Genant, HK. Quantitative bone mineral analysis. In: Resnick D, ed. Diagnosis of bone and joint disorders, 3rd ed. Philadelphia; WB Saunders; 1995:1854–1884.

Jergas M, Glüer C-C. Assessment of fracture risk by bone density measurements. *Semin Nucl Med* 1997;27:261–275.

Kanis JA, Delmas P, Burckhardt P, Cooper C, Torgerson D. Guidelines for diagnosis and management of osteoporosis. *Osteoporosis Int* 1997;7:390–406.

Kanis JA, Melton JL III, Christiansen C, Johnston CC, Khaltaev N. The diagnosis of osteoporosis. *J Bone Miner Res* 1994;9:1137–1141.

Krolner B, Nielsen SP. Bone mineral content of the lumbar spine in normal and osteoporotic women: cross-sectional and longitudinal studies. *Clin Sci* 1982;62:329–336.

Krolner B, Nielsen SP. Measurement of bone mineral contents (BMC) of the lumbar spine, I: Theory and application of a new two-dimensional dual photon attenuation method. *Scand J Clin Lab Invest* 1980;40:653–663.

Lai KC, Goodsitt MM, Murano R, Chesnut CH. A comparison of two dual-energy x-ray absorptiometry systems for spinal bone mineral measurement. *Calcif Tissue Int* 1992;50:203–208.

Lang P, Steiger P, Faulkner K, Glaer C, Genant HK. Osteoporosis. Current techniques and recent developments in quantitative bone densitometry. *Radiol Clin North Am* 1991;29:49–76.

Lenchik L, Rochmis P, Sartoris DJ. Perspective. Optimized interpretation and reporting of dual X-ray absorptiometry (DXA) scans. *AJR Am J Roentgenol* 1998;17:1509–1520.

Lenchik L, Sartoris SJ. Current concepts in osteoporosis. *AJR Am J Roentgenol* 1998;168:905–911.

Lomoschitz FM, Grampp S, Henk CB, Linnau KF, Kresta CR, Resch H, Imhof H. Comparison of imaging-guided and non-imaging guided quantitative sonography of the calcaneus with dual X-ray absorptiometry of the spine and femur. *AJR Am J Roentgenol* 2003;180:1111–1116.

Majumdar S, Genant HK. High resolution magnetic resonance imaging of trabecular structure. *Eur Radiol* 1997;7[Suppl 2]:S51–S55.

Mazess RB. Bone densitometry of the axial skeleton. *Orthop Clin North Am* 1990;21:51–63.

Mazess RB, Barden HS. Measurement of bone by dual-photon absorptiometry (DPA) and dual-energy x-ray absorptiometry (DEXA). *Ann Chir Gynaecol* 1988;77:197–203.

Miller PD, Bonnick SL, Rosen CJ. Consensus of an international panel on the clinical utility of bone mass measurement in the detection of low bone mass in the adult population. *Calcif Tissue Int* 1996;58:207–214.

Nelson DA, Brown EB, Flynn MJ, Cody DD, Shaffer S. Comparison of dual photon and dual energy x-ray bone densitometers in a clinical setting. *Skeletal Radiol* 1991;20:591–595.

Nilas L, Borg J, Gotfredsen A, Christiansen C. Comparison of single- and dual-photon absorptiometry in postmenopausal bone mineral loss. *J Nucl Med* 1985;26:1257–1262.

Pacifici R, Susman N, Carr PL, Birge SJ, Avioli LV. Single and dual energy tomographic analysis of spinal trabecular bone: a comparative study in normal and osteoporotic women. *J Clin Endocrinol Metab* 1987;640:209–214.

Passariello R, Albanese CV, Kvasnovà M. Bone densitometry in the clinical practice. *Eur Radiol* 1997;7[Suppl 2]:S2–S10.

Pullan BR, Roberts TE. Bone mineral measurement using an EMI scanner and standard methods: a comparative study. *Br J Radiol* 1978;51:24–28.

Reinbold WD, Genant HK, Reiser UJ, Harris ST, Ettinger B. Bone mineral content in early-postmenopausal osteoporotic women and postmenopausal women: comparison of measurement methods. *Radiology* 1986;160:469–478.

Resnick D, Niwayama G. Osteoporosis. In: Resnick D, ed. *Diagnosis of bone and joint disorders*, vol 5, 3rd ed. Philadelphia: WB Saunders; 1995.

Reynolds WA, Karo JJ. Radiographic diagnosis of metabolic bone disease. *Orthop Clin North Am* 1972;3:521–543.

Rosenberg AE. The pathology of metabolic bone disease. *Radiol Clin North Am* 1991;29:19–36.

Ross PD, Wasnich RD, Vogel JM. Precision errors in dual-photon absorptiometry related to source age. *Radiology* 1988;166:523–527.

Rupich R, Pacifici R, Delabar C, Susman N, Avidi LV. Lateral dual energy radiography: new technique for the measurement of L3 bone mineral density. *J Bone Miner Res* 1989;4:S194.

Ryan PJ. Overview of role of BMD measurements in managing osteoporosis. *Semin Nucl Med* 1997;27:197–209.

Sartoris DJ. Clinical value of bone densitometry. *AJR Am J Roentgenol* 1994;163:133–135.

Sartoris DJ. Coding and reimbursement issues for dual-energy x-ray absorptiometry. *AJR Am J Roentgenol* 1994;163:137–139.

Sartoris DJ, Resnick D. Dual energy radiographic absorptiometry for bone densitometry: current status and prospective. *AJR Am J Roentgenol* 1989;152:241–246.

Scientific Advisory Board of the Osteoporosis Society of Canada. Clinical practice guidelines for the diagnosis and management of osteoporosis. *Can Med Assoc J* 1996;155:1113–1133.

Slemenda CW, Johnston CC. Bone mass measurement: which site to measure? *Am J Med* 1988;84:643–645.

Slosman DO, Rissoli R, Donath A, Bonjour J-P. Vertebral bone mineral density measured laterally by dual-energy x-ray absorptiometry. *Osteoporosis Int* 1990;1:23–29.

Staron RB, Greenspan R, Miller TT, Bilezikian JP, Shane E, Haramati N. Computerized bone densitometric analysis: operator-dependent errors. *Radiology* 1999;211:467–470.

Svendsen OL, Marslew U, Hassager C, Christiansen C. Measurements of bone mineral density of the proximal femur by two commercially available dual-energy x-ray absorptiometric systems. *Eur J Nucl Med* 1992;19:41–46.

Virtama P, Helelä T. Radiographic measurements of cortical bone: variations in a normal population between 1 and 90 years of age. *Acta Radiol* 1969;7[Suppl]:268–293.

Wahner HW, Dunn WL, Brown ML, Morin RL, Riggs BL. Comparison of dual-energy x-ray absorptiometry and dual photon absorptiometry for bone mineral measurements of the lumbar spine. *Mayo Clin Proc* 1988;63:1075–1084.

Wilson CR, Collier BD, Carrera GF, Jacobson DR. Acronym for dual-energy x-ray absorptiometry. *Radiology* 1990;176:875–876.

CHAPTER 27

OSTEOPOROSIS, RICKETS, AND OSTEOMALACIA

Osteoporosis

Osteoporosis is a generalized metabolic bone disease characterized by insufficient formation or increased resorption of bone matrix that results in decreased bone mass. Although there is a reduction in the amount of bone tissue, the tissue present is still fully mineralized. In other words, the bone is quantitatively deficient but qualitatively normal.

Osteoporosis has a variety of possible causes and consequently manifests in a number of different forms (Table 27.1). The basic distinction in osteoporosis is between those types that are *generalized* or *diffuse,* involving the entire skeleton, and those that are *localized* to a single region or bone (*regional*) (Fig. 27.1). The basic distinction between possible causes is between those that are *congenital* and those that are *acquired.*

Generalized Osteoporosis

Certain radiographic features are common to virtually all forms of osteoporosis, regardless of their specific cause. There are always some diminution of cortical thickness and decrease in the number and thickness of the spongy bone trabeculae (Fig. 27.2). These changes

are more prominent in non-weight-bearing segments and those not subject to stress. The first sites affected by osteoporosis, as well as the ones that are best demonstrated on radiographic study, are the periarticular regions, where the cortex is anatomically thinner (Fig. 27.3). In the long bones, the thickness of the cortices decreases, the bones become brittle, and there is increased clinical incidence of fractures, particularly of the proximal femur (Fig. 27.4), the proximal humerus, the distal radius, and the ribs.

Besides quantitative computed tomography (QCT) and other methods of evaluating osteoporosis (discussed in detail in Chapter 26), some simple methods using conventional radiography have been developed.

The analysis of the trabecular pattern of the bones has been emphasized as an effective method to evaluate osteoporosis, since patterns of trabecular loss correlate well with increasing severity of osteoporosis.

In the femur, these changes may be evaluated using the Singh index, which is based on the trabecular architecture of the proximal femur—namely, the pattern of the principal compressive group of trabeculae, the secondary compressive group of trabeculae, and the principal tensile group of trabeculae (Fig. 27.5 and Table 27.2). The trabecular pattern of the proximal end of the femur is an excellent indicator of the severity of the osteoporosis. Singh has shown that tra-

Table 27.1 **Causes of Osteoporosis**

Generalized (Diffuse)		Localized (Regional)
Genetic (Congenital)	*Deficiency States*	
Osteogenesis imperfecta	Scurvy	Immobilization (cast)
Gonadal dysgenesis:	Malnutrition	Disuse
Turner syndrome (XO)	Anorexia nervosa	Pain
Klinefelter syndrome	Protein deficiency	Infection
(XXY)	Alcoholism	Reflex sympathetic dystrophy
Hypophosphatasia	Liver disease	syndrome (Sudeck atrophy)
Homocystinuria	*Neoplastic*	Transient regional osteoporosis:
Mucopolysaccharidosis	Myeloma	Transient osteoporosis of the hip
Gaucher disease	Leukemia	Regional migratory osteoporosis
Anemias:	Lymphoma	Idiopathic juvenile osteoporosis
Sickle-cell syndromes	Metastatic disease	Paget disease (hot phase)
Thalassemia	*Iatrogenic*	
Hemophilia	Heparin-induced	
Christmas disease	Dilantin-induced	
Endocrine	Steroid-induced	
Hyperthyroidism	*Miscellaneous*	
Hyperparathyroidism	Involutional	
Cushing syndrome	(senescent/post-	
Acromegaly	menopausal)	
Estrogen deficiency	Amyloidosis	
Hypogonadism	Ochronosis	
Diabetes mellitus	Paraplegia	
Pregnancy	Weightlessness	
	Idiopathic	

Figure 27.1 **Target sites of osteoporosis.**

Figure 27.2 Generalized osteoporosis. An 82-year-old man presented with generalized osteoporosis. Anteroposterior **(A)** and lateral **(B)** radiographs of the left knee reveal increased radiolucency of bones, thinning of the cortices, and sparse trabecular pattern. These changes are more effectively demonstrated on axial CT sections obtained through the proximal tibia **(C)** and distal femur **(D)**, as well as on reformatted coronal image of the distal femur **(E)**.

Figure 27.3 Periarticular osteoporosis. Anteroposterior **(A)** and lateral **(B)** radiographs of an ankle reveal sparse trabecular pattern and increase radiolucency in the subchondral areas.

Figure 27.4 Osteoporosis complicated by a fracture. An 85-year-old woman with advanced postmenopausal osteoporosis sustained an intertrochanteric fracture of the left femur, as seen on this anteroposterior radiograph. Note the thinning of the cortex and the increased radiolucency of the bones.

Figure 27.5 The Singh trabecular index. (A) The trabecular pattern of the proximal end of the femur is an excellent indicator of the severity of the osteoporosis. **(B)** The trabecular arcades important to the Singh trabecular index. Confluence of principal tensile, principal compressive, and secondary compressive trabeculae in the femoral neck forms a triangular region of radiolucency, the Ward triangle. The principal tensile trabeculae are more important than the secondary trabeculae, the compressive trabeculae are more important than the tensile trabeculae. Bone loss occurs in order of increasing importance. (Modified from Singh M, et al., 1970, with permission.)

Table 27.2 **The Five Major Groups of Trabeculae**

1. Principal Compressive Group
   - Extend from medial cortex of femoral neck to superior part of femoral head
   - Major weight-bearing trabeculae
   - In normal femur are the thickest and most densely packed
   - Appear accentuated in osteoporosis
   - Last to be obliterated
2. Secondary Compressive Group
   - Originate at the cortex, near the lesser trochanter
   - Curve upward and laterally toward the greater trochanter and upper femoral neck
   - Characteristically thin and widely separated
3. Principal Tensile Group
   - Originate from the lateral cortex, inferior to the greater trochanter
   - Extend in an arch-like configuration medially, terminating in the inferior portion of the femoral head
4. Secondary Tensile Group
   - Arise from the lateral cortex below the principal tensile group
   - Extend superiorly and medially to terminate after crossing the middle of the femoral neck
5. Greater Trochanter Group
   - Composed of slender and poorly defined tensile trabeculae
   - Arise laterally below the greater trochanter
   - Extend upward to terminate near the greater trochanter's superior surface

becular loss occurs in a predictable sequence that can be used to grade the severity of osteopenia. He recognized that the compressive trabeculae were more essential than the tensile trabeculae, and that the peripherally located trabeculae were more vital than central ones.

Six radiologic grades have been defined according to the trabecular pattern (Fig. 27.6).

In early osteoporosis, both the compressive and tensile trabeculae are accentuated because of initial resorption of the randomly oriented trabeculae, and thus the radiolucency of the Ward triangle becomes more prominent. With increasing severity of osteoporosis, the tensile trabeculae are reduced in number and regress from the medial femoral border to the lateral. When trabecular resorption increases, the outer portion of the principal tensile trabeculae opposite the greater trochanter disappear, opening the Ward triangle laterally. As osteoporosis increases in severity, resorption of all trabeculae occur, with the exception of those in the principal compressive group. In ad-

vanced osteoporosis, the principal compressive component is the last to be involved, a process manifested by a decrease in the number and length of individual trabeculae. Eventually, the upper femur may be completely devoid of all trabecular markings.

The other major area in which osteoporotic changes are evaluated is the axial skeleton, particularly the spine. This is especially true in osteoporosis associated with aging, i.e., *involutional* (senescent and postmenopausal) *osteoporosis*, in which the vertebral bodies are particularly vulnerable. Initially, there is a relative increase in the density of the vertebral end plates due to resorption of the spongy bone, causing what is called an "empty box" appearance (Fig. 27.7). Later, there is an overall decrease in density with a loss of any trabecular pattern, creating a "ground glass" appearance. A typical feature of vertebral involvement in osteoporosis is biconcavity of the body, which exhibits a "fish mouth" appearance ("codfish vertebrae") (Fig. 27.8). This presentation results from expansion of the disks, leading to arch-like in-

SINGH INDEX—RADIOLOGIC GRADES

Grade 6
all normal trabecular groups visible; proximal end of femur completely occupied by cancellous bone

Grade 5
principal tensile and compressive trabeculae accentuated; Ward triangle prominent

Grade 4
principal tensile trabeculae reduced in number but still can be traced from lateral cortex to femoral neck

Grade 3
break in continuity of principal tensile trabeculae opposite greater trochanter

Grade 2
only principal compressive trabeculae can be seen; all tensile trabeculae have been resorbed

Grade 1
principal compressive trabeculae markedly reduced in number

Figure 27.6 **Singh index—radiologic grades.** (Modified from Singh M, et al., 1970, with permission.)

dentations on both superior and inferior margins of the weakened vertebral bodies. In advanced stages, there is complete collapse of the vertebral body associated with a wedge-shaped deformity. In the thoracic spine this leads to increased kyphosis.

Of special interest in generalized osteoporosis are the three major varieties of *iatrogenic osteoporosis. Heparin-induced osteoporosis* may develop after long-term, high-dose daily heparin treatment (more than 10,000 units). Precisely how this type of osteoporosis is initiated and develops is not clearly understood, although osteoclastic stimulation and osteoblastic inhibition with suppressed endochondral ossification have been implicated as potential causes. Spontaneous fractures of the vertebrae, ribs, and femoral neck are noted on radiographic studies. *Dilantin-induced osteoporosis* occasionally develops after prolonged use of phenytoin (Dilantin). The vertebral column and ribs are usually affected, and fractures are a common complication.

Steroid-induced osteoporosis, occurring either during the course of Cushing syndrome or iatrogenically during treatment with various corticosteroids, is characterized by decreased bone formation and increased bone resorption. Although the axial skeleton is most often affected, the appendicular skeleton may also be involved. In the spine, considerable thickening and sclerosis of the vertebral end plates occur without a concomitant change in the anterior and posterior vertebral margins.

Osteoporosis associated with neoplastic processes is discussed in Chapter 16.

Localized Osteoporosis

Transient regional osteoporosis is a collective term for a group of conditions that have one feature in common: rapidly developing osteoporosis that usually affects the periarticular regions and has no definite etiology like trauma or immobilization. It is a self-limiting and reversible disorder, of which three subtypes have been described.

Figure 27.8 Involutional osteoporosis. Biconcavity, or "codfish vertebrae," seen here on the lateral view of the thoracolumbar spine in an 80-year-old woman with osteoporosis, results from weakness of the vertebral end plates and intravertebral expansion of nuclei pulposi.

Transient osteoporosis of the hip is seen predominantly in pregnant women and in young and middle-aged men. Its primary manifestation is local osteoporosis involving the femoral head and neck and the acetabulum. *Regional migratory osteoporosis,* which affects the knee, the ankle, and the foot, is mainly seen in men in their fourth and fifth decades. This migratory condition is characterized by pain and swelling around the affected joints. It develops rapidly and subsides in about 6 to 9 months; there may be subsequent recurrence and involvement of other joints. *Idiopathic juvenile osteoporosis* is commonly seen during or just before puberty, and typically regresses spontaneously. Skeletal involvement is often symmetrical and is generally juxtaarticular in location. It is frequently associated with pain and the presence of vertebral body compression fractures.

Localized osteoporosis secondary to immobilization in a cast or due to disuse of a painful limb is discussed in Chapter 4. Sudeck atrophy (reflex sympathetic dystrophy syndrome) may also occur as a complication of fractures (see Fig. 4.52).

Rickets and Osteomalacia

Whereas in osteoporosis the fundamental change is decreased bone mass, in rickets (which occurs in children) and osteomalacia (which occurs in adults) the essential bone abnormality is faulty mineralization (calcification) of the bone matrix. If adequate amounts of

Figure 27.7 Involutional osteoporosis. Lateral radiograph of the lumbar spine of an 89-year-old woman demonstrates a relative increase in the density of the vertebral end plates and resorption of the trabeculae of spongy bone, creating an "empty box" appearance. This is commonly seen in involutional osteoporosis.

Table 27.3 **Etiology of Rickets and Osteomalacia**

Nutritional Deficiency
Vitamin D
  Dietary
  Insufficient sunlight
  Impaired synthesis
Calcium
Phosphorus
Absorption Abnormalities
Gastric surgery
Intestinal surgery (bypass)
Gastric disorders (obstruction)
Intestinal disorders (sprue)
Biliary diseases
Renal Disorders
Renal tubular disorders:
  Proximal tubular lesions (failure of absorption of inorganic phosphate, glucose, amino acids)
  Distal tubular lesions (renal tubular acidosis)
  Combined proximal and distal tubular lesions
Renal osteodystrophy
Miscellaneous
Associated with:
  Wilson disease
  Fibrogenesis imperfecta
  Fibrous dysplasia
  Neurofibromatosis
  Hypophosphatasia
  Neoplasm

ization in the provisional zone of calcification is reflected in widening of the growth plate and cupping and flaring of the metaphysis, which appears disorganized and "frayed" (Fig. 27.10 and 27.11; see also Fig. 26.6). In the secondary ossification centers of the epiphysis, similar changes are seen; the bone becomes radiolucent, with loss of sharpness at the periphery, and bowing deformities frequently occur (Fig. 27.12).

Vitamin D-Resistant Rickets

This condition is found in older children (those above 30 months of age), and four distinct types have been reported. *Classic vitamin D-resistant* (or hypophosphatemic) *rickets*, also known as *familial vitamin*

Figure 27.9 Target sites of rickets.

calcium and phosphorus are not available, proper calcification of osteoid tissue cannot occur.

In the past, the most common cause of rickets and osteomalacia was *deficient intake* of vitamin D, which is responsible for calcium and phosphorus homeostasis and for maintenance of proper bone mineralization. Now, however, the major causes include *inadequate intestinal absorption*, resulting in loss of calcium and phosphorus through the gastrointestinal tract in patients who have gastric, biliary, or enteric abnormalities or have undergone gastrectomy or other gastric surgery; *renal tubular disorders* (proximal and/or distal tubular lesions frequently leading to renal tubular acidosis); and *renal osteodystrophy* secondary to renal failure, which results in loss of calcium through the kidneys. Several other conditions associated with osteomalacia have been identified, such as neurofibromatosis, fibrous dysplasia, and Wilson disease, but the exact relationship between the underlying disorder and osteomalacia is still unclear (Table 27.3).

Rickets

Infantile Rickets

Found mainly in infants between 6 and 18 months of age, infantile rickets is characterized by generalized demineralization of the skeleton, which leads to bowing deformities in weight-bearing bones when infants begin to stand and walk. Infants with early rickets are restless and sleep poorly. Closing of the fontanelles is delayed. The earliest physical sign is softening of the cranial vault (craniotabes). Enlargement of the cartilage at the costochondral junction produces a prominence known as "rachitic rosary." The serum values of calcium and phosphorus are low, and that of alkaline phosphatase is increased.

The key radiographic features are observed in the metaphysis and the epiphysis—the regions where growth is most active—particularly at the distal ends of the radius, ulna, and femur, as well as at the proximal ends of the tibia and fibula (Fig. 27.9). Deficient mineral-

Figure 27.10 Rickets. (A), (B) Dorsovolar radiograph of both hands of an 8-year-old boy with untreated dietary rickets shows osteopenia of the bones, widening of the growth plates of the distal radius and ulna, and flaring of the metaphyses, all typical features of this condition.

Figure 27.11 Rickets. Anteroposterior radiograph of the knee in a 4-year-old boy shows widening of the growth plates of the distal femur and proximal tibia secondary to lack of mineralization in the provisional zone of calcification. Note also cupping and flaring of the metaphyses.

Figure 27.12 Rickets. Lateral radiograph of the lower leg of a 3-year-old girl with vitamin D-deficiency rickets shows increased bone radiolucency, widening of the growth plates, cupping and flaring of the metaphyses, and blurring of the outline of the secondary ossification centers, all radiographic hallmarks of this condition. Note also bowing of the tibia and fibula, a frequent feature of rickets.

D-resistant rickets, is a congenital disorder that is transmitted as a sex-linked dominant trait. It is characterized by hypophosphatemia and normal levels of serum calcium. Patients are short, stocky, and bow-legged. Ectopic calcifications and ossifications in the axial and the appendicular skeleton, along with occasional sclerotic changes, are among the identifying radiographic findings. *Vitamin D-resistant rickets with glycosuria* is characterized by an abnormal resorptive mechanism

for glucose and inorganic phosphate. *Fanconi syndrome* is characterized by a defect in the proximal renal tubules and deficient resorption of phosphate, glucose, and several amino acids. *Acquired hypophosphatemic syndrome* manifests in late adolescence or early adulthood; it is probably of toxic etiology.

The radiographic findings in all four types of vitamin D-resistant rickets are similar to those in infantile rickets. Bowing of the legs and shortening of the long bones, however, are more pronounced, and occasionally the bones appear sclerotic (Fig. 27.13).

Osteomalacia

Osteomalacia, which results from the same pathomechanism as rickets, occurs only after bone growth has ceased, and hence the term refers to changes in the cortical and trabecular bone of the axial and appendicular skeleton. It is most often caused by faulty absorption of fat-soluble vitamin D from the gastrointestinal tract secondary to malabsorption syndrome. It may also result from dysfunction of the proximal renal tubules, resulting in so-called renal osteomalacia. The most common clinical presentation of this condition is bone pain and muscle weakness.

Histologically, osteomalacia is characterized by excessive quantities of inadequately mineralized bone matrix (osteoid) coating the surfaces of trabeculae in spongy bone and lining the haversian canals in the cortex.

Radiographically, osteomalacia presents with generalized osteopenia, and multiple, bilateral, and often symmetric radiolucent lines are seen in the cortex perpendicular to the long axis of the bone; they are referred to as "pseudofractures" or Looser zones (Fig. 27.14, see also Fig. 26.5). These defects, which represent cortical stress fractures filled with poorly mineralized callus, osteoid, and fibrous tissue, are common along the axillary margins of the scapulae, the inner margin of the femoral neck, the proximal dorsal aspect of the ulnae, the ribs, and the pubic and ischial rami (Fig. 27.15). The condition, described by Milkman and known as "Milkman syndrome," is a mild form of osteomalacia in which the pseudofractures are particularly numerous.

Renal Osteodystrophy

A skeletal response to long-standing renal disease, renal osteodystrophy (also referred to as "uremic osteopathy") is usually associated with chronic renal failure due to glomerulonephritis or pyelonephritis. The condition is also seen in patients who are on dialysis or who have undergone renal transplantation.

Two main mechanisms, acting in unison but varying in severity and proportion, are responsible for bony changes associated with this condition: secondary hyperparathyroidism and abnormal vitamin D metabolism. The secondary hyperparathyroidism is provoked by phosphate retention and leads to depression of serum calcium, which in turn stimulates release of parathormone from parathyroid glands. The abnormal vitamin D metabolism is affected by renal insufficiency, since the kidney is the source of an enzyme, 25-OH-D-1 α-hydroxylase, which converts the inactive vitamin D from 25-hydroxyvitamin D (25-OH-D) to active 1,25-dihydroxyvitamin D (1,25 $(OH)_2D$). Only this most potent, physiologically active form of vitamin D is responsible for calcium and phosphorus homeostasis and for maintenance of proper bone mineralization.

The major radiographic manifestations of renal osteodystrophy are those associated with rickets, osteomalacia, and secondary hyperparathyroidism. Rickets and osteomalacia secondary to renal osteodystrophy are seldom seen in its pure form; usually there are superimposed changes typical of secondary hyperparathyroidism (Fig. 27.16). Increased bone radiolucency and cortical thinning may be present (Fig. 27.17), but Looser zones are very uncommon. In most patients, some sclerotic changes develop in the bones. Slipped epiphyses may be seen in advanced uremic disease.

Figure 27.13 Vitamin D-resistant rickets. (A) Anteroposterior radiograph of the femora of a 9-year-old girl with vitamin D-resistant (hypophosphatemic) rickets shows lateral bowing and shortening of both bones. There is also evidence of sclerotic changes, which are occasionally seen in this condition. **(B)** The knees and lower legs of the same patient show a bowing deformity of the tibiae and fibulae, as well as widening and deformity of the growth plates about the knee and the distal femora and tibiae.

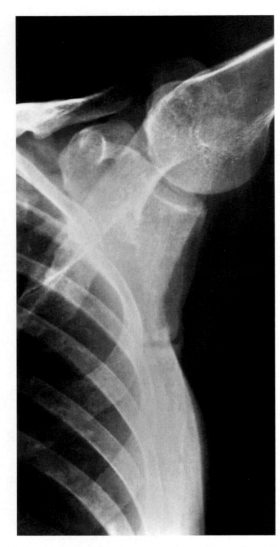

Figure 27.14 Osteomalacia. Anteroposterior radiograph of the left shoulder of a 25-year-old woman with osteomalacia caused by malabsorption syndrome shows a radiolucent cleft perpendicular to the cortex of the scapula. Such defects, known as pseudofractures (Looser zones), are almost pathognomonic for osteomalacia (see also Fig. 26.5).

Figure 27.15 Target sites of osteomalacia.

Figure 27.16 Renal osteodystrophy. A 13-year-old boy with posterior urethral valves and secondary renal failure exhibited radiographic changes typical of renal osteodystrophy, encompassing a mixture of osteomalacia and secondary hyperparathyroidism. Anteroposterior radiograph of the pelvis shows sclerotic changes in the bones and characteristic widening of the sacroiliac joints. The multiple cystic defects in the proximal femora indicate secondary hyperparathyroidism.

Figure 27.17 Renal osteodystrophy. Anteroposterior **(A)** radiograph of the knees and dorsovolar **(B)** radiograph of the wrist of a 6-year-old boy with chronic pyelonephritis reveals osteopenic bones and thin cortices. (Courtesy of Dr. Philip E. S. Palmer, Davis, California.)

PRACTICAL POINTS TO REMEMBER

Osteoporosis

[1] Osteoporosis is characterized by:
- insufficient formation or increased resorption of bone matrix, resulting in decreased bone mass
- increased radiolucency of bone and thinning of the cortices on standard radiography.

[2] The target sites of osteoporotic changes are:
- the axial skeleton (spine and pelvis)
- the periarticular regions of the appendicular skeleton.

[3] The analysis of the trabecular pattern in the proximal end of femur (Singh index) is an effective method of evaluating osteoporosis, since patterns of trabecular loss correlate well with increasing severity of osteoporosis.

[4] In the spine, characteristic radiographic features that indicate the severity of osteoporotic involvement are:
- "empty box" appearance (early stage)
- "codfish vertebrae"
- multiple wedge-shaped fractures (advanced stage).

[5] There are several noninvasive methods available that allow accurate measurements of bone mineral density in patients with osteoporosis. The most effective technique is DEXA, which uses photons produced from a low-dose energy source. The other effective method is quantitative computed tomography (QCT) for measuring the lumbar spine mineral content.

Rickets and Osteomalacia

[1] Rickets (in children) and osteomalacia (in adults) are the result of faulty mineralization (calcification) of the bone matrix.

[2] On radiographic examination, rickets is characterized by:
- generalized osteopenia
- bowing deformities of the long bones, particularly the femur and tibia
- widening of the growth plate (secondary to deficient mineralization in the provisional zone of calcification) and cupping or flaring of the metaphysis, particularly in the proximal humerus, distal radius and ulna, and distal femur.

[3] The radiographic findings in vitamin D-resistant rickets are similar to those in infantile rickets. Bowing deformities and shortening of the long bones are, however, more pronounced.

[4] Radiographically, osteomalacia is characterized by:
- generalized osteopenia
- symmetric radiolucent lines in the cortex (Looser zones or pseudofractures).

[5] Renal osteodystrophy, usually associated with chronic renal failure due to glomerulonephritis or pyelonephritis, represents a skeletal response to long-standing renal disease. The major radiographic manifestations are those associated with rickets, osteomalacia, and secondary hyperparathyroidism, with predominance of osteosclerosis, bone resorption, and bowing deformities.

SUGGESTED READINGS

Arnstein AR. Regional osteoporosis. *Orthop Clin North Am* 1972;3:585–600.

Beaulieu JG, Razzano D, Levine RB. Transient osteoporosis of the hip in pregnancy. Review of the literature and a case report. *Clin Orthop* 1976;115:165–168.

Cotton GE, Van Puffelen P. Hypophosphatemic osteomalacia secondary to neoplasia. *J Bone Joint Surg* 1986;68:129–133.

Cumming WA. Idiopathic juvenile osteoporosis. *Can Assoc Radiol J* 1970;21:21–26.

Dunn AW. Senile osteoporosis. *Geriatrics* 1967;22:175–180.

Eggleston DE, Bartold K, Abghari R. Recognition of renal osteodystrophy on bone imaging. *Clin Nucl Med* 1986;11:543–544.

Gillespy T III, Gillespy MP. Osteoporosis. *Radiol Clin North Am* 1991;29:77–84.

Greenfield GB. Roentgen appearance of bone and soft tissue changes in chronic renal disease. *AJR Am J Roentgenol* 1972;116:749–757.

Griffith GC, Nichols G Jr, Asher JD, Flanagan B. Heparin osteoporosis. *JAMA* 1965;193: 91–94.

Houang MTW, Brenton DP, Renton P, Shaw DG. Idiopathic juvenile osteoporosis. *Skeletal Radiol* 1978;3:17–23.

Hunder GG, Kelly PJ. Roentgenologic transient osteoporosis of the hip. A clinical syndrome? *Ann Intern Med* 1968;68:539–552.

Jaworski AFG. Pathophysiology, diagnosis, and treatment of osteomalacia. *Orthop Clin North Am* 1972;3:623–652.

Jones G. Radiological appearance of disuse osteoporosis. *Clin Radiol* 1969;20:345–353.

Kaplan FS. Osteoporosis: pathophysiology and prevention. *Clin Symp* 1987;39:1–32.

Lang P, Steiger P, Faulkner K, Glüer C, Genant H. Osteoporosis: current techniques and recent developments in quantitative bone densitometry. *Radiol Clin North Am* 1991;29:49–76.

Mankin HJ. Rickets, osteomalacia, and renal osteodystrophy—Part I. *J Bone Joint Surg [Am]* 1974;56A:101–128.

Mankin HJ. Rickets, osteomalacia, and renal osteodystrophy—Part II. *J Bone Joint Surg [Am]* 1974;56A:352–386.

Mayo-Smith W, Rosenthal DI. Radiographic appearance of osteopenia. *Radiol Clin North Am* 1991;29:37–47.

McCarthy JT, Kumar R. Behavior of the vitamin D endocrine system in the development of renal osteodystrophy. *Semin Nephrol* 1986;6:21–30.

Milkman LA. Pseudofractures (hunger osteopathy, late rickets, osteomalacia). *AJR Am J Roentgenol* 1930;24:29–37.

Murphey MD, Sartoris DJ, Quale JL, Pathria MN, Martin NL. Musculoskeletal manifestations of chronic renal insufficiency. *Radiographics* 1993;13:357–379.

Parfitt AM. Renal osteodystrophy. *Orthop Clin North Am* 1972;3:681–698.

Parfitt AM, Chir B. Hypophosphatemic vitamin D refractory rickets and osteomalacia. *Orthop Clin North Am* 1971;3:653–680.

Pitt MJ. Rachitic and osteomalacic syndromes. *Radiol Clin North Am* 1981;19:581–598.

Pitt MJ. Rickets and osteomalacia. In Resnick D, ed. *Bone and joint imaging.* Philadelphia: WB Saunders; 1989:589–602.

Pitt MJ. Rickets and osteolamalacia are still around. *Radiol Clin North Am* 1991;29: 97–118.

Resnick DL. Fish vertebrae. *Arthritis Rheum* 1982;25:1073–1077.

Resnick D, Deftos LJ, Parthemore JG. Renal osteodystrophy: magnification radiography of target sites of absorption. *AJR Am J Roentgenol* 1981;136:711–714.

Resnick D, Niwayama G. Subchondral resorption of bone in renal osteodystrophy. *Radiology* 1976;118:315–321.

Riggs BL, Melton JM. Involutional osteoporosis. *N Engl J Med* 1986;314:1676–1686.

Sackler JP, Liu L. Case reports: heparin-induced osteoporosis. *Br J Radiol* 1973;46: 548–550.

Singh M, Nagrath AR, Maini PS. Changes in trabecular pattern of the upper end of the femur as an index of osteoporosis. *J Bone Joint Surg [Am]* 1970;52A:457–467.

Singh M, Riggs BL, Beabout JW, Jowsey J. Femoral trabecular-pattern index for evaluation of spinal osteoporosis. *Ann Intern Med* 1972;77:63–67.

Walton J. Familial hypophosphatemic rickets: a declination of its subdivisions and pathogenesis. *Clin Pediatr* 1976;15:1007–1012.

HYPERPARA-THYROIDISM

Pathophysiology

Hyperparathyroidism, also known as generalized osteitis fibrosa cystica or Recklinghausen disease of bone, is the result of overactivity of the parathormone-producing parathyroid glands. Increased production of this hormone is secondary to either gland hyperplasia (9% of cases) or adenoma (90%); only in very rare instances (1%) does hyperparathyroidism occur secondary to parathyroid carcinoma. Excessive secretion of parathormone, which acts on the kidneys and on bone, leads to disturbances in calcium and phosphorus metabolism, resulting in hypercalcemia, hyperphosphaturia, and hypophosphatemia. Renal excretion of calcium and phosphate is increased, and serum levels of calcium are elevated, while those of phosphorus are reduced. Serum levels of alkaline phosphatase are also elevated.

Hyperparathyroidism can be divided into primary, secondary, and tertiary forms. The classic form of the disorder, *primary hyperparathyroidism,* is marked by increased secretion of parathormone resulting from hyperplasia, adenoma, or carcinoma of the parathyroid glands. Primary hyperparathyroidism is usually associated with hypercalcemia. Women are affected about three times as often as men, and the condition is most often seen in the patient's third to fifth decade. *Secondary hyperparathyroidism* is caused by increased secretion of parathyroid hormone in response to a sustained hypocalcemic state. Usually the fundamental cause of parathyroid gland hyperfunction is impaired renal function. Hyperphosphatemia due to renal failure results in chronic hypocalcemia, which in turn promotes increased parathyroid secretion. Although secondary hyperparathyroidism is usually hypocalcemic, it may be normocalcemic as an adaptive response to the hypocalcemic state. *Tertiary hyperparathyroidism* represents a transformation from a hypocalcemic to a hypercalcemic state. The parathyroid glands "escape" from the regulatory effect of serum calcium levels. Patients in whom this escape occurs are usually receiving kidney hemodialysis; they are considered to have autonomous hyperparathyroidism.

Although primary hyperparathyroidism is traditionally synonymous with the hypercalcemic form of the disorder, some patients nonetheless may have normal or even reduced serum calcium levels. For this reason, Reiss and Canterbury proposed an alternative method of classifying hyperparathyroidism based on serum calcium levels. In this system, hyperparathyroidism is considered either hypercalcemic, normocalcemic, or hypocalcemic.

In order to understand the clinical, pathologic, and radiologic manifestations of hyperparathyroidism, knowledge of the interrelated roles of parathyroid hormone and vitamin D in the metabolization of calcium is essential.

Physiology of Calcium Metabolism

Serum concentrations of calcium are maintained within a narrow normal physiologic range (2.20 to 2.65 mmol/L or 8.8 to 10.6 mg/dL) by the intestines and kidneys, the major sites of classic negative feedback mechanisms that balance calcium intake and excretion. The bones also contribute to preserving calcium homeostasis and, since they represent approximately 99% of elemental calcium in the human body, are considered to be a calcium reservoir. Essential to these mechanisms involving a variety of hormones is the action of parathyroid hormone (PTH), a polypeptide hormone whose secretion is induced by a decrease in the level of calcium in the extracellular fluid. In primary hyperparathyroidism, there is inappropriate oversecretion of PTH in the presence of elevated serum calcium levels, while secondary hyperparathyroidism is marked by appropriate PTH production in response to chronic hypocalcemia.

PTH works to increase serum calcium concentrations by several means. Predominant among these is conserving calcium in the kidneys by promoting both increased reabsorption of calcium and increased excretion of phosphates in the distal renal tubules. PTH also promotes release of calcium and phosphorus from bone by increasing the number and activity of osteoclasts, resulting in bone resorption, although the exact mechanism by which this occurs is not fully understood. Finally, although PTH has been shown to have no direct effect on intestinal calcium absorption, it plays a role in stimulating vitamin D metabolism, with subsequent increased absorption of calcium and phosphorus by the intestines.

Both of the forms of vitamin D in the human body—ergocalciferol (vitamin D_2), a synthetic compound and frequent food additive; and cholecalciferol (vitamin D_3), formed predominantly in the skin from 7-dehydrocholesterol by the action of ultraviolet light—are metabolized to 25-hydroxyvitamin D in the liver. The critical step in the metabolism of vitamin D occurs in the kidneys, where 25-hydroxyvitamin D undergoes hydroxylation to its most active form, 1,25-dihydroxyvitamin D, and an inactive metabolite, 24,25-dihydroxyvitamin D. This step is catalyzed by the renal enzyme 1-α-hydroxylase, which is synthesized in the kidneys under the stimulation of PTH in the presence of decreased serum calcium and phosphate levels. This gives the kidneys a unique central role in the metabolism of vitamin D. 1,25-dihydroxyvitamin D is the primary mediator of calcium and phosphorus absorption in the small intestine. The kidneys also have the ability to switch between producing the active and inactive forms of vitamin D, yielding a fine control of calcium metabolism.

The symptoms of hyperparathyroidism are related to hypercalcemia, skeletal abnormalities, and renal disease. Hypercalcemia produces weakness, muscular hypotonia, nausea, anorexia, constipation, polyuria, and thirst. The skeletal abnormalities most commonly seen are generalized osteopenia and foci of bone destruction, which are commonly referred to as brown tumors. These pseudotumors represent areas of fibrous scarring in which osteoclasts collect, blood decomposes, and cysts form. The most common sites of involvement are the mandible, clavicle, ribs, pelvis, and femur. Also, subchondral and subperiosteal bone resorption is invariably present. Kidney involvement results in nephrocalcinosis, impairment of renal function, and uremia.

Figure 28.1 Major target sites of hyperparathyroidism.

Radiographic Evaluation

The major target sites in the skeletal system for hyperparathyroidism are the shoulder, the hand, the vertebrae, and the skull (Fig. 28.1). Standard radiography is usually sufficient to demonstrate its characteristic features: generalized osteopenia; subperiosteal, subchondral, and cortical bone resorption; brown tumors; and soft-tissue and cartilage calcifications. Subperiosteal resorption is particularly well demonstrated on radiographs of the hands, where it usually affects the radial aspects of the middle phalanges of the middle and index fingers (Fig. 28.2; see also Fig. 26.7). Commonly, subchondral bone resorp- tion is present resulting in depression of overlying articular cartilage (Fig. 28.3). Also characteristic of this condition is resorption of the acromial ends of the clavicle (Fig. 28.4). Intracortical resorption is manifested by longitudinal striations, a finding known as "tunneling," which can be most clearly appreciated on magnification studies (see Fig. 26.9). Another characteristic feature is loss of the lamina dura around the tooth socket, which normally is seen as a thin sharp white line surrounding the peridental membrane that attaches the tooth to bone (Fig. 28.5). In the skull, there is a characteristic mottling of the

Figure 28.2 Primary hyperparathyroidism. Dorsovolar radiograph of the left hand of a 42-year-old man with primary hyperparathyroidism caused by hypertrophy of the parathyroid glands shows typical subperiosteal resorption affecting primarily the radial aspects of the middle phalanges of the middle and index fingers.

Figure 28.3 Primary hyperparathyroidism. Subchondral bone resorption is present at the head of the second metacarpal (*arrow*). Note also subperiosteal resorption at the proximal and distal phalanges (*open arrows*).

Figure 28.4 Primary hyperparathyroidism. Anteroposterior radiograph of the shoulder of a 36-year-old woman with primary hyperparathyroidism shows resorption of the acromial end of the right clavicle.

Figure 28.5 Primary hyperparathyroidism. Radiograph of the lower second molar tooth in a patient with primary hyperparathyroidism shows loss of the lamina dura around the tooth socket.

Figure 28.6 Primary hyperparathyroidism. Lateral radiograph of the skull of the patient seen in Figure 28.2 demonstrates a decrease in the overall density of the bone and a granular appearance of the vault—the so-called salt-and-pepper skull.

vault, which yields a "salt-and-pepper" appearance (Fig. 28.6). Localized destructive changes in bones affected by hyperparathyroidism take the form of cyst-like lesions of various sizes, commonly referred to as brown tumors. The jaw, pelvis, and femora are the usual sites for these lesions, but they may be found in any part of the skeleton (Fig. 28.7).

In secondary hyperparathyroidism, other characteristic features may be present in addition to the radiographic abnormalities just discussed. A generalized increase in bone density occurs, particularly in younger patients. In the spine, this change is reflected in dense sclerotic bands seen adjacent to the vertebral end plates, giving the vertebrae a sandwich-like appearance. This phenomenon is termed "rugger-jersey" spine because the sclerotic bands form horizontal stripes resembling those of rugby shirts (Fig. 28.8). However, it must be kept in mind in the evaluation of hyperparathyroidism that osteosclerotic changes may also occur as a manifestation of healing, either spontaneously or as a result of treatment. Deposition of calcium in fibrocartilage, articular cartilage, and soft tissue is common, and vascular calcifications are much more frequent in patients with secondary hyperparathyroidism (Fig. 28.9).

Complications

Both primary and secondary hyperparathyroidism may be complicated by pathologic fractures, which usually occur in the ribs and

Figure 28.7 Primary hyperparathyroidism. Anteroposterior radiograph of the lower legs of the same patient seen in Figure 28.4 shows multiple lytic lesions (brown tumors) in both tibiae.

Figure 28.8 Secondary hyperparathyroidism. A 17-year-old boy with chronic renal failure developed secondary hyperparathyroidism. Lateral radiograph of the lumbar spine demonstrates sclerotic bands adjacent to the vertebral end plates—the so-called Rugger-Jersey spine.

Figure 28.9 Secondary hyperparathyroidism. Posteroanterior radiograph of the distal forearms and hands of a 48-year-old woman shows evidence of soft-tissue and vascular calcifications, characteristic findings in secondary hyperparathyroidism. Note also diffuse osteopenia.

vertebral bodies. Hyperparathyroidism arthropathy, another frequent complication, has been discussed in more detail in Chapter 15. Slipped capital femoral or humeral epiphysis may also be observed on occasion. The involvement of ligaments and tendons results in capsular and ligamentous laxity, which may lead to joint instability. Occasionally, spontaneous tendon avulsion has been observed, a phenomenon attributed to the direct effect of parathyroid hormone on connective tissue. Even less frequently intraarticular crystal deposition (calcium pyrophosphate dihydrate) in cartilage, capsule, and synovium may occur, which may lead to the pseudogout syndrome.

PRACTICAL POINTS TO REMEMBER

[1] The typical radiographic changes of primary (hypercalcemic) hyperparathyroidism include:
  • generalized osteopenia
  • subperiosteal, subchondral, and cortical resorption
  • resorption of the acromial end of the clavicle
  • a "salt-and-pepper" appearance of the skull
  • cyst-like lesions (brown tumors) of varying sizes.
[2] Subperiosteal resorption of bone is best demonstrated on a dorsovolar radiograph of the hands, since these changes characteristically occur on the radial aspects of the middle phalanges of the middle and index fingers.
[3] Subchondral resorption of bone is most commonly seen in the sacroiliac, sternoclavicular, and acromioclavicular joints.
[4] Cortical resorption (tunneling) is best appreciated on magnification radiography of the hand or long bones.
[5] Secondary hyperparathyroidism (due to renal disease) is typified radiographically by:
  • a generalized increase in bone density
  • sclerotic bands adjacent to the vertebral end plates, known as "rugger-jersey" spine
  • soft-tissue calcifications.
[6] The most common complications of hyperparathyroidism include pathologic fractures (vertebral bodies, ribs), metabolic arthropathies, and slipped epiphyses (femoral and humeral).

SUGGESTED READINGS

Beale MG, Salcedo JR, Ellis D, Rao DD. Renal osteodystrophy. *Pediatr Clin North Am* 1976;23:873–884.

Brecht-Krauss D, Kusmierek J, Hellwig D, Adam WE. Quantitative bone scintigraphy in patients with hyperparathyroidism. *J Nucl Med* 1987;28:458–461.

Broadus AE. Primary hyperparathyroidism. *J Urol* 1989;141:723–728.

Brown TW, Genant HK, Hattner RS, Orloff S, Potter DE. Multiple brown tumors in a patient with chronic renal failure and secodary hyperparathyroidism. *AJR Am J Roentgenol* 1977;128:131–134.

Bywaters EGL, Dixon ASJ, Scott JT. Joint lesions of hyperparathyroidism. *Ann Rheum Dis* 1963;22:171–187.

De Graaf P, Schicht IM, Pauwels EKJ, te Velde J, de Graeff J. Bone scintigraphy in renal osteodystrophy. *J Nucl Med* 1978;19:1289–1296.

Genant HK, Heck LL, Lanzl LH, Rossmann K, Vander Horst J, Paloyan E. Primary hyperparathyroidism: a comprehensive study of clinical, biochemical and radiographic manifestations. *Radiology* 1973;109:513–524.

Greenfield GB. Roentgen appearance of bone and soft tissue changes in chronic renal disease. *AJR Am J Roentgenol* 1972;116:749–757.

Hayes CW, Conway WF. Hyperparathyroidism. *Radiol Clin North Am* 1991;29:85–96.

Hooge WA, Li D. CT of sacroiliac joints in secondary hyperparathyroidism. *J Can Assoc Radiol* 1981;31:42–44.

Jensen PS, Kliger AS. Early radiographic manifestations of secondary hyperparathyroidism associated with chronic renal disease. *Radiology* 1977;125:645–652.

Kricun ME, Resnick D. Patellofemoral abnormalities in renal osteodystrophy. *Radiology* 1982;143:667–669.

Massry S, Ritz E. The pathogenesis of secondary hyperparathyroidism of renal failure. *Arch Intern Med* 1978;138:853–856.

Murphey MD, Sartoris DJ, Quale JL, Pathria MN, Martin NL. Musculoskeletal manifestations of chronic renal insufficiency. *Radiographics* 1993;13:357–379.

Pugh DG. Subperiosteal resorption of bone: a roentgenologic manifestation of primary hyperparathyroidism and renal osteodystrophy. *AJR Am J Roentgenol* 1951;66: 577–586.

Reiss E, Canterbury JM. Spectrum of hyperparathyroidism. *Am J Med* 1974;56:794–799.

Resnick D. Erosive arthritis of the hand and wrist in hyperparathyroidism. *Radiology* 1974;110:263–269.

Resnick D. The "rugger jersey" vertebral body. *Arthritis Rheum* 1981;24:1191–1192.

Resnick D, Deftos LJ, Parthemore JG. Renal osteodystrophy: magnification radiography of target sites of absorption. *AJR Am J Roentgenol* 1981;136:711–714.

Resnick D, Niwayama G. Parathyroid disorders and renal osteodystrophy. In: *Diagnosis of bone and joint disorders,* vol 4, 2nd ed. Philadelphia: WB Saunders;1988: 2219–2285.

Resnick D, Niwayama G. Subchondral resorption of bone in renal osteodystrophy. *Radiology* 1976;118:315–321.

Richardson ML, Pozzi-Mucelli RS, Kanter AS, Kolb FO, Ettinger B, Genant HK. Bone mineral changes in primary hyperparthyroidism. *Skeletal Radiol* 1986;15:85–95.

Roche CJ, O'Keeffe DP, Lee WK, Duddalwar VA, Torreggiani WC, Curtis JM. Selections from the buffet of food signs in radiology. *Radiographics* 2002;22:1369–1384.

Rossi RL, ReMine SG, Clerkin EP. Hyperparathyroidism. *Surg Clin North Am* 1985; 65:187–209.

Shapiro R. Radiologic aspects of renal osteodystrophy. *Radiol Clin North Am* 1972; 10:557–568.

Sly WM, Mittal AK. Bone scan in chronic dialysis patients with evidence of secondary hyperparathyroidism and renal osteodystrophy. *Br J Radiol* 1975;48:878–884.

Sundaram M, Joyce PF, Shields JB, Riaz MA, Sagar S. Terminal tufts of the hands: site for earliest changes of renal osteodystrophy in patients on maintenance hemodialysis. *AJR Am J Roentgenol* 1979;133:25–29.

Sundaram M, Phillipp SR, Wolverson MK, Riaz MA, Rae BJ. Ungual tufts in the follow-up of patients on maintenance hemodialysis. *Skeletal Radiol* 1980;5:247–249.

Teplick JG, Eftekhari F, Haskin ME. Erosion of the sternal ends of the clavicle: a new sign of primary and secondary hyperparathyroidism. *Radiology* 1974;113:323–326.

Weller M, Edeiken J, Hodes PJ. Renal osteodystrophy. *AJR Am J Roentgenol* 1968; 104:354–363.

Wittenberg A. The rugger jersey spine sign. *Radiology* 2004;230:491–492.

PAGET DISEASE

Pathophysiology

Paget disease, a relatively common bone disorder, is a chronic, progressive disturbance in bone metabolism that primarily affects older persons. It is slightly more common in men than in women (3:2), with an average age of onset between 45 and 55 years, although the disease has been known to occur in young adults. The prevalence of Paget disease varies considerably in different parts of the world, reaching its greatest incidence in Great Britain, Australia, and New Zealand.

The precise nature of Paget disease and its etiology are still unknown. Sir James Paget named the disease *osteitis deformans* in the belief that the basic process was infectious in origin. Other etiologies have also been proposed, such as neoplastic, vascular, endocrinologic, immunologic, traumatic, and hereditary. Recent ultrastructural studies and the discovery of giant multinucleated osteoclasts containing microfilaments in the affected cytoplasm, as well as intranuclear inclusion bodies, suggest a viral etiology. Some investigators have obtained immunocytologic evidence identifying the particles as analogous to those from the measles group virus material. Other immunologic studies have demonstrated viral antigens in affected cells identical to those from the respiratory syncytial virus. The most recent research indicates a paramyxovirus as an etiologic factor.

Whatever the fundamental cause of Paget disease, its basic pathologic process has to do with the balance between bone resorption and appositional new bone formation. There is disordered and extremely active bone remodeling, secondary to both osteoclastic bone resorption and osteoblastic bone formation in a characteristic mosaic pattern, which is the histologic hallmark of this condition. Biochemically, the increase in osteoblastic activity is reflected in elevated levels of serum alkaline phosphatase, which can rise to extremely high values. Similarly, the increase in osteoclastic bone resorption is reflected in high urinary levels of hydroxyproline, which is formed as a result of collagen breakdown.

The skeletal abnormalities seen in Paget disease are frequently asymptomatic and may be an incidental finding on radiographic examination or at autopsy. When the changes are symptomatic, clinical manifestations are often related to complications of the disease, such as deformity of the long bones, warmth in the involved extremity, periosteal tenderness and bone pain, fractures, secondary osteoarthritis, neural compression, and sarcomatous degeneration. The distribution of a lesion varies from monostotic involvement to widespread disease. The following bones, in order of decreasing frequency, are most often affected: the pelvis, femur, skull, tibia, vertebrae, clavicle, humerus, and ribs (Fig. 29.1). The fibula is involved only in exceptional cases.

Radiologic Evaluation

The radiographic features of Paget disease correspond to the pathologic processes in the bone and depend on the stage of the disorder. In the early phase, the *osteolytic* or *hot phase,* active bone resorption is evident as a radiolucent wedge or an elongated area with sharp borders that destroys both the cortex and cancellous bone as it advances along the shaft. The terms frequently used to describe this phenomenon are "advancing wedge," "candle flame," and "blade of grass"

Paget Disease

Figure 29.1 Major target sites of Paget disease.

(Fig. 29.2). In flat bones such as the calvarium or the iliac bone, an area of active bone destruction known as osteoporosis circumscripta appears as a purely osteolytic lesion (Fig. 29.3). In the skull, most commonly affected sites are the frontal and occipital bones; both inner and outer calvarial tables are involved, but the former is usually more extensively affected.

In the *intermediate* or *mixed phase,* bone destruction is accompanied by new bone formation, with the latter process tending to predominate. Bone remodeling appears radiographically as thickening of the cortex and coarse trabeculation of cancellous bone (Fig. 29.4). In the pelvis, cortical thickening and sclerosis of the iliopectineal and ischiopubic lines are present. Pubic rami and ischia may enlarge. In the spine, the thin cortex of the vertebral body, which disappears in

the hot phase, is later replaced by broad, coarsely trabeculated bone, forming what appears to be a "picture frame" around the body (Fig. 29.5). In the skull, focal patchy densities with a "cotton-ball" appearance are characteristic (Fig. 29.6).

In the *cool* or *sclerotic phase,* a diffuse increase of bone density occurs together with enlargement and widening of the bone and marked cortical thickening, with blurring of the demarcation between cortex and spongiosa (Fig. 29.7). Bowing of long bones may become a striking feature (Fig. 29.8). Similar changes are observed in the skull, where obliteration of the diploic space is also a typical feature (Fig. 29.9).

It is important to remember that, since in the long bones Paget disease starts at one articular end and advances to the other, all three

Figure 29.2 Osteolytic phase of Paget disease. (A) Anteroposterior radiograph of the lower leg of a 68-year-old woman shows an advancing wedge of osteolytic destruction in the midportion of the tibia (*arrow*). **(B)** Magnification study of the mid-femur in another patient shows the purely osteolytic phase of Paget disease. In both examples, the lesion resembles a blade of grass or a candle flame. **(A** from Sissons HA, Greenspan A, 1986, with permission.)

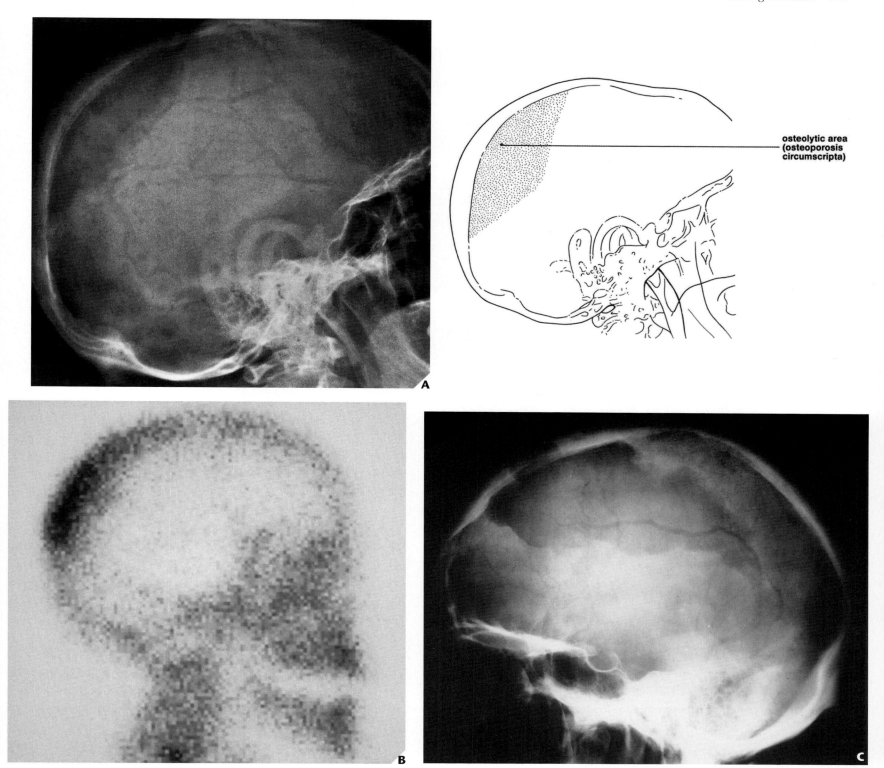

Figure 29.3 Osteolytic phase of Paget disease. (A) Lateral radiograph of the skull of a 60-year-old man shows an osteolytic lesion in the parieto-occipital area. This sharply demarcated defect, known as osteoporosis circumscripta, represents a hot phase of the disease. **(B)** Radionuclide bone scan shows a characteristic localized increased uptake of the radiopharmaceutical tracer resulting in the appearance of a "yarmulke" sign. **(C)** Lateral radiograph of the skull of a 65-year-old woman reveals osteoporosis circumscripta in the fronto-parietal area.

Figure 29.4 Intermediate phase of Paget disease. (A) In the intermediate phase, seen here affecting the tibia in a 62-year-old woman, thickening of the cortex and a coarse trabecular pattern in the medullary portion of the bone are characteristic features. Note the anterior bowing. **(B)** In another patient, an 81-year-old woman, intermediate phase is seen in the pubic and ischial bones. **(C)** Mixed phase affecting the proximal phalanx of the middle finger (*arrows*) is seen in a 67-year-old woman with monostotic Paget disease.

A

B

Figure 29.5 Intermediate phase of Paget disease. (A) Involvement of the lumbar spine in the mixed phase can be recognized by the "picture frame" appearance of the vertebral bodies created by dense sclerotic bone on the periphery and greater radiolucency in the center. Note the partial replacement of vertebral end plates by coarsely trabeculated bone. **(B)** In another patient, the "picture frame" appearance of the vertebral body of L-2 marks the intermediate phase of Paget disease. **(A** from Sissons HA, Greenspan A, 1986, with permission.)

Figure 29.6 Intermediate phase of Paget disease. Focal patchy densities in the skull, having a "cotton ball" appearance, are typical of the intermediate phase of Paget disease as seen in this radiograph of a 68-year-old woman.

Figure 29.7 Cool phase of Paget disease. In the cool phase, there is considerable thickening of the cortex and bone deformity. **(A)** The pelvic cavity, seen here in an 80-year-old woman, may assume a triangular appearance. **(B)** Involvement of a long bone, in this case the distal humerus of a 60-year-old woman, exhibits marked cortical thickening, narrowing of the medullary cavity, and a coarse trabecular pattern. **(C)** Similar changes are present in the tibia in a 72-year-old man. **(D)** Anteroposterior radiograph of the skull of an 82-year-old woman reveals typical changes of the cool phase of Paget disease. (**A** and **B** from Sissons HA, Greenspan A, 1986, with permission.)

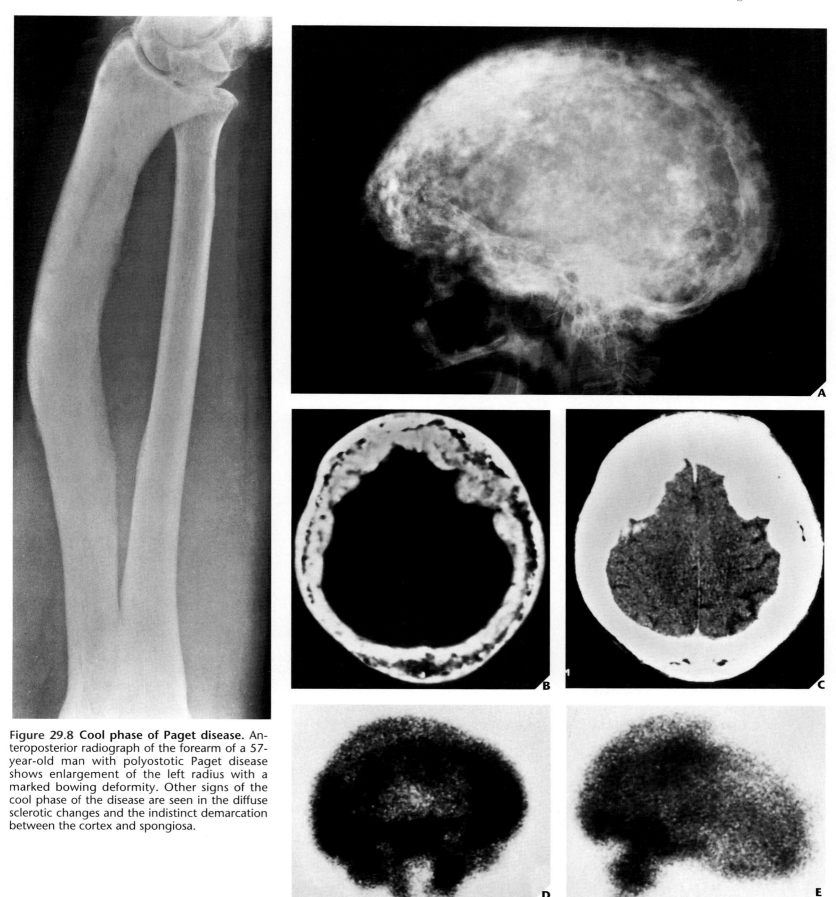

Figure 29.8 Cool phase of Paget disease. Anteroposterior radiograph of the forearm of a 57-year-old man with polyostotic Paget disease shows enlargement of the left radius with a marked bowing deformity. Other signs of the cool phase of the disease are seen in the diffuse sclerotic changes and the indistinct demarcation between the cortex and spongiosa.

Figure 29.9 Cool phase of Paget disease. (A) Lateral radiograph of the skull of an 80-year-old woman demonstrates numerous coalescent densities associated with thickening and sclerosis of the cranial vault and base of the skull. CT sections clearly demonstrate predominant involvement of the inner table with marked diminution of the diploic space **(B)** and thickening of the cranial vault **(C)**. **(D)**, **(E)** Scintigraphy demonstrates markedly increased uptake of radiopharmaceutical.

phases of the disorder may coexist in the same bone (Fig. 29.10A). Likewise, different phases may coexist in the flat bones or in the spine (Fig. 29.10B).

Magnetic resonance imaging is occasionally employed to demonstrate cortical and intramedullary involvement better, and to exclude (or confirm) extension of the process into the soft tissues. In general, the pagetic bone exhibits unhomogeneous signal intensity. On T1-weighted sequences intermediate-to-low signal intensity is usually noted. On T2 weighting the signal may be either high, intermediate, or low, depending on the stage of the disease and degree of fibrosis and sclerosis (Figs. 29.11 and 29.12).

Differential Diagnosis

Several conditions may mimic Paget disease, while the disease itself may be mistaken for other pathologic processes; for example, involvement of a single bone can be mistaken for monostotic fibrous dysplasia, and a uniform increase in osseous density may mimic lymphoma or metastatic cancer. The rugger-jersey appearance of the spine in secondary hyperparathyroidism may resemble Paget vertebra (see Fig. 28.8). Vertebral hemangioma also looks very much like Paget vertebra on a radiograph, except that the vertebral body is not enlarged and the vertebral end plates are well outlined (see Fig. 20.43B).

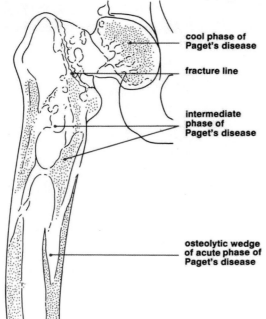

cool phase of Paget's disease

fracture line

intermediate phase of Paget's disease

osteolytic wedge of acute phase of Paget's disease

Figure 29.10 Coexistence of different phases of Paget disease. (A) Anteroposterior radiograph of the proximal half of the femur of a 77-year-old woman demonstrates all three phases of the disorder. The cool phase is seen in the femoral head, the intermediate phase in the proximal shaft, and the hot phase, represented by an osteolytic wedge of resorption, in the medial cortex more distally. **(B)** In another patient, a 54-year-old man, intermediate phase is seen in the vertebra L-3 (*arrow*), whereas the L-4 reveals a cool phase (*open arrow*).

Figure 29.11 MRI of Paget disease. (A) Anteroposterior radiograph of the left distal femur shows typical appearance of Paget disease: enlargement of the bone, cortical thickening, and sclerosis and coarse trabecular pattern of cancellous bone. **(B)**, **(C)** Two coronal T1-weighted (SE; TR 500/TE 20 msec) MR images demonstrate cortical thickening (*arrow*) and low-signal coarse cancellous trabeculae. **(D)** Coronal T2-weighted (SE; TR 2000/TE 80 msec) MRI shows heterogeneous signal in the femoral condyles.

Figure 29.12 MRI of Paget disease. Sagittal T1-weighted (SE; TR 500/TE 20 msec) MR image of the lumbar spine shows involvement of the vertebra by Paget disease.

However, the condition that bears the most striking resembalance to Paget disease is familial idiopathic hyperphosphatasia, also called "juvenile Paget disease" (see Figs. 30.1 and 30.2). In this condition, unlike Paget disease, the articular ends of the bone may not be affected.

Complications

Pathologic Fractures

Of the numerous complications observed in patients with Paget disease, the most common are pathologic fractures in the long bones. They may resemble partial or incomplete stress fractures, appearing radiographically as multiple short horizontal radiolucent lines on the convex aspect of the cortex (Fig. 29.13). True complete fractures are referred to as "banana-type" because of the horizontal direction of the fracture line as it traverses the affected bone (Fig. 29.14), and they have also been compared with crushed rotten wood or chalk. Fractures are more likely to occur during the osteolytic or hot phase, and they are frequently the main presenting manifestation of Paget disease.

Degenerative Joint Disease

The development of degenerative joint disease is a common complication of Paget disease. This secondary form of osteoarthritis usually occurs in the knee and hip articulations, where the characteristic changes are present, including joint space narrowing and osteophyte formation. Involvement of the acetabulum may be complicated by acetabular protrusio (Fig. 29.15).

Neurologic Complications

The neurologic complications of Paget disease are secondary to involvement of the vertebral column and skull. Collapse of a vertebral body, for example, causes extradural spinal canal block, which may lead to paraplegia (Fig. 29.16). Severe involvement of the bony spinal canal may lead to spinal stenosis, the presence of which can be effectively demonstrated by computed tomography (CT) (Fig. 29.17). Basilar invagination due to softening of the skull may lead to encroachment on the foramen magnum and neurologic deficit.

Neoplastic Complications

Benign or malignant giant cell tumors, single or multiple, may complicate Paget disease. The usual sites of these tumors are the calvarium and the iliac bone.

The development of a bone sarcoma is a serious but rare complication of Paget disease; the incidence is less than 1%. Osteosarcoma is by far the most common histologic type (Fig. 29.18), followed by fibrosarcoma, malignant fibrous histiocytoma, chondrosarcoma, and lymphoma, with the pelvis, femur, and humerus at highest risk for development of malignant transformation. The main radiographic features of this complication are development of a lytic lesion at the site of Paget disease, cortical breakthrough, and formation of a soft-tissue mass (Fig. 29.19); a periosteal reaction is rare. There is often a pathologic fracture as well. The radiographic appearance of Paget sarcoma must be distinguished from that of metastases of a primary carcinoma of the kidney (Fig. 29.20), breast, or prostate. The metastatic deposit may be lodged in either unaffected or pagetic bone. The prognosis for patients with sarcomatous degeneration of Paget disease is poor; the mean survival time usually does not exceed 6 to 8 months. Occasionally, an osteosarcoma in pagetic bone may metastasize to other bones and soft tissues, but metastases to the lung, liver, and adrenals are much more likely.

Orthopedic Management

Because of the variable clinical presentation of Paget disease, decisions regarding therapy must be based on the particular manifestations in each patient. The goal of the medical treatment is the control and relief of pain, rather than restitution of normal bone quality. The role of the orthopedic surgeon in the management of Paget disease is to evaluate and treat the cause of a patient's pain, to assess and manage any deformities, and to provide therapy for pathologic fractures and tumors developing in pagetic bone. The radiologist contributes to these aims by providing essential information. For instance, CT is useful for demonstrating spinal stenosis, which frequently leads to neurologic symptoms in patients with Paget disease (see Fig. 29.17). Radionuclide imaging is also a valuable technique, particularly for determining the skeletal distribution of the disease (see Fig. 26.10).

Treatment consists of inhibiting osteoclastic activity by calcitonin, a 32-amino-acid hormone secreted by the C cells of the thyroid gland, and oral administration of biphosphonates, which bind to areas of high bone turnover, decreasing bone resorption. The main action of biphosphonates is decreasing osteoclastic activity. The most frequently used drugs in this group include etidronate, pamidronate, alendronate, and tiludronate. Administration of plicamycin, previously called mithramycin, inhibits RNA synthesis and has a potent cytotoxic effect on osteoclasts. The serum alkaline phosphatase determination and the 24-hour urinary hydroxyproline measurement were the main indicators of the response of the disease to medical treatment, however, the recently developed biochemical markers of bone resorption and formation allow a more accurate assessment of disease activity and response to therapy.

Surgical intervention is indicated for treatment of pathologic fractures, advanced, disabling arthritis, and extreme bowing deformities of the long bones. Stress or pseudofractures, which occur most often in the tibia and proximal femur, are treated by bracing and protection from weight bearing for a period of several months. Complete fractures are treated either with intramedullary rods or with compression plates and screws. For arthritic complications, which are particularly frequent in the hip and knee articulations, total joint replacement is usually performed.

Figure 29.14 Pathologic fracture in Paget disease. A 62-year-old man with monostotic Paget disease affecting the right tibia sustained a pathologic fracture. Note that the fracture line traverses the area of active, osteolytic bone destruction. (From Sissons HA, Greenspan A, 1986, with permission.)

Figure 29.13 Stress fractures in Paget disease. Numerous stress fractures, seen in the lateral cortex of the femur in an 80-year-old man with advanced Paget disease, are the most frequent complications of this condition.

Figure 29.15 Secondary osteoarthritis in Paget disease. A 75-year-old woman with long-standing polyostotic Paget disease had been reporting progressive pain in her right hip for 1 year. Anteroposterior radiograph demonstrates advanced osteoarthritis and acetabular protrusio. (From Sissons HA, Greenspan A, 1986, with permission.)

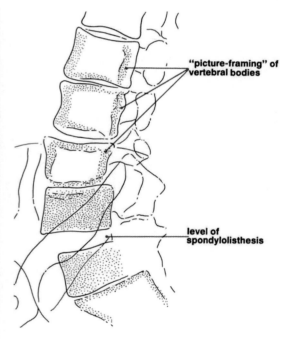

Figure 29.16 **Pathologic fracture in Paget disease.** A 60-year-old man with polyostotic Paget disease presented with lower back pain and neurologic symptoms. Anteroposterior **(A)** and lateral **(B)** radiographs of the lumbar spine show a pathologic compression fracture of L-3 with encroachment on the spinal canal, which was the source of his symptoms. (From Sissons HA, Greenspan A, 1986, with permission.)

Figure 29.17 **Spinal complications in Paget disease.** An 84-year-old man with extensive polyostotic Paget disease for many years developed degenerative spondylolisthesis and spinal stenosis. Anteroposterior **(A)** and lateral **(B)** radiographs of the lumbar spine show Paget disease in the cool phase. Second-degree degenerative spondylolisthesis is seen at the L4-5 level. **(C)** CT section through L-5 demonstrates narrowing of the spinal canal characteristic of spinal stenosis, the major cause of most neurologic symptoms in Paget disease.

Figure 29.18 Paget sarcoma. A 70-year-old woman with Paget disease affecting her left hemipelvis had a rare complication, sarcomatous degeneration. **(A)** Radiograph of the pelvis shows extensive involvement of the left ilium, pubis, and ischium by Paget disease. There is also destruction of the cortex and a large soft-tissue mass accompanied by bone formation, typical findings for osteosarcoma. **(B)** CT scan demonstrates the soft-tissue mass more clearly.

Figure 29.19 MRI of Paget sarcoma. (A) Coronal T1-weighted (SE; TR 500/TE 20 msec) MR image shows Paget disease affecting the distal femur. Destruction of the cortex and soft-tissue mass are well demonstrated. Axial T2-weighted **(B)** and coronal STIR sequences **(C)** confirm the presence of a soft-tissue mass (*arrows*), thus corroborating the diagnosis of malignant transformation.

Figure 29.20 Metastases in Paget disease. Anteroposterior radiograph of the pelvis of a 55-year-old woman with Paget disease for 10 years shows extensive osteolytic destruction of the right ilium, ischium, and pubis secondary to metastatic renal cell carcinoma (hypernephroma). Note the typical involvement of the pelvis by Paget disease. This metastatic lesion should not be mistaken for Paget sarcoma.

PRACTICAL POINTS TO REMEMBER

[1] The histologic hallmark of Paget disease is a mosaic pattern of disorderly and active bone remodeling secondary to osteoclastic resorption and osteoblastic formation.

[2] The characteristic radiographic features of Paget disease of bone include:
- involvement of at least one articular end of a long bone
- thickening of the cortex and enlargement of the affected bone
- a coarse trabecular pattern to the spongiosa
- bowing deformities of the long bones
- a "picture-frame" appearance of a vertebral body.

[3] Particular radiographic changes in Paget disease are related to the stage of the disorder. In the acute (hot) phase, a radiolucent osteolytic area is seen
- in the calvarium or in a flat bone, where it is known as "osteoporosis circumscripta"
- in a long bone, where it appears as an advancing wedge of active disease, resembling a candle flame or a blade of grass.

[4] Radionuclide bone scan, which invariably shows increased uptake of the tracer in bones affected by Paget disease, is effective in determining the distribution of the lesion.

[5] The most frequent complication of Paget disease is pathologic fracture, either incomplete stress fractures or "banana-type" complete fractures.

[6] The most serious complication of Paget disease is sarcomatous degeneration. Radiographically, it can be recognized by:
- osteolytic bone destruction at the site of the pagetic lesion
- cortical breakthrough
- a soft-tissue mass.

Malignant transformation must be distinguished from metastatic lesions to pagetic bone from a primary carcinoma of the lung, breast, kidney, gastrointestinal tract, or prostate.

[7] Paget disease must be distinguished from:
- "juvenile Paget disease" (familial idiopathic hyperphosphatasia)
- van Buchem disease (hyperostosis corticalis generalisata)
- vertebral hemangioma
- rugger-jersey spine seen in secondary hyperparathyroidism
- lymphoma
- extensive osteoblastic metastases.

SUGGESTED READINGS

Adkins MC, Sundaram M. Radiologic case study: insufficiency fracture of the acetabular roof in Paget's disease. *Orthopedics* 2001;24:1019–1020.

Altman RD, Bloch DA, Hochberg MC, Murphy WA. Prevalance of pelvic Paget's disease of bone in the United States. *J Bone Miner Res* 2000;15:461–465.

Anderson DC. Paget's disease of bone is characterized by excessive bone resorption coupled with excessive and disorganized bone formation. *Bone* 2001;29:292–293.

Bahk YW, Parh YH, Chung SK, Chi JG. Bone pathologic correlation of multimodality imaging in Paget's disease. *J Nucl Med* 1995;36:1421–1426.

Bank YW, Park YH, Chung SK. Bone pathologic correlation of multimodality imaging in Paget's disease. *J Nucl Med* 1995;36:1421–1426.

Barry HC. *Paget's disease of bone.* London: Livingstone; 1969.

Basle MF, Chappard D, Rebel A. Viral origin of Paget's disease of bone? *Presse Med* 1996;25:113–118.

Birch MA, Taylor W, Fraser WD, Ralston SH, Hart CA, Gallagher JA. Absence of paramyxovirus RNA in cultures of pagetic bone cells and in pagetic bone. *J Bone Miner Res* 1994;9:11–16.

Boutin RD, Spitz DJ, Newman JS, Lenchik L, Steinbach LS. Complications in Paget disease at MR imaging. *Radiology* 1998;209:641–651.

Brandolini F, Bacchini P, Moscato M, Bertoni F. Chondrosarcoma as a complicating factor in Paget's disease of bone. *Skeletal Radiol* 1997;26:497–500.

Brown JP, Chines AA, Myers WR, Eusebio RA, Ritter-Hrncirik C, Hayes CW. Improvement of pagetic bone lesions with risedronate treatment: a radiologic study. *Bone* 2000;26:263–267.

Chapman GK. The diagnosis of Paget's disease of bone. *Aust N Z J Surg* 1992; 62: 24–32.

Clarke CR, Harrison MJ. Neurological manifestations of Paget's disease. *J Neurol Sci* 1978;38:171–178.

Colarintha P, Fonseca AT, Salgado L, Vieira MR. Diagnosis of malignant change in Paget's disease by T1-201. *Clin Nucl Med* 1996;21:299–301.

Conrad GR, Johnson AW. Solitary adenocarcinoma metastasis mimicking sarcomatous degeneration in Paget's disease. *Clin Nucl Med* 1997; 22: 300–302.

Delmas PD, Meunier PJ. The management of Paget's disease of bone. *N Engl J Med* 1997;336:558–566.

Edeiken J, Dalinka M, Karasick D. Paget disease (osteitis deformans): metabolic and dystrophic bone disease. In: *Edeiken's roentgen diagnosis of diseases of bone,* vol 2, 4th ed. Baltimore: Williams & Wilkins; 1990:1231–1259.

Fenton P, Resnick D. Metastases to bone affected by Paget's disease: a report of three cases. *Int Orthop* 1991;15:397–399.

Firooznia HF. Paget's disease. In: Firooznia HF, Golimbu C, Rafii M, Rauschning W, Weinreb J, eds. *MRI and CT of the musculoskeletal system.* St. Louis: Mosby-Year Book; 1992:176–181.

Berquist TH. *MRI of the musculoskeletal system,* 3rd ed. Philadelphia: Lippincott-Raven; 1996:920–922.

Fogelman I. Bone scanning in Paget's disease. In: Freeman LM, ed. *Nuclear medicine annual.* New York: Raven Press; 1991:99–128.

Fogelman I, Carr D. A comparison of bone scanning and radiology in the assessment of patients with symptomatic Paget's disease. *Eur J Nucl Med* 1980;5:417–421.

Fogelman I, Ryan PJ. Bone scanning in Paget's disease. In: Collier BD Jr, Fogelman I, Rosenthall L, eds. *Skeletal nuclear medicine.* St. Louis, MO: CV Mosby; 1996: 171–181.

Frame B, Marel GM. Paget's disease: a review of current knowledge. *Radiology* 1981;141:21–24.

Fraser WD. Paget's disease of bone. *Curr Opin Rheumatol* 1997;9:347–354.

Frassica FJ, Sim FH, Frassica DA, Wold LE. Survival and management considerations in postirradiation osteosarcoma and Paget's osteosarcoma. *Clin Orthop* 1991;270:120–127.

Greditzer HG III, McLeod RA, Unni KK, Beabout JW. Bone sarcomas in Paget disease. *Radiology* 1983;146:327–333.

Greenspan A. A review of Paget's disease: radiologic imaging, differential diagnosis, and treatment. *Bull Hosp Jt Dis* 1991;51:22–33.

Greenspan A. Paget's disease: current concept, radiologic imaging, and treatment. *Recent Adv Orthop* 1993;1:32–48.

Greenspan A, Norman A, Sterling AP. Precocious onset of Paget's disease—a report of three cases and review of the literature. *Can Assoc Radiol J* 1977;28:69–72.

Guyer PB, Chamberlain AT. Paget's disease of bone in South Africa. *Clin Radiol* 1988;39:51–52.

Guyer PB, Clough PW. Paget's disease of bone: some observations on the relation of the skeletal distribution to pathogenesis. *Clin Radiol* 1978;29:421–426.

Hadjipavlou A, Lander P, Srolovitz H, Enker IP. Malignant transformation in Paget disease of bone. *Cancer* 1992;70:2802–2808.

Hadjipavlou AG, Gaitanis IN, Kontakis GM. Paget's disease of the bone and its management. *J Bone Joint Surg [Br]* 2002;84B:160–169.

Haibach H, Farrell C, Dittrich FJ. Neoplasms arising in Paget's disease of bone: a study of 82 cases. *Am J Clin Pathol* 1985;83:594–600.

Hosking D, Meunier PJ, Ringe JD, Reginster JY, Gennari C. Paget's disease of bone: diagnosis and management. *BMJ* 1996;312:491–495.

Hutter RVP, Foote FW Jr, Frazell EL, Francis KC. Giant cell tumors complicating Paget's disease of bone. *Cancer* 1963;16:1044–1056.

Huvos AG, Butler A, Bretsky SS. Osteogenic sarcoma associated with Paget's disease of bone: a clinicopathologic study of 65 patients. *Cancer* 1983;52:1489–1495.

Kaufmann GA, Sundaram M, McDonald DJ. Magnetic resonance imaging in symptomatic Paget's disease. *Skeletal Radiol* 1991;20:413–418.

Kelly JK, Denier JE, Wilner HI, Lazo A, Metes JJ. MR imaging of lytic changes in Paget disease of the calvarium. *J Comput Assist Tomogr* 1989;13:27–29.

Kim CK, Estrada WN, Lorberboym M, Pandit N, Religioso DG, Alaxi A. The "mouse face" appearance of the vertebrae in Paget's disease. *Clin Nucl Med* 1997;22:104–108.

Krane SM. Paget's disease of bone. *Clin Orthop* 1977;127:24–36.

Kumar A, Poon PY, Aggarwal S. Value of CT in diagnosing nonneoplastic osteolysis in paget disease. *J Comput Assist Tomogr* 1993;17:144–146.

Kunin JR, Strouse PJ. The "yarmulke" sign of Paget's disease. *Clin Nucl Med* 1991;16: 788–789.

Lander PH, Hadjipavlou AG. A dynamic classification of Paget's disease. *J Bone Joint Surg [Br]* 1986;68B:431–438.

Lentle BC, Russell AS, Heslip PG, Percy JS. The scintigraphic findings in Paget's disease of bone. *Clin Radiol* 1976;27:129–135.

Maldague B, Malghem J. Dynamic radiological patterns of Paget's disease of bone. *Clin Orthop* 1987;217:126–151.

McKenna RJ, Schwinn CP, Soong KY, Higinbotham NI. Osteogenic sarcoma arising in Paget's disease. *Cancer* 1964;17:42–66.

McKillop JH, Fogelman I, Boyle IT, Greig WR. Bone scan appearance of a Paget's osteosarcoma: failure to concentrate EHDP. *J Nucl Med* 1977;18:1039–1040.

Meunier PJ, Vignot E. Therapeutic strategy in Paget's disease of bone. *Bone* 1995;17:489S–491S.

Milgram JW. Orthopedic management of Paget's disease of bone. *Clin Orthop* 1977;127:63–69.

Milgram JW. Radiographical and pathological assessment of the activity of Paget's disease of bone. *Clin Orthop* 1977;127:43–54.

Miller C, Rao VM. Sarcomatous degeneration of Paget disease in the skull. *Skeletal Radiol* 1983;10:102–106.

Mills BG, Frausto A, Singer FR, Ohsaki Y, Demulder A, Roodman GD. Multinucleated cells formed in vitro from Paget's bone marrows express viral antigens. *Bone* 1994;15:443–448.

Mirra JM. Pathogenesis of Paget's disease based on viral etiology. *Clin Orthop* 1987;217: 162–170.

Mirra JM, Brien EW, Tehranzadeh J. Paget's disease of bone: review with emphasis on radiologic features. Part I. *Skeletal Radiol* 1995;24:163–171; 173–184.

Mirra JM, Gold RM: Giant cell tumor containing viral-like intranuclear inclusions, in association with Paget's disease. Case report. *Skeletal Radiol* 1982;8:67–70.

Moore TE, Kathol MH, El-Koury GY, Walker CW, Gendall DW, Whitten CG. Unusual radiologic features of Paget's disease of bone. *Skeletal Radiol* 1994;23:257–260.

Nicholas JJ, Srodes CH, Herbert D, Hoy RJ, Peel RL, Goodman MA. Metastatic cancer in Paget's disease of bone: a case report. *Orthopedics* 1987;10:725–729.

Noor M, Shoback D. Paget's disease of bone: diagnosis and treatment update. *Curr Rheumatol Rep* 2000;2:67–73.

Paget J. On a form of chronic inflammation of bones (osteitis deformans). *Med Chir Trans* 1877;60:37–64.

Pande KC, Ashford RU, Dey A, Kayan K, McCloskey EV, Kanis JA. Atypical familial Paget's disease of bone. *Joint Bone Spine* 2001;68:257–261.

Potter HG, Schneider R, Ghelman B, Healey JH, Lane JM. Multiple giant cell tumors and Paget disease of bone: radiographic and clinical correlations. *Radiology* 1991;180:261–264.

Resnick D. Paget's disease of bone: current status and a look back to 1943 and earlier. *AJR Am J Roentgenol* 1988;150:249–256.

Resnick D, Niwayama G. Paget's disease. In: Resnick D, ed. *Diagnosis of bone and joint disorders*, 4th ed. Philadelphia: WB Saunders; 2002:1947–2000.

Resnik C. Paget disease of bone: the uncomplicated and the complicated. *Radiologist* 1999;6:1–11.

Roberts MC, Kressel HY, Fallon MD, Zlatkin MB, Dalinka MK. Paget disease: MR imaging findings. *Radiology* 1989;173:341–345.

Rosenbaum HD, Hanson DJ. Geographic variation in the prevalence of Paget's disease of bone. *Radiology* 1969;92:959–963.

Ryan PJ, Fogelman I. Paget's disease—five years follow-up after pamidronate therapy. *Br J Rheumatol* 1994;33:98–99.

Schajowicz F, Santini Araujo E, Berenstein M. Sarcoma complicating Paget's disease of bone: a clinicopathological study of 62 cases. *J Bone Joint Surg [Br]* 1983;65B: 299–307.

Serafini AN. Paget's disease of the bone. *Semin Nucl Med* 1976;6:47–58.

Siris ED. Paget's disease of bone. *J Bone Miner Res* 1998;13:1061–1065.

Sissons HA. Epidemiology of Paget's disease. *Clin Orthop* 1966;45:73–79.

Sissons HA, Greenspan A. Paget's disease. In: Taveras JM, Ferrucci JT, eds. *Radiology— imaging, diagnosis, intervention*, vol. 5. Philadelphia: JB Lippincott; 1986:1–14.

Smith J, Botet YF, Yeh SDJ. Bone sarcoma in Paget's disease: a study of 85 patients. *Radiology* 1984;152:583–590.

Smith SE, Murphey MD, Motamedi K, Mulligan ME, Resnik CS, Gannon FH. From the Archives of the AFIP. Radiologic spectrum of Paget disease of bone and its complications with pathologic correlation. *Radiographics* 2002; 22: 1191–1216.

Som PM, Hermann G, Sacher M, Stollman AL, Moscatello AL, Biller HF. Paget disease of the calvaria and facial bones with an osteosarcoma of the maxilla: CT and MR findings. *J Comput Assist Tomogr* 1987;11:887–890.

Sundaram MG, Khanna G, el-Khoury GY. T1-weighted MR imaging for distinguishing large osteolysis of Paget's disease from sarcomatous degeneration. *Skeletal Radiol* 2001;30:378–383.

Sy WM. *Gamma images in benign and metabolic bone diseases,* vol I. Boca Raton, FL: CRC Press; 1981:58–60.

Tehranzadeh J, Fung Y, Donohue M, Anavim A, Pribram HW. Computed tomography of Paget disease of the skull versus fibrous dysplasia. *Skeletal Radiol* 1998;27: 664–672.

Vellenga CJ, Bijvoet OLM, Pauwels EKJ. Bone scintigraphy and radiology in Paget's disease of bone: a review. *Am J Physiol Imaging* 1988;3:154–168.

Wallace E, Wong J, Reid IR. Pamidronate treatment of the neurologic sequelae of pagetic spinal stenosis. *Arch Intern Med* 1995;155:1813–1815.

Waxman AD, McKee D, Siemsen JK, Singer FR. Gallium scanning in Paget's disease of bone: effect of calcitonin. *AJR Am J Roentgenol* 1980;134:303–306.

Wellman HN, Schauwecker D, Robb JA, Khairi MR, Johnston CC. Skeletal scintimaging and radiography in the diagnosis and management of Paget's disease. *Clin Orthop* 1977;127:55–62.

Wick MR, Siegal GP, Unni KK, McLeod RA, Greditzer HG III. Sarcomas of bone complicating osteitis deformans (Paget's disease): fifty years' experience. *Am J Surg Pathol* 1981;5:47–59.

Wittenberg K. The blade of grass sign. *Radiology* 2001;221:199–200.

Yu T, Squires F, Mammone J, DiMarcangelo M. Lymphoma arising in Paget's disease. *Skeletal Radiol* 1997;26:729–731.

Zlatkin MB, Lander PH, Hadjipavlou AG, Levine JS. Paget disease of the spine: CT with clinical correlation. *Radiology* 1986;160:155–159.

MISCELLANEOUS METABOLIC AND ENDOCRINE DISORDERS

Familial Idiopathic Hyperphosphatasia

Familial idiopathic hyperphosphatasia is a rare autosomal-recessive disorder affecting young children, generally within their first 18 months and exhibiting a striking predilection for those of Puerto Rican descent. The condition is associated with progressive bone deformities. Clinically, it is characterized by painful bowing of the limbs, muscular weakness, abnormal gait, pathologic fractures, spinal deformities, loss of vision and hearing, elevation of serum alkaline phosphatase, and an increase in the amount of leucine aminopeptidase.

Radiographic Evaluation

Increased turnover of bone and skeletal collagen demonstrated by radionuclide bone scan is a characteristic finding in familial idiopathic hyperphosphatasia. Its radiographic features are typical. Although this disorder has no relationship to classic Paget disease, it is often re-

ferred to as "juvenile Paget disease," and it exhibits similar radiographic features. The long bones are increased in size, showing thickening of the cortex and a coarse trabecular pattern (Fig. 30.1). Likewise, bowing deformities are common, as are involvement of the pelvis and skull (Fig. 30.2). However, unlike Paget disease, the epiphyses are usually not affected.

Differential Diagnosis

A few conditions exist similar to familial idiopathic hyperphosphatasia that belong to the general group of endosteal hyperostoses, or hyperostosis corticalis generalisata. In particular, an autosomal-recessive form of these disorders, van Buchem disease, although classified as chronic hyperphosphatasia tarda, is in fact a distinct dysplasia. Its onset is later than that of congenital hyperphosphatasia, and the age of patients ranges from 25 to 50 years. The major radiographic finding is a symmetric thickening of the cortices of the long and short tubular

Figure 30.1 Familial idiopathic hyperphosphatasia. (A) Anteroposterior radiograph of the shoulder and arm of a 12-year-old Puerto Rican boy reveals marked thickening of the cortex of the humerus and coarsening of the bony trabeculae, resembling pagetic bone. **(B)** Radiograph of the hands shows sclerotic changes in the bones and a marked narrowing of the medullary cavity of the metacarpals and phalanges. **(C)** Anteroposterior radiograph of the skull of a 30-year-old man shows calvarial thickening and sclerosis resembling that of Paget disease. **(D)** Magnification study reveals marked thickening of the inner table and widening of the diploë.

Figure 30.2 Familial idiopathic hyperphosphatasia. (A) Radiograph of a 4-year-old boy demonstrates marked bowing of the long bones of the lower extremity, a striking feature of familial idiopathic hyperphosphatasia. **(B)** Anteroposterior film of the pelvis shows the coarse trabecular pattern and cortical thickening typical of this condition. Note that the epiphyses are not affected. **(C)** Lateral radiograph of the skull demonstrates thickening of the tables and a "cotton ball" appearance of the cranial vault, similar to that of Paget disease. **(B** from Sissons HA, Greenspan A, 1986, with permission.)

Figure 30.3 The most clearly revealing target sites of acromegaly.

bones. The femora are not bowed, and the articular ends are spared. The cranial bones show marked thickening of the vault and the base. Serum alkaline phosphatase levels are elevated, but calcium and phosphorus levels are normal.

Acromegaly

Increased secretion of growth hormone (somatotropin) by the eosinophilic cells of the anterior lobe of the pituitary gland, as a result of either hyperplasia of the gland or a tumor, leads to acceleration of bone growth. If this condition develops before skeletal maturity (i.e., while the growth plates are still open), then it results in gigantism;

development after skeletal maturity results in acromegaly. The onset of symptoms is usually insidious, and the involvement of certain target sites in the skeleton is typical (Fig. 30.3). Gradual enlargement of the hands and feet as well as exaggeration of facial features are the earliest manifestations. The characteristic facial changes result from overgrowth of the frontal sinuses, protrusion of the jaw (prognathism), accentuation of the orbital ridges, enlargement of the nose and lips, and thickening and coarsening of the soft tissues of the face.

Radiographic Evaluation

Radiographic examination reveals a number of characteristic features of this condition. A lateral view of the skull demonstrates thickening of the cranial bones and increased density. The diploë may be obliterated. The sella turcica, which houses the pituitary gland, may or may not be enlarged. The paranasal sinuses become enlarged (Fig. 30.4) and the mastoid cells become overpneumatized. The prognathous jaw, one of the obvious clinical features of this condition, is apparent on the lateral view of the facial bones.

The hands also exhibit revealing radiographic changes. The heads of the metacarpals are enlarged, and irregular bony thickening along the margins, simulating osteophytes, may be seen. Increase in the size of the sesamoid at the metacarpophalangeal joint of the thumb may be helpful in evaluating acromegaly. Values of the sesamoid index (determined by the height and width of this ossicle measured in millimeters) greater than 30 in women and greater than 40 in men suggest acromegaly; however, generally the dividing line between normal and abnormal values is not sharp enough to allow individual borderline cases to be diagnosed on the basis of this index alone. Characteristic changes are also seen in the distal phalanges; their bases enlarge and the terminal tufts form spur-like projections. The joint spaces widen as a result of hypertrophy of articular cartilage (Fig. 30.5), and hypertrophy of the soft tissues may also occur, leading to the development of square, spade-shaped fingers.

Evaluation of the foot on the lateral view allows an important measurement to be made, the heel-pad thickness. This index is determined by the distance from the posteroinferior surface of the os calcis to the nearest skin surface. In a normal 150-pound subject, the heel-pad thickness should not exceed 22 mm. For each additional 25 pounds of body weight, 1 mm can be added to the basic value; thus,

Figure 30.4 Acromegalic skull. Lateral radiograph of the skull of a 75-year-old woman with acromegaly shows marked enlargement of the frontal sinuses, prominent supraorbital ridges, and thickening of the frontal bones.

Figure 30.5 Acromegalic hand. Dorsovolar radiograph of the hand of a 38-year-old woman shows characteristic overgrowth of the terminal tufts and spur-like projections. The bases of the terminal phalanges are also enlarged, and the radiographic joint spaces are widened.

24 mm would be the highest normal value for a 200-pound person. If the heel-pad thickness is greater than the established normal value, then acromegaly is a strong possibility (Fig. 30.6), and determination of growth hormone level by immunoassay is called for.

The spine in acromegaly may also reveal identifying features. A lateral view of the spine may disclose an increase in the anteroposterior diameter of a vertebral body, as well as scalloping or increased concavity of the posterior vertebral margin (Fig. 30.7). Although the exact mechanism of this phenomenon is not known, bone resorption has been implicated as a potential cause. Other conditions have also been associated with posterior vertebral scalloping (Table 30.1). In addition, thoracic kyphosis is often increased in spinal acromegaly and lumbar lordosis is accentuated. The invertebral disk space may be wider than normal because of overgrowth of the cartilaginous portion of the disk.

The articular abnormalities seen in acromegaly are the result of a frequent complication, degenerative joint disease, which is in turn the result of overgrowth of the articular cartilage and subsequent inadequate nourishment of abnormally thick cartilage. The combination of joint space narrowing, osteophytes, subchondral sclerosis, and formation of cyst-like lesions is similar to the primary osteoarthritic process.

Gaucher Disease

Classification

Gaucher disease is a familial inherited disturbance of unknown cause transmitted as an autosomal-recessive trait. It is a metabolic disorder characterized by the abnormal deposition of cerebrosides (glycolipids) in the reticuloendothelial cells of the spleen, liver, and bone marrow. These altered macrophages, called *Gaucher cells,* are the histologic hallmark of the disease. The disease results from numerous mutations at the genetic locus encoding the enzyme glucocerebrosidase (glucosylceramidase cerebroside β-glucosidase) that lead to the defective activity of lysosomal hydrolase. It is classified into three distinct categories:

Stage I: The *nonneuronopathic,* or *adult type,* is the most common form, occurring mainly in Ashkenazi Jews. Onset is in the patient's first or second decade, and the individuals affected usually live normal life spans. Bone abnormalities and hepatosplenomegaly characterize this form of the disease.

Stage II: The *acute neuronopathic* form is lethal within the patient's first year. This type apparently has no predilection for any ethnic group.

Stage III: The *subacute juvenile neuronopathic* form begins in the latter part of the first year and follows a malignant course similar to that of type II. Patients experience mental retardation and seizures and usually die by the end of their second decade of life.

increased heel-pad thickness

Figure 30.6 Acromegalic foot. Lateral radiograph of the foot of a 58-year-old man shows a heel-pad thickness of 38 mm, far above normal for this patient who weighs only 140 pounds. This measurement corresponds to the shortest distance between the calcaneus and the plantar aspect of the heel.

Figure 30.7 Acromegalic spine. Lateral radiograph of the thoracolumbar spine of a 49-year-old woman with acromegaly demonstrates posterior vertebral scalloping, a phenomenon apparently caused by bone resorption.

The presenting clinical features of patients depend on the type of disease they have. The adult form of the disorder (type I) is the most common and typically presents with abdominal distention secondary to splenomegaly. Recurrent bone pain is a sign of skeletal involvement, and acute severe bone pain together with swelling and fever

Table 30.1 Causes of Scalloping in Vertebral Bodies

Increased Intraspinal Pressure
Intradural neoplasms
Intraspinal cysts
Syringomyelia and hydromyelia
Communicating hydrocephalus
Dural Ectasia
Marfan syndrome
Ehlers-Danlos syndrome
Neurofibromatosis
Bone Resorption
Acromegaly
Congenital Disorders
Achondroplasia
Morquio disease
Hunter syndrome
Osteogenesis imperfecta (tarda)
Physiologic Scalloping

(From Mitchell GE, et al., 1967, with permission.)

Figure 30.8 Gaucher disease. Anteroposterior radiograph of a 12-year-old boy with adult-type Gaucher disease shows the Erlenmeyer-flask deformity of both lower femora, secondary to medullary expansion. Note the thinning of the cortex caused by diffuse osteoporosis.

suggests acute pyogenic osteomyelitis. This clinical complex, which is the result of ischemic necrosis of bone, has been called "aseptic osteomyelitis." Pingueculae may be present in the eyes, and the skin may acquire a brown pigmentation. Epistaxis or other hemorrhages caused by thrombocytopenia may occur. The diagnosis is made by demonstrating characteristic gaucher cells in bone marrow aspirate or in a biopsy specimen from the liver.

Radiologic Evaluation

The radiographic examination in Gaucher disease reveals characteristic findings. There is a diffuse osteoporosis that is frequently associated with medullary expansion. In the ends of the long bones, this phenomenon is referred to as the "Erlenmeyer flask" deformity (Fig. 30.8 and Table 30.2). Localized bone destruction assuming a honeycomb appearance is also typically seen (Fig. 30.9); gross osteolytic destruction is usually limited to the shafts of the long bones. Moreover, sclerotic changes are common, occurring secondary to a repair pro-

Table 30.2 Causes of Erlenmeyer's-Flask Deformity

Gaucher disease
Niemann-Pick disease
Fibrous dysplasia
Sickle-cell anemia
Thalassemia
Multiple cartilaginous exostoses
Ollier disease (enchondromatosis)
Albers-Schönberg disease (osteopetrosis)
Engelmann disease (progressive diaphyseal dysplasia)
Pyle disease (metaphyseal dysplasia)
Pycnodysostosis
Lead poisoning

Figure 30.9 Gaucher disease. Destructive changes, seen here in the proximal right humerus of a 52-year-old woman with the adult form of the disease, may assume a honeycomb appearance.

cess or bone infarctions (Fig. 30.10). Medullary bone infarction and a periosteal reaction may lead to a bone-within-bone phenomenon, which may resemble osteomyelitis (Fig. 30.11). Recently, Hermann and associates conducted a study of 29 patients with type I Gaucher disease using MRI to determine the usefulness of this technique in the evaluation of bone marrow involvement. The results of this investigation suggest that MRI is a valuable noninvasive modality in this respect to assess disease activity. Apparently, the patients with decreased signal intensity within bone marrow on both T1-weighted and T2-weighted images, but showing a relative increase in signal intensity from T1 weighting to T2 weighting can be considered to have an "active process" that correlates well with their symptoms.

Complications

The most common complication of Gaucher disease is osteonecrosis of the femoral head and occasionally of the femoral condyles (Fig. 30.12). Superimposition of degenerative changes is also a frequent finding that necessitates surgery. Pathologic fractures are common, and they may involve the long bones as well as the spine. The most serious complication (although fortunately a rare one) is malignant transformation at the site of bone infarcts.

Treatment

Enzyme replacement therapy using placental derived alglucerase or recombinant (i.e., imuglucerase) preparations has resulted in hematologic improvement and resolution of hepatosplenomegaly. In some patients, signs of skeletal regeneration have also been reported.

Tumoral Calcinosis

Pathophysiology

First described by Inclan and coworkers in 1943, tumoral calcinosis is characterized by the presence of single or multiple periarticular lobulated cystic masses containing chalky material. Their formation is the result of the deposition of calcium salt in the soft tissues about the joints—the shoulders (particularly near the scapula), hips, and elbow joints—as well as on the extensile surfaces of the limbs. The masses are painless and usually occur in children and adolescents. Blacks are affected more frequently than other racial groups, with most cases of tumoral calcinosis reported from Africa and New Guinea. Because the cause is unknown, the diagnosis is one of exclusion. Other causes of soft-tissue calcifications, such as secondary hyperparathyroidism, hypervitaminosis D, gout and pseudogout, myositis ossificans, paraarticular chondroma, and calcinosis circumscripta, must be excluded before the diagnosis of tumoral calcinosis can be made.

Radiographic Evaluation

Radiographic examination usually reveals well-demarcated and lobulated calcific masses that are circular or oval and located about the joints (Fig. 30.13). They vary in density; some are lacy and amorphous, and others are almost bone-like in appearance. Only in very rare instances is the calcific deposit located within the joint capsule.

Figure 30.10 Gaucher disease. Anteroposterior radiograph of the right distal femur of a 29-year-old man demonstrates medullary infarction of the bone and endosteal and periosteal reactions secondary to reparative processes.

Figure 30.11 **Gaucher disease.** Lateral radiograph of the distal femur in a 28-year-old woman shows extensive medullary infarction and periosteal new bone formation, producing a bone-within-bone appearance.

Figure 30.12 **Gaucher disease complicated by osteonecrosis.** (A) Anteroposterior radiograph of the pelvis of an 11-year-old Ashkenazi Jew with non-neuronopathic Gaucher disease shows osteonecrosis of the left femoral head, a common complication of this disorder. (B) Anteroposterior radiograph of the right knee of a 25-year-old man with Gaucher disease demonstrates osteonecrotic changes of the medial and lateral femoral condyles. Note also the extensive bone infarction of the proximal tibia.

Figure 30.13 Tumoral calcinosis. A 66-year-old black subject had multiple bumps about the wrists and elbows since childhood. Dorsovolar **(A)** and lateral **(B)** radiographs of the wrists demonstrate calcific masses located on the dorsal aspect just beneath the skin. **(C)** Anteroposterior radiograph of the right elbow shows similar tumoral accumulation of calcium on the anteromedial aspect.

Treatment

Surgical excision of the calcified masses is the most effective form of treatment, although attempts to treat this disorder with low-calcium and low-phosphate diets and phosphate-combining antacids have had some success.

Hypothyroidism

Pathophysiology

Hypothyroidism is a syndrome encountered in infants and children, resulting from a deficiency of the thyroid hormones thyroxine and triiodothyronine, either during fetal life (cretinism) or early childhood (juvenile myxedema or juvenile hypothyroidism). The deficiency may be primary, caused by disease of the thyroid gland, or secondary, caused by lack of thyroid-stimulating hormone (TSH) produced by the pituitary gland. The major target sites are the growth plates and epiphyses, best-demonstrated in the hands and the hips (Fig. 30.14). The key symptoms and signs include lethargy, constipation, an enlarged tongue, abdominal distention, and dry skin. The manifestations are typically less severe when the deficiency occurs in early childhood as an acquired disease than when it is congenital.

Radiographic Evaluation

The fundamental radiographic feature in both forms of hypothyroidism is delayed skeletal maturation with stunting of bone growth leading to dwarfism. In particular, the appearance of the secondary ossification centers is greatly delayed, as a dorsovolar radiograph of the hand may demonstrate (Fig. 30.15). Epiphyses ossify from numerous ossification centers, thereby acquiring a fragmented appearance and on occasion appearing abnormally dense (Fig. 30.16). This process may be mistaken for osteonecrosis, as seen in Legg-Calvé-Perthes disease (see Fig. 32.26), or for certain dysplasias, such as dysplasia epiphysealis punctata, also known as Conradi disease. Underpneumatization of the sinuses and mastoids are also typical radiographic findings associated with hypothyroidism.

Complications

One of the common complications of hypothyroidism is the development of slipped femoral capital epiphysis. The radiographic findings of this condition are described in Chapter 32.

Scurvy

Pathophysiology

Barlow disease, as scurvy is also known, results from a deficiency of ascorbic acid (vitamin C). The function of vitamin C is to maintain intracellular substances of mesenchymal derivation, such as connective tissue, osteoid tissue in bones, and dentin in the teeth. In infants, primary deficiency is caused most commonly by failure to supplement the diet with vitamin C, whereas in adults it is usually caused by food idiosyncrasies or an insufficient diet. Deficiency of vitamin C causes a hemorrhagic tendency, leading to subperiosteal bleeding and abnormal function of osteoblasts and chondroblasts. The latter results in defective osteogenesis.

Radiographic Evaluation

The characteristic bone lesions of scurvy are caused by cessation of endochondral bone ossification caused by failure of the osteoblasts to form osteoid tissue. Continuing osteoclastic resorption without adequate formation of new bone yields the appearance of osteoporosis, with generalized osteopenia and thinning of the cortices. Deposition of calcium phosphate continues in whatever osteoid tissue is formed,

so that an area of increased density develops adjacent to the growth plate. Such areas have been called the "white lines of scurvy" (Fig. 30.17). A ring of increased density is also seen around the secondary centers of ossification, a finding known as a Wimberger ring sign. Fractures of the metaphysis are common, producing a "corner" sign or "Pelkan beak" (Fig. 30.17). Increased capillary fragility leads to subperiosteal and soft-tissue bleeding and the formation of hematomas, which may trigger a periosteal reaction (Fig. 30.18). In adults, the bleeding may extend into the joints.

Differential Diagnosis

Scurvy should be differentiated from "battered child syndrome," congenital syphilis, and leukemia. In battered child syndrome, char-

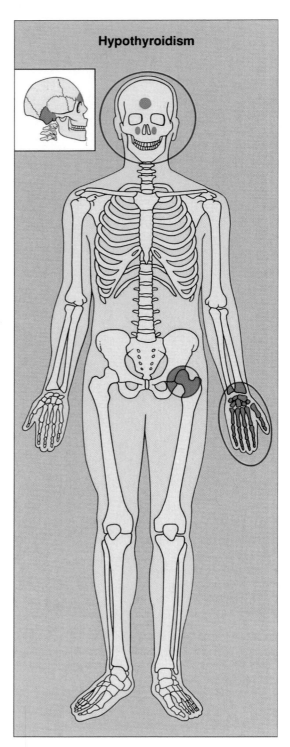

Figure 30.14 **Target sites of hypothyroidism.**

Figure 30.15 Juvenile hypothyroidism. (A) Dorsovolar radiograph of the right hand of a 13-year-old boy with juvenile hypothyroidism demonstrates skeletal immaturity; the bone age is approximately 8 years. Note the fragmented secondary ossification centers of the distal ulna and distal phalanges. In fact, they represent separated foci of ossification. **(B)** The hand of a healthy boy of the same age is shown for comparison.

Figure 30.16 Congenital hypothyroidism. Anteroposterior radiograph of the pelvis of a 5-year-old girl with congenital hypothyroidism (cretinism) shows pseudofragmentation of both capital femoral epiphyses. This process may be mistaken for Legg-Calvé-Perthes disease.

Figure 30.17 Scurvy. (A) and **(B)** Anteroposterior radiographs of the lower legs of an 8-month-old infant shows the typical skeletal changes of scurvy. Note the dense segment adjacent to the growth plate ("white line of scurvy"), the ring of increased density around the secondary ossification centers of the distal femora and proximal tibiae (Wimberger ring sign), and the beaking of the metaphysis of both tibiae (Pelkan beak). A periosteal reaction secondary to subperiosteal bleeding is also noted.

subperiosteal hemorrhage and periostitis

Wimberger's ring sign

white line of scurvy

Figure 30.18 Scurvy. Lateral radiograph of the right leg of a 10-month-old infant with subperiosteal bleeding secondary to scurvy shows a marked periosteal reaction in the distal femoral diaphysis. A peripheral ring of increased density and central radiolucency, the Wimberger ring sign, is evident in the posteriorly displaced ossification center of the distal femoral epiphysis and in the proximal tibial epiphysis. Note also "white line" in the tibial metaphysis.

acteristic metaphyseal corner fractures and fractures in different healing stages are characteristic. In congenital syphilis, the epiphyseal centers are normal. In leukemia, radiolucent metaphyseal bands are common, but fractures and epiphysiolysis are not part of the disorder.

PRACTICAL POINTS TO REMEMBER

Familial Idiopathic Hyperphosphatasia

[1] Two conditions of similar radiographic presentation are familial idiopathic hyperphosphatasia ("juvenile Paget disease") and autosomal-recessive form of hyperostosis corticalis generalisata, van Buchem disease. The radiographic features of these disorders, similar to those of Paget disease, are:
  * cortical thickening and a coarse trabecular pattern to the spongiosa
  * sparing of the articular ends of bones (unlike classic Paget disease).

Acromegaly

[1] In the diagnosis and evaluation of acromegaly, the following radiographic projections have specific value:
  * lateral view of the skull to evaluate the thickness of the cranial vault, the size of the paranasal sinuses, and prognathism
  * dorsovolar view of the hands to evaluate the sesamoid index and detect changes of the distal tufts
  * lateral view of the foot to measure the heel-pad thickness
  * lateral view of the spine to evaluate the intervertebral disk spaces and the posterior margins of the vertebral bodies.

[2] One of the frequent complications of acromegaly is degenerative joint disease (osteoarthritis) secondary to undernourished hypertrophied articular cartilage.

Gaucher Disease

[1] Gaucher disease is a metabolic disorder characterized by the abnormal deposition of cerebrosides (glycolipids) in the reticuloendothelial system.

[2] Characteristic radiographic features of Gaucher disease include:
  * Erlenmeyer flask deformity of the distal femora
  * osteonecrosis of the femoral heads

- medullary bone infarction of the long bones, frequently associated with periosteal reaction
- generalized osteopenia.

[3] MRI is a noninvasive technique to assess disease activity.

Tumoral Calcinosis

[1] Tumoral calcinosis, a condition seen predominantly in blacks, consists of multiple cystic, calcium-containing masses about the large joints (shoulders, hips, and elbows).

[2] The diagnosis of tumoral calcinosis is one of exclusion: other causes of soft-tissue calcifications, such as secondary hyperparathyroidism, hypervitaminosis D, and juxtacortical myositis ossificans, must be excluded.

Hypothyroidism

[1] The fundamental radiographic feature of hypothyroidism (cretinism and juvenile myxedema) is retarded skeletal maturation, which is best demonstrated on a dorsovolar view of the hand.

[2] Other characteristic radiographic features of hypothyroidism include:
- a fragmented appearance of the ossification centers of the epiphyses
- increased density of both epiphyses and metaphyses.

[3] In the femoral heads, these features may mimic osteonecrosis (Legg-Calvé-Perthes disease) or dysplasia epiphysealis punctata (Conradi disease).

Scurvy

[1] The characteristic radiographic changes seen in scurvy (deficiency of vitamin C) include:
- generalized osteopenia
- "white lines of scurvy" adjacent to the growth plate
- Wimberger ring sign, representing increased density around ossification centers
- the "corner" sign or "Pelkan beak," representing metaphyseal fractures
- periosteal reaction secondary to subperiosteal bleeding.

[2] Conditions that should be differentiated from scurvy include:
- battered child syndrome
- congenital syphilis
- leukemia.

SUGGESTED READINGS

Albright F. Changes simulating Legg Perthes disease (osteochondritis deformans juvenilis) due to juvenile myxoedema. *J Bone Joint Surg* 1938;20:764–769.

Amstutz HC. The hip in Gaucher's disease. *Clin Orthop* 1973;90:83–89.

Amstutz HC, Carey EJ. Skeletal manifestations and treatment of Gaucher's disease. Review of twenty cases. *J Bone Joint Surg [Am]* 1966;48A:670–679.

Beighton P, Goldblatt J, Sachs S. Bone involvement in Gaucher disease. In: Desnick RJ, Gatt S, Grabowski GA, eds. *Gaucher disease: a century of delineation and research.* New York: Alan R Liss; 1982:107–129.

Beutler E. Gaucher disease. Review article. *N Engl J Med* 1991;325:1354–1360.

Bishop AF, Destovet JM, Murphy WA, Gilula LA. Tumoral calcinosis: case report and review. *Skeletal Radiol* 1982;8:269–274.

Bourke JA, Heslin DJ. Gaucher's disease: roentgenologic changes over 20 years interval. *AJR Am J Roentgenol* 1965;94:621–630.

Cremin BJ, Davey H, Goldblatt J. Skeletal complications of type I Gaucher disease: the magnetic resonance features. *Clin Radiol* 1990;42:244–247.

Desnick RJ. Gaucher disease (1882–1982): centennial perspectives on the most prevalent Jewish genetic disease. *Mt Sinai J Med* 1982;49:443–455.

Detenbeck LC, Tressler HA, O'Duffy JD, Randall, RV. Peripheral joint manifestations of acromegaly. *Clin Orthop* 1973;91:119–127.

Duncan TR. Validity of sesamoid index in diagnosis of acromegaly. *Radiology* 1975;115:617–619.

Feldman RH, Lewis MM, Greenspan A, Steiner GC. Tumoral calcinosis in an infant. A case report. *Bull Hosp Jt Dis Orthop Inst* 1983;43:78–83.

Goldblatt J, Sachs S, Beighton P. The orthopedic aspects of Gaucher disease. *Clin Orthop* 1978;137:208–214.

Grabowski GR. Gaucher disease. *Adv Hum Genet* 1993;21:341–377.

Grenfield GB. Bone changes in chronic adult Gaucher's disease. *AJR Am J Roentgenol* 1970;110:800–807.

Hermann G. Skeletal manifestation of type 1 Gaucher disease—an uncommon genetic disorder. *Osteol Közlem* 2001;10:141–148.

Hermann G, Goldblatt J, Levy RN, Goldsmith SJ, Grabowski GA. Gaucher's disease type I. Assessment of bone involvement by CT and scintigraphy. *AJR Am J Roentgenol* 1986;147:943–948.

Hermann G, Shapiro RS, Abdelwahab IF, Grabowski G. MR imaging in adults with Gaucher disease type I: evaluation of marrow involvement and disease activity. *Skeletal Radiol* 1993;22:247–251.

Hernandez RJ, Poznanski AK. Distinctive appearance of the distal phalanges in children with primary hypothyroidism. *Radiology* 1979;132:83–84.

Hernandez RJ, Poznanski AW, Hopwood NJ. Size and skeletal maturation of the hand in children with hypothyroidism and hypopituitarism. *AJR Am J Roentgenol* 1979;133:405–408.

Hirsch M, Mogle P, Barkli Y. Neonatal scurvy. *Pediatr Radiol* 1976;4:251–253.

Horev G, Kornreich L, Hadar H, Katz K. Hemorrhage associated with bone crisis in Gaucher disease identified by magnetic resonance imaging. *Skeletal Radiol* 1991;20:479–482.

Inclan A, Leon P, Camejo MG. Tumoral calcinosis. *JAMA* 1943;121:490–495.

Israel O, Jershalmi J, Front D. Scintigraphic findings in Gaucher disease. *J Nucl Med* 1986;27:1557–1563.

Kho KM, Wright AD, Doyle FH. Heel-pad thickness in acromegaly. *Br J Radiol* 1970;43:119–125.

Kinsella RA Jr, Back DK. Thyroid acropachy. *Med Clin North Am* 1968;52:393–398.

Kleinberg DL, Young IS, Kupperman HS. The sesamoid index. An aid in the diagnosis of acromegaly. *Ann Intern Med* 1966;64:1075–1078.

Lacks S, Jacobs RP. Acromegalic arthropathy: a reversible rheumatic disease. *J Rheumatol* 1986;13:634–636.

Lafferty FW, Reynolds ES, Pearson OH. Tumoral calcinosis: a metabolic disease of obscure etiology. *Am J Med* 1965;38:105–118.

Lang EK, Bessler WT. The roentgenologic features of acromegaly. *AJR Am J Roentgenol* 1961;86:321–328.

Lanir A, Hadar H, Cohen I, et al. Gaucher disease: assessment with MR imaging. *Radiology* 1986;161:239–244.

Layton MW, Fudman EJ, Barkan A, Braunstein EM, Fox IH. Acromegalic arthropathy: characteristics and response to therapy. *Arthritis Rheum* 1988;31:1022–1027.

Levin B. Gaucher's disease: clinical and roentgenologic manifestations. *AJR Am J Roentgenol* 1961;85:685–696.

Lin SR, Lee KR. Relative value of some radiographic measurements of the hand in the diagnosis of acromegaly. *Invest Radiol* 1971;6:426–431.

Manaster BJ, Anderson TM Jr. Tumoral calcinosis: serial images to monitor successful dietary therapy. *Skeletal Radiol* 1982;8:123–125.

Mankin HJ, Rosenthal DI, Xavier R. Current concepts review. Gaucher disease – new approaches to an ancient disease. *J Bone Joint Surg [Am]* 2001;83A:748–760.

Mass M, van Kuijk C, Stoker J, Hollak CE, Akkerman EM, Aerts JFMG, den Heeten GJ. Quantification of bone involvement in Gaucher disease: MR imaging bone marrow burden score as an alternative to Dixon quantitative chemical shift MR imaging—initial experience. *Radiology* 2003;229:554–561.

McNulty JF, Pim P. Hyperphosphatasia. Report of a case with a 30-year follow-up. *AJR Am J Roentgenol* 1972;115:614–618.

Melmed S. Acromegaly. *N Engl J Med* 1990;322:966–977.

Mitchell GE, Lourie H, Berne AS. The various causes of scalloped vertebrae and notes on their pathogenesis. *Radiology* 1967;89:67–74.

Nerubay J, Pilderwasser D. Spontaneous bilateral distal femoral physiolysis due to scurvy. *Acta Orthop Scand* 1984;55:18–20.

Palmer PES. Tumor calcinosis. *Br J Radiol* 1966;39:518.

Randall RV. Acromegaly and gigantism. In DeGroot LJ, ed. *Endocrinology,* 2nd ed. Philadelphia: WB Saunders; 1989:330–350.

Riggs BL, Randall RV, Wahner HW, Jowsey J, Kelly PJ, Singh M. The nature of the metabolic bone disorder in acromegaly. *J Clin Endocrinol Metab* 1972;34:911–918.

Rosenthal DI, Scott JA, Barranger J, et al. Evaluation of Gaucher disease using magnetic resonance imaging. *J Bone Joint Surg [Am]* 1986;68A:802–808.

Scanlon GT, Clemett AR. Thyroid acropachy. *Radiology* 1964;83:1039–1042.

Sissons HA, Greenspan A. Paget's disease. In: Taveras JM, Ferrucci JT, eds. *Radiology—imaging, diagnosis, intervention.* Philadelphia: JB Lippincott; 1986:1–14.

Smit GG, Schmaman A. Tumoral calcinosis. *J Bone Joint Surg [Br]* 1967;49B:698–703.

Steinbach HL, Feldman R, Goldberg MG. Acromegaly. *Radiology* 1959;72:535–549.

Steinbach HL, Russell W. Measurement of the heel-pad as an aid to diagnosis of acromegaly. *Radiology* 1964;82:418–423.

Stuberg JL, Palacios E. Vertebral scalloping in acromegaly. *AJR Am J Roentgenol* 1971;112:397–400.

Torres-Reyes E, Staple TW. Roentgenographic appearance of thyroid acropachy. *Clin Radiol* 1970;21:95–100.

Van Buchem FSP, Hadders HN, Hansen JF, Woldring MG. Hyperostosis corticalis generalisata. Report of seven cases. *Am J Med* 1962;33:387–397.

Van Buchem FSP, Hadders HN, Ubbens R. An uncommon familial systemic disease of the skeleton: hyperostosis corticalis generalisata familiaris. *Acta Radiol* 1955;44:109–120.

Zimram A, Gelbart T, Westwood B, Grabowski G, Beutler E. High frequency of the Gaucher disease mutation at nucleotide 1226 among the Ashkenazi Jews. *Am J Hum Genet* 1991;49:855–859.

Zubrow AB, Lane JM, Parks JS. Slipped capital femoral epiphysis occurring during treatment for hypothyroidism. *J Bone Joint Surg [Am]* 1978;60A:256–258.

CONGENITAL AND DEVELOPMENTAL ANOMALIES

RADIOLOGIC EVALUATION OF SKELETAL ANOMALIES

Classification

The conditions discussed in this part comprise disturbances in skeletal formation, development, growth, maturation, and modeling. Some of these anomalies arise during fetal development, such as congenital absence of a whole or part of a limb, supernumerary digits in a hand or foot, or fused digits, and are obvious at the time the baby is born. Some may begin to develop during fetal life but become apparent later in childhood, such as Hurler syndrome (gargoylism) or osteogenesis imperfecta tarda. Other anomalies, such as certain sclerosing dysplasias, develop after birth because of a genetic predisposition and become manifest later in life.

Congenital anomalies can be classified in various ways, but because of their complexity a full and detailed classification of these disorders is beyond the scope of this chapter. To simplify the variety of classifications, which are constantly changing and expanding, the congenital anomalies may be divided from the pathologic point of view into those involving disturbances of bone formation, bone growth, and bone maturation and modeling (Table 31.1). Anomalies of bone formation include the *complete failure of a bone to form* and *faulty formation* of bones, which may manifest in a decreased number of bones (agenesis and aplasia) (Fig. 31.1A) or in the number of supernumerary bones (polydactyly) (Fig. 31.1B,C). Anomalies of formation may

also be encountered in aberrations involving bone *differentiation,* which include pseudoarthroses (Fig. 31.2A) and bone fusions (syndactyly and synostosis) (Fig. 31.2B). Disturbances in bone growth may lead to *aberrations in the size or shape* of bones. These may manifest in undergrowth (hypoplasia or atrophy) (Fig. 31.3A,B), in overgrowth (hypertrophy or gigantism) (Fig. 31.3C), or deformed growth, such as congenital tibia vara (see Fig. 32.40). Anomalies related to bone growth may also be exhibited in abnormalities affecting the *motion in a joint,* such as contractures, subluxations, and dislocations (Fig. 31.4). Among the last group of congenital anomalies affecting the skeletal system are those exhibiting aberrations in bone *growth, maturation, and modeling,* as manifest in the various dysplasias (Fig. 31.5).

A second simple classification system is anatomic and based on the affected region of the body. This system comprises anomalies of the shoulder girdle and upper limb, pelvis and lower limb, spine, and the skeleton in general.

Radiologic Imaging Modalities

Radiologic examination is essential for the accurate diagnosis of many congenital and developmental anomalies, which in some instances (such as osteopoikilosis or osteopathia striata) are totally asymptomatic

Table 31.1 **Simplified Classification of Congenital Anomalies of the Skeletal System**

Anomalies of Bone Formation	**Anomalies of Bone Maturation and Modeling**
Complete failure of formation (agenesis, aplasia)	Failure of endochondral bone maturation and modeling
Faulty formation	Failure of intramembranous bone maturation and modeling
Decreased number of bones	Combined failure of endochondral and intramembranous bone maturation and modeling
Increased number of bones	**Constitutional Diseases of Bone**
Faulty differentiation	Abnormalities of cartilage and/or bone growth and development (osteochondrodysplasias)
Pseudoarthrosis	Malformation of individual bones, isolated or in combination (dysostoses)
Fusion (synostosis, coalition, syndactyly)	Idiopathic osteolyses
Anomalies of Bone Growth	Chromosomal aberrations and primary metabolic abnormalities
Aberrant size	
Undergrowth (hypoplasia, atrophy)	
Overgrowth (hypertrophy, gigantism)	
Aberrant shape (deformed growth)	
Aberrant fit (subluxation, dislocation)	

Figure 31.1 Anomalies of bone formation. Congenital anomalies related to disturbances in bone formation may be seen in the complete failure of a bone to form, as shown on this film in a 1-year-old girl with sacral agenesis (**A**), and in a 26-year-old woman with bilateral agenesis of the fibulae (**B**) or in formation of supernumerary bones, as seen in this 12-year-old boy with polydactyly in both hands (**C**), and in this 3-year-old girl with polydactyly in the right foot (**D**). *(continued)*

Figure 31.1 **Anomalies of bone formation.** *Continued.*

Figure 31.2 **Anomalies of bone formation.** Congenital anomalies related to bone division may manifest in congenital pseudoarthrosis, seen here involving the left radius in a 4-year-old boy (**A**); in full fusion of digits (syndactyly), seen here in a 1-year-old boy (**B**) who, in addition, has polydactyly; in partial fusion (synostosis) of two bones, seen here affecting the proximal radius and ulna in a 6-year-old girl (**C**); or in coalition, seen in the complete fusion of the lunate and triquetrum bones in a 33-year-old man (**D**) and in the fusion of the calcaneus and navicular bones (*arrow*) in a 21-year-old man (**E**). *(continued)*

Figure 31.2 **Anomalies of bone formation.** *Continued.*

Figure 31.3 Anomalies of bone growth. Congenital anomalies related to the size of bones may manifest in hypoplasia, as seen here in the right thumb of a 4-year-old girl (**A**), and in the proximal femur of a 7-month-old boy with proximal femoral focal deficiency (**B**), or in congenital brachydactyly, shown here in both hands of a 25-year-old woman (**C**). Overgrowth may also be encountered, as in this case of macrodactyly (megalodactyly) involving the first two digits of the left foot of a 12-year-old girl (**D**).

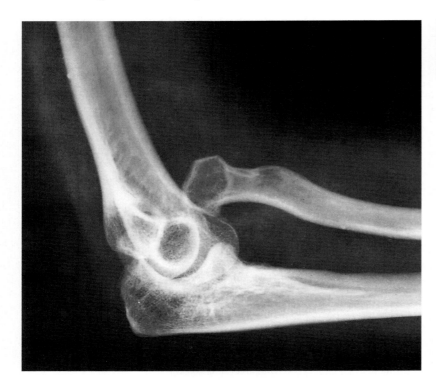

Figure 31.4 Anomaly of bone growth. Congenital dislocation of the radial head, seen here in a 35-year-old woman, is an anomaly related to aberrant bone growth leading to a condition affecting the motion of a joint. Note the hypoplasia and abnormal shape of the radial head, an important feature differentiating this condition from traumatic dislocation.

Figure 31.5 Anomaly of bone development and maturation. (A) Osteopetrosis (Albers-Schönberg disease), seen here in the spine, pelvis, and both femora of a 28-year-old man, is a congenital anomaly related to the development and maturation of bone. The persistence of immature spongiosa packing the marrow cavity results in the dense marble-like appearance of the bones. **(B)** Osteopoikilosis, seen here affecting the pelvis and proximal femora of a 21-year-old man, is a developmental anomaly of endochondral bone formation, where islands of secondary spongiosa fail to resorb and remodel.

and only revealed on radiographs obtained for other purposes. It also plays an important part in monitoring the progress of treatment. In many instances the results of therapy, whether conservative or surgical, can be assessed only on the basis of the proper radiologic examination.

The radiologic imaging modalities most frequently used in diagnosing congenital malformations of the bones and joints are the following:

1. Conventional radiography, including standard and special projections
2. Arthrography
3. Myelography
4. Computed tomography (CT)
5. Radionuclide imaging (scintigraphy, bone scan)
6. Ultrasound
7. Magnetic resonance imaging (MRI)

In most instances, the diagnosis can be made on the standard radiographic projections specific for the anatomic site under investigation. As in most other orthopedic conditions, radiographs should be obtained in at least two projections at 90 degrees to one another (Fig. 31.6, see also Fig. 4.1). Supplemental views, however, are sometimes necessary for a full evaluation of an anomaly, particularly those affecting complex structures such as the ankle and foot (Fig. 31.7). Weight-bearing views of the foot should be obtained whenever possible.

Ancillary imaging techniques play an important role in the evaluation of many congenital and developmental conditions. Myelography, for example, is still valuable for detecting anomalies of the spine (Fig. 31.8). In congenital dislocations, particularly in the hip, arthrography remains an essential technique (Fig. 31.9); it is also effective in demonstrating developmental anomalies affecting the articular cartilage and menisci of the knee, as in Blount disease (Fig. 31.10). CT examination is particularly valuable in the evaluation of congenital hip dislocations. Apart from providing important interpretive data about this complex anomaly, including demonstration of details of the relationship between the acetabulum and the femoral head, CT provides an accurate assessment of the degree of reduction of the head after treatment, often disclosing very subtle abnormalities not detected by radiography or arthrography of the hip (Fig. 31.11). A further application of CT is seen in its ability to measure the angle of anteversion of the femoral head, that is, the degree of anterior torsion of the femoral head and neck from the coronal plane (Figs. 31.12 and 31.13). Three-dimensional CT reformatted images may be helpful in global visualization of spinal deformities (Figs. 31.14 and 31.15).

Other ancillary techniques also have important functions in the evaluation of skeletal anomalies. Radionuclide bone scan, for instance, is particularly effective in detecting silent sites of skeletal abnormality in various developmental dysplasias (Fig. 31.16). Ultrasound has only recently come to be used in the diagnosis of congenital skeletal abnormalities, including hip dysplasia and dislocation. It is effective in assessing the position of the femoral head in the acetabulum, as well as the status of the cartilaginous acetabular roof and other cartilaginous structures such as the limbus that cannot be demonstrated on the standard radiographs (Fig. 31.17). This technique also

Figure 31.6 Clubfoot deformity. Dorsoplantar **(A)** and lateral **(B)** radiographs of the foot of a 7-year-old boy are sufficient to demonstrate all the components of congenital equinovarus deformity of the foot (clubfoot), namely, the equinus position of the heel, the varus position of the hindfoot, and the adduction and varus deformity of the forefoot.

Figure 31.7 Talocalcaneal coalition. Posterior tangential (Harris-Beath) projection of both calcanei in a 23-year-old woman demonstrates bony fusion at the level of the middle facet of both subtalar joints, a diagnostic feature of a talocalcaneal coalition.

Figure 31.8 Diastematomyelia. A myelogram of a 9-year-old girl demonstrates a filling defect in the center of the contrast-filled thecal sac, caused by a fibrous spur attached to the vertebral body. This finding is diagnostic of diastematomyelia, a rare congenital anomaly of the vertebrae and spinal cord. Note the associated increase in the interpedicular distances.

Figure 31.9 Congenital hip dislocation. (A) Standard anteroposterior radiograph of the right hip of a 7-year-old girl who was treated conservatively for congenital hip dislocation demonstrates persistent complete dislocation. **(B)** Arthrography was performed to evaluate the cartilaginous structures of the joint. In addition to a deformed cartilaginous limbus, the ligamentum teres appears thickened and contrast medium has accumulated in the stretched capsule. The thickened ligamentum teres frustrated several previous attempts at closed reduction.

Figure 31.10 **Blount disease. (A)** Anteroposterior radiograph of the knee of a 4-year-old boy demonstrates congenital tibia vara (Blount disease). **(B)** Double-contrast arthrogram of the knee shows hypertrophy of the medial meniscus and thick non-ossified cartilage at the medial aspect of the proximal tibial epiphysis.

Figure 31.11 **Congenital hip dislocation. (A)** Anteroposterior radiograph of the pelvis in a 1-year-old girl demonstrates congenital dislocation of the left hip. After conservative management with a Pavlik harness, a contrast arthrogram **(B)** was performed to evaluate the results of treatment. The femoral head appears to be well seated in the acetabulum. Note the smoothness of the Shenton-Menard line (see Fig. 32.8A). **(C)** CT section, however, demonstrates persistence of posterolateral subluxation.

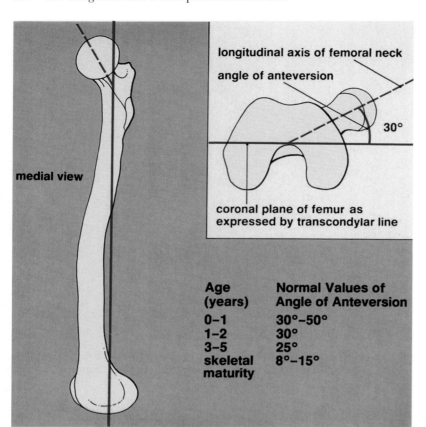

Figure 31.12 Anteversion of the femoral head. The angle of anteversion of the femoral head represents the degree of anterior torsion of the femoral head and neck from the coronal plane. It is determined by the angle formed between the longitudinal axis of the femoral neck and the coronal plane of the femur as expressed by a transcondylar line (see Fig. 31.13).

Figure 31.13 CT determination of the angle of version of the femoral head. To obtain the angle of version of the femoral head on CT examination, the patient is supine, with the lower extremities in the neutral position, the feet taped together, and the knees taped to the table. Preferably, a single scanogram is obtained that includes both hips and knees on the same film; however, separate films may be obtained **(A)**, **(B)** if the patient is too tall. In the latter case, care should be taken not to move the patient between the two takes. On a section through the femoral neck and the upper portion of the greater trochanter **(C)**, a line is drawn through the femoral neck, using the femoral head and greater trochanter as guides. The angle that this line forms with the horizontal line (the level of the CT table) determines the *relative* angle of anteversion (or retroversion) of the femoral head. On the CT section through the femoral condyles at the intercondylar notch **(D)**, a line is drawn through the posterior margins of the condyles, and the angle formed by this line and the horizontal line determines the degree of internal or external rotation of the extremities. From these two measurements, a *true* angle of version (anteversion or retroversion) is calculated. If the knee is in internal rotation, as in the present case, the sum of both angles yields the degree of anteversion. If the knee is in external rotation, the angle obtained at the knee must be subtracted from the angle at the hip, yielding the degree of version. *(continued)*

relative angle of version

angle of internal rotation

Figure 31.13 *Continued.* **CT determination of the angle of version of the femoral head.**

Figure 31.14 Congenital kyphoscoliosis. Three-dimensional CT reformatted images of the spine of a 4-year-old boy with congenital kyphoscoliosis in frontal (**A**) and lateral (**B**) orientation are effective in global demonstration of spinal deformity.

Figure 31.15 Congenital hemivertebra. Frontal **(A)** and lateral **(B)** views of three-dimensional CT reformatted images of the lumbar spine of a 5-year-old girl with congenital dextroscoliosis reveal a hemivertebra (*arrows*) wedged between L-3 and L-4.

Figure 31.16 Melorheostosis. A 9-year-old boy had a deformity of the left foot since birth, which was diagnosed as a clubfoot. **(A)** Dorsoplantar radiograph of the foot demonstrates the clubfoot deformity, together with sclerotic changes in the phalanges of the great toe, the first and second metatarsals, the first and second cuneiforms, the talus, and the calcaneus. Such changes are typical of melorheostosis, a form of sclerosing dysplasia. **(B)**, **(C)** On bone scan, the extent of skeletal involvement is indicated by increased uptake of radiopharmaceutical not only in the foot but also in the left tibia, which is confirmed on a subsequent radiograph of the left leg **(D)**.

Figure 31.16 **Melorheostosis.** *Continued.*

Figure 31.17 **Ultrasound of congenital hip dysplasia. (A)** Coronal ultrasound of the left hip in a newborn boy shows normal relationship of the femoral head and acetabulum (*FH,* femoral head; *C,* cartilaginous acetabulum; *B,* bony acetabulum; *T,* triradiate cartilage; *g,* gluteus muscle; *IL,* ilium; *S,* superior; *LAT,* lateral; *MED,* medial). **(B)** Coronal ultrasound of the left hip in a newborn girl shows dysplastic acetabulum and laterally subluxated femoral head (Courtesy of Dr. E. Gerscovich, Sacramento, CA).

offers a noninvasive method of examining the infant hip, which might otherwise require arthrography. In addition, ultrasound does not expose the patient to ionizing radiation.

MRI is ideally suited to evaluate congenital and development anomalies of the spine because all structures, including neural components, are shown simultaneously. Because MRI evaluation is mainly an assessment of neuroanatomic development, spin-echo T1-weighted images are usually obtained (Fig. 31.18). However, anomalies affecting the spinal cord and thecal sac are best seen on T2-weighted images because of high contrast of the spinal fluid. These sequences can be quite effective in demonstrating, for example, spinal dysraphism and diastematomyelia (Fig. 31.19).

Figure 31.18 MRI of hypoplasia of the odontoid. (A) Sagittal T1-weighted MR image (SE; TR 800/TE 20 msec) demonstrates a hypoplastic odontoid, which arises from a normal second vertebral body. The anterior arch of the first cervical vertebra is not visualized because of fusion to the occiput. **(B)** Coronal T1-weighted (SE; TR 800/TE 20 msec) MR image confirms that the second cervical vertebral body is normal but only a rudimentary odontoid process has formed. The atlas has fused with the occiput so that there are no occipital condyles (From Beltran J, 1990, with permission).

Figure 31.19 MRI of diastematomyelia. (A) Axial proton density (FSE; TR 5000/TE 16 msec Ef) MR image in a 17-year-old girl with spina bifida and diastematomyelia shows a split spinal cord at the level of T-12. **(B)** Sagittal T2-weighted (FSE; TR 3000/TE 133 msec Ef) MR image shows a low-signal fibous septum within a markedly expanded thecal sac. The spinal fluid exhibits high signal intensity.

PRACTICAL POINTS TO REMEMBER

[1] Congenital anomalies comprise disturbances in bone formation, bone growth, and bone maturation and modeling.

[2] Although most congenital and developmental anomalies can be diagnosed on standard radiographs, the use of ancillary techniques should be considered, such as:
- radionuclide bone scan, particularly in determining the distribution of sites of involvement in various dysplasias
- CT examination, particularly in the evaluation of congenital hip dislocation and determining the angle of version of the femoral head
- 3D CT, particularly in the evaluation of spinal deformities
- Ultrasound, particularly in the evaluation of congenital hip dysplasia
- MRI, particularly in the evaluation of abnormalities of the spine, thecal sac, and spinal cord.

[3] Special projections may be required for the evaluation of anomalies of complex structures such as the ankle and foot.

[4] The results and progress of treatment of various congenital disorders, especially congenital hip dislocation, can best be monitored by ultrasound and CT examinations.

SUGGESTED READINGS

Bailey JA. *Disproportionate short stature: diagnosis and management*. Philadelphia: WB Saunders; 1973.

Barksy AJ. Macrodactyly. *J Bone Joint Surg [Am]* 1967;49A:1255–1266.

Beighton P, Cremin B, Faure C, et al. International nomenclature of constitutional diseases of bone. *Ann Radiol* 1984;27:275.

Beltran J. *MRI: musculoskeletal system*. Philadelphia: JB Lippincott; 1990.

Berkshire SB, Maxwell EN, Sams BF. Bilateral symmetrical pseudoarthrosis in a newborn. *Radiology* 1970;97:389–390.

Boal DKB, Schwenkter EP. The infant hip: assessment with real-time US. *Radiology* 1985;157:667–672.

Brower JS, Wootton-Gorges SL, Costouros JG, Boakes J, Greenspan A. Congenital diplopodia. *Pediatr Radiol* 2003;33:797–799.

Carlson DH. Coalition of the carpal bones. *Skeletal Radiol* 1981;7:125–127.

Cleveland RH, Gilsanz V, Wilkinson RM. Congenital pseudoarthrosis or the radius. *AJR Am J Roentgenol* 1978;130:955–957.

Eich GF, Babyn P, Giedion A. Pediatiric pelvis: radiographic appearance in various congenital disorders. *Radiographics* 1992;12:467–484.

Gerscovich EO. Infant hip in developmental dysplasia: facts to consider for a successful diagnostic ultrasound examination. *Applied Radiol* 1999;28:18–25.

Graf R. New possibilities for the diagnosis of congenital hip joint dislocation by ultrasonography. *J Pediatr Orthop* 1983;3:354–359.

Graham CB. Assessment of bone maturation: methods and pitfalls. *Radiol Clin North Am* 1972;10:185–202.

Grissom LE, Harcke HT. Imaging in developmental dysplasia of the hip. *Imaging* 1992;4:79–85.

Hotston S, Carthy H. Lumbosacral agenesis: a report of three new cases and a review of the literature. *Br J Radiol* 1982;55:629–633.

International nomenclature of constitutional diseases of bone. *AJR Am J Roentgenol* 1978;131:352–354.

Kulik SA, Clanfon TO. Tarsal coalition. *Foot Ankle Int* 1996;17:286–296.

Newman JS, Newberg AH. Congenital tarsal coalition: multimodality evaluation with emphasis on CT and MR imaging. *Radiographics* 2000;20:321–332.

O'Rahilly R, Gardner E, Gray DJ. The skeletal development of the hand. *Clin Orthop* 1959;13:42–50.

Page LK, Post MJD. Spinal dysraphism. In Post MJD, ed. *Computed tomography of the spine*. Baltimore: Williams & Wilkins; 1984.

Reed MH, Genez B. Hands. In: Reed MH, ed. *Pediatric skeletal radiology*. Baltimore: Williams & Wilkins; 1992:584–625.

Rubin P. *Dynamic classification of bone dysplasias*. Chicago: Year Book Medical Publishers; 1972.

Sharma BG. Duplication of the clavicle with triplication of the coracoid process. *Skeletal Radiol* 2003;32:661–664.

Smith CF. Current concepts review—tibia vara (Blount's disease). *J Bone Joint Surg [Br]* 1982;64B:630–632.

Walker HS, Lufkin RB, Dietrich RB, Peacock WJ, Flannigan BD, Kangarloo H. Magnetic resonance of the pediatric spine. *Radiographics* 1987;7:1129–1152.

Wechsler RJ, Karasick D, Schweitzer ME. Computed tomography of talocalcaneal coalition: imaging techniques. *Skeletal Radiol* 1992;21:353–358.

Wechsler RJ, Schweitzer ME, Deely DM, Horn BD, Pizzutillo PD. Tarsal coalition: depiction and characterization with CT and MR imgaing. *Radiology* 1994;193:447–452.

Zaleske DJ. Development of the upper limb. *Hand Clin* 1985;1:383–390.

ANOMALIES OF THE UPPER AND LOWER LIMBS

Anomalies of the Shoulder Girdle and Upper Limbs

Congenital Elevation of the Scapula

Sprengel deformity, as congenital elevation of the scapula is also known, may be unilateral or bilateral. It is marked by the appearance of a scapula that is small, high in position, and rotated with its inferior edge pointing toward the spine—features that are easily identified on an anteroposterior view of the shoulder or chest (Fig. 32.1). The finding of a congenitally elevated scapula is important because of this condition's frequent association with other anomalies, such as scoliosis, rib anomalies, and fusion of the cervical or upper thoracic vertebrae, known as Klippel-Feil syndrome (Fig. 32.2). Furthermore, there is sometimes a bony connection between the elevated scapula and one of the vertebrae (usually the C-5 or C-6 vertebra), creating what is known as the omovertebral bone (Fig. 32.3).

Madelung Deformity

This developmental anomaly of the distal radius and carpus, originally described by the German surgeon Otto Madelung in 1879, usually manifests in adolescent girls presenting with pain in the wrist and decreased range of motion but with no history of previous trauma or infection. Today, the term *Madelung deformity* is often used to describe a variety of conditions in the wrist marked by premature fusion of the distal physis of the radius, with consequent deformity of the distal ulna and wrist. From the etiologic viewpoint, these abnormalities can be divided into posttraumatic deformities, dysplasias, and idiopathic conditions. A genetic cause has also been proposed. Association with mesomelic dwarfism (e.g., dyschondrosteosis) and a mutation on the X chromosome (e.g., Turner syndrome) has also been described. The posttraumatic deformity may occur after repetitive injury or after a single event that disrupts the growth of the distal radius. Among the bone dysplasias associated with Madelung deformity are multiple hereditary cartilaginous exostoses, Ollier disease, achondroplasia, multiple epiphyseal dysplasia, and the mucopolysaccharidoses including Hurler and Morquio syndromes.

On physical examination, the hand is translated volarly to the long axis of the forearm and there is dorsal subluxation of the ulna. A decreased range of motion limits supination, dorsiflexion, and radial deviation, but pronation and palmar flexion are usually preserved.

Figure 32.1 Sprengel deformity. Anteroposterior radiograph of the left shoulder of a 1-year-old boy demonstrates a high position of the left scapula typical of Sprengel deformity.

elevated
scapula

Figure 32.2 Klippel-Feil syndrome and Sprengel deformity. Anteroposterior radiograph of the left shoulder of a 13-year-old boy with Klippel-Feil syndrome shows an elevated scapula *(arrow)*.

Figure 32.3 Klippel-Feil syndrome and Sprengel deformity. Posteroanterior radiograph of the cervical and upper thoracic spine in a 37-year-old woman with Sprengel deformity associated with Klippel-Feil syndrome (fusion of the cervical vertebrae) shows the omovertebral bone connecting the elevated right scapula and the C-5 vertebra.

fused cervical
vertebrae

elevated right
scapula

omovertebral
bone

Table 32.1 **Radiographic Criteria for the Diagnosis of Madelung Deformity**

Changes in the Radius	*Changes in the Ulna*
Double curvature (medial and dorsal)	Dorsal subluxation
Decrease in bone length	Increased density (hypercondensation and distortion) of the ulnar head
Triangular shape of the distal epiphysis	Increase in bone length
Premature fusion of the medial part of the distal physis, associated with medial and volar angulation of the articular surface	*Changes in the Carpus*
	Triangular configuration with the lunate at the apex
Focal radiolucent areas along the medial border of bone	Increase in distance between the distal radius and the ulna
Exostosis at the distal medial border	Decrease in carpal angle

(Modified from Dannenberg M, et al. 1939, with permission.)

The radiographic criteria for the diagnosis of Madelung deformity were proposed by Dannenberg and colleagues (Table 32.1). The posteroanterior and lateral projections of the distal forearm and wrist are sufficient to demonstrate any of the abnormalities associated with this deformity (Fig. 32.4).

Surgical treatment of Madelung deformity is indicated for pain relief and cosmetic improvement. A variety of procedures are available. These include ligament release (Vickers physiolysis), wedge osteotomy, Carter-Ezaki dome osteotomy, and radioscaphocapitate arthrodesis. Occasionally, a Darrach or a Suavé-Kapandji procedure is indicated.

Anomalies of the Pelvic Girdle and Hip

An overview of the most effective radiographic projections and radiologic techniques for evaluating the most common anomalies of the pelvic girdle and hip is presented in Table 32.2.

Congenital Hip Dislocation (Developmental Dysplasia of the Hip)

The hip joint is the most frequent site of congenital dislocations. The condition occurs with an incidence of 1.5 per 1,000 births, and eight-times more often in girls than in boys. In unilateral dislocation, the left hip is involved twice as often as the right, and bilateral dislocation occurs in more than 25% of affected children. More frequently encountered in white than in black persons, the condition is very common in Mediterranean and Scandinavian countries; it is almost unknown in China, which may be explained in part by the Chinese custom of carrying the infant on the mother's back with its hips flexed and abducted.

The criteria for the diagnosis of congenital dislocation of the hip (CDH) include physical and radiographic findings. Certain clinical signs have been identified that are helpful in the evaluation of newborns and infants for possible CDH (Table 32.3).

Figure 32.4 Madelung deformity. (A) Posteroanterior radiograph of the left wrist of a 21-year-old woman shows a decrease in the length of the radius, the distal end of which has assumed a triangular shape. This is associated with a triangular configuration of the carpus, with the lunate at the apex wedged between the radius and ulna. **(B)** Lateral radiograph demonstrates dorsal subluxation of the ulna.

Table 32.2 **Most Effective Radiographic Projections and Radiologic Techniques for Evaluating Common Anomalies of the Pelvic Girdle and Hip**

Projection/Technique	Crucial Abnormalities	Projections/Technique	Crucial Abnormalities
Congenital Hip Dislocation		*Legg-Calvé-Perthes Disease*	

Anteroposterior of pelvis and hips	Determination of:
	  Hilgenreiner Y-line
	  Acetabular index
	  Perkins-Ombredanne line
	  Shenton-Menard line (arc)
	  Center-edge (C-E) angle
	    of Wiberg
	  Ossification center of capital
	    femoral epiphysis
		Anteroposterior and frog-lateral of hips	Osteonecrosis of femoral head as indicated by crescent sign and subchondral collapse
			Gage sign
			Subluxation of femoral head
			Horizontal orientation of growth plate
			Calcifications lateral to epiphysis
			Cystic changes in metaphysis

	Relations of femoral head and acetabulum	Arthrography	Incongruity of hip joint Thickness of articular cartilage
Anteroposterior of hips in abduction and internal rotation	Andrén-von Rosen line	Radionuclide bone scan	Decreased uptake of isotope (earliest stage) Increased uptake of isotope (late stage)

Arthrography	Congruity of the joint
	Status of:
	  Cartilaginous limbus (limbus thorn)
	  Ligamentum teres
	  Zona orbicularis
		Computed tomography and magnetic resonance imaging	Incongruity of hip joint
			Osteonecrosis

		Slipped Capital Femoral Epiphysis	
Computed tomography (alone or with arthrography)	Relations of femoral head and acetabulum Superior, lateral, or posterior subluxation	Anteroposterior of hips	Loss of Capener triangle sign Periarticular osteoporosis Widening and blurring of growth plate Decreased height of femoral epiphysis Absence of intersection of epiphysis by line tangent to lateral cortex of femoral neck Herndon hump Chondrolysis (complication)

Ultrasound	Position of femoral head in acetabulum
	Status of:
	  Acetabular roof
	  Cartilaginous limbus		

Developmental Coxa Vara			
Anteroposterior of pelvis and hips	Varus angle of femoral neck and femoral shaft	Frog-lateral of hips	Absence of intersection of epiphysis by line tangent to lateral cortex of femoral neck Actual slippage (displacement) of femoral epiphysis
Proximal Femoral Focal Deficiency			
Anteroposterior of hip and proximal femur	Shortening of femur Superior, posterior, and lateral displacement of proximal femoral segment	Radionuclide bone scan and magnetic resonance imaging	Osteonecrosis (complication)
Arthrography	Nonossified femoral head		

Table 32.3 **Clinical Manifestations of Congenital Dislocation of the Hip**

Limited abduction of the flexed hip (due to shortening andcontraction of hip adductors)
Increase in depth or asymmetry of the inguinal or thigh skin folds
Shortening of one leg
Allis or Galeazzi sign*—lower position of knee of affected side when knees and hips are flexed (due to location of femoral head posterior to acetabulum in this position)
Ortolani "jerk" sign ("clunk of entry" or reduction sign)
Barlow test ("clunk of exit" or dislocation sign)
Telescoping or pistoning action of thighs* (due to lack of containment of femoral head within acetabulum)
Trendelenburg test*—dropping of normal hip when child, standing on both feet, elevates unaffected limb and bears weight on affected side (due to weakness of hip abductors)
Waddling gait*

* This finding can occur in older children.

Figure 32.5 Congenital hip dysplasia. Anteroposterior radiograph of the pelvis of a 1-year-old boy shows a slightly flattened acetabulum and delayed appearance of the ossification center for the right femoral epiphysis; that of the left epiphysis is normally centered over the triradiate cartilage.

Figure 32.7 Congenital hip dislocation. Anteroposterior radiograph of the pelvis of a 2-year-old boy demonstrates complete superolateral dislocation of the right hip. Note the abnormal position of the center of ossification in relation to the acetabulum compared with the normal left hip.

Radiographic Evaluation

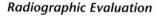Each of the stages of CDH—dysplasia of the hip, subluxation of the hip, and dislocation of the hip—has a characteristic radiographic presentation. The term *congenital hip dysplasia,* first introduced by Hilgenreiner in 1925, refers to delayed or defective development of the hip joint leading to a deranged articular relationship between an abnormal acetabulum and a deformed proximal end of the femur (Fig. 32.5). The condition is considered a precursor of subluxation and dislocation of the hip, although some authorities use the term "developmental dysplasia of the hip" (DDH) to denote all stages of CDH. In *congenital subluxation of the hip,* there is an abnormal relationship between the femoral head and the acetabulum, but the two are in contact (Fig. 32.6). *Congenital dislocation of the hip,* however, is marked by the femoral head's complete loss of contact with the acetabular cartilage; the proximal femur is displaced most often superiorly, but lateral, posterior, and posterolateral dislocation may also be seen (Fig. 32.7).

Measurements

In contrast to an adult hip, the relationship between the femoral head and the acetabulum in a newborn's hip cannot be assessed by direct

Figure 32.6 Congenital hip dysplasia. Anteroposterior radiograph of the pelvis of a 1-year-old girl shows congenital superolateral subluxation of the left hip. Note the slightly smaller size of the left femoral epiphysis.

visualization because the femoral head is not ossified, and as a cartilaginous body it is not visible on standard films. The ossification center first appears between the ages of 3 and 6 months, and a delay in its appearance should be viewed as an indication of congenital hip dysplasia. The neck of the femur must therefore be used for ascertaining this relationship. The anteroposterior view of the pelvis serves as the basis for determining several indirect indicators of the relationship between the femoral head and acetabulum. To obtain accurate measurements, however, proper positioning of the infant is imperative; the lower extremities should be extended in the neutral position and longitudinally aligned, whereas the central ray should be directed toward the midline, slightly above the pubic symphysis, to ensure the symmetry of both halves of the pelvis. The measurements used to evaluate the relation of the femoral head to the acetabulum are the following (Fig. 32.8):

1. The *Hilgenreiner line* or *Y-line,* which is drawn through the superior part of the triradiate cartilage, is itself a valuable indicator of femoroacetabular relations and serves as the basis for all other indicators.
2. The *acetabular index,* which is an angle formed by a line tangent to the acetabular roof and the Y-line, cannot alone be diagnostic of dislocation, because it can occasionally exceed 30 degrees in normal subjects. Generally, however, values greater than 30 degrees are considered abnormal and indicate impending dislocation. Some investigators propose that only angles in excess of 40 degrees are significant.
3. The *Perkins-Ombredanne line,* which is drawn perpendicular to the Y-line through the most lateral edge of the ossified acetabular cartilage, is helpful in determining subluxation and dislocation of the hip. The intersection of this line with the Y-line creates four quadrants; normally, the medial aspect of the femoral neck or the ossified capital femoral epiphysis falls in the lower medial quadrant.
4. The *Shenton-Menard line,* which forms a smooth arc through the medial aspect of the femoral neck and the superior border of the obturator foramen, may be interrupted in subluxation or dislocation of the hip. Even under normal circumstances, however, the arc may not be smooth if the radiograph is obtained with the hip in external rotation and adduction.
5. The *Andrén–von Rosen line,* which is drawn on a radiograph obtained with the hips abducted 45 degrees and internally rotated, describes the relation of the longitudinal axis of the femoral shaft to the acetabulum (Fig. 32.9). In dislocation or subluxation of the hip, this line bisects or falls above the anterosuperior iliac spine.

Figure 32.8 Measurements helpful to evaluate the relation of the femoral head to the acetabulum. (A) The *Hilgenreiner line* or *Y-line* is drawn through the superior part of the triradiate cartilage. In normal infants, the distance represented by a line *(ab)* perpendicular to the Y-line at the most proximal point of the femoral neck should be equal on both sides of the pelvis, as should the distance represented by a line *(bc)* drawn coincident with the Y-line medially to the acetabular floor. In infants aged 6 to 7 months, the mean value for the distance *(ab)* has been determined to be 19.3 ± 1.5 mm; the distance for *(bc)* is 18.2 ± 1.4 mm. The *acetabular index* is an angle formed by a line drawn tangent to the acetabular roof from point *(c)* at the acetabular floor on the Y-line. The normal value of this angle ranges from 25 to 29 degrees. The *Shenton-Menard line* is an arc running through the medial aspect of the femoral neck and the superior border of the obturator foramen. It should be smooth and unbroken. **(B)** The *Perkins-Ombredanne line* is drawn perpendicular to the Y-line through the most lateral edge of the ossified acetabular cartilage, which actually corresponds to the anteroinferior iliac spine. In normal newborns and infants, the medial aspect of the femoral neck or the ossified capital femoral epiphysis falls in the lower inner quadrant. The appearance of either of these structures in the lower outer or upper outer quadrant indicates subluxation or dislocation of the hip.

After the capital femoral epiphysis achieves full ossification at approximately 4 years of age, a diagnosis of gross displacement can usually be made without difficulty. The evaluation of subtle hip dysplasias, however, can be aided by another parameter of the relation of the femoral head to the acetabulum, the *center-edge (C-E) angle of Wiberg* (Fig. 32.10). Determination of this angle is most useful after full ossification of the femoral head, because its relationship to the acetabulum is then fully established.

Arthrography and Computed Tomography

Aside from conventional radiography, hip arthrography is the most useful technique for evaluating CDH. During the procedure, films are routinely obtained with the hip in the neutral (Fig. 32.11A) and frog-lateral positions (Fig. 32.11B), as well as in abduction, adduction, and internal rotation. In subluxation, the femoral head lies lateral to just below the margin of the acetabular cartilaginous labrum, and the joint capsule is usually loose (Fig. 32.12). In complete dislocation, the femoral head lies superior and lateral to the edge of the labrum (Fig. 32.13). Deformities may also be encountered in the cartilaginous limbus, a structure lying between the femoral head and the acetabulum. In advanced stages, it may be inverted and hypertrophied, thus making the reduction impossible. Moreover, the portion of the capsule lying medial to the femoral head is usually constricted to form an isthmus with a "figure-eight" appearance.

Computed tomography (CT), either alone (Fig. 32.14) or with arthrography, is also a frequently used modality in the evaluation of CDH. In subluxation or dislocation, the congruity of the acetabulum and the femoral head, which is normally centered over the triradiate cartilage, is disturbed (Fig. 32.15). CT has proved to be the most accurate technique for determining the degree of subluxation or dislocation. It is also an essential modality for monitoring the progress of CDH treatment.

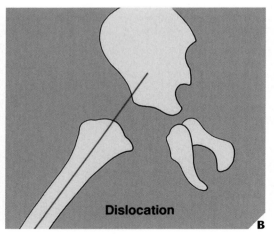

Figure 32.9 The Andrén-von Rosen line. (A) With at least 45 degrees of hip abduction and internal rotation, the line is drawn along the longitudinal axis of the femoral shaft. In normal hips, it intersects the pelvis at the upper edge of the acetabulum. **(B)** In subluxation or dislocation of the hip, the line bisects or falls above the anterosuperior iliac spine.

Age (years)	Lowest Normal Value of C–E Angle
5–8	19°
9–12	12°–25°
13–20	26°–30°

Figure 32.10 Angle of Wiberg. The center-edge (C-E) angle of Wiberg is helpful in evaluating the development of the acetabulum and its relation to the femoral head. A baseline is projected, connecting the centers of the femoral heads. The C-E angle is formed by two lines originating in the center of the femoral head, one drawn perpendicular to the baseline into the acetabulum, and the other connecting the center of the femoral head with the superior acetabular lip. Values below the lowest normal value given for each age group indicate hip dysplasia.

Ultrasound

In recent years, ultrasound has become one of the most effective techniques to diagnose and evaluate congenital hip dysplasia. It is performed with the patient at rest, and during motion and stress. A lateral approach is widely used, with the infant supine or in the lateral decubitus position. Scanning is performed in the coronal plane with the hips extended or flexed (see Fig. 31.17). In the axial plane, the thighs are in 90 degrees of flexion, and images are obtained with and without stress. The bony and cartilaginous components of the hip joint are well demonstrated on the displayed images, and acetabular coverage of the femoral head can be assessed. In addition, the slope of the acetabulum α-angle) can be measured with respect to the iliac line. An angle of 60 degrees or more is normal. An angle 50 to 60 degrees is considered physiologic before age 3 months, but needs to be followed-up by repeat studies. Values less than 50 degrees are abnormal at any age. A second angle (β-angle) is formed by the iliac line and a line drawn from the labrum to the transition point between the iliac bone and the bony acetabulum. This measurement is indicative of the acetabular cartilaginous roof coverage and is secondary in significance to the α-angle. The smaller the β-angle, the less the cartilaginous coverage because of a better acetabular bony containment of the femoral head. The dynamic study, first described by Harcke in 1984, incorporates the use of real-time ultrasound visualization of the hip joint. The purpose of this

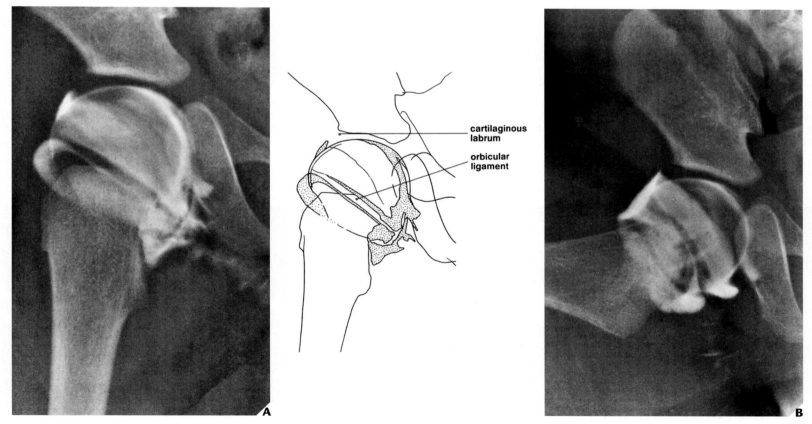

cartilaginous labrum

orbicular ligament

Figure 32.11 Normal hip arthrogram. (A) Arthrogram of the right hip in the neural position in a 5-month-old boy shows contrast medium accumulating in the large recesses medial and lateral to the constriction produced by the orbicular ligament. Note the smoothness and even thickness of the cartilage covering the femoral head. **(B)** On the frog-lateral view, contrast medium is seen outlining the edge of the cartilaginous labrum. The ligamentum teres can be seen medial to the femoral head, extending from the inferior portion of the acetabulum.

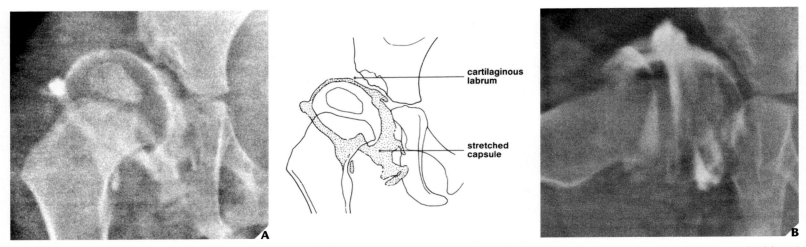

Figure 32.12 Arthrogram of congenital hip dysplasia. (A) Arthrogram of the right hip in the neutral position in a 1-year-old girl with congenital subluxation of the hip shows the typical displacement of the hip lateral to butt below the acetabular labrum. There is accumulation of contrast agent in the stretched capsule, and the ligamentum teres is elongated. **(B)** In the frog-lateral position, the head moves more deeply into the acetabulum, but subluxation is still present.

Figure 32.13 Arthrogram of congenital hip dislocation. (A) Anteroposterior radiograph of the right hip in an 8-year-old girl demonstrates complete superolateral dislocation of the femoral head. Note the shallow acetabulum. **(B)** Arthrogram of the hip shows a deformed cartilaginous limbus and stretching of the ligamentum teres. The femoral head lies superior and lateral to the edge of the cartilaginous labrum. Note the accumulation of contrast agent in the loose joint capsule.

Figure 32.14 Normal CT of the hips. Axial section of both hips in a 19-month-old infant shows good congruity of the acetabula and femoral heads, which are centered over the triradiate cartilage.

Figure 32.15 CT of congenital hip dislocation. Axial section through the proximal femora and hips of a 6-month-old boy shows posterolateral dislocation of the left hip. The right hip is normal.

technique is to demonstrate the instability. It is performed in the transverse flexion projection and consists of a Barlow maneuver to try to displace, sublux, or dislocate an apparently well-seated femoral head.

Recently, three-dimensional (3D) sonographic evaluation of developmental dysplasia of the hip has been attempted. This technique permits evaluation of the bony and fibrocartilaginous acetabulum and its relationship to the femoral head in a global fashion (*gestalt*) without the need for detailed acetabular angle measurements. The information obtained can be stored for later review, analysis, and additional reconstructions with different parameters. The computer-generated sagittal-plane image offers a unique view of the hip that is unobtainable with conventional sonography (Fig. 32.16). The generated spa-

Figure 32.16 Ultrasound of congenital hip dysplasia. (A) On the coronal 3D ultrasound image of the left hip in a 3-day-old girl (lower left) the acetabulum (*A*) appears shallow, and subluxation of the femoral head can be observed at the intersection of the ilium (*I*) line with the medial third of lthe femoral head (*FH*). On the reconstructed axial image *(upper left)*, the femoral head is subluxated but still in contact with the acetabulum. On the sagittal image *(upper right)*, only the peripheral segment of femoral head is visualized. **(B)** A sagittal image of a normal left hip *(left)* is shown for comparison. Note that femoral head (*FH*) is centered over the ilium line (*I*). A sagittal image of a subluxated head *(right)* clearly shows distortion of femoral head–ilium line relationship. (From Gerscovich EO, et al., 1994, with permission.)

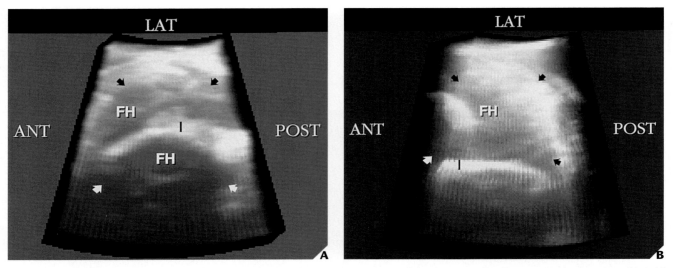

Figure 32.17 Three-dimensional ultrasound of congenital hip dysplasia. (A) Craniocaudal projection (bird's-eye view) of a normal left hip shows the ilium (*I*) projecting over the midportion of the femoral head (*FH*) (*arrows* outline its contour). **(B)** Craniocaudal projection of a subluxated left hip shows that the ilium (*I*) projects over the medial portion of the femoral head (*FH*) (*arrows* outline its contour). The femoral head is laterally displaced. (From Gerscovich EO, et al., 1994, with permission.)

Figure 32.18 Treatment of congenital hip dysplasia. (A) Anteroposterior radiograph of the pelvis in a 1-year-old boy demonstrates the typical appearance of congenital dislocation of the left hip. **(B)** After conservative treatment with a Pavlik harness at age 2, there is still subluxation. Note the broken Shenton-Menard arc. At age 3, after further conservative treatment by skin traction and application of a spica cast, there is almost complete reduction of subluxation, as demonstrated by contrast arthrography **(C)**. **(D)** CT scan, however, demonstrates some minimal residual lateral displacement of the femoral head, as evidenced by the medial accumulation of contrast.

tial-revolving image likewise yields an informative craniocaudal (bird's eye) view of the infant hip (Fig. 32.17). The 3D appearance of the revolving image is enhanced by the transparency of the reconstruction, in contrast to the contour reconstructions available with 3D CT.

Classification

Dunn has proposed a classification of CDH based primarily on the shape of the acetabular margins, the gross contour of the femoral head, and whether there is eversion or inversion of the limbus:

Type I   This is usually seen in neonates. The changes along the acetabular margins are mild. The femoral head, which is anteverted but spherically normal, is not completely covered by acetabular cartilage. This may lead to variable instability, particularly in extension and adduction of the hip. The labrum may also be deformed.

Type II   The hips are subluxed, and the cartilaginous labrum shows eversion. The femoral head is normally anteverted but shows a loss of sphericity. The acetabulum is shallower than in type I, and the failure of the acetabular roof to ossify laterally leads to an increased acetabular angle.

Type III   There is significant deformity of the acetabulum and femoral head, which is posterosuperiorly dislocated, leading to the formation of a false acetabulum by eversion of the labrum. The limbus is hypertrophied, and the ligamentum teres is elongated and pulled, bringing with it the transverse acetabular ligament. This situation compromises the acetabular space, precluding complete reduction.

Treatment

The principle behind conservative treatment is to reduce the dislocation of the femoral head, by means of a flexion-abduction maneuver, for a period sufficient enough to permit proper growth of the head and acetabulum, which in turn ensures a congruent and stable hip joint. This approach is usually taken in the very early stages of CDH and in infants younger than age 2 years; it includes splinting, such as with the Frejka splint or Pavlik harness, as well as various traction procedures (Fig. 32.18). Colonna or buck skin traction is usually used in children 2 months to 12 years of age, with a well-padded spica cast applied simultaneously to the unaffected side. Interval radiographs are obtained to monitor the progress of the traction and the descent of the femoral head. A system for this purpose, composed of various traction "stations," has been described by Gage and Winter (Fig. 32.19). It

has been reported that the achievement of "station +2" by means of skeletal traction, before further treatment by open or closed reduction, is associated with a far smaller frequency of osteonecrosis of the femoral head.

When the conservative approach fails, the child is too old for conservative treatment, or the abnormalities are too extensive, then surgical management is indicated. Radiologic assessment of the hip, in which CT examination plays the leading role, is mandatory before surgical intervention because it provides the surgeon with excellent images of the anatomy of the hip, particularly the size of the femoral head, its relation to the acetabulum, and the acetabular configuration. The information regarding these structures may contraindicate the use of certain surgical procedures.

Several surgical techniques are now used for treatment of congenital hip dysplasia. Their common goal is to achieve better coverage of the femoral head. These surgical procedures can be divided into four categories: shelf operations, in which bone grafts are used to extend the acetabular roof; acetabuloplasties, in which the acetabular roof is mobilized and turned down; pelvic osteotomies, in which the acetabulum is redirected; and pelvic displacement osteotomies, in which the femoral head is positioned beneath the displaced bony portion of the pelvis. *Capsulorrhaphy* consists of removal of the excess of the stretched joint capsule, combined with a femoroplasty and/or acetabuloplasty. *Femoral varus derotational osteotomy* is performed to correct an excessive anteversion of the neck and valgus deformity. It involves a varus angulation of the proximal femur, with or without rotation, to redirect the femoral head into the acetabulum. The most popular procedure is the *Salter osteotomy* of the innominate bone, which may be combined with simultaneous derotational varus osteotomy of the femoral neck. It is usually performed in children aged 1 to 6 years. The principle of this technique is to redirect the abnormal orientation of the acetabulum, which in children with CDH faces more anterolaterally, thus rendering the hip stable only in abduction, flexion, and internal rotation. This redirection is accomplished by displacing the entire acetabulum anterolaterally and downward, without changing its shape or capacity, by means of a triangular bone graft (Fig. 32.20). *Pemberton osteotomy* is an incomplete transiliac osteotomy, hinging the anterolateral acetabular roof on the flexible triradiate cartilage. This procedure is indicated when there is an elongated, dysplastic acetabulum; however, it should be performed only in children younger than age 7 years when there is flexibility in the triradiate cartilage and when growth remains for remodeling of the joint surfaces. *Steele triple innominate osteotomy* is usu-

Station	Position
− 1	medial aspect of femoral metaphysis above Hilgenreiner line
0	metaphysis between Hilgenreiner line and the normal position relative to the contralateral femur
+ 1	metaphysis directly opposite that of contralateral, normal hip
+ 2	metaphysis distal to that of normal hip

Hilgenreiner line

line denoting normal position of contralateral femur

Figure 32.19 The Gage and Winter system. This measurement of stations for monitoring the progress of treatment by traction and the descent of the femoral head is based on the position of the proximal femoral metaphysis relative to the ipsilateral acetabulum and the contralateral normal hip.

Figure 32.20 Salter osteotomy. (A) Anteroposterior radiograph of the pelvis in a 7-year-old girl with CDH shows persistent superolateral subluxation of the left hip following conservative treatment. Note the anterolateral orientation of the acetabulum in comparison with the normal right hip. **(B)** Postoperative film after Salter osteotomy through the supra-acetabular portion of the iliac bone shows the acetabulum displaced anterolaterally and downward; a triangular bone graft, taken from the anterolateral aspect of the ilium, is secured by two Steinmann pins at the site of the osteotomy. **(C)** Four years later, the femoral head is completely covered by the acetabulum. Because of a valgus configuration of the femoral neck, the patient may yet require a varus derotational osteotomy.

ally indicated for children older than age 6 to 8 years who have an immobile symphysis pubis. In addition to Salter osteotomy, osteotomies of the inferior and superior pubic rami are performed. The acetabulum is brought forward and rotated in the frontal plane, avoiding external rotation. The *Chiari pelvic osteotomy* is usually reserved for older children. This is a displacement osteotomy that essentially provides a shelf or buttress to limit further proximal subluxation of the femoral head. This procedure displaces the femoral head medially and increases the weight-bearing surface of the head by producing an overhanging superior acetabular ledge. This technique may also be combined with a varus derotational osteotomy of the femoral neck. *Ganz osteotomy*, also known as *Bernese periacetabular osteotomy*, is usually performed in older children and adolescents, and occasionally in adults. The principle behind the procedure is to allow anterior and lateral rotation and medialization of the hip without violation of the posterior column of the hemipelvis. Osteotomies are performed around the acetabulum (complete osteotomy of the pubis and biplanar osteotomy of the ilium); however, the cut through the posterior column of the ischium is incomplete. The acetabular fragment is ro-

tated anteriorly and laterally (maintaining anteversion) and is then medialized. This procedure provides excellent femoral head coverage and acetabular mobility.

Complications

Conservative and surgical management of CDH may be complicated by osteonecrosis of the femoral head, redislocation, infection, sciatic nerve injury, or early fusion of the growth plate caused by prolonged casting. The most frequent late complication of untreated and treated CDH is degenerative joint disease.

Proximal Femoral Focal Deficiency

Proximal femoral focal deficiency (PFFD) is a congenital anomaly characterized by dysgenesis and hypoplasia of variable segments of the proximal femur. The defect ranges in severity from femoral shortening associated with a varus deformity of the neck to the formation of only a small stub of distal femur.

Classification and Radiographic Evaluation

Several classifications of PFFD have been proposed. The one offered by Levinson and colleagues, which is based on the severity of the abnormalities involving the femoral head, femoral segment, and acetabulum, is the most practical from the prognostic point of view:

Type A The femoral head is present, and the femoral segment is short. There is a varus deformity of the femoral neck. The acetabulum is normal.

Type B The femoral head is present, but there is an absence of bony connection between it and the short femoral segment. The acetabulum exhibits dysplastic changes.

Type C The femoral head is absent or represented only by an ossicle. The femoral segment is short and tapered proximally. The acetabulum is severely dysplastic.

Type D The femoral head and acetabulum are absent. The femoral segment is rudimentary, and the obturator foramen is enlarged.

Conventional radiography is usually sufficient to make a diagnosis of proximal femoral focal deficiency. The femur is short, and the proximal segment is displaced superior, posterior, and lateral to the iliac crest; ossification of the femoral epiphysis is invariably delayed (Fig. 32.21). Arthrography is useful in the evaluation of this anomaly, particularly in its classification, because early in infancy the nonossified femoral head and acetabulum can be outlined adequately with a positive contrast agent (Fig. 32.21C). This technique is also helpful in distinguishing proximal femoral focal deficiency from the occasionally similar presentations of congenital dislocation of the hip.

Treatment

Several surgical procedures are used to correct this anomaly, including amputation. One limb-sparing procedure involves conversion of the knee to a hip joint by flexing it 90 degrees and fusing the femur to the pelvis. Another technique, developed by Borggreve in 1930 and called the "turn-about" procedure or "rotation-plasty" after an improvement by Van Nes, converts the foot into the knee joint; the limb is then fitted with a leg prosthesis.

Legg-Calvé-Perthes Disease

Legg-Calvé-Perthes disease, also known as coxa plana, is the name applied to osteonecrosis (ischemic necrosis) of the proximal epiphysis of

Figure 32.21 Proximal femoral focal deficiency. (A) Anteroposterior radiograph in an 18-month-old boy who had a short right leg demonstrates a varus configuration at the right hip joint, the absence of an ossification center for the proximal femoral epiphysis, and shortening of the femur—the classic radiographic features of proximal femoral focal deficiency. **(B)** A coned-down view of the right hip shows superior, posterior, and lateral displacement of the proximal femoral segment in relation to the acetabulum. **(C)** Arthrography was performed to classify the abnormality, and the presence of the femoral head in the acetabulum and the absence of any defect in the femoral neck was found, making this a type A focal deficiency.

Figure 32.22 Legg-Calvé-Perthes disease. A 5-year-old boy presented with pain in the right hip for several months. **(A)** Anteroposterior radiograph of the pelvis and hips shows advanced Legg-Calvé-Perthes disease affecting the right hip, where osteonecrosis and collapse of the capital femoral epiphysis are apparent, as are extensive changes in the metaphysis. Note the lateral subluxation in the hip joint. The left hip is normal. **(B)** Three years later, the left hip also became involved. Note the progression of osteonecrotic changes in the right femoral epiphysis.

Radiologic Evaluation

Radiologic examination is essential for diagnosing Legg-Calvé-Perthes disease and for identifying its prognostic signs. Conventional radiography is adequate for evaluating most of the features of the disease (Fig. 32.22), whereas arthrography helps in the assessment of acetabular congruity, the thickness of the articular cartilage, and the degree of subluxation (Fig. 32.23). The earliest indication of Legg-Calvé-Perthes disease is demonstrated on radionuclide bone scan by a decreased uptake of tracer in the hips caused by a deficient blood sup-

ply. However, with progression of the disease, an increased uptake is seen, which reflects reparative processes.

The earliest radiographic sign of Legg-Calvé-Perthes disease is periarticular osteoporosis and periarticular soft-tissue swelling, with distortion of the pericapsular and iliopsoas fat planes. There may also be a discrepancy in the size of the ossification centers of the capital epiphyses. Later, lateral displacement of the affected ossification center produces widening of the medial aspect of the joint; the presence of the crescent sign (which at times may be detected only on the frog-lateral projection of the hip) (Fig. 32.24), or of radiolucent fissures in the epiphysis, indicates progression of the disease. At a more advanced stage, flattening and sclerosis of the capital epiphysis become apparent and are associated with an increased density of the femoral head secondary to necrosis of the bone, microfractures, and reparative changes known as "creeping substitution." A vacuum phenomenon may occasionally be seen, caused by nitrogen gas released into the fissures in the capital epiphysis. Cystic changes may also be en-

the femur. It occurs five times more often in boys than in girls, usually between the ages of 4 and 8 years. Its appearance at an early age is usually associated with a better prognosis. Either hip can be affected, and bilateral involvement, which is successive rather than simultaneous, is seen in approximately 10% of cases (Fig. 32.22). The clinical symptoms consist of pain, limping, and limitation of motion. Not infrequently, the pain is localized not to the involved hip but to the ipsilateral knee. It is a self-limiting disorder that eventually heals, but because of the progressive deformity it produces in the shape of the femoral head and neck, it often leads to precocious osteoarthritis of the hip joint. The cause of this anomaly has been the subject of debate. Some investigators consider it a type of idiopathic osteonecrosis, but trauma or repeated microtrauma may play a role in compromising the circulation of blood to the femoral capital epiphysis. Trueta has suggested that the blood supply to the femoral head is deficient between the ages of 4 and 8 years, and that this might be a factor in the development of the condition.

Figure 32.23 Arthrogram of Legg-Calvé-Perthes disease. A 6-year-old boy presented with progressive pain in the right hip joint and a limp for the previous 8 months. **(A)** Anteroposterior radiograph shows a dense, flattened, and deformed femoral epiphysis, with subchondral collapse and fragmentation, diffuse metaphyseal changes, broadening of the femoral neck, and lateral subluxation—all characteristic features of Legg-Calvé-Perthes disease. **(B)** Contrast arthrogram demonstrates flattening of the articular cartilage at the lateral aspect of the femoral head and a relatively smooth contour of the cartilage at the anteromedial aspect. The pulling of the contrast medially indicates lateral subluxation.

Figure 32.24 Legg-Calvé-Perthes disease. Frog-lateral view of the right hip of a 7-year-old girl shows the crescent sign, one of the earliest radiographic features of osteonecrosis.

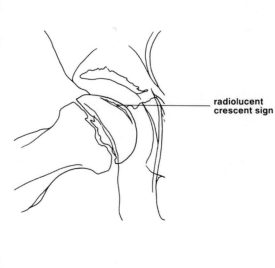

radiolucent crescent sign

countered in the metaphyseal segment. Later, there may be broadening of the femoral neck. Throughout the course of the disease, the joint space is remarkably well preserved because the articular cartilage is not affected. Only in the end stage of Legg-Calvé-Perthes disease, when secondary osteoarthritis develops, does the joint become compromised as in primary degenerative joint disease.

The Moss technique is used to determine the degree of deformity of the femoral head. This consists of overlaying the anteroposterior radiograph of the hip with a template having concentric circles spaced 2 mm apart. If the concentricity of the femoral head deviates by more than two of the 2-mm circles, then the result is rated "poor"; deviation equal to one 2-mm circle is "fair," and no deviation is rated "good." Lateral subluxation can be measured by means of the center-edge angle of Wiberg (Fig. 32.12). It must be stressed that both measurements do not correlate well with development of secondary osteoarthritis, the main complication of Legg-Calvé-Perthes disease.

Several investigators have recently stressed the applicability of MRI for early detection of Legg-Calvé-Perthes disease and for evaluation of cartilaginous and synovial changes. This technique has also proved valuable for determination of the cartilaginous shape of the femoral head. MRI allows preoperative and postoperative assessment of containment of the femoral head and enables its medial aspect to be visualized. The advantages of MRI over arthrography are noninvasiveness, the ability to obtain images in several imaging planes (i.e., axial, coronal, and sagittal), and lack of exposure to the side effects of radiation and injection of intraarticular contrast.

Classification

Several classification systems and prognostic indicators have been developed for the evaluation of Legg-Calvé-Perthes disease. Walderström proposed a three-stage system based on the progression of the osteonecrotic process. The first stage is marked by changes in the blood supply to the femoral epiphysis, with secondary alteration in the shape and density of the femoral head. In the second stage, revascularization takes place, and necrotic bone is replaced by new bone (creeping substitution). The third stage represents a healing phase of the disease in which reconstruction of the femoral epiphysis may result either in congruency of the joint or in incongruency because of deformity of the femoral head (coxa magna), with a predisposition to degenerative changes.

The Catterall classification, which has better prognostic value, divides this anomaly into four groups based on radiographic findings:

Group 1   The anterior portion of the epiphysis is involved; there is no evidence of subarticular collapse or fragmentation of the femoral head. The prognosis is good, and patients do well even without treatment, particularly those younger than age 8 years.

Group 2   The anterior portion of the epiphysis is more severely affected, but the medial and lateral segments are still preserved. Small cystic changes may be seen in the metaphysis (Fig. 32.25). The prognosis is worse than that of patients in group 1, but healing may occur, particularly in children younger than 5 years.

Group 3   The entire epiphysis appears dense, yielding a "head-within-a-head" phenomenon. The changes are more generalized, and the neck becomes widened. The prognosis is poor, and more than 70% of patients require surgical intervention.

Group 4   There is marked flattening and "mushrooming" of the femoral head, eventually leading to its complete collapse; the metaphyseal changes are extensive (Fig. 32.26). The prognosis is much worse than in the previous groups.

Figure 32.25 Legg-Calvé-Perthes disease. Anteroposterior radiograph of the right hip of a 9-year-old boy demonstrates a more advanced stage of disease (Catterall group 2). Note the central defect in the femoral head, with preservation of the lateral and medial buttresses.

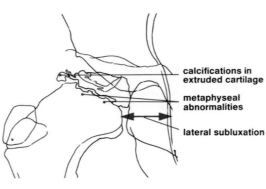

calcifications in
extruded cartilage

metaphyseal
abnormalities

lateral subluxation

Figure 32.26 Legg-Calvé-Perthes disease. Anteroposterior film of the right hip of an 8-year-old girl with advanced disease (Catterall group 4) shows increased density and fragmentation of the entire femoral head. "Head-at-risk" signs are apparent in the metaphyseal changes and the lateral subluxation. Calcifications lateral to the epiphysis represent extruded cartilage and indicate pressure on the head from the lateral edge of the acetabulum.

Subsequently, Catterall improved this classification by introducing four "head-at-risk" signs that signify a poor prognosis; these features can be demonstrated on an anteroposterior projection of the hip joint:

1. Gage sign—a radiolucent, V-shaped osteoporotic segment in the lateral portion of the femoral head (Fig. 32.27)
2. Calcification lateral to the epiphysis, representing extruded cartilage and indicating pressure on the head from the lateral edge of the acetabulum (see Fig. 32.26)
3. Lateral subluxation of the femoral head (see Fig. 32.26)
4. Horizontal inclination of the growth plate, indicating physeal growth closure (see Fig. 32.22B).
5. Recently, Murphy and Marsh added a fifth sign to this group of indicators—diffuse metaphyseal changes (see Fig. 32.23A).

Patients in any of the four groups who have two or more "head-at-risk" signs have a significantly worsened prognosis. Moreover, the prognosis is poor when the disease is in a late stage at the time of diagnosis and when the patient is older than age 6 years.

Differential Diagnosis

The differential diagnosis of this condition should include other causes of osteonecrosis and fragmentation of the femoral head, which may be seen, for example, in hypothyroidism, Gaucher disease, and sickle-cell anemia.

Treatment

The treatment of Legg-Calvé-Perthes disease is individualized on the basis of the clinical and radiographic findings, including the age of onset, the range of motion in the hip joint, the extent of femoral head involvement, and the presence or absence of femoral deformity and lateral subluxation. Although some authorities have suggested eliminating weight-bearing to prevent deformity of the femoral head, prevention requires measures that maintain the femoral head within the acetabulum (containment), thereby preventing extrusion and subluxation, as well as obtaining a full range of motion in the hip joint. In this respect, Salter advocates full weight-bearing together with containment methods of treatment. To minimize synovitis and its sequelae of pain and stiffness, a combination of nonweight-bearing, traction, treatment with nonsteroidal antiinflammatory agents, and gentle range-of-motion exercises is used to enhance molding of the femoral head by the acetabulum. The surgical treatment consists of femoral (varus derotational) or pelvic (innominate bone) osteotomy, aimed at covering the femoral head with the acetabulum.

Slipped Capital Femoral Epiphysis

Slipped capital femoral epiphysis (SCFE) is a disorder of adolescence in which the femoral head gradually slips posteriorly, medially, and inferiorly with respect to the neck. Boys are affected more often than girls are, and children of both sexes with this disorder are often overweight. In boys, the left hip is involved twice as often as the right, whereas in girls both hips are affected with equal frequency. Bilateral involvement occurs in 20% to 40% of patients.

Although the specific cause of SCFE is obscure, its onset, which is usually insidious and without a history of trauma, commonly coincides with the growth spurt at puberty. Studies by Harris have suggested that an imbalance between growth hormone and sex hormones weaken the growth plate, rendering it more vulnerable to the shearing forces of weight bearing and injury.

Regardless of its cause, SCFE represents a Salter-Harris type I fracture (see Fig. 4.28) through the growth plate of the proximal femur.

Figure 32.27 Legg-Calvé-Perthes disease. A V-shaped radiolucent defect in the lateral aspect of the physis (Gage sign), indicating a "head-at-risk," is demonstrated in this 7-year-old girl.

This comes about through posterior, medial, and inferior displacement of the capital epiphysis, resulting in a varus deformity in the hip joint and external rotation and adduction of the femur. Pain in the hip, or occasionally the knee, is often the presenting symptom of this condition, and physical examination may reveal shortening of the involved extremity and limitation of abduction, flexion, and internal rotation in the hip joint.

Radiologic Evaluation

The radiographic abnormalities that may be seen in SCFE depend on the degree of displacement of the capital epiphysis. The anteroposterior radiograph of the hip, supplemented by a frog-lateral view, is usually sufficient to make a correct diagnosis. Several diagnostic indicators of SCFE have been identified on the anteroposterior projection of the hip (Fig. 32.28). The triangle sign of Capener may be of value in recognizing early SCFE. On a plain film of the normal adolescent hip, an intracapsular area at the medial aspect of the femoral neck is seen overlapping the posterior wall of the acetabulum, creating a dense triangular shadow; in most cases of SCFE, this triangle is lost (Fig. 32.29). In a later stage, periarticular osteoporosis becomes apparent, as do widening and blurring of the physis and a decrease in height of the epiphysis (see Fig. 32.29). Moreover, as the disease progresses, slippage of the capital epiphysis can be identified by the absence of an intersection of the epiphysis with a line

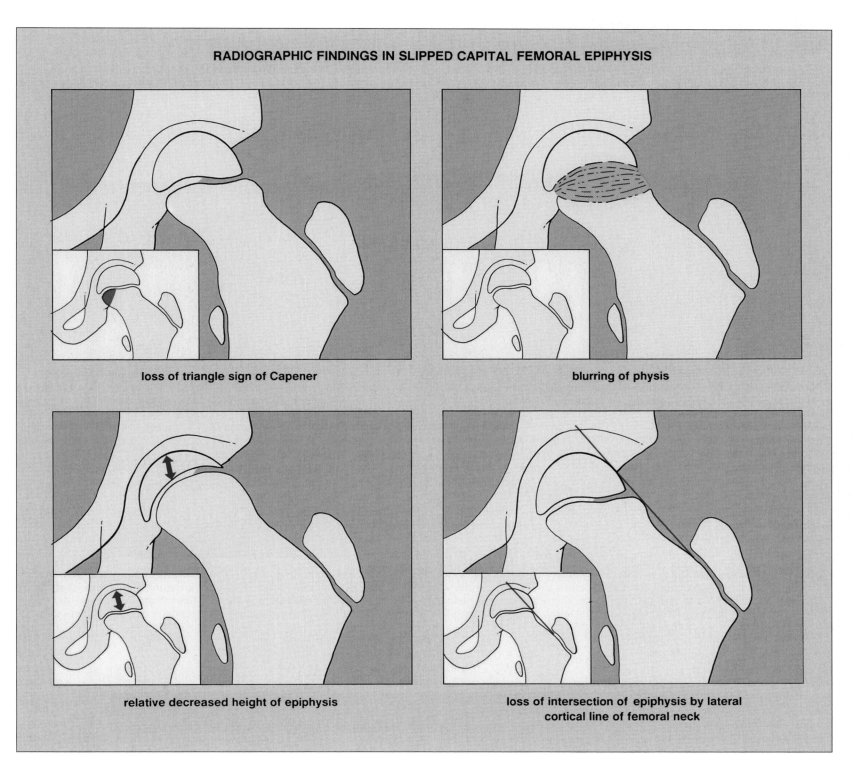

RADIOGRAPHIC FINDINGS IN SLIPPED CAPITAL FEMORAL EPIPHYSIS

loss of triangle sign of Capener

blurring of physis

relative decreased height of epiphysis

loss of intersection of epiphysis by lateral cortical line of femoral neck

Figure 32.28 Slipped capital femoral epiphysis. Various radiographic findings have been identified as diagnostic clues to slipped capital femoral epiphysis. The insets show the normal appearance.

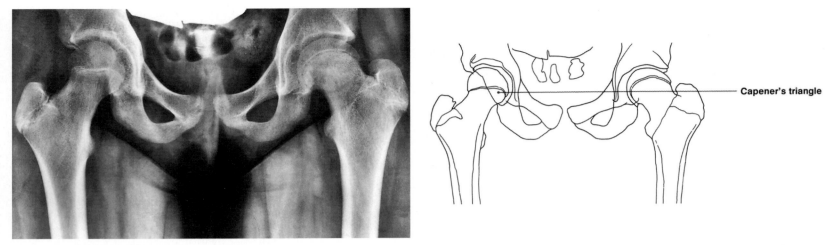

Figure 32.29 Slipped capital femoral epiphysis. Anteroposterior radiograph of the hips of a 12-year-old girl shows the absence of a triangular density in the area of overlap of the medial segment of the femoral metaphysis with the posterior wall of the acetabulum (Capener sign). The triangle is clearly seen in the normal right hip.

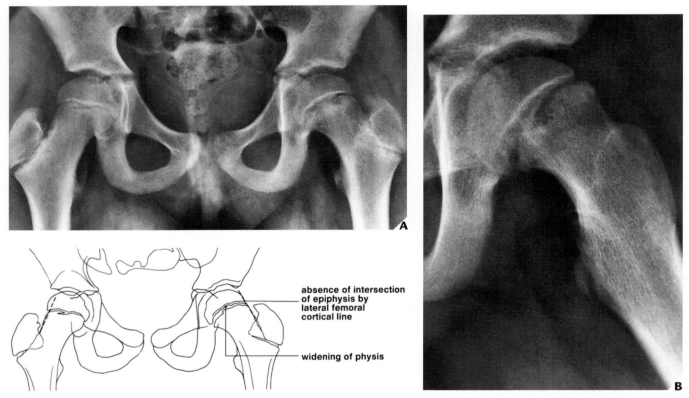

Figure 32.30 Slipped capital femoral epiphysis. A 9-year-old girl presented with pain in the left hip and knee for 4 months. On physical examination, there was slight limitation of abduction and internal rotation in the hip joint. **(A)** Anteroposterior radiograph of the pelvis demonstrates a minimal degree of periarticular osteoporosis of the left hip, widening of the growth plate, and a slight decrease in the height of the epiphysis. Note the lack of intersection of the epiphysis by the lateral cortical line of the femoral neck. **(B)** Frog-lateral view of the left hip shows posteromedial slippage of capital epiphysis.

Herndon's hump

Figure 32.31 Slipped capital femoral epiphysis. (A) A 14-year-old boy with a 14-month history of chronic pain in the left hip was examined by a pediatrician because of significant foreshortening of the left leg and a limp. Frog-lateral view of the left hip shows changes typical of chronic slipped capital femoral epiphysis. There is a moderate degree of osteoporosis and a remodeling deformity of the femoral neck, known as a Herndon hump. **(B)** Anteroposterior radiograph of the right hip of a 20-year-old man who had a slipped capital femoral epiphysis treated with pins demonstrates a Herndon hump *(open arrow)* and secondary osteoarthritis.

drawn tangent to the lateral cortex of the femoral neck (Fig. 32.30). The frog-lateral projection of the hip reveals slippage more readily (Fig. 32.30B), and comparison radiographs of the opposite side are helpful. Chronic stages of this disorder exhibit reactive bone formation along the superolateral aspect of the femoral neck, along with remodeling; this creates a protuberance and broadening of the femoral neck, which gives it a "pistol-grip" appearance known as a Herndon hump (Fig. 32.31). At times, SCFE occurs as a result of acute trauma, in which case it is known as a transepiphyseal fracture (Fig. 32.32).

Occasionally, SCFE is evaluated with MRI. This technique, in addition to findings revealed by radiography, may show a bone marrow edema of the affected femur (Fig. 32.33).

Treatment and Complications

SCFE is treated surgically by closed or open reduction of the slippage and internal fixation using various types of nails, wires, and pins to prevent further slippage and to induce closure of the physis. One of

the complications of treatment is inadvertent penetration of the articular cartilage of the femoral head by a Knowles pin during placement. Lehman and colleagues have introduced a cannulated pin that prevents this complication by allowing contrast medium to be injected during surgery to determine proper placement of the pin in the femoral head on fluoroscopy. Other complications may be encountered that are not necessarily related to surgical treatment. Chondrolysis is observed in approximately 30% to 35% of patients with SCFE and is much more common in black patients than in white. It usually occurs within 1 year of the slippage and may be evident by gradual narrowing of the joint space (Fig. 32.34). Osteonecrosis secondary to the precarious blood supply to the femoral head and the vulnerability of the epiphyseal vessels has been reported in approximately 25% of patients with SCFE (Fig. 32.35). Secondary osteoarthritis may also occur, and it can be recognized by a typical narrowing of the joint space, subchondral sclerosis, and marginal osteophyte formation (Fig. 32.36; see also Fig. 32.31B). A severe varus deformity of the femoral neck, known as coxa vara, may also be encountered.

Figure 32.32 Slipped capital femoral epiphysis. Anteroposterior radiograph of the left hip of a 13-year-old boy who was thrown from a car in an automobile accident shows acute slippage of the femoral epiphysis. This injury represents a Salter-Harris type I fracture through the growth plate.

Figure 32.33 MRI of slipped capital femoral epiphysis. (A) Coronal T1-weighted MRI of the hips in a 14-year-old boy shows slipped femoral epiphysis on the left side (*arrow*). The right hip is normal. **(B)** Coronal T2-weighted fat-suppressed image reveals joint effusion (*arrows*) and marrow edema in the metaphysis (*open arrow*).

Figure 32.34 Complication of slipped capital femoral epiphysis. Anteroposterior radiograph of the left hip of a 13-year-old girl who 1 year earlier had been treated for slipped capital femoral epiphysis shows narrowing of the joint secondary to chondrolysis, a complication of this condition.

Figure 31.35 Complication of slipped capital femoral epiphysis. A 12-year-old boy with a slipped left capital femoral epiphysis was treated by the insertion of three Knowles pins into the femoral head **(A)**. Six months later, a repeat film **(B)** shows minimal flattening of the weight-bearing segment of the femoral epiphysis, an early sign suggesting osteonecrosis. The pins were removed. **(C)** On a film obtained 1 year later, there is an increase in density of the femoral head together with fragmentation of the epiphysis and subchondral collapse, features of advanced osteonecrosis.

Anomalies of the Lower Limbs

An overview of the most effective radiographic projections and radiologic techniques for evaluating common anomalies of the lower limb and foot is presented in Table 32.4.

Congenital Tibia Vara

Congenital tibia vara, or Blount disease, as this developmental anomaly is also known, predominantly affects the medial portion of the proximal tibial growth plate, as well as the medial segments of the tibial metaphysis and epiphysis, resulting in a varus deformity at the knee joint. The cause of this disorder is unknown. Bateson has demonstrated convincingly that Blount disease and physiologic bowleg deformity are part of the same condition, which is influenced by early weight-bearing and racial factors. On the basis of a study of South African black children, among whom there is an increased incidence of Blount disease (as there is in Jamaica), Bathfield and Beighton have suggested that its cause might be related to the custom of mothers carrying children on their backs. The child's thighs are abducted and flexed, and the flexed knees gripping the mother's waist are forced to assume a varus configuration.

Two forms of Blount disease have been identified: *infantile tibia vara*, which is usually bilateral and affects children younger than age 10 years, with onset most commonly between ages 1 and 3 years; and *adolescent tibia vara*, which is usually unilateral and occurs in children between the ages of 8 and 15 years. The course of the adolescent form of the disease is less severe and its incidence less frequent than in the infantile form. Regardless of its variants, Blount disease must be

differentiated from other causes of tibia vara, such as those seen as sequelae to trauma.

Radiographic Evaluation and Differential Diagnosis

Radiologically, the early stages of Blount disease are marked by hypertrophy of the nonossified cartilaginous portion of the tibial epiphysis and hypertrophy of the medial meniscus, which represent compensatory changes secondary to growth arrest at the medial aspect of the physis. As the metaphysis and growth plate become depressed, the cartilage decreases in height. In advanced stages of the disease, there is premature fusion of the growth plate on the medial side, which can be demonstrated effectively by conventional tomography (Fig. 32.37). The presence of fusion is important information for surgical planning, because either resection of the bony bridge or epiphysiodesis (fusion of the physis) would be required in addition to the corrective osteotomy. Double-contrast arthrography is also a valuable technique in the radiologic evaluation of Blount disease, because it permits visualization of nonossified cartilage of the medial plateau (Fig. 32.38) and associated abnormalities of the medial meniscus (Fig. 32.39).

In most cases, it is also possible to distinguish Blount disease radiographically, particularly in its advanced stage, from developmental bowing of the legs. In Blount disease, the medial aspect of the tibial metaphysis is characteristically depressed, exhibiting an abrupt angulation and formation of a beak-like prominence, which is associated with cortical thickening of the medial aspect of the tibia. Similar changes are seen in the medial aspect of the tibial epiphysis. Because of the sharp angulation of the metaphysis and adduction of the diaphysis, the tibia assumes a varus configuration (Fig. 32.40). In most instances, the lateral cortex of the tibia remains relatively straight. In developmental bowleg

Figure 32.36 Complication of slipped capital femoral epiphysis. Frog-lateral radiograph of the right hip of a 14-year-old boy who had acute slippage of the capital epiphysis at age 9 demonstrates narrowing of the joint space and osteophytosis, characteristic features of a secondary osteoarthritic process. Note the presence of a Herndon hump.

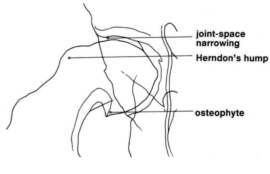

Table 32.4 Most Effective Radiographic Projections and Radiologic Techniques for Evaluating Common Anomalies of the Lower Limb and Foot

Projection/Technique	Crucial Abnormalities	Projections/Technique	Crucial Abnormalities
Congenital Tibia Vara		**Congenital/Developmental Planovalgus Foot**	
Anteroposterior of knees	Depression of medial tibial metaphysis with beak formation	Anteroposterior of foot	Medial projection of axial line through the talus
	Varus deformity of tibia	Lateral of foot	Flattening of longitudinal arch
Conventional tomography	Premature fusion of tibial growth plate	**Congenital Vertical Talus**	
Arthrography	Hypertrophy of:	Lateral of foot	Vertical position of talus
	Nonossified portion of epiphysis		Talonavicular dislocation
	Medial meniscus		Boat-shaped or Persian-slipper appearance of foot
Genu Valgum		With forced plantar flexion	Possibility of reduction of dislocation
Anteroposterior of knees	Valgus deformity	Anteroposterior of foot	Flat-foot deformity
			Medial displacement of talus
Infantile Pseudoarthrosis of the Tibia			Abduction of forefoot
Anteroposterior and lateral of tibia	Bowing of tibia	**Calcaneonavicular Coalition**	
	Pseudoarthrosis	Lateral or medial oblique (45°) of foot and computed tomography	Fusion of calcaneus and navicular bone
Dysplasia Epiphysealis Hemimelica		**Talocalcaneal Coalition**	
Anteroposterior and lateral of ankle (or other affected joint)	Unilateral bulbous deformity of distal tibial (or any affected) epiphysis	Medial oblique (15°) of foot	Fusion of talus and calcaneus
		Lateral of foot	Talar beak
Talipes Equinovarus		Posterior tangential of calcaneus and computed tomography	Fusion or deformity of middle facet of subtalar joint
Anteroposterior of foot	Varus position of hindfoot	Subtalar arthrography	Cartilaginous or fibrous bridge
	Adduction and varus position of forefoot	**Talonavicular Coalition**	
	Kite anteroposterior talocalcaneal angle (<20°)	Lateral of foot	
	Talus-first metatarsal (TFM) angle (>15°)	Computed tomography	Fusion of talus and navicular bone
	Metatarsal parallelism		
Lateral of foot (weight-bearing or with forced dorsiflexion)	Equinous position of the heel		
	Talocalcaneal subluxation		
	Kite lateral talocalcaneal angle (<35°)		

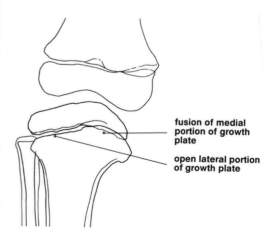

Figure 32.37 Blount disease. (A) Anteroposterior radiograph of the right knee of an 8-year-old girl shows the typical changes of congenital tibia vara. There is, in addition, a possible fusion of the medial portion of the growth plate. **(B)** Conventional tomogram confirms the presence of a bony bridge in the medial aspect of the physis. Treatment of this condition would require either epiphysiodesis or bridge resection in addition to corrective valgus osteotomy of the tibia.

fusion of medial portion of growth plate

open lateral portion of growth plate

normal medial
meniscus

contrast in inferior
meniscal recess

hypertrophied
nonossified
cartilage

Figure 32.38 Blount disease. (A) Anteroposterior radiograph of the right knee of a 10-year-old boy demonstrates the classic appearance of this condition, as evident in the depression of the medial metaphysis associated with a beak formation and slanting of the medial tibial epiphysis. **(B)** Spot film of an arthrogram shows contrast outlining the thickened nonossified cartilage of the medial tibial plateau. In this case, the medial meniscus shows no abnormalities.

Figure 32.39 Blount disease. Fluoroscopic spot film of a knee arthrogram in a 4-year-old girl shows hypertrophy of the medial aspect of the proximal tibial cartilage and an enlarged medial meniscus.

Figure 32.40 Blount disease. (A) Anteroposterior radiograph of the right knee of a 4-year-old girl with unilateral congenital tibia vara shows depression of the medial tibial metaphysis associated with a beak formation and medial slant of the tibial epiphysis. **(B)** The left knee is normal.

deformity, however, a gentle bilateral bowing is noted in the medial and lateral femoral and tibial cortices; the growth plates appear normal, and depression of the tibial metaphysis with a beak formation is absent (Fig. 32.41). Physiologic bowing resolves to straight alignment without treatment as ambulation increases, with the reversal usually beginning at approximately age 18 months. Both conditions, however, may be associated with internal tibial torsion. Developmental bowing usually persists for approximately 18 to 24 months, and in most affected children, it decreases progressively, although bowing may occasionally progress with skeletal maturation. Blount disease can be differentiated from rickets on the basis of ossification of the metaphyses and the absence of widening of the growth plate (see Figs. 27.12 and 27.13).

Classification

Based on the progression of radiographic changes in Blount disease, Langeskjöld divided congenital tibia vara into six stages as a guideline for prognosis and treatment:

Stage I   A varus deformity of the tibia, associated with irregularity of the growth plate and a small beak at the medial metaphysis; usually seen in children from 2 to 3 years of age.

Figure 32.41 Developmental bowleg deformity. Weight-bearing (standing) anteroposterior film of the legs of a 3-year-old boy demonstrates bowleg deformity of the femora and a varus configuration of the knees. However, there are no signs of Blount disease; both proximal tibial metaphyses and growth plates are normal, although there is associated internal torsion of both tibiae and thickening of the medial femoral and tibial cortices, which is frequently seen in this condition.

Stage II   A definite depression of the medial portion of the metaphysis, associated with slanting of the medial aspect of the epiphysis; usually seen in children from 2 to 4 years of age.

Stage III   Progression of the varus deformity and a very prominent beak, with occasional fragmentation of the medial portion of the metaphysis; seen in children between ages 4 and 6 years.

Stage IV   Marked narrowing of the growth plate and severe slanting of the medial aspect of the epiphysis, which shows an irregular border; usually seen in children between ages 5 and 10 years.

Stage V   Marked deformity of the medial epiphysis, which is separated into two parts by a clear band, the distal part having a triangular shape; seen in children between 9 and 11 years of age.

Stage VI   A bony bridge between the epiphysis and metaphysis and possible fusion of the triangular fragment of the separated medial epiphysis to the metaphysis; seen in children between ages 10 and 13 years.

Stages V and VI represent phases of irreparable structural damage.

Recently, Smith introduced a simplified classification of Blount disease in an attempt to relate the grade of deformity to the need for treatment. His scheme comprises four grades: grade A, potential tibia vara; grade B, mild tibia vara; grade C, advanced tibia vara; and grade D, physeal closure.

Treatment

Blount disease is usually treated conservatively with braces. If the deformity continues to progress despite such treatment, a high valgus tibial osteotomy may be required to achieve normal alignment of the limb; usually, correction of a rotary deformity requires an osteotomy of the proximal fibula as well. Arthrography may be required before surgery to determine the status of the tibial articular cartilage, information helpful in planning the degree of angular correction necessary to eliminate the deformity.

Dysplasia Epiphysealis Hemimelica

Trevor-Fairbank disease (or tarsoepiphyseal aclasis) is a developmental disorder characterized by asymmetric cartilaginous overgrowth of one or more epiphyses in the lower extremity, with a decided preference for the distal tibial epiphysis and the talus. The lesion is characteristically found on one side of the affected limb, hence the name "hemimelica." Its cause is unknown, and there is no definite familial or hereditary predilection. Males are affected three-times as often as females. Pathologically, the lesion shows similarity to an osteochondroma, and for this reason it is occasionally referred to as "epiphyseal" or "intraarticular osteochondroma." Clinically, there is deformity and restricted motion of the affected joint, and pain, particularly around the ankle, is the most frequent presenting symptom in adults.

Radiographic Evaluation and Treatment

A diagnosis of Trevor-Fairbank disease can be established through radiographic examination. It typically presents with an irregular, bulbous overgrowth of the ossification center or epiphysis on one side, resembling an osteochondroma (Fig. 32.42). Occasionally, the other ossification centers, particularly at the knee, may be similarly affected in the same individual.

Treatment for the condition is individualized according to the amount of deformity and pain; usually, surgical resection of the lesion is required. Recurrence is common.

Talipes Equinovarus

Clubfoot is a congenital deformity comprising four elements: (a) an equinus position of the heel; (b) a varus position of the hindfoot; (c) adduction and a varus deformity of the forefoot; and (d) talonavicular subluxation. Before the ossification of the navicular bone at 2 to 3

Figure 32.42 Trevor-Fairbank disease. A 12-year-old girl presented with pain and limitation of motion in the ankle joint. Anteroposterior **(A)** and lateral **(B)** radiographs of the ankle demonstrate deformity and enlargement of the medial malleolus, talus, and navicular bone, features typical of dysplasia epiphysealis hemimelica. Note that the growth disturbance is limited to the medial side of the ankle and foot. (A: from Norman A, Greenspan A, 1982, with permission.)

years of age, only the first three elements can be verified radiographically.

Measurements and Radiographic Evaluation

A sound knowledge of the anatomy of the foot is essential to understanding and properly describing the various foot abnormalities involved in this disorder (see Fig. 10.2). Certain lines and angles drawn on dorsoplantar and lateral radiographs of the foot are helpful in identifying the deformity. The most useful of these are the Kite angles and the talus-first metatarsal (TFM) angle (Fig. 32.43). In the clubfoot deformity, the Kite anteroposterior talocalcaneal angle is less than 20 degrees, the lateral angle is less than 35 degrees, and the TFM angle is greater than 15 degrees (Fig. 32.44). In addition to these measurements, there are other alignments in the normal infant's foot that are disrupted in the clubfoot deformity. For example, the anteroposterior view of the normal foot reveals the parallel alignment of the metatarsal bones, which in the clubfoot deformity converge proximally. Likewise, in the determination of the Kite anteroposterior talocalcaneal angle, the lines of the angle normally intersect the first and fourth metatarsals; in the clubfoot anomaly, these lines fall lateral to the normal points. It is important to note that rendering accurate measurements of these various angles requires a carefully standardized technique for obtaining the anteroposterior and lateral views of the foot, because slight changes in position can alter the relationship of the bones. Whenever possible, both projections should be obtained in weight-bearing positions. With infants in whom this is not possible, an anteroposterior view is obtained with the infant seated and the knees held together; the sagittal plane of the leg must be at a right angle to the radiographic cassette, on which the infant's feet are secured. When a weight-bearing lateral view is not possible, the infant's knee should be held in flexion and the foot held in dorsiflexion.

Treatment

Most clubfoot deformities can be corrected with conservative treatment using various manipulations and casts. The necessary degree of correction can be determined from the lines and angles described previously. If complete correction cannot be achieved with conservative treatment, then surgical release is usually performed and intraoperative radiography is used to confirm the results (Fig. 32.45). Radiographic evaluation is also essential after surgery to monitor the patient's progress. The most common complication of surgery for a clubfoot is related to overcorrection, which results in a "rocker-bottom" flat-foot deformity.

Congenital Vertical Talus

Congenital vertical talus, as its name denotes, consists of primary dislocations in the talonavicular and talocalcaneal joints, with the talus assuming a vertical position and pointing plantarly and medially. This anomaly, which occurs more often in males than in females, is usually diagnosed in the first few weeks after birth. The foot is usually in dorsiflexion, and a prominent bulge is present on the plantar surface in the midtarsal region. The entire foot may assume a "boat-shaped" or "Persian-slipper" configuration.

Radiographic Evaluation

Radiographic examination, particularly the lateral projection, is diagnostic. The talus is seen in a vertical position, and in children aged 2 to 3 years the fully ossified navicular bone makes talonavicular dislocation

Figure 32.43 The Kite measurements. (A) The Kite anteroposterior talocalcaneal angle and the talus-first metatarsal (TFM) angle are determined on a weight-bearing dorsoplantar radiograph of the foot. The Kite angle is the intersection of two lines: One line *(a)* drawn through the longitudinal axis of the talus normally intersects the first metatarsal bone; a second line *(b)* drawn through the longitudinal axis of the calcaneus usually intersects the fourth metatarsal. The angle of intersection of these lines normally ranges from 20 to 40 degrees; an angle less than 20 degrees indicates a varus position of the hindfoot. The TFM angle is determined on the same radiograph by a line *(c)* drawn through the longitudinal axis of the first metatarsal and intersecting line *(a)*. The values of this angle normally range between 0 and −20 degrees; positive values indicate adduction of the forefoot. **(B)** The Kite lateral talocalcaneal angle is determined on a weight-bearing lateral radiograph of the ankle and foot by the intersection of lines drawn through the longitudinal axes of the talus and calcaneus (lines parallel to the inferior borders of these two bones). Normally, this angle measures between 35 and 50 degrees; an angle less than 35 degrees indicates an equinus deformity of the heel.

TFM angle
(0 – −20°)

Kite anteroposterior
talocalcaneal angle (20° – 40°)

A

Kite lateral talocalcaneal angle (35°– 50°)

B

obvious (Fig. 32.46). The presence of talonavicular dislocation differentiates this condition from the developmental flat-foot deformity. Before ossification of the navicular bone occurs, congenital vertical talus can be identified on the lateral projection by a slight equinus position of the calcaneus, by widening of the calcaneocuboid joint, and by a valgus position of the forefoot, which is dorsiflexed at the midtarsal joint. The longitudinal arch is reversed, and the entire foot assumes a "rocker-bottom" configuration (Fig. 32.47A). The dorsoplantar projection characteristically reveals medial displacement of the distal talus and abduction of the forefoot (Fig. 32.47B). It is important to obtain a lateral view with the foot in forced plantar flexion to see whether the dislocation can be reduced (Fig. 32.48), because on the basis of this finding, the surgeon can decide not only between conservative and surgical treatment but also on the type of operation to perform.

Treatment

Most cases of congenital vertical talus require surgical correction of the deformity by soft-tissue release, reduction of the dislocation, and pinning of the talus to the navicular bone (Fig. 32.49). In children older than age 6 years, the navicular bone is resected. Radiographic confirmation of the correction is essential.

Tarsal Coalition

Tarsal coalition refers to the fusion of two or more tarsal bones to form a single structure. This fusion may be complete or incomplete, and the bridge may be fibrous (syndesmosis), cartilaginous (synchondrosis), or osseous (synostosis). Various bones may be affected, but most commonly the coalition occurs between the calcaneus and navicular bone, less frequently between the talus and calcaneus, and least often between the calcaneus and cuboid bone. At times, more than two bones may be affected. Despite its occurrence at birth, signs and symptoms of tarsal coalition rarely develop before the patient's sec-

ond or third decade. Pain, particularly associated with prolonged walking or standing, is a typical presenting symptom. On physical examination, peroneal muscular spasm and restricted joint mobility (the so-called peroneal spastic foot) are revealed.

Although the clinical presentation usually suggests the correct diagnosis, radiographic examination is diagnostic. The primary sign of tarsal coalition is evidence of fusion. Secondary signs may also be present, representing adaptive alterations of the affected and adjacent bones and articulations.

Calcaneonavicular Coalition

The best projection for demonstrating this type of fusion is either lateral or a 45-degree medial oblique view of the foot (Fig. 32.50), although conventional tomography may at times be useful. The secondary signs include hypoplasia of the talus head.

Talonavicular Coalition

This rare type of tarsal coalition is best seen on the lateral radiograph of the foot or on CT examination (Fig. 32.51).

Talocalcaneal Coalition

Because osseous fusion of the talus and calcaneus most often occurs at the level of the sustentaculum tali and the middle facet of the subtalar joint, it can effectively be demonstrated on oblique and Harris-Beath (posterior tangential) projections (Fig. 32.52); occasionally, tomography or CT examination may also be useful (Figs. 32.53 and 32.54). In suspected cartilaginous or fibrous union that is not readily demonstrated on radiographs, secondary changes should be sought, such as close apposition of the articular surfaces of the middle facet of the subtalar joint, eburnation and sclerosis of the articular margins, and broadening or rounding of the lateral process of the talus. Moreover, a C-shaped continuous line extending from the talus to the sustentaculum tali (the so-called C sign, originally described by Lateur et al. in

Figure 32.44 Clubfoot deformity. (A) Dorsoplantar radiograph of the left foot of a 12-year-old boy demonstrates a varus position of the hindfoot, as determined by the Kite anteroposterior talocalcaneal angle, as well as adduction of the forefoot, as indicated by the abnormal values of the TFM angle (see Fig. 32.43A). **(B)** On the lateral projection, an equinus position of the heel is evident from the determination of the Kite lateral talocalcaneal angle (see Fig. 32.43B).

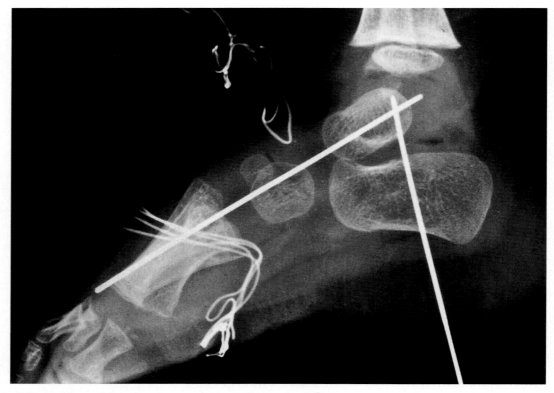

Figure 32.45 Treatment of the clubfoot deformity. Intraoperative radiograph of the foot of a 2-year-old girl was obtained to verify the degree of correction of a clubfoot. After soft-tissue release (Achilles tendon lengthening and a posterior ankle joint syndesmotomy), two Kirschner wires were passed across the talonavicular and subtalar joints to stabilize the hindfoot. Note the correction of the equinus deformity, as determined by the horizontal position of the calcaneus and the normal value of the Kite lateral talocalcaneal angle (compare with Fig. 32.44B).

Figure 32.46 Congenital vertical talus. Lateral radiograph of the foot of a 12-year-old boy with neglected congenital vertical talus shows obvious dislocations in the talonavicular and talocalcaneal articulations. Note the hourglass deformity of the talus and the wedging of the navicular bone.

Figure 32.47 Congenital vertical talus. (A) Lateral radiograph of the foot of a 2-year-old boy demonstrates the vertical position of the talus and the equinus position of the calcaneus. Note the flattening of the longitudinal arch and the alignment of the third cuneiform bone with the talar neck. **(B)** Dorsoplantar film shows the talus pointing medially; the navicular bone is not yet ossified. Note the soft-tissue bulge at the medial aspect of the foot.

Figure 32.48 Congenital vertical talus. (A) Lateral radiograph of the foot of a 2-year-old girl shows the vertical orientation of the talus, as well as talonavicular dislocation, although the navicular bone is not ossified. **(B)** Forced plantar flexion of the foot does not reduce the dislocation.

Figure 32.49 Congenital vertical talus. (A) Preoperative radiograph of the foot of a 2-year-old girl shows the longitudinal axis of the talus in continuity with that of the tibia. **(B)** Intraoperative film demonstrates satisfactory reduction of the talonavicular dislocation.

Figure 32.50 Calcaneonavicular coalition. (A) A 45-degree medial oblique projection of the foot of an 18-year-old man demonstrates solid osseous bridge between the calcaneus and navicular bones. **(B)** In another patient a lateral view demonstrates a similar osseous fusion of these two bones.

Figure 32.51 Talonavicular coalition. Axial (**A**) and reformatted sagittal (**B**) CT sections show a solid osseous fusion of the talus and navicular bones *(arrows)* in a 17-year-old boy.

Figure 32.52 Talocalcaneal coalition. (**A**) Oblique projection of the hindfoot of a 12-year-old boy shows obliteration of the middle facet of the subtalar joint. Note the prominent talar beak. (**B**) A Harris-Beath view confirms the osseous talocalcaneal coalition.

talocalcaneal coalition

1994) is visible on lateral radiographs of the ankle. This line is created by the combined shadows of the talar dome and the fused facets of the subtalar joint, together with a prominent inferior outline of the sustentaculum. In addition, the so-called absent middle facet sign, which refers to the lack of visualization of the middle facet of the subtalar joint on standing lateral view of the ankle and originally described by Harris in 1955, may be helpful in diagnosing this anomaly. A common secondary sign of talocalcaneal coalition is an osseous excrescence at the dorsal aspect of the talus, forming what is called a talar beak (see Figs. 32.52A and 32.53A), which is seen in the osseous, chondrus, and fibrous types of coalition. It is important to keep in mind, however, that a similar hypertrophy of the talar ridge may be seen in other conditions as well; for example, it may be related to abnormal capsular and ligamentous traction associated with degenerative changes in the talonavicular joint (Fig. 32.55).

Figure 32.53 CT of talocalcaneal coalition. A 25-year-old man presented with pain in his left foot that was particularly pronounced after prolonged walking or standing. **(A)** Lateral radiograph of the left foot shows sclerotic changes in the middle facet of the subtalar joint, narrowing of the posterior talocalcaneal joint space, and a prominent talar beak—features suggesting tarsal coalition. **(B)** Coronal CT section clearly demonstrates narrowing of the middle facet joint space and a bony bridge. The normal right foot is shown for comparison.

Figure 32.54 CT of talocalcaneal coalition. A coronal CT scan in a 12-year-old boy with right foot pain shows an osseous talocalcaneal coalition at the site of the middle subtalar facet. The left foot is normal.

Figure 32.55 Talonavicular osteoarthritis. (A) Lateral radiograph of the foot of a 61-year-old woman demonstrates a talar beak and degenerative changes in the talonavicular joint. The middle and posterior facets of the subtalar joint appear normal. **(B)** A Harris-Beath view shows no evidence of tarsal coalition.

Demonstration of nonosseous forms of tarsal coalition may require subtalar arthrography. Similarly, when the clinical presentation is unclear and standard radiographs are equivocal, radionuclide bone scan may help localize the site of coalition by an increased uptake of radiopharmaceutical, although this is a nonspecific finding.

PRACTICAL POINTS TO REMEMBER

Anomalies of the Shoulder Girdle and Upper Limbs

[1] Congenital elevation of the scapula (Sprengel deformity) is frequently accompanied by other anomalies, most commonly Klippel-Feil syndrome (fusion of the cervical or upper thoracic vertebrae).

[2] A Madelung deformity can be effectively evaluated on the posteroanterior and lateral projections of the distal forearm and wrist. The constant findings include:
- a decreased radial and an increased ulnar length
- medial and dorsal bowing of the radius
- a triangular configuration of the carpal bones with the lunate at the apex.

Anomalies of the Pelvic Girdle and Hip

[1] Congenital dislocation of the hip is bilateral in more than 50% of affected children; therefore, in apparently unilateral cases the unaffected hip should be carefully examined.

[2] Several lines and angles can be drawn on an anteroposterior radiograph of the pelvis and hips to help determine congenital dislocation of the hip:
- the Hilgenreiner Y-line
- the Perkins-Ombredanne line
- the Andrén-von Rosen line
- the Shenton-Menard arc
- the acetabular index
- the center-edge (C-E) angle of Wiberg.

[3] In addition to standard radiography, the radiologic evaluation of congenital dislocation of the hip requires arthrography and CT scan, which is particularly valuable in monitoring the results of treatment.

[4] Ultrasound is a highly effective technique to diagnose and evaluate congenital hip dysplasia. The bony and cartilaginous components of the hip joint are well demonstrated, and acetabular coverage of the femoral head can be assessed.

[5] 3D ultrasound of the infant hip offers a unique image in the sagittal plane and allows evaluation of the joint from the craniocaudal (bird's eye) view.

[6] Before conservative or surgical treatment, skin or skeletal traction is applied to bring the dislocated femoral head to "station +2" to avoid osteonecrosis of the femoral head. The Gage and Winter traction stations are determined by the position of the proximal femoral metaphysis (femoral neck) relative to the ipsilateral acetabulum and contralateral normal hip.

[7] Proximal femoral focal deficiency (PFFD) can mimic congenital hip dislocation. Arthrography is helpful in distinguishing these anomalies by demonstrating:
- presence of the femoral head in the acetabulum in type A
- a defect in the femoral neck in type B
- the absence of the femoral head in types C and D.

[8] Legg-Calvé-Perthes disease (coxa plana) represents osteonecrosis (ischemic necrosis) of the proximal epiphysis of the femur. The radiologic evaluation of this condition includes:
- a radionuclide bone scan, particularly in the early stages
- standard radiography
- contrast arthrography
- MRI.

[9] The most frequently encountered radiographic findings in Legg-Calvé-Perthes disease include:
- periarticular osteoporosis
- increased density and flattening of the capital epiphysis
- a crescent sign
- fissuring and fragmentation of the epiphysis
- cystic changes in the metaphysis and broadening of the femoral neck
- lateral subluxation in the hip joint.

[10] A femoral "head-at-risk" in Legg-Calvé-Perthes disease is defined by five radiographic signs indicating a poor prognosis:
- a radiolucent, V-shaped defect in the lateral portion of the femoral head (Gage sign)
- calcifications lateral to the femoral epiphysis
- lateral subluxation of the femoral head
- a horizontal orientation of the growth plate
- diffuse metaphyseal cystic changes.

[11] A slipped capital femoral epiphysis is a Salter-Harris type I fracture through the physis, which is best demonstrated on the frog-lateral projection. Important diagnostic clues include:
- loss of the triangle sign of Capener
- decreased height of the epiphysis
- widening and blurring of the growth plate
- lack of intersection of the epiphysis by the lateral cortical line of the femoral neck.

Anomalies of the Lower Limbs

[1] Congenital tibia vara (Blount disease) can be differentiated from developmental bowing of the legs by its characteristic presentation with depression of the medial tibial metaphysis associated with abrupt angulation and the formation of a beak-like prominence on the metaphysis.

[2] Dysplasia epiphysealis hemimelica (Trevor-Fairbank disease) most often affects the ankle joint. The radiographic hallmark of this lesion, which histologically resembles osteochondroma, is an irregular bulbous overgrowth of one side of the ossification center or epiphysis.

[3] The clubfoot deformity is recognized radiographically by:
- an equinous position of the heel
- a varus position of the hindfoot
- adduction and a varus position of the forefoot
- talonavicular subluxation.

[4] In the evaluation of the clubfoot deformity, certain angles and lines drawn on the anteroposterior and lateral radiographs of the foot are helpful:
- the Kite anteroposterior and lateral talocalcaneal angles
- the talus–first metatarsal angle
- the extension of lines drawn through the longitudinal axis of the talus and the calcaneus.

[5] Proper positioning of the feet is a crucial factor in the radiographic evaluation of infants and small children. Weight-bearing films should be obtained whenever feasible; in small infants, the foot should be pressed against the radiographic cassette.

[6] Congenital vertical talus can be distinguished from developmental flat foot by the presence of dislocation in the talonavicular and talocalcaneal articulations.

[7] In tarsal coalition, the most common cause of the so-called peroneal spastic foot deformity, fusion of the affected bones (usually the talus and calcaneus or calcaneus and navicular bone) may be:
- fibrous (syndesmosis)
- cartilaginous (synchondrosis)
- osseous (synostosis).

[8] The radiologic evaluation of tarsal coalition includes:
- standard radiographs in the lateral projection (which reveals the most frequently encountered secondary sign of this condition, the formation of a talar beak), as well as in Harris-Beath and oblique projections
- conventional and computed tomography
- subtalar arthrography.

SUGGESTED READINGS

Alasaarela E, Koivukangas J. Evaluation of image quality of ultrasound scanners in medical diagnostics. *J Ultrasound Med* 1990;9:23–34.

Artz TD, Lim WN, Wilson PD, Levine DB, Salvati EA. Neonatal diagnosis, treatment and related factors of congenital dislocation of the hip. *Clin Orthop* 1975;110: 112–136.

Barlow TG. Early diagnosis and treatment of congenital dislocation of the hip. *J Bone Joint Surg [Br]* 1962;44B:292–301.

Barnes JM. Premature epiphysial closure in Perthes' disease. *J Bone Joint Surg [Br]* 1980;62B:432–437.

Bateson EM. Non-rachitic bowleg and knock-knee deformities in young Jamaican children. *Br J Radiol* 1966;39:92.

Bateson EM. The relationship between Blount's disease and bow legs. *Br J Radiol* 1968;41:107–114.

Bathfield CA, Beighton PH. Blount disease. A review of etiological factors in 110 patients. *Clin Orthop* 1978;135:29–33.

Bellyei A, Mike G. Weight bearing in Perthes' disease. *Orthopedics* 1991;14:19–22.

Bennett JT, Mazurek RT, Cash JD. Chiari's osteotomy in the treatment of Perthes' disease. *J Bone Joint Surg [Br]* 1991;73B:225–228.

Bick U, Müller-Leisse C, Tröger J. Ultrasonography of the hip in preterm neonates. *Pediatr Radiol* 1990;20:331–333.

Bloomberg TJ, Nuttall J, Stocker DJ. Radiology in early slipped femoral capital epiphysis. *Clin Radiol* 1978;29:657–667.

Blount WP. Tibia vara. Osteochondrosis deformans tibiae. *J Bone Joint Surg* 1937;19: 1–29.

Bluemm RG, Falke TH, Ziedses des Plantes BG Jr, Steiner RM. Early Legg-Perthes disease (ischemic necrosis of the femoral head) demonstrated by magnetic resonance imaging. *Skeletal Radiol* 1985;14:95–98.

Boeree NR, Clarke NMP. Ultrasound imaging and secondary screening for congenital dislocation of the hip. *J Bone Joint Surg [Br]* 1994;76B:525–533.

Bos CF, Bloem JL, Obermann WR, Rozing PM. Magnetic resonance imaging in congenital dislocation of the hip. *J Bone Joint Surg [Br]* 1988;70B:174–178.

Boyer DW, Mickelson MR, Ponseti IV. Slipped capital femoral epiphysis—long-term follow-up study of 125 patients. *J Bone Joint Surg [Am]* 1981;63A:85–95.

Brown RR, Rosenberg ZS, Thornhill BA. The C sign: more specific for flatfoot deformity than subtalar coalition. *Skeletal Radiol* 2001;30:84–87.

Buchanan JR, Greer RB III, Cotter JM. Management strategy for prevention of avascular necrosis during treatment of congenital dislocation of the hip. *J Bone Joint Surg [Am]* 1981;63A:140–146.

Caffey J, Ames R, Silverman WA. Contradiction of the congenital dysplasia-predislocation hypothesis of congenital dislocation of the hip through a study of the normal variation in acetabular angles at successive periods in infancy. *Pediatrics* 1956;17: 632–641.

Calhoun JD, Pierret G. Infantile coxa vara. *AJR Am J Roentgenol* 1972;115:561–568.

Catterall A. *Legg-Calvé-Perthes' disease.* New York: Churchill Livingstone; 1982.

Catterall A. The natural history of Perthes' disease. *J Bone Joint Surg [Br]* 1971;53B:37–53.

Cheema JI, Grissom LE, Harcke HT. Radiographic characteristics of lower-extremity bowing in children. *Radiographics* 2003;23:871–880.

Chiari K. Beckenosteotomie zur Pfannendachplastik. *Wien Med Wochenschr* 1953;103: 707–714.

Chiari K. Medial displacement osteotomy of the pelvis. *Clin Orthop* 1974;98:55–71.

Chung SMK. *Hip disorders in infants and children.* Philadelphia: Lea & Febiger; 1981.

Clancy M, Steel HH. The effect of an incomplete intertrochanteric osteotomy on Legg-Calvé-Perthes disease. *J Bone Joint Surg [Am]* 1985;67A:213–216.

Clarke NMP, Harcke HT, McHugh R, Lee MS, Borns PF, MacEwen GD. Real-time ultrasound in the diagnosis of congenital dislocation and dysplasia of the hip. *J Bone Joint Surg [Br]* 1985;67B:406–412.

Coleman SS. *Congenital dysplasia and dislocation of the hip.* St. Louis: CV Mosby; 1978: 1–39.

Coleman SS. Diagnosis of congenital dysplasia of the hip in the newborn infant. *JAMA* 1956;162:548–554.

Condon VR. Radiology of practical orthopaedic problems. *Radiol Clin North Am* 1972; 10:203–223.

Conway JJ, Cowell HR. Tarsal coalition: clinical significance and roentgenographic demonstration. *Radiology* 1969;92:799–811.

Craig JG, van Holsbeeck M, Zaltz I. The utility of MR in assessing Blount disease. *Skeletal Radiol* 2002;31:208–213.

Crim JR, Kjeldsberg KM. Radiographic diagnosis of tarsal coalition. *AJR Am J Roentgenol* 2004;182:323–328.

Crutcher JP, Staheli LT. Combined osteotomy as a salvage procedure for severe Legg-Calvé-Perthes disease. *J Pediatr Orthop* 1992;12:151–156.

Dalinka MK, Coren G, Hensinger R, Irani RN. Arthrography in Blount's disease. *Radiology* 1974;113:161–164.

Dannenberg M, Anton JI, Spiegel MB. Madelung's deformity. Consideration of its roentgenological diagnostic criteria. *AJR Am J Roentgenol* 1939;42:671.

DeRosa GP, Feller N. Treatment of congenital dislocation of the hip: management before walking age. *Clin Orthop* 1987;225:77–85.

Deutsch AL, Resnick D, Campbell G. Computed tomography and bone scintigraphy in the evaluation of tarsal coalition. *Radiology* 1982;144:137–140.

DiPietro MA. Pediatric musculoskeletal and spinal sonography. In: Van Holsbeeck M, Introcaso JH, eds. *Musculoskeletal ultrasound.* St. Louis: Mosby-Year Book; 1991: 177–206.

Dunn PM. The anatomy and pathology of congenital dislocation of the hip. *Clin Orthop* 1976;119:23–27.

Dunn PM. Perinatal observations on the etiology of congenital dislocation of the hip. *Clin Orthop* 1976;119:11–22.

Egund N, Wingstrand H. Legg-Calvé-Perthes disease: imaging with MR. *Radiology* 1991;179:89–92.

Evans IK, Deluca PA, Gage JR. A comparative study of ambulation-abduction bracing and varus derotation osteotomy in the treatment of severe Legg-Calvé-Perthes disease in children over 6 years of age. *J Pediatr Orthop* 1988;8:676–682.

Eyring EJ, Bjornson DR, Peterson CA. Early diagnostic and prognostic signs in Legg-Calvé-Perthes disease. *AJR Am J Roentgenol* 1965;93:382–387.

Fairbank TJ. Dysplasia epiphysealis hemimelica (tarso-epiphysial aclasis). *J Bone Joint Surg [Br]* 1956;38B:237–257.

Felman AH, Kirkpatrick JA Jr. Madelung's deformity: observations in 17 patients. *Radiology* 1969;93:1037–1042.

Freiberger RH, Hersh A, Harrison MO. Roentgen examination of the deformed foot. *Semin Roentgenol* 1970;5:341.

Fulford GE, Lunn PG, Macnicol MF. A prospective study of nonoperative and operative management for Perthes disease. *J Pediatr Orthop* 1993;13:281–285.

Gage JR, Winter RB. Avascular necrosis of the capital femoral epiphysis as a complication of closed reduction of congenital dislocation of the hip. A critical review of twenty years' experience at Gillette Children's Hospital. *J Bone Joint Surg [Am]* 1972;54A:373–388.

Gallagher JM, Weiner DS, Cook AJ. When is arthrography indicated in Legg-Calvé-Perthes disease? *J Bone Joint Surg [Am]* 1983;65A:900–905.

Ganz R, Klave K, Vinh TS, Mast JW. A new periacetabular osteotomy for the treatment of hip dysplasias. Technique and preliminary results. *Clin Orthop* 1988;232:26–36.

Gerscovich EO. A radiologist's guide to the imaging in the diagnosis and treatment of developmental dysplasia of the hip. I. General considerations, physical examination as applied to real-time sonography and radiology. *Skeletal Radiol* 1997;26: 386–397.

Gerscovich EO. A radiologist's guide to the imaging in the diagnosis and treatment of developmental dysplasia of the hip. II. Ultrasonography: anatomy, technique, acetabular angle measurements, acetabular coverage of femoral head, acetabular cartilage thickness, three-dimensional technique, screening of newborns, study of older children. *Skeletal Radiol* 1997;26:447–456.

Gerscovich EO, Greenspan A, Cronan MS, Karol LA, McGahan JP. Three-dimensional sonographic evaluation of developmental dysplasia of the hip: preliminary findings. *Radiology* 1994;190:407–410.

Goldman AB. Hip arthrography in infants and children. In: Freiberger RH, Kaye JJ, eds. *Arthrography.* New York: Appleton-Century-Crofts; 1979:217–235.

Goldman AB, Schneider R, Martel W. Acute chondrolysis complicating slipped capital femoral epiphysis. *AJR Am J Roentgenol* 1978;130:945–950.

Graf R. New possibilities for the diagnosis of congenital hip joint dislocations by ultrasonography. *J Pediatr Orthop* 1983;3:354–359.

Graf R. The diagnosis of congenital hip-joint dislocation by the ultrasonic compound treatment. *Arch Orthop Trauma Surg* 1980;97:117–133.

Greenhill BJ, Hugosson C, Jacobsson B, Ellis RD. Magnetic resonance imaging study of acetabular morphology in developmental dysplasia of the hip. *J Pediatr Orthop* 1993;13:314–317.

Grissom LE, Harcke HT, Kumar SJ, Bassett GS, MacEwen GD. Ultrasound evaluation of hip position in the Pavlik harness. *J Ultrasound Med* 1988;7:1–6.

Harcke HT. Screening newborns for developmental dysplasia of the hip: the role of sonography. *AJR Am J Roentgenol* 1994;162:395–397.

Harcke HT, Clarke NM, Lee MS, Boms PF, MacEwen GD. Examination of the infant hip with real-time ultrasonography. *J Ultrasound Med* 1984;3:131–137.

Harcke HT, Grissom LE. Performing dynamic sonography of the infant hip. *AJR Am J Roentgenol* 1990;155:837–844.

Harcke HT, Kumar SJ. The role of ultrasound in the diagnosis and management of congenital dislocation and dysplasia of the hip. *J Bone Joint Surg [Am]* 1991;73A:622–628.

Harris RI. Rigid valgus foot due to talocalcaneal bridge. *J Bone Joint Surg* 1955;37: 169–182.

Harris WR. The endocrine basis for slipping of the upper femoral epiphysis. An experimental study. *J Bone Joint Surg [Br]* 1950;32B:5–11.

Haveson SB. Congenital flatfoot due to talonavicular dislocation (vertical talus). *Radiology* 1959;72:19–25.

Hensinger RN. Congenital dislocation of the hip: treatment in infancy to walking age. *Orthop Clin North Am* 1987;18:597–616.

Herring JA. Current concepts review. The treatment of Legg-Calvé-Perthes disease. A critical review of the literature. *J Bone Joint Surg [Am]* 1994;76A:448–458.

Herring JA, Neustadt JB, Williams JJ, Early JS, Browne RH. The lateral pillar classification of Legg-Calvé-Perthes disease. *J Pediatr Orthop* 1992;12:143–150.

Herzenberg JE, Goldner JL, Martinez S, Silverman PM. Computerized tomography of talocalcaneal tarsal coalition: a clinical and anatomic study. *Foot Ankle* 1986;6: 2730–288.

Hillmann JS, Mesgarzadeh M, Revesz G, Bonakdarpour A, Clancy M, Betz RR. Proximal femoral focal deficiency: radiologic analysis of 49 cases. *Radiology* 1987; 165:769–773.

Holen KJ, Terjesen T, Tegnader A, Bredland T, Salther OD, Eik-Nes SH. Ultrasound screening for hip dysplasia in newborns. *J Pediatr Orthop* 1994;14:667–673.

Ingman AM, Paterson DC, Sutherland AD. A comparison between innominate osteotomy and hip spica in the treatment of Legg-Calvé-Perthes' disease. *Clin Orthop* 1982;163:141–147.

Jones D. An assessment of the value of examination of the hip in the newborn infant. *J Bone Joint Surg [Br]* 1977;59B:318–322.

Kamhi E, MacEwen GD. Treatment of Legg-Calvé-Perthes disease. *J Bone Joint Surg [Am]* 1975;57A:651–654.

Keller MS, Weiss AA. Sonographic guidance for infant hip reduction under anesthesia. *Pediatr Radiol* 1988;18:174–175.

Kelly FB Jr, Canale ST, Jones RR. Legg-Calvé-Perthes disease. Long-term evaluation of non-containment treatment. *J Bone Joint Surg [Am]* 1980;62A:400–407.

Kendig RJ, Evans GA. Biologic osteotomy in Perthes disease. *J Pediatr Orthop* 1986;6:278–284.

Kettelkamp DB, Campbell CJ, Bonfiglio M. Dysplasia epiphysealis hemimelica. A report of fifteen cases and a review of the literature. *J Bone Joint Surg [Am]* 1966;48A:746–766.

Kiepurska A. Late results of treatment in Perthes' disease by a functional method. *Clin Orthop* 1991;272:76–81.

Kim SH. Signs in imaging. The C sign. *Radiology* 2002;223:756–757.

Kite NH. *The clubfoot.* New York: Grune & Stratton; 1964.

Kleiger B, Mankin HJ. A roentgenographic study of the development of the calcaneus by means of the posterior tangential view. *J Bone Joint Surg [Am]* 1961;43A:961–969.

Kruse RW, Guille JT, Bowen JR. Shelf arthroplasty in patients who have Legg-Calvé-Perthes disease. A study of long-term results. *J Bone Joint Surg [Am]* 1991;73A:1338–1347.

Langeskjöld A. Tibia vara (osteochondrosis deformans tibiae): a survey of seventy-one cases. *Acta Chir Scand* 1952;103:1–22.

Langeskjöld A, Riska EB. Tibia vara (osteochondrosis deformans tibiae). *J Bone Joint Surg [Am]* 1964;46A:1405–1420.

Lateur LM, Van Hoe LR, Van Ghillewe KV, Gryspeerdts SS, Baert AL, Dereymaeker GE. Subtalar coalition: diagnosis with the C sign on lateral radiograph of the ankle. *Radiology* 1994;193:847–851.

Legg AT. An obscure affection of the hip-joint. *Boston Med Surg J* 1910;162:202–204.

Lehman WB. Decision-making in Legg-Calvé-Perthes disease. *Orthop Rev* 1984;13:78–90.

Lehman WB. *The clubfoot.* Philadelphia: JB Lippincott; 1980.

Lehman WB, Atar D, Grant AD. Pelvic osteotomies in children. *Bull NY Acad Med* 1992;68:483–496.

Lehman WB, Grant A, Rose D, Pugh J, Norman A. A method of evaluating possible pin penetration in slipped capital femoral epiphysis using a cannulated internal fixation device. *Clin Orthop* 1984;186:65–70.

Lehman WB, Grant AD, Nelson J, Robbins H, Milgram J. Hospital for Joint Diseases' Traction System for preliminary treatment of congenital dislocation of the hip. *J Pediatr Orthop* 1983;3:104–107.

Lehman WB, Lubliner J, Rosen C, Grant A. Observations on the use of computerized axial tomography in the management of congenital dislocation of the hip. *Bull Hosp Jt Dis Orthop Inst* 1985;45:21–28.

Lehman WB, Menche D, Grant A, Norman A, Pugh J. The problem of evaluating in situ pinning of slipped capital femoral epiphysis: an experimental model and a review of 63 consecutive cases. *J Pediatr Orthop* 1984;4:297–303.

Leitch JM, Paterson DC, Foster BK. Growth disturbance in Legg-Calvé-Perthes disease and the consequences of surgical treatment. *Clin Orthop* 1991;262:178–184.

Levinson ED, Ozonoff MB, Royen PM. Proximal femoral focal deficiency (PFFD). *Radiology* 1977;125:197–203.

Liu PT, Roberts CC, Chivers FS, et al. "Absent middle facet": a sign on unenhanced radiography of subtalar joint coalition. *AJR Am J Roentgenol* 2003;181:1565–1572.

Lloyd-Roberts GC, Catterall A, Salamon PB. A controlled study of the indications for and the results of femoral osteotomy in Perthes disease. *J Bone Joint Surg [Am]* 1976;58B:31–36.

Lowe HG. Necrosis of articular cartilage after slipping of capital femoral epiphysis. Report of six cases with recovery. *J Bone Joint Surg [Br]* 1970;52B:108–118.

Lysack JT, Fenton PV. Variations in calcaneonavicular morphology demonstrated with radiography. *Radiology* 2004;230:493–497.

Marks DS, Clegg J, Al-Chalabi AN. Routine ultrasound screening for neonatal hip instability. *J Bone Joint Surg [Br]* 1994;76B:534–538.

Martinez AG, Weinstein SL, Dietz FR. The weight-bearing abduction brace for the treatment of Legg-Perthes disease. *J Bone Joint Surg [Am]* 1992;74A:12–21.

Masciocchi C, D'Archivio C, Barile A, et al. Talocalcaneal coalition: computed tomography and magnetic resonance imaging diagnosis. *Eur J Radiol* 1992;15:22–25.

Maxted MJ, Jackson RK. Innominate osteotomy in Perthes disease: a radiological survey of results. *J Bone Joint Surg [Br]* 1985;67B:399–401.

McClure JG, Raney RB. Anomalies of the scapula. *Clin Orthop* 1975;110:22–31.

McEwan DW, Dunbar JS. Radiologic study of physiologic knock knees in childhood. *J Can Assoc Radiol* 1958;9:59.

McNally EG. Posteromedial subtalar coalition: imaging appearances in the three cases. *Skeletal Radiol* 1999;28:961–965.

Meehan PL, Angel D, Nelson JM. The Scottish Rite abduction orthosis for the treatment of Legg-Perthes disease. A radiographic analysis. *J Bone Joint Surg [Am]* 1992;74A:2–12.

Morin C, Harcke HT, MacEwen GD. The infant hip: real-time US assessment of acetabular development. *Radiology* 1985;157:673–677.

Mose K. Methods of measuring in Legg-Calvé-Perthes disease with special regard to the prognosis. *Clin Orthop* 1980;150:103–109.

Murphy RP, Marsh HO. Incidence and natural history of "head at risk" factors in Perthes' disease. *Clin Orthop* 1978;132:102–107.

Murphy SB, Simon SR, Kijewski PK, Wilkinson RH, Griscom NT. Femoral anteversion. *J Bone Joint Surg [Am]* 1987;69A:1169–1176.

Newman JS, Newberg AH. Congenital tarsal coalition: multimodality evaluation with emphasis on CT and MR imaging. *Radiographics* 2000;20:321–332.

Nielsen JB. Madelung's deformity. A follow-up study of 26 cases and a review of the literature. *Orthop Scand* 1977;48:379–384.

Norman A, Greenspan A. Bone dysplasia. In: Jahss MH, ed. *Disorders of the foot*, vol 1. Philadelphia: WB Saunders; 1982.

Novick GS. Sonography in pediatric hip disorders. *Radiol Clin North Am* 1988;26: 29–53.

Ogden JA, Conlogue GJ, Phillips MS, Bronson ML. Sprengel's deformity. Radiology of the pathologic deformation. *Skeletal Radiol* 1979;4:204–211.

Ogden JA, Moss HL. Pathologic anatomy of congenital hip disease. In: Weill UH, ed. *Progress in orthopaedic surgery*, vol 2. *Acetabular dysplasia in childhood*. New York: Springer-Verlag; 1978.

Paterson DC, Leitch JM, Foster BK. Results of innominate osteotomy in the treatment of Legg-Calvé-Perthes disease. *Clin Orthop* 1991;266:96–103.

Pavlik A. Die funktionelle Behand-lungmethode mittels Riemenbügel als Prinzip der konservativen Therapie bei angeborenen Hüftgelenks verrenkungen der Säuglinge. *Z Orthop* 1958;8:341–352.

Perpich M, McBeath A, Kruse D. Long-term follow-up of Perthes disease treated with spica casts. *J Pediatr Orthop* 1983;3:160–165.

Phillips WE II, Burton EM. Ultrasonography of development displacement of the infant hip. *Appl Radiol* 1995;24:25–32.

Pineda C, Resnick D, Greenway G. Diagnosis of tarsal coalition with computed tomography. *Clin Orthop Relat Res* 1986;208:282–288.

Pinto MR, Peterson HA, Berquist TH. Magnetic resonance imaging in early diagnosis of Legg-Calvé-Perthes disease. *J Pediatr Orthop* 1989;9:19–22.

Rab GT. Preoperative roentgenographic evaluation for osteotomies about the hip in children. *J Bone Joint Surg [Am]* 1981;63A:306–309.

Rab GT. Surgery for developmental dysplasia of the hip. In: Chapman MW, ed. *Operative orthopaedics*, 2nd ed. Philadelphia: JB Lippincott; 1993:3101–3112.

Ramsey PL, Lasser S, MacEwen GD. Congenital dislocation of the hip. Use of the Pavlik harness in the child during the first six months of life. *J Bone Joint Surg [Am]* 1976;58A:1000–1004.

Resnick D. Talar ridges, osteophytes, and beaks: a radiologic commentary. *Radiology* 1984;151:329–332.

Robbins H. Naviculectomy for congenital vertical talus. *Bull Hosp Jt Dis Orthop Inst* 1976;37:77–97.

Robinson HJ Jr, Putter H, Sigmond MB, O'Connor S, Murray KR. Innominate osteotomy in Perthes disease. *J Pediatr Orthop* 1988;8:426–435.

Rosendahl K, Markestad T, Lie RT. Ultrasound in the early diagnosis of congenital dislocation of the hip: the significance of hip stability versus acetabular morphology. *Pediatr Radiol* 1992;22:430–433.

Rush BH, Bramson RT, Ogden JA. Legg-Calvé-Perthes disease: detection of cartilaginous and synovial change with MR imaging. *Radiology* 1987;167:473–476.

Sakellariou A, Sallomi D, Janzen DL, Munk PL, Claridge RJ, Kiri VA. Talocalcaneal coalition: diagnosis with the C-sign on lateral radiographs of the ankle. *J Bone Joint Surg [Br]* 2000;82B:574–578.

Salter RB. Current concepts review. The present status of surgical treatment for Legg-Perthes disease. *J Bone Joint Surg [Am]* 1984;66A:961–966.

Salter RB. Etiology, pathogenesis and possible prevention of congenital dislocation of the hip. *Can Med Assoc J* 1968;98:933–945.

Salter RB. Legg-Perthes disease. The scientific basis for methods of treatment and their indications. *Clin Orthop* 1980;150:8–11.

Salter RB. Role of innominate osteotomy in the treatment of congenital dislocation and subluxation of the hip in the older child. *J Bone Joint Surg [Am]* 1966;48:1413–1439.

Salter RB, Thompson GH. Legg-Calvé-Perthes disease. The prognostic significance of the subchondral fracture and a two-group classification of the femoral head involvement. *J Bone Joint Surg [Am]* 1984;66A:479–489.

Sartoris DJ, Resnick DL. Tarsal coalition. *Arthritis Rheum* 1985;28:331–338.

Scham SM. The triangular sign in the early diagnosis of slipped capital femoral epiphysis. *Clin Orthop* 1974;103:16–17.

Sellers DS, Sowa DT, Moore JR, Weiland AJ. Congenital pseudoarthrosis of the forearm. *J Hand Surg [Am]* 1988;13A:89–93.

Siebenrock KA, Schöll E, Lottenbach M, Ganz R. Bernese periacetabular osteotomy. *Clin Orthop* 1999;363:9–20.

Smith CF. Tibia vara (Blount's disease). *J Bone Joint Surg [Am]* 1982;64A:630–632.

Soboleski DA, Babyn P. Sonographic diagnosis of developmental dysplasia of the hip: importance of increased thickness of acetabular cartilage. *AJR Am J Roentgenol* 1993;161:839–842.

Sohn C, Grotepass J. 3-dimensional organ image using ultrasound. *Ultraschall Med* 1990;11:295–301.

Sohn C, Lenz GP, Thies M. 3-dimensional ultrasound image of the infant hip. *Ultraschall Med* 1990;11:302–305.

Sponseller PD, Desai SS, Millis MB. Comparison of femoral and innominate osteotomies for the treatment of Legg-Calvé-Perthes disease. *J Bone Joint Surg [Am]* 1988;70A:1131–1139.

Sprengel W. Die angeborne Verschiebung des Schulterblattes nach oben. *Arch Klin Chir* 1891;42:545.

Steel HH. Triple osteotomy of the innominate bone. *J Bone Joint Surg [Am]* 1973;55A:343–350.

Stulberg SD, Cooperman DR, Wallensten R. The natural history of Legg-Calvé-Perthes disease. *J Bone Joint Surg [Am]* 1981;63A:1095–1108.

Sutherland DH, Greenfield R. Double innominate osteotomy. *J Bone Joint Surg [Am]* 1977;59A:1082–1091.

Suzuki S, Kasahara Y, Futami T, Ushikubo S, Tsuchiya T. Ultrasonography in congenital dislocation of the hip. *J Bone Joint Surg [Br]* 1991;73B:879–883.

Tachdjian MO. *Congenital dislocation of the hip.* New York: Churchill Livingstone; 1982:20–25.

Tachdjian MO. Reflections on complex problems of the hip in the adolescent. *Bull Hosp Jt Dis Orthop Inst* 1985;45:1–20.

Taniguchi A, Tanaka Y, Kadono K, Takakura Y, Kurumatani N. C sign for diagnosis of talocalcaneal coalition. *Radiology* 2003;228:501–505.

Terjesen T, Rundén TO, Johnsen HM. Ultrasound in the diagnosis of congenital dysplasia and dislocation of the hip joints in children older than two years. *Clin Orthop* 1991;262:159–169.

Tillema DA, Golding JSR. Chondrolysis following slipped capital femoral epiphysis in Jamaica. *J Bone Joint Surg [Am]* 1971;53A:1528–1540.

Tönnis D. Normal values of the hip joint for the evaluation of x-rays in children and adults. *Clin Orthop* 1976;119:39–47.

Tredwell SJ. Davis L. A prospective study of congenital dislocation of the hip. *J Pediatr Orthop* 1989;9:386–390.

Trevor D. Tarso-epiphyseal aclasis: a congenital error of epiphyseal development. *J Bone Joint Surg [Br]* 1950;32B:204–213.

Trueta J. Normal vascular anatomy of the human femoral head during growth. *J Bone Joint Surg [Br]* 1957;39B:358.

Waldenström H. The first stages of coxa plana. *J Bone Joint Surg* 1938;20:559–566.

Walter RS, Donaldson JS, Davis CL, et al. Ultrasound screening of high-risk infants. A method to increase early detection of congenital dysplasia of the hip. *Am J Dis Child* 1992;146:230–234.

Walters R, Simons S. Joint destruction—a sequel of unrecognized pin penetrations in patients with slipped capital femoral epiphysis. In: *The Hip Society: Proceedings of the 8th Open Scientific Meeting.* St. Louis: CV Mosby; 1980:145.

Wechsler RJ, Karasick D, Schweitzer ME. Computed tomography of talocalcaneal coalition: imaging techniques. *Skeletal Radiol* 1992;21:353–358.

Weinstein SL. Natural history of congenital hip dislocation (CDH) and hip dysplasia. *Clin Orthop* 1987;225:62–76.

Weishaupt D, Exner GU, Hilfiker PR, Hodler J. Dynamic MR imaging of the hip in Legg-Calvé-Perthes disease: comparison with arthrography. *AJR Am J Roentgenol* 2000;174:1635–1637.

Wenger DR, Bomar JD. Human hip dysplasia: evolution of current treatment concepts. *J Orthop Sci* 2003;8:264–271.

Wynne-Davies R. Acetabular dysplasia and familial joint laxity: two etiological factors in congenital dislocation of the hip. *J Bone Joint Surg [Br]* 1970;52B:704–716.

Yamamuro T, Ishida K. Recent advances in the prevention, early diagnosis, and treatment of congenital dislocation of the hip in Japan. *Clin Orthop* 1984;184:34–40.

CHAPTER 33

SCOLIOSIS AND ANOMALIES WITH GENERAL AFFECT ON THE SKELETON

Scoliosis

Regardless of its cause (Fig. 33.1), scoliosis is defined as a lateral curvature of the spine occurring in the coronal plane. This fact differentiates it from kyphosis, a posterior curvature of the spine in the sagittal plane, and lordosis, an anterior curvature of the spine also in the sagittal plane (Fig. 33.2). If the curve occurs in both coronal and sagittal planes, then the deformity is called kyphoscoliosis. Besides a lateral curvature, scoliosis may also have a rotational component in which vertebrae rotate toward the convexity of the curve.

Idiopathic Scoliosis

Idiopathic scoliosis, which constitutes almost 70% of all scoliotic abnormalities, can be classified into three groups. The *infantile* type, of which there are two variants, occurs in children younger than age 4 years; it is seen predominantly in boys, and the curvature usually occurs in the thoracic segment with its convexity to the left. In the *resolving* (benign) variant, the curve commonly does not increase beyond 30 degrees and resolves spontaneously, requiring no treatment. The *progressive* variant carries a poor prognosis, with the potential for severe deformity unless aggressive treatment is initiated early in the process. *Juvenile idiopathic scoliosis* occurs equally in boys and girls from the ages of 4 to 9 years. By far, the most common type of idiopathic scoliosis, comprising 85% of cases, is the *adolescent* form, seen predominantly in girls from 10 years of age to the time of skeletal maturity. The thoracic or thoracolumbar spine is most often involved, and the convexity of the curve is to the right (Fig. 33.3). Although the cause of this type is unknown, it has been postulated that a genetic factor may be at work and that idiopathic scoliosis is a familial disorder.

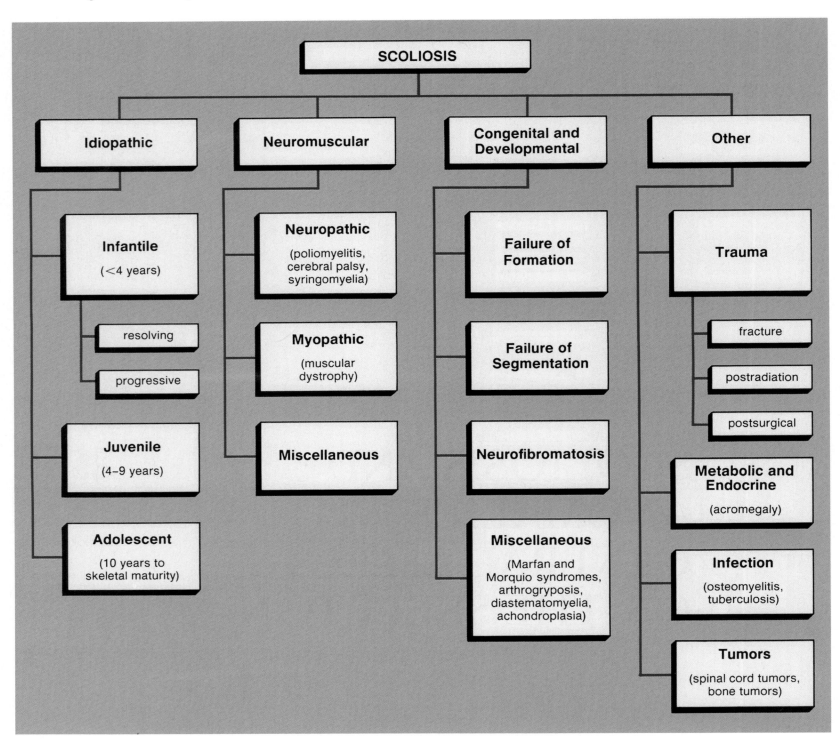

Figure 33.1 **General classification of scoliosis on the basis of cause.**

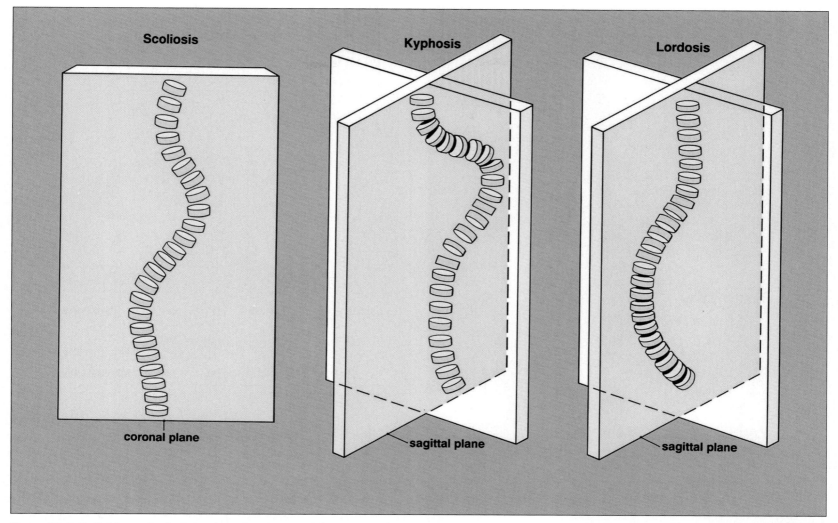

Figure 33.2 Definitions. Scoliosis is a lateral curvature of the spine in the coronal (frontal) plane. Kyphosis is a posterior curvature of the spine and lordosis an anterior curvature, both occurring in the sagittal (lateral) plane.

Congenital Scoliosis

Congenital scoliosis is responsible for 10% of the cases of this deformity. It may generally be classified into three groups, according to MacEwen (Fig. 33.4): those resulting from a *failure in vertebral formation*, which may be partial or complete (Fig. 33.5); those caused by a *failure in vertebral segmentation*, which may be asymmetric and unilateral or symmetric and bilateral; and those resulting from a *combination* of the first two. The effects of congenital scoliosis on balance and support result in faulty biomechanics throughout the skeletal system.

Miscellaneous Scolioses

Several other forms of scoliosis having a specific cause may develop, including neuromuscular, traumatic, infections, metabolic, and secondary to tumors, among others. Their discussion is beyond the scope of this text.

Radiologic Evaluation

The radiographic examination of scoliosis includes standing anteroposterior and lateral radiographs of the entire spine; a supine anteroposterior film centered over the scoliotic curve (Figs. 33.3 and 33.5), which is used for the various measurements of spinal curvature and vertebral rotation (discussed below); and anteroposterior radiographs obtained with the patient bending laterally to each side for evaluation of the flexible and structural components of the curve. Care should be

taken to include the iliac crests in at least one of these radiographs for a determination of skeletal maturity (see Figs. 33.14 and 33.15).

Ancillary techniques, such as conventional tomography and computed tomography (CT), may be required for evaluating congenital lesions such as segmentation failures. Intravenous urography (pyelography, IVP) is essential in congenital scoliosis for evaluating the presence of associated anomalies of the genitourinary tract (Fig. 33.6). Magnetic resonance imaging (MRI) is the technique of choice to evaluate associated abnormalities of the spinal cord and the nerve roots.

An overview of the radiographic projections and radiologic techniques used in the evaluation of scoliosis is presented in Table 33.1.

Measurements

To evaluate the various types of scoliosis, certain terms (Fig. 33.7) and measurements must be introduced. Measurement of the severity of a scoliotic curve has practical application not only in the selection of patients for surgical treatment but also in monitoring the results of corrective therapy. Two widely accepted methods of measuring the curve are the Lippman-Cobb (Fig. 33.8) and Risser-Ferguson techniques (Fig. 33.9). The measurements obtained by these methods, however, are not comparable. The values yielded by the Lippman-Cobb method, which determines the angle of curvature only by the ends of the scoliotic curve, depending solely on the inclination of the end vertebrae, are usually greater than those given by the Risser-Ferguson method. This also applies to the percentages of correction as determined by the two methods; the more favorable correction percentage is obtained by the

Figure 33.3 Idiopathic scoliosis. Anteroposterior radiograph of the spine in a 15-year-old girl shows the typical features of idiopathic scoliosis involving the thoracolumbar segment. The convexity of the curve is to the right; a compensatory curve in the lumbar segment has its convexity to the left.

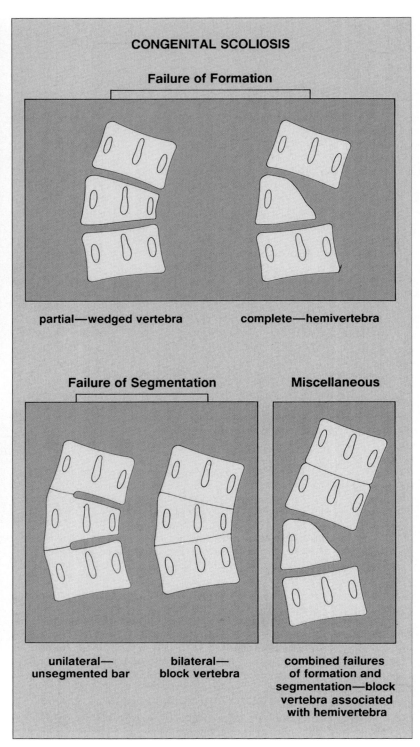

Figure 33.4 Classification of congenital scoliosis on the basis of cause. (Modified from MacEwen GD, et al., 1968; Winter RB, et al., 1968.)

Figure 33.5 Congenital scoliosis. Antero-posterior radiograph of the lumbosacral spine in a 22-year-old man demonstrates scoliosis caused by hemivertebrae, a complete unilateral failure of formation. Note the deformed L-3 vertebra secondary to the faulty fusion of the hemivertebra on the left side, where two pedicles are evident. The resulting scoliosis has its convex border to the left. An associated anomaly is also apparent from the presence of the so-called transitional lumbosacral vertebra.

fused hemivertebra

transitional lumbosacral vertebra

anomalous transverse process

Figure 33.6 Congenital scoliosis. (A) Supine antero-posterior radiograph of the thoracolumbar spine in a 13-year-old girl shows congenital scoliosis secondary to block vertebrae consisting of a fusion of L1-3. **(B)** IVP demonstrates only the left kidney, an example of renal agenesis. Congenital scoliosis is frequently associated with urinary tract anomalies.

A

B

Table 33.1 **Standard Radiographic Projections and Radiologic Techniques for Evaluating Scoliosis**

Projection/Technique	Demostration	Projections/Technique	Demostration
Anteroposterior	Lateral deviation Angle of scoliosis (by Risser-Ferguson and Lippman-Cobb methods and scoliotic index) Vertebral rotation (by Cobb and Moe methods)	*Conventional and Computed Tomography*	Congenital fusion of vertebrae Hemivertebrae
Of vertebra	Ossification of ring apophysis as determinant of skeletal maturity	*Myelography*	Tethering of cord
		Magnetic Resonance Imaging	Abnormalities of nerve roots Compression and displacement of thecal sac Tethering of cord
Of pelvis	Ossification of iliac crest apophysis as determinant of skeletal maturity	*Intravenous Urography*	Associated anomalies of genitourinary tract (in congenital scoliosis)
Lateral bending	Flexibility of curve Amount of reduction of curve		
Lateral	Associated kyphosis and lordosis		

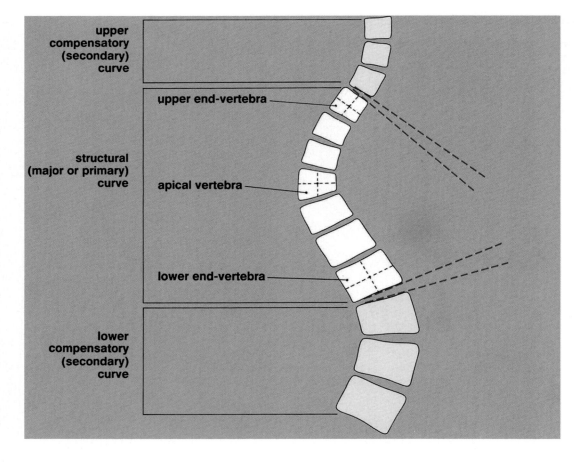

upper compensatory (secondary) curve

upper end-vertebra

structural (major or primary) curve

apical vertebra

lower end-vertebra

lower compensatory (secondary) curve

Figure 33.7 Terminology used in describing the scoliotic curve. The end-vertebrae of the curve are defined as those that tilt maximally into the concavity of the structural curve. The apical vertebra, which shows the most severe rotation and wedging, is the one whose center is most laterally displaced from the central line. The center of the apical vertebra is determined by the intersection of two lines, one drawn from the center of the upper and lower end plates and the other from the center of the lateral margins of the vertebral body. The center should not be determined by diagonal lines through the corners of the vertebral body.

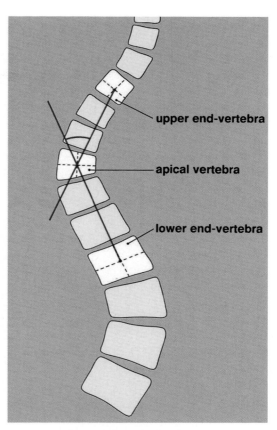

Figure 33.8 Lippman-Cobb method. In the Lippman-Cobb method of measuring the degree of scoliotic curvature, two angles are formed by the intersection of two sets of lines. The first set of lines, one drawn tangent to the superior surface of the upper end-vertebra and the other tangent to the inferior surface of the lower end-vertebra, intersects to form angle *(a)*. The intersection of the other set of lines, each drawn perpendicular to the tangential lines, forms angle *(b)*. These angles are equal, and either may serve as the measurement of the degree of scoliosis.

Figure 33.9 Risser-Ferguson method. In the Risser-Ferguson method, the degree of scoliotic curvature is determined by the angle formed by the intersection of two lines at the center of the apical vertebra, the first line originating at the center of the upper end-vertebra and the other at the center of the lower end-vertebra.

Lippman-Cobb method. The latter method, which has been adopted and standardized by the Scoliosis Research Society, classifies the severity of scoliotic curvature into seven groups (Table 33.2).

Another technique for measuring the degree of scoliosis, introduced by Greenspan and colleagues in 1978, uses a "scoliotic index." Designed to give a more accurate and comprehensive representation of the scoliotic curve, this technique measures the deviation of each involved vertebra from the vertical spinal line as determined by points at the center of the vertebra immediately above the upper end-vertebra of the curve and at the center of the vertebra immediately below the lower end-vertebra (Fig. 33.10). Its most valuable feature is that it minimizes the influence of overcorrection of the end vertebrae in the measured angle, a frequent criticism of the Lippman-Cobb technique. Furthermore, short segments or minimal curvatures, often difficult to measure with the currently accepted methods, are easily measurable with this technique.

Recently, computerized methods for measuring and analyzing the scoliotic curve have been introduced. Although more accurate than the manual methods, they require more sophisticated equipment and are more time consuming than the methods described above.

In addition to the measurement of scoliotic curvature, the radiographic evaluation of scoliosis also requires the determination of other factors. Measurement of the degree of *rotation of the vertebrae* of the involved segment can be obtained by either of two methods currently in use. The Cobb technique for grading rotation uses the position of the spinous process as a point of reference (Fig. 33.11). On the normal anteroposterior radiograph of the spine, the spinous process appears at the center of the vertebral body if there is no rotation. As the degree of rotation increases, the spinous process migrates toward the convexity of the curve. The Moe method, also based on the mea-

surements obtained on the anteroposterior projection of the spine, uses the symmetry of the pedicles as a point of reference, with the migration of the pedicles toward the convexity of the curve determining the degree of vertebral rotation (Fig. 33.12).

The final factor in the evaluation of scoliosis is the determination of *skeletal maturity*. This is important for both the prognosis and treatment of scoliosis, particularly the idiopathic type, because there is a potential for significant progression of the degree of curvature as long as skeletal maturity has not been reached. Skeletal age can be determined by comparison of a radiograph of a patient's hand with the standards for different ages available in radiographic atlases. It can also be assessed by radiographic observation of the ossification of the apophysis of the vertebral ring (Fig. 33.13) or, as is often performed, from the ossification of the iliac apophysis (Figs. 33.14 and 33.15).

Table 33.2 Lippman-Cobb Classification of Scoliotic Curvature

Group	Angle of Curvature (Degrees)
I	<20
II	21–30
III	31–50
IV	51–75
V	76–100
VI	101–125
VII	>125

Figure 33.10 Scoliotic index. In the measurement of scoliosis using the scoliotic index, each vertebra (a–g) is considered an integral part of the curve. A vertical spinal line (xy) is first determined whose endpoints are the centers of the vertebrae immediately above and below the upper and lower end-vertebrae of the curve. Lines are then drawn from the center of each vertebral body perpendicular to the vertical spinal line (aa', bb', . . . gg'). The values yielded by these lines represent the linear deviation of each vertebra; their sum, divided by the length of the vertical line (xy) to correct for radiographic magnification, yields the scoliotic index. A value of zero denotes a straight spine; the higher the scoliotic index, the more severe the scoliosis.

$$\frac{aa' + bb' + cc' + \ldots gg'}{xy} = \text{scoliotic index (corrected for magnification)}$$

Figure 33.11 Cobb spinous-process method. In the Cobb spinous-process method for determining rotation, the vertebra is divided into six equal parts. Normally, the spinous process appears at the center. Its migration to certain points toward the convexity of the curve marks the degree of rotation.

Figure 33.12 Moe pedicle method. The Moe pedicle method for determining rotation divides the vertebra into six equal parts. Normally, the pedicles appear in the outer parts. Migration of a pedicle to certain points toward the convexity of the curve determines the degree of rotation.

Figure 33.13 Skeletal maturity. Determination of skeletal maturity from ossification of the vertebral ring apophysis.

Figure 33.14 Skeletal maturity. The ossification of the iliac apophysis is helpful in determining skeletal age. Progression of the apophysis in this 14-year-old girl with idiopathic scoliosis has been completed, but the lack of fusion with the iliac crest indicates continuing skeletal maturation.

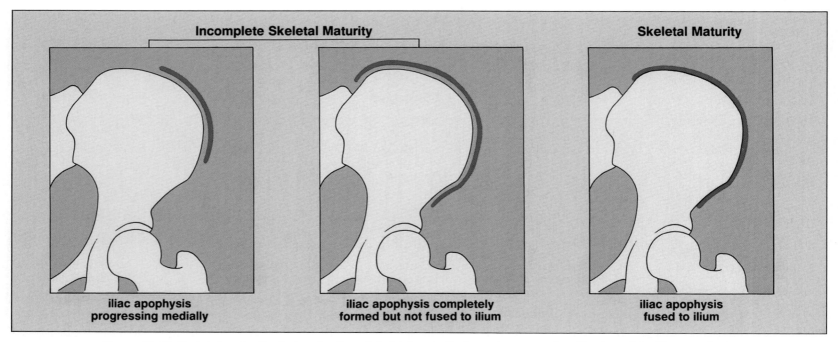

Incomplete Skeletal Maturity

iliac apophysis
progressing medially

iliac apophysis completely
formed but not fused to ilium

Skeletal Maturity

iliac apophysis
fused to ilium

Figure 33.15 **Skeletal maturity.** Determination of skeletal maturity from the status of ossification of the iliac apophysis.

Treatment

Various surgical procedures are available for the treatment of scoliosis. The main objective of surgery is to balance and fuse the spine to prevent the deformity from progressing; its secondary objective is to correct the scoliotic curve to the extent of its flexibility. Determining the level of fusion depends on several factors, including the cause of the scoliosis and the age of the patient, as well as the pattern of the scoliotic curve and the extent of vertebral rotation as evaluated during the radiographic examination of the patient.

Spinal fusion is now commonly accompanied by internal fixation of the spine to provide stability. One of the most popular methods for internal fixation is the Harrington-Luque technique (Wisconsin segmental instrumentation), using square-ended distraction rods and wire loops inserted through the bases of the spinous processes and connected to two contoured paravertebral rods (Fig. 33.16). The procedure involves decortication of the laminae and spinous processes, obliteration of the posterior facet joints by removal of the cartilage, and the placement of an autogenous bone graft from the iliac crest along the concave side of the curve. The hooks of the distraction rods are inserted under the laminae at the upper and lower ends of the curve. The prebent stainless-steel paravertebral rods (Luque rods or L-rods) are anchored into the spinous process or pelvis, depending on the location of the curve; wires, passed through the base of the spinous process at each level of the spine to be fused, are then fixed to the L-rods. Variations in this technique have been used with L-rod instrumentation alone, which involves the use of sublaminar wires fixed to the rods, or a combination of Harrington distractors and wires fixed to them. Recently, Cotrel-Dubousset spinal instrumentation using knurled rods has gained popularity. Fixation is achieved via pediculotransverse double-hook purchase at several levels. The two knurled rods are additionally stabilized by two transverse traction devices. The Dwyer technique, involving anterior fixation of the spine and obliteration of the intervertebral disks, is also used in the surgical treatment of scoliosis but more often in the paralytic types of the deformity.

The postoperative radiographic evaluation of internal fixation by the Harrington-Luque technique should focus on: (a) whether the hooks of the Harrington rod are properly anchored with their brackets on the laminae of the superior and inferior vertebrae of the fused segment; (b) whether a hook has separated or been displaced; and (c) whether the rods and wires are intact. Moreover, evidence of pseudoarthrosis of the fused vertebrae should be sought when the postoperative loss of correction exceeds 10 degrees; a range of 6 to 10 degrees of loss of correction is ordinarily seen. The evaluation of pseudoarthrosis may require conventional tomography in addition to the standard projections. Tomography may also be needed within 6 to 9 months after surgery to demonstrate suspected nonunion of the bone engrafted on the concave side of the curve. Union of the graft with the spinal segment should appear solid; tomography may demonstrate radiolucent defects suggesting nonunion. Other complications involving the instrumentation may occur, such as fracture of a distraction rod or of a wire cable or screw, or excessive bending of the rods. Usually, these are easily demonstrated on standard radiographs.

Anomalies with General Affect on the Skeleton

Table 33.3 presents an overview of radiographic projections and radiologic techniques most effective for evaluating congenital and developmental anomalies exhibiting general affect on the skeleton.

Neurofibromatosis

Originally considered a disorder of neurogenic tissue (nerve-trunk tumors), neurofibromatosis (also called von Recklinghausen disease) is now believed to be a hereditary dysplasia that may involve almost every organ system of the body. It is transmitted as an autosomal-dominant trait, with more than 50% of cases reporting a family history of neurofibromatosis. Sessile or pedunculated skin lesions (mollusca fibrosa) are an almost constant finding, and café au lait spots occur in more than 90% of patients. The latter lesions have a smooth border that has been likened to the coast of California; this distinguishes them from the café au lait spots seen in fibrous dysplasia, which have rugged "coast of Maine" borders. Plexiform neurofibromatosis is a diffuse involvement of the nerves, associated with elephantoid masses of soft tissue (elephantiasis neuromatosa) and localized or generalized enlargement of a part or all of a limb. Patients with these manifestations are particularly prone to malignant tumors (see Fig. 22.33).

Skeletal abnormalities are often encountered in neurofibromatosis; at least 50% of patients demonstrate some bony changes, most com-

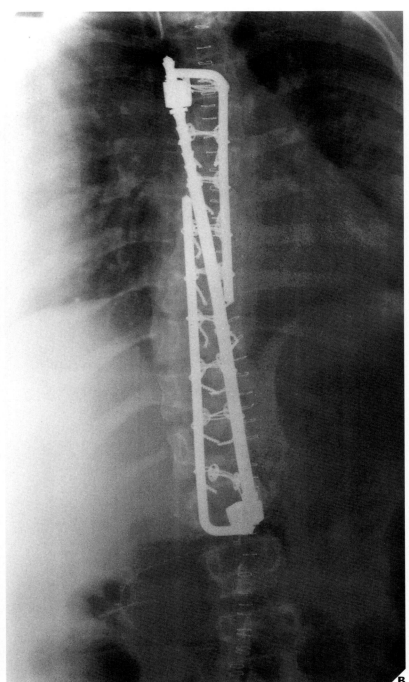

Figure 33.16 Treatment of scoliosis. (A) Preoperative anteroposterior radiograph of the lumbar spine in a 15-year-old girl shows idiopathic dextroscoliosis. **(B)** Postoperative film shows the placement of the Harrington distractor and two Luque rods. Note the multiple wires fixed into the prebent L-rods.

Table 33.3 Most Effective Radiographic Projections and Radiologic Techniques for Evaluating Common Anomalies with General Affect on the Skeleton

Projection/Technique	Crucial Abnormalities	Projection/Technique	Crucial Abnormalities
Arthrogryposis		*Morquio-Brailsford Disease*	

Anteroposterior, lateral, and oblique of affected joints	Multiple subluxations and dislocations
	Fat-like lucency of soft tissues
	Cubital and popliteal webbing
		Anteroposterior and lateral of spine
		Anteroposterior:
		  Of pelvis
		  Of hips
			Oval or hook-shaped vertebrae with central beak
			Overconstriction of iliac bodies
			Wide iliac flaring
			Dysplasia of proximal femora

Down Syndrome		*Hurler Syndrome*	

Anteroposterior:
  Of pelvis and hips
  Of ribs
Dorsovolar of both hands
 	
Lateral of cervical spine
Tomography (lateral) of cervical spine (C-1, C-2)
	Hip dysplasia
	11 pairs of ribs
	Clinodactyly and hypoplasia of fifth fingers
	Atlantoaxial subluxation
	Hypoplastic odontoid
		Anteroposterior and lateral:
		
		  Of spine
		
		  Of skull
		
		Anteroposterior of pelvis
			Rounding and lower beaking of vertebral bodies
			Recessed hooked vertebra at apex of kyphoscoliotic curve
			Frontal bossing
			Synostosis of sagittal and lambdoidal sutures
			Thickening of calvarium
			J-shaped sella turcica
			Flaring of iliac wings
			Constriction of inferior portion of iliac body
			Shallow, obliquely oriented acetabula

Neurofibromatosis			

Anteroposterior, lateral, and oblique of long bones
Anteroposterior:
 	
  Of ribs
  Of lower cervical/upper thoracic spine
Oblique of cervical spine
Lateral of thoracic/lumbar spine
Myelography
 	
Computed tomography
Magnetic resonance imaging
	Pit-like erosions
	
	Pseudoarthrosis of distal tibia and fibula
	Rib notching
	Scoliosis
	Kyphoscoliosis
	Enlarged neural foramina
	Posterior vertebral scalloping
	Intraspinal neurofibromas
	Increased volume of enlarged subarachnoid space
	Localized dural ectasia
	Complications (e.g., sarcomatous degeneration)
		Osteopetrosis
		Anteroposterior and lateral:
		  Of long bones
		  Of spine
		Anteroposterior of pelvis
			
			Increased density (osteosclerosis)
			Bone-in-bone appearance
			"Rugger-jersey" vertebral bodies
			Ring-like pattern of normal and abnormal bone in ilium

		Pycnodysostosis	
		Anteroposterior and lateral of long bones Dorsovolar of hands Lateral of skull	Increased density (osteosclerosis) Resorption of terminal tufts (acro-osteolysis) Wormian bones Persistence of anterior and posterior fontanelles Obtuse (fetal) angle of mandible
Osteogenesis Imperfecta			
Anteroposterior, lateral, and oblique of affected bones Lateral of skull Anteroposterior and lateral of thoracic/lumbar spine	Osteoporosis Bowing deformities Trumpet-like metaphysis Fractures Wormian bones Kyphoscoliosis	*Osteopoikilosis* Anteroposterior of affected bones	 Dense spots at the articular ends of long bones
Achondroplasia		*Osteopathia Striata*	

Anteroposterior:
  Of upper and lower extremities
 	
  Of pelvis
 	
  Of spine
 	
Lateral of spine
 	
Dorsovolar of hands
 	
Computed tomography
	Shortening of tubular bones, particularly humeri and femora
	Rounded iliac bones
	Horizontal orientation of acetabular roofs
	Small sciatic notches
	Narrowing of interpedicular distance
	Short pedicles
	Posterior scalloping of vertebral bodies
	Short, stubby fingers
	Separation of middle finger ("trident" appearance)
	Spinal stenosis
		Anteroposterior of affected bones
		
		Progressive Diaphyseal Dysplasia
		Anteroposterior of long bones (particularly lower limbs)
		
		Melorheostosis
		Anteroposterior and lateral of affected bones
			Dense striations, particularly in metaphysis
			
			Symmetric fusiform thickening of cortex
			Sparing of epiphyses
			
			Asymmetric, wavy hyperostosis (like dripping candle wax)
			Ossifications of periarticular soft tissues

some ancillary techniques may be useful. Myelography is particularly valuable for demonstrating the increased volume of the enlarged subarachnoid space and the localized dural ectasia extending into the scalloped defects in the vertebral bodies; with the introduction of MRI, this modality became more prevalent in investigation of the aforementioned abnormalities.

Osteogenesis Imperfecta

Osteogenesis imperfecta, also known as fragilitas ossium, is a congenital, non-sex-linked, hereditary disorder that manifests in the skeleton as a primary defect in the bone matrix. It is characterized by bone fragility resulting from abnormal quality and/or quantity of type I collagen. Depending on the type of osteogenesis imperfecta, the inheritance of the disorder can be autosomal-dominant, autosomal-

Figure 33.17 Neurofibromatosis. Anteroposterior radiograph of the lower legs of an 11-year-old girl with neurofibromatosis shows pit-like erosions in the upper tibiae and fibulae, a common finding in this condition.

monly extrinsic, pit-like cortical erosions resulting from direct pressure by adjacent neurofibromas. This is commonly seen in the long bones (Fig. 33.17) and ribs. The long bones often exhibit bowing deformities, and pseudoarthroses, seen in approximately 10% of cases, most commonly occur in the lower tibia and fibula (Fig. 33.18).

This type of false joint formation must be differentiated from congenital pseudoarthrosis. Moreover, the long bones are the site of lesions that were once considered to represent intraosseous neurofibromas; these cyst-like radiolucencies are now regarded as lesions representing fibrous cortical defects and nonossifying fibromas, associated with neurofibromatosis. Whittling of the bones is also a typical feature of neurofibromatosis (Fig. 33.19).

The spine is the second most common site of skeletal abnormalities in neurofibromatosis. Scoliosis or kyphoscoliosis, which characteristically involves a short segment of the vertebral column with acute angulation, commonly occurs in the lower cervical or upper thoracic spine. Widening of the intervertebral foramina in the cervical segment may also occur, resulting from dumbbell-shaped neurofibromas arising in spinal nerve roots (Fig. 33.20). In the thoracic and lumbar segments, scalloping of the posterior border of vertebral bodies is another characteristic feature (Fig. 33.21). Although most of these abnormalities can easily be diagnosed with conventional radiography,

Figure 33.18 Neurofibromatosis. Lateral radiograph of the right lower leg of an 11-year-old boy with generalized neurofibromatosis demonstrates anterior bowing of the distal tibia and fibula, associated with pseudoarthrosis. Note the pressure erosions in the middle third of the tibial diaphysis.

Figure 33.19 Neurofibromatosis. Lateral radiograph of the lower leg and foot of a 37-year-old woman with plexiform neurofibromatosis shows whittling of the calcaneus and marked hypertrophy of the soft tissues (elephantiasis).

Figure 33.20 Neurofibromatosis. Oblique radiograph of the cervical spine in a 26-year-old man demonstrates widening of the upper neural foramina secondary to "dumbbell" neurofibromas arising in the spinal nerve roots.

dominant with new mutation, or autosomal-recessive. Looser, in 1906, divided this condition into two forms, "congenita" and "tarda," and suggested that they are expressions of the same disease. Osteogenesis imperfecta congenita (Vrolik disease) has been classified as the more severe form, which is evident at birth and marked by bowing of the upper and lower extremities in an infant who is either stillborn or does not survive the neonatal period. The more benign osteogenesis imperfecta tarda (Ekman-Lobstein disease), in which there is a normal life expectancy, may show fractures present at birth, but these more often appear later in infancy. This condition is also associated with other manifestations, such as deformities of the extremities, blue sclerae, laxity of ligaments, and dental abnormalities.

Classification

In general, four major clinical features characterize osteogenesis imperfecta: (a) osteoporosis with abnormal bone fragility; (b) blue sclera; (c) defective dentition (dentinogenesis imperfecta); and (d) presenile onset of hearing impairment. Other clinical features also may be seen, among them ligamentous laxity and hypermobility of joints, short stature, easy bruising, hyperplastic scars, and abnormal temperature regulation. The earlier classification of osteogenesis imperfecta into two types, congenita and tarda, failed to reflect the complexity and heterogenous nature of this disorder. The new classification proposed by Sillence and colleagues in 1979, and later revised, is based on phenotypic features and the mode of inheritance.

Figure 33.21 Neurofibromatosis. Lateral spot-film of the lower thoracic spine in a 29-year-old woman shows scalloping of the posterior border of the T-12 vertebra, a common manifestation of this condition.

Currently, four major types of osteogenesis imperfecta and their subtypes are recognized:

Type I   This most common type of the disorder is a relatively mild form, with autosomal-dominant inheritance. Bone fragility is mild to moderate and osteoporosis is invariably present. Sclera are distinctly blue and hearing loss or impairment is a common feature. Stature is normal or near normal. Wormian bones are present. The two subtypes are distinguished by the presence of normal teeth (subtype IA) or dentinogenesis imperfecta (subtype IB).

Type II This is the fetal or perinatal lethal form of the disorder. This form demonstrates an autosomal-dominant inheritance with new mutation. The very severe nature of generalized osteoporosis, bone fragility, and severe intrauterine growth retardation results in death in the fetal or early perinatal period. Of those infants who survive, 80% to 90% die by 4 weeks of age. All patients in this group have radiologic features typical of osteogenesis imperfecta. In addition, the sclera are blue and the face has a triangle shape caused by soft craniofacial bones and a beaked nose. The calvarium is large relative to the face, and the skull shows a marked lack of mineralization as well as wormian bones. Limbs are short, broad, and angulated. Three subtypes, A, B, and C, are marked by differences in the appearance of the ribs and the long bones. In subtype A, the long bones are broad and crumpled and the ribs are broad, with continuous beading. In subtype B, the long bones also are broad and crumpled, but the ribs show either discontinuous beading or no beading. Subtype C is characterized by thin fractured long bones and ribs that are thin and beaded.

Type III This is a severe progressive form and represents a rare autosomal-dominant inheritance with new mutations. Bone fragility and osteopenia are considerable, leading with age to multiple fractures and severe progressive deformity of the long bones and spine. Bone abnormalities are generally less severe than in type II and more severe than in types I or IV. Sclera are normal, although pale blue or gray at birth, but the color changes through infancy and early childhood until it is normal by adolescence or adulthood. The calvarium is large, thin, and poorly ossified; wormian bones are present.

Type IV This is also a rare type of osteogenesis imperfecta and is inherited as an autosomal-dominant trait. Characteristically, osteoporosis, bone fragility, and deformity are present, but they are very mild. Sclera are usually normal. The incidence of hearing impairment is low and is even lower than in type I.

Radiologic Evaluation

The radiologic features of osteogenesis imperfecta are easily identified on standard radiographs. Severe osteoporosis, deformities of the bones, and thinning of the cortices are consistently observed features. The bones are also attenuated and gracile, with a trumpet-shaped appearance to the metaphysis (Fig. 33.22). Other typical skeletal abnormalities are seen in the skull, where wormian bones are a recognizable feature (Fig. 33.23), and in the spine, where severe kyphoscoliosis may develop from a combination of osteoporosis, ligamentous laxity, and posttraumatic deformities (Fig. 33.24). In children with a severe degree of disorder, the metaphyses and epiphyses of the long bones may exhibit numerous scalloped radiolucent areas with sclerotic margins (Fig. 33.25). This appearance is referred to as "popcorn calcifications," and it may be the result of traumatic fragmentation of the growth plate. The pelvis is invariably deformed, and acetabular protrusio is a frequent finding (Fig. 33.26).

Differential Diagnosis

Occasionally, osteogenesis imperfecta may be misdiagnosed as child abuse and vice versa. Patient and family history, physical examination,

Figure 33.22 Osteogenesis imperfecta. Lateral view of the leg of a 12-year-old boy with type III disease demonstrates thinning of the cortices and anterior bowing of the tibia and fibula. Note the trumpet-shaped appearance of the tibial metaphysis.

diagnostic imaging, and the clinical course of the abnormalities all contribute to the distinction of this condition from child abuse. The keys to distinguishing osteogenesis imperfecta from child abuse are: (a) the presence of blue sclera or abnormal teeth in osteogenesis imperfecta (OI); (b) investigation of clinical and family history (invariably positive in OI); (c) physical examination; and (d) radiologic examination for detection of wormian bones and osteoporosis in OI, and metaphyseal corner fractures and "bucket-handle" fractures that are highly specific and virtually pathognomonic features of child abuse. Several other features are also specific for child abuse, including multiple rib fractures, especially posterior rib fractures near or at the costovertebral junction; multiple fractures and/or multiple fractures showing different stages of healing; and sternal or scapular fractures, especially of the acromion. Transverse, oblique, or spiral fractures of a long bone with normal mineralization in the absence of any previous history, especially in a nonambulatory infant, are also highly suggestive of child abuse. The key to diagnosis of either condi-

Figure 33.23 CT of osteogenesis imperfecta. Axial CT sections of the skull **(A)** through the frontal and parietal bones and **(B)** through the vertex show sutural (wormian) bones.

Figure 33.24 MRI of osteogenesis imperfecta. (A) Sagittal T2-weighted MR image of the thoracic spine in a 13-year-old boy with osteogenesis imperfecta shows compression fractures of several vertebral bodies associated with kyphosis and compression of the spinal cord. **(B)** Sagittal T2-weighted MRI of the lumbar spine demonstrates multiple vertebral fractures and dural ectasia.

Figure 33.25 Osteogenesis imperfecta. Anteroposterior radiograph of the left leg of a 12-year-old boy with a type III osteogenesis imperfecta shows "popcorn calcifications" at the articular ends of the long bones. A Rush pin has been placed in the tibia because of a pathologic fracture.

Figure 33.26 Osteogenesis imperfecta. Marked deformity of the pelvis, seen here in a 27-year-old woman, is a consistent finding in osteogenesis imperfecta tarda. Note the bilateral acetabular protrusio and the pathologic fracture of the right femur.

tion is the correlation of clinical history, physical examination, family history, and radiologic findings.

Treatment

There is no specific treatment for osteogenesis imperfecta other than correction of the deformities it produces and the prevention of fractures. The condition, however, tends to improve spontaneously at puberty, with cessation or a decrease in the number of fractures. The limb deformities are corrected by various types of osteotomies, with the popular method being the Sofield ("shish kabob") technique, in which the deformed bones are osteotomized in a fragmentation procedure, cut into short segments, and then realigned by threading them onto a rigid or expandable rod (Fig. 33.27). The most common complications of this treatment are rod breakage, refracture of the bone at the end of the metallic device, and pseudoarthrosis.

Achondroplasia

Achondroplasia is a hereditary autosomal-dominant anomaly that begins in utero caused by a failure in endochondral bone formation and that affects the growth and development of cartilage. Its most prominent effect is short-limb, rhizomelic (disproportional) dwarfism. The hands and feet are short and stubby; the trunk is relatively long, with the chest flattened in the anteroposterior dimension; and the lower limbs are often bowed, producing a characteristic waddling gait. The head is large, with prominent frontal bossing, a depressed nasal bridge, and a "scooped-out" facial appearance.

Radiographically, achondroplasia exhibits distinctive features. As is typical in rhizomelic dwarfism, the tubular bones of the limbs are shortened, with the proximal segments (humeri and femora) more severely affected than the distal portions of the extremities (radius, ulna, tibia, and fibula); the growth plates assume a V-shaped configu-

ration (Fig. 33.28). In the hand, the fingers are short and stubby, with the middle finger separated from the others, giving the hand a "trident," appearance (Fig. 33.29). Identifying features of this disorder may also be encountered in the spine and pelvis. The spine exhibits a characteristic narrowing of the interpedicular distance and short pedicles, which often result in spinal stenosis; scalloping of the posterior aspect of the vertebral bodies is also a common finding (Fig. 33.30). In the pelvis, which is short and broad, the iliac bones are rounded, lacking the normal flaring; the acetabular roofs are horizontally oriented; and the sciatic notches are small. These features together give the hemipelvis the appearance of a ping-pong paddle. The shape of the inner contour of the pelvis has also been likened to a champagne glass (Fig. 33.31).

The most serious complication of achondroplasia is related to the spinal stenosis secondary to the typically short pedicles. Patients with the disease also occasionally have herniation of the nucleus pulposus. CT and MRI are the procedures of choice for confirming these two complications.

It is important to note that there are two other conditions resembling achondroplasia, but they differ from it in the severity of their symptoms and in radiographic presentation. *Hypochondroplasia* is a mild form of chondrodystrophy, in which the skeletal abnormalities are less severe than in achondroplasia. The skull is unaffected. *Thanatophoric dwarfism*, conversely, is thought to be a severe form of achondroplasia. It is lethal either in utero or within hours to days after birth.

Mucopolysaccharidoses

The mucopolysaccharidoses constitute a group of hereditary disorders having in common an excessive accumulation of mucopolysaccharides secondary to deficiencies in specific enzymes. Although sev-

Figure 33.27 Treatment of osteogenesis imperfecta. A 10-year-old boy with severe long bone deformities sustained a pathologic fracture of the right femur. **(A)** A single intramedullary Kirschner wire was inserted, and union was achieved. However, there is still marked lateral bowing of the femur. **(B)** Postoperative film after a Sofield osteotomy shows the bony segments of the femur realigned on a rigid rod.

Figure 33.28 Achondroplasia. Anteroposterior radiograph of the lower legs of a 12-year-old boy shows the short, broad tibiae characteristic of this disorder; the fibulae are relatively longer. The epiphyses about the knee joints have a V-shaped configuration and appear recessed into the trumpet-like metaphyses. (From Norman A, Greenspan A, 1982, with permission.)

Figure 33.29 Achondroplasia. Typical appearance of a hand in a 3-year-old girl. Note short metacarpals and short phalanges of the fingers.

Figure 33.30 Achondroplasia. (A) Anteroposterior radiograph of the thoracolumbar spine in a 2-year-old boy shows progressive narrowing of the interpedicular distance of the lumbar vertebrae in a caudal direction. **(B)** Lateral radiograph reveals the short pedicles and posterior vertebral scalloping.

Figure 33.31 Achondroplasia. Anteroposterior radiograph of the pelvis of a 13-year-old boy shows the classic manifestations of this condition. The iliac bones are rounded, lacking their normal flaring, and the acetabular roofs are horizontal—features rendering the appearance of a ping-pong paddle. Note also the "champagne-glass" inner contour of the pelvic cavity.

Table 33.4 Classification of the Mucopolysaccharidoses (MPS)

Designated Number	Eponym	Genetic and Clinical Characteristics
MPS I-H	Hurler syndrome (gargoylism)	Autosomal-recessive Corneal clouding, mental retardation, hepatosplenomegaly, cardiomegaly Urinary excretion of dermatan and heparan sulfates Deficiency of α-L-iduronidase enzyme
MPS I-S	Scheie syndrome	Autosomal-recessive Corneal clouding, normal mental development, pigeon chest, prominent clavicles and scapulae, stiff joints, carpal tunnel syndrome, flattening of the vertebral bodies, aortic valve disease, inguinal and umbilical hernias
MPS I-H/S	Hurler-Scheie compound syndrome	Urinary excretion of same product as in MPS I-H, and same enzyme deficiency
MPS II	Hunter syndrome (mild and severe variants)	Sex-chromosome-linked recessive disorder (males only) Mild mental retardation, absence of corneal clouding Urinary excretion of same product as in MPS I-H Deficiency of iduronate sulfatase
MPS III	Sanfilippo syndrome (A, B, and C variants)	Autosomal-recessive Progressive mental retardation, motor overactivity, coarse facial features Urinary excretion of heparan sulfate Deficiency of heparan-N-sulfatase
MPS IV	Morquio-Brailsford disease (type A, classic; type B, milder abnormalities)	Autosomal-recessive Short-trunk dwarfism; characteristic posture with knock knees, lumbar lordosis, and severe pectus carinatum; corneal opacities; impaired hearing; hepatosplenomegaly Urinary excretion of keratan sulfate Deficiency of galactosamine-6-sulfate sulfatase
MPS V	Redesignated MPS I-S	
MPS VI	Maroteaux-Lamy syndrome	Autosomal-recessive Normal intelligence, short stature, lumbar kyphosis; hepatosplenomegaly, joint contractures Urinary excretion of dermatan sulfate Deficiency of arylsulfatase B
MPS VII	Sly syndrome	Autosomal-recessive Growth and mental retardation, hepatosplenomegaly, pulmonary infections Urinary excretion of heparan and dermatan sulfates Deficiency of β-glucoronidase
MPS VIII	DiFerrante syndrome	Probably genetic trait Short stature Urinary excretion of keratan and heparan sulfates Deficiency of glucosamine-6-sulfate sulfatase

eral distinctive types of mucopolysaccharidoses have been delineated (Table 33.4), each with distinctive clinical and radiologic features, a specific diagnosis of any of these conditions is made on the basis of the patient's age at onset, the level of neurologic stunting, the amount of corneal clouding, and other clinical features. With the exception of Morquio-Brailsford disease, all the mucopolysaccharidoses are marked by excessive urinary excretion of dermatan and heparan sulfate.

The mucopolysaccharidoses exhibit common radiographic findings. These include osteoporosis, oval or hook-shaped vertebral bodies, and an abnormal configuration of the pelvis, with overconstriction of the iliac bodies and wide flaring of the iliac wings. The tubular bones are shortened and dysplastic changes are evident in the proximal femoral epiphyses (Fig. 33.32). The mucopolysaccharidoses, however, do show variations in these radiographic abnormalities; Hurler syndrome, for example, exhibits a characteristic rounding of the vertebral end plates on the lateral projection; the vertebral bodies appear oval in shape but frequently there is a dorsolumbar gibbous with a hypoplastic hook-shaped, recessed vertebral body.

Fibrodysplasia Ossificans Progressiva (Myositis Ossificans Progressiva)

Fibrodysplasia ossificans progressiva is a rare systemic autosomal-dominant disorder with variable expressivity and complete penetrance.

The gene responsible has recently been mapped to chromosome 17q21-22, and another study has localized it to chromosome 4q21-31. In most cases, only a single family member is affected. This suggests the involvement of a sporadic mutation.

The primary histopathologic abnormality is in the connective tissues. Most patients are affected early in life (from birth to age 5 years), and there is no sex predominance. The earliest clinical symptom is the appearance of painful nodules and masses in the subcutaneous tissue, particularly around the head and neck, with associated stiffness and limitation of movement. Subsequently, excessive ossification of muscles, ligaments, and fascia occur, with the predominant sites of involvement in the head and neck, the dorsal paraspinal muscles, the shoulder girdles, and the hips. Involvement of intercostal musculature interferes with respiration.

Clinically, the condition progresses from the shoulder girdle to the upper arms, spine, and pelvis. The natural history is one of remissions and exacerbations; death secondary to respiratory failure caused by constriction of the chest wall is an almost inevitable outcome. No effective treatment is known to date.

Radiologic Evaluation

Abnormalities of the thumb and great toe are present at birth and precede the soft-tissue ossification. The characteristic radiologic changes consist of agenesis, microdactyly, or congenital hallux valgus, occasionally with fusion at the metacarpophalangeal or metatarsopha-

Figure 33.32 Morquio-Brailsford disease. The classic features of this disease are present in radiographic studies of a 3-year-old boy. **(A)** Radiograph of the right arm shows foreshortening and deformity of the humerus, radius, and ulna, with an irregular outline of the metaphyses. **(B)** Anteroposterior film of the pelvis and hips shows flaring of the iliac wings and constriction of the iliac bodies. The narrowing of the pelvis at the level of the acetabula, which are distorted, produces a characteristic "wine-glass" appearance. Note the fragmentation of the ossification centers in the femoral heads and the broadening of the femoral necks, with subluxation in the hip joints and a coxa valga deformity. *(continued)*

Figure 33.32 Morquio-Brailsford disease. *Continued.* **(C)** The legs show deformities in the epiphyses of the femora and tibiae, as well as foreshortening of these bones. **(D)** Anteroposterior radiograph of the spine shows marked kyphoscoliosis. The vertebrae are grossly deformed and flat (platyspondylia), and the ribs are wide but with narrow vertebral ends, giving them a characteristic "canoe-paddle" appearance. Note the pronounced osteoporosis.

langeal joints (Fig. 33.33A). Short big toes and short thumbs may be associated with clinodactyly of the fifth finger, as well as with brachydactyly. In the soft tissues, extensive ossifications are seen, along with bridging bony masses in the cervical and thoracic spine, the thorax, and the extremities (Fig. 33.33B). Involvement of the insertions of ligaments and tendons occasionally produces bony excrescences mimicking exostoses. Joint ankylosis results most often from ossification of the surrounding soft tissue, but a true intra-articular fusion may occur (Fig. 33.33C). CT provides accurate anatomic localization of preosseous lesions. MRI, particularly contrast-enhanced studies, may further characterize soft-tissue abnormalities. Early-stage lesions exhibit low signal intensity on T1-weighted sequences and high signal on T2-weighted images, accompanied by marked homogeneous enhancement on post-gadolinium studies.

Histopathology

The pathologic abnormalities are similar to those of myositis ossificans circumscripta, but the zoning phenomenon of centripetal ossifi-

cation is absent. The earliest histologic changes are edema and inflammatory exudate, followed by mesenchymal proliferation and formation of a large mass of collagen. This collagen is capable of accepting the deposition of calcium salts. Eventually, the lesion is transformed into irregular masses of lamellar and woven bone.

Sclerosing Dysplasias of Bone

The sclerosing bone dysplasias are a group of developmental anomalies that reflect disturbances in the formation and modeling of bone, most commonly as a result of inborn errors in metabolism. A common defect in many of these disorders is reflected in a failure of cartilage and/or bone to resorb during the process of skeletal maturation and remodeling. One defect in many cases involves the resorption capabilities of osteoclasts in the presence of normal osteoblastic activity. In other instances, the defect lies in excessive bone formation by osteoblasts, which may occur in the presence of normal or diminished osteoclastic activity. These basic errors in metabolism most commonly

Figure 33.32 Morquio-Brailsford disease *Continued.* **(E)** Lateral film of the spine demonstrates hyperlordosis in the lumbar segment and kyphosis at the thoracolumbar junction. Note the shape of the vertebral bodies, with the characteristic irregular outline of the end plates and central tongue-like or beak-like projections in the lumbar segment.

arise during the processes of endochondral and intramembranous ossification. All sclerosing dysplasias share the common feature of excessive bone accumulation resulting in the radiographic appearance of increased bone density. Norman and Greenspan have developed a classification of these disorders based on the site of failure, whether endochondral or intramembranous, in skeletal development and maturation. Recently, Greenspan expanded and modified this classification (Table 33.5). The approach reflected in this classification is focused on target sites of involvement and pathomechanism of these dysplasias.

Osteopetrosis

An inherited disorder, osteopetrosis (also called Albers-Schönberg disease or marble-bone disease) involves a failure in resorption and remodeling of bone formed by endochondral ossification. The result is an excessive accumulation of primary spongiosa (calcified cartilage matrix) in the medullary portion of flat bones and long and short tubular bones, as well as in the vertebrae. Until recently, two variants have been described. The infantile "malignant" autosomal-recessive form is recognized at birth or in early childhood, and if not treated by

bone marrow transplantation it is frequently fatal because of severe anemia secondary to substantial quantities of cartilage and immature bone packing the marrow cavity. The "benign" autosomal-dominant adult form, which is marked by sclerosis of the skeleton, is compatible with a long lifespan. More recent reports describe what appear to be additional variants of this developmental anomaly, which illustrate the heterogeneity of inheritance of osteopetrosis: intermediate-recessive type and autosomal-recessive type with tubular acidosis.

The radiographic hallmark of this disorder, as of all sclerosing bone dysplasias, is increased bone density. The radiographic examination also reveals a lack of differentiation between the cortex and the medullary cavity and occasionally a bone-in-bone appearance. The long and short tubular bones exhibit a club-like deformity and splaying of their ends secondary to a failure in remodeling (Figs. 33.34 and 33.35). The same failure in the spine results in a characteristic sandwich-like appearance of the vertebral bodies (Fig. 33.36). Osteopetrosis may occur in a cyclic pattern, with intervals of normal growth. This produces alternating bands of normal and abnormal bone in a ring-like pattern, which is particularly well demonstrated in the metaphysis of long bones and in flat bones such as the pelvis and scapula (Fig. 33.37).

Figure 33.33 Myositis ossificans progressiva. A 28-year-old man with fibrodysplasia ossificans progressiva diagnosed at age 3 years. **(A)** Microdactyly of the great toe is a frequent feature of this disorder. **(B)** Lateral radiograph of the elbow shows extensive ossification in the soft tissues, bridging the distal humerus to the radius and ulna. **(C)** Massive ossification around the hip accompanies the ankylosis of the hip joint.

Table 33.5 **Classification of Sclerosing Dysplasias of Bone**

I. *Dysplasias of Endochondral Bone Formation*
 • Affecting primary spongiosa (immature bone)
  Osteopetrosis (Albers-Schönberg disease)
   Autosomal-recessive type (lethal)
   Autosomal-dominant type
   Intermediate-recessive type
   Autosomal-recessive type with tubular
    acidosis (Sly disease)
  Pycnodysostosis (Maroteaux-Lamy disease)
 • Affecting secondary spongiosa (mature bone)
  Enostosis (bond island)
  Osteopoikilosis (spotted bone disease)
  Osteopathia striata (Voorhoeve disease)
II. *Dysplasias of Intramembranous Bone Formation*
  Progressive diaphyseal dysplasia
   (Camurati-Engelmann disease)
  Hereditary multiple diaphyseal sclerosis
   (Ribbing disease)
  Endosteal hyperostosis (hyperostosis
   corticalis generalisata)
   Autosomal-recessive form
    van Buchem disease
    Sclerosteosis (Truswell-Hansen disease)
   Autosomal-dominant form
    Worth disease
    Nakamura disease

III. *Mixed Sclerosing Dysplasias (Affecting Both Endochondral and Intramembranous Ossification)*
 • Affecting predominantly endochondral ossification
   Dysosteosclerosis
   Metaphyseal dysplasia (Pyle disease)
   Craniometaphyseal dysplasia
 • Affecting predominantly intramembranous ossification
   Melorheostosis
   Progressive diaphyseal dysplasia with skull base involvement
    (Neuhauser variant)
   Craniodiaphyseal dysplasia
 • Coexistence of two or more sclerosing bone dysplasias (overlap
  syndrome)
   Melorheostosis with osteopoikilosis and osteopathia striata
   Osteopathia striata with cranial sclerosis (Horan-Beighton
    syndrome)
   Osteopathia striata with osteopoikilosis and cranial sclerosis
   Osteopathia striata with generalized cortical hyperostosis
   Osteopathia striata with osteopetrosis
   Osteopoikilosis with progressive diaphyseal dysplasia

From Greenspan A, 1991, with permission.

Figure 33.34 Osteopetrosis. Dorsovolar film of both hands of a 7-year-old boy shows the dense sclerotic bones lacking differentiation between the cortex and medullary cavity that are characteristic of this condition. The metacarpals appear club-like because of a failure in bone remodeling.

Figure 33.35 Osteopetrosis. Anteroposterior radiograph of the legs of a 10-year-old girl shows a uniform increase in bone density in the epiphyses, metaphyses, and diaphyses, with a lack of distinction between the cortical and medullary portions of the bones. The trabecular pattern is completely obliterated by the accumulation of immature bone. Note the splaying deformity of the distal femora and proximal tibiae as a result of remodeling failure.

Figure 33.36 Osteopetrosis. Lateral radiograph of the thoracolumbar spine in a 14-year-old boy demonstrates the characteristic sandwich-like or "rugger-jersey" appearance seen in this disorder. Note the overall increase in bone density.

Figure 33.37 Osteopetrosis. Radiographic examination of a 12-year-old girl demonstrates the cyclic pattern of this dysplasia. In the pelvis (**A**), alternating bands of normal (radiolucent) and abnormal (sclerotic) bone are arranged in a ring-like pattern in both iliac wings. In both legs (**B**), the alternating sclerotic and radiolucent bands are seen in the distal diaphyses and metaphyses of the tibiae and fibulae (*arrows*).

Fractures are a frequent complication of osteopetrosis caused by brittle bones.

Pycnodysostosis (Pyknodysostosis)

Pyknodysostosis (Maroteaux-Lamy disease) is an inherited autosomal-recessive disorder whose skeletal manifestations result from a failure of resorption of primary spongiosa. Patients with this disease, like the artist Toulouse-Lautrec, have a disproportionately short stature, which becomes evident in early childhood. Unlike patients with osteopetrosis, however, those with pyknodysostosis are usually asymptomatic; a pathologic fracture may be the occasion of its discovery.

Radiographically, pyknodysostosis presents with the increased bone density common to all sclerosing bone dysplasias. Moreover, in the skull, there is persistence of the anterior and posterior fontanelles, wormian bones, and an obtuse angle to the ramus of the mandible (Fig. 33.38). The features distinguishing this disease from osteopetrosis are hypoplasia of the distal phalanges of the fingers and toes and resorption of the terminal tufts of the distal phalanges (Fig. 33.39). The latter feature, known as acro-osteolysis, may, however, also be seen in a variety of other conditions (see Table 14.3).

Enostosis, Osteopoikilosis, and Osteopathia Striata

When endochondral ossification proceeds normally, but mature bony trabeculae coalesce and fail to resorb and remodel, the resulting developmental anomalies are referred to as enostosis (bone island), osteopoikilosis, or osteopathia striata. The exact mode of inheritance of each is not known, but all three are probably transmitted as autosomal-dominant traits. The most common and mildest of the three is enostosis (Figs. 33.40 and 33.41), which is asymptomatic; it is important, however, to differentiate this condition from an osteoid osteoma (see Figs. 16.19 and 17.8B) and from osteoblastic bone metastasis. Osteopoikilosis (osteopathia condensans disseminata, or "spotted-bone" disease) is also an asymptomatic disorder, and it is characterized by multiple bone islands symmetrically distributed and clustered near the articular ends of a bone (Fig. 33.42). Although radiography is usually sufficient to make a diagnosis, questionable cases may require

Figure 33.38 Pyknodysostosis. Lateral radiograph of the skull and facial bones of an 8-year-old shows persistence of the anterior and posterior fontanels and the obtuse (fetal) angle of the mandible, common manifestations of this disorder. (Courtesy of Dr. W.E. Berdon, New York, NY.)

Figure 33.39 Pyknodysostosis. Dorsovolar projection of both hands of a 9-year-old boy shows resorption of the terminal phalangeal tufts (acro-osteolysis), a feature differentiating this condition from osteopetrosis. (Courtesy of Dr. J. Dorst, Baltimore, MD.)

Figure 33.40 Enostosis. Anteroposterior radiograph of the right hip of a 10-year-old boy who was examined for an injury to the hip reveals, as an incidental finding, a giant bone island in the femoral neck, which was completely asymptomatic.

Figure 33.41 Enostosis. Anteroposterior **(A)** radiograph of the knee and CT section **(B)** through the proximal tibia demonstrate a bone island, displaying characteristic brush border. **(C)** In another patient CT section through the knee joint shows a giant bone island in the medial femoral condyle.

Figure 33.42 Osteopoikilosis. (A) Anteroposterior radiograph of the shoulder of a 34-year-old man who had pain in his right shoulder after an automobile accident shows no fracture or dislocation. However, multiple sclerotic foci representing lesions of osteopoikilosis are apparent, scattered near the articular ends of the scapula and humerus. A subsequent bone survey showed extensive involvement of the skeleton, especially the hands, wrists **(B)**, and hips **(C)**.

radionuclide imaging, which is diagnostic. In osteopoikilosis, a bone scan is relatively normal, unlike in metastatic disease, which invariably shows an increased uptake of radiopharmaceutical.

Histologically, both enostoses and the lesions of osteopoikilosis are characterized by foci of compact bone scattered in the spongiosa, with prominent cement lines and occasionally haversian systems. Clinically, osteopoikilosis must be distinguished from more severe disorders such as mastocytosis and tuberous sclerosis, as well as from osteoblastic metastatic lesions.

Osteopathia striata, the least common disorder in this group, is an asymptomatic lesion marked by fine or coarse linear striations, chiefly in the long bones and at sites of rapid growth such as the knee (Fig. 33.43) and shoulder. Several authors postulate a relationship between this disorder and osteopoikilosis; some suggest that it is in fact a variant of osteopoikilosis.

Progressive Diaphyseal Dysplasia

Failure of bone resorption and remodeling at the sites of intra membranous ossification (such as the cortex of tubular bones, the vault of the skull, the mandible, or the mid-segment of the clavicle) is the abnormality typically noted in progressive diaphyseal dysplasia, also

called Camurati-Engelmann disease. Like enostosis, osteopoikilosis, and osteopathia striata, this is an autosomal-dominant disorder with considerable variability of expression. Clinically, it is characterized by growth retardation, muscle wasting, pain and weakness in the extremities, and a waddling gait.

Because of its striking tendency toward symmetric involvement of the extremities, with characteristic sparing of the epiphysis and metaphysis (the sites of endochondral ossification), progressive diaphyseal dysplasia is recognized radiographically by symmetric fusiform thickening of the cortices of the long bone shafts, particularly in the lower extremities (Fig. 33.44).

A familial disorder similar to progressive diaphyseal dysplasia, described by Ribbing and later by Paul, is generally asymptomatic and exhibits limited asymmetric involvement, usually only of the long bones, especially the tibia and the femur. Known as *hereditary multiple diaphyseal sclerosis*, this condition is generally believed to be the same disorder as Camurati-Engelmann disease (Fig. 33.45). Radiography reveals focal sclerosis largely caused by formation of endosteal and periosteal new bone. These findings can be confirmed by CT. Scintigraphy shows increased uptake of ^{99m}Tc-methylene diphosphonate at the sites of radiographic abnormalities. Histopathologic features are not

Figure 33.43 Osteopathia striata. Anteroposterior radiograph of the right knee of a 14-year-old girl who had a history of trauma reveals, as an incidental finding, fine linear striations in the diaphysis and metaphysis of the distal femur and proximal tibia; the epiphyses, however, are spared.

Figure 33.44 Camurati-Engelmann disease. Anteroposterior radiograph of the hips and upper femora of an 8-year-old boy shows symmetric fusiform thickening of the cortices. Note that only the sites of intramembranous bone formation are affected, whereas the sites of endochondral bone formation are spared. (Courtesy of Dr. W.E. Berdon, New York, NY.)

Figure 32.45 Ribbing disease. Anteroposterior **(A)** and lateral **(B)** radiographs of the right lower leg in an asymptomatic 32-year-old man show features of hereditary multiple diaphyseal sclerosis (Ribbing disease). Note the slightly irregular circumferential thickening of the cortex of tibia.

Figure 33.46 Melorheostosis. A 28-year-old man presented with pain in the right elbow and an enlargement of the middle finger of his right hand. **(A)** Lateral radiograph of the elbow demonstrates a flowing hyperostosis of the anterior cortex of the distal humerus, typical of melorheostosis. Note the bridging of the joint by the lesion and the involvement of the coronoid process of the ulna. **(B)** The radiograph of the right femur shows involvement of only the anterolateral aspect of the bone. **(C)** Dorsovolar radiograph of the right hand shows marked hypertrophy of the middle digit. The cortices (the sites of intramembranous ossification) are involved, as are the articular ends of the bones (the sites of endochondral ossification). This is characteristic of mixed sclerosing dysplasias.

specific. Reactive cortical thickening is present, with variable formation of woven bone and fibrosis. One study revealed increased numbers of osteocytes per unit area compared with normal bone, as well as focal increases in plump osteoblastic rimming. Haversian systems were normal to markedly reduced in size. Although they are usually nonspecific, pathologic findings can aid in excluding other diagnoses, e.g., infection.

Melorheostosis

A rare condition of unknown cause, melorheostosis (Leri disease) shows no evidence of hereditary features. It belongs to a group of bone disorders called the mixed sclerosing dysplasias, which combine characteristics of both endochondral and intramembranous failure of ossification. The presenting symptom is pain intensified by activity. Limitation of joint motion and stiffness are common, due to contractures, soft-tissue fibrosis, and periarticular bone formation in the soft tissues. It may be monostotic (*forme fruste*) or polyostotic, affecting an entire limb.

Standard radiography is sufficient to make a diagnosis. The lesion is characterized by a wavy hyperostosis that resembles melted wax dripping down the side of a candle, the feature from which the disease derives its name (Greek *melos*-[member]; *rhein*-[flow]); moreover, only one side of the bone is usually involved (Fig. 33.46). Associated joint abnormalities are also well delineated on standard radiographs. The involvement of soft tissues is not rare, and the ossified masses are often present around the hip and knee joints (Fig. 33.47). CT effectively reveals involvement of the cortex and the medullary cavity (Fig. 33.48A). MRI shows low signal intensity localized to the affected areas on all pulse sequences (Figs. 33.48B,C and 33.49). This technique is also helpful for imaging of soft tissue involvement. In one study reported by Judkiewicz and associates, soft tissue masses were heterogeneous on all MRI pulse sequences with

Figure 33.47 Melorheostosis. (A) Anteroposterior radiograph of the right knee in a 46-year-old woman shows ossifications of the soft tissues at the lateral aspect of the knee joint. The femoral cortex is also affected *(arrow)*. **(B)** A radiograph of the left knee in a 25-year-old woman shows involvement of the medial femoral cortex extending into the soft tissues *(arrows)*.

Figure 33.48 CT and MRI of melorheostosis. (A) CT section through the middle segment of tibia in a 30-year-old woman shows involvement of the anterior cortex and anteromedial portion of medullary cavity. **(B)** An axial T1-weighted (spin-echo, TR 800/TE 16 msec) MRI shows the lesion to be of low signal intensity, which is the same as the cortical bone. The uninvolved bone marrow exhibits high signal similar to the subcutaneous fat. **(C)** A sagittal T2-weighted (fast spin-echo, TR 3000/TE 108 msec Ef) MR image shows that the lesion remains of low signal intensity *(open arrows)*. *Arrowheads* point to the medullary involvement.

Figure 33.49 MRI of melorheostosis. A coronal T1-weighted (SE; TR 800/TE 20 msec) MR image of the knee in a 20-year-old man shows decreased signal activity of the ossific mass attached to the femoral condyle (*arrow*) as well as in the medullary foci of melorheostosis (*open arrows*).

signal void in areas corresponding to mineralization on conventional radiographs. Most of the soft tissue masses exhibited ill-defined margins, were contiguous or adjacent to areas of osseous hyperostosis, and demonstrated enhancement after administration of gadolinium-DTPA. Radionuclide bone scan can determine other sites of skeletal involvement by demonstrating abnormal uptake of radiopharmaceutical (see Fig. 31.16). Microscopic examination of melorheostotic specimens reveals nonspecific, hyperostotic periosteal bone formation with thickened trabeculae and fibrotic changes in the marrow spaces. The bone appears primitive and consists largely of primary haversian systems, particularly on the periosteal surface, that are almost completely obliterated by the deposition of sclerotic, thickened, and somewhat irregular lamellae. Islands of cartilage in periarticular lesions have been described, with evidence of both endochondral and intramembranous bone formation within the cellular fibrous tissue, and osteoblastic activity along the margins of osteons.

Treatment. The disorder is chronic and occasionally debilitating. Conservative treatment with biphosphonate (pamidronate) infusion has been tried occasionally, with mixed results. Surgical treatment consists of soft-tissue procedures such as tendon lengthening, excision of fibrous and osseous tissue, fasciotomy, and capsulotomy. Other procedures include corrective osteotomies, excision of hyperostotic bone, and even amputations in severely affected and painful limbs caused by vascular ischemia. Recurrences are common.

Other Mixed Sclerosing Dysplasias

The most common of the other mixed sclerosing dysplasias is the coexistence of melorheostosis, osteopathia striata, and osteopoikilosis. The radiographic features of this "overlap syndrome" are a combination of each of these three dysplasias (Fig. 33.50), a phenomenon suggesting a common pathogenetic mechanism.

The discussion of other sclerosing dysplasias, listed in Table 33.5, is beyond the scope of this text.

Figure 33.50 Mixed sclerosing dysplasia. These radiographic studies in an 18-year-old man demonstrate the coexistence of melorheostosis with osteopoikilosis and osteopathia striata. **(A)** Anteroposterior film of the right hemipelvis and hip shows the wavy hyperostosis typical of melorheostosis affecting the iliac bone and proximal femur. Anteroposterior **(B)** and lateral **(C)** radiographs of the knee demonstrate the linear striations characteristic of osteopathia striata in the distal femur and proximal tibia, as well as the focal densities that are the identifying feature of osteopoikilosis. (From Norman A, Greenspan A, 1986, with permission.)

PRACTICAL POINTS TO REMEMBER

Scoliosis

[1] Congenital scoliosis may result from:
- a failure of vertebral formation, which may be unilateral and partial (wedged vertebra) or unilateral and complete (hemivertebra)
- a failure of segmentation, which may be unilateral (unsegmented bar) or bilateral (block vertebra)
- failures of both formation and segmentation.

[2] Idiopathic scoliosis, the most prevalent type of scoliosis (70%), can be divided into infantile (M>F), juvenile (M=F), and adolescent (M<F) categories. In the last type, the structural (major) curve is located in the thoracic or thoracolumbar segment, with its convexity to the right.

[3] In the evaluation of scoliosis, the shape of the curve usually indicates the variant, so that:
- an S-shaped curve is common in idiopathic scoliosis
- a C-shaped curve indicates the neuromuscular variant
- scoliosis marked by a sharply angled short spinal segment is most commonly congenital in origin (e.g., neurofibromatosis, hemivertebra).

[4] The scoliotic curve is described as composed of:
- a structural (major or primary) curve demarcated by upper and lower (transitional) end-vertebrae
- compensatory (secondary) curves proximal and distal to the transitional vertebrae
- an apical vertebra showing the most rotation and wedging, and whose center is most displaced from the central spinal line.

[5] Several methods for measuring the scoliotic curve are available:
- the Lippmann-Cobb method, in which the angle is determined only by the inclination of the end-vertebrae of the curve
- the Risser-Ferguson method, which utilizes three points as determinants of the curve—the centers of the upper and lower end-vertebrae and of the apical vertebra
- the scoliotic index method, which measures the deviation of each vertebra in the scoliotic curve from the central spinal line.

[6] To ensure accuracy in determining the degree of correction of a scoliotic curve, the same measuring points should be used in comparing the pretreatment and posttreatment curvature, even if the end-vertebrae have changed their locations.

[7] The rotation of a vertebral body can be evaluated on the anteroposterior radiograph by:
- the Cobb method, which uses the position of the spinous process as a point of reference
- the Moe method, which uses the pedicles as points of reference.

[8] The determination of skeletal maturity, an important factor in the prognosis and treatment of congenital scoliosis, may be made by:
- comparison of a radiograph of a patient's wrist and hand with standards in radiographic atlases
- evaluation of the ossification of the vertebral ring apophysis or iliac crest apophysis.

Anomalies with General Affect on the Skeleton

[1] The skeletal abnormalities frequently encountered in neurofibromatosis include:
- extrinsic cortical erosions
- pseudoarthroses, particularly in the tibia and fibula
- short segment kyphoscoliosis marked by acute angulation in the lower cervical and upper thoracic spine
- enlarged neural foramina and scalloping of the posterior aspect of vertebral bodies.

[2] Malignant transformation to sarcoma is the most serious complication of the plexiform variant of neurofibromatosis.

[3] The radiographic hallmarks of osteogenesis imperfecta, a disorder characterized by excessive fragility of the bones, include:
- severe osteoporosis
- thinning of the cortices
- sutural (Wormian) bones
- bone deformities, such as trumpet-shaped metaphyses
- "popcorn calcifications" at the articular ends of long bones
- kyphoscoliosis
- multiple fractures.

[4] Radiographically, achondroplasia is characterized by:
- rhizomelic (disproportional) dwarfism
- a configuration of the hemipelves resembling ping-pong paddles and a "champagne-glass" appearance of the inner pelvic contour
- narrowing of the interpedicular distance in the lumbar spine (spinal stenosis)
- scalloping of the posterior aspect of vertebral bodies
- "trident" appearance of the hand.

[5] The various disorders constituting the mucopolysaccharidoses share common radiographic features:
- osteoporosis
- oval or hook-shaped vertebral bodies
- an abnormal configuration of the pelvis
- shortened tubular bones.

[6] Fibrodysplasia ossificans progressiva (myositis ossificans progressiva) is characterized by extensive ossifications of the muscular structures and subcutaneous tissues, leading to joint ankylosis and constriction of the chest wall. Congenital abnormalities of the thumb and great toe (agenesis, microdactyly, etc.) should alert the radiologist to the possibility of this severely crippling disorder.

[7] The sclerosing bone dysplasias share the radiographic feature of increased bone density.

[8] The radiographic hallmarks of osteopetrosis and pycnodysostosis, disorders related to the failure of endochondral ossification, are:
- a uniformly increased bone density
- the absence of remodeling
- obliteration of the boundary between the medullary cavity and cortex.

Pathologic fractures are common.

[9] The specific changes characteristic of pycnodysostosis include:
- acro-osteolysis
- obtuse angle of the mandible
- persistence of the fontanelles
- wormian (sutural) bones.

[10] Enostosis, osteopoikilosis, and osteopathia striata, conditions also related to a failure of endochondral ossification, are characterized radiographically by:
- foci of sclerotic, mature bone in the medullary cavity (enostosis and osteopoikilosis)
- fine linear striations (osteopathia striata) at sites of rapid bone growth.

[11] Progressive diaphyseal dysplasia and hereditary multiple diaphyseal sclerosis, conditions related to the failure of intramembranous ossification, are recognized radiographically by thickening of the cortices of the long bones. The articular ends of the bones are, as a rule, not affected.

[12] Melorheostosis, a mixed sclerosing bone dysplasia marked by failure of endochondral and intramembranous ossification, is recognized radiographically by a flowing hyperostosis ("wax drippings") associated with involvement of the surrounding soft tissues and joint.

SUGGESTED READINGS

Aaro S, Dahlborn M. The longitudinal axis rotation of the apical vertebra, the vertebral, spinal, and rib cage deformity in idiopathic scoliosis studied by computer tomography. *Spine* 1981;6:567–572.

Ablin DS, Greenspan A, Reinhart M, Grix A. Differentiation of child abuse from osteogenesis imperfecta. *AJR Am J Roentgenol* 1990;154:1035–1046.

Abrahamson MN. Disseminated asymptomatic osteosclerosis with features resembling melorheostosis, osteopoikilosis and osteopathia striata. *J Bone Joint Surg [Am]* 1968; 50A:991–996.

Andersen PE Jr, Bollerslev J. Heterogeneity of autosomal dominant osteopetrosis. *Radiology* 1987;164:223–225.

Bailey JA II. Orthopedic aspects of achondroplasia. *J Bone Joint Surg [Am]* 1970;52A: 1285–1301.

Balkissoon ARA, Hayes CW. Case 14: intramedullary osteosclerosis. *Radiology* 1999;212: 708–710.

Barnes PD, Brody JD, Jaramillo D, Akbar JU, Emans JB. Atypical idiopathic scoliosis: MR imaging evaluation. *Radiology* 1993;186:73–738.

Bauze RJ, Smith R, Francis JO. A new look at osteogenesis imperfecta. *J Bone Joint Surg [Br]* 1975;57B:2–12.

Beals RK. Endosteal hyperostosis. *J Bone Joint Surg [Am]* 1976;58A:1172–1173.

Beighton P. *Inherited disorders of the skeleton.* Edinburgh: Churchill Livingstone; 1978.

Beighton P, Cremin BJ. *Sclerosing bone dysplasias.* New York: Springer-Verlag; 1984.

Beighton P, Cremin BJ, Hamersma H. The radiology of sclerosteosis. *Br J Radiol* 1976; 49:934–939.

Bhullar TPS, Portinaro NMA, Benson MKD. The measurement of angular deformity: an extended role for the "Cobbometer". *J Bone Joint Surg [Br]* 1995;77B:506–507.

Bridges AJ, Hsu K-C, Sing A, Churchill R, Miles J. Fibrodysplasia (myositis) ossificans progressiva. *Semin Arthritis Rheum* 1994;24:155–164.

Bridwell KH. Spinal instrumentation in the management of adolescent scoliosis. *Clin Orthop* 1997;335:64–72.

Brien EW, Mirra JM, Latanza L, Dedenko A, Luck J Jr. Giant bone island of femur. Case report, literature review, and its distinction from low grade osteosarcoma. *Skeletal Radiol* 1995;24:546–550.

Brown RR, Steiner GC, Lehman WB. Melorheostosis: case report with radiologic-pathologic correlation. *Skeletal Radiol* 2000;29:548–552.

Callahan BC, Georgopoulos G, Eilert RE. Hemivertebral excision for congenital scoliosis. *J Pediatr Orthop* 1997;17:96–99.

Campbell CJ, Papademetriou T, Bonfiglio M. Melorheostosis. A report of the clinical roentgenographic and pathological findings in fourteen cases. *J Bone Joint Surg [Am]* 1968;50A:1281–1304.

Camurati M. Di un raro caso di osteite simmetrica ereditaria degli arti inferiori. *Chir Organi Mov* 1922;6:662–665.

Carlson DH. Osteopathia striata revisited. *J Can Assoc Radiol* 1977;28:190–192.

Caron KH, DiPietro MA, Aisen AM, Heidelberger KP, Phillips WA, Martel W. MR imaging of early fibrodysplasia ossificans progressiva. *J Comput Assist Tomogr* 1990;14: 318–321.

Chanchairujira K, Chung CB, Lai YM, Haghighi P, Resnick D. Intramedullary osteosclerosis: imaging features in nine patients. *Radiology* 2001;220:225–230.

Cobb JR. Outline for the study of scoliosis. *AAOS Instructional Course Lectures* 1948;5:261–275.

Coccia PF, Krivit W, Cervenka J, et al. Successful bone-marrow transplantation for infantile malignant osteopetrosis. *N Engl J Med* 1980;302:701–708.

Connor J, Evans DA. Fibrodysplasia ossificans progressiva: the clinical features and natural history of 34 patients. *J Bone Joint Surg [Br]* 1982;64B:76–83.

Connor J, Evans DA. Genetic aspects of fibrodysplasia ossificans progressiva. *J Med Genet* 1982;19:35–39.

Cremin BJ, Beighton P. Osteopetrosis and other sclerosing bone dysplasias. In: Cremin BJ, Beighton P, eds. *Bone dysplasias of infancy: a radiological atlas.* New York: Springer; 1978:101.

Cremin B, Connor J, Beighton P. The radiological spectrum of fibrodysplasia ossificans progressiva. *Clin Radiol* 1982;33:499–508.

D'Addabbo A, Macarini L, Rubini G, Rubini D, Salzillo F, Lauriero F. Correlation between bone imaging and the clinical picture in two unsuspected cases of progressive diaphyseal dysplasia (Engelmann's disease). *Clin Nucl Med* 1993;18:324–328.

D'Agostino AN, Soule EH, Miller RH. Sarcomas of the peripheral nerves and somatic soft tissues associated with multiple neurofibromatosis (von Recklinghausen's disease). *Cancer* 1963;16:1015–1027.

Davis DC, Syklawer R, Cole RL. Melorheostosis on three-phase bone scintigraphy. Case report. *Clin Nucl Med* 1992;17:561–564.

Deacon P, Flood BM, Dickson RA. Idiopathic scoliosis in three dimensions: a radiographic and morphometric analysis. *J Bone Joint Surg [Br]* 1984;66B:509–512.

Demas PN, Soteranos GC. Facial-skeletal manifestations of Engelmann's disease. *Oral Surg Oral Med Oral Pathol* 1989;68:686–690.

De Vits A, Keymeulen B, Bossugt A, Somers G, Verbruggen LA. Progressive diaphyseal dysplasia (Camurati-Engelmann's disease). Improvement of clinical signs and of bone scintigraphy during pregnancy. *Clin Nucl Med* 1994;19:104–107.

Diard F. Imaging of scoliosis. *Rev Prat* 1993;43:1420–1431.

Dickson JM. An eleven-year clinical investigation of Harrington instrumentation: a preliminary report on 578 cases. *Clin Orthop* 1973;93:113–130.

Dickson RA. Early-onset idiopathic scoliosis. In: Weinstein SL, ed. *The pediatric spine: principles and practice.* New York: Raven Press; 1994:421–430.

Donáth J, Poór G, Kiss C, Fornet B, Genant H. Atypical form of active melorheostosis and its treatment with biphosphonate. *Skeletal Radiol* 2002;31:709–713.

Dorst JP. Mucopolysaccharidosis IV. *Semin Roentgenol* 1973;8:218–219.

Drummond DS. Neuromuscular scoliosis: recent concepts. *J Pediatr Orthop* 1996;16: 281–283.

Eastman JR, Bixler D. Generalized cortical hyperostosis (van Buchem disease): nosologic considerations. *Radiology* 1977;125:297–304.

Eggli KD. The mucopolysaccharidoses. In: Taveras JM, Ferrucci JT, eds. *Radiology—diagnosis, imaging, intervention,* vol 5. Philadelphia: JB Lippincott; 1986:1–13.

Elmore SM. Pycnodysostosis. A review. *J Bone Joint Surg [Am]* 1967; 49A:153–158.

Engelmann G. Ein Fall von Osteopathia hyperostotica (sclerotisans) multiplex infantilis. *Fortschr Geb Rontgenstr* 1929;39:1101–1106.

Evans SC, Edgar MA, Hall-Craggs MD, et al. MRI of "idiopathic" juvenile scoliosis: a prospective study. *J Bone Joint Surg [Br]* 1996;78B:314–317.

Fairbank HAT. *An atlas of general affections of the skeleton.* Baltimore: Williams & Wilkins; 1951.

Fairbank HAT. Melorheostosis. *J Bone Joint Surg [Br]* 1948;30B:533–543.

Fairbank HAT. Osteopathia striata. *J Bone Joint Surg [Br]* 1948;30B:117.

Fairbank HAT. Osteopoikilosis. *J Bone Joint Surg [Br]* 1948;30B:544–546.

Falvo KA, Root L, Bullough PG. Osteogenesis imperfecta: clinical evaluation and management. *J Bone Joint Surg [Am]* 1974;56A:783–793.

Figueiredo UM, James JIP. Juvenile idiopathic scoliosis. *J Bone Joint Surg [Br]* 1981;63: 61–66.

Fujimoto H, Nishimura G, Tsumurai Y, Nosaka K, Kanisawa S, Ohba S, Tanaka Y. Hyperostosis generalisata with striations of the bones: report of a female case and a review of the literature. *Skeletal Radiol* 1999;28:460–464.

Furia JP, Schwartz HS. Hereditary multiple diaphyseal sclerosis: a tumor simulator. *Orthopedics* 1990;13:1267–1274.

Gehweiler JA, Bland WR, Carden TS Jr, Daffner RH. Osteopathia striata—Voorhoeve's disease: Review of the roentgen manifestations. *AJR Am J Roentgenol* 1973;118: 450–455.

Gelman MI. Autosomal dominant osteosclerosis. *Radiology* 1977;125:289–296.

George K, Rippstein JA. A comparative study of the two popular methods of measuring scoliotic deformity of the spine. *J Bone Joint Surg [Am]* 1961;43A:809.

Gertner JM, Root L. Osteogenesis imperfecta. *Orthop Clin North Am* 1990;21:151–162.

Goldstein LA, Waugh TR. Classification and terminology of scoliosis. *Clin Orthop* 1973;93:10–22.

Green AE, Ellswood WH, Collins JR. Melorheostosis and osteopoikilosis with a review of the literature. *AJR Am J Roentgenol* 1962;87:1096–1111.

Greenspan A. Bone island (enostosis): current concept—a review. *Skeletal Radiol* 1995; 24:111–115.

Greenspan A. Sclerosing bone dysplasias—a target-site approach. *Skeletal Radiol* 1991;20:561–583.

Greenspan A, Azouz EM. Bone dysplasia series. Melorheostosis: review and update. *Canad Assoc Radiol J* 1999;50:324–330.

Greenspan A, Klein MJ. Giant bone island. *Skeletal Radiol* 1996;25:67–69.

Greenspan A, Pugh JW, Norman A, Norman RS. Scoliotic index: a comparative evaluation of methods for the measurement of scoliosis. *Bull Hosp Jt Dis Orthop Inst* 1978;39:117–125.

Greenspan A, Stadalnik RC. Bone island: scintigraphic findings and their clinical application. *Can Assoc Radiol J* 1995;46:368–379.

Greenspan A, Steiner G, Knutzon R. Bone island (enostosis): clinical significance and radiologic and pathologic correlations. *Skeletal Radiol* 1991;20:85–90.

Greenspan A, Steiner G, Sotelo D, Norman A, Sotelo A, Sotelo-Ortiz F. Mixed sclerosing bone dysplasia coexisting with dysplasia epiphysealis hemimelica (Trevor-Fairbank disease). *Skeletal Radiol* 1986;15:452–454.

Griffiths DL. Engelmann's disease. *J Bone Joint Surg [Br]* 1956;38B:312–326.

Gundry CR, Heithoff KB. Imaging evaluation of patients with spinal deformity. *Orthop Clin North Am* 1994;15:247–264.

Hagiwara H, Aida N, Machida J, Fujita K, Okuzumi S, Nishimura G. Contrast-enhanced MRI of an early preosseous lesion of fibrodysplasia ossificans progressiva in a 21-month-old boy. *AJR Am J Roentgenol* 2003;181:1145–1147.

Hoppenfeld S. *Scoliosis: a manual of concept and treatment.* Philadelphia: JB Lippincott; 1967.

Hopper WC Jr, Lovell WW. Progressive infantile idiopathic scoliosis. *Clin Orthop* 1977;126:26–32.

Hopwood JJ, Morris CP. The mucopolysaccharidoses: diagnosis, molecular genetics and treatment. *Mol Biol Med* 1990;7:381–404.

Hundley JD, Wilson FC. Progressive diaphyseal dysplasia. Review of the literature and report of seven cases in one family. *J Bone Joint Surg [Am]* 1973;55A:461–474.

Hurt RL. Osteopathia striata—Voorhoeve's disease: report of a case presenting features of osteopathia striata and osteopetrosis. *J Bone Joint Surg [Br]* 1953;35B:89–96.

Jacobson HG. Dense bone—too much bone: radiological considerations and differential diagnosis. Part I. *Skeletal Radiol* 1985;13:1–20.

Judkiewisz AM, Murphey MD, Resnik CS, Newberg AH, Temple HT, Smith WS. Advanced imaging of melorheostosis with emphasis on MRI. *Skeletal Radiol* 2001;30:447–453.

Kaftori JK, Kleinhaus U, Naveh Y. Progressive diaphyseal dysplasia (Camurati-Engelmann): radiographic follow-up and CT findings. *Radiology* 1987;164:777–782.

Kaplan FS, McCluskey W, Hahn G, Tabas JA, Muenke M, Zasloff MA. Genetic transmission of fibrodysplasia ossificans progressiva. Report of a family. *J Bone Joint Surg [Am]* 1993;75:1214–1220.

Kaufmann HJ. Classification of the skeletal dysplasias and the radiologic approach to their differentiation. *Clin Orthop* 1976;114:12–17.

Kennedy JG, Donahue JR, Aydin H, Hoang BH, Huvos A, Morris C. Metastatic breast carcinoma to bone disguised by osteopoikilosis. *Skeletal Radiol* 2003;32:240–243.

Kim HW, Weinstein SL. Spine update. The management of scoliosis in neurofibromatosis. *Spine* 1997;22:2770–2776.

Klatte EC, Franken EA, Smith JA. The radiographic spectrum in neurofibromatosis. *Semin Roentgenol* 1976;11:17–33.

Kleinman PK. Differentiation of child abuse and osteogenesis imperfecta: medical and legal implications. *AJR Am J Roentgenol* 1990;154:1047–1048.

Kleinman RG, Csongradi JJ, Rinsky LA, Bleck EE. The radiographic assessment of spinal flexibility in scoliosis: a study of the efficacy of the prone push film. *Clin Orthop* 1983;162:47–53.

Kobayashi H, Kotoura Y, Hosono M, Tsuboyama T, Shigeno C, Konishi J. A case of melorheostosis with a 14-year-old follow-up. *Eur Radiol* 1995;5:651–653.

Korovessis PG, Stamatakis MV. Prediction of scoliotic Cobb angle with the use of the scoliometer. *Spine* 1996;21:1661–1666.

Kozlowski K, Nicol R, Hopwood JJ. A clinically mild case of mucopolysaccharidosis type I—Scheie syndrome (case report). *Eur Radiol* 1995;5:561–563.

Kumar R, Murphy WA, Whyte MP. Progressive diaphyseal dysplasia (Engelmann disease): scintigraphic-radiographic-clinical correlations. *Radiology* 1981;140:87–92.

Lagier R, Mbakop A, Bigler A. Osteopoikilosis: a radiological and pathological study. *Skeletal Radiol* 1984;11:161–168.

Langer LO Jr, Baumann PA, Gorlin RJ. Achondroplasia. *AJR Am J Roentgenol* 1967;100:12–26.

Lenke LG, Betz RR, Harms J, Bridwell KH, Clements DH, Lowe TG, Blanke K. Adolescent idiopathic scoliosis. A new classification to determine extent of spinal arthrodesis. *J Bone Joint Surg [Am]* 2001;83A:1169–1181.

Lenke LG, Bridwell KH, Blanke K, Baldus C, Weston J. Radiographic results of arthrodesis with Cotrel-Dubousset instrumentation for the treatment of adolescent idiopathic scoliosis. A five to ten-year follow-up study. *J Bone Joint Surg [Am]* 1998;80:807–814.

Léri A, Joanny J. Une affection non décrite des os. Hyperostose en coulée sur toute la longueur d'un membre ou mélorhéostose. *Bull Mem Soc Med Hop Paris* 1922;46:1141.

Lonstein JE, Carlson JM. The prediction of curve progression in untreated idiopathic scoliosis during growth. *J Bone Joint Surg [Am]* 1984;66A:1061–1071.

MacEwen GD, Conway JJ, Miller WT. Congenital scoliosis with a unilateral bar. *Radiology* 1968;90:711–715.

Mahoney J, Achong DM. Demonstration of increased bone metabolism in melorheostosis by multiphase bone scanning. *Clin Nucl Med* 1991;16:847–848.

Maiocco B, Deeney VF, Coulon R, Parks PF Jr. Adolescent idiopathic scoliosis and the presence of spinal cord abnormalities. *Spine* 1997;22:2537–2541.

Marchesi DG, Transfeldt EE, Bradford DS, Heithoff KB. Changes in intervertebral rotation after Harrington and Luque instrumentation for idiopathic scoliosis. *Spine* 1992;17:775–780.

Maroteaux P, Lamy M. La pycnodysostose. *Presse Med* 1962;70:999–1002.

Maroteaux P, Lamy M. The malady of Toulouse-Lautrec. *JAMA* 1965;191:715–717.

McKusick V. *Hereditary disorders of connective tissue*, 4th ed. St. Louis: CV Mosby; 1972.

McMaster MJ. Infantile idiopathic scoliosis: can it be prevented? *J Bone Joint Surg [Br]* 1983;65B:612–617.

Millner PA, Dickson RA. Idiopathic scoliosis: biomechanics and biology. *Eur Spine J* 1996;5:362–373.

Mishra GK, Mishra M, Vernekar J, Tehrai M, Patel BR. Progressive diaphyseal dysplasia: Engelmann's disease. *Indian Pediatr* 1987;24:1052–1054.

Moser FG, Mangiardi JR, Kantrowitz AB. Device for accurate localization of vertebrae before spinal surgery. *AJR Am J Roentgenol* 1996;166:626–627.

Murray DW, Bulstrode CJ. The development of adolescent idiopathic scoliosis. *Eur Spine J* 1996;5:251–257.

Murray RO, McCredie J. Melorheostosis and the sclerotomes: a radiological correlation. *Skeletal Radiol* 1979;4:57–71.

Nash CL Jr, Moe JH. A study of vertebral rotation. *J Bone Joint Surg [Am]* 1969;51A:223–229.

Nasu K, Kuroki Y, Nawano S, et al. Thoracic cage extent of melorheostosis depicted by multislice CT. *Skeletal Radiol* 2002;31:464–466.

Neufeld E, Muenzer J. The mucopolysaccharidoses. In: Scriver CR, Beaudet MC, Sly WS, Valle D, eds. *The metabolic basis of inherited disease*, 6th ed. New York: McGraw-Hill; 1989:1565–1587.

Neuhauser EBD, Schwachman H, Wittenberg M, Cohen J. Progressive diaphyseal dysplasia. *Radiology* 1948;51:11–22.

Norman A. Myositis ossificans and fibrodysplasia ossificans progressiva. In: Taveras JM, Ferrucci JT, eds. *Radiology—diagnosis, imaging, intervention*, vol 5. Philadelphia: JB Lippincott; 1986.

Norman A, Greenspan A. Bone dysplasias. In: Jahss MH, ed. *Disorders of the foot and ankle: medical and surgical management*, vol 1, 2nd ed. Philadelphia: WB Saunders; 1991:754–770.

Norman A, Greenspan A. Sclerosing dysplasias of bone. In: Taveras JM, Ferrucci JT, eds. *Radiology—diagnosis, imaging, intervention*, vol 5. Philadelphia: JP Lippincott; 1986:1–18.

Oestreich AE, Young LW, Poussaint TY. Scoliosis *circa* 2000: radiologic imaging perspective. I. Diagnosis and pretreatment evaluation. *Skeletal Radiol* 1998;27:591–605.

Oestreich AE, Young LW, Poussaint TY. Scoliosis *circa* 2000: radiologic imaging perspective. II. Treatment and follow-up. *Skeletal Radiol* 1998;27:651–656.

Omeroglu H, Ozekin O, Biçimoglu A. Measurement of vertebral rotation in idiopathic scoliosis using the Perdriolle torsionmeter: a clinical study on intraobserver and interobserver error. *Eur Spine J* 1996;5:167–171.

Onitsuka H. Roentgenologic aspects of bone islands. *Radiology* 1977;123:607–612.

Ozonoff M. *Pediatric orthopaedic radiology*. Philadelphia: WB Saunders; 1979.

Palmer PES, Thomas JEP. Case reports. Osteopetrosis with unusual changes in the skull and digits. *Br J Radiol* 1958;31:705–708.

Paul LW. Hereditary, multiple diaphyseal sclerosis (Ribbing disease). *Radiology* 1953;60:412–416.

Pollack S, Naveh Y, Katz R. Immunological investigations in two families with progressive diaphyseal dysplasia. *J Rheumatol* 1989;16:1259–1262.

Raffaelli P, Ronzini MF. Camurati-Engelmann's disease: a case report. *Ital J Orthop Traumatol* 1988;14:267–271.

Reinig JW, Hill SC, Fang M, Marini J, Zasloff MA. Fibrodysplasia ossificans progressiva: CT appearance. *Radiology* 1986;159:153–157.

Resnick D, Nemcek AA Jr, Haghighi P. Spinal enostoses (bone islands). *Radiology* 1983;147:373–376.

Rhys R, Davies AM, Mangham DC, Grimer RJ. Sclerotome distribution of melorheostosis and multicentric fibromatosis. *Skeletal Radiol* 1998;27:633–636.

Ribbing S. Hereditary, multiple, diaphyseal sclerosis. *Acta Radiol* 1949;31:522–536.

Riccardi VM. Von Recklinghausen's neurofibromatosis. *N Engl J Med* 1981;305:1617–1627.

Robinson EF, Wade WD. Statistical assessment of two methods of measuring scoliosis before treatment. *Can Med Assoc J* 1983;129:839–841.

Rubin P. *Dynamic classification of bone dysplasias*. Chicago: Year Book Medical Publishers; 1964:325–349.

Sanders JO, Herring JA, Browne RH. Posterior arthrodesis and instrumentation in the immature (Risser-grade-0) spine in idiopathic scoliosis. *J Bone Joint Surg [Am]* 1995;77A:39–45.

Scheie HG, Hambrick GW Jr, Barness LA. A newly recognised forme fruste of Hurler's disease (gargoylism): the Sanford R Gifford lecture. *Am J Ophthalmol* 1962;53:753–769.

Schwartz A, Ramos R. Neurofibromatosis and multiple nonossifying fibromas. *AJR Am J Roentgenol* 1980;135:617–619.

Scott H, Bunge S, Gal A, Clarke L, Morris CP, Hopwood JJ. The molecular genetics of mucopolysaccharidosis type I: diagnostic, clinical and biological implications. *Hum Mutat* 1995;6:288–302.

Seeger LL, Hewel KC, Yao L, et al. Ribbing disease (multiple diaphyseal sclerosis): imaging and differential diagnosis. *AJR Am J Roentgenol* 1996;167:689–694.

Shafritz AB, Shore EM, Gannon FH, et al. Overexpression of an osteogenic morphogen in fibrodysplasia ossificans progressiva. *N Eng J Med* 1996;335:555–561.

Shier CK, Krasicky GA, Ellis IB, Kottamasu SR. Ribbing's disease: radiographic-scintigraphic correlation and comparative analysis with Engelmann's disease. *J Nucl Med* 1987;28:244–248.

Shufflebarger HL, Clark CE. Fusion levels and hook patterns in thoracic scoliosis with Cotrel-Dubousset instrumentation. *Spine* 1990;15:916–920.

Sillence DO. Osteogenesis imperfecta: an expanding panorama of variants. *Clin Orthop* 1981;159:11–25.

Sillence DO, Senn A, Danks DM. Genetic heterogeneity in osteogenesis imperfecta. *J Med Genet* 1979;16:101–116.

Silverman BJ, Greenbarg PE. Internal fixation of the spine for idiopathic scoliosis using square-ended distraction rods and lamina wiring (Harrington-Luque technique). *Bull Hosp Jt Dis Orthop Inst* 1984;44:41–55.

Silverman FN. Achondroplasia. *Semin Roentgenol* 1973;8:142–143.

Singleton EB, Thomas JR, Worthington WW, Hild JR. Progressive diaphyseal dysplasia (Engelmann's disease). *Radiology* 1956;67:233–240.

Slone RM, MacMillan M. Montgomery WJ, Heare M. Spinal fixation. 2. Fixation techniques and hardware for the thoracic and lumbar spine. *Radiographics* 1993;13:521–544.

Slucky AV, Engelking B, Shufflebarger HL. A simple method for improving vertebral visualization on a scoliosis series lateral radiograph. *Spine* 1995;20:2570–2571.

Smith J. Giant bone islands. *Radiology* 1973;107:35–36.

Sparkes RS, Graham CB. Camurati-Engelmann disease: genetics and clinical manifestations with a review of the literature. *J Med Genet* 1972;9:73–85.

Spieth ME, Greenspan A, Forrester DM, Ansari AN, Kimura RL, Siegel ME. Radionuclide imaging in forme fruste of melorheostosis. *Clin Nucl Med* 1994;19:512–515.

Spranger JW. Mucopolysaccharidosen. In: Schwiegk H, ed. *Handbuch der inneren Medizin*, 5th ed. New York: Springer-Verlag; 1974:212–215.

Spranger JW, Langer LO Jr, Wiederman HR. *Bone dysplasias. An atlas of constitutional disorders of skeletal development*. Philadelphia: WB Saunders; 1974.

Stegman KF, Peterson JC. Progressive hereditary diaphyseal dysplasia. *Pediatrics* 1957;20:966–974.

Stevenson RE, Howell RR, McKusick VA, et al. The iduronidase-deficient mucopolysaccharidoses: clinical and roentgenographic features. *Pediatrics* 1976;57:111–122.

Stokes IA. Three-dimensional terminology of spinal deformity. *Spine* 1994;19:236–248.

Taitz LS. Child abuse and osteogenesis imperfecta. *BMJ* 1987;295:1082–1083.

Thompson SB, Eales W. Clinical considerations and comparative measures of assessing curvature of the spine. *J Med Eng Technol* 1994;18:143–147.

Thomsen MN, Schneider U, Weber M, Johannisson R, Niethard FU. Scoliosis and congenital anomalies associated with Klippel-Feil syndrome types I-III. *Spine* 1997;22:396–401.

Transfeldt EE. Complications of treatment. In: Lonstein JE, Bradford DS, Winter RB, Ogilvie JW, eds. *Moe's textbook of scoliosis and other spinal deformities*, 3rd ed. Philadelphia: WB Saunders; 1995:451–481.

Urbaniak JR, Schaefer WW, Stalling FH III. Iliac apophyses: prognostic value in idiopathic scoliosis. *Clin Orthop* 1976;116:80–85.

van Buchem FSP. Hyperostosis corticalis generalisata: eight new cases. *Acta Med Scand* 1971;189:257–267.

van Buchem FSP, Hadders HN, Hansen JF, Woldring MG. Hyperostosis corticalis generalisata: report of seven cases. *Am J Med* 1962;33:387–397.

van Buchem FSP, Hadders HN, Ubbens R. An uncommon familial systemic disease of the skeleton: hyperostosis corticalis generalisata familiaris. *Acta Radiol [Diagn]* 1955;44:109–120.

Vanhoenacker FM, Balemans W, Tan GJ, et al. Van Buchem disease: lifetime evolution of radioclinical features. *Skeletal Radiol* 2003;32:708–718.

Van Hul W, Balemans W, Van Hul E, et al. Van Buchem disease (hyperostosis corticalis generalisata) maps to chromosome 17q12-q21. *Am J Hum Genet* 1998;62:391–399.

Vaughan JJ, Winter RB, Lonstein JE. Comparison of the use of supine bending and traction radiographs in the selection of the fusion area in adolescent idiopathic scoliosis. *Spine* 1996;21:2469–2473.

Walker GF. Mixed sclerosing bone dystrophies. Two case reports. *J Bone Joint Surg [Br]* 1964;46B:546–552.

Ward M, Betz RR, Clements DH, Cole BA. Prevalence of segmental wire breakage using Contrel-Dubousset instrumentation in the management of idiopathic scoliosis. *Spine* 1997;22:406–407.

Warkany J. Dwarfs and other little people: an overview. *Semin Roentgenol* 1973;8:135–138.

Weiss IR. Measurement of vertebral rotation: Perdriolle versus Raimondi. *Eur Spine J* 1995;4:34–38.

Whyte MP, Murphy WA, Siegel BA. ^{99m}Tc-pyrophosphate bone imaging in osteopoikilosis, osteopathia striata and melorheostosis. *Radiology* 1978;127:439–443.

Whyte MP, Murphy WA, Fallon MD, Hahn TJ. Mixed-sclerosing-bone-dystrophy: report of a case and review of the literature. *Skeletal Radiol* 1981;6:95–102.

Winter RB. Congenital spine deformity. In: Bradford DS, Lonstein JE, Moe JH, Ogilvie JW, Winter RB, eds. *Moe's textbook of scoliosis and other spinal deformities,* 2nd ed. Philadelphia: WB Saunders; 1987:233–270.

Winter RB, Haven JJ, Moe JH, Lagaard SM. Diastematomyelia and congenital spinal deformities. *J Bone Joint Surg [Am]* 1974;56A:27–39.

Winter RB, Moe JH, Eilers VE. Congenital scoliosis. A study of 234 patients treated and untreated. *J Bone Joint Surg [Am]* 1968;50A:1.

Worth HM, Wollin DG. Hyperostosis corticalis generalisata congenita. *J Can Assoc Radiol* 1966;17:67–74.

Wynne-Davies R, Fairbank TJ. *Atlas of general affections of the skeleton, Fairbank's atlas of general affections of the skeleton,* 2nd ed. New York: Churchill Livingstone; 1976.

Yaghmai I. Spine changes in neurofibromatosis. *Radiographics* 1986;6:261–285.

Young LW, Oestreich AE, Goldstein LA. Roentgenology in scoliosis: contribution to evaluation and management. *AJR Am J Roentgenol* 1970;108:778–795.

Ziran N, Hill S, Wright ME, Kovacs J, Robey PG, Wientroub S, Collins MT. Ribbin disease: radiographic and biochemical characterization, lack of response to pamidronate. *Skeletal Radiol* 2003;31:714–719.

FIGURE CREDITS

The following figures were reproduced with permission, in addition to those so indicated in the text.

Figures 7.35, 9.32, 9.44, 29.11, 29.12, and 29.19 from Berquist TH, ed. *MRI of the musculoskeletal system, 3rd ed.* Philadelphia: Lippincott-Raven Publishers, 1997.

Figure 10.14B modified from Berquist TH, ed. *Radiology of the foot and ankle.* New York: Raven Press, 1989.

Figures 9.31, 9.43, 9.74, 9.75, and 13.30 from Bloem JL, Sartoris DJ, eds. *MRI and CT of the musculoskeletal system. A text-atlas.* Baltimore: Williams & Wilkins, 1992.

Figure 11.21B from Chapman MW, Madison M, eds. *Operative orthopaedics, vol 4, 2nd ed.* Philadelphia: JB Lippincott, 1993.

Figures 10.69, 10.70B, and 10.81 from Deutsch AL, Mink JH, Kerr R, eds. *MRI of the foot and ankle.* New York: Raven Press, 1992.

Figures 6.40, 7.24, 7.89, and 9.62 from Deutsch AL, Mink JH, eds. *MRI of the musculoskeletal system: A teaching file, 2nd ed.* Philadelphia: Lippincott-Raven Publishers, 1997.

Figures 16.22, 16.34, 16.41C, 17.16, 17.19, 18.24, 21.6B, 22.4D, 22.37, 23.1, 23.12, 23.13, and 23.17 from Greenspan A, Remagen W. *Differential diagnosis of tumors and tumor-like lesions.* Philadelphia: Lippincott-Raven Publishers, 1998.

Figure 7.73 from Higgins CB, Hricak H, Helms CA, eds. *Magnetic resonance imaging of the body, 3rd ed.* Philadelphia: Lippincott-Raven Publishers, 1997.

Figures 5.25, and 5.47 from Steinbach LS, Tirman PFJ, Peterfy CG, Feller JF, eds. *Shoulder magnetic resonance imaging.* Philadelphia: Lippincott-Raven Publishers, 1998.

Figures 5.51B-C 5.56, 5.57, 7.22, 7.88, 9.33, 9.54, 9.76, 9.80, 9.81, 10.58, 10.63, 13.12, 13.13, 13.31, 13.32, and 13.40 from Stoller DW, *MRI in orthopaedics and sports medicine.* Philadelphia: JB Lippincott, 1993.

INDEX

Page numbers in *italics* indicate figures; those followed by "t" indicate tables.